Dictionary of
Biological Psychology

Dictionary of
Biological Psychology

Edited by Philip Winn

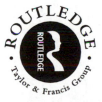

ROUTLEDGE
ROUTLEDGE
Taylor & Francis Group

London and New York

First published 2001
by Routledge
11 New Fetter Lane, London EC4P 4EE

Simultaneously published in the USA and Canada
by Routledge
29 West 35th Street, New York, NY 10001

Routledge is an imprint of the Taylor & Francis Group
© 2001 Routledge

Typeset in Sabon by Taylor & Francis Books Ltd
Printed and bound in Great Britain by TJ International Ltd,
Padstow, Cornwall

British Library Cataloguing in Publication Data
A catalogue record for this book is available from the British Library

Library of Congress Cataloging in Publication Data
Dictionary of Biological Psychology / edited by Philip Winn.
p.cm.
Includes bibliographical references and index.
1. Psychology. I. Winn, Philip, 1954–
QP360.D52 2001
612.8'03—dc21
00–059241

ISBN 0–415–13606–7

Contents

Editorial board

List of contributors

Note: unattributed entries were written by the editor

John P. Aggleton
School of Psychology, Cardiff University, Wales

Marlene Behrmann
Department of Psychology, Carnegie-Mellon University, USA

Kent C. Berridge
Department of Psychology, University of Michigan at Ann Arbor, USA

Charles D. Blaha
Department of Psychology, Macquarie University, Australia

T. V. P. Bliss FRS
National Institute for Medical Research, Mill Hill, London, England

Charlotte Bonardi
Department of Psychology, University of York, England

Eric M. Bowman
School of Psychology, University of St Andrews, Scotland

Oliver J. Braddick
Department of Psychology, University College London, England

Jasper Brener
Department of Psychology, SUNY at Stony Brook, USA

Richard E. Brown
Department of Psychology, Dalhousie University, Canada

Verity J. Brown
School of Psychology, University of St Andrews, Scotland

Daniel N. Bub
Department of Psychology, University of Victoria, Canada

Richard W. Byrne
School of Psychology, University of St Andrews, Scotland

David P. Carey
Department of Psychology, University of Aberdeen, Scotland

Patricia S. Churchland
Department of Philosophy, University of California at San Diego, USA

Andrew M. Colman
Department of Psychology, University of Leicester, England

Chris Cullen
Department of Psychology, University of Keele, England

Anne Cutler
Max Planck Institute for Psycholinguistics, Nijmegen, Netherlands

Graham Davies
Department of Psychology, University of Leicester, England

Michael Davis
Department of Psychiatry, Emory University, USA

Paul Dean
Department of Psychology, University of Sheffield, England

John E. Dowling
Department of Molecular and Cellular Biology, Harvard University, USA

Stephen B. Dunnett
School of Biosciences, Cardiff University, Wales

Jos J. Eggermont
Departments of Physiology & Biophysics, and Psychology, University of Calgary, Canada

Howard Eichenbaum
Department of Psychology, Boston University, USA

Howard H. Ellenberger
Department of Basic Medical Sciences, CCPM, San Francisco, USA

Robert P. Erickson
Departments of Psychological and Brain Sciences, and Neurobiology, Duke University, USA

Barry J. Everitt
Department of Experimental Psychology, University of Cambridge, England

David L. Ferster
Department of Neurobiology and Physiology, Northwestern University, USA

Stanley B. Floresco
Department of Neuroscience, University of Pittsburgh, USA

Jonathan K. Foster
Department of Psychology, University of Western Australia, Australia

Keith B. J. Franklin
Department of Psychology, McGill University, Canada

Christopher Frith FRS
Wellcome Department of Cognitive Neurology, Institute of Neurology, London, England

Elaine Funnell
Department of Psychology, Royal Holloway, University of London, England

Richard L. Gregory FRS
Department of Psychology, University of Bristol, England

Geoffrey Hall
Department of Psychology, University of York, England

Francesca G. Happé
Social, Genetic and Developmental Psychiatry Research Centre, Institute of Psychiatry,
  Kings College, London, England

David W. Heeley
School of Psychology, University of St Andrews, Scotland

L. Jacob Herberg
Department of Neuropathology, Institute of Neurology, London, England

Marion M. Hetherington
Department of Psychology, University of Dundee, Scotland

J. Allan Hobson
Department of Psychiatry, Harvard University, USA

Jill M. Hooley
Department of Psychology, Harvard University, USA

David A. Hopkins
Department of Anatomy and Neurobiology, Dalhousie University, Canada

Ian P. Howard
Department of Psychology, York University, Canada

Fiona M. Inglis
Department of Neurology, Yale University School of Medicine, USA

Wendy L. Inglis
Department of Experimental Psychology, University of Cambridge, England

Malcolm A. Jeeves CBE FRSE
School of Psychology, University of St Andrews, Scotland

Derek W. Johnston
School of Psychology, University of St Andrews, Scotland

Barbara E. Jones
Montreal Neurological Institute, McGill University, Canada

Robert G. Kalb
Department of Neurology, Yale University School of Medicine, USA

Ann E. Kelley
Department of Psychiatry, University of Wisconsin at Madison, USA

Barry Keverne FRS
Sub-Department of Animal Behaviour, Department of Zoology, University of Cambridge, England

Roger J. Keynes
Department of Anatomy, University of Cambridge, England

A. Simon Killcross
School of Psychology, University of Cardiff, Wales

Stefan Köhler
Department of Psychology, University of Western Ontario, Canada

Malcolm D. MacLeod
School of Psychology, University of St Andrews, Scotland

Jennifer A. Mangels
Department of Psychology, Columbia University, USA

Aubrey W. G. Manning
School of Biology, University of Edinburgh, Scotland

Keith Matthews
Department of Psychiatry, University of Dundee, Scotland

Michael McCloskey
Department of Cognitive Science, Johns Hopkins University, USA

Mitul Mehta
Department of Psychiatry, University of Cambridge, England

A. David Milner FRSE
Department of Psychology, University of Durham, England

Donald E. Mitchell
Psychology Department, Dalhousie University, Canada

Ian J. Mitchell
School of Psychology, University of Birmingham, England

Charlotte C. Mitchum
Department of Neurology, University of Maryland, USA

Akira Miyake
Department of Psychology, University of Colorado at Boulder, USA

Richard G. M. Morris FRSE FRS
Department of Neuroscience, University of Edinburgh, Scotland

Kathy T. Mullen
Department of Ophthalmology, McGill University, Canada

Jenni A. Ogden
Department of Psychology, University of Auckland, New Zealand

Karalyn E. Patterson
MRC Cognition and Brain Sciences Unit, University of Cambridge, England

James G. Pfaus
Department of Psychology, Concordia University, Canada

Dennis P. Phillips
Department of Psychology, Dalhousie University, Canada

David C. Plaut
Department of Psychology, Carnegie-Mellon University, USA

Douglas D. Rasmusson
Department of Physiology and Biophysics, Dalhousie University, Canada

Catherine L. Reed
Department of Psychology, University of Denver, USA

Ian C. Reid
Department of Psychiatry, University of Dundee, Scotland

Patricia A. Reuter-Lorenz
Department of Psychology, University of Michigan at Ann Arbor, USA

Rosalind Ridley
Department of Experimental Psychology, University of Cambridge, England

Trevor W. Robbins
Department of Experimental Psychology, University of Cambridge, England

Robert D. Rogers
Department of Psychiatry, University of Oxford, England

Michael D. Rugg FRSE
Institute of Cognitive Neuroscience, University College London, England

Benjamin Rusak FRSC
Department of Psychology, Dalhousie University, Canada

Barbara J. Sahakian
Department of Psychiatry, University of Cambridge, England

John D. Salamone
Department of Psychology, University of Connecticut at Storrs, USA

Kazue Semba
Department of Anatomy and Neurobiology, Dalhousie University, Canada

Keith T. Sillar
School of Biology, University of St Andrews, Scotland

Peter J. B. Slater FRSE
School of Biology, University of St Andrews, Scotland

Robert J. Snowden
School of Psychology, University of Cardiff, Wales

Larry R. Squire
Department of Psychiatry, University of California at San Diego, USA

James R. Stellar
Department of Psychology, Northeastern University, USA

Petra Stoerig
Institut für Experimentelle Psychologie, Heinrich-Heine-Universität Düsseldorf, Germany

Richard C. Tees
Department of Psychology, University of British Columbia, Canada

Daniel Tranel
Department of Neurology, University of Iowa, USA

Christopher Tyler
The Smith-Kettlewell Eye Research Institute, San Francisco, USA

Mark A. Ungless
Ernest Gallo Clinic and Research Center, University of California at San Francisco, USA

Lawrence M. Ward
Department of Psychology, University of British Columbia, Canada

Jasper Ward-Robinson
School of Psychology, University of Cardiff, Wales

Roger J. Watt
Department of Psychology, University of Stirling, Scotland

Ian Q. Whishaw FRSC
Department of Psychology and Neuroscience, University of Lethbridge, Canada

Donald M. Wilkie
Department of Psychology, University of British Columbia, Canada

Philip Winn
School of Psychology, University of St Andrews, Scotland

Jeremy M. Wolfe
Center for Ophthalmic Research, Brigham and Women's Hospital, Boston, USA

Andrew W. Young
Department of Psychology, University of York, England

Introduction

Over the last twenty years or so, the neurosciences – brain sciences – have had an increasing influence on psychology. It is taken as axiomatic by very many psychologists and neuroscientists that psychological processes such as perception, memory and attention are at root brain processes, and as such are to be best explained in terms of the underlying brain systems and processes that operate them. It is not the purpose of this book to judge this development, though it is unequivocally a product of it. Because psychological processes are increasingly thought of as being biological in nature, there has been a steady incorporation into the psychological literature of terms drawn from a variety of biological sciences. As such, in order to understand modern psychology, it is increasingly necessary to use an eclectic vocabulary drawn from many places – biology, information theory, computer science, the neurosciences, among many others – as well as the technical language of psychology and its various disciplines. These words are not 'jargon', a term carrying connotations of clumsiness and artificiality and which is generally thought to be an obstacle to understanding. The terms defined in this Dictionary do not fall into this class. Rather, the words collected here describe clearly real things – anatomical structures, psychological processes, cell functions and so on. What creates difficulty in their use is that they are drawn from such disparate sources and that they are unfamiliar to many students of psychology.

This Dictionary has been prepared primarily with undergraduates in mind, though it is also intended for postgraduates and active research scientists: keeping up with the entire vocabulary is too much for most of us. I know from my own experience as a teacher in St Andrews that the words I use can obstruct learning. Here, as in all Scottish universities, students spend their first two years of study taking a variety of subjects. The students to whom I teach biological psychology – whom I hope to interest in biological psychology – come from a variety of intellectual backgrounds. Some may be students of biological sciences, but the majority are not. Indeed, many have had only minimal experience of natural sciences of any sort. This is not uncommon in universities across the world. Psychology is amongst the most popular of all degree subjects, attracting students from a wider variety of backgrounds than most other disciplines. Nevertheless, whatever their background, in order to come to as complete an understanding of psychology as possible, all students have to wrestle with biological psychology, and all therefore have to deal with the words biological psychologists use. This Dictionary is an attempt to collect technical terms of relevance to biological psychology – defined in the widest sense possible – so that anyone interested has access to a reference work that will guide them though the literature. No other publication does this adequately: medical dictionaries are medical, not psychological, biological dictionaries likewise; dictionaries of general psychology omit too much necessary neuroscience. To understand biological psychology, one needs a dictionary of biological psychology.

Every day, when I walk into St Mary's Quad on my way to the School of Psychology in St Andrews, I pass through gates which bear the legend *in principio erat verbum* – 'in the beginning was the word' – the sublime opening of St John's Gospel. It is my hope, and that of the editorial team who have prepared this Dictionary, that students of psychology – indeed, anyone interested in this subject – will find that understanding the words that make up biological psychology will lead to a richer and more comprehensive understanding of it. Armed with understanding of the words, I hope that the subject itself will become more accessible and will interest new students as much as it has interested me.

Philip Winn

How to use this dictionary

Organization: the entries are (of course) arranged alphabetically. The one point of interest to note is that entries which describe chemicals that begin with a number – 6-hydroxydopamine for example – are listed alphabetically by the first letter, *excluding* the number. 6-hydroxydopamine is therefore found under 'H' for hydroxydopamine.

Cross referencing: terms in SMALL CAPITALS appear as entries elsewhere in the Dictionary. Please note several things about these cross-references: first, they operate in two directions. That is, they are picked out in small capitals so that the reader can look them up elsewhere in the Dictionary, and so that a reader who has been referred on can more easily find the term within an entry. Second, some of the cross-references refer only to entries that simply say '*see elsewhere*'. In these instances, all that one needs to know about a particular term is contained within the entry referred to. Third, the cross-references are not exhaustive: there are terms, relatively familiar ones such as POSTERIOR or HUNGER, that often appear in entries without being cross-referenced. To have picked all of these out in small capitals on every occasion would have been distracting, and such entries are therefore only cross-referenced when it is particularly relevant to do so.

Spelling: this Dictionary follows English conventions for the most part. For example, it uses *centre* rather than *center*; and discussion is typically of NORADRENALINE rather than NOREPINEPHRINE (the entry for which simply refers the reader to the noradrenaline entry). However, the American NEURON is preferred to the English *neurone*, this being now the most popular spelling. Words such as *capitalize* are presented with a z rather than an s – -ize not -ise. Entries are all presented in the singular, except those instances where the plural is the more commonly encountered expression.

Abbreviations: a Glossary of Abbreviations is included. Within the text I have tried for the most part to avoid using abbreviations, because they tend to confuse readers unfamiliar with an area of study. As Greek letters are commonly used to discriminate different forms of things (OPIATE RECEPTORS for example) a table of these is included with the Glossary of Abbreviations.

Drugs, neurochemicals and neurotransmitter receptors: included in this Dictionary are entries describing a number of DRUGS. Both particular drugs and pharmacological terms relating to features or properties of drugs (for example DRUG IONIZATION and TOLERANCE) are included. The drugs included are the most well known, principally because of their value in either experiments or therapeutic regimes. Entries covering classes of drugs (for example BENZODIAZEPINES or ANTIPSYCHOTIC DRUGS) are also present. However, readers should be aware that drug development occurs continuously and that there are many more drugs of interest to biological psychology than can be included in a work such as this. Entries covering all the main NEUROTRANSMITTERS are present, as are entries concerning the chemicals concerned with the METABOLISM of neurotransmitters. There are also entries describing both RECEPTORS in general and specific classes of neurotransmitter receptors (for example, ACETYLCHOLINE RECEPTORS). Again, readers should be aware that neurotransmitter receptors nomenclature is the subject of debate and continual refinement. For further information concerning new drugs and receptors, readers should consult the following works of reference: Reynolds J.E.F. (1996) *Martindale: The Extra Pharmacopoeia*, 31st edn, Royal Pharmaceutical Society: London. (This is a frequently revised reference work which first appeared in 1883. It lists drugs and medicines for the benefit of physicians and pharmacists.) *Trends in Pharmacological Sciences Receptor Supplement*: the journal *Trends in Pharmacological Sciences* produces an annual supplement classifying receptors and ion channels. The 1999 edition (the 10th) was compiled by S.P.H. Alexander and J.A. Peters.

Neuroanatomy: included in this Dictionary are entries describing a number of neuroanatomical structures of interest to biological psychologists. Readers are advised to consult an appropriate stereotaxic atlas in order to obtain a better understanding of the three dimensional relations between these various structures. The entry STEREOTAXIC ATLAS contains references to commonly used atlases.

Positions and directions: there are several entries describing positions. The entry PLANES OF SECTION describes these, as do several particular entries (for example, ANTERIOR, POSTERIOR, DORSAL, VENTRAL, LATERAL, MEDIAL). There are also a number of terms that combine these, especially in describing structures in the brain: *dorsolateral* for example is a combination of dorsal and lateral that describes a relative position. There are no obvious rules for the combination of terms: for example, dorsal and lateral combine to form both *dorsolateral* (as in DORSOLATERAL PREFRONTAL CORTEX) and *laterodorsal* (as in LATERODORSAL TEGMENTAL NUCLEUS). All of these many combinations are not listed: the reader should understand that such combinations can be made in a very flexible manner and search the Dictionary for the necessary elements.

Weights and measures: this Dictionary follows the convention of using metric measures; *see* SI UNITS for discussion of WEIGHTS AND MEASURES.

Orders of magnitude: many terms used are qualified by a prefix indicating an order of magnitude. Metres and grams, for example, are often expressed as *kilo*metres, *micro*grams and so on. All the possible prefixes used to indicate different orders of magnitude are listed in the entry SI UNITS.

Correspondence

In compiling this Dictionary I have tried to be as comprehensive as possible, but there are bound to be some terms missing. If you think an essential term is missing, or if you find that the definitions given are not helpful enough, please let me know, so that future editions can be revised. Comments should be sent to me at the School of Psychology, University of St Andrews, St Andrews, Fife KY16 9JU, Scotland, or by email at pw@st-andrews.ac.uk.

References

A number of entries have particular references associated with them. These often point to a seminal paper – either contemporary or historical – or to a helpful review. On other occasions, textbooks are referred to. This is often the case with very broad topics, when the entry here can only give a synoptic view rather than the detailed description offered by a textbook. In preparing this Dictionary, I have found the following texts particularly useful:

Campbell NA, Reece JB and Mitchell LG (1999) *Biology*, 5th edition, Addison-Wesley: Menlo Park CA.

Carlson N.R. (1998) *Physiology of Behaviour*, 6th edition, Allyn & Bacon: Boston

Cooper J.R., Bloom F.E. and Roth R.H. (1996) *The Biochemical Basis of Neuropharmacology*, Oxford University Press: New York.

Davison G.C. and Neale J.M. (2001) *Abnormal Psychology*, 8th edition, John Wiley & Sons: New York.

Feldman R.S., Meyer J.S. and Quenzer L.F. (1997) *Principles of Neuropsychopharmacology*, Sinauer Associates Inc. Sunderland, MA.

Finger S. (1994) *Origins of Neuroscience*, Oxford University Press: New York.

Kandel E.R., Schwartz J.H. and Jessell T.M. (2000) *Principles of Neural Science*, 4th edition, McGraw-Hill Inc.

McFarland D. (1999) *Animal Behaviour*, 3rd edition, Longman: Harlow, UK.

Paxinos G. (1995) *The Rat Nervous System*, 2nd edition, Academic Press: San Diego.

Rosenzweig M.R., Leiman A.L. and Breedlove S.M., (1999) *Biological Psychology*, Sinauer Associates Inc.: Sunderland, MA.

I have also consulted three more general Dictionaries while preparing this one. I used *The Macmillan Dictionary of Psychology* by Stuart Sutherland (2nd edition, 1995, Macmillan Press, Basingstoke) as a general guide to psychology; *Stedman's Medical Dictionary* (24th edition, 1982, Williams and Wilkins, Baltimore) as a source of information about medical terms; and *The Chambers Dictionary* (1998 edition, Chambers Harrap Publishers, Edinburgh) as my basic guide to English vocabulary and etymology.

Acknowledgements

I want to express my gratitude to five groups of people: first, the staff at Routledge: Fiona Cairns, the commissioning editor whose brainchild this Dictionary is, Colville Wemys, Denise Rea, Dominic Shryane, Tarquin Acevedo (production editor) and Anna Hodson (copy editor), all of whom patiently suffered my lack of speed in preparing material; second, the members of the editorial board, for agreeing to serve and for their invaluable help in preparing this Dictionary; third, all the contributors whose enthusiasm sustained it through a long and difficult creation – especially those (Verity Brown, Anne Cutler, David Heeley, Fiona Inglis and Keith Matthews) to whom I repeatedly returned requesting more entries; fourth, colleagues in St Andrews and elsewhere who suffered my questions and corrected my errors – particularly James Ainge, Helen Alderson, Bob Cywinski, Trisha Jenkins, Sue Kilcoyne, Mary Latimer, Mel Lyon, Malcolm MacLeod, Ronan O'Carroll, Michael Oram, Patrick Pallier, Gerry Quinn and Scott Zahm; and finally, Jane, Paul, Dorothy and Alexander, who endured my tiredness and absences, and whom I could not have managed without.

Abbreviations

Please note the following points when consulting the Glossary of Abbreviations:

i.   It is not exhaustive: it is intended as a guide to abbreviations frequently encountered in biological psychology. In particular, many abbreviations for anatomical structures are not included. Readers should refer to a good STEREOTAXIC ATLAS for anatomical abbreviations.

ii. Many terms have more than one abbreviation; there are relatively few universally agreed abbreviations.

iii. The same abbreviation may be used to mean different things: LH for example can be LATERAL HYPOTHALAMUS, LEARNED HELPLESSNESS or LUTEINIZING HORMONE. The context in which an abbreviation is used provides a strong clue as to meaning.

iv. Case is often important, especially in units of measurement, chemistry and pharmacology – see, for example, Na (SODIUM) and NA (NORADRENALINE). Equally, case is often unimportant: STn and STN can both be used to indicate the SUBTHALAMIC NUCLEUS.

v.   Only symbols for ELEMENTS commonly encountered in biological psychology are listed here. The entry PERIODIC TABLE OF THE ELEMENTS gives details of a website that describes fully all the elements and their symbols.

vi. There are conventions – not always observed – in the naming of anatomical parts. Lower case letters are typically used for abbreviating the names of fibre pathways (for example, scp is the SUPERIOR CEREBELLAR PEDUNCLE) while upper case letters are used for structures (GP is the GLOBUS PALLIDUS for instance). When abbreviating the term NUCLEUS many authors will use lower case (for example, subthalamic nucleus becomes STn) though this is not a standard practice. CRANIAL NERVES are typically indicated by Roman numerals (I–XII) not Arabic (1–12).

vii. For GENES and PROTEINS there is a convention to follow: the names of genes are written in italics, the proteins they code for are not. For example, cfos (in italics and a lower case f) is a gene; Fos (not italicized and with capital F) is the protein coded by that gene.

viii. All the terms below are defined in this Dictionary. Abbreviations are listed alphabetically by abbreviation rather than the thing for which the abbreviation stands; abbreviations beginning with numbers are listed separately at the start.

Glossary of abbreviations

2-DG	2-deoxy-D-glucose
3-MT	3-methoxytyramine
5,7-DHT	5,7-dihydroxytryptamine
5-HIAA	5-hydroxyindoleacetic acid
5-HT	5-hydroxytryptamine (serotonin)
5-HTP	5-hydroxytryptophan
6-OHDA	6-hydroxydopamine
7-OHDPAT	7-hydroxydipropylaminotetralin
8-OHDPAT	8-hydroxydipropylaminotetralin
A1 – A15	adrenaline, noradrenaline, dopamine cell groups (see CLASSIFICATION OF DAHLSTRÖM AND FUXE)
ABC	avidin-biotin complex (see IMMUNOHISTOCHEMISTRY)
Acb	nucleus accumbens (*also* NAC; NAcc; NAS)
ACE	angiotensin converting enzyme
acetyl Co A	acetyl coenzyme A
ACh	acetylcholine
AChE	acetylcholinesterase
AChR	acetylcholine receptors
aCSF	artificial cerebrospinal fluid (see CEREBROSPINAL FLUID)
ACTH	adrenocorticotropic hormone
ADH	antidiuretic hormone
ADHD	attention deficit hyperactivity disorder
ADP	adenosine diphosphate
AF64A	acetylethylcholine mustard hydrochloride
Ag	silver
AI	artificial intelligence
Al	aluminium (aluminum)
ALS	amyotrophic lateral sclerosis (Lou Gehrig's disease)
AMPA	alpha-amino-3-hydroxy-5-methylisoxazole-4-propionic acid
AMPT	alpha-methyl-para-tyrosine
ANN	artificial neural network
ANP	atrial natriuretic peptide

ANS	autonomic nervous system
AP5	2-amino-5-phosphonovaleric acid (*also* APV)
apo E	apolipoprotein E
APV	2-amino-5-phosphonovaleric acid (*also* AP5)
ATP	adenosine triphosphate
Au	gold
AVP	arginine vasopressin
B1–B9	serotonin cell groups (see CLASSIFICATION OF DAHLSTRÖM AND FUXE)
BAT	brown adipose tissue
BBB	blood brain barrier
BDI	Beck depression inventory
BDNF	brain derived neurotrophic factor
BDZ	benzodiazepine
BEAM	brain electrical activity mapping
BLA	basolateral nucleus of the amygdala (see AMYGDALA)
B_{max}	maximum concentration of available binding sites
BNP	brain natriuretic peptide
BNST	bed nucleus of the stria terminalis
BSE	bovine spongiform encephalopathy
BuChE	butyrylcholinesterase
CA	catecholamine
Ca	calcium
Ca^{2+}	calcium ions
CANTAB	Cambridge automated neurological test battery
CAT	choline acetyltransferase (*also* ChAT)
CAT	computerized axial tomography (*also* CT)
CBT	cognitive-behavioural therapy
CCK	cholecystokinin
Cdk	cyclin dependent kinase (see CELL DIVISION)
cDNA	complementary DNA
CEA	central nucleus of the amygdala (see AMYGDALA)
Cg 1–3	cingulate cortex
CGRP	calcitonin gene related peptide
Ch	choline
Ch1–Ch8	cholinergic cell groups (entered under CH1–CH8)
ChAT	choline acetyltransferase (*also* CAT)
CJD	Creutzfeldt-Jakob disease
Cl	choline
Cl⁻	chloride ions
CNF	ciliary neurotrophic factor
CNP	C-type natriuretic peptide
CNQX	6-cyano-7-nitroquinoxaline-2,3-dione
CNS	central nervous system
CO	carbon monoxide
CO_2	carbon dioxide

COase	cytochrome oxidase
COMT	catechol-O-methyl-transferase
COS	carbonyl sulphide
CPG	central pattern generator
CPP	conditioned place preference
CR	conditioned response
CRF	conditioned reinforcer (-ment)
CRF	corticotropin releasing factor
CRH	corticotropin releasing hormone
CS	conditioned stimulus
CS_2	carbon disulphide
CSF	cerebrospinal fluid
CT	computerized axial tomography (*also* CAT)
CTB	cholera toxin subunit B
D1 – D5	D1 – D5 dopamine receptors
DA	dopamine
DAB	diaminobenzidene (see IMMUNOHISTOCHEMISTRY)
DAG	diacylglycerol
dB	decibel
DBH	dopamine beta hydroxylase
DFP	diisopropylfluorophosphate
DHMA	3,4-dihydroxymandelic acid
DHPA	3,4-dihydroxyphenylacetaldehyde
DHPG	3,4-dihydroxyphenylglycol
DHPGA	3,4-dihydroxyphenylglycoacetaldehyde
DMI	desmethylimipramine
DNA	deoxyribonucleic acid
DNAB	dorsal noradrenergic bundle
DNQX	6,7-dinitroquinoxaline-2,3-dione
DOPA	dihydroxyphenylalanine (see L-DOPA)
DOPAC	3,4-dihydroxyphenylacetic acid
DRL	differential reinforcement of low rates
DRO	differential reinforcement of other behaviour
DSM	diagnostic and statistical manual (of the American Psychiatric Association)
DSP4	N-2-chloroethyl-N-ethyl-2-bromobenzylamine
EAA	excitatory amino acid
EC50	effective concentration, 50%
ECG	electrocardiogram
ECT	electroconvulsive therapy
ED50	effective dose, 50%
EEG	electroencephalogram
ELISA	enzyme linked immunoabsorbent assay
EM	electron microscopy
EMG	electromyogram

EOG	electrooculogram
EPSP	excitatory postsynaptic potential
ERG	electroretinogram
ERP	event related potential
ESB	electrical brain stimulation
FAS	foetal alcohol syndrome
Fe	iron
FGF	fibroblast growth factor
FI	fixed interval (see SCHEDULES OF REINFORCEMENT)
fMRI	functional magnetic resonance imaging
FR	fixed ratio (see SCHEDULES OF REINFORCEMENT)
FSH	follicle stimulating hormone
FW	formula weight
GABA	gamma amino butyric acid
GABA A/B/C	GABA receptors
GABA-T	GABA transaminase
GAD	glutamic acid decarboxylase
GFAP	glial fibrillary acidic protein
GH	growth hormone
Glu	glutamate
Gly	glycine
GnRH	gonadatropin releasing hormone
GP	globus pallidus
GTP	guanosine triphosphate
H	histamine
H	hydrogen
H^+	hydrogen ions
H_2O	water
HLA	human leukocyte antigen
HO	heme oxygenase
HPA	hypothalamo-pituitary axis
HPC	hippocampus
HPLC	high performance liquid chromatography
HRP	horseradish peroxidase
HVA	homovanillic acid
IAA	inhibitory amino acid
ibo	ibotenic acid
IC50	inhibitory concentration, 50%
ICD10	International Statistical Classification of Diseases, Injuries and Causes of Death, 10th edition
ICSA	intracranial self-administration
ICSS	intracranial self-stimulation
IEG	immediate early gene

IgG	immunoglobulin G (see also IgA *etc.*)
im	intramuscular (injection)
ip	intraperitoneal (injection)
IP3	inositol 1,4,5-triphosphate
IPSP	inhibitory postsynaptic potential
IQ	intelligence quotient
ITI	intertrial interval
iv	intravenous (injection)
IVSA	intravenous self-administration
K	potassium
K$^+$	potassium ions
kai	kainic acid
LAMP	limbic system associated membrane protein
LC	locus coeruleus
LD50	lethal dose, 50%
L-DOPA	L-3,4-dihydroxyphenylalanine
LDTg	laterodorsal tegmental nucleus
Leu	leucine
LGn	lateral geniculate nucleus
LH	lateral hypothalamus
LH	learned helplessness
LH	luteinizing hormone
LHA	lateral hypothalamic area (see LATERAL HYPOTHALAMUS)
LHRH	luteinizing hormone releasing hormone
LI	latent inhibition
Li	lithium
LIA	large amplitude irregular activity
LiCl	lithium chloride
LNNB	Luria Nebraska neuropsychological test battery
LSD	lysergic acid diethylamide
LTD	long term depression
LTP	long term potentiation
M	molar (-ity)
mAChR	muscarinic acetylcholine receptors
MAO	monoamine oxidase
MAO-A	monoamine oxidase A
MAO-B	monoamine oxidase B
MAOI	monoamine oxidase inhibitor
MCA	middle cerebral artery
MD	mediodorsal nucleus of the thalamus
MDMA	3,4 methylenedioxymethamphetamine
ME	myalgic encephalitis (chronic fatigue syndrome)
MEA	midbrain extrapyramidal area
mfb	medial forebrain bundle

Mg	magnesium
Mg^{2+}	magnesium ions
MGn	medial geniculate nucleus
MHC	major histocompatibility complex
MHPA	3-methoxy-4-hydroxyphenylacetaldehyde
MHPG	3-methoxy-4-hydroxyphenylglycol
MHPGA	3-methoxy-4-hydroxyphenylglycoaldehyde
mol	mole (see MOLARITY)
MPP+	1-methyl-4-phenylpyridinium ion (see MPTP)
MPTP	1-methyl-4-phenyl-1,2,3,6-tetrahydropyridine
MRI	magnetic resonance imaging
mRNA	messenger RNA
MSG	monosodium glutamate
MSH	melanocyte stimulating hormone
MST	medial superior temporal region (see MOTION PERCEPTION)
MT	middle temporal region
MW	molecular weight
nA	nanoamp
NA	noradrenaline
Na	sodium
Na$^+$	sodium ions
NAC	nucleus accumbens (*also* Acb; NAcc; NAS)
NAcc	nucleus accumbens (*also* Acb; NAC; NAS)
nAChR	nicotinic acetylcholine receptors
NaCl	sodium chloride (saline)
NADPH	nicotinamide adenine dinucleotide phosphate (see NADPH DIAPHORASE)
NaOH	sodium hydroxide
NAS	nucleus accumbens septi (*also* Acb; NAC; NAcc)
NBM	nucleus basalis of Meynert
NBQX	6-nitro-sulfamoyl-benzo(f)-quinoxaline-2,3-dione
NE	norepinephrine
NGF	nerve growth factor
NMDA	N-methyl-D-aspartate
NMN	normetanephrine
nmol	nanomol (see MOLARITY)
NMR	nuclear magnetic resonance imaging
NO	nitric oxide
NOS	nitric oxide synthase
NPT	nocturnal penile tumescence
NPY	neuropeptide Y
NPYY	neuropeptide YY
nSOL	nucleus of the solitary tract
NTPP	nucleus tegmenti pedunculopontinus (*equivalent to* PPT, PPTg)
O	oxygen
OB	olfactory bulb

OCD	obsessive compulsive disorder
OPCA	olivopontocerebellar atropy
OT	olfactory tubercle
OVLT	organum vasculosum of the lamina terminalis
PAG	periaqueductal gray
PAP	peroxidase-antiperoxidase (see IMMUNOHISTOCHEMISTRY)
Pb	lead
PCP	1-(1-phenylcyclohexy-1)piperidine; phencyclidine; angel dust
PCPA	para-chlorophenylalanine
PCR	polymerase chain reaction labelling
PD	Parkinson's disease
PDP	parallel distributed processing
PEA	phenylethylamine
PET	positron emission tomography
PFC	prefrontal cortex
PFCx	prefrontal cortex
PGO	pons-geniculate-occipital (see PGO WAVES)
PHA-L	*phaseolus vulgaris* leucoagglutinin
PKA	protein kinase A
PKC	protein kinase C
PKU	phenylketonuria
PMS	premenstrual syndrome (see PREMENSTRUAL TENSION)
PMT	premenstrual tension
PNMT	phenylethanolamine-N-methyltransferase
PNS	peripheral nervous system
POMC	proopiomelanocortin
PPA	pedunculopontine area (see PEDUNCULOPONTINE TEGMENTAL NUCLEUS)
PPI	prepulse inhibition
PPT	pedunculopontine tegmental nucleus (*also* PPTg, TPP, NTPP)
PPTg	pedunculopontine tegmental nucleus (*also* PPT, TPP, NTPP)
PR	progressive ratio (see SCHEDULES OF REINFORCEMENT)
PRAE	partial reinforcement acquisition effect
PREE	partial reinforcement extinction effect
PrP	prion protein
PSP	progressive supranuclear palsy
PTSD	post-traumatic stress disorder
PVN	paraventricular nucleus (of the hypothalamus *or* the thalamus)
QTL	quantitative trait loci
Quin	quinolinic acid
Quis	quisqualic acid
rCBF	regional cerebral blood flow
REM	rapid eye movement sleep
RER	rough endoplasmic reticulum
RIA	radioimmunoassay

RNA	ribonucleic acid
rRNA	ribosomal RNA
RSA	rhythmic slow activity
RT	reaction time
SI	primary somatosensory cortex
SII	secondary somatosensory cortex
SAS	supervisory attentional system
sc	subcutaneous (injection)
SC	superior colliculus
SCN	suprachiasmatic nucleus
scp	superior cerebellar peduncle
SDAT	senile dementia of the Alzheimer type
SDLT	senile dementia of the Lewy body type
SER	smooth endoplasmic reticulum
shh	sonic hedgehog
SIDS	sudden infant death syndrome
SMA	supplementary motor area
SN	substantia nigra
SNc	substantia nigra pars compacta
SNr	substantia nigra pars reticulata
SNRI	selective noradrenaline reuptake inhibitor
SNRI	serotonin and noradrenaline reuptake inhibitor
SOD	superoxide dismutase
SON	supraoptic nucleus of the hypothalamus
SP	substance P
SPECT	single photon emission tomography
SPTg	subpeduncular tegmental nucleus
SQUID	superconducting quantum interference device
SSRI	selective serotonin reuptake inhibitor
SST	somatostatin
STn	subthalamic nucleus
STP	short term potentiation
STS	superior temporal sulcus
STX	saxitoxin
T3	triiodothyronine
T4	thyroxine
TD50	toxic dose, 50%
TEA	tetraethylammonium
TEO	temporal occipital area (see TEO)
TH	tyrosine hydroxylase (*also* TOH)
THA	tetrahydroaminacridine
THC	tetrahydro-cannabis
TI	therapeutic index
TIA	transient ischaemic attack

TNF	tumour necrosis factor
TOH	tyrosine hydroxylase (*also* TH)
TRH	thyrotropin releasing hormone
Trk	tyrosine kinase (receptors)
TRn	thalamic reticular nucleus
tRNA	transfer RNA
TSH	thyroid stimulating hormone
TTX	tetrodotoxin
UR	unconditioned response
US	unconditioned stimulus
VA-VL	ventroanterior-ventrolateral nuclei of the thalamus (see THALAMUS)
VCNP	C-type natriuretic peptide
VI	variable interval (see SCHEDULES OF REINFORCEMENT)
VIP	vasoactive intestinal polypeptide
VP	ventral pallidum
VMH	ventromedial hypothalamus
VMn	ventromedial nucleus (of the hypothalamus)
VNAB	ventral noradrenergic bundle
VR	variable ratio (see SCHEDULES OF REINFORCEMENT)
VTA	ventral tegmental area of Tsai (see VENTRAL TEGMENTAL AREA)
WAIS	Wechsler adult intelligence scale
WGA-HRP	wheat germ agglutinated horseradish peroxidase (see TRACT TRACERS)
WISC	Wisconsin card sorting task
w/v	weight/volume (see PERCENT SOLUTION)
w/w	weight/weight (see PERCENT SOLUTION)
Zn	zinc

Greek letters

Lower case	Upper case	Name	English equivalent
α	A	alpha	a
β	B	beta	b
γ	Γ	gamma	g
δ	Δ	delta	d
ϵ	E	epsilon	e – as in *red*
ζ	Z	zeta	z
η	H	eta	e – as in *tree*
θ or ϑ	Θ	theta	th
ι	I	iota	i
κ	K	kappa	k
λ	Λ	lambda	l
μ	M	mu	m
ν	N	nu	n
ξ	Ξ	xi	x – ks
o	O	omicron	o – as in *got*
π	Π	pi	p
ρ	P	rho	r
σ or ς	Σ	sigma	s
τ	T	tau	t
υ	Υ	upsilon	u
ϕ	Φ	phi	ph
χ	X	chi	kh
ψ	Ψ	psi	ps
ω	Ω	omega	o – as in *bone*

A

A fibres These are FIBRES involved in the sensation of PAIN. A-delta (δ) fibres are small myelinated (see MYELIN) fibres; A-alpha (α) and A-beta (β) fibres are larger than delta and are also myelinated. The delta fibres, like the unmyelinated C FIBRES, come from cell bodies in the DORSAL ROOT GANGLIA.They are UNIPOLAR NEURONS: the AXON takes information into layers 1 and 5 of the DORSAL HORN of the spinal cord (from where information is sent to the BRAINSTEM and THALAMUS). The DENDRITE brings information in from nociceptors. The A-alpha and A-beta fibres project to layer 4 of the dorsal horn and bring information in from MECHANORECEPTORS. For further information, see PAIN.

a- (an-) Prefix indicating complete absence. The prefix dys- indicates a partial loss. Thus for example AKINESIA is an absence of movement and DYSKINESIA a partial loss of movement.

A1–A12, B1–B9 A1–A12 are catecholamine-containing cell groups in the central nervous system; B1–B9 are serotonin-containing; see CLASSIFICATION OF DAHLSTRÖM AND FUXE.

abducens nerve The sixth cranial nerve (see CRANIAL NERVES); controls activity of the musculature of the eyes.

Abercrombie correction Formula applied to estimates of cell counts in brain sections that corrects for cells extending across more than one histological section.

See also: histology; stereology

STEPHEN B. DUNNETT

ablation Removal of tissue. The term LESION is now much more commonly used to refer to the surgical removal of tissue.

abnormal illness behaviour Abnormal illness behaviour is regarded by Pilowsky, who has popularized the concept, as a maladaptive way of experiencing, perceiving, evaluating or responding to one's health status despite being offered an accurate explanation of one's health from an appropriate person. Persons displaying abnormal illness behaviour are often described as hypochondriacal. It is usually measured using the Illness Behaviour Questionnaire.

Reference

Pilowsky, I. (1993) Dimensions of illness behaviour as measured by the Illness Behaviour Questionnaire: a replication study. *Journal of Psychosomatic Research* 37: 53–62.

DEREK W. JOHNSTON

absence seizure Absence seizure, also known as PETIT MAL SEIZURE, is a generalized non-convulsive seizure characterized by the symmetrical appearance of spike-and-wave discharges in the cortical ELECTROENCEPHALOGRAM(EEG) at a frequency of 3 per second. The seizure starts and ends abruptly, lasting for 2 to 10 seconds. Consciousness is lost during this period but returns almost immediately when the abnormal EEG stops. The seizure is often associated with rolling up of the eyes and blinking. The characteristic spike-and-wave pattern is thought to be generated through the interaction of non-specific thalamic neurons and cortical neurons.

See also: epilepsy

KAZUE SEMBA

absolute refractory period The period following an ACTION POTENTIAL during which it is impossible to elicit a second action potential. This property is the result of the activation and inactivation of sodium currents during an action potential. The voltage-sensitive SODIUM CHANNELS cannot be activated (opened) while they are still inactivated from the previous action potential. Since sodium inactivation is dependent on DEPOLARIZATION, the cell membrane must be sufficiently repolarized for this inactivation to be removed. Only then can a new action potential be produced by a new depolarizing stimulus. The absolute refractory period imposes an upper limit on the frequency with which action potentials can occur.

DOUGLAS D. RASMUSSON

absorption *see* digestion

abstinence Derived from the term 'abstain' which has a Latin root: *abs*: from, and *temetum*: strong wine. Abstinence indicates refraining or withdrawing from something; typically to do with the denial (either forced or voluntary) of something carrying POSITIVE REINFORCEMENT. Abstinence may be unpleasant: in extreme cases it leads to a state known as WITHDRAWAL SYNDROME, or, as it is often called, abstinence syndrome. In Western societies the most commonly experienced form of this involves individuals giving up smoking TOBACCO, though NICOTINE abstinence is not as serious a condition as can occur with other drugs.

abstinence syndrome *see* withdrawal syndrome

abuse potential A term used in PSYCHOPHARMACOLOGY and drug development research to denote the potential a drug has to become abused (used in a manner that deviates from the approved medical or social patterns within a given culture). It is important to establish the abuse potential of compounds that are prescribed for therapeutic purposes, particularly for newly developed drugs. Often the abuse potential of a compound will be determined in the drug SELF-ADMINISTRATION test in animals; if the drug is self-administered, it has abuse potential.

ANN E. KELLEY

acalculia Impairment in the ability to perform simple arithmetic calculations; also used more broadly to refer to any deficit in the ability to use numbers, whether or not calculation is affected. The term DYSCALCULIA is synonymous in most usages (although in the strictest sense acalculia refers to an inability to calculate or use numbers, whereas dyscalculia implies impairment without complete abolition of the ability). Acalculia may result from brain injury or disease (for instance, STROKE, head trauma, ALZHEIMER'S DISEASE), in which case the deficit is referred to as an acquired acalculia. In developmental acalculias children with no obvious neurological abnormalities have difficulty learning to use numbers or calculate, despite normal educational opportunities.

Number use and calculation require a wide variety of cognitive processes. For example, solving a written multiplication problem involves, among other abilities, comprehending the multiplication sign, recognizing the digits in the problem, recalling the sequence of steps for performing multidigit multiplications, retrieving arithmetic facts from memory and writing the digits of the answer. Disruption or abnormal development of any processes required for a numerical skill will result in impairment on that skill, with the specific form of impairment depending upon what particular processes are affected. As a consequence, both acquired and developmental acalculias take many different forms. Some forms of acalculia stem from impairment in basic processes required for comprehending or producing numerals (for example, 2047 or two thousand forty-seven). These deficits may be quite selective, affecting some aspects of numeral comprehension or production while sparing other aspects. For example, comprehension of numerals may be disrupted while ability to produce numerals remains intact, or vice versa; and processing of numerals in digit form (arabic numerals) may be impaired while processing of numerals in word form (verbal numerals) remains intact, or vice versa. In some instances the deficits may be even more specific. Several researchers have described well-educated adults who, after suffering brain damage, were intact in comprehending and producing verbal numerals (such as six thousand seven hundred), and in comprehending arabic numerals (6700) yet were impaired in producing arabic numerals (for example writing 6700 as 6000700). This pattern of impairment suggests that the cognitive processes required for producing arabic numerals are at least partially distinct from the processes for comprehending them, and from those for processing verbal numerals. Other comparably selective numeral-processing deficits have also been reported. These deficits have provided a major source of evidence for proposing and testing theories of the cognitive representations and processes involved in normal number processing.

Impairments affecting numeral comprehension or production processes will lead to deficits in calculation tasks requiring the impaired processes. For example, impaired comprehension of arabic digits will disrupt performance on arithmetic problems presented in digit form. However, arithmetic performance may also be impaired by disruption or abnormal development of cognitive processes specific to calculation. For example, both developmental and acquired deficits in recalling arithmetic table facts (such as $6 \times 7 = 42$) have been reported. Individuals suffering from arithmetic fact retrieval deficits may show normal comprehension and production of numerals, and may have no difficulty remembering the sequence of steps for solving multidigit arithmetic problems. However, these individuals have difficulty learning table facts (in the case of developmental deficits) or recalling previously well-learned facts (acquired deficits). In solving problems they may laboriously work out each required table fact (for instance, in solving 758×4, adding four 8s to obtain 32, then adding four 5s to get 20, and so forth), or may make errors in attempting to remember the facts (recalling 28 as the answer to 4×8 for instance). In contrast, other individuals show normal ability to retrieve arithmetic facts, but are selectively impaired in learning or remembering multidigit calculation

procedures. These individuals make errors in which the individual table facts are recalled accurately, but the problem-solving process is disrupted in some way (for example, $758 \times 4 = 282032$, resulting from writing each retrieved product in its entirety, rather than writing the 1s digit and carrying the 10s digit). These selective impairments have been taken as evidence that the cognitive representations and processes for recalling arithmetic table facts are at least partially separate from those for carrying out calculation procedures.

In addition to impairments specifically affecting numeral comprehension, numeral production, or calculation processes, acalculias can result from disruption of more general cognitive abilities required for a wide range of cognitive functions. For example, in spatial acalculia some general spatial deficit leads to impairment in appreciating or using the spatial arrangement of numbers in a problem, or in producing the digits of the answer in the appropriate spatial positions. Also, at least some deficits in comprehending or producing verbal numerals are not specific to numerals, but represent manifestations of more general language deficits.

See also: mathematics and the brain

MICHAEL McCLOSKEY

acamprosate *see* alcoholism

accessory nerve The eleventh cranial nerve (see CRANIAL NERVES): involved in the control of swallowing and movement of the head and shoulders.

accessory olfactory bulb The accessory olfactory bulb lies behind the main OLFACTORY BULB. While the main olfactory bulb projects to the THALAMUS and CORTEX, the accessory olfactory bulb projects to the AMYGDALA and HYPOTHALAMUS, making direct contact with structures concerned with primary motivated behaviours (see PRIMARY MOTIVATION) such as FEEDING and SEXUAL BEHAVIOUR, and responses to STRESS. Its input comes principally from the VOMERONASAL NERVE, which comes from the VOMERONASAL ORGAN; see OLFACTION.

accessory optic system This is a subcortical element of the VISUAL SYSTEM that has been little studied. Most studies in vision are directed to the cortex (see VISUAL CORTEX) and THALAMUS (see LATERAL GENICULATE NUCLEUS) but the evolutionarily older subcortical systems (see SUPERIOR COLLICULUS and RETINOHYPOTHALAMIC SYSTEM) are probably very much more active than is commonly supposed. From the RETINA, two accessory optic pathways can be traced, the inferior and superior accessory optic tracts. These are crossed pathways that run in parallel (until the terminal regions) with the OPTIC NERVE fibres that innervate the superior colliculus and lateral geniculate nucleus. The inferior accessory optic tract terminates in a part of the MIDBRAIN tegmentum known as the MEDIAL TERMINAL NUCLEUS. The superior accessory optic tract terminates here also (most notably in the basal parts of the nucleus) as well as in two nuclei located close by, the dorsal and lateral terminal nuclei. The superior and inferior fibres also project to the NUCLEUS OF THE OPTIC TRACT, slightly anterior to the lateral terminal nucleus and lateral and anterior to the medial terminal nucleus. Very little work has been carried out to determine the functions of this system, though it is thought to be involved in the ability to maintain GAZE (see Ariel & Tusa, 1992).

References

Ariel M. & Tusa R.J. (1992) Spontaneous nystagmus and gaze-holding ability in monkeys after intravitreal picrotoxin injections. *Journal of Neurophysiology* 67: 1124–1132.

Davson H. (1990) *Physiology of the Eye*, 5th edn, Macmillan: London.

Hart W.M. Jr (1992) *Adler's Physiology of the Eye*, 9th edn, Mosby Year Book: St Louis MO.

accommodation The adjustment of the eye to achieve a sharply focused image on the RETINA for different viewing distances. In humans and other mammals this is achieved by the action of the ciliary muscle which alters the shape of the lens. Maximum accommodative effort is required to focus on near objects. Viewing a near object binocularly requires convergence (to minimize RETINAL DISPARITY) as well as accommodation (to minimize blur), and the neural control systems for these two responses are closely coupled. The sensed degree of accommodation provides a weak cue for DEPTH PERCEPTION for nearby objects.

See also: refractive error; vergence

OLIVER J. BRADDICK

acetaldyde Primary metabolite of ALCOHOL, created by the action of acetaldehyde dehydrogenase on alcohol in the liver. Highly toxic, it is quickly broken down to acetate by aldehyde dehydrogenase. Acetate combines with coenzyme A to form ACETYL COA which is decomposed further to produce carbon dioxide, water and 7 calories per gram of alcohol.

Reference

Feldman R.S., Meyer J.S. & Quenzer L.F. (1997) *Principles of Neuropsychopharmacology*, Sinauer Associates: Sunderland MA.

acetate (acetic acid) *see* alcohol

acetic acid (acetate) *see* alcohol

acetyl CoA Shortened form of ACETYL COENZYME A: see ACETYLCHOLINE; ALCOHOL.

acetyl coenzyme A The neurotransmitter ACETYLCHOLINE is synthesized from ACETYL COENZYME A (acetyl CoA) and CHOLINE, a reaction catalyzed by the enzyme CHOLINE ACETYLTRANSFERASE. Acetyl CoA is formed in the MITOCHONDRIA of most cells. In cholinergic neurons, it is transported out of mitochondria for use in synthesizing acetylcholine.

acetylcholine (ACh) Acetylcholine is a small-molecule NEUROTRANSMITTER synthesized from ACETYL COENZYME A and CHOLINE. The term CHOLINERGIC is used to describe a neuron that contains acetylcholine. The synaptic (*see* SYNAPSE) action of ACh is mediated by muscarinic and NICOTINIC ACETYLCHOLINE RECEPTORS, and unbound ACh is inactivated by ACETYLOCHLINESTERASE. ACh is used as a transmitter by all somatic MOTOR NEURONS as well as a subpopulation of autonomic neurons. Main cholinergic cell groups in the brain include neurons in the BASAL FOREBRAIN projecting to the CORTEX, neurons in the MESOPONTINE tegmentum innervating the THALAMUS and BRAINSTEM, and the large interneurons in the striatum. The cholinergic projection neurons are implicated in LEARNING, MEMORY, ATTENTION, AROUSAL and REM SLEEP.

See also: Ch1–Ch8

KAZUE SEMBA

acetylcholine receptors (cholinergic receptors) Acetylcholine (ACh) binds to two receptor subtypes: nicotinic and muscarinic receptors. Nicotinic ACh receptors are LIGAND-gated receptors; muscarinic ACh receptors are G PROTEIN coupled. Both types of receptor are found in the brain and spinal cord and in the sympathetic and parasympathetic nervous systems. ACh receptors have been implicated in many CNS processes, from learning and memory, through the control of eating and drinking to reward processes.

Nicotinic receptors – so-called because they are the receptors that bind the drug NICOTINE – are made from four GLYCOPROTEIN subunits (alpha, beta, gamma and delta): two of the alpha subunits are present with one of each of the others. These five units cluster in such a way that a small pore can be created through which ions can travel (an ION CHANNEL). Activation of the receptor causes influx of Na^+ and K^+ ions into neurons, depolarizing the neuron and generating a fast EXCITATORY POSTSYNAPTIC POTENTIAL. Both alpha subunits must be occupied by ACh for ion channel opening to occur; binding at these sites shows positive co-operativity. Muscarinic receptors – so-called because they bind muscarine, the poison found in *Amanita muscaris* mushrooms (fly agaric) – are found in different subtypes, M1–M5, identified by their differential binding of cholinergic drugs and by the genes that code for them (the *m1 – m5* genes). M1, M3 and M5 receptors stimulate phosphatidylinosiotol and increase CYCLIC AMP actions (see SECOND MESSENGERS) among other things. They activate Ca^{2+}-dependent K^+ and Cl^- currents. Activation of M2 and M4 receptors in contrast inhibits adenylate cyclase activity and inhibits Ca^{2+} currents. In the CNS, the effects of muscarinic activation are mostly excitatory, though the effects of ACh at muscarinic receptors may have rather more neuromodulatory functions. For example, action at muscarinic receptors in the cortex enhances excitatory responses to other inputs onto the same neuron.

See also: muscarinic acetylcholine receptors; nicotinic acetylcholine receptors; depolarization

acetylcholinesterase (AChE) The enzyme that inactivates ACETYLCHOLINE by hydrolyzing it to CHOLINE and ACETIC ACID. This degradation and the diffusion out of the SYNAPTIC CLEFT are the main mechanisms for terminating the synaptic action of acetylcholine. AChE is a specific cholinesterase with high affinity for acetylcholine as a substrate, whereas BUTYRYLCHOLINESTERASE, also called a non-specific cholinesterase or PSEUDOCHOLINESTERASE, degrades butyrylcholine preferentially. AChE is a sugar-containing GLYCOPROTEIN made up of one or more subunits. Various molecular forms of AChE exist, including globular and asymmetric forms, and are classified into hetero- and homomeric families. AChE is present in CHOLINERGIC as well as certain non-cholinergic neurons.

KAZUE SEMBA

achromatic mechanisms *see* opponent process theory of colour vision

achromatopsia The inability to distinguish different hues despite normally pigmented cells in the RETINA and despite normal VISUAL ACUITY and normal form discrimination is referred to as achromatopsia, cortical colour blindness or central achromatopsia. It is distinguished from COLOUR ANOMIA in which colours, although recognized, cannot be named. Patients may describe their world as devoid of colour and containing only black, white and grey and may be impaired on all sectors of the colour spectrum (on the Farnsworth–Munsell 100-Hue test; Farnsworth, 1957) although distant hue contrasts (on the Ishihara colour plates; Ishihara, 1983) may still be discriminated. Full-field achromatopsia following bilateral lesions in the region of the occipitotemporal junction (where the occipital and temporal lobes meet) in the lingual and fusiform gyri is possible but rare. Hemiachromatopsia occurs after lesions to the CONTRALATERAL occipitotemporal region but the most common form, quadrantachromatopsia, is generally accompanied by a QUADRANTANOPSIA (or a more circumscribed SCOTOMA) following lesions to the inferior bank of the CALCARINE FISSURE particularly on the left. Neuroimaging studies with normal subjects performing a colour search task have shown activation in the same region of the lingual and fusiform gyri, the putative human area V4, shown to be damaged by the lesions. There are a number of neurobehavioural deficits which frequently accompany achromatopsia, including ACQUIRED DYSLEXIA, VISUAL AGNOSIA and PROSOPAGNOSIA. Acquired dyslexia, usually of the PURE ALEXIA variety occurs following lesions to the left OCCIPITAL LOBE. Visual agnosia, in which patients may fail to recognize certain objects presented in the visual modality, may also be observed with the achromatopsic deficit. Finally, prosopagnosia may be present because of the close proximity of areas involved in FACE PERCEPTION to the V4 area on the fusiform gyrus.

References

Farnsworth, D. (1957) *Farnsworth–Munsell 100-hue Test for Colour Vision* Munsell Colour Company: Baltimore.

Ishihara, S. (1983) *Ishihara's Test for Colour Blindness*, Kanehara: Tokyo.

MARLENE BEHRMANN

acid (from Latin, *acidus*: sour) The term acid has multiple meanings. The more relevant scientific uses are: (1) in respect of taste (see TASTE PERCEPTION), acid means sour or sharp, as the etymology suggests. (2) In biology and chemistry, an acid is a substance that increases the hydrogen ION (H^+) content of a solution. In water, hydrochloric acid (HCl), for example, dissociates into hydrogen ions (H^+) and CHLORIDE ions (Cl^-) (see Campbell, Reece & Mitchell, 1999). (3) In the language of the street 'acid' refers to the dangerous HALLUCINOGEN LSD (LYSERGIC ACID DIETHYLAMIDE).

See also: alkali; amino acids; base; neurotransmitters; pH

References

Campbell N.A., Reece J.B. & Mitchell L.G. (1999) *Biology*, 5th edn, Addison-Wesley: Menlo Park CA.

acid fuchsin A novel STAIN used in HISTOLOGY that only reacts with a NEURON that is functionally compromised or dying.

acoustic spectrum The acoustic spectrum of a sound is the average distribution of sound pressure across frequency and is usually represented on double logarithmic axes because of the large dynamic range of the auditory system and the logarithmic representation of frequency on the BASILAR MEMBRANE. The sound pressure is commonly expressed in decibels (dB); 6 dB represents a factor 2 in sound pressure. Zero dB sound-pressure-level (SPL) corresponds approximately to the level of a 1000 Hz tone that is just audible to normal hearing human adults. The maximum of the dynamic range of hearing is 120 dB SPL, a level that is painful.

JOS J. EGGERMONT

acquired dyslexia Disorders of READING following brain damage in individuals who were previously normal readers. Disorders are classified as peripheral or central. Peripheral disorders affect the ability to process the visual forms of written words. Central disorders affect the ability to understand and read aloud written words.

The three types of peripheral dyslexia are NEGLECT DYSLEXIA, ATTENTIONAL DYSLEXIA and PURE ALEXIA. Neglect dyslexia affects the processing of letters at one end of the written word, usually on the left. Complete words on the left side of text may be omitted also. Neglect dyslexia is usually accompanied by SPATIAL NEGLECT in which there is a general lack of awareness of objects on one side of space, usually the left. ATTENTIONAL DYSLEXIA is a rare disorder affecting the ability to attend to individual letters in a written word, although the complete word and the letters presented individually can be identified. In PURE ALEXIA (or LETTER-BY-LETTER READING) complete written word forms cannot be recognized. Instead, each letter is identified separately and often named alphabetically, before the word can be recognized. Reading is slow, and short words are read faster than long words.

The three types of central dyslexias are DEEP DYSLEXIA, PHONOLOGICAL DYSLEXIA and SUR-

FACE DYSLEXIA. Deep dyslexia destroys the ability to pronounce novel letter strings; function words cannot be read aloud; and abstract words are read poorly. Concrete words, and words with imageable meanings, are read best. Reading errors include SEMANTIC ERRORS, in which a written word is confused with one related in meaning, and visual errors, in which a written word is confused with a word of similar appearance. PHONOLOGICAL DYSLEXIA particularly affects the ability to pronounce novel letter strings. The ability to read previously familiar words may be spared or partly impaired. Grammatical words (see GRAMMAR) and abstract words can be read, sometimes as successfully as imageable and concrete words. Visual errors occur, but not semantic errors. SURFACE DYSLEXIA affects the ability to pronounce and comprehend previously familiar words with irregular spelling–sound correspondences, for example *pint*, and affects less frequent words most. These words are often mispronounced using more regular pronunciations. Familiar words with regular spelling–sound correspondences, such as *mint*, are pronounced most successfully. The ability to pronounce novel letter strings is either normal or only partly impaired.

Different patterns of brain damage are associated with different forms of acquired dyslexia. Neglect dyslexia is associated with lesions in the PARIETAL LOBE in the hemisphere which processes the side of space affected (the right hemisphere in the case of left-sided neglect). Attentional dyslexia arises with lesions in the left parietal lobe. Pure alexia occurs when posterior lesions prevent visually presented material reaching the LANGUAGE areas. The reading that does occur is thought by some researchers to be processed in the subdominant hemisphere. The central dyslexias are associated with damage to the language areas of the TEMPORAL LOBE and parietal lobe of the LEFT HEMISPHERE. The remaining reading abilities in phonological and surface dyslexia are supported by impaired dominant hemisphere processes, but the residual reading in deep dyslexia has been argued to take place in the subdominant hemisphere.

The processing deficits underlying the peripheral dyslexias arise in the early visual–perceptual processing stages. Neglect dyslexia is commonly viewed as a deficit in ATTENTION to a particular side of space affecting the letters that fall within that area. But sometimes the deficit affects the initial letters of the word, irrespective of the spatial area in which they appear. Attentional dyslexia may arise when the ability to change the size of the attentional window from the space of a whole word to that of single letters is affected. Pure alexia is thought to occur when letters in the word cannot be processed in parallel. Theories of the processing deficits underlying different forms of acquired dyslexia have been explained in terms of models of normal reading. The model that accounts best for acquired dyslexia proposes a LEXICON (or word store) of written (or orthographic – see ORTHOGRAPHY) forms of words and a lexicon of spoken (or phonological – see PHONOLOGY) forms of words. These lexica allow familiar orthographic and phonological word forms to be understood via pathways to the semantic system in which word meanings are stored. Deep dyslexia is thought to arise when only this route is available for reading. Orthographic word forms are also linked directly to phonological word forms. Phonological dyslexia is thought to arise when only the direct lexical pathway and the semantic pathway are available for reading. A further sub-lexical reading process analyses the written letter string into letter groups and links these to sounds producing a novel phonological sequence. Surface dyslexia is thought to arise when the lexical reading pathways are damaged and the sub-lexical reading process is used in support.

The prognosis for peripheral reading disorders is quite good, but central disorders usually endure, although effective treatments, based on preserved abilities, have proved successful in some cases of deep and surface dyslexia.

Reference

Ellis, A.W. (1993) *Reading, Writing and Dyslexia*, 2nd edn, Lawrence Erlbaum: Hove.

ELAINE FUNNELL

acquired reading disorder The term acquired reading disorder can be taken to be synonymous with ACQUIRED DYSLEXIA; it is therefore a term that can also be applied to the categories of dyslexia that come under this general heading: see DYSLEXIA for a description of these.

See also: agraphia

acquisition A period of LEARNING. The acquisition stage of an experiment allows the subject to discover the consequences associated with the occurrence of a specific event or carrying out a particular action. Acquisition can be measured objectively by monitoring the subject's behaviour across a number of sessions, the acquisition period being complete when the subject reaches a predetermined level of performance.

WENDY L. INGLIS

acquisition of a novel response An alternative description of the procedure of responding with CONDITIONED REINFORCEMENT: a novel response is required to obtain a conditioned reinforcer.

acquisition of language by non-human primates Since the 1970s several research projects have introduced PRIMATES of various species to certain modes of non-verbal communication: natural SIGN LANGUAGE, invented systems of symbols to be communicated via a keyboard, plastic chips to be arranged in sequence. Many apes have achieved an impressive ability to use these systems to acquire food and other rewards. The most recent general assessment (Wallman, 1992) is however that there is no compelling evidence that the apes have acquired the ability to encode propositions syntactically (in contrast to human children who demonstrate such ability from the beginning of multiword utterance production).

See also: grammar

Reference

Wallman, J. (1992) *Aping Language*, Cambridge University Press: Cambridge.

ANNE CUTLER

acrocentric chromosome A chromosome in which the CENTROMERE, the region in which the two chromatids are joined, is situated towards one end of the chromosome, producing two short arms and two long arms.

FIONA M. INGLIS

across-fibre pattern theory In the across-fibre pattern theory of NEURAL CODING it is maintained that information is carried by the relative amounts, or pattern, of activity across many neurons. A good analogy is that of a matrix of light bulbs in a movie marquee, with each bulb representing one NEURON. The message is given by the pattern of bulbs that are on, and neurally a message is given in the pattern of activity across neurons. This theory has economic power in that, as a marquee may display many different messages, a population of neurons may carry many different messages. However a neuron is not an on-or-off device like a bulb, but can assume many levels of activity. Thus the amount of information carried by a neural population is indeed large. If 13 neurons each have 10 possible levels of activity, they will support 10 000 000 000 different patterns, or neural messages; this approximates the number of neurons in the human brain. This theory has empirical support. Typically neurons function as 'marquee' ensembles since wide varieties of stimuli are represented by the same population. For example, colour-sensitive neurons respond to nearly all wavelengths, so wavelength must be encoded across them. Similarly taste, temperature, vestibular, auditory, somaesthetic, kinesthetic and olfactory neurons each respond to many different stimuli within their domains, and motor neurons each participate in wide ranges of movement. Thus the marquee ensemble analogy holds for these systems. And a brain, as a marquee, can function with considerable loss of its units. The economic power of this theory would be useful in all neural functions, especially those with high information content (many messages), adding at least memory and complex cognitive processes along with emotional and motivational states to the above systems. Modern approaches to neural coding, including PARALLEL PROCESSING, DISTRIBUTED PROCESSING and ENSEMBLE CODING, incorporate the idea of across-fibre patterning. The terms ACROSS-NEURON PATTERNING and ACROSS-UNIT PATTERNING are identical to across-fibre patterning. This theory is in strong contrast with the other major coding position, the LABELLED-LINE THEORY, since the latter holds that each neuron carries its own distinct message unaffected by the overall pattern of activity in which it is imbedded. In the labelled-line theory, the number of possible messages would equal the number of neurons.

See also: connectionism; neural networks; parallel vs. serial processing

ROBERT P. ERICKSON

across-neuron patterning *see* across-fibre pattern theory

across-unit patterning *see* across-fibre pattern theory

ACTH *see* adrenocorticotropic hormone

actin *see* muscles

action potential A stereotyped change in electrical potential across the MEMBRANE of a neuron or muscle cell as a result of stimulation. The occurrence of an action potential is dependent on the cell being depolarized (see DEPOLARIZATION) past the point called the THRESHOLD. Once the threshold is reached, a positive feedback loop initiates a sequence of depolarization and repolarization that is independent of the initial cause. This allows an action potential to maintain the same amplitude as it travels (or propagates) along the cell membrane. In the case of neurons, this property allows information to be encoded in terms of the rate of firing of action potentials. This information can then be carried without change from one part of the nervous system to another via the neuron's axon. An action potential is also called a spike. The simultaneous occurrence of many action potentials in a peripheral nerve or muscle is recorded as a COMPOUND ACTION POTENTIAL.

An action potential is dependent on the presence of SODIUM CHANNELS that are sensitive to membrane voltage. Depolarization of the membrane opens these channels rapidly (sodium activation) and closes them slowly (sodium inactivation). The initial opening allows positive sodium ions to flow into the cell, which depolarizes the membrane more; this

depolarization in turn opens more sodium channels. At the point where the positive feedback effect of the inflowing sodium ions cannot be stopped (the threshold) the action potential is initiated. The membrane voltage becomes positive inside the cell as the membrane potential approaches the equilibrium potential for sodium. This large depolarization is terminated by progressive sodium inactivation as well as by the opening of voltage-dependent POTASSIUM CHANNELS which permits potassium ions to flow out of the cell. The slower time course of potassium activation often produces a HYPERPOLARIZATION at the end of the action potential. Voltage-dependent sodium channels cannot be reopened until sodium inactivation is complete. This results in an ABSOLUTE REFRACTORY PERIOD which limits the frequency of action potentials. The absolute refractory period is followed by a relative refractory period, during which a second action potential can be initiated if a stronger stimulus is applied. In other words, the threshold is raised during the relative refractory period.

Propagation of the action potential along the axon results from the fact that the depolarization at one point on the membrane produces passive spread of current in surrounding membrane. Therefore this adjacent membrane will also be depolarized and it too will produce an action potential when it reaches threshold. The movement of an action potential along the cell membrane is therefore analogous to the burning of a fuse. The rate of action potential propagation, or conduction velocity, is dependent on two factors: the internal axonal resistance and the membrane resistance. Conduction velocity is indirectly proportional to the internal resistance, which is primarily determined by the diameter of the axon. In a manner analogous to water flow in a pipe, the smaller the diameter of the axon the greater will be the resistance and consequently the slower the conduction velocity. Membrane resistance affects the velocity in the opposite manner: the greater the membrane resistance the greater the velocity. This is because the greater membrane resistance prevents the current generated by the action potential from leaking out through the membrane. Greater current therefore travels along the axon and is better able to depolarize the next segment of the axon. The membrane resistance is primarily determined by the presence or absence of MYELIN. The NODES OF RANVIER are the regions between myelinated segments and are characterized by a high density of voltage-sensitive sodium channels. The high resistance underlying the myelin and the high density of sodium channels at the nodes of Ranvier allows the action potential to 'jump' from one node to the next. This type of action potential conduction is therefore called SALTATORY and is much faster than can be obtained by increasing the axonal diameter.

Diseases that affect conduction velocity can impair sensory and/or motor function because information cannot travel from one end of neuron to the other. This can be due to damage to the neurons themselves or to loss of myelin (DEMYELINATION). Peripheral neuropathies, associated with diabetes and many other diseases, can cause pain or loss of sensation in various parts of the body . The more peripheral parts of the body (hands and feet) are most affected by these diseases because the axons to and from the hands and feet travel the longest distances and are therefore the most easily affected. Other types of peripheral demyelination may result from viral infection (for instance, Guillain–Barr disease). The major demyelinating disease of the central nervous system is MULTIPLE SCLEROSIS.

See also: all-or-none; neuropathology; sodium-potassium pump

DOUGLAS D. RASMUSSON

action tremor *see* tremor

activation (i) *Neural systems*: Activation refers to increased activity within neural systems and can be used at the level of the individual NEURON, in terms of activation of a POSTSYNAPTIC membrane, or it could be at the level of entire neural systems. Activation at the level of the individual neuron occurs when an impulse arrives at a PRESYNAPTIC membrane. NEUROTRANSMITTERS are released into the SYNAPTIC CLEFT and bind to RECEPTORS on the postsynaptic membrane, leading to the opening of ion channels (see ION CHANNEL) and postsy-

naptic membrane activation. Each synaptic terminal produces a slow, weak and graded synaptic potential. This could be an EXCITATORY POSTSYNAPTIC POTENTIAL (EPSP)or INHIBITORY POSTSYNAPTIC POTENTIAL (IPSP), depending on the neurotransmitter and ionic channels involved. In the central nervous system, postsynaptic neurons can be activated with EPSPs and IPSPs from adjacent synaptic terminals. The activation caused by a single synapse is usually not sufficient for the postsynaptic neuron to fire (see FIRING). A stronger activation signal requires SUMMATION of activity, either by addition of a number of postsynaptic potentials (spatial summation), or by increasing the frequency of discharge of individual synapses (temporal summation). Activation by a GLUTAMATE-containing neuron always results in excitation of the postsynaptic membrane; GABA release leads to inhibition. In all but the simplest organisms, activation of individual neurons is not sufficient to perform the integrative and regulatory actions of the nervous system; in the vertebrate nervous system this occurs through the activation of millions of synapses grouped into specific networks. For instance, when groups of long-axoned CHOLINERGIC and MONOAMINERGIC neurons located in the brainstem – and belonging to the ASCENDING RETICULAR ACTIVATING SYSTEM (ARAS) – fire, one result is the activation of networks of neurons in the THALAMUS and CEREBRAL CORTEX. The type of activation seen in the cortex depends on the pattern of activity in component networks of the ARAS, and the resulting balance of excitation and inhibition in target neural systems. In the cortex, activation can be measured using an ELECTROENCEPHALOGRAM (EEG). Levels of activation in different neural systems, during performance of particular tasks, can be compared by using imaging techniques, such as positron emission tomography (see PET) or magnetic resonance imaging. Just as activation at the postsynaptic membrane can result in excitation or inhibition, high levels of activation in a particular neural system measured by imaging techniques may be excitatory or inhibitory. An additional way of measuring activation in neural systems is through the use of EVENT-RELATED POTENTIALS.

(ii) *Behaviour*: Behavioural activation refers to heightened motor output. As behavioural activation may be a sign of increased AROUSAL, it is often used synonymously with this, though such use should be avoided; see also ALERTNESS; MOTOR READINESS.

WENDY L. INGLIS AND VERITY J. BROWN

activational effect of steroid hormones A property of steroid HORMONES, usually contrasted with the ORGANIZATIONAL EFFECTS OF STEROID HORMONES. Organizational effects of steroid hormones occur during development and have long-term effects. Activational effects in contrast occur during adulthood and have short-term effects. For example, increasing levels of TESTOSTERONE will activate a male rat's interest in female rats, causing him to display typical SEXUAL BEHAVIOUR. In the long term steroids organize; in the short term they activate.

activation-synthesis hypothesis *see* dreaming

active avoidance Avoidance behaviour occurs when organisms behave in such a way as to decrease the probability of an AVERSIVE STIMULUS being presented or encountered. Avoidance is distinguished from ESCAPE by the occurrence of the aversive event; escape occurs when the animal escapes from or terminates an aversive stimulus, whereas avoidance occurs when the animal avoids the aversive stimulus altogether. Active avoidance is characterized by the animal actively engaging in a response that delays or cancels the presentation of an aversive stimulus.

JOHN D. SALAMONE

active sleep *see* REM sleep

active transport The process whereby a molecule or ION is moved across a cell membrane against a concentration or electrical gradient. Active transport is characterized by the expenditure of energy released from the breakdown of ADENOSINE TRIPHOSPHATE (ATP) by a protein that spans the membrane. The most important use of active transport in the nervous system is the SODIUM–POTASSIUM PUMP which restores the ionic balance of these ions following an ACTION POTENTIAL. Active transport is also used for reuptake of neurotransmitters. Another important use of active transport is the CALCIUM pump which maintains intracellular calcium at very low levels by pumping calcium out of the cell or into intracellular stores.

DOUGLAS D. RASMUSSON

acuity A measure of the finest spatial detail which can be signaled by the visual system, often referred to as the 'resolving power'. It must be distinguished from sensitivity to light intensity or to contrast – these determine the limits on the smallest isolated bright or dark target that can be detected. The finest black/white grating pattern which can be distinguished from a uniform grey field is about 50 cycles per degree when viewing with the central FOVEA under optimal conditions – a value close to the limits set both by optical blur in the retinal image, and the spacing of the PHOTORECEPTOR mosaic. Acuity is reduced with increasing eccentricity in the VISUAL FIELD or with lower levels of illumination. Judgements of alignment and separation show HYPERACUITY; that is, the VISUAL SYSTEM can convey positional information at a finer scale than the spatial detail it can resolve.

There are many different types of standardized tests of acuity, some of which are a key part of the clinical assessment of the visual system (see 6/6 NOTATION; SNELLEN LETTERS). Performance on many of these tasks is limited by the optical properties of the eye itself (see GRATING ACUITY). However, in other cases, such as the ability to detect a misalignment of two thin lines (known as vernier acuity) it has been convincingly proved that performance is a reflection of the manner in which the visual nervous system operates rather than being limited by the eye's optics.

See also: amblyopia; contrast sensitivity

OLIVER J. BRADDICK AND DAVID W. HEELEY

acupuncture Acupuncture is an ancient Chinese method of healing which involves inserting needles into the skin at specific points on the body. It was described by Chi Po in the second century BC. The principles of traditional acupuncture are derived from the theory of natural law (Tao) described by the Laotse in the fifth century BC. This theory holds that nature is governed by the balance of two opposing forces, yin and yang, and that natural objects are composed of five elements – wood, fire, earth, metal and water. Yin and yang are manifested in any naturally occurring pair of opposites such as heat (yang) and cold (yin), or day (yang) and night (yin). In medical theory each major organ is identified with one of the five elements, and there is continuous dynamic interaction between the organs. In the healthy individual these interactions are in balance and there is an unobstructed flow of vital energy (Qi). When the balance is disturbed the flow of Qi is impeded, and this is manifested as illness. The purpose of needling is to restore an unobstructed flow of Qi. The 361 traditional acupuncture points are located on imaginary longitudinal lines which connect a yin organ and its corresponding yang organ, and are the flow paths of the vital energy.

In scientific medicine acupuncture has been used and studied primarily as a treatment for chronic pain. The PAIN-inhibiting effect of acupuncture can be demonstrated in animals as well as in human patients. It can be evoked by needling or electrical stimulation of many areas of the body surface, not just the traditional acupuncture points. Scientific investigations suggest the phenomenon can be explained by the GATE CONTROL THEORY OF PAIN. The pain-relieving effects of acupuncture depend on the stimulation of SOMATOSENSORY nerves, and are mediated by ENDORPHINS and MONOAMINE NEUROTRANSMITTERS in the central nervous system. The efficacy of acupuncture treatment for pain is difficult to estimate because there is no adequate control for PLACEBO ANALGESIA, and there has been great variability in the placement of needles and in the duration and frequency of treatment in clinical trials. Clinical trials of acupuncture for low back pain, muscle pain and arthritic pain suggest 50% to 80% of patients obtain some relief of pain. In 50% of patients pain returns within 6 months. Known complications are broken needles, infection from non-sterile needles, vasovagal symptoms and premature labour.

KEITH B. J. FRANKLIN

acute A brief or rapid event, in contrast to a longer lasting challenge or event, which is referred to as CHRONIC. For instance, one could measure an acute response to a single injection of a drug or examine the chronic response to long-term drug administration.

acute confusional state An organic state characterized by diminution of CONSCIOUSNESS, usually associated with a global impairment of cognitive function. The syndrome is often accompanied by abnormalities of MOOD, PERCEPTION (commonly in the form of visual HALLUCINATION) and behaviour. There are many causes, ranging from infection to alcohol withdrawal. Onset is rapid, and resolution quickly follows effective treatment of the precipitating illness.

IAN C. REID

acute stress disorder A disruption to behaviour and cognitive processing produced by acute STRESS. Acute stress disorder is a category recognized by DSM-IV though it must be borne in mind that almost everyone will at one time or another show an acute stress disorder. Contrast this with POST-TRAUMATIC STRESS DISORDER: similar features can appear in both, but in post-traumatic stress disorder the signs and symptoms are more severe and prolonged.

ad libitum (ad lib) Freely available. Experimental animals are often maintained on an ad lib food and water regime, when both are freely available all the time.

adaptation (i) *Perception*: Adaptation is a nearly universal property of neural systems. Prolonged stimulation leads to steady decline in responsivity. Adaptation has also been demonstrated behaviourally in studies of human spatial vision and has been a key technique in developing the concept of SPATIAL FREQUENCY CHANNELS. Exposure to a high contrast visual stimulus has been shown to lead to a number of transitory perceptual changes such as decreases in sensitivity and changes in the visual appearance of subsequently viewed patterns. Close analysis of these effects lead to the development of the multiple-channel theory of spatial vision. An unresolved issue is the exact cause of the contrast adaptation (or more precisely, HABITUATION), which may be due either to reductions in the concentration of some essential metabolite or the result of alterations in the neural organisation of visually responsive neurons.

(ii) *Evolution*: SPECIES tend to evolve whose individuals are well fitted to the challenges of their environment: this process is called ADAPTATION. It depends upon the existence of heritable variation between individuals, yet its mechanism – differential death – inexorably uses up this variation; see NATURAL SELECTION.

DAVID W. HEELEY AND RICHARD W. BYRNE

addiction The process or state in which an organism needs the presence of a DRUG (including ALCOHOL) to function normally. The concept and definition of addiction has undergone considerable evolution throughout recent history. Central to this process has been the role of volition or 'will' of the addicted individual and of personal responsibility. Before the nineteenth century, addictions were generally considered as vice, sin, or moral failings. It was recognized that certain substances led to undesirable 'habits,' but it was generally thought that drinking, for example, was something over which the individual had ultimate control; that is, drinking to excess was an individual choice. The notion that ALCOHOLISM (and eventually, drug addiction) was more like a disease than wilful immoral behaviour has its roots in the nineteenth century. Thomas Trotter wrote in 1804 that 'the habit of drunkenness is a disease of the mind'. In this century, the MEDICAL MODEL (or the DISEASE MODEL) of alcoholism and other drug addictions has been most influential. The addict is viewed as a patient with a disease, in need of medical or psychiatric treatment. Detractors of this view argue that that the disease concept has actually caused addictive behaviour to increase because it excuses uncontrolled behaviours and allows people to interpret their lack of control as the expression of a disease they can do nothing about. However, there is now strong evidence that many addictive drugs, including COCAINE, alcohol, HEROIN, AMPHETAMINE and NICOTINE can exert powerful long-term effects on the biochemical and molecular machinery of the brain. It is believed that many of these neuroadaptive phenomena (for example, long-lasting changes in GENE EXPRESSION and the SECOND MESSENGERS system) underlie the intense craving and relapse to drug use characteristic of addiction. Thus, while free choice is certainly involved in the decision to initiate drug-taking behaviour, the emotional and cognitive distress associated with dependence is in large part out of the individual's control once the process of addiction has started.

Traditionally, the appearance of a physical WITHDRAWAL SYNDROME was essential in determining if someone was 'addicted' to a substance. For example, some years ago cocaine was not thought to be addictive because users experienced no apparent withdrawal syndrome during abstinence from the drug. Today, physical signs of addiction are still important but not necessary for diagnosis. Several internationally accepted diagnostic criteria exist for drug dependence. The DSM-IV (Diagnostic and Statistical Manual of the American Psychiatric Association) criteria for psychoactive substance dependence emphasize clusters of symptoms or behavioural manifestations that clearly indicate distress or disability. These criteria reflect behavioural changes that would be considered as extremely undesirable in all cultures. There are three basic characteristics to this set of criteria: (1) loss of control over the use of the substance, (2) impairment in daily functioning and continued use of substance despite adverse consequences and (3) physical or emotional adaptation to the drug, such as in the development of tolerance or a withdrawal syndrome. The problem of defining drug abuse has also been considered by the World Health Organization (WHO), from the point of view of public health policy. The WHO model was instrumental in formulating the 'dependence syndrome' concept, which has gradually come to replace the terms 'drug addiction' and 'drug abuse'. In 1981, the WHO committee defined the DEPENDENCE SYNDROME as 'a cluster of physiological, behavioural, and cognitive phenomena in which the use of a substance or a class of substances takes on a much higher priority for a given individual than other behaviours that once had higher value'. A central descriptive characteristic of the dependence syndrome is the desire (often strong, sometimes overpowering) to take drugs, alcohol or TOBACCO. This model also emphasizes the high frequency of maladaptive behaviours, loss of control and neglect of alternative pleasures or interests in favour of substance use. Incorporated into the WHO definition is the concept of NEUROADAPTATION, in which the constant presence of the drug somehow induces long-lasting changes in the brain.

As is clear from both the DSM-IV and WHO criteria, modern concepts of drug addiction tend to emphasize the behaviour of the individual and the adverse consequences of such behaviour; they do not attempt to explain the dependence. These definitions fall within the framework of psychiatry and public health, and reflect current society's general acceptance of drug dependence as a medical problem or disease.

Reference

Kelley A.E. (1995) Psychoactive substance use disorders. In *Abnormal Psychology*, eds. D. J. Rosenhan & M. E. P. Seligman, Norton: New York.

ANN E. KELLEY

adenine A nucleotide (see DNA).

adenohypophysis; neurohypophysis The pituitary gland, at the base of the brain, below the HYPOTHALAMUS, was thought of in ancient times as a channel through which unpleasant fluids could drain away from the brain. (Pituitary is derived from *pituita*, Latin for phlegm.) The pituitary gland is not really one structure but two: the ADENOHYPOPHYSIS (anterior pituitary) and NEUROHYPOPHYSIS (posterior pituitary) regulate different HORMONES, are controlled independently and are derived from different embryonic tissues. The neurohypophysis is embryologically part of brain: it is essentially neural tissue. The adenohypophysis is not – it is a 'real' gland. Both adenohypophysis and neurohypophysis are connected to the brain by the INFUNDIBULUM (or pituitary stalk), a collection of axons and blood vessels communicating between pituitary and hypothalamus, sheathed in connective tissue. Importantly though, the axons only communicate with the neurohypophysis – posterior pituitary – and the blood vessels only communicate with the adenohypophysis – anterior pituitary. Hor-

mones are liberated from the adenohypophysis and neurohypophysis in two different ways. (1) The hormones arginine VASOPRESSIN and oxytoxin are synthesized by MAGNOCELLULAR neurons in the paraventricular and supraoptic nuclei of the hypothalamus. These neurons send their axons down through the infundibulum into the neurohypophysis, where they liberate oxytocin and vasopressin into capillaries, which carry these hormones out around the body. (2) The HYPOTHALAMIC-PITUITARY PORTAL SYSTEM (also known as the hypothalamic–hypophyseal portal system) is based on the blood vessels supplied by the hypophyseal artery to an area called the MEDIAN EMINENCE, at the base of the hypothalamus, above the pituitary. It is a system containing a dense network of capillaries, into which axons from a variety of neuroendocrine neurons in the hypothalamus can release hormones. The capillaries of the hypothalamo-pituitary portal system flow to the adenohypophysis. Cells within the adenohypophysis synthesize and release various hormones (including GROWTH HORMONE, PROLACTIN and ACTH among others) whose release is triggered by the hormones and releasing factors carried in the hypothalamo-pituitary portal system. Thus the neurohypophysis has direct neural contact with the hypothalamus, while the adenohypophysis communicates with the hypothalamus through the intermediate actions of the blood stream, in the shape of the hypothalamo-pituitary portal system.

Note that there is also an INTERMEDIATE LOBE OF THE PITUITARY, situated between the neurohypophysis and the adenohypophysis. It contains cells that secrete ENDORPHIN and melanocyte-stimulating hormone and appears to be innervated by DOPAMINE fibres from the hypothalamus (suggesting that it is more closely related to the neurohypophysis than to the adenohypophysis). There is also a small pars tuberalis, an extension of the adenohypophysis along the infundibulum: this is differentially developed across species. In the rat it is quite small, but in other species – sheep for instance – it is quite large.

See also: hypothalamo-pituitary axis

adenoma *see* tumour

adenosine A PURINE nucleoside with a variety of cellular functions, found in a variety of locations around the body. In brain it is synthesized from adenosine 5'-monophosphate and inactivated principally by REUPTAKE into synaptic terminals. There are several receptor subtypes, G PROTEIN coupled: A_1, A_{2A}, A_{2B} and A_3, the distributions of which in brain differ. Adenosine is thought to interact with a variety of other neurotransmitter systems, most notably cholinergic (see CHOLINE) systems. Adenosine inhibits the firing of CHOLINERGIC involved in ATTENTION and AROUSAL. It has also been suggested that the stimulants THEOPHYLLINE and CAFFEINE (found in tea and coffee) are adenosine antagonists and that their stimulant properties can be accounted for by suppression of the inhibitory actions of adenosine on cholinergic neurons.

See also: psychomotor stimulants

adenosine diphosphate (ADP) *see* adenosine triphosphate

adenosine triphosphate (ATP) Cells work: they engage in mechanical work (such as muscle cell contraction); transport (moving molecules across various kinds of MEMBRANE for example); and they do chemical work, powering chemical reactions that do not happen of their own accord. This work requires fuel, and it is this that ATP provides. ATP, when subject to hydrolysis (the addition of water) breaks down: a phosphate molecule leaves ATP (which thus becomes adenosine diphosphate, ADP). This breakdown liberates ENERGY. If the reaction occurred in a test tube this energy would be present as heat. Heat in cells is clearly not a good thing, so cells use another molecule to capture the phosphate that is liberated from ATP in water (a process said to involve a phosphorylated intermediate). This process is simply a means for transferring the phosphate molecule from ATP to a target molecule without generating unwanted heat energy. The donation of a phosphate molecule by ATP is reciprocated: the product, ADP, can acquire phosphate molecules to become ATP again, a process known as the ATP cycle. This cycle is tremendously powerful: a single muscle cell can recycle all its ATP – all 10 million molecules of it – in about 60 seconds (see Campbell *et al.* for a clear exposition of the functions and properties of ATP).

Reference

Campbell N.A., Reece J.B. & Mitchell L.G. (1999) *Biology*, 5th edn, Addison-Wesley: Menlo Park CA.

adenovirus A complex type of VIRUS with a double strand of DNA.

See also: gene transfer in the CNS

adenylate cyclase An enzyme found in many cells in the nervous system that converts the energy substrate molecule ADENOSINE TRIPHOSPHATE (ATP) to CYCLIC AMP (see SECOND MESSENGERS). Also known as adenylyl cyclase, it alters the phosphate groups on the ATP and requires the cofactor magnesium (Mg^{2+}). It is a critical part of the intracellular biochemical signalling mechanisms in many neurons. Via a certain type of proteins bound in the neuronal membrane called G PROTEIN, the neurotransmitter is able to influence the levels of adenylate cyclase. For example, via a stimulatory G protein which is linked to the transmitter receptor, transmitters such as NORADRENALINE and DOPAMINE are able to increase the production of adenylate cyclase. The regulation of adenylate cyclase by NEUROTRANSMITTERS has a wide array of influences on neuronal activity and function. It is now known that there are multiple forms of this enzyme that differ slightly in structure and interactions with G proteins.

ANN E. KELLEY

adequate stimulus A normal (that is, appropriate) STIMULUS that is above threshold for detection is said to be an adequate stimulus. An INADEQUATE STIMULUS is not simply one that is below threshold for detection, but may be one that is inappropriate for a particular modality. For example, rubbing one's eyes can stimulate the visual system.

adhesion molecules Literally, molecules that aid in securing cells together. GLYCOPROTEIN molecules often serve in this way; see GROWTH CONE for an example of adhesion molecules in action.

adipocyte *see* adipose tissue

adipose Adipose tissue is fat; normal body fat is white. Brown fat – BROWN ADIPOSE TISSUE – is involved in NON-SHIVERING THERMOGENESIS.

adipose tissue (from Latin, *adepis*: soft fat) Adipose tissue is what is more commonly known as fat; adiposity is a term indicating fatness. Adipose tissue (which is white – BROWN ADIPOSE TISSUE has a different function) consists of a matrix of CONNECTIVE TISSUE in which are held adipose cells (also called ADIPOCYTES). These cells contain TRIGLYCERIDES, which may be metabolized and released by adipocytes when there are ENERGY demands on the organism. Adipocytes have a necessary relation to adiposity. There are two factors that are important in this: one is the number of adipocytes that are present, and the second is their size (that is, how much fat each adipocyte actually contains). The number of adipocytes present in an organism is probably set initially by genetic factors but it has been shown that sustained periods of overfeeding can lead to adipocyte HYPERPLASIA. Controlling the size of adipocytes is relatively straightforward – reducing fat intake will do this – but reducing adipocyte number is harder to do, requiring very lengthy periods of intake restriction. There is another important question about the regulation of adipocytes: is fat storage regulated or merely a consequence of energy intake? Is the surplus energy that is neither used straightaway nor consumed in thermogenesis simply stored or are there active mechanisms governing adiposity? Until recently no identifiable signal from adipose tissue to brain mechanisms controlling intake could be detected, but the recent discovery of LEPTIN has suggested that there may indeed by a signal from adipocytes to the HYPOTHALAMUS that allows for regulation of adiposity.

See also: body weight; digestive system; feeding; insulin; obesity

adipsia The absence of DRINKING.

adjuvant (from Latin, *ad*: to, *juvare*: to help) An agent, often without significant independent effect, given in combination with another in order to promote its effectiveness.

ADP Adenosine diphosphate; see ADENOSINE TRIPHOSPHATE.

adrenal gland (from Latin, *ad*: to, *renes*: kidneys) The adrenal gland, situated (as the name indicates) immediately next to the kidneys, is involved in STRESS and OSMOREGULATION. The adrenal gland is composed of two distinct components: the adrenal cortex (the outer portion or shell of the adrenal gland) and the adrenal medulla (the inner portion or core of the adrenal gland). The adrenal gland is related to the tissue of the nervous system, being derived from NEURAL CREST cells which, having moved into position, can develop either into cells capable of releasing HORMONES in the adrenal medulla, or into sympathetic neurons (see SYMPATHETIC NERVOUS SYSTEM). The differentiation of neural crest cells into either of these is chemically controlled: in the presence of GLUCOCORTICOIDS, neural crest cells develop into adrenal medulla cells; in the presence of NERVE GROWTH FACTOR they develop into sympathetic neurons.

Stress triggers activity in the HYPOTHALAMUS, which then generates activity in the adrenal gland by two routes. A neural signal, relayed from the hypothalamus via the sympathetic nervous system, promotes release of ACETYLCHOLINE in the adrenal medulla, which in turn stimulates the release of the catecholamine neurotransmitters, ADRENALINE and NORADRENALINE (also known as, respectively, EPINEPHRINE and NOREPINEPHRINE). Adrenaline and noradrenaline are released from the adrenal medulla into the blood to produce several effects: increased breakdown of GLYCOGEN to GLUCOSE (to fuel 'FIGHT-OR-FLIGHT'), increases in blood pressure, RESPIRATION and METABOLISM, and alteration of the pattern of blood flow, with decreasing digestive activity and a concomitant increase in alertness. Stressors also generate an ENDOCRINE response from the hypothalamus. Activation causes the hypothalamus to trigger release of ADRENOCORTICOTROPIC HORMONE (ACTH) from the anterior PITUITARY GLAND. ACTH activates the adrenal cortex, causing release of MINERALOCORTICOIDS (such as ALDOSTERONE) which act to retain sodium and water by the kidneys, and increase blood pressure (see OSMOREGULATION). Glucocorticoids such as cortisol are also released by the adrenal cortex, leading to conversion of fats and proteins to glucose (again helping fuel 'fight or flight') and suppression of the IMMUNE SYSTEM. The endocrine response to stress by the adrenal cortex, being dependent on diffusion of ACTH from the pituitary gland, is of course much slower than the response made by the adrenal medulla, which is under very fast neural control. In addition to a role in stress and osmoregulation, the adrenal gland also appears to have the capacity to produce STEROID HORMONES related to SEXUAL BEHAVIOUR: the adrenal cortex produces ANDROGENS (such as TESTOSTERONE), ESTROGENS (such as ESTRADIOL) and PROGESTINS (such as PROGESTERONE). These are all made in greater quantities in the GONADS. Exactly what function adrenal SEX HORMONES have is unclear.

Loss of the adrenal gland – either by disease or by surgical removal (ADRENALECTOMY) – has significant physiological effects, the most pressing of which is an inability to retain sodium. Adrenalectomized animals have to be given additional salt in their water or food in order to maintain sodium levels. Adrenalectomy produces a specific loss of GRANULE CELLS from the HIPPOCAMPUS, a unique event: no other neurons in the brain are damaged by adrenalectomy (see Sloviter et al., 1993). It is thought that glucocorticoids might act as nerve growth factors in the developing hippocampus. Their function in the adult hippocampus is uncertain. In addition, some of the effects psychological of AMPHETAMINE are thought to be mediated, directly or indirectly, via an action on catecholamine release from the adrenal gland (see Martinez et al., 1980)

See also: chromaffin cells; Cushing's disease

References

Campbell N.A., Reece J.B. & Mitchell L.G. (1999) *Biology*, 5th edn, Addison-Wesley: Menlo Park CA.

Martinez J.L., Jensen R.A., Messing R.B., Vasquez B.J., Soumireu-Mourat B., Geddes D., Liang K.C. & McGaugh J.L. (1980) Central and peripheral actions of amphetamine on memory storage. *Brain Research* 182: 157–166.

Sloviter R.S., Dean E. & Neubort S. (1993) Electron microscopic analysis of adrenalect-
omy induced hippocampal granule cell degeneration in the rat – apoptosis in the adult central nervous system. *Journal of Comparative Neurology* 330: 337–351.

adrenalectomy Removal of the ADRENAL GLAND.

adrenaline (adrenergic) A monoamine that is primarily synthesized in the ADRENAL GLAND, specifically the CHROMAFFIN CELLS of the adrenal medulla. Also known as epinephrine, it is synthesized from NORADRENALINE (or norepinephrine) by the enzyme PHENYLETHANOLAMINE-N-METHYLTRANSFERASE (PNMT). Experiments in the early part of the twentieth century suggested that nerves of the SYMPATHETIC NERVOUS SYSTEM stimulated the heart and constricted blood vessels by a hormonal substance acting on the effector organs. When the adrenal medulla is excited by sympathetic activity, adrenaline is released into the circulatory system and quickly reaches many target organs, such as the heart, lungs and blood vessels. Along with the neurotransmitter noradrenaline, it has an important role in increasing oxygen delivery to muscles and brain, preparing the body for STRESS or FIGHT-OR-FLIGHT situations. The term ADRENERGIC is used to describe a neuron that contains adrenaline.

ANN E. KELLEY

adrenergic Relating to the neurotransmitter ADRENALINE. For instance, a neuron that synthesizes and releases adrenaline is said to be adrenergic.

adrenoceptors These are receptors for both NORADRENALINE (NOREPINEPHRINE) and ADRENALINE (EPINEPHRINE). They are found in the CENTRAL NERVOUS SYSTEM and on a variety of tissues innervated by the PERIPHERAL NERVOUS SYSTEM. All the various subtypes of adrenoceptor are coupled to G PROTEINS. Adrenoceptors are discriminated broadly into two types: ALPHA RECEPTORS (α receptors) and BETA RECEPTORS (β receptors). Alpha receptors tend to be found in the CENTRAL NERVOUS SYSTEM, beta receptors in the rest of the body, though this dissociation is by no means absolute. Both types, alpha and beta, are divided into subclasses. The table on page 18 shows the subclasses of adrenoceptor, the relative potency of noradrenaline and adrenaline, and the main locations of the receptors. Note also that it was once thought that alpha-2 receptors had an exclusively PRESYNAPTIC location. This is not longer thought to be the case. Adrenoceptors of all sorts can be found at both pre- and POSTSYNAPTIC sites, and may act as AUTORECEPTORS.

The following table (on page 19) indicates some of the drugs that have been used as AGONISTS or ANTAGONISTS at adrenoceptors. Note that it is unusual to find a drug that has an action exclusively at one type of RECEPTOR: in most cases selectivity for a receptor subtype is relative. The agonists and antagonists listed here, unless otherwise specifically noted, show strong selectivity for the receptors indicated, though this selectivity may not necessarily be absolute.

Reference

Feldman R., Meyer J.S. & Quenzer L.F. (1997) *Principles of Neuropsychopharmacology*, Sinauer Press: Sunderland MA.

adrenocorticotropic hormone (ACTH) One of the HORMONES liberated from the ADENOHYPOPHYSIS (anterior PITUITARY GLAND) following stimulation by CORTICOTROPIN-RELEASING FACTOR (CRF). In turn it stimulates release of STEROID HORMONES (principally GLUCOCORTICOIDS) from the adrenal cortex (see ADRENAL GLAND) and is important in a variety of processes, including resistance to infection (see IMMUNE SYSTEM) and reactions to a wide variety of types of STRESS. Prolonged release of ACTH in the face of stress leads to elevations in glucocorticoids that in turn promote HYPERGLYCAEMIA, HYPERINSULINAEMIA, increased GASTRIC ACID secretion (and the consequent formation of ulcers) and impairs immune functioning.

See also: endocrine glands

adrenomedullin see calcitonin gene-related peptide (CGRP)

aerobic Requiring the presence of free OXYGEN.

Adrenoceptor potency and location

SUBTYPE	RELATIVE POTENCY	LOCATION
alpha 1A	NA > adrenaline	HIPPOCAMPUS, PONS, MEDULLA OBLONGATA, SPINAL CORD
alpha 1B	NA = adrenaline	CEREBRAL CORTEX, THALAMUS, HYPOTHALAMUS, CEREBELLUM
alpha 1D	NA = adrenaline	HEART
alpha 2A	adrenaline > NA	LOCUS COERULEUS, AMYGDALA, hippocampus, thalamus
alpha 2B	adrenaline >NA	thalamus, KIDNEY
alpha 2C	adrenaline > NA	locus coeruleus, amygdala, hippocampus, thalamus, SUBSTANTIA NIGRA, STRIATUM
beta 1	NA > adrenaline	receptors for SYMPATHETIC NERVOUS SYSTEM actions of noradrenaline; also cerebral cortex
beta 2	adrenaline > NA	receptors in tissues for HORMONE-like actions of adrenaline and noradrenaline; also cerebellum
beta 3	NA = adrenaline	BROWN ADIPOSE TISSUE; ADIPOSE TISSUE
beta 4	NA > adrenaline	uncertain as yet

Drugs acting at adrenoceptors

alpha 1 receptors:	*agonists*:	PHENYLEPHRINE, METHOXAMINE, CIRAZOLINE
	antagonists:	WB4101, PRAZOSIN, PHENOXYBENZAMINE, CORYNANTHINE
alpha 2 receptors:	*agonists*:	ALPHA-METHYL-NORADRENALINE, CLONIDINE, OXY-METAZOLINE, B-HT920, UK14,304
	antagonists:	YOHIMBINE, RAUWOLSCINE, IDAZOXAN
beta receptors:	*agonists*:	ISOPROTERONOL, ALBUTEROL (also called SALBUTAMOL)
	antagonists:	PROPRANOLOL, ALPRENOLOL, PINDOLOL
	(these two groups are non-selective with respect to beta receptor subtypes)	
beta 1 receptors:	*agonists*:	DENOPAMINE, XAMOTEROL
	antagonists:	ATENOLOL, BISOPEROL
beta 2 receptors	*agonists*:	PROCATEROL, SULFONTEROL
	antagonists:	ICI-118,551
beta 3 receptors:	*agonists*:	CL-316,243

AESOP A model of CLASSICAL CONDITIONING that extends the RESCORLA–WAGNER THEORY. SOP was the first extension (SOP being an acronym for standard operating procedure), with AESOP (affective extension SOP). AESOP is a real time model that attempts to account for LEARNING and performance of a task.

Reference

Domjan M. (1993) *Domjan and Burkhard's The principles of learning and behaviour*, 3rd edn, Brooks Cole: Pacific Grove CA.

aestivation The opposite of HIBERNATION: aestivation is a period of dormancy during the summer months, typically in response to oppresive heat or drought conditions.

aetiology (US: etiology) (from Greek, *aitiologia* – *aitia*: cause, *logos*: discourse) The study of the causes of events, most particularly in the context of medicine: the causes of diseases.

AF-64A A neurotoxin, ethylcholine mustard aziridinium ion, an irreversible LIGAND for the choline REUPTAKE system. AF-64A has been proposed as an agent capable of producing selective loss of CHOLINERGIC neurons or, if not loss of neurons, at least reduced cholinergic function. It has not been widely used,

because it often has been found to produce CAVITATION in tissue. This non-selective toxic property has been difficult to separate from the selective. It has been suggested that at very low concentrations AF-64A is selective for the high affinity CHOLINE uptake system, which is specifically found on cholinergic neurons, while higher concentrations affect both high and low affinity choline uptake systems (the low affinity system being present on a wide variety of cells). The success of selective neurotoxins such as 6-HYDROXYDOPAMINE stimulated a great interest in the possibility of finding a lesioning agent selective for cholinergic neurons. However, the non-selective effects of AF-64A have very seriously inhibited its use.

References

Hanin I. (1990) AF64A-induced cholinergic hypofunction, in Aquilonius S.-M. & Gillberg P.-G. (eds) *Progress in Brain Research*, vol. 84, pp. 289–299, Elsevier Science Publishers, B.V.

affect The term affect has been regarded as synonymous with the term EMOTION: an AFFECTIVE DISORDER such as DEPRESSION is one of emotion or mood; *see* MOOD for further discussion.

affective disorder Broad term referring to a group of related psychiatric disorders in which disturbance of MOOD is a core feature – referred to as MOOD DISORDERS in ICD10 and DSM-IV. Includes pathological DEPRESSION and elevation of mood (MANIA).

See also: bipolar disorder; manic depression; monoamine hypothesis of depression; seasonal affective disorder; unipolar depression

IAN C. REID

afferent (from Latin, *afferens* – *ad*: to, *ferre*: carry) Moving toward or inward. Afferent projections (often simply, 'the afferents') of a brain structure are the neurons that project to that structure from another one.

See also: efferent

affinity Affinity is a measure of the strength with which a RECEPTOR molecule and LIGAND interact. Receptor molecule and ligand are used here in their most general sense rather than specifically referring to neurotransmitter molecules and neurotransmitter receptors (see NEUROTRANSMITTERS). Of course, neurotransmitters and drugs vary in their affinity for the receptor molecules to which they bind, but other systems also show varying degrees of affinity: REUPTAKE mechanisms for example can show varying degrees of affinity. A bimodal distribution is often implied when discussing affinity: reuptake is often divided into high and low affinity for instance.

afterdischarge A series of ACTION POTENTIAL reactions produced in a neuron by a single stimulus. This usually consists of a high-frequency burst of action potentials. Many neurons in the central nervous system show afterdischarges as a result of their intrinsic membrane properties. This may allow a short stimulus to have a more prolonged effect in some parts of the central nervous system. Afterdischarge may also be seen in abnormal states such as EPILEPSY and may be indicative of excessive excitatory or decreased inhibitory influences on the neuron.

DOUGLAS D. RASMUSSON

aftereffect The residual and brief effect of a sensory STIMULUS after it has been removed.

See also: afterimage

afterimage Following exposure to a prolonged and/or intense pattern of light, the afterimage is a continuing visual sensation corresponding to the stimulated areas of the RETINA. This is believed to reflect prolonged photochemical events following pigment bleaching in the PHOTORECEPTORS, which both generate a neural signal (giving a bright sensation on a dark background) and reduce sensitivity (hence a dark sensation on a bright background). The afterimage is fixed on the retina, and so like any stabilized image, appears to fade even before the pigment has regenerated.

OLIVER J. BRADDICK

ageing Colloquially this term refers to those changes which occur in later life, but ageing more accurately refers to the changes which occur in any living system over its total lifespan. Where people are concerned, societies divide lifespan in various different ways. For example, one Western social framework sees life as progressing through the stages of infancy, childhood, adolescence and adulthood. The latter may be further divided into early adulthood, middle adulthood and old age. Age may also be defined in terms of biological and psychological markers. These various markers of maturity may be attained at different stages of one's life. Therefore, knowing someone's chronological age may only provide a broad indication of their physical and psychological capabilities.

Psychologically, ageing is characterized by a decline in some sensory and cognitive capacities. Research has demonstrated that central cognitive changes may account for a substantial proportion of behavioural differences which occur in old age. One important distinction is that between 'fluid' and 'crystallized' INTELLIGENCE. Fluid intelligence is broadly synonymous with on-line mental agility. On average, performance on tests which draw heavily on these capacities tend to decline from around one's early 20s onwards. By contrast, crystallized intelligence is broadly synonymous with knowledge and performance on tasks which load heavily on this capacity tends to increase or remain stable over the lifespan. Some of the age-related decline in fluid intelligence which occurs may occur because older adults have problems spontaneously organizing, structuring or attending to novel information in their environment.

One general hallmark of psychological ageing is that differences in performance between individuals tend to become exaggerated, as the influences of an individual's specific personal history make their mark. Therefore, it is problematic to attempt to delineate hard-and-fast rules about the capacity of a particular individual at a specific age. A general characteristic of old age is that performance becomes slower on many tasks, whether these are conducted at home or in the laboratory. There is considerable debate in the research literature concerning the extent of this slowing in information processing. However, data indicates that the peripheral (sensory and/or motor) processing speed of older adults is in the region of 1.0–1.5 times slower than that of younger adults whereas central slowing rates indicate retardation in the region of 1.5–2.0 times that of young controls. It has been argued by some (for instance Salthouse, 1985) that all of the deficits in psychological processes which occur in old age may be explained in terms of generic cognitive slowing, though this remains controversial. From a neuropsychological perspective, it has been suggested that older individuals' pattern of cognitive performance (their relative inflexibility) may be closely related to deficits in frontal lobe functioning which occur as we age.

In terms of MEMORY and LEARNING capacity, older people seem to have problems in actively processing information held in short-term memory, in rehearsing supra-span list lengths and/or in transferring material into long-term storage. In long-term memory, free recall performance is generally more impaired than cued recall recognition in old age, suggesting that old people may have problems in generating and/or using appropriate retrieval cues to access information held in the long-term store. Overlearned and familiar information, well rehearsed motor skills and implicit memory tend to be retained well into old age, although there is often difficulty in learning new facts and acquiring new skills. However, once information has been encoded into long-term memory, it does not seem to be forgotten more rapidly than by younger people. Thus, the general observation that old people spend more time talking about events which occurred in their youth than those which occurred more recently may be at least partly due to problems in encoding new information into long-term memory, rather than in retaining such material. However, as with younger people, learning in older people can be facilitated through active rather than passive learning of to-be-remembered materials.

Personality changes have also been noted anecdotally in old age, with many old people complaining of psychosocial isolation and loneliness. By contrast, observers often comment upon the greater self-centredness which may become apparent in some older people. Antisocial tendencies and personality traits suppressed or inhibited during working life may become more apparent after retirement. However, these proposed changes have proven somewhat elusive when investigated experimentally. It has also been suggested that behaviour in old age becomes dominated by routine and habit. However, there is little evidence that ageing *per se* is responsible for personality changes which occur across the lifespan. Rather, the literature indicates a basic stability of adult personality traits which are differentially responsive to significant life events and environmental conditions across the lifespan.

References

Craik F. & Salthouse T. (1992) *The Handbook of Ageing and Cognition*, Lawrence Erlbaum: New Jersey.

Salthouse T. A. (1985) *A Theory of Cognitive Ageing*, Elsevier: Amsterdam.

JONATHAN K. FOSTER

agenesis A term referring to the failure of development of any anatomical region during embryonic development. The term DYSGENESIS is sometimes used to denote diminished development, as distinct from the absence, of a region. Regional agenesis of the nervous system may result from a variety of genetic mutations, affecting diverse developmental processes such as neuronal proliferation, NEU-

RONAL MIGRATION and axon guidance. In humans it is exemplified by agenesis of the CORPUS CALLOSUM (see CALLOSAL AGENESIS).

ROGER J. KEYNES

agenesis of the corpus callosum *see* callosal agenesis

ageusia (ageustia) The loss of gustatory sensation. GUSTATION is the term used to describe the sense of taste: ageusia is literally, not tasting.

See also: sapid

aggression (from Latin, *ad*: to, *gradi*: step) Aggression strictly refers to the act of making a first attack, or initiating a quarrel or fight, but it is used as an all-embracing term to cover a variety of states in animal behaviour relating to ATTACK and DEFENCE. Virtually all species engage in aggressive behaviour, the most common causes being to do with mate selection and the establishment of social status, recruitment and defence of territory (or other resources) and the capture of prey.

Aggressive behaviour can take a variety of forms. For example, much aggression involves *threat behaviours* in which various postures are taken or gestures made as forms of ritualized DISPLAY – and which may be followed by *submissive behaviours*. Such threatening and submissive actions serve to establish DOMINANCE between animals and often involve little or no actual FIGHTING. Threatening behaviours may also be followed by the production of species typical defensive behaviours, which might involve the production of ALARM CALLS to warn a CONSPECIFIC. Defence can take many forms, from straightforward ESCAPE by running away (see EXPLOSIVE MOTOR BEHAVIOUR) to the adoption of hostile defensive positions (hedgehogs for example curl up into prickly balls) or FREEZING, the adoption of an immobile posture held to avoid detection. The form of attack is also species typical, but two rather different classes can be differentiated: one is RAGE, involving the production of noise and threatening gestures, while the other form of attack is much quieter. Predation typically involves a stealthy attack (in rodents and other small animals it is often referred to as QUIET BITING ATTACK) in which the production of

noise or gesture would alert the prey and initiate their escape or defence reactions. SOCIAL BEHAVIOUR is also important in both defence and attack. Many animals live in groups – herds, flocks or shoals – which can be organized for effective defence. The behaviour of animals in herds, flocks or shoals can show an apprently remarkable degree of co-ordination, individuals seeming to act as one to avoid capture, and generating what is known as PREDATOR CONFUSION. (A good example of this is the movement of a herd of zebras – their movement as a group, combined with their striped pattern, is disorientating for predators.) Such group behaviour, while superficially complicated, is easily maintained by following simple rules: keep a more-or-less fixed distance from the animal adjacent and move in whatever direction it goes. These rules, and an additional one that prompts scattering when a predator strikes (followed by immediate group re-formation) allow large numbers of animals to avoid predation on the principle of 'unity is strength'. On the other hand, by operating in a co-ordinated manner predators such as big cats or wolves, for example, can work to attack animals much larger than any of the individual predators. Some predators working socially have developed procedures for grouping their prey and attacking *en masse*: humpbacked whales for example engage in complex patterns of activity involving different functions for different members of the attacking group, that enable them to corral shoals of fish, driving them to the waters' surface where they are devoured.

The neural and physiological mechanisms involved in aggression are not wholly clear. It is apparent that threats generate activity in the AUTONOMIC NERVOUS SYSTEM (see FIGHT-OR-FLIGHT) which serves to provide ENERGY for highly activated behaviour. HORMONES are also involved: in rodents, CASTRATION can reduce aggression, the administration of exogenous TESTOSTERONE serving to restore appropriate aggressive behaviour. Female sex hormones are also implicated, aggression by females being closely related to PREGNANCY. Female baboons for example have been shown to display higher levels of aggression during ovulation and when female mice are at their most receptive they appear to be least aggressive. Both male mice and male primates have been reported to show INFANTICIDE (of the offspring of others, not their own) which appears to be related to the hormonal state of females (usually females with whom they wish to mate but who have issue by other males). Explanations for infanticide typically engage arguments about the establishment of an individual's reproductive success.

Neural mechanisms involved in aggression are widespread: there is no single site in the brain that controls aggression. Systems implicated in the control of FEEDING and FORAGING are involved, as are the neuronal systems involved in FEAR. It is also clear that BRAINSTEM mechanisms are involved in the production of appropriate species-typical defence reactions. The PERIAQUEDUCTAL GREY and nearby structures in the PONS and MEDULLA can, when stimulated, elicit defensive behaviours. It is useful when considering aggression to think in terms of rodents. Rats in the wild live in a hostile world: prey and predators need to be dealt with promptly by appropriate attack and defence behaviours. One likely mechanism involves the SUPERIOR COLLICULUS, a structure with direct input from the RETINA and direct output to brainstem motor systems. This structure is able to make a rapid analysis of visual input (the INFERIOR COLLICULUS can make a similar analysis of auditory input) and to initiate appropriate motor activities at very high speed. Stimulation of the superior colliculus, or the structures to which it is monosynaptically connected (such as the CUNEIFORM NUCLEUS) can elicit rapid defensive behaviours in rodents, including explosive motor behaviour (running away at speed). For rodents, overhead threat (the recognition of stimuli passing close above them, as birds of prey do) is a potent elicitor of escape. Of course, if time permits, more detailed analyses of incoming sensory data can be made, allowing the opportunity for FOREBRAIN systems involved in sensory analysis, LEARNING and MEMORY to be used.

Aggression is evidently a complex phenomenon. Virtually all species show aggression in some form, and it is beyond doubt that hormonal states, autonomic activation and complex neural systems throughout the central nervous system are involved in it. There is always a temptation to ascribe human aggression to simple biological causes, but it is a temptation that should be resisted. While it is likely that aggression and violence by humans has biological antecedents – the influence of hormones for example – it is also clear that humans have elaborate social systems to channel and control aggression and that as willful, self-aware, autonomous creatures, humans have to accept responsibility for their own actions. An example of this differentiation between humans (and indeed PRIMATES) and other animals comes from studies of overcrowding. Research indicated that overcrowding in rodent colonies could lead to heightened aggression, and it was assumed that this would be universally true. Recent research has shown that this is not the case (see de Waal *et al.*, 2000). The appropriate suppression of antisocial biological urges is something that people must learn to do.

See also: conflict; social behaviour

Reference

de Waal F.B.M., Aureli F. & Judge P.G. (2000) Coping with overcrowding. *Scientific American* 282: 54–59.

agnosia Agnosia implies a failure in gaining access to some kind of stored knowledge or object-specific representation. The term is due to Freud and taken from the Greek, meaning 'without knowledge'. The disorder is produced by neurological damage, and may be confined to one modality (for example, an auditory or tactile agnosia may co-occur with intact visual identification) unless there is general disturbance of conceptual SEMANTIC MEMORY, in which case meaning will no longer be fully accessed from all sensory channels. Such generalized failure to derive a fully specified meaning can be observed in dementing diseases like ALZHEIMER'S DEMENTIA. Furthermore, agnosia may be restricted to LANGUAGE as opposed to non-verbal material. For these cases, the term necessarily implies a modality-specific disorder; word meaning, for example, may not be accessed for a spoken utterance, but readily interpreted if the written form of the word is presented.

VISUAL AGNOSIA can be the result of a deficit that interferes with the ability to derive, by accessing an internal description of the object's physical structure, a representation that is constant regardless of changes in the conditions under which an object is viewed (see APPERCEPTIVE AGNOSIA). Cases with damage to the right PARIETAL LOBE may experience difficulty identifying objects viewed under conditions that obscure or distort critical features, despite the evident preservation of lower-level visual abilities. Objects that are unevenly illuminated, with potentially misleading contours, are problematic for such individuals relative to objects with more habitual shading, as are photographs of common objects taken from an unusual viewpoint.

Agnosia may also occur when normal access to meaning is prevented by neurological injury (see ASSOCIATIVE AGNOSIA). COLOUR AGNOSIA is the failure to correctly classify colours despite intact COLOUR VISION. Agnosia can be more pronounced for objects (or words) in certain categories. Most typically, the class affected is that of biological kinds, while identification of man-made objects is relatively spared. However, the reverse phenomenon has also been reported. The difficulty that some cases experience with biological objects cannot be simply attributed to subtle effects of object familiarity. Brain damage to regions of the TEMPORAL LOBE can affect identification of common fruits and vegetables like banana or tomato, but not complicated, unusual objects like bagpipes or windmill. Some authors have been tempted to suggest that CATEGORY-SPECIFIC AGNOSIA reflects a distinction between biological and man-made objects at the level of stored structural representations that provide the entry point to meaning from vision, an interpretation that provides little basis for understanding why, say, the agnosic can easily recognize and draw from memory the shape of a lightbulb but not a pear. An alternative explanation is that object classification depends on both functional and perceptual knowledge that are dissociable by brain damage. Identifying the members of biological classes may require more perceptual than functional distinctions in semantic memory, and if this knowledge is selectively impaired, recogni-

tion of these exemplars will be worse than artefacts. Finally, some authors have argued that category specific agnosia is the outcome of a general disturbance in the mapping between object structure and meaning, leading to misclassification when exemplars are both physically similar and have similar conceptual attributes, a situation most often encountered for biological objects. This account, however, does not accommodate the observation that in some (albeit very rare) cases of agnosia, the more affected categories appear to be those incorporating man-made objects rather than biological.

Nevertheless, at least one kind of agnosia for biological objects does appear to reflect an inability to map objects with overlapping structural characteristics (say, objects like banana, carrot, cucumber and zucchini that share similar values on dimensions like thickness, curvature and tapering) to conceptual and even episodic memory when the memory attributes are very similar. Man-made objects from the same category (for example, articles of clothing) tend to have non-overlapping shape dimensions (compare pants, shoes, sweater) and differ more widely in conceptual attributes, and for these kind of exemplars the agnosia does not prevent correct mapping between the object's form and meaning. Other subtypes of central agnosia, even though they resemble each other superficially, undoubtedly require a different interpretation; for some cases, the disturbance appears to emerge prior to the classification of each object as a familiar physical exemplar. But damage beyond this point and closer to the activation of stored conceptual representations would produce errors that reflect the organization of membership within particular semantic categories. The memory representations for biological objects must maintain distinctions between a large number of exemplars with very similar attributes, and their organization may well have different properties than the organization of man-objects, where the members of a category are less highly correlated in terms of perceptual and conceptual characteristics. Damage to meaning affects various classes of object differentially as a direct consequence of their particular representation in LONG-TERM MEMORY.

See also: prosopagnosia

DANIEL N. BUB

agonist An agonist is a DRUG or chemical that is able to bind to a RECEPTOR and activate it, producing an appropriate response which may involve changes in ION CHANNEL opening or closing, activation of SECOND MESSENGERS and changes in neuronal FIRING. An agonist effectively mimics whatever effect the natural LIGAND for a receptor has. Such agonists are called DIRECT AGONISTS. It is important to note that receptors may have multiple binding sites present on them: the principal site is that at which the neurotransmitter binds, but there may be other sites at which neuromodulators or co-transmitters bind (see NEUROMODULATION). An INDIRECT AGONIST is one which binds to a site on receptor other than the main biding site for the ligand. In doing so it interferes with the action of the receptor, facilitating actions there. An INVERSE AGONIST is a molecule that binds to a site on the receptor other than the main binding site to produce an effect opposite to that of the agonist: essentially it binds to the same receptor yet has an opposite effect to the agonist – it is a functional ANTAGONIST. A PARTIAL AGONIST is one which is unable to produce a maximal effect, whatever concentration is applied.

See also: antagonist; competitive–noncompetitive binding

agoraphobia (from Greek, *agora*: marketplace, *phobos*: fear) A fear of open places; often an accompaniment to PANIC disorder. It is made manifest by typical symptoms of panic or PHOBIA: shortness of breath, cardiac palpitations, trembling, dizziness, NAUSEA and choking, numbness, tingling and chest pain; DEPERSONALIZATION and DEREALIZATION are often present also. DSM-IV indicates that the change in behaviour brought about by agoraphobia must be sufficient to cause a restriction of the sufferer's daily life.

See also: claustrophobia

agrammatism A form of APHASIA in which GRAMMAR is disturbed: words may be used appropriately but grammatical construction into coherent sentences is absent. It might be considered a form of NON-FLUENT APHASIA.

agranular cortex The agranular cortex refers to the motor areas of the CEREBRAL CORTEX that lack the internal granular layer (layer 4). These areas are characterized by the presence of a type of giant (50–80 μm) pyramidal neuron, called a BETZ CELL, in layer 5. These and the smaller pyramidal neurons contribute their axons to the corticospinal tract, a major descending motor pathway. The agranular cortex is one of the five cytoarchitectonic (see CYTOARCHITECTURE) types of the cerebral cortex that were identified by von Economo (1876–1931) on the basis of relative development of granule and pyramidal cell layers.

See also: granular cortex; motor cortex

KAZUE SEMBA

agraphia (from Greek, *a*: not, *graphein*: to write) Agraphia (or dysgraphia) is an acquired disorder of WRITING and/or SPELLING. It typically results from damage to the LANGUAGE areas of the dominant cerebral hemisphere. In peripheral dysgraphias, the impairment may be restricted to letter formation, such that the subject retains the ability to spell words orally. In central DYSGRAPHIC syndromes, spelling knowledge itself is affected. The different patterns of central dysgraphia have been classified and named largely by analogy with similar patterns of ACQUIRED READING DISORDER. In SURFACE DYSGRAPHIA, atypical correspondences between a word's sound and its spelling cause particular problems and result in regularization errors (for example spelling *yacht* as *yot*). In PHONOLOGICAL DYSGRAPHIA, familiar words – including those with atypical correspondences – may be spelled correctly, but the patient has problems spelling novel stimuli such as unfamiliar words and non-words. In DEEP DYSGRAPHIA, there is a severe deficit in generating plausible spellings of novel items, and the patient's success with known words is modulated by word meaning: words with abstract meanings are particularly vulnerable, and even concrete, imageable words are subject to semantic errors such as *yacht* being transformed to *ship*.

Reference

Ellis A.W. (1993) *Reading, Writing and Dyslexia*, 2nd edn, Lawrence Erlbaum: Hove.

ELAINE FUNNELL AND KARALYN E. PATTERSON

AIDS-related dementia Encephalopathy which may progress to DEMENTIA associated with HIV (human immunodeficiency virus) infection. Sometimes termed AIDS dementia complex (ADC). HIV infects both CNS immune cells and glial cells such as astrocytes leading to brain scarring, ATROPHY and DEMYELINATION. The dementia arises from a progressive, global decline in cognitive function, which may be heralded by personality change, apathy, poor concentration and loss of MEMORY. Overall, there is evidence of cognitive slowing, with delay abnormalities in the P300 (see EVOKED POTENTIALS). Neuropsychological testing reveals a SUBCORTICAL DEMENTIA pattern, while magnetic resonance imaging may detect cortical atrophy, in addition to ventricular enlargement and white matter hyperintensities indicating demyelination. The encephalopathy may occur without sufferers meeting criteria for 'full blown' acquired immune deficiency syndrome (AIDS), though 50–75% of HIV-positive patients who develop dementia die within 6 months. It has been estimated that while some degree of encephalopathy may be very common at some stage in HIV sufferers, the ADC is more rare, affecting 4–6% of HIV positive individuals in European studies. Recent epidemiological investigations suggest that ADC risk is greater in intravenous drug abusers, in older patients and in women. The risk of ADC appears to increase as indices of healthy immune cell function (the primary infection targets of the virus, such as T4 lymphocyte count) fall. It remains controversial as to whether treatments which may have an impact on the development of AIDS and its complications (such as zidovudine) protect in any way against ADC. HIV infection can affect the central nervous system in a variety of ways: the disorder may lead to opportunistic brain infections (such as toxoplasmosis and cryptococcal MENINGITIS) or brain cancers. Alternatively, early symptoms of encephalopathy may be mistaken for depression. It is therefore important that treatable conditions be distinguished from encephalopathy.

IAN C. REID

akinesia (from Greek, *a-*: not, *kinesis*: motion) Lack of movement. It is one of the common symptoms of PARKINSON'S DISEASE. Animal models suggest that in this case akinesia is caused by loss of DOPAMINE-containing neurons from the SUBSTANTIA NIGRA, leading to a decrease in dopaminergic transmission in the CAUDATE–PUTAMEN (dorsal STRIATUM). Rats which have received 6-HYDROXYDOPAMINE lesions of the NIGROSTRIATAL DOPAMINE SYSTEM have difficulties initiating movement.

See also: bradykinesia

WENDY L. INGLIS

alarm calls *see* animal communication

albedo (diffuse reflection coefficient) *see* luminance

albuterol A non-selective beta-NORADRENALINE receptor AGONIST (also known as SALBUTAMOL); see ADRENOCEPTORS.

alcohol Alcohol is a rather general term for a class of hydrocarbon compounds, and is widely used as a cleansing agent (for example to wipe the skin before an injection is made). But in everyday talk (and, for the most part, in PSYCHOPHARMACOLOGY) 'alcohol' is taken to refer to fermented drinks that contain ethanol (alternatively known as ethyl alcohol). Consumption of these gives rise to a variety of psychological states: alcohol is a PSYCHOACTIVE substance that can act as a SEDATIVE or ANXIOLYTIC, or induce EUPHORIA. Evidence suggests that the practice of producing alcohol for consumption is about 6000 years old, and societies in all places and at all times appear to have discovered means for producing alcoholic drinks. Consumption is world-wide, with the exception, of course, of Moslem countries: the denial of alcohol use appears to represent an example of how humans can consciously and volitionally deny themselves the use of a substance that, when made available to animals, is always accepted. Alcohol is absorbed rapidly by the body and is metabolized, mostly in the liver. There are three stages in its metabolism: ethanol is converted by alcohol dehydrogenase to acetaldehyde; acetaldehyde is quickly converted, by a process involving aldehyde dehydrogenase, to acetic acid (acetate). Acetate passes out of the liver into the bloodstream. Here it combines with acetyl CoA (acetyl coenzyme A – which is also involved in the synthesis of acetylcholine) and is finally broken down to produce carbon dioxide, water and to produce 7 calories per gram of alcohol. Excessive alcohol intake very rapidly induces body weight gain, amongst a raft of adverse effects on the brain, heart and on behaviour (see ALCOHOLISM) and as with any other addictive agent (see ADDICTION; SUBSTANCE ABUSE), TOLERANCE can develop and absence provoke WITHDRAWAL SYMPTOMS. Low to moderate doses can have benefit; higher doses unambiguously do not.

The effects of alcohol on the brain are not especially well understood. It appears to have a generalized effect on neuronal membranes, interfering with the lipids in the membranes themselves, as well as affecting ION CHANNEL activity. Alcohol has also been associated with changes in the function of a variety of neurotransmitter systems, including GABA, DOPAMINE, acetylcholine, SEROTONIN, NORADRENALINE and OPIOID PEPTIDE systems.

See also: foetal alcohol syndrome

Reference

Feldman R., Meyer J.S. & Quenzer L.F. (1997) *Principles of Neuropsychopharmacology*, Sinauer Associates: Sunderland MA.

alcohol abuse Alcohol use disorder associated with excessive alcohol intake, which may lead to alcohol DEPENDENCE, with social, physical and psychological damage.

See also: addiction; alcoholism

IAN C. REID

alcohol dehydrogenase *see* alcohol

alcoholism General term encompassing ALCOHOL ABUSE and ALCOHOL DEPENDENCE (DSM-IV). Classified as 'mental and behavioural disorders due to alcohol' in ICD 10. ALCOHOL abuse and dependence are the commonest forms of substance abuse in the Western world (affecting 10% of women and 20% of men in the USA at some time in their lives). Inappropriate use of alcohol constitutes an enormous healthcare problem, and is associated with considerable social disruption, physical ill health and premature death. As a result, alcohol-related difficulties represent an enormous financial burden (estimated at $150 billion per year in the USA).

Pharmacologically, alcohol acts as a CNS depressant. The acute effects of alcohol range from mild disinhibition in low doses to respiratory failure and death in overdose. Intermediate levels result in the depression of motor function, disruption of emotional function, and the development of a state of STUPOR. In the UK, limits to safe drinking have been proposed, which when exceeded place the drinker at increased risk of physical harm. For women, this is 14 units of alcohol per week, for men, 21 units. One unit of alcohol is roughly equivalent to a single standard measure of spirits, or one glass of wine, or half a pint of regular strength beer.

Patterns of alcohol misuse vary, ranging from 'binge drinking', where large amounts of alcohol are consumed in individual sessions with abstinence in between, to continuous intoxication. While acute intoxication may by itself lead to health risk via accidents, falls, fights and in some climates, hypothermia, repeated alcohol misuse risks dependence and physical harm from the toxic effects of alcohol on the body. Repeated alcohol consumption results in increasing tolerance, both as a consequence of neural changes and up-regulation of the liver enzymes which metabolise alcohol. Physical dependence is revealed by withdrawal effects on stopping drinking. Symptoms include restlessness, tremulousness, nausea, anxiety and sweating. More severe effects include DELIRIUM TREMENS (the DTs), characterized by an ACUTE CONFUSIONAL STATE, often with visual HALLUCINATION. If this condition is untreated it may prove fatal, with repeated epileptic seizures supervening. Other physical effects of chronic alcohol abuse result in liver damage (cirrhosis) and increased risk of gastrointestinal cancers. Direct toxic effects on the brain may result in cortical atrophy, and an alcohol-associated DEMENTIA. Malnutrition, which often accompanies excessive drinking, leads to a deficiency of vitamin B1 (thiamine), which if untreated may result in the WER-NICKE–KORSAKOFF SYNDROME, a devastating organic state characterized by permanent AMNESIA.

A range of treatments for alcoholism is available. Medical intervention may be necessary for detoxification of dependent patients, with the provision of gradually decreasing doses of an ANTICONVULSANT and B-complex vitamins to prevent delirium tremens and Wernicke–Korsakoff syndrome respectively. Although a return to controlled drinking is advocated by some authorities, a consensus is emerging that complete abstinence is a more sensible and effective therapeutic goal. Psychotherapeutic approaches may be necessary to maintain abstinence. Some patients find attendance at Alcoholics Anonymous helpful. Drugs may sometimes be useful – DISULFRAM acts by interrupting the metabolic pathway for alcohol and results in the accumulation of the toxic metabolite acetaldehyde, so that drinking alcohol becomes extremely unpleasant – and potentially dangerous. More recently, acamprosate, which has a similar structure to the neurotransmitter GABA, has been used to maintain abstinence in abstinent alcoholics by reducing alcohol craving. It is believed to activate inhibitory GABA RECEPTORS and to antagonize the action of EXCITATORY AMINO ACIDS such as GLUTAMATE. Further study is necessary to determine the true potential of the drug.

See also: addiction

IAN C. REID

aldehyde An aldehyde is a molecule produced by OXIDATION of ALCOHOL; the term is a reduction of alcohol dehydrogenatum – alcohol without hydrogen. ALIPHATIC ALDEHYDES – aliphatic means fatty or oily – are aldehydes combined with methane derived organic compounds

aldehyde dehydrogenase *see* alcohol; dopamine

aldehyde reductase *see* noradrenaline

aldosterone A mineralocorticoid (one of the classes of STEROID HORMONES) important in OSMOREGULATION and SODIUM APPETITE.

See also: adrenal gland

alertness A cognitive state of readiness for information processing, which is characterized by a subjective sense of attentiveness and mental energy. Cognitive performance is optimal when alertness is greatest, but there is a cost to the organism in maintaining a state of high alertness and therefore high alertness can be maintained for only a limited time. Alertness is phasic, related to diurnal rhythms, but can be modulated by cognitive factors. Alertness is related to AROUSAL, but can be distinguished from it. Arousal refers to a physiological state that impacts on cognition by its influence on alertness. For example, as the body is aroused by danger in preparation for FIGHT-OR-FLIGHT, the cognitive status is raised to one of high alertness. It is possible, however, to be aroused without increased alertness and, conversely, it is possible to be highly alert but not highly aroused. Alertness is also related to VIGILANCE and MOTOR READINESS. Vigilance and motor readiness describe states of expectation or preparedness for processing specific information or making specific responses, respectively. However, although high alertness is required for vigilance and readiness, the two terms are not synonymous, as not being in a state of vigilance or readiness does not imply a subject is not alert.

VERITY J. BROWN

alexia Traditionally, a severe form of ACQUIRED READING DISORDER, contrasting with DYSLEXIA, a milder form. Nowadays, the terms ALEXIA and DYSLEXIA are used interchangeably.

ELAINE FUNNELL

alexithymia An impairment in the ability verbally to express internal feelings.

See also: alexia; emotion

alien hand The expression ALIEN HAND is used in two ways: (i) in certain conditions in which there is loss of MOTOR CONTROL, such as PARKINSON'S DISEASE, the term alien hand may be used to describe a hand over which a patient does not have proper control; (ii) more commonly, the term is used to describe a condition in which patients believe their hand not to be under their own control and it may appear to act of its own volition. For example, an individual may turn a television set on, only to have their alien hand turn it off again, despite the individual wanting the set on. It is thought to be due to disruption of circuitry in the FRONTAL LOBE; it has been seen also after commissurotomy (see COMMISSURE).

alimentary canal *see* digestive system

aliphatic aldehyde *see* aldehyde; stereochemical theory of odour discrimination

alizarin red *see* stain

alkali (alkaline) *see* base

alkaloids Alkaloids are chemicals produced by plants. They have a common chemical structure: they contain nitrogen, are formed from AMINO ACIDS and have a pH greater than 7 – that is, they are ALKALIS (see BASE). Many alkaloids are dangerously neuroactive or have psychoactive properties: CURARE and ERGOT are two examples of alkaloids.

See also: belladonna alkaloids

all-or-none A property of an ACTION POTENTIAL describing the fact that once THRESHOLD has been reached the amplitude is not dependent on the size of the stimulus, but on the properties of the underlying ION CHANNEL. If threshold is reached, the action potential proceeds to its full amplitude (all), but if threshold is not reached, the action potential does not occur (none) and the change in membrane potential dissipates. This principle does not mean that all action potentials are the same size, even in the same neuron, as changes in the ionic environment may cause changes in the absolute size or shape of the action potential.

DOUGLAS D. RASMUSSON

allele A particular variation of a GENE, for example, the 'red' or 'brown' alleles of the gene for hair colour. With the exception of sex CHROMOSOMES, DIPLOID organisms have two alleles for each gene, since they inherit one set of chromosomes from each parent. Alleles may be dominant or recessive. Dominant alleles will be expressed rather than recessive ones, although a recessive allele will be expressed if both alleles inherited are recessive. If different

alleles are co-dominant, a mixture of the two characteristics will be observed.

FIONA M. INGLIS

allergy An allergy is an extreme reaction to an ANTIGEN present in the environment: antigens that produce an allergic reaction are called allergens. The most common allergies – hay fever for example, an allergic reaction to specific types of plant pollen – involve IgE antibodies (see ANTIBODY) interacting with MAST CELLS, producing exaggerated release of HISTAMINE (which is why antihistamines are the most common anti-allergy drugs). Typical symptoms of allergy include runny nose (rhinitis), watering eyes, and contraction of smooth muscles (which can, in very extreme cases produce difficulties with BREATHING).

It is of particular interest to biological psychologists to note that animals can often induce allergic reactions in people. Of special concern is laboratory animal allergy, an allergic reaction to a protein in rat urine. This protein will contaminate the rats' bedding and can become airborne in the dust present in labs. It is estimated that as many as one in three lab workers will show some form of allergic reaction to rats. The mildest forms are skin rash (urticaria – nettle rash) which requires direct contact with the rat and breaking of the skin (which can be caused just by the rats' tail brushing across one's wrist while holding a rat). More severe forms involve rhinitis and breathing difficulties. Medication to combat these symptoms is available, but there is no long-term cure for the condition.

allesthesia The mislocalization of sensory stimulation to a corresponding site on the opposite side of the body. First identified in the tactile modality and termed ALLOCHIRIA, a history of terminological confusion is associated with allesthesia (see Meador *et al.*, 1991). Visual and auditory allesthesia are also well documented. Allesthesia can occur with various pathologies including hysteria, myelopathy, damage to parietal and/or occipital cortex and often accompanies contralateral neglect.

Reference
Meador K.J., Allen M.E., Adams R.J. &

Loring D.W. (1991). Allochiria vs. allesthesia: is there a misperception? *Archives of Neurology* 48: 546–549.

PATRICIA A. REUTER-LORENZ

allied reflexes Reflexes are relatively simple automatic actions, not requiring significant degrees of information processing. The concept of allied reflexes describes the notion that individually identifiable reflexes can group together in order to generate coherent patterns of action. By grouping reflexes together it enables an individual REFLEX to trigger automatically all of the others with which it is allied: prompting performance of an individual reflex can trigger a more complex behavioural chain. Patients with PARKINSON'S DISEASE who show AKINESIA have been encouraged to walk normally simply by having them swing their arms in the normal way one does when walking. This action appears able to trigger all of the components of behaviour that collectively make up normal walking.

Reference

Teitelbaum P., Pellis V.C. & Pellis S.M. (1990) Can allied reflexes promote the integration of a robot's behaviour? In *From Animals to Animats*, ed. J.-A. Meyer & S.W. Wilson, pp. 97–104. MIT Press: Cambridge MA.

allocentric (from Greek, *allos*: other) Allocentric means literally centred on the other – that is, not on the self (which is referred to as EGOCENTRIC). Allocentric is a term used in referring to an animal's SPATIAL BEHAVIOUR. Cue responses (in which movements guided by an external cue, such as a landmark) and place responses (in which an animal's target is out of its immediate perception, and NAVIGATION to which requires a COGNITIVE MAP) can both be described as allocentric.

allocentric space; egocentric space Allocentric space and egocentric space are means of dividing space and generating, formally or informally, the positional co-ordinates of things, living and inanimate, in SPACE. Allocentric space is defined with reference to arbitrarily defined points: for example, where Fisher and Donaldson's patisserie is in relation to the University Library. One might know where both of these things are and define space

with reference to them. Allocentric space is frequently defined in terms of objects and provides a fixed set of reference points for NAVIGATION around the world. In contrast, egocentric space is space defined with reference to ones own body position, and therefore constantly changes as one moves around the world. Allocentric space provides a map of the world ('Where is Fisher and Donaldson's in relation to the University Library?'); egocentric space is ones personal positional reference scheme ('How can I get to Fisher and Donaldson's from here?').

See also: spatial behaviour

allochiria *see* allesthesia

allocortex The allocortex is the oldest part of the CEREBRAL CORTEX, in terms of evolution. Unlike the NEOCORTEX it contains only three layers of neurons (see CORTICAL LAYERS). Included in the allocortex are the PYRIFORM CORTEX, OLFACTORY BULB, OLFACTORY TUBERCLE, the DIAGONAL BAND OF BROCA, the SEPTAL NUCLEI, AMYGDALA and hippocampal formation and dentate gyrus (see HIPPOCAMPUS). Allocortex is also known as the archipallium or RHINENCEPHALON (meaning olfactory brain); the hippocampal formation and dentate gyrus are also known as the ARCHICORTEX while the pyriform cortex is also called the PALAEOCORTEX. These terms – archipallium, rhinencephalon, archicortex and palaeocortex – might still be found in older literature but are rarely used terms now. Closely associated with the allocortex (and often combined with it in the rather vague term LIMBIC CORTEX) is the JUXTALLOCORTEX.

See also: nucleus accumbens

allograft An allograft is a graft of tissue within the same species (rat to rat, human to human and so on); a XENOGRAFT is a graft between different species; see TRANSPLANTATION.

allometry (from Greek, *allos*: other, *metron*: measure) Allometry is the comparative measurement of the growth and size of parts of an organisms body in relation either to other parts of the same organisms body, or to the same body part in a CONSPECIFIC or indeed in another SPECIES. In terms of the nervous system, there has been considerable interest in the development and size of the HIPPOCAMPUS in animals which place a high demand on SPATIAL MAPPING and accurate NAVIGATION, such as FOOD-STORING BIRDS (the hypothesis being that such animals should have larger hippocampi). Similarly the ENCEPHALIZATION QUOTIENT and related measures have attempted to assess INTELLIGENCE across species with reference to brain size; see NERVOUS SYSTEM.

allomones *see* pheromones

allostasis (from Greek, *allo*: other, *stasis*: stopped, stationary) Allostasis means stability through change. It is a process contrasted to HOMEOSTASIS, which is all to do with the maintenance of constancy in living processes. Allostasis highlights mechanisms of anticipation, expectation and an animal's readiness to adapt (through both behaviour and by manipulation of physiology) to circumstances as they develop. Allostasis is an adaptive process in which LEARNING and dynamic change are emphasized, in contrast to homeostasis.

Reference

Schulkin J., McEwen B.S. & Gold P.W. (1994) Allostasis, amygdala and anticipatory angst. *Neuroscience and Biobehavioral Reviews* 18: 385–396.

allosteric (from Greek, *allos*: other, *stereos*: solid) Allosteric relates to a binding site, referred to as an ALLOSTERIC SITE, and engages a process called ALLOSTERIC BINDING. Binding at an allosteric site changes the structure of the molecule possessing the site, such that the molecule can no longer function properly. For example, some molecules may regulate the activity of certain enzymes by binding to allosteric sites. The effect of the binding is to change the shape and function of the enzyme, leading to a change (either an increase or a decrease) in its activity. For example, the synthesis of ACETYLCHOLINE involves the binding of the component parts, ACETYL COENZYME A and CHOLINE, to a molecule of the enzyme CHOLINE ACETYLTRANSFERASE. But acetylcholine itself can bind to choline acetyltransferase at an allosteric site. This action changes the conformation of choline acetyltransferase, reducing its activity. This allosteric binding

therefore operates to regulate enzyme activity and hence control the production of acetylcholine. Many other examples of this can be found.

allosteric binding *see* allosteric

allosteric site *see* allosteric

allothetic navigation; idiothetic navigation Allothetic navigation involves the use of external cues: animals can learn about the relationships between permanent or semi-permanent objects in space and use this information to guide their movements around the world. Idiothetic navigation uses self-generated information: information from the VESTIBULAR SYSTEM, MUSCLES and joints, the flow of sensory information and animals' own sense of TIMING can all be used for this.

See also: allocentric space; dead reckoning; egocentric space; navigation; path integration

alogia Alogia is a failure of speech production, including poverty of SPEECH PRODUCTION (that is, the amount of speech is low) and poverty in the content of speech (that is, a very restricted vocabulary is used, speech often consisting of only monosyllabic utterances). It is a feature of negative symptom SCHIZOPHRENIA.

alpha and beta conditioning During CLASSICAL CONDITIONING or PAVLOVIAN CONDITIONING, a to-be-conditioned stimulus (CS) is presented contiguously with an unconditioned stimulus (UCS). Following pairing of these two stimuli, conditioned responding (CR; conditioned response) to the CS is measured. If a change in responding is observed, it may be concluded that CONDITIONING has occurred. Depending on the type of CR measured, this conditioning is typically referred to as either alpha or beta conditioning. During alpha conditioning, a response is measured which the CS elicited before conditioning. Pairing of the CS and the UCS acts to quantitatively change the nature of the CR. For example, a novel mild stimulus such as a tone, or light, will elicit some aversive responses such as withdrawal, freezing, and increases in AROUSAL. If that stimulus is now paired with a strong noxious stimulus, it will be observed that the mild stimulus subsequently elicits enhanced withdrawal, prolonged freezing, and increased arousal. In contrast, during beta conditioning the nature of the CR changes qualitatively, in that it will come to resemble some aspect of the response elicited by the UCS. Traditionally, it is necessary to provide evidence that conditioning is the result of the pairing of the CS and UCS, and not simply the effects of receiving the stimuli *per se*. One way to test this is to present a separate group of subjects with the same stimuli in an unpaired fashion (for example, several minutes apart). If no change in responding is observed following unpaired training, then it may be concluded that conditioning was observed in the group which received paired stimuli. Alpha and beta conditioning are ubiquitous phenomena, and have been observed in a variety of species, ranging from molluscs to mammals. It has often been suggested that conditioning, in general, provides animals with the ability to detect causal relationships, and thereby learn which stimuli predict important events. Moreover, it is now generally recognized that conditioning is a far more sophisticated and powerful form of learning than previously thought (for example, see BLOCKING).

MARK A. UNGLESS

alpha herpes virus *see* tract tracers

alpha male When DOMINANCE ranks are stable amongst pairs of individuals in a group, for each sex there is usually one individual who is dominant to all others. This is called the alpha individual (sometimes the others are termed beta, gamma and so on). In monkeys and apes, where males are at least as large as females, the alpha male is usually the most dominant individual of the group; in certain PRIMATES and various other social animals, the alpha female may be the most dominant.

RICHARD W. BYRNE

alpha motor neuron *see* muscle spindle

alpha receptor *see* adrenoceptors

alpha waves Alpha waves constitute the 8–12 Hz component of the cortical EEG (see ELECTROENCEPHALOGRAM). In humans, alpha waves dominate the EEG when the subject is sitting still with the eyes closed, and are most prominent in the occipital cortex. They can be blocked by gross bodily movements. Alpha-like EEG activities have been recorded from the sensory and motor cortices in a variety of species including human, baboon, cat and rat, and these are called mu rhythm, wicket rhythm, *rythme en arceau*, *rythme de veille immobile* and sensorimotor rhythm. All these EEG activities are likely to share common thalamocortical rhythm-generating mechanisms.

See also: theta waves

KAZUE SEMBA

alpha-methyl-5-hydroxytryptamine An agonist at the $5HT_{2A}$, $5HT_{2B}$, $5HT_{2C}$, $5HT_3$ and $5HT_4$ receptors (see SEROTONIN RECEPTORS).

alpha-methyl-noradrenaline An alpha 2 noradrenaline receptor AGONIST (see ADRENOCEPTORS).

alpha-methyl-para-tyrosine (AMPT) A drug that blocks TYROSINE HYDROXYLASE activity, consequently preventing synthesis of the CATECHOLAMINE neurotransmitters DOPAMINE, NORADRENALINE and ADRENALINE.

alprazolam A benzodiazepine drug: it has similar actions to CLONAZEPAM, but has high lipid solubility and is absorbed quickly.

alprenolol A non-selective beta NORADRENALINE receptor ANTAGONIST (see ADRENOCEPTORS).

alternation learning Learning to make a response that is opposite to the one previously made. Alternation learning can be carried out in a MAZE or an OPERANT environment such as a SKINNER BOX, although different neural processes may be involved with each. In the highly spatial setting of mazes, rats have a strong tendency to SPONTANEOUS ALTERNATION; in operant situations, rats more commonly show WIN–STAY, LOSE–SHIFT tendencies. The HIPPOCAMPUS is likely to be very important for LEARNING and MEMORY in both settings, although alternation learning in the operant environment may be more dependent on attentional processes (see ATTENTION). In some studies, a delay is inserted between trials (see DELAYED ALTERNATION). Traditionally, a T

MAZE or Y MAZE has been used for spatial alternation learning. In this, a hungry rat is placed in the start box, from which it enters the stem of the maze. At the other end of the stem, the rat has a choice of entering one of the two arms. Often, ACQUISITION consists of two stages: in the first, one arm will be blocked off and the rat is forced to enter the open arm and allowed to eat the food pellets placed in the well at the end of the arm; in the second, the rat is allowed a free choice of arms, but food pellets are only found in the arm not visited in the previous trial. Following acquisition, rats are tested on continuous alternation: on the first trial, the rat is forced to enter one arm, but on subsequent trials, the rewarded arm would always be the opposite arm to the one chosen on the previous trial. For alternation learning in an operant chamber, rats would be trained first to press a lever when a light was illuminated above it, for a reward such as a food pellet or sucrose solution. Following acquisition of the lever-press response during illumination of the signal light, a choice of two levers would be presented on each trial, with a light above each one. The initial trial would be rewarded regardless of which lever was pressed, but on the following trials, the 'correct' response – the one which resulted in reward – would always be a response on the opposite lever to the one which was previously pressed.

WENDY L. INGLIS

alternative splicing Also known as RNA EDITING (see GENE).

altricial mammals *see* maternal behaviour

altruism Modern, intimate studies of animal behaviour have repeatedly shown that nature is not always 'red in tooth and claw'. Individuals help each other: to avoid predation (sounding alarms, joining in co-operative defence, sometimes risking their lives for others), to hunt prey together, to rear offspring co-operatively, or to construct elaborate nests or burrows by working together. In many cases, the net result of an animal's behaviour benefits other individuals more than itself, or considerable costs are borne which outweigh personal benefit: behaviour of this kind is called altruism.

Popular presentations often suggest that altruism evolved because, although disadvantageous for the individual, it benefits the group, population or species. However, NATURAL SELECTION operates by differential selection among individuals relative to other individuals, not among competing groups. (The only exception is where the mutual fate of all group members is so intertwined that it can be treated as a single individual.) Thus, altruism presents a problem for evolutionary explanation.

The solution has come from advances in theoretical biology, developing the implications of natural selection for social organisms (see SOCIOBIOLOGY). All cases of animal altruism can now be explained as (concealed) individual benefit, kin selection, or reciprocal altruism. For instance, giving an alarm call was formerly regarded as self-sacrificing behaviour, subjugating the individual's chance of escape for the good of its companions. Many cases are now known where, in complete contrast, alarm giving reduces predation likelihood. The ability to give an energetically costly alarm (for example, the 'stotting' display of deer or antelope) advertises to predators that the individual is particularly healthy and vigorous. In other cases, alarm giving does reduce the individual's survival chances, often only slightly, but increases those of some of its kin. Ground squirrels, for instance, alarm call significantly more often when kin are in hearing, even if the kin are not direct descendants. In a sense, these explanations demystify altruism to the point where it is no longer altruism in the everyday sense. Indeed, it would seem impossible for natural selection to produce altruism of the everyday sort, since that would always confer selective disadvantage. There is a larger issue here than semantics, because the explanations offered by sociobiology for animal altruism can also apply to humans. Few would seriously doubt that some part of a mother's deep protective love of her child, and willingness for extreme self-sacrifice on its behalf, have some genetic component. Most people, in most societies, have some equivalent of the 'blood is thicker than water' belief, and would have little hesitation in attributing many of their actions to relatedness. At the other extreme, humans evidence a number of behaviours which appear contrary to natural selection in that they systematically reduce the likelihood of descendants (for instance, risking one's life to save a stranger from death, religious martyrdom, lifetime chastity, homosexuality, suicide). Only the most enthusiastic sociobiologists attempt to explain such actions by GENE inheritance.

RICHARD W. BYRNE

aluminium (Al; in the United States, aluminum, with no second -i-) A metal, it is of most significance in biological psychology (other than for its general laboratory use in foil sheets) as a potential environmental cause of ALZHEIMER'S DEMENTIA. The brains of Alzheimer patients were reported, at AUTOPSY, to contain abnormally high concentrations of aluminium and it was at one time thought possible that aluminium from cookware – pots and pans, cutlery – could be accumulating in the brains of Alzheimer patients. Doubts have been cast over this finding however and it is no longer regarded as a likely cause of this disease.

alveus *see* fimbria

Alzheimer's dementia A form of DEMENTIA distinguished by characteristic neuropathological changes. Originally described by Alois Alzheimer(1864–1915) in 1906, the condition is the commonest of the dementias, accounting for 50% to 60% of all dementing illnesses. The incidence of the disorder increases with age: approximately 5% of 65-year-olds and 25% of those aged 85 or older suffer from the condition. As the proportion of elderly people in the population increases, so does the prevalence of Alzheimer's disease. Patients with Alzheimer's disease display marked progressive, global cognitive impairment, with memory loss as a prominent feature. An intensely disabling disease, leading to significant impairment in occupational and social function, self-care and ultimately death, Alzheimer's dementia places an enormous burden on sufferers, their families and society.

Neuropathologically, cortical ATROPHY with VENTRICULAR ENLARGEMENT is observed. There is marked loss of TEMPORAL LOBE volume, which can be detected on COMPUTERIZED AXIAL TOMOGRAPHY (CAT) scanning. Histological examination reveals neuronal loss, senile PLAQUES (which contain an abnormal deposition of AMYLOID protein), and neurofibrillary TANGLES. Though the diagnosis is usually made on clinical grounds, valid confirmation can only be obtained *post mortem*.

The cause of Alzheimer's disease is not fully understood, though genetic factors are increasingly recognized as playing an important role. A very small proportion of suffers have an early-onset AUTOSOMAL DOMINANT inherited form of the condition. They either carry a mutation of a gene coding for amyloid protein precursor on chromosome 21, or mutations of genes coding for proteins known as the PRESENILINS (chromosomes 1 or 14). The abnormalities appear to lead to ultimately to the deposition of the abnormal amyloid protein. However, most Alzheimer's dementia sufferers have a sporadic (non-inherited) form of the condition, with later onset than the autosomal dominant form. In a significant proportion of patients – perhaps 60% – the condition is associated with the inheritance of a certain allelic form of the APOLIPOPROTEIN E (apoE) gene, apoE4. Carriers of the apoE2 allele may be protected from the disease. Those who are HOMOZYGOUS for the E4 allele show a very strong likelihood of developing the disease by age 75. Precisely how the apoE4 gene exerts its effects is unknown. It has been suggested that the E4 form may influence aggregation of amyloid protein. Environmental factors have also been suggested to be implicated in the aetiology of Alzheimer's disease, including ALUMINIUM toxicity and head injury.

Numerous deficits of NEUROTRANSMITTERS have been described in Alzheimer's disease, particularly in noradrenergic and cholinergic systems. It has been suggested that there is a specific degeneration of the cholinergic neuron cell bodies in the NUCLEUS BASALIS OF MEYNERT in the FOREBRAIN, and reductions in concentrations of ACETYLCHOLINE and CHOLINE ACETYLTRANSFERASE (an important enzyme involved in the synthesis of acetylcholine) have been observed *post mortem* in brains from patients with Alzheimer's disease.

CHOLINOMIMETIC drugs, which enhance the activity of the cholinergic system, such as inhibitors of ACETYLCHOLINESTERASE (AChE) which reduce the breakdown of acetylcholine, have been developed for use in Alzheimer's disease. Unfortunately, they have very limited efficacy, and are of little value to advanced cases. At present, there is no curative treatment for the disorder.

IAN C. REID

amacrine cells Amacrine cells are interneurons located in the inner nuclear layer of the RETINA. They lack axons, but through their dendrites modify signal transmission from BIPOLAR CELLS TO GANGLION CELLS. The input to amacrine cells comes from axons of bipolar cells as well as from dendrites of other amacrine cells. Their output is directed to ganglion cells, other amacrine cells, and axons of bipolar cells, thus forming complex feedback, feed-forward, and reciprocal networks. Amacrine cells use GABA, GLYCINE, ACETYLCHOLINE and DOPAMINE as neurotransmitters, and some of these transmitters are co-localized in the same cell.

See also: horizontal cells; neurotransmitters; retinal cell layers

KAZUE SEMBA

amantadine A drug that stimulates release of the neurotransmitter DOPAMINE, through mechanisms that are as yet unclear. It is used in the treatment of PARKINSON'S DISEASE, especially when the disease is in its early stages.

amblyopia A deficit in visual ACUITY, usually of one eye, not correctable by spectacles and not associated with visible pathology of the eye. Amblyopia results from STRABISMUS (cross eyes), ANISOMETROPIA (difference in focus between eyes), or deprivation of a sharp retinal image (for instance, by CATARACT). The deficit continues even if these problems are corrected, because the eye has become functionally ineffective due to competitive interactions with the other eye in establishing connections in VISUAL CORTEX. Experiments on visually deprived animals, and clinical experience, indicate that these effects depend on the balance of stimulation during a CRITICAL PERIOD in early life.

See also: visual development

OLIVER J. BRADDICK

amenorrhoea (US: amenorrhea) Absence or failure of menstruation (see MENSTRUAL CYCLE). The menstrual cycle is typically, in humans, a 28-day period, though there is considerable individual variation in this. Absolute loss of menstruation can occur for a variety of reasons. For example, significantly reduced food intake, either through unavoidable starvation or that associated with ANOREXIA NERVOSA, produces amenorrhoea.

amiloride A drug that blocks SODIUM CHANNELS in cell membranes; see SALT and SWEETNESS.

amine hormones see hormones – classification

amine An amine is a derivative of ammonia in which hydrocarbon radicals have replaced one or more of the hydrogen atoms ammonia possesses (see BIOGENIC AMINE).

aminergic Relating to any neurotransmitter that is an AMINE (including the CATECHOLAMINE transmitters DOPAMINE, NORADRENALINE and ADRENALINE; the INDOLEAMINE transmitter SEROTONIN; HISTAMINE and even such transmitters as OCTOPAMINE). It is a very broad category. For instance, any NEURON that synthesizes and releases a neurotransmitter that is a MONOAMINE or BIOGENIC AMINE is said to be aminergic.

amino acids Technically, amino acids are organic molecules that have at least one carboxyl and at least one amino groups. There are, for adult human beings, eight ESSENTIAL AMINO ACIDS which are not synthesized within the body and must be supplied from the diet. (For infants there is a ninth essential amino acid, histidine.) Amino acids are the basic building units of PROTEINS and PEPTIDES. From a neuroscientific perspective however, possibly the most important function of amino acids is in NEUROTRANSMITTERS.

amino acid neurotransmitters Amino acids can function as NEUROTRANSMITTERS, typically engaged in FAST NEUROTRANSMISSION. They are divided into two groups: EXCITATORY

AMINO ACIDS (principally GLUTAMIC ACID and ASPARTIC ACID) and INHIBITORY AMINO ACIDS (principally GABA and GLYCINE, though TAURINE may also be an inhibitory amino acid neurotransmitter).

aminoglycosides Certain aminoglycosides (for example KANAMYCIN) serve as OTOTOXIC DRUGS (see NERVE DEAFNESS).

amitryptiline An antidepressant drug (one of the TRICYCLICS) that works by blocking the REUPTAKE of monoamines from the SYNAPTIC CLEFT.

See also: depression

Ammon's horn An old term for the HIPPO-CAMPUS introduced in the eighteenth century after a mythological Egyptian god called Amun Kneph. Other writers also likened the curious shape of this structure, occupying the floor of the lateral ventricle (see VENTRICLES) of the human brain, to a ram's horn. A curious feature of hippocampal terminology is that although Ammon's Horn and its original Latin name *cornu Ammonis* are rarely used nowadays, cell fields within the hippocampus continue to refer to this heritage. CA3 pyramidal cells project prominently to CA1 cells whose axons, in turn, provide the major output of the hippocampus (see CA1–CA3).

RICHARD G. M. MORRIS

amnesia Failure of learning and MEMORY (see AMNESIC SYNDROME).

IAN C. REID

amnesic syndrome Failure of MEMORY function, usually permanently, following brain damage. Deficits are restricted to memory function, in the setting of clear consciousness, with intellectual abilities unimpaired (in contrast to the memory failure associated with global dysfunction encountered in DEMENTIA). Sufferers experience a marked ANTEROGRADE AMNESIA (failure to learn new material), with variable RETROGRADE AMNESIA (failure to remember events that occurred prior to the brain insult). Memory for episodes (see EPISODIC MEMORY, DECLARATIVE MEMORY) is grossly and specifically impaired. Amnesics retain certain memory capacities, however, such as

PERCEPTUAL LEARNING, PROCEDURAL LEARNING and PRIMING effects. IMMEDIATE MEMORY is also unaffected. The syndrome may follow either bilateral TEMPORAL LOBE damage (for example, after HERPES ENCEPHALITIS, neurosurgical damage – see H.M.) or damage to the DIENCEPHALON (for example, KORSAKOFF'S SYNDROME – see DIENCEPHALIC AMNESIA). Crucial structures appear to be the HIPPOCAMPUS in the temporal lobe and the DORSOMEDIAL NUCLEUS OF THE THALAMUS or MAMMILLARY BODIES in the diencephalon.

IAN C. REID

amnestic aphasia Impaired word-finding ability. From a classical framework in which aphasic symptoms (see APHASIA) are attributed to a loss of the capacity for abstract behaviour. It refers specifically to an inability to associate an object with its arbitrary label, or name.

CHARLOTTE C. MITCHUM

amniocentesis A technique for sampling amniotic fluid (see AMNIOTIC EGG) from within the UTERUS of a pregnant female. Examination of chemicals in the fluid withdrawn can reveal whether there are any abnormalities in the developing foetus. Present in the fluid will also be cells from the developing foetus. These can be captured, cultured (see TISSUE CULTURE) and analysis of them made (as for example for detecting DOWN SYNDROME).

amnion *see* amniotic egg

amniotic egg Embryos of mammals, birds and reptiles (the AMNIOTIC VERTEBRATES, in contrast to the ANAMNIOTIC VERTEBRATES) possess four membranes: the AMNION, yolk sac, allantois and CHORION. The amnion is a fluid-filled sac that offers physical protection (buffering the developing EMBRYO against movement); the yolk sac has nutritive functions; the allantois has disposal functions; and the chorion is involved in gas exchange. In mammals, the egg is embedded in the maternal body. In reptiles and birds, the embryo and all four membranes are held in a shell.

See also: twin studies

amniotic vertebrates *see* anamniotic vertebrates

amodal completion *see* pattern completion

AMPA Alpha-amino-3-hydroxy-5-methylisox-azole-4-propionic acid: an EXCITOTOXIN frequently used to produce lesions in experimental animals and the definitive AGONIST at a class of GLUTAMATE RECEPTORS.

amphetamine Amphetamines and chemically related compounds of the beta-phenylethyl-amine family are in the pharmacological class of PSYCHOMOTOR STIMULANTS, which also includes methylphenidate and COCAINE. Amphetamine was synthesized in 1887 by Edeleano and introduced commercially first as a bronchial decongestant in 1932 ('benzedrine') and later as a treatment for NARCOLEPSY and for weight control. In the war-time years it was used commonly by the military to enhance vigilance and later by the general population for similar purposes. However, in the 1950s and 1960s it became evident that amphetamines were potentially dangerous drugs of abuse with psychotic side-effects. It has recently been claimed that chronic use of high doses of amphetamine can cause permanent neuronal damage in experimental animals. Following observations made in the 1930s, the psychomotor stimulant methylphenidate ('Ritalin') is much used in the USA as a medication for ATTENTION-DEFICIT DISORDER and hyperactivity syndromes in children.

Amphetamine exists in two stereoisomeric forms, D and L amphetamine, the former being much more potent. Methamphetamine is more potent still than the D form. It resembles the plant product cathinone in chemical structure. Amphetamines produce their pharmacological effects by a combination of actions as an indirect CATECHOLAMINE AGONIST; it releases DOPAMINE and (probably) NORADRENALINE, as well as blocking the REUPTAKE of both of these neurotransmitters into the presynaptic cell, and probably at higher doses acting as a MONO-AMINE OXIDASE inhibitor. Thus, by a combination of these three actions it enhances the concentrations of these catecholamine neurotransmitters in the SYNAPTIC CLEFT. The mechanisms of action of the different psychomotor stimulant drugs differ subtly. Whereas amphetamine appears to displace cytoplasmic neurotransmitter via its action on the synaptic VESICULAR TRANSPORTER, both cocaine and methylphenidute work mainly by inhibiting the monoamine (reuptake) transporter on the presynaptic terminal.

In behavioural terms, amphetamine increases central and sympathetic arousal and desynchronizes (see SYNCHRONY/DESYNCHRONY) the ELECTROENCEPHALOGRAM (EEG) in humans, inhibiting SLEEP. It is a mild anorectic (see ANOREXIA) agent but can produce euphoric subjective responses (see EUPHORIA) which contribute to ABUSE POTENTIAL. At high, generally repeated doses, it has been shown to produce symptoms that are difficult to distinguish from those of paranoid SCHIZOPHRENIA, and which can be antagonized by the same NEUROLEPTIC drugs used in the treatment of schizophrenia. For this reason, the behavioural effects of amphetamine have been considered as a model psychosis, the existence of which provides support for a DOPAMINE HYPOTHESIS OF SCHIZOPHRENIA.

Many of the behavioural effects of amphetamine in humans resemble those found in experimental animals. At low doses amphetamine enhances spontaneous locomotor activity in the rat, and at larger doses leads to a syndrome of behavioural STEREOTYPY in which the same response is repeated over and over again at a high rate. In rats, this is often manifested as repeated head movements (including sniffing), but other responses can also become stereotyped. In monkeys, stereotyped GROOMING and even social behaviour are observed. In humans stereotypy can also be observed as grooming: repetitive picking of the skin because of tactile hallucinations of infestation by ants or other insects has been noted. It can however also take a more symbolic form and even be expressed, for example, in the thinking patterns of amphetamine addicts and in their artwork.

In experimental animals, amphetamine may increase responding for food even though it is anorectic, leading to suggestions that it increases the reinforcing or rewarding value of stimuli associated with food (and other rewards) – that is, it enhances the power of the conditioned reinforcer. Amphetamine will also increase responding for, and apparently reduce the rewarding threshold of, ELECTRICAL STIMULATION OF THE BRAIN via implanted electrodes.

The clear demonstration of its own rewarding properties is its self-adminstration via intravenous catheters by experimental animals (see INTRAVENOUS SELF-ADMINISTRATION). A good deal is now known about the neural mediation of the behavioural effects of amphetamine, much of which occurs via effects on the mesotelencephalic dopamine system from its origins in the midbrain to innervate structures such as the NUCLEUS ACCUMBENS (or ventral STRIATUM) and the CAUDATE–PUTAMEN or dorsal striatum. Thus, for example, the stereotyped oral behaviour and head movements induced in rats by large doses of the drug are known to depend on the integrity of the NIGROSTRIATAL DOPAMINE SYSTEM that projects to the dorsal striatum, whereas the locomotor hyperactivity is blocked by dopamine depletion from the ventral striatum. Amphetamine has been shown to be reinforcing to rats when it is self-administered directly into the nucleus accumbens, and loss of dopamine there attenuates self-adminstration behaviour. Thus, it appears that the rewarding and potentially addictive effects of amphetamine result from effects on the nucleus accumbens. Much less is known about the neural basis of its effects in man, but recent neuroimaging studies of the effects of cocaine and methylphenidate suggest that subjective effects of the drugs can be correlated with actions in structures such as the striatum and the thalamus.

See also: addiction

Reference

Feldman R., Meyer J.S. & Quenzer L.F. (1997) *Principles of Neuropsychopharmacology*, Sinauer Associates: Sunderland MA.

TREVOR W. ROBBINS

amplitude Strength of a STIMULUS or a behaviour as separate from its timing characteristics such as frequency or duration. In brain stimulation studies, amplitude would be the stimulation current. In acoustical studies, it would be the sound intensity. In behavioural studies, amplitude typically refers to response strength such as the force applied in a specific motor act (for instance, a startle reaction).

JAMES R. STELLAR

ampulla *see* vestibular system

amusia An inability to sing, or play a musical instrument properly, or to perceive music, these previously having been intact functions; a condition similar to APHASIA but specific for music rather than LANGUAGE. See also MUSIC AND THE BRAIN.

amygdala The amygdala is a key component of the LIMBIC SYSTEM and has an important role in EMOTION. This brain structure, which is named after its fanciful resemblance to an almond, lies in the anterior medial portion of each TEMPORAL LOBE. It is composed of approximately a dozen nuclei each with a distinctive pattern of cytoarchitectural, histochemical and connectional features. These nuclei are often divided into a basolateral group and a corticomedial group. The basolateral group contains many cortical like cells and its nuclei have dense connections with sensory association and limbic cortical areas. The corticomedial group is more closely linked with hypothalamic and olfactory regions (see HYPOTHALAMUS; OLFACTION). The central nucleus of the amygdala has features of both groups but is unique in having many connections with subcortical AUTONOMIC centres. Other subcortical connections of the amygdala include dense projections to the NUCLEUS BASALIS OF MEYNERT, the ventral STRIATUM, and the DORSOMEDIAL NUCLEUS OF THE THALAMUS. The amygdala also has a complex array of intrinsic connections and is noteworthy for the enormous range of NEUROTRANSMITTERS and neuromodulators that are present within the structure.

The amygdala has a variety of functions (Aggleton, 2000), and while most attention has focused on its role in emotion it can also modulate different aspects of motivation (such as feeding, drinking, and sexual behaviour). Damage to this structure can decrease emotional reactivity, as seen in the KLÜVER–BUCY SYNDROME, and severely disrupt social behaviour. These changes, which are very dramatic in monkeys, are less evident in humans. Experimental studies indicate that the amygdala is involved in the formation of stimulus–affect associations, and the evidence for this is especially convincing for aversive stimuli (see

FEAR). The structure is also important for the identification of affective states in others, and research on people with bilateral amygdala damage has revealed a selective loss of the ability to recognize expressions of fear. The structure may also facilitate learning about events that are associated with highly emotional or arousing experiences. Finally, the amygdala contributes more generally to LEARNING by enabling the formation of STIMULUS–REINFORCER ASSOCIATIONS.

Reference

Aggleton J.P. (ed.) (2000) *The Amygdala: A Functional Analysis*, Oxford University Press: Oxford.

JOHN P. AGGLETON

amylin *see* calcitonin gene-related peptide

amyloid Amyloid, also called BETA AMYLOID PROTEIN (the standard abbreviation is Aβ), is a PEPTIDE of about 4,000 molecular weight made of between 40 and 42 AMINO ACIDS. It forms part of a larger PROTEIN known as BETA AMYLOID PRECURSOR PROTEIN (abbreviated as APP). Amyloid can be visualized by histological (see HISTOLOGY) stains such as Congo red and thioflavine S, or by IMMUNOHISTOCHEMISTRY. Amyloid is water-insoluble, self-aggregating, and resistant to further degradation. The function of amyloid is not exactly clear, but it is a MEMBRANE protein thought to be involved in the inhibition of PROTEOLYSIS or possibly in CELL growth or adhesion. It is the main component of the neuritic (see NEURITE) or senile PLAQUES seen in ALZHEIMER'S DEMENTIA (and indeed in the brains of other patients groups; see for example DOWN SYNDROME). Although amyloid-containing plaques are neuropathological hallmarks of Alzheimer's dementia, how they lead to typical neuronal loss and dementia is not well understood.

KAZUE SEMBA

amyloid precursor protein *see* amyloid

amyotrophic lateral sclerosis Progressive loss of motor neurons from the anterior horn of the SPINAL CORD and, in the later stages of the disease, from the motor nuclei of the CRANIAL NERVES and CEREBRAL CORTEX. Degeneration of the spinal CORTICOSPINAL TRACTS (lateral sclerosis) and associated muscle wasting (amyotrophy) account for its name. In the USA the condition is also associated with the name of Lou Gehrig, a sports personality, and in the UK with the well-known figure of Stephen Hawking, astrophysicist and best-selling author.

The disease usually presents in middle age with limb weakness and FASCICULATION – fleeting contractions of isolated muscle bundles, visible in one muscle after another. A paradoxical increase in the strength of tendon reflexes coupled with weakness and wasting of the same limb is a distinctive feature. The paradox is accounted for by the loss of spinal (lower motor) neurons being accompanied by loss of inhibitory input from cortical (upper motor) neurons. As the disease progresses, gradual involvement of cranial nerve nuclei (that is, progressive BULBAR palsy) leads to increasing difficulty with swallowing and speech, but eye movement, sphincter control and intellect are usually preserved.

The cause of ALS remains unknown. Evidence for the involvement of a virus, dietary toxins or autoimmune processes is weak. About 10% of cases are familial, showing AUTOSOMAL DOMINANT inheritance, and of these about one-fifth carry one of many identified mutations affecting the gene (SOD1) that encodes the enzyme copper/zinc SUPEROXIDE DISMUTASE. This enzyme is thought to confer protection against oxidative damage by free radicals, but the harmful effects of the mutant gene product are also likely to result from a gain in function that causes it to act as an oxidant in its own right. The role of OXIDATIVE STRESS in sporadic (non-familial) ALS has not been clearly established. Other possible contributory factors include endogenous EXCITOTOXINS, especially the amino acid neurotransmitter GLUTAMATE. Excessive extracellular concentrations of this compound in the spinal cord are thought to result in harmful transmembrane inward currents of calcium ions (Ca^{2+}); certain glutamate antagonists (for instance, riluzole) have accordingly been approved for the long-term treatment of ALS but their efficacy and the rationale for their use have been questioned. Therapeutic trials with intrathecal injections of ciliary neurotrophic factor, a NEUROTROPHIN, have met with limited success. Supportive treatment of advanced ALS with artificial feeding, assisted breathing, synthesized phonation and computerized communication has reached a high degree of sophistication but may not be unreservedly welcomed by those involved.

L. JACOB HERBERG

anabolism; anabolic; anabolite *see* metabolism

anaerobic Not requiring the presence of free OXYGEN.

anaesthesia Loss of sensation resulting from pharmacological depression of nerve function caused by administration of a DRUG or by other medical interventions, or from neurological dysfunction usually by damage to a nerve or receptor. Somewhat arbitrary divisions have been established describing various stages of clinical anaesthesia: stage I (ANALGESIA), initial period immediately following administration of the anaesthetic and up to loss of consciousness; stage II (delirium), period extending from the loss of CONSCIOUSNESS to the beginning of surgical anaesthesia and characterized by increases in muscle tone, irregular breathing, incontinence, hypertension, and TACHYCARDIA, including disquieting behaviours such as excitable movements and vocalizations; stage III (surgical anaesthesia), period extending from the second stage to cessation of spontaneous respiration and subdivided into four planes (1–4) in order of increasing depth of anaesthesia that are related to changes in respiration, eyeball movements, reflexive tone, and pupil size; stage IV (medullary depression), period following plane 4 of stage III beginning with failure of systemic circulation and ending typically in the death of the subject.

Satisfactory general anaesthesia for the purpose of surgical intervention should result in at least four effects on the individual: (1) motionlessness in response to strong stimuli produced by surgery, (2) suppression of autonomic responses (for example, tachycardia, HYPERTENSION, LACRIMATION), (3) lack of pain (analgesia), and (4) lack of recall (AMNESIA). Phenomena 1 and 4 comprise the main traditional indicators of satisfactory anaesthesia and

loss of consciousness in human subjects. These responses include a complete lack of organized movement made by the subject in response to surgical stimuli (such as an incision), a complete lack of awareness in the form of non-reflexive movement to stimuli, and loss of recall of intraoperative events following recovery. Other indicators of anaesthetic-induced unconsciousness are retrospective phenomena and include priming in which behaviour has been changed by intraoperative stimuli, but the subject does not have any post-operative memory of the priming stimuli. Achieving all of these criteria is thought to imply complete unconsciousness during anaesthesia and represents accepted methodological practice in clinical anaesthesiology. Nevertheless, several issues remain as to whether these phenomena represent the most reliable means of assessing consciousness at different levels of anaesthesia (see Kulli & Koch, 1991). This is particularly true in the case of general anaesthesia in animals.

The existence of consciousness in non-human subjects remains a topic of considerable debate in the field of COGNITIVE NEUROSCIENCE. The same behavioural and cognitive phenomena used to assess awareness or recall in humans treated with anaesthetics do not apply easily to laboratory animals. Thus, in addition to the cognitive phenomena noted above, several neurophysiological criteria have been explored as potential indicators of depth of anaesthesia. These diagnostic procedures include ELECTROENCEPHALOGRAM (EEG) and sensory-EVOKED POTENTIALS recordings from the cortex. Initial efforts have assessed the spectrum of EEG which has been observed to vary in a MONOTONIC, DOSE-DEPENDENT fashion in response to various anaesthetics. For example, increasing the dosage of non-specific anaesthetics decreases the EEG signal from 20 Hz to 6 Hz and below. However, the degree of variability in the EEG record associated with the various non-specific agents makes this an unreliable measure of the depth of anaesthetic-induced unconsciousness. This variability in the EEG is further evident for receptor-specific anaesthetics and a reliable index has yet to be described. However, a more promising approach has involved the monitoring of evoked potentials from the surface of the cortex following presentation of different sensory stimuli. For example, middle latency auditory-evoked potentials resembling 3–5 cycles of a 40 Hz wave have been recorded in humans and cats under various anaesthetic agents. The barbiturate THIOPENTAL induces a decrease of 10 Hz in these oscillations or abolishes them altogether. Non-specific VOLATILE ANAESTHETICS such as HALOTHANE dose-dependently decreases the auditory-evoked 40 Hz wave. However, receptor-specific anaesthetics (such as FENTANYL, KETAMINE, or BENZODIAZEPINES) appear to have minimal effects on these oscillations. These evoked responses have also been correlated with periods of spontaneous movements and movements associated with verbal commands in patients under anaesthesia. As such, several investigators (see Kulli & Koch, 1991) have concluded that the presence of 40 Hz signals serve to confirm the presence of consciousness in anaesthetic-treated subjects. A number of theories have been put forward as to the significance of 40 Hz cortical waves and depth of anaesthesia. The most prominent theory states that these oscillations may be acting as a clock to provide a temporal framework for sensory processing within and across different modalities. Thus, these oscillations serve to link transiently together activity of several areas of the cortex involved in coherently perceiving the various qualities and aspects of its surrounding. Without this bridge the nervous system may lose temporal coherency of incoming sensory stimuli, possibly resulting in a loss of consciousness.

Reference

Kulli J. & Koch C. (1991) Does anaesthesia cause loss of consciousness? *Trends in Neurosciences* 14: 6–10.

CHARLES D. BLAHA

anaesthetics Drugs that reversibly depress neuronal function with accompanying loss of pain perception (ANALGESIA) and/or other sensations (anti-nociceptive; see NOCICEPTION). Drugs that induce a state of ANAESTHESIA fall into three main categories. (1) General: an agent that abolishes CONSCIOUSNESS and perception of all sensations. (2) Local: an agent whose anaesthetic action is limited to an area

of the body determined by the site of its application. (3) Topical: a LOCAL ANAESTHETIC applied directly to the area to be anaesthetised, usually the mucous membranes or the skin.

Two main classes of general anaesthetics are non-specific agents that depress excitable tissue at all levels of the CNS and receptor-specific agents that have an action at specific neurotransmitter receptor sites in the CNS. Non-specific agents include inhalational VOLATILE ANAESTHETICS (including HALOTHANE, enflurane, methoxyflurane and isoflurane) and other agents (such as NITROUS OXIDE, CHLOROFORM, cyclopropane, and diethyl ETHER). Volatile anaesthetics are combined typically with an ADJUVANT such as nitrous oxide to induce clinical (human) anaesthesia. The mechanisms of action for these compounds remain unknown but is thought to involve a dose-dependent reduction in the metabolic rates of certain neurons in the CNS. In contrast to non-specific anaesthetics, general anaesthesia can be produced only with a combination of several receptor-specific agents. The main component is either one of the opioid NARCOTICS (such as FENTANYL) or one of the BARBITURATES (for instance THIOPENTAL) to induce sedation, analgesia, and reduced autonomic response, and may be given in combination with a BENZODIAZEPINE (for example DIAZEPAM) to decrease awareness during NARCOSIS. Opioid analgesics may also be combined with NEUROLEPTIC compounds to reduce motor activity and ANXIETY together with CURARE-like agents to suppress movement. Compounds used almost exclusively in experimental animal research to induce surgical anaesthesia include urethane, CHLORAL HYDRATE, CHLORALOSE, XYLAZINE, and KETAMINE. The second and third category of anaesthetics include the short-acting local anaesthetics (for instance LIDOCAINE, PROCAINE and COCAINE) and long-acting ION CHANNEL NEUROTOXINS (such as TETRODOTOXIN and saxitoxin). These drugs are used mainly to interrupt nerve transmission of pain sensations when applied locally to nerve tissue in appropriate concentrations. Local anaesthetics act selectively at the level of the neuronal cell body to prevent transient increases in sodium ion channel permeability and to reduce potassium permeability at rest.

The cell THRESHOLD of excitation is increased resulting in a blockade of both the generation and the conduction of any ACTION POTENTIAL.

See also: dissociative anaesthetics; endorphins; enkephalins; gate theory of pain; opiates; opium; sedative

CHARLES D. BLAHA

analgesia (from Greek, *an*: not, *algeein*: to feel pain) Analgesia is a reduction in the sensation of PAIN, without inducing SLEEP or unconsciousness. Analgesics are drugs that induce analgesia: many drugs have analgesic properties, ranging from MORPHINE through to aspirin. Testing drugs for their analgesic properties is difficult, since it necessarily involves inflicting pain and looking for a reduction in response to it when drugs are given. With rats, various tests have been used: the TAIL-FLICK TEST involves warming a part of the rat's tail (a focused heat lamp is typically used) and the latency to flick the tail away measured. The hot-plate test involves measuring escape latency from a hot plate and the related FLINCH–JUMP TEST involves passing electric current through a grid floor and monitoring rats' flinching and jumping responses. Inflicting pain on an animal and measuring responses to it is clearly an issue that requires careful ethical consideration. Evaluation of alternative methods that could be used, and careful consideration of the likely costs and benefits of an experiment, has to be made. It is worth remembering though that the management of pain in both human and veterinary practice remains an enormous challenge to physicians and that methods to alleviate pain still require considerable improvement.

See also: drug; gate control theory of pain

anamniotic vertebrates The anamniotic vertebrates are fish and amphibia. They lack an amnion, the innermost membrane surrounding the embryos of reptiles, birds and mammals, the AMNIOTIC VERTEBRATES.

anandamide (from Sanskrit, *ananda*: bliss) The natural LIGAND for TETRAHYDROCANNABINOL receptors.

anarthria An inability to produce speech, caused either by damage to neural mechanisms or by damage to the physical machinery of SPEECH PRODUCTION.

androgen insensitivity syndrome *see* gender

androgens A set of SEX HORMONES, including TESTOSTERONE, secreted from the ADRENAL GLAND and the TESTES.

See also: corticosteroids; endocrine glands; hormones; hormones – classification; organization effects of steroid hormones

anencephaly (from Greek, *an*: without, ENCEPHALON: brain). Literally this means without a brain, though in fact this is a little inaccurate. Anencephaly is an exceptionally severe disorder of development in which the CEREBRAL HEMISPHERES and DIENCEPHALON and elements of the MIDBRAIN do not develop. The condition is not lethal but does produce profound impairment.

anergasia Loss of function; descriptive of the loss of function that might occur in any of many conditions.

anergia Literally, loss of ENERGY; descriptive of an individual suffering from an inability to generate actions.

aneurysm (from Greek, *ana*: up, *eurys*: wide) Aneurysm can refer to any abnormal enlargement, but in medical practice it refers to an abnormal dilation of an ARTERY, which may burst. In the brain this is likely to lead to neurological impairment (see ISCHAEMIA; STROKE).

angel dust (PCP) One the commonest of several street names for the abused synthetic drug phencyclidine (PCP) [1-(1-phenylcyclo-hexy-1)piperidine]. PCP was originally synthesized and developed as an anaesthetic agent, but unpleasant psychomimetic side effects led to its withdrawal. The drug acts by binding in the calcium ion channel associated with the NMDA RECEPTOR, a subclass of the EXCITATORY AMINO ACIDS receptor complex, and interferes with GLUTAMATE-mediated DOPAMINERGIC regulation. Use leads to disorientation, drowsiness and HALLUCINATION. PCP has been used as a drug of abuse in the USA – more rarely in the UK – for the last 30 years, and DSM-IV includes a criteria for coding PCP intoxication. Physical

DEPENDENCE is rare, but psychological dependence is common. The effects of PCP have been considered a useful model for SCHIZOPHRENIA. KETAMINE is a related, clinically available anaesthetic.

See also: addiction; anaesthetics

IAN C. REID

angioma *see* tumour

angiotensin Angiotensin II is a PEPTIDE with a variety of functions, though it is best known for its role in OSMOREGULATION. Indeed, angiotensin II is perhaps the most potent DIPSOGEN (a chemical that stimulates drinking) known to exist. When the kidneys detect a loss of blood flow, cells there secrete a substance called RENIN into the blood. Renin is an enzyme that converts ANGIOTENSINOGEN (which is always present in the blood) to ANGIOTENSIN I. This is further converted by the enzyme ANGIOTENSIN CONVERTING ENZYME (ACE) to the highly active molecule ANGIOTENSIN II which has an action on the brain, leading quickly to release of VASOPRESSIN. Vasopressin is synthesized by the magnocellular neurons of the paraventricular and supraoptic nuclei of the HYPOTHALAMUS: axons from these neurons travel to the NEUROHYPOPHYSIS (posterior pituitary) where they release vasopressin directly into the bloodstream. Vasopressin acts on the kidneys to prevent further water loss. Angiotensin II also has an action on the ADRENAL GLAND to stimulate ALDOSTERONE secretion, and stimulates contraction of blood vessels to increase blood pressure (see BLOOD). Because of this action, angiotensin converting enzyme inhibitors have been developed as a potent drug for the control of HYPERTENSION.

The angiotensin system in the blood was initially described by James Fitzsimons in the 1960s, but later studies have shown that all components of the angiotensin II formation pathway are also present in the brain. Like many other peptides that are found in the body, angiotensin II and its associated enzymes also appears to operate within NEUROTRANSMITTERS in the central nervous system. Angiotensin II is for example thought to be colocalized with DOPAMINE neurons and has an action in the STRIATUM. Angiotensin convert-ing enzyme is also found in the striatum, and administration of angiotensin converting enzyme inhibitors appears to stimulate dopamine activity.

angiotensin I *see* angiotensin; osmoregulation

angiotensin II *see* angiotensin; osmoregulation

angiotensin converting enzyme *see* angiotensin; osmoregulation

angiotensinogen *see* angiotensin; osmoregulation

angular gyrus A gyrus that sits at the junction of the PARIETAL LOBE and OCCIPITAL LOBE; it is thought to be involved in LANGUAGE functions, most notably verbal visual images. It has also been implicated as a substrate for oculomotor deficits, such as those that occur in BALINT'S SYNDROME.

anhedonia Hedonia means a state or condition of PLEASURE. Anhedonia is therefore characterized by the absence of pleasure. Anhedonia is often listed as a symptom of DEPRESSION, and this is meant to describe the lack of responsiveness to normally pleasurable stimuli in depressed individuals. Although it is sometimes suggested that a DOPAMINE ANTAGONIST or depletion of dopamine could produce anhedonia, and blunt the pleasurable effects of stimuli such as food, there is also considerable evidence against this idea.

JOHN D. SALAMONE

anhedonia hypothesis The anhedonia hypothesis (or general anhedonia model) concerns the functions of DOPAMINE in the NUCLEUS ACCUMBENS. It takes as its basis the hypothesis that dopamine activation in the nucleus accumbens is critical for the perception of REWARD and that the absence of dopamine will lead to ANHEDONIA and extinction of appropriate reward-related responding. Both natural reinforcers (such as food and water) and artificial reinforcers such as drugs (see ADDICTION; REINFORCEMENT) are suggested to operate through this system. This model has been of considerable value but there are now several findings that suggest it might not be entirely correct. For example, nucleus accumbens dopamine appears to be activated by both POSI-

TIVE REINFORCEMENT and NEGATIVE REINFOR-
CEMENT; and depletion of dopamine from the
nucleus accumbens does not necessarily lead to
reduction in food intake. Hypotheses that have
developed from the anhedonia hypothesis have
suggested that accumbens dopamine might be
involved in the allocation of responding to
stimuli rather than in the perception of reward
per se.

References

Berridge K.C. (1996) Food reward: brain substrates of wanting and liking. *Neuroscience
and Biobehavioral Reviews* 20: 1–25.

Salamone J.D., Cousins M.S. & Snyder B.J.
(1997) Behavioral functions of nucleus accumbens dopamine: empirical and conceptual problems with the anhedonia
hypothesis. *Neuroscience and Biobehavioral
Reviews* 21: 341–359.

animal communication For us, the most
obvious means of communication is through
LANGUAGE, which remains a resolutely human
attribute (see ACQUISITION OF LANGUAGE BY
NON-HUMAN PRIMATES). There are however a
variety of non-linguistic means through which
members of species communicate with each
other. The table below summarizes the effectiveness of different means of communication.

Much of animal communication involves
RITUALIZATION – patterns of behaviour that
have become established during the course of
EVOLUTION. For example, the interactions between offspring and parent in the presentation
of food can be ritualized: gull chicks are called
from cover by parents, the chick then pecking
at the parents beak to initiate the regurgitation
of food. However, probably the most famous
example of ritualized communication is the
dance performed by honey bees, first described
by Karl Von Frisch (1886–1982 – co-winner,
with Konrad Lorenz and Niko Tinbergen of
the 1973 Nobel Prize for Medicine). On
returning to the hive from a FORAGING trip,
honey bees perform one of two different types
of dance to indicate the presence of food. The
dance is preceded by the returning bee beating
its wings and releasing a pheromone to attract
attention if it has found a food source worth
recruiting. A relationship between the quality
of the food source and food availability has
been noted – in high summer when food is
plentiful bees are more selective in their foraging. A simple round dance indicates that food
is very close by; the waggle dance contains
more complex information. The angle at which
the body is held from vertical indicates the
angle of the sun in relation to the food source
while the duration of the dance corresponds to
the foods' distance from the hive. The scent
that the returning bee brings back provides a
further indication of the location of the new
food supply. It has been suggested also that
bees can use other forms of information – the
emission of sounds, gravity, odours, or even
light polarization for example – in addition to
their ritualized dances, and it is clear that
CIRCADIAN RHYTHMS influence dance production. It is also worth noting first, that there are
variations in the dances between different types
of honey bee in different locations (see also

Animal communication channels

	Signal channel			
	Chemical	Auditory	Visual	Tactile
Range	Long	Long	Intermediate	Short
Rate of change	Slow	Fast	Fast	Fast
Ability to overcome obstruction	Good	Good	Bad	Bad
Ease with which it can be located	Variable	Intermediate	High	High
Energy cost	Low	High	Low	Low
Examples:	PHEROMONES	BIRDSONG	GESTURE	GROOMING

Source: Adapted from McFarland (1999)

CULTURE); and second, that these apparently innate forms of communication are followed by adaptive activity, as the bees learn (see LEARNING) and remember (see MEMORY) where food is. COURTSHIP – the interaction that precedes the pairing off of mates (however transiently) and COPULATION – is also often ritualized, involving patterns of DISPLAY. Display is a complex phenomenon, involving interpretation of situations and the production of appropriate behaviour before, during and after the display. GESTURE (that is, the production of specific movements) and POSTURE (the way in which the body is held) are both important features of display, and auditory events may also play a part (see for example, BIRDSONG). Similarly, TERRITORIAL BEHAVIOUR may involve ritualized displays of AGGRESSION which communicate to conspecifics that they should depart.

VOCALIZATION is an important part of animal communication, involved in many aspects of behaviour. For example, ALARM CALLS in social animals serve to warn conspecifics of intruders – typically predators – in a group's territory. DISTRESS CALLS serve to indicate warnings either to conspecifics or to parents. Distress and alarm calls often have similar physical characteristics, and can serve similar functions. *Separation distress calls* are common among the young of many mammalian species and appear to be available to infants immediately after birth. Neonatal humans separated from their mothers begin crying in a way that indicates a recognition (at some level) of separation: when the infant is restored to contact with the mother crying stops.

Non-verbal communication is important also to humans: much information is communicated by BODY LANGUAGE (gesture and posture) and by facial expressions (see FACE PERCEPTION). Charles Darwin (1809–1882) wrote extensively about the nature of facial expression, which it has been thought might reflect universal principles of human non-verbal communication. However, it is clear that much of human non-verbal communication is learned, driven by culture.

See also: social behaviour

Reference

McFarland D. (1999) *Animal Behaviour*, 3rd edn, Addison Wesley Longman: Harlow UK.

animal models The experimental study of animal behaviour and neurobiology in an effort to explore the neural basis of human PSYCHOPATHOLOGY by analogy. Animal models offer the opportunity to exert control over many of the variables which epidemiological research suggests may be influential in the aetiology of psychiatric and neurological disorder, for example, GENOTYPE, early social experience (see SOCIAL ISOLATION) and magnitude, type and duration of environmental STRESS. Physical and pharmacological manipulation of brain function is a core feature. Certain species also offer a relatively short life span, permitting developmental study within a feasible time-scale.

Animal models are used in a variety of ways: these include efforts to predict the efficacy of experimental treatments; or to investigate pathophysiological processes. An example of the former would be the use of the PORSOLT TEST, in which the time rats spend trying to escape from a beaker of water is measured, which (perhaps surprisingly) predicts the ANTIDEPRESSANT activity of novel compounds. An example of the latter would be bilateral destruction of the hippocampus in primates and measurement of effects on LEARNING tasks in an effort to determine the role of the hippocampus in MEMORY. Which of these approaches is the more valuable is difficult to determine. The use of animals in tests to screen new therapeutic strategies (both pharmacological and surgical) is the more widely publicized and can sometimes appear rather odd to the layman (as with the Porsolt test) though there is always a logic to the test. The use of animals in research to understand basic biological processes is less publicized but is possibly of more benefit: medics and veterinary surgeons cannot deal with bodies unless they have an understanding of how those bodies work.

There has been considerable debate about the morality of using animals in research. This has focused on a number of points, including whether or not it is ethical to use animals in research (regardless of the value of the research) (see ANIMAL WELFARE); and whether or not animal models can reveal anything meaningful about the human condition (that is, does the research have any value?). Some have argued that animal research is misleading and wasteful, pointing to differences in the physiology of humans and animals commonly studied in laboratories. On the other hand, others have argued that this is not the case and that animal experimentation is critical to both medicine and biology. This debate is explored in a series of reviews in a recent edition of *Scientific American*.

References

Barnard N.D. & Kaufman S.R. (1997) Animal research is wasteful and misleading. *Scientific American* 276: 64–66.

Botting J.H. & Morrison A.R. (1997) Animal research is vital to medicine. *Scientific American* 276: 67–69.

Mukerjee M. (1997) Trends in animal research. *Scientific American* 276: 70–77.

Rowan A.N. (1997) The benefits and ethics of animal research. *Scientific American* 276: 63.

IAN C. REID AND PHILIP WINN

animal models of anxiety Animal models of ANXIETY attempt to mimic various aspects of the AETIOLOGY, symptomatology and treatment of human anxiety disorders with the aim of providing a better understanding of, and more successful treatments for, these clinical conditions. There are many different animal models of anxiety, some examining UNCONDITIONED BEHAVIOUR, others making use of PAVLOVIAN CONDITIONING and INSTRUMENTAL CONDITIONING procedures. Each of the different models has its own merits, and each has a degree of predictive validity – that is, the ability to accurately predict which drugs are likely to be beneficial in the treatment of human clinical anxiety disorders, and equally important, which are not.

Models based on unconditioned behaviour commonly employ a test environment that is designed to induce a level of anxiety in the laboratory animal (most commonly in rats or mice). As such behaviours are held to be more natural to the animal than those observed in models which employ Pavlovian or instrumental conditioning procedures, they are often perceived as possessing a high level of etholo-

gical validity. Models based on unconditioned behaviours include extremely simple tests examining the behaviour of animals in an OPEN FIELD, in simple social interactions with a CONSPECIFIC, or in ELEVATED MAZES. The most typical form of elevated maze is the elevated plus maze, in which anxiety is measured by examining the proportion of time spent on the two arms of the maze which are open, relative to the amount of time spent on the two safer, enclosed arms. Following drug treatment, increased activity in the open field, increased SOCIAL BEHAVIOUR, or increased time spent on the open arms of the plus maze are all indicative of ANXIOLYTIC potential. However, care must be taken to avoid the potentially confounding influence of drugs which merely alter locomotor activity, such as AMPHETAMINE. Such drugs may decrease indices of anxiety in these tests, but are not in fact anxiolytic.

Models examining conditioned behaviours rely on fear conditioning to imbue a CONDITIONED STIMULUS or test environment with the ability to evoke FEAR or anxiety. One general class of model involves simple PAVLOVIAN FEAR conditioning in which a conditioned stimulus predicts the onset of an aversive event such as mild FOOTSHOCK. This fear conditioning may then be assessed in a variety of ways, including the development of conditioned freezing, the skeletal muscle rigour and immobility produced by presentation of an aversive conditioned stimulus, conditioned suppression, or fear-potentiated startle. Decreases in any of these measures of conditioned fear following drug treatment would be indicative of anxiolytic potential. A second class of conditioned fear model involves instrumental conditioning, usually in the form of avoidance learning. In these procedures animals either produce an active response or withhold some prepotent response in order to terminate, or avoid presentation of, an aversive event. Examples of active response procedures include ACTIVE AVOIDANCE in which a locomotor response is required to terminate and avoid signalled footshock and SIDMAN AVOIDANCE which requires production of repeated, timed responses to avoid unsignalled footshock. Procedures requiring the inhibition of a response include

PASSIVE AVOIDANCE and punishment or conflict procedures such as CONDITIONED PUNISHMENT, GELLER–SEIFTER CONFLICT and VOGEL CONFLICT. In each of these cases, a response that is usually present, such as locomotor activity and exploration, lever-pressing for food, or licking for water must be inhibited in order to avoid presentation of an aversive event. Anxiety is inferred from the degree to which an animal is successful in avoiding or terminating shocks, and hence a decrease in this success following drug treatment suggests that anxiety has been reduced. These conditioning procedures are again not without their problems. There can be unwanted interactions with the ability of drugs to increase or decrease general activity. In the case of behaviours that examine the disruption of appetitive behaviour, changes in hunger or thirst motivation can influence the outcome. Finally, drugs that directly influence the learning processes underlying the induction of conditioned fear may also disrupt performance in these tasks, without necessarily having an anxiolytic effect.

Animal models of anxiety have been of great utility in the development of novel anxiolytic drugs for human treatment. Hence, in addition to the continuing refinement of 'classical' BENZODIAZEPINE anxiolytics such as CHLORDIAZEPOXIDE (VALIUM) and MIDAZOLAM (Hypnovel) to produce treatments with fewer sedative, mnemonic and muscle relaxant side-effects, alternative classes of drug which influence serotonergic systems, such as buspirone and ipsapirone (both PARTIAL AGONISTS at the 5-HYDROXYTRYPTAMINE 1A receptor) have also been developed. The development of more sophisticated test batteries which examine a wide variety of animal models of anxiety, including both unconditioned and conditioned behaviours, and an ever more comprehensive understanding of the neural and even molecular basis of fear and anxiety through the use of advanced behavioural and neuroscientific techniques, are contributing to the continuing progress in the development of treatments for clinical anxiety disorders in humans.

See also: aversive conditioning

A. SIMON KILLCROSS

animal welfare Animal welfare is of general concern, beyond the narrow scope of biological psychology. All animals should be treated in a humane manner. Legislation in the United Kingdom and elsewhere governs, amongst many other things, the care of animals, their sale and transport, and the protection of endangered species. In many countries there is legislation specifically to protect the welfare of laboratory animals. Such legislation typically covers the maintenance of animals, the scientific procedures that can be applied, and the nature and location of the places where animals can be bred, kept and tested.

Legislation in the United Kingdom (the Animals [Scientific Procedures] Act 1986) lays down, for each SPECIES, appropriate measures for such things as housing (both the nature of the housing – each species should be kept in an environment appropriate to its natural behaviour – and the density of occupation), temperature, humidity and maintenance regimes – the delivery of food and water, how often bedding should be refreshed and cages cleaned, how often a veterinary surgeon must inspect the animals, and so on. In addition to these things, legislation also specifies such things as the institutional management structures and the record-keeping needed, and requires independent inspectors to monitor all aspects of laboratory animal maintenance and use. The manner in which animals should be destroyed on completion of experimentation is also regulated. The legislation specifies who can undertake which regulated procedures on laboratory animals, weighing what is done against the likely benefit that might accrue to medicine, veterinary science and basic science. Scientists in the United Kingdom are obliged to practise the three Rs: replacement, refinement and reduction. That is, they are required by law always to consider replacing living animals with alternatives (TISSUE CULTURE methods or computer simulations for example); to refine the techniques used; and to reduce the numbers of animals used.

Animal welfare is an issue that arouses considerable passion, as do questions about the natures and rights of animals. Discussion of animal rights is necessarily complex, involving legal and moral problems that are beyond the scope of this entry. That humans can confer some kinds of rights on animals is beyond doubt: we can confer legal rights on whatever we wish, even abstractions. For example, limited liability companies have certain rights, statutorily enforceable. In this sense, animals have been conferred rights: legislation in the United Kingdom and elsewhere lays down the conditions under which laboratory animals must be kept, which in effect gives animals rights. Further, Parliament in New Zealand and several states in the United States of America have debated whether to give extensive rights, more or less equal to those enjoyed by all citizens, to chimpanzees and other apes. But all of these are essentially benefactions granted by humans to animals to ensure humane and proper treatment. Do animals have natural rights independent of social and legal structures? This is a much more vexed problem that raises questions about the nature of rights. For example, are there such things as natural rights, or do rights merely represent consensus among humans to do or not to do certain things? Is it necessary, in order to enjoy rights, to be cognizant of them and to accept responsibilities and duties that are entailed? Consult a philosopher about rights; Warnock (1998) provides a sensible starting point.

See also: environmental enrichment

Reference

Warnock M. (1998) *An Intelligent Person's Introduction to Ethics*, Duckworth: London.

animat Animat is a generic term given to simulated animals and autonomous robots: in essence, animats are artificial animals. The exchange of ideas and information between scientists working with ARTIFICIAL INTELLIGENCE and those in the natural sciences – including neuroscience, psychology and ETHOLOGY – will promote advances in all disciplines concerned with adaptive behaviour in changing environments of both natural and artificial systems. For a general introduction to animats, see Meyer & Wilson.

Reference

Meyer J.-A. & Wilson S.W. (1991) *From Animals to Animats*, MIT Press: Cambridge MA.

anion A negatively charged ION.

anisometropia A difference in focus between the eyes; see AMBLYOPIA.

anlage Effectively a synonym for PRIMORDIUM – the rudimentary tissue or cells from which a structure develops.

See also: neural tube

annexins *see* mobilization

annulospiral ending *see* muscle spindle

anode A positively charged metallic ELECTRODE towards which anions migrate in an electrolytic cell or tissue medium in which it is placed.

See also: anion; cathode

CHARLES D. BLAHA

anomia Anomia is an acquired disorder of naming. Like most disorders, anomia is a matter of degree: that is, anomic patients rarely fail completely in naming, and their success is often significantly related to one or more factors, such as the familiarity of the object/concept, the frequency of the word used to name it, the age at which the term was learned, the length and/or complexity of the word, and so on. PURE ANOMIA is a disorder limited to word retrieval, and can be distinguished from anomia attributable to other underlying causes, such as deficits in OBJECT RECOGNITION, semantic knowledge, phonological or articulatory processes (see SPEECH PERCEPTION; SPEECH PRODUCTION) and so forth. There are some documented cases of selective anomia for a particular class of names (for example, names of people, places or objects) or from a particular modality of presentation (for example, naming an object in response to seeing it, or touching it without seeing it, or being given a verbal description of it). Such category-specific or modality-specific anomias are however rare, with the majority of anomic patients having difficulties in naming under all of these conditions.

The symptoms of anomia are: a failure to find words; the use of a more general word (for instance *place* instead of *kitchen*); circumlocutions (such as a description of the meaning of the word rather than the name – for instance a *chair* becomes *you sit on it*); and a variety of errors. These errors are referred to as PARAPHASIAS and may take various forms. In VERBAL PARAPHASIA an incorrect word is substituted that is unrelated to the correct word; SEMANTIC PARAPHASIAS substitute a word related in meaning (for example *dog* named as *cat*), and PHONEMIC PARAPHASIAS occur when a word is mispronounced (for example *boat* as *bat* or *broat*). Subjects who make phonemic paraphasias often make several attempts at naming the word, suggesting that they recognize that the pronunciation is wrong. A mispronunciation that is not related to the target is called a NEOLOGISM (for example *horse* named as *sprod*). In connected speech which includes affixed words, such as *dancing, rider*, only the root morphemes (that is *dance, ride*) are neologized; the affixes *ing* and *er* are spared. Subjects who make numerous neologisms in speech are referred to as showing JARGON APHASIA.

Anomia is affected by the frequency of the word in the language, and the age at which the word is acquired. Less common words, and those acquired later, are most vulnerable. This follows the pattern observed in normal subjects who are slower to name less common words and words that appear later in the vocabulary. Anomia can arise from a number of underlying causes. A pure anomia arises when a word in the LEXICON of spoken word forms is either damaged, or cannot be retrieved. SEMANTIC ANOMIA arises when there is a disorder of SEMANTIC MEMORY: semantic paraphasias are produced frequently, and particular semantic categories (such as fruit and vegetables, or proper names) may be affected.

PHONEMIC CUEING is a technique used to assist in the production of spoken words. The initial phoneme of the word is provided which may then prompt the word to be produced. The technique is successful in cases where the spoken lexical form is intact but cannot be retrieved. In cases of semantic anomia, the initial phoneme of a word related semantically to the target will sometimes evoke a semantic paraphasia (for example the initial phoneme /t/ will prompt the word *tiger* to a picture of a *lion*). Treatment with phonemic cueing, based on the subject's knowledge of the initial letter of the word, have had most success. is most successful in cases of pure anomia. To date, methods using semantic cueing and computer generated phonemic cueing have had most success.

Reference

Ellis A.W. & Young A.W. (1996) *Human Neuropsychology*, Psychology Press: Hove UK.

ELAINE FUNNELL

anomic aphasia A major clinical syndrome of APHASIA (Goodglass & Kaplan, 1983). Patients classified as anomic aphasic produce fluent speech with relatively preserved grammatical structure. The primary feature is ANOMIA which usually is most pronounced for nouns and may affect other content words. Mild impairment of language comprehension is inclusive in the syndrome. Patients classified with WERNICKE'S APHASIA may evolve to anomic aphasia as comprehension skills are recovered. Lesions associated with anomic aphasia are rarely focal and tend to comprise multiple small lesion sites that are remote from one another.

Reference

Goodglass, H. & Kaplan, E. (1983) *The Assessment of Aphasia and Related Disorders*, 2nd edn, Lea & Febiger: Philadelphia.

CHARLOTTE C. MITCHUM

anorectic agent A drug that suppresses eating; an APPETITE suppressant. In the past, AMPHETAMINE and FENFLURAMINE have both been prescribed as anorectic drugs. True suppression of appetite, as opposed to the induction of activities or states competitive with feeding, is difficult to achieve.

See also: anorexia; feeding

anorexia An absence of eating. It is a term generally used in reference to an absence of eating in humans, especially in the condition ANOREXIA NERVOSA. Absence of eating in experimental animals following treatment of some kind is more often referred to as APHAGIA.

anorexia nervosa Psychiatric disorder involving significant loss of weight. Anorexia is derived from Greek, *an*: loss or absence, *orexia*: longing or desire. However, anorexia nervosa is defined on the basis of BODY WEIGHT not loss of APPETITE. The World Health Organization and the American Psychiatric Association agree on the following clinical criteria: maintenance of weight below expected for age and height by 15% or failure to gain weight during a period of growth; self-induced weight loss; body image disturbance in that there is a pathological fear of being or becoming fat; endocrine disorder manifest as AMENORRHOEA (loss of menses) in postmenarchal women or decreased sexual interest and potency in men. The term ANOREXIA NERVOSA was first used by William Gull in 1873, although the first medical description of anorexia nervosa is credited to Richard Morton in 1689, who described two cases of 'nervous consumption' in a woman aged 18 and a boy aged 16. Both share with modern accounts significant loss of weight caused by self-starvation in the absence of any primary organic aetiology.

Weight loss is achieved in anorexia nervosa principally by dietary restriction and high levels of exercise. Dietary restriction in anorexia nervosa differs from restrained eating both in the degree and rigidity of restriction imposed (see also RESTRAINED AND UNRESTRAINED EATING). However, some patients with anorexia nervosa also rid themselves of calories using the same purgation methods found in BULIMIA NERVOSA such as self-induced vomiting, fasting, abuse of diuretics and/or laxatives either following binge eating episodes or in the absence of such episodes. Therefore, two main subtypes of anorexia nervosa are recognized – the restricting subtype and the bulimic/purging subtype. Important differences in impulse control, and history of OBESITY are evident between the two subtypes, with the bulimic subtype associated with higher levels of impulsivity, substance abuse, having a higher premorbid weight and family history of obesity. The prognosis of the bulimic/purging subtype is worse than that for the restricting subtype. Anorexia nervosa is characterized by an intense desire to achieve or maintain thinness, to this end, behaviours are focused on losing or maintaining weight. The physical consequences of both the drastic loss of weight and the self-imposed restrictive eating practices are severe. Complications arise in all major organ systems (endocrine, cardiovascular, pulmonary, gastrointestinal, bone, renal, metabolic, haematological, dermatological and neurological). The mortality rate is high in anorexia nervosa – estimated at 18% – and similar to that observed in other psychiatric syndromes such as AFFECTIVE DISORDER and SCHIZOPHRENIA. Anorexia nervosa occurs almost exclusively in developed, industrialized countries and in women (5% of anorexics are male). Diagnoses of anorexia nervosa have been recorded across the lifespan from 7 to 70 years, however, the typical age of onset is adolescence. In the general population, the incidence (new cases) of anorexia nervosa is between 5.0 and 8.1 per 100 000 whereas the prevalence (actual number) of anorexia nervosa is estimated at 280 per 100 000 of the at-risk population. Certain groups appear to have a higher incidence of anorexia nervosa such as ballet dancers and fashion models.

It is recognized from studies of starvation such as those conducted by Ancel Keys that certain overlapping features exist between the physiological consequences of semi-starvation and psychological features of anorexia nervosa such as intense preoccupation with food and eating. Since a period of dieting generally predates the development of anorexia nervosa, dieting may play a critical role in the onset of anorexia nervosa. However, no single cause of anorexia nervosa has been identified, rather a multifactorial model is generally accepted to account for aetiology. Thus, dieting alongside other precipitating events or experiences may contribute to the development of anorexia nervosa in individuals who are vulnerable (predisposed), but dieting alone is not sufficient to produce the illness. Risk factors that may contribute to the development of anorexia nervosa span individual, family and sociocultural domains. Individual risk factors include genetic predisposition (history of psychiatric illness), stress, low self-esteem, body dissatisfaction, anxiety or feelings of ineffectiveness and physical factors such as the changes experienced during puberty. Family risk factors include history of psychopathology, specific family dynamics and eating disturbances in parents and siblings. The sociocultural climate contributes to the overvalued notion of seeking slimness whilst rejecting and stigmatizing obesity. Factors that contribute to the maintenance of anorexia nervosa include distorted cognitions, low self-esteem, physiological and psychological concomitants of starvation. Therefore, in the multidisciplinary treatment of anorexia nervosa there are two main stages of the therapeutic process. First of all, immediate medical stabilization is necessary using refeeding and pharmacological therapies. In the longer term, objectives such as nutritional management, building self-esteem, and challenging overvalued ideas about thinness are achieved by psychotherapy.

Failure to maintain weight at a normal or expected level characterizes anorexia nervosa. Significant morbidity and mortality are linked to this illness. It is not simply a 'slimmer's disease' but is caused by a myriad of factors. Treatments focus on weight gain, improving self-esteem and body image.

See also: body image; eating disorders

MARION M. HETHERINGTON

anosagnosia The unilateral disturbance of body schema and subsequent unawareness of one's disability in the absence of a primary sensory deficit is referred to as anosagnosia. This occurs following a brain LESION, usually to the PARIETAL CORTEX, and is related to SOMATOPARAPHRENIA in which a patient may deny ownership of a body part such as a limb and claim that the body part belongs to someone else. Anosagnosia often co-occurs with HEMISPATIAL NEGLECT and, as with neglect, can be ameliorated through the use of caloric stimulation. Anosagnosia can extend to a number of deficits including the unawareness of a SCOTOMA, of blindness, of a HEMIPLEGIA or of AMNESIA.

MARLENE BEHRMANN

anosmia Anosmia is a condition which deprives an individual of the sense of smell. It is invariably related to a peripheral dysfunction at the receptor level. In humans, KALLMANN'S SYNDROME is characterized by anosmia together with HYPOGONADISM. This dysfunctional relationship is brought about during

development by AGENESIS of the OLFACTORY NERVES and a failure of cells to migrate from the olfactory placode and generate GONADO-TROPHIN-RELEASING HORMONE neurons in the HYPOTHALAMUS. SPECIFIC ANOSMIAS may also occur to a subset of odorants. Some 90 specific anosmias have been reported and human twin studies support the view that these are also genetically determined.

BARRY KEVERNE

anosodiaphoria A lack of concern about a (typically neurological) problem, while remaining aware of it. It may follow a period of explicit denial of the existence of a problem. Anosodiaphoria is typically contrasted with ANOSAGNOSIA, the lack of awareness of a problem.

anoxia An inadequate supply of OXYGEN to the brain. Brain structures are particularly vulnerable to interruptions in oxygen supply. Areas most affected include the HIPPOCAMPUS, GLOBUS PALLIDUS and the WATERSHED AREAS OF CORTEX such as the occipito-parietal and occipito-temporal regions, and medial temporal cortex. Common causes of cerebral anoxia include suffocation, strangulation, CARBON MONOXIDE poisoning, cardiac arrest and improper ANAESTHETIC use. Posterior cerebral structures can be particularly susceptible to anoxic events, leading to AGNOSIA and AMNESIA, and failures in EXECUTIVE FUNCTIONS are also a possible outcome.

Reference

Wilson B.A. (1996) Cognitive functioning of adult survivors of cerebral hypoxia. *Brain Injury* 10: 863–874.

DAVID P. CAREY

antabuse *see* disulfram

antagonist An antagonist is a DRUG or chemical that binds to a RECEPTOR and blocks it, preventing it operating normally. It may be a COMPETITIVE ANTAGONIST (also known as SURMOUNTABLE ANTAGONIST) (that is, they compete with the natural LIGAND and AGONIST for receptor occupancy) or it may be an unsurmountable antagonist – agonists at whatever concentration cannot overcome these. An IRREVERSIBLE ANTAGONIST is one which remains bound to receptors for very long periods, up to and including forever.

antagonistic muscles *see* muscles

anterior Forward; at the front. Anterior is contrasted to POSTERIOR, at the back. The terms ROSTRAL (front) and CAUDAL (back) are synonymous with anterior and posterior.

anterior aphasia *see* Broca's aphasia

anterior cingulate cortex That portion of the CINGULATE CORTEX which is located within the FRONTAL LOBE (the remainder being in the PARIETAL LOBE). It is believed to be involved in the processing of ATTENTION.

VERITY J. BROWN

anterior commissure The anterior commissure is a small compact bundle of fibres that interconnect FOREBRAIN structures involved in OLFACTION and other functions. It crosses the MIDLINE immediately anterior to the columns of the FORNIX, and consists of two, roughly U-shaped pathways. The small anterior pathway, greatly reduced in humans, interconnects olfactory structures on the two sides, and this pathway is thought to be involved in the efferent control of neuronal activity in the OLFACTORY BULB. The larger posterior part forms the bulk of the anterior commissure. It passes laterally and caudally and interconnects regions of the middle and inferior temporal gyri (see GYRUS; TEMPORAL LOBE).

KAZUE SEMBA

anterior lobe *see* cerebellum – anatomical organization

anterior olfactory nucleus *see* olfactory system

anterior pituitary *see* adenohypophysis; pituitary gland

anterograde (from Latin, *anterior*: previous, *gressus*: to go) To progress onwards or forwards. ANTEROGRADE AMNESIA is a failure of memory that progresses forwards in time from a defined event; an ANTEROGRADE TRACER is a tracing agent (see TRACT TRACERS) that moves from cell body to terminal.

See also: retrograde

anterograde amnesia Polysensory failure to learn and subsequently remember new material, usually in the setting of organic brain disease. Anterograde amnesia is a core feature of the AMNESIC SYNDROME.

IAN C. REID

anterograde tracers *see* tract tracers

anterograde transport Movement of a chemical from CELL BODY to AXON TERMINAL within a neuron; the opposite is of course RETROGRADE TRANSPORT.

anterolateral system One of the principal SOMATOSENSORY PATHWAYS, also known as the SPINOTHALAMIC TRACT. It originates in the DORSAL HORN, neurons crossing to the CONTRALATERAL side before ascending to innervate sites in the RETICULAR FORMATION, PONS and MEDULLA, MIDBRAIN and, of course, the THALAMUS (the ventral posterior lateral nucleus, posterior nuclei of the thalamus, and intralaminar thalamic nuclei). The information transmitted relates mostly to PAIN and TEMPERATURE, though some TACTILE information is transmitted also (giving therefore some overlap with the DORSAL COLUMN – MEDIAL LEMNISCAL SYSTEM). Early stages of the pathway are divided into two components known as the ventral spinothalamic tract and the lateral spinothalamic tract. These originate in different parts of the spinal cord, but combine to form a single fibre pathway to the brain.

anthropomorphism The attribution of human characteristics to animals. When animals behave in an apparently human way, people have a tendency to describe their actions in terms which imply an understanding of the thoughts, intentions and emotions behind them. Although occasionally useful, this can be very misleading without expert knowledge of a species. Anthropomorphic tendencies probably result from our innate ability to recognize patterns of behaviour in those around us for appropriate social interaction.

See also: emotion

WENDY L. INGLIS

anti- Prefix meaning against or in opposition to. For instance, anti-histamines counteract the effects of HISTAMINE.

anti-anxiety drug *see* anxiolytic

antibody *see* immune system; monoclonal antibody; polyclonal antibody

anticholinergic A drug that antagonizes (see ANTAGONIST) the effects of the neurotransmitter ACETYLCHOLINE.

anticholinesterase A drug that inhibits or prevents the effects of the enzyme ACETYLCHOLINESTERASE.

anticipatory phase *see* appetitive vs. consummatory phases

anticodon *see* codon

anticonvulsant A DRUG that reduces or prevents convulsions (abnormal electrical activity; see SEIZURES) in the brain. Many sedative drugs are also effective anticonvulsants. Drugs that are effective anticonvulsants generally either enhance inhibitory mechanisms in the brain (primarily through GABA RECEPTORS) or reduce excitatory transmission via interaction with GLUTAMATE receptors, sodium or calcium channels (see ION CHANNEL). Anticonvulsant drug treatment is needed to control seizure activity in disorders such as EPILEPSY, and also for acute treatment of conditions that may be associated with seizures, such as viral infection, drug or ALCOHOL withdrawal, drug overdose, febrile seizures, brain damage, or poisoning. Commonly used anticonvulsant drugs include PHENYTOIN (Dilantin), SODIUM VALPROATE (Depakene) CARBAMAZEPINE (Tegretol), PHENOBARBITAL and BENZODIAZEPINES.

ANN E. KELLEY

antidepressant Term usually applied to chemical treatments for DEPRESSION, though also applies to other physical treatments, such as ELECTROCONVULSIVE THERAPY (ECT). Chemical antidepressants were first recognized by clinical observation in the late 1950s and early 1960s amongst substances being developed for other purposes: the MONOAMINE OXIDASE INHIBITORS (MAOIs), for example, emerged from a group of drugs targeted at tuberculosis. The earliest of the modern antidepressant agents used in clinical practice today were thus discovered, rather than designed.

Antidepressants are broadly classified in terms of their chemical structure or mode of action. Most act in some way to increase the availability of monoamines at the SYNAPTIC CLEFT (see MONOAMINE HYPOTHESIS OF DEPRESSION). The MAOIs (for example phenelzine, tranylcypromine) act in the main by inhibiting irreversibly the enzyme MONOAMINE OXIDASE (MAO), which catalyses the breakdown of monoamines intracellularly. Consequently, the amount of monoamine available for synaptic transmission is increased. Because the drugs act systemically, MAO in the gut is also disabled and the dietary substance TYRAMINE is permitted to enter the circulation in abnormally high amount. Intake of foodstuffs containing tyramine (such as mature cheeses) must be restricted in patients taking MAOIs. A newer, reversible inhibitor of MAO, moclobemide, has lessened the danger of such interactions. The TRICYCLICS (such as AMITRIPTYLINE and IMIPRAMINE), named after their structure, block the reuptake of monoamines from the synaptic cleft with varying degrees of selectivity. Many have other pharmacological actions, such as ANTICHOLINERGIC effects, which contribute to their side-effect profile. Tricyclics are potentially cardiotoxic, and may be lethal in overdose. The newer selective serotonin reuptake inhibitors SSRIs (for instance PROZAC) and serotonin and noradrenaline reuptake inhibitors SNRIs have a more specific reuptake blocking activity (for SEROTONIN, and serotonin and NORADRENALINE respectively), and though not free from side-effects themselves, may be better tolerated than the older tricyclics. They are safer if taken in overdose. At present, they are considerably more expensive. There are also effective 'atypical' antidepressants which neither block monoamine reuptake, nor inhibit MAO, such as the alpha 2 ADRENOCEPTOR antagonist, mianserin.

Chemical antidepressants are very effective in depressive disorder. DOUBLE BLIND STUDIES indicate that most of the wide variety of antidepressants are equally effective, with 70% of depressed patients responding. Tricyclics may, however, be more effective than MAOIs and SSRIs in particularly severe depressive illnesses. For reasons that remain poorly understood, all antidepressants take between 14 and 21 days to exert their therapeutic action.

IAN C. REID

antidiuretic hormone *see* vasopressin

antidromic (from Greek, *anti*: against, *dromos*: a course) Antidromic refers to the ability of an axon to conduct ACTION POTENTIAL in the reverse direction to that normally occurring. The opposite of antidromic is ORTHODROMIC.

antidromic activation Activation, induced experimentally (by electrical stimulation for example) or occurring naturally (see for example MIGRAINE), that induces ACTION POTENTIAL to run in reverse along an axon. It is the opposite of ORTHODROMIC ACTIVATION, which is the induction of action potentials flowing in the correct direction.

antiemetic *see* vomiting

antigen *see* immune system

antigravity muscles This is an alternative term for the EXTENSOR MUSCLES. We use extensors to sit up; quadrupeds lift their feet using FLEXOR MUSCLES, and push them back down with extensors. Activation of the extensor is therefore working against gravity, flexor activation is working with gravity.

antihistamine A drug used to counter the effects of HISTAMINE; typically given to combat allergic reactions, antihistamines have a SEDATIVE effect that is mediated through an action on the CENTRAL NERVOUS SYSTEM.

antihypertensive A drug that reduces HYPERTENSION.

antiparkinsonian The general name given to any treatment administered to relieve the symptoms of PARKINSON'S DISEASE. The earliest treatments for Parkinson's disease were ANTICHOLINERGIC drugs: belladonna alkaloids were used, acting to block MUSCARINIC ACETYLCHOLINE RECEPTORS. In the very early stages of Parkinsonism these are often still given, but their long-term use is of less value. Early treatment is often now achieved using AMAN-

TADINE, which increases the synthesis and release of the neurotransmitter DOPAMINE. However, most typically L-DOPA, a precursor of dopamine (which is deficient in the CAUDATE NUCLEUS and PUTAMEN of Parkinsonian patients) is used to provide symptomatic relief. L-DOPA can be converted to dopamine in the brain, replacing absent endogenous dopamine. L-DOPA represented the first systematic REPLACEMENT THERAPY – an effort to replace by pharmacological means neurotransmitter that was absent from the brain, preventing it working normally. It is decarboxylated in the brain to dopamine by amino acid decarboxylase, but peripheral decarboxylase inhibitors are given with L-DOPA because decarboxylation can also occur in other tissues. The vast majority of Parkinsonian patients are prescribed L-DOPA but eventually (after 3 to 5 years) the effects begin to wear off, giving way to the ON-OFF EFFECTS, so-called because the effects of the drug become increasingly delicately poised between a full 'on' effect – symptomatic relief – and 'off', with all the signs and symptoms of Parkinsonism present. These response fluctuations become worse, limiting the value of the medication. Dopamine receptor agonists such as BROMOCRIPTINE, PERGOLIDE and LISURIDE (which all affect D2 DOPAMINE receptors to a greater degree than D1) are often used as an adjunct to L-DOPA therapy, rarely being used alone. DEPRENYL (available commercially as Selegiline) which inhibits MONOAMINE OXIDASE action, is also used in conjunction with L-DOPA.

Reference

Feldman R.S., Meyer J.S. & Quenzer L.F. (1997) *Principles of Neuropsychopharmacology*, Sinauer Associates: Sunderland MA.

antipsychotic The antipsychotic drugs are those given to combat PSYCHOSIS, but in general it is taken as read that by antipsychotic one is referring to a drug given to treat the SIGNS AND SYMPTOMS of SCHIZOPHRENIA. The terms MAJOR TRANQUILLIZER and NEUROLEPTIC are to all intents and purposes synonymous with the term antipsychotic: antipsychotic is used for preference. The first antipsychotic to be given was CHLORPROMAZINE. In the 1940s Henri Laborit (1914–1995), a French surgeon, administered this to patients about to undergo surgery, in order to reduce STRESS. He hypothesized that the drug's calming effect could have benefit in treating schizophrenic patients. It was tested for this property and found to be very successful. Other members of the class of drugs – the PHENOTHIAZINES – to which chlorpropmazine belongs were also found to have antipsychotic properties. From a class of drugs related to the phenothiazines, the THIOXANTHINES, were derived the BUTYROPHENONES. Included in this group are HALOPERIDOL and SPIROPERIDOL. The phenothiazines and butyrophenones are commonly used to treat schizophrenia. There are also the so-called ATYPICAL ANTIPSYCHOTIC drugs (or ATYPICAL NEUROLEPTICS) which are members of other classes: for example, SULPIRIDE (a benzamine), MOLINDONE (similar to SEROTONIN) and PIMOZIDE (a diphenylbutylpiperidine). CLOZAPINE has also been used as an antipsychotic. Antipsychotic drugs are generally characterized as being antagonists at DOPAMINE receptors (see ANTAGONIST). Studies have shown striking correlations between the ability of a drug to bind to dopamine receptors (particularly D2 dopamine receptors) and antipsychotic potency. This relationship has been very influential in generating the DOPAMINE HYPOTHESIS OF SCHIZOPHRENIA. However, clozapine is a marked exception to this general rule. Although it has an antagonistic effect at dopamine receptors, it also has a variety of other properties. Despite this lack of specificity it is a widely used antipsychotic, with more power to combat the negative symptoms of schizophrenia that the phenothiazines or butyrophenones. It does have other unwanted effects that limit its use.

Antipsychotic medication has had an enormous beneficial effect. Prior to their introduction there were no successful therapies with which to treat schizophrenia (see PSYCHOSURGERY). Some argued that antipsychotic drugs merely provided a 'chemical straitjacket', effectively imprisoning patients by sedation, rendering them incapable of independent action. But sedative drugs have no therapeutic benefit in schizophrenia, while the use of antipsychotic drugs has enabled countless numbers of patients to be treated as outpatients rather than as long-stay hospital patients. The increasing admission rates to psychiatric units that occurred in the 1940s and 50s, when mental illness was increasingly recognized as deserving medical attention, fell away dramatically following the introduction of antipsychotic drugs. They are not however without side-effects. Prolonged use of antipsychotic medication can lead to conditions resembling PARKINSON'S DISEASE and to TARDIVE DYSKINESIA. It is also clear that many patients will relapse into further episodes of schizophrenia despite using antipsychotic medication. However, the use of antipsychotic drugs offers the best relief available from schizophrenia.

Reference

Feldman R.S., Meyer J.S. & Quenzer L.F. (1997) *Principles of Neuropsychopharmacology*. Sinauer Associates: Sunderland MA.

antisaccade Eye movement made in a task where targets appear suddenly on either side of the visual field, and the subject is instructed to look to the opposite side. Such a SACCADE requires a higher-level control mechanism than the response of fixating directly on the target. Errors or delays in antisaccades are generally believed to occur when control mechanisms in the FRONTAL LOBE fail to inhibit this prepotent response, and have been used to evaluate the neurological basis of PARKINSON'S DISEASE, SCHIZOPHRENIA, and other conditions.

OLIVER J. BRADDICK

antisense A complementary sequence to that of DNA (deoxyribonucleic acid) or RNA (ribonucleic acid) which encodes for a GENE. Genomic DNA is composed of two complementary DNA strands. Gene activation leads to the production of RNA, which is homologous to one strand of the DNA. This strand is known as the sense strand, while the other is the antisense strand. The antisense strand actually forms the template for RNA production. Each antisense OLIGONUCLEOTIDE will bind tightly to part of the RNA, and may be used experimentally to block GENE EXPRESSION, or to measure gene expression.

See also: *in situ* hybridization

FIONA M. INGLIS

antiserum *see* serum

anus *see* digestive system

anxiety A term to describe the physiological and psychological response to a perceived threat that can represent either a biologically appropriate adaptive response to impending challenge or a pathological state whereby there is a contextually and temporally inappropriate activation of bodily defence systems. When anxiety is chronic and appears to be dissociated from defined threat events, it is generally considered to be abnormal and to merit psychological or psychopharmacological (see PSYCHOPHARMACOLOGY) therapeutic intervention. Contextually appropriate anxiety is considered as an integral component of the FIGHT-OR-FLIGHT response. The main clinical features of anxiety can be divided into two categories, cognitive and physiological. Typical cognitive features include apprehension, perception of impending threat and constant vigilance for danger. Typical physical features include increased AUTONOMIC NERVOUS SYSTEM activity with elevated heart rate, respiratory rate and blood pressure. There is also an elevated release of stress hormones from the adrenal glands, such as ADRENALINE and cortisol (see CORTICOSTERONE).

There are three major subdivisions of the so-called clinical anxiety disorders, although anxiety symptoms are ubiquitous throughout the entire range of psychiatric diagnoses. (1) GENERALIZED ANXIETY is a term used to describe a global, non-specific, persistent anxiety without the specific features of PANIC disorder or PHOBIA. (2) Panic disorder is characterized by recurrent attacks of acute, severe and overwhelming anxiety accompanied by sensations of breathlessness, cardiac palpitations and dizziness. There is often an acute fear of losing consciousness, or even of dying. Such attacks may become associated with specific predictive stimuli such as places, leading to marked anticipatory fear and an avoidance of these locations. (3) PHOBIC ANXIETY is that generated by very specific stimuli in an irrational, involuntary manner, leading to significant avoidance behaviour. Common phobic stimuli include spiders and social situations. Clinically,

there is significant overlap among the three categories of disorder.

Anxiety symptoms appear to be mediated by a complex neural circuitry that includes multiple components of the LIMBIC SYSTEM. Enquiry into the neural basis of anxiety has traditionally taken three main approaches. First, to investigate the mechanism of action of drugs known to suppress or alleviate anxiety symptoms. Second, to develop ANIMAL MODELS OF ANXIETY or of FEAR (see CONDITIONED FEAR) which are sensitive to the ANXIOLYTIC (anxiety reducing) effects of drugs. Third, to describe the neural pathways and chemical systems activated by fear stimuli and to develop specific drugs to act on those systems. Advances in brain imaging techniques have added a further option for the detection of which structures and chemical systems are activated by fear stimuli in humans. For example, changes in cerebral blood flow patterns and some structural changes have been demonstrated in the anterior TEMPORAL LOBE, specifically in the PARAHIPPOCAMPAL GYRI, in panic disorder patients when anxiety is experimentally induced. Similarly, the ORBITOFRONTAL CORTEX has been identified as a likely site for pathology in patients with OBSESSIVE–COMPULSIVE DISORDER, a clinical syndrome that is considered by many to represent a specific type of anxiety disorder. The amygdaloid complex also appears to be a critical substrate for the mediation of fear and anxiety. Anatomically, the AMYGDALA is well placed to integrate many of the physiological responses typical of states of fear or anxiety, with prominent projections to the HYPOTHALAMUS, LOCUS COERULEUS, the VENTRAL TEGMENTAL AREA (VTA) and multiple BRAINSTEM nuclei involved in autonomic control. Electrical stimulation of the central nucleus of the amygdala elicits complex behavioural and autonomic responses that closely resemble those observed during states of fear. Furthermore, a LESION of the central nucleus of the amygdala can lead to an abolition of the integrated behavioural and physiological responses to stimuli which have previously been paired with aversive events, a so-called CONDITIONED EMOTIONAL RESPONSE. However, amygdala lesions do not closely mimic the effects of anxiolytic drugs.

Animal models of anxiety are conventionally grouped into those which are based on PUNISHMENT, reward reduction, or those with an ethological perspective. Typical tests based on punishment include the GELLER–SEIFTER CONFLICT test, where an aversive stimulus, e.g. an electric shock, is used to suppress a rewarded behaviour, such as lever-pressing for food. A typical test based on reward reduction is that of the negative contrast, where two rewards of differing magnitude are juxtaposed and the response to the reduction is measured. The most widely used ethologically based tests include the ELEVATED MAZE where patterns of activity on the apparatus are deemed to reflect competition between EXPLORATION and avoidance. Each of these tests appear to detect anxiolytic drug action quite reliably (see BENZODIAZEPINE).

See also: affective disorder; behaviour therapy; cognitive behavioural therapy; post-traumatic stress disorder; startle reflex

Reference

Bloom F.E. & Kupfer D.J. (eds.) (1994) *Psychopharmacology: The Fourth Generation of Progress*, Raven Press: New York.

KEITH MATTHEWS

anxiogenic Generic term for any DRUG that has the property of increasing ANXIETY. The best-known is BETA CARBOLINE (also known as harmaline), a drug that is a partial inverse agonist (see AGONIST) at BENZODIAZEPINE-binding sites on GABA RECEPTORS.

anxiolytic Generic term for a heterogenous group including any DRUG that has the property of reducing ANXIETY. The group includes both substances in therapeutic use and recreational drugs. In the latter category, NICOTINE and ALCOHOL have anxiolytic effects amongst their other actions. Many anxiolytic substances are drugs with ABUSE POTENTIAL. In therapeutic use, the principal anxiolytics are of the BENZODIAZEPINE type. The MAJOR TRANQUILLIZERS, such as CHLORPROMAZINE are occasionally used in very severe anxiety. Beta adrenergic blocking drugs, such as PROPRANOLOL may be used to attenuate the physical effects of anxiety and PANIC. Drugs with ANTIDEPRESSANT effects also have anxiolytic

properties and may be particularly useful in the treatment of panic disorder.

IAN C. REID

aorta *see* blood

apathy (from Greek, *a*: not, *pathos*: feeling) A state of apathy is a state in which an individual is EMOTION-less and lacking in DRIVE. It is a state all individuals feel from time to time, but in a pathological manifestation it is characteristic of a number of MOOD disorders, and is associated with the negative symptoms of SCHIZOPHRENIA.

aphagia The absence of eating. It is a term generally used in reference to an absence of eating in experimental animals following treatment of some kind. Absence of eating in humans is more often referred to as ANOREXIA, most notably in the condition ANOREXIA NERVOSA.

aphasia Impairment in the human capacity to use LANGUAGE for communication. Aetiology is associated with brain pathology. Acute onset may follow cerebrovascular accident (known commonly as STROKE) or traumatic brain injury (CLOSED HEAD INJURY). Insidious origin may result from damage to the central nervous system secondary to infection, HYDROCEPHALUS, progressive (dementing) disease, toxicity, intracranial tumour and metabolic and nutritional disorder. The diagnosis of aphasia excludes language impairments associated with psychiatric disorders or primary sensory deficits. The clinical term aphasia encompasses a wide range of language-based symptoms of brain pathology. Symptoms differ widely among patients, and severity of impairments range from mild to severe. Nevertheless, classification by syndromes derived by typical clustering of aphasia symptoms is standard in clinical practice (Goodglass & Kaplan, 1983). Approximately 80% of patients diagnosed with aphasia will evince a pattern consistent with one of seven 'cortical' syndromes (Helm-Estabrooks & Albert, 1991). These include BROCA'S APHASIA, WERNICKE'S APHASIA, CONDUCTION APHASIA, ANOMIC APHASIA, TRANSCORTICAL MOTOR APHASIA, TRANSCORTICAL SENSORY APHASIA and GLOBAL APHASIA. There are also subcortical aphasia syndromes described for the locus of the aphasia-producing brain lesion. These loci include portions of the BASAL GANGLIA and the THALAMUS. It is important to note that aphasia classification by subtype is based on clinical symptoms, not on brain lesion type or location. Indeed, symptom correlation with brain pathology is imperfect. Aphasia-producing lesions typically are accompanied by concomitant right-sided weakness since the left cerebral hemisphere is language-dominant in a majority of the general population. Uncommon forms of aphasia are expressed in patients with atypical cerebral dominance (suggested by left-handedness or ambidexterity), history of a previous brain LESION, DRUG ABUSE or ANOXIA. A complete medical history is crucial to the accurate interpretation of aphasia symptoms.

Clinical diagnosis of aphasia type is based on the pattern of results obtained with testing of the cognitive tasks of naming, conversational speech, auditory comprehension and repetition. Naming is impaired to some degree in nearly all aphasic patients. A disorder purely of naming is more accurately termed ANOMIA and can occur independently of other aphasic symptoms. Naming impairments sometimes are associated with specific types of words, such as proper names, words of certain semantic or grammatical categories, and often are more pervasive for words that occur infrequently in the language than for more common words. The method of assessing naming can also influence patient performance (for instance, naming of pictures or objects upon confrontation vs. reciting from memory words that conform to a particular category or start with a particular letter). Speech fluency is generally divisible into fluent and non-fluent although these descriptors represent ends of a continuum. Objective measures of fluency are obtained by examining the length of the phrases uttered (in number of words), the ratio of content words to function words used (underuse of content words is associated with fluent aphasia whereas underuse of functions is associated with NON-FLUENT APHASIA), and the occurrence of PARAPHASIA in speech attempts. Quantitative fluency rating scales typically are included in formal aphasia tests (Goodglass & Kaplan, 1983). The PROSODY (melody and intonation) of speech patterns and ease of motor speech production (articulatory agility) contribute subjectively to clinical descriptions of speech fluency.

Absolute preservation of auditory comprehension is rarely observed in aphasia. Clinical assessment of auditory comprehension requires a range of testing, and the interpretation of test results requires some experience. Testing encompasses a variety of stimuli ranging widely in length (single words, phrases, sentences and paragraphs) and complexity. The distinction between a primary memory deficit and an impairment of auditory comprehension may be particularly difficult in some cases. In many types of aphasia, auditory comprehension and speech production are not equated in severity and the relative asymmetry can contribute to clinical classification. The preservation of auditory comprehension relative to speech production is observed in Broca's, transcortical motor, conduction and anomic aphasias. The opposing pattern – speech production preserved relative to auditory comprehension – is notable in Wernicke's and transcortical sensory types of aphasia. Repetition ability is also a clinically important factor. An inability to repeat heard speech is an important component of differential diagnosis among the aphasia classifications. The relative preservation of repetition skills is the key symptom to distinguish transcortical motor from Broca's aphasia; transcortical sensory from Wernicke's aphasia; and anomic from conduction aphasia, respectively.

Clinical classification of aphasia into subtype is common in clinical practice. Nevertheless, it is important to note that diagnosis of an aphasia type does not necessarily lead to a particular therapeutic plan. Therapy for aphasia is based only in part on the constellation and severity of symptoms. The needs, goals and prognostic directives of individual patients and their families contribute importantly to the development of a language-based cognitive/communication therapy plan.

See also: dysphasia

References

Goodglass H. & Kaplan E. (1983) *The Assessment of Aphasia and Related Disorders*, 2nd edn, Lea & Febiger: Philadelphia.

Helm-Estabrooks N. & Albert M.L. (1991) *Manual of Aphasia Therapy*, Pro-ed: Austin.

CHARLOTTE C. MITCHUM

aphemia An impairment of SPEECH PRODUCTION: speech becomes very laboured, pronunciation occurring slowly, syllable by syllable.

See also: aphasia

apical dendrite Pyramidal neurons in the CEREBRAL CORTEX have apical dendrites which rise to the outer surface of the cortex and shorter BASAL DENDRITES which spread out horizontally.

See also: dendrite; neuron

Aplysia Work with the marine mollusc, or sea slug, *Aplysia*, pioneered by Eric Kandel (joint winner of the Nobel Prize for Medicine, 2000) and his colleagues, has provided us with some of most fundamental insights currently available into the nature of neural mechanisms underlying LEARNING and MEMORY (see, e.g., Kandel, 1979). The nervous system of *Aplysia* (also referred to as the 'sea-hare' because of its ear-like tentacles and hunched posture during feeding), is relatively simple, compared to the vertebrate nervous system, and offers many technical advantages for the neurobiologist. For instance, it contains only thousands of neurons, many of which are large enough to be identified individually (or as small groups). Moreover, *Aplysia* exhibits many forms of learning, including HABITUATION, SENSITIZATION and CLASSICAL CONDITIONING.

Reference

Cohen T.E., Kaplan S.W., Kandel E.R. and Hawkins R.D. (1997) A simplified preparation for relating cellular events to behaviour: mechanisms contributing to habituation, dishabituation and sensitization of the Aplysia gill-withdrawal reflex. *Journal of Neuroscience* 17: 2886–2899.

Kandel E (1979) *Behavioral Biology of Aplysia*, W.H. Freeman: San Francisco.

MARK A. UNGLESS

apnoea (from Greek, *a*: not, *pnoie*: breath) An absence of breathing, usually transient. (If not transient, death can result.) Apnoea is associated with dysfunction in the brain mechanisms regulating breathing (see BREATHING, NEURAL CONTROL OF) and with SLEEP dysfunction (see SLEEP APNOEA).

See also: central apnoea; obstructive apnoea

apolipoprotein E The gene for apolipoprotein E (*apoE*) has three major alleles: *apoE2*, *apoE3* and *apoE4*. Possession of the *apoE4* allele appears to place individuals at risk for late onset Alzheimer's dementia (see ALZHEIMER'S DEMENTIA for further information about this). Apolipoprotein itself is a GLYCOPROTEIN: beyond the central nervous system it is involved in the transport through the blood of CHOLESTEROL and TRIGLYCERIDES. Within the nervous system it is found in astrocytes and in the cytoplasm of neurons. Damage to the brain increases levels of apolipoprotein E dramatically, suggesting that it may be involved in the processes of repair and regeneration after injury.

apomorphine An agonist at dopamine receptors, with preference for D2 over D1 dopamine receptors (see D1–D5 DOPAMINE RECEPTORS). It has been widely used in psychopharmacological studies as a drug capable of stimulating dopamine receptors, and its effects are often contrasted with those of AMPHETAMINE, which promotes release of dopamine rather than directly stimulating receptors (see, for example, ROTATION). It is a derivative of MORPHINE and, like morphine, induces nausea and vomiting in humans (but not rodents, which do not vomit). It is therapeutically used as an emetic (see EMESIS) in cases of poisoning.

apoptosis Apoptosis (literally the falling of petals) refers to a specific form of cell death. It is an active process, that is, it requires the dying cell to synthesize proteins which act to dismantle the cell. The process, which can be referred to as cell suicide, represents a form of naturally occurring cell death or PROGRAMMED CELL DEATH. Apoptosis appears to be the default condition which operates unless specific external signals are present.

During the process of apoptosis the cell shrinks whilst its cellular and nuclear membranes remain intact. This ensures that the cellular and nuclear contents are retained until the dead cell can be cleared by phagocytosis. This process minimizes the disruption that the death of a cell has on surrounding cells. Apoptosis is thus in marked contrast to death by NECROSIS where cells die in a passive way and their intracellular contents are showered on neighbouring cells. The non-disruptive and selective nature of apoptosis has caused it to be described as an 'altruistic' form of cell death. The process of apoptosis is further characterized by condensation of chromatin, fragmentation of DNA in to bands of roughly equal length and the lack of an inflammatory response.

Apoptosis of neurons occurs on a massive scale during the early development of the vertebrate nervous system, the process accounting for the loss of around 50% of all neurons produced. This process is regulated by TROPHIC FACTORS that prevent the initiation of apoptosis in neurons which receive sufficient quantities of these survival factors. It is hypothesized that competition amongst developing neurons for limited supplies of trophic factors released from target neurons ensures the elimination of excess neurons and those which have made inappropriate connections. Apoptosis requires *de novo* TRANSCRIPTION and TRANSLATION. It can accordingly be prevented by the administration of drugs which inhibit the synthesis of RNA or protein. The molecular mechanisms that control apoptosis involve the interaction of death genes and survival genes. The majority of research into this field has been conducted in the nematode, *CAENORHABDITIS ELEGANS*. In this roundworm transcription of the genes *ced-3* and *ced-4* is required for cell to die whilst transcription of *ced-9* acts to keep cells alive. The mammalian counterpart to *ced-9* is *bcl-2*, over expression of which results in a form of lymphoma. Continuous expression of the IMMEDIATE EARLY GENE *c-fos* is also implicated in the triggering of apoptosis.

Apoptosis may also account for the pathological loss of neurons seen under a variety of circumstances including ISCHAEMIA, HYPOGLYCAEMIA and TRAUMA. Therapeutic approaches to the treatment of such conditions are being developed which are based on preventing neuronal apoptosis. These approaches include raising the levels of trophic factors and the increasing the expression of protective genes such as *bcl-2*.

IAN J. MITCHELL

apperceptive agnosia The term apperceptive agnosia implies a deficit in sub-components of the visual system responsible for the ability to derive, by accessing an internal description of the object's physical structure, a representation that is constant regardless of the observer's initial viewing conditions. Relevant cases, given this conceptualization, must have intact form discrimination and figure and ground synthesis, at least for tasks that do not require access to an internal description of an object's structure. Failure on these lower-level perceptual tasks leading to a disorder of object recognition are referred to as 'PSEUDAGNOSIA' by some researchers So, for example, apperceptive agnosics should demonstrate normal ability to judge whether two similar forms (say, triangles with straight or slightly curved lines) are the same or different, and they must be able to detect the presence of a degraded form (for instance, an X) against a background of visual noise, a task which does not depend on object identification for accurate performance.

A variety of experiments have shown that neurological cases with damage to the right PARIETAL LOBE may experience difficulty identifying objects viewed under conditions that obscure or distort critical features, despite the evident preservation of lower level visual abilities. Objects that are unevenly illuminated, with potentially misleading contours, are problematic for such individuals relative to objects with more habitual shading, as are photographs of common objects taken from an unusual viewpoint. How can the functional deficit responsible for apperceptive agnosia be further analysed? One suggestion capitalizes on the conjecture that perceptual classification requires that the major and minor axis of the object be derived from the image, and that apperceptive agnosia is due to a failure in extracting this information when the available image is foreshortened. Impaired recognition, however, may occur for objects even though the major axis has not been foreshortened. Thus, an alternative explanation assumes that deficit in apperceptive agnosia affects a RIGHT

HEMISPHERE system maintaining sets of hierarchically organized distinctive features as well as the spatial relations between them. If this system has been rendered inefficient by neurological damage, more features need to be available in the image before a critical number can be extracted for identification, and poor performance occurs when the visible surfaces of the object are obscured.

DANIEL N. BUB

appetite An appetite is a desire to slake a perceived need of whatever nature. Typically it is a term used in relation to SEXUAL BEHAVIOUR, and more particularly FEEDING. It is distinct from HUNGER, which is generally used to indicate a need for food, where appetite indicates a desire for food. APPETITE SUPPRESSANTS are drugs given to as part of BODY WEIGHT control programmes to suppress the desire for food (FENFLURAMINE and AMPHETAMINE have both been used) though whether they have an effect on a specific process or appetite or produce effects incompatible with eating is uncertain.

See also: eating disorders; orexigenic; satiety; specific appetites

appetite suppressants *see* appetite

appetitive conditioning A category of behavioural change elicited as a direct response to appetitive environmental events. A term to describe LEARNING contingencies (see CONTINGENCY) where the REINFORCER is inferred to convey pleasant or pleasurable hedonic consequences. Appetitive stimuli or reinforcers are those eliciting approach behaviour and contact. Typically, such stimuli will increase the probability of repetition of the responses upon which they are contingent. This is the converse of AVERSIVE CONDITIONING procedures, where the reinforcer is inferred to convey unpleasant consequences for the subject.

See also: classical conditioning; instrumental conditioning; reinforcement

Reference
Dickinson A. (1980) *Contemporary Animal Learning Theory*, Cambridge University Press: Cambridge.

KEITH MATTHEWS

appetitive reinforcement *see* appetitive vs. consummatory phases; instrumental conditioning; positive reinforcement

appetitive vs. consummatory phases The distinction between appetitive and consummatory relates to different phases of a sequence of actions in response to presentation of an appetitive stimulus (that is, a POSITIVE REINFORCEMENT, in contrast to a NEGATIVE REINFORCEMENT [an AVERSIVE STIMULUS]). The appetitive phase (alternatively called the ANTICIPATORY PHASE) involves approach to and anticipation of the STIMULUS; the consummatory phase involves the actual acquisition and use of the stimulus (eating for example, if the stimulus is food). In SEXUAL BEHAVIOUR, the terms proceptive and RECEPTIVE are used more or less synonymously with appetitive and consummatory. Female rats typically display behaviours such as hopping and darting towards and away from a male rat. Male rats will attempt to sniff the female and maintain contact with her. The consummatory phase involves COPULATION. Measurement of DOPAMINE release in the NUCLEUS ACCUMBENS and CAUDATE–PUTAMEN during the appetitive and consummatory parts of sexual behaviour suggests that the nucleus accumbens is selectively involved in processing REWARD related information, the caudate–putamen being more concerned with motor processing. (see Daamsma *et al.*, 1992).

See also: appetitive conditioning; aversive conditioning; classical conditioning; instrumental conditioning; reinforcement

Reference
Daamsma G., Pfaus J.G., Wenkstern D., Phillips A.G. & Fibiger H.C. (1992) Sexual behaviour increases dopamine transmission in the nucleus accumbens and striatum of male rats: comparison with novelty and locomotion. *Behavioural Neuroscience* 106: 181–191.

apraxia (from Greek, *a*: not, *praxis*: action) Apraxia (a term coined by P. Stendal in 1871) therefore means no action. It is not used in this strict sense. Now it is used to describe all sorts of missing or inappropriate actions of the hands that cannot be clearly attributed to frank motor impairment, sensory loss, or other more primary motor deficits on the one hand, or to lack of comprehension or motivation on the other. Numerous forms of apraxia have been described, the definitions of which vary from author to author. Henry Hecaen described four major forms of apraxia. These are IDEOMOTOR APRAXIA (an impairment limited to single gestures such as brushing to teeth or waving goodbye), IDEATIONAL APRAXIA (an impairment in performing a complex act, such as making tea, but in which the individual elements are executed correctly), CONSTRUCTIONAL APRAXIA (in which the spatial organization or drawing or assembling objects is disturbed) and DRESSING APRAXIA (an inability to dress oneself correctly). Some authors classify these kinds of apraxia in relation to instructions. For example, a patient may be asked to perform an act or only required to copy an act. There are a variety of other apraxias that are defined by the body part that is impaired, such as the fingers, mouth, trunk, lower limbs, and the body more generally. Many apraxias are bilateral in that they occur in both hands, but apraxia can be limited to one hand or one side of the body. Apraxia is usually assessed by relatively informal tests in which a patient is told to wave a flag, perform a series of arm movements, or assemble objects. There have been some attempts to develop more formal tests such as the Kimura box test, in which a subject pushes a button, pulls a lever, or pushes on a bar. In the test individual movements can be examined or a subject can be asked to make a series of movements. The earliest and most comprehensive theory of apraxia was articulated by Liepmann in the 1920s. Liepmann's best-known patient was an imperial councillor. His right arm was not paralysed, its muscular power was preserved, and it performed most of the movements of daily life. In contrast, when the patient was asked to perform with his right hand such gestures as pointing to his nose, making a fist, or showing how to use a harmonica or a brush, he failed completely. Even though he made movements indicating that he understood the instructions, he could not make the appropriate movements. If the right arm was held by the observer, all of the movements were carried out by the left arm.

When the gesture required the coordinated use of both hands, the right hand prohibited the execution of the gesture, even while the left hand was responding correctly. For example, when the patient attempted to pour water into a glass, the left hand took the pitcher in order to pour while the right hand was bringing the glass to the mouth. Since neither the comprehension of the instructions nor the motor execution itself was defective, the difficulty that produced the apraxia had to be located at another level. Liepmann placed it between the sensory memories (which understood the instructions) and the motor memories (which allowed the patient to transform the instructions into an action). Liepmann proposed that there was damage to the LEFT HEMISPHERE in an area that received projections from left hemisphere language area and carried them to the motor cortex of the left hemisphere that in turn controls the right hand. The death of the imperial councillor allowed the hypothesis to be verified. These anatomical observations formed the basis for Liepmann's theory that apraxia results from lesions to the LEFT HEMISPHERE. In order to explain apraxia in the left hand, Liepmann proposed that apraxia could also occur in the fibres of the CORPUS CALLOSUM, connecting the left and right hemisphere, were additionally damaged. Liepmann also proposed that a number of apraxias can occur, each of which most likely results from damage to a specific locus of the left hemisphere. Liepmann's proposal that the left hemisphere plays a special role in apraxia is confirmed by Milner and colleagues' studies of patients who have received SODIUM AMOBARBITAL injections of either the left or right carotid artery, which anaesthetizes the IPSILATERAL hemisphere. They taught patients a series of complex arm movements prior to the injections. Only injections into the speaking left hemisphere disrupted the movements, even when movements were to be performed with the ipsilateral limb (controlled by the contralateral motor cortex that had not received an injection). The proposal that the left hemisphere plays a special role in performing skilled movements also figures in Kimura's proposal that LANGUAGE and skilled movements (see SKILL LEARNING) have a special relation. She proposes that skilled gestures, controlled by the left hemisphere, eventually evolved into sound based language. One problem faced by the left hemisphere theory is that circumscribed cortical excisions do not typically result in lasting impairments on tests of PRAXIS. Thus, it is possible that subcortical structures, including the thalamus and basal ganglia, are also involved in producing the symptoms. The corpus callosum may also play a special role. Milner & Kolb studied the ability of four patients, in whom the corpus callosum had been severed as a treatment for epilepsy, to copy meaningless sequences of arm or facial movements with either the left or the right hand. The patients were very impaired at copying the movements, even when compared to patients with left hemisphere lesions. Thus, although the cortex of the left hemisphere may play a special role in the control of skilled movements, subcortical structures of the left hemisphere as well as the corpus callosum and possibly even areas of the right hemisphere can also be involved.

Reference
Kolb B. & Whishaw I.Q. (1955) *Fundamentals of Human Neuropsychology*, W.H. Freeman: San Francisco.

IAN Q. WHISHAW

aprosodia (Also known as aprosody.) PROSODY is a feature of LANGUAGE and is concerned with the accent, stress and rhythm of speech. Aprosodia involves difficulties with such things, and is seen different forms. MOTOR APROSODIA involves poor expression of prosody but no difficulty in interpreting it in others. Motor aprosody is associated with damage to the posterior inferior FRONTAL LOBE. SENSORY APROSODIA on the other hand involves normal expression of prosody but difficulty in comprehension of it in others; this is associated with damage to the right posterior inferior PARIETAL LOBE and the posterior superior TEMPORAL LOBE.

AP5 (Or, less commonly, APV) This is 2-amino-5-phosphonovaleric acid: it is a competitive ANTAGONIST at NMDA RECEPTORS and has been widely used in research on amino acid NEUROTRANSMITTERS.

aqueduct of Sylvius Also known as the CEREBRAL AQUEDUCT; see VENTRICLES.

aqueous humour The fluid that lies between the CORNEA and the LENS in the EYE.

arachidonic acid A FATTY ACID associated with PHOSPHOLIPIDS in MEMBRANES. It can undergo a variety of transformations: its derivatives are the eicosanoids (see EICOSANOID), some of which may function as SECOND MESSENGERS.

arachnoid membrane *see* meninges

arachnoid trabeculae *see* meninges

arborization (from Latin, *arbor*: tree) Arborization is used to refer to the spreading out of neuronal processes, particularly dendrites (see PROCESS; DENDRITE) which branch in a tree-like manner.

archicerebellum *see* cerebellum

archicortex *see* allocortex; cerebral cortex

archistriatum Archaic term that refers to the AMYGDALA.

See also: neostriatum; palaeostriatum

arcuate fasciculus (from Latin, *fasciculus*: a little bundle) A fibre connection that allows information to be conveyed from WERNICKE'S AREA to BROCA'S AREA; see APHASIA; LANGUAGE; TRANSCORTICAL SENSORY APHASIA.

arcuate nucleus of the hypothalamus The arcuate nucleus is a small, arc-shaped nucleus in the ventral part of the HYPOTHALAMUS, immediately adjacent to the third ventricle. It has attracted attention recently because it is the principal source of NEUROPEPTIDE Y in the hypothalamus and contains receptors for the peptide LEPTIN. These are both associated with the control of FEEDING and BODY WEIGHT. It is also the source of the TUBEROINFUNDIBULAR DOPAMINE SYSTEM and synthesizes ENDORPHINS.

arcuate sulcus A major SULCUS on the outer surface, and relatively posterior, in the FRONTAL LOBE; see PREFRONTAL CORTEX.

area postrema A small nucleus within the BRAINSTEM which monitors the status of the VISCERA and the physiological conditions ('internal milieu') important to energy balance. The area postrema sits exposed at the bottom of the fourth VENTRICLE, forming part of the roof of the brainstem. It receives extensive projections directly from sensory neurons of the VAGUS NERVE, the tenth cranial nerve, which contains both parasympathetic command neurons and sensory or afferent neurons. The sensory neurons of the vagus convey signals from receptors in the stomach, intestines, liver, kidneys, heart, and other internal organs. The area postrema thus acts as an entry point to the brain for this information and for its first stage of integrative processing. A variety of physiological reflexes controlled by the brainstem, carried out by the autonomic nervous system, rely on the neural signals received by the area postrema. In addition, the area postrema is the initial level of processing for ascending vagal signals related to HUNGER, THIRST, and other motivational states (see MOTIVATION) that are required by neural structures in the FOREBRAIN, such as the HYPOTHALAMUS, in order to control motivated behaviour. Beyond its role as a neural relay, the area postrema also is able itself to detect the presence of certain chemical substances within the blood or CEREBROSPINAL FLUID because as a CIRCUMVENTRICULAR ORGAN it is one of the few parts of the brain to lack a BLOOD–BRAIN BARRIER. In this way the area postrema acts directly to monitor the chemical status of the organism, possibly detecting the presence of poisons or nutrients, in addition to monitoring indirectly through its sensory neural projections. Lesions of the area postrema have sometimes been called a 'central vagotomy' because they eliminate the brain's capacity to monitor physiological status through the vagus nerve. But lesions also do more than simply eliminate vagus input. Area postrema lesions also impair the independent chemical detection function ordinarily provided by this nucleus. For example, area postrema lesions prevent the detection of poisons in the blood such as LITHIUM CHLORIDE, which becomes toxic at high concentrations. This can be seen via the psychological procedure known as taste aversion conditioning. Ordinarily an intravenous injection of lithium chloride that is given to a rat after a meal of a

novel food will produce a conditioned avoidance of that food when the rat encounters it in the future. If a lesion of the area postrema has been made in the rat previously, however, the effect of lithium chloride is blocked and no conditioned aversion is formed.

KENT C. BERRIDGE

area TE A term used synonymously with INFERIOR TEMPORAL CORTEX (or INFEROTEMPORAL CORTEX).

areas VI–V5 The terms V1 to V5 refer to a system of classification of some of the areas of cortex thought to be involved in visual perception. Area V1 is the PRIMARY VISUAL CORTEX and is also referred to as area 17 or STRIATE CORTEX. It was termed V1 (visual area 1) as it was the first to be discovered and is the largest of the areas. The area of cortex surrounding V1 (termed EXTRA- or PRESTRIATE CORTEX and contained in the BRODMANN'S AREAS 18 and 19) contains numerous other areas (at least 25) that appear to be implicated in visual processing. The first four of these to be defined and studied in the Old World monkey were given the labels V2, V3, V4 and V5 though the latter is often referred to as MT (MIDDLE TEMPORAL REGION) due to its homologue in the New World monkey that had already received considerable attention when V5 was first defined. These areas where first discovered through anatomical techniques that examined projections from V1 to pre-striate cortex. Areas discovered later seem to have abandoned this numbering scheme in favour of more descriptive terms (such as ventral interparietal, among others).

Areas V1–V5 each contain an orderly topographic map of the visual world (though it is somewhat less orderly in area V5) thus inviting the question of why the cortex should need to reproduce this map several times? The initial and still popular answer appears to be that each of the areas may be more specialized for some aspect of vision (such as colour, motion, depth) or visual task (such as saccadic eye movements; see SACCADE) – hence the hypothesis of 'one-area-one-function'. Based upon the early work of Zeki and others it was suggested that V2 analyses STEREOSCOPIC DEPTH, V4 colour information (see COLOUR VISION) and

V5 motion information (see MOTION PERCEP-TION). A less extreme version of the separatist debate holds that there are TWO VISUAL STREAMS that have differing specialities. One stream is suggested to process motion information and spatial location (sometimes termed the 'where' stream) and involves area V5 whereas the other is suggested to process colour and form and may involve area V4 (sometimes termed the 'what' stream)

The 'one-area-one-function' hypothesis now has little credence. For example in area V2 staining for CYTOCHROME OXIDASE has shown a system of thick and thin stripes which have differing anatomical connections and the functional properties of the cells within the stripes differ with those outside (and differ between thick and thin stripes). Thus information about colour, motion, form and depth all appear to be represented within this area suggesting a possible role in their integration. In area V3 there also appears to be a convergence of information and many of this area's properties appear to resemble those of V2 and some resemble those of V5. It has therefore been suggested that this area may have some role in processing dynamic form. Early recordings from area V4 suggested that nearly all its cells were sensitive to the chromatic properties of stimuli, however subsequent work showed that this property was no more prevalent than in area V1. Likewise lesions of the area do not bring about complete loss of colour vision but more subtle deficits involving colour constancy. Other deficits have been found in the animal's ability to learn new visual tasks which may relate to the 'attentional' modulation of cells' responses that have been demonstrated in the alert animal. The cells of area V5 are nearly all motion-sensitive; damage to area V5 does cause a specific (if somewhat transient) loss of motion perception and stimulation of the area can invoke the perception of motion. Thus this area does appear to be a 'motion area'.

In humans the task of identifying and locating these areas is well under way. Recent studies have used FUNCTIONAL NEUROIMAGING techniques in conjunction with special stimuli in order to map these regions. One technique involves presenting stimuli that selectively excite the horizontal meridian or the vertical meridian and thus obtaining maps of the representation of these meridians. From these, and knowledge of organization of the areas in macaques, the boundaries between areas have been identified and labelled. The second technique involves designing stimuli that will specifically target a certain area (again based on findings from the macaque) such as, for example, a coloured stimulus to activate area V4 and a moving one to activate area V5.

ROBERT J. SNOWDEN

arecoline see parasympathomimetic drugs

arginine An amino acid: the L ISOMER (L-arginine) is the precursor from which NITRIC OXIDE is synthesized. Arginine vasopressin is the form of that hormone found in most mammals (see VASOPRESSIN for discussion of this).

arhythmia (Also spelt arrhythmia.) An irregularity of rhythm; a term most commonly used in relation to the heart beat, in which arhythmia may be caused by (for example structural problems in the heart itself (for example a valve dysfunction) or by changes in the neural control of heart beat; see BLOOD.

aromatase An enzyme that converts ANDROGENS to ESTROGENS (including the conversion of TESTOSTERONE to ESTRADIOL). Aromatase is found in high concentrations in the OVARIES and in the BRAIN and is important in shaping masculine copulatory responses.

See also: aromatic; sex hormones; sexual behaviour

aromatic L-amino acid decarboxylase see dopamine; noradrenaline

aromatic In everyday language, aromatic means possessing an aroma, a distinctive odour; in biochemistry, aromatic refers to benzene derivatives, a closed-chain class of organic compounds. Aromatization is a term given to the process of rendering a molecule aromatic. For example, AROMATASE is an enzyme that converts testosterone to estradiol. Aromatics are the opposite of the aliphatic (or fatty) compounds, open-chain organic molecules derived from methane; see for example ALIPHATIC ALDEHYDES; FATTY ACIDS.

arousal A general state of alertness. During wakefulness, arousal mechanisms have been said to increase or decrease the efficiency of information processing by the CEREBRAL CORTEX. The relationship between arousal and level of performance is not straightforward however, and is traditionally described by an inverted-U shaped function known as the YERKES–DODSON LAW. This indicates that increased arousal may not always be facilitatory to behaviour, which may be because very high levels of arousal are harder to control or coordinate in neural terms. In some circumstances, arousal is thought to provide added intensity to emotional or motivationally salient (see MOTIVATION) stimuli. In other situations, arousal level may determine not whether a response occurs, but what type of behaviour is performed. For instance, in studies with rats, feeding may occur at one level of arousal, while FIGHT-OR-FLIGHT occurs at another.

As a general rule, level of arousal increases throughout the day and can be modified by a number of different stimuli. Sensory input (particularly noise) increases arousal, as do incentives (see INCENTIVE), unsatisfied biological drives (such as HUNGER, THIRST and SEXUAL BEHAVIOUR), and stimulants (such as AMPHETAMINE, CAFFEINE and NICOTINE). For instance, there is enough caffeine in a few cups of coffee to produce an increased capacity for sustained intellectual effort and decreased reaction times. Sensory deprivation and SLEEP deprivation can also reduce levels of arousal. The interactions between these different modulators on level of arousal are complex and poorly understood. In some cases it is clear that deterioration in performance due to a 'de-arousing' stressor can be compensated for by the application of an 'arousing' stressor. However, it is also clear that in general there is no simple arithmetical interaction, since arousal is not a unitary process.

Measurement of arousal level is not straightforward. Some indices, such as increased heart rate, also occur during exertion due to the need for additional OXYGEN in muscle tissue. A quantitative measure of arousal can be extrapolated from an analysis of the different frequencies of electrical activity present in the cortical ELECTROENCEPHALOGRAM (EEG): a fast 'desynchronized' EEG is typical of a state of high arousal. Although EEG desynchrony (see SYNCHRONY/DESYNCHRONY) is also characteristic of REM SLEEP (rapid eye movement sleep) – hence the term PARADOXICAL SLEEP – arousal is clearly dissociable from this by taking into account parallel changes in neck muscle tone (see ELECTROMYOGRAM), since this measure is high during waking and negligible during REM sleep.

From a physiological perspective, arousal is thought to occur as a result of increased activity within the ASCENDING RETICULAR ACTIVATING SYSTEM (ARAS) of the brain: interactions of the ARAS with many highly distinct cortical and subcortical systems are important for the coordination of arousal processes specific to external circumstances and internal needs. The complex projection systems of the different neurotransmitters within the ARAS imply that different stimuli will interact with specific neurochemical sub-components and modify arousal in unique ways. For instance, many centrally acting stimulants, including amphetamine and caffeine, have their principal arousing actions through the NORADRENERGIC sub-component of the ARAS at a number of different locations in the forebrain, notably the thalamus, hypothalamus and cortex. Nicotine, on the other hand, acts through the CHOLINERGIC sub-component of the ARAS, having potential arousing effects at nicotinic receptors in the THALAMUS, BASAL FOREBRAIN and cortex. TAIL-PINCH studies in rats have also demonstrated the powerful, but non-specific, role of DOPAMINE in arousal processes: if food is present, the rat will eat; if water is present, it drinks; presence of rat pups invokes maternal behaviour; and the presence of females induces sexual behaviour; three pinches a day in the presence of food can cause a rat to overeat until it is obese (see OBESITY). Such evidence, alongside the anatomical organisation of the DOPAMINERGIC projection system, suggests that arousal in dopaminergic terms is to intensify the impact of motivationally salient stimuli. However, despite the involvement of widespread brain nuclei in arousal processes, a focal point is clearly the thalamus, which modifies sensory, motor and motivational information *en route* to different specialized regions of the cortex. At the level of these thalamic synapses, there are clear similarities in physiological terms between attention and arousal functions.

WENDY L. INGLIS

arterenol *see* noradrenaline

arteriole *see* blood

arteriosclerosis (from Greek, *arteria*: artery, *sklerosis*: hardening) Literally, hardening of the arteries.

See also: atherosclerosis

arteritis Inflammation of an artery: see STROKE

artery *see* blood

articulatory loop The articulatory loop – also referred to as the 'phonological loop' – is one of the subsystems postulated in Alan Baddeley's multicomponent model of WORKING MEMORY. It is specialized for the temporary storage of verbal information and consists of two subcomponents, a PHONOLOGICAL STORE and an articulatory REHEARSAL process. The phonological store can hold speech-based information, subject to a rapid decay. The articulatory rehearsal process can refresh the decaying representation by reading it off and feeding it back to the store. It also serves to convert visually presented information (such as written words) into phonological codes and register them into the phonological store.

This two-component structure is consistent with the results from recent neuroimaging studies indicating that the passive storage and active rehearsal of verbal information may depend on separable neural circuits, the former being more dependent on a posterior portion of the brain and the latter on an anterior portion (see Smith & Jonides, 1997). The distinction also serves to explain various experimental findings on MEMORY SPAN performance. For example, the rapid decay in the phonological store can explain the phonological similarity effect, the disadvantage of similar sounding items (for example, P-G-V-C-T) over dissimilar ones (for example, K-Y-B-R-W) in immediate serial recall (that is, similar items have fewer distinguishing features available than dissimilar items, hence, more vulnerable to decay). In contrast, the time-based nature of rehearsal can explain the word length effect, the larger memory span for shorter words like *boat* than longer words like *refrigerator* – longer words require more time to rehearse, hence, more susceptible to decay.

A popular method for studying the articulatory loop is to ask subjects to repeatedly articulate common words (for example, *the*) while they are performing a target cognitive task. The rationale behind this articulatory suppression technique is that concurrent articulation occupies the articulatory rehearsal component and thereby disrupts the performance of any cognitive task that implicates the articulatory loop. Recent studies using this and other methodologies (for instance, neuropsychological studies of brain-damaged patients with a selective verbal SHORT-TERM MEMORY impairment) suggest that the evolutionary significance of the articulatory loop may be to serve as a language-acquisition device. While its role in LANGUAGE comprehension and production seems to be rather minor (particularly among adults), it has been shown to play an essential role in the acquisition of spoken and written language among children (such as vocabulary acquisition and learning to read) (see Gathercole & Baddeley, 1993 for review).

See also: central executive; memory deficits; phonology

References

Gathercole S.E. & Baddeley, A.D. (1993) *Working Memory and Language*, Erlbaum: Hillsdale NJ.
Smith E.E. & Jonides, J. (1997) Working memory: a view from neuroimaging. *Cognitive Psychology* 33: 5–42.

AKIRA MIYAKE

artificial intelligence Artificial intelligence (AI) is concerned with building something that will exhibit behaviour we call intelligent (see INTELLIGENCE). It only became feasible on any scale with the development of computers in the 1950s. Initial work was dominated by a particular idea of what was intelligent, which influenced both the problems selected and the methods of solution. Many of the problems involved high-level formal reasoning – for example how to produce mathematical proofs or to play chess. It was hoped these would be amenable to general problem-solving methods, in which the initial question and the solution were seen as points in a multidimensional space, the task being to find a path between them. This approach therefore focused on techniques for representing problems in such spaces, for searching through them, and for classifying the points within them. Important achievements include EXPERT SYSTEMS which use production systems as local rules-of-thumb for navigating through search spaces, and have been employed for example in the diagnosis of bacterial infections.

It has become apparent that there is an important trade-off between search and classification. In the case of chess, for example, the most primitive classification of a position would be whether it was checkmate or not; in checkmate, one side has won by definition. With this as its only classification method, a computer program would need to keep searching through a given sequence of moves until a checkmate position was reached. If however a predictive classification were possible (for example, one side has overwhelming material advantage), the particular moves between the classified position and checkmate would not have to be examined. In general, the better the classification the shorter the search.

The reason for stressing this trade-off is that computers can search very much more rapidly than people. It is thus an option for chess-playing programs to use 'brute force' (among other tools) to play well, whereas expert human players must rely on limited search but sophisticated methods of classification. This potential DOUBLE DISSOCIATION between artificial and natural intelligence has important implications for psychology. Many tasks that people do well seem to have some resemblance to the classification of chess positions: these include FACE PERCEPTION, motor coordination, and understanding the meaning of sentences. In each case, the problem appears to be solved by simultaneously considering many factors, no single one of which is decisive (factors sometimes referred to as multiple soft constraints). Ironically, these sorts of problem that humans deal with effortlessly have proved more difficult to solve artificially than certain formal reasoning tasks that many people fail to solve at all (Crevier, 1993). The impact of this realization has been heightened by the investigation of new kinds of program in which instructions are effectively carried out by a number of processors simultaneously, rather than by a single processor one step at a time. Neural nets use such PARALLEL DISTRIBUTED PROCESSING, and it has been argued that their connectionist architecture (see CONNECTIONISM) performs more like people than do traditional programs in artificial intelligence.

There has consequently arisen a wide-ranging debate about the nature of intelligence which addresses very deep questions concerning thought and consciousness in both people and machines. In particular, the precise role of rules and symbols in human cognition is proving the subject of polemic. From the practical standpoint, a number of different lines of enquiry can be loosely grouped under the head of artificial intelligence. These include: (1) The manufacture of devices that work commercially (for example, for translating text from one language to another) regardless of whether the method adopted is like that used by people, (2) the refinement of rule-based architectures for generic problem-solving as models of human cognition, (3) the acquisition of very large knowledge data-bases. It seems that people often solve problems with multiple soft constraints by using extensive knowledge about the problem area. This knowledge is acquired by interaction with the world, so interest has focused on making computers that can interact similarly. These are usually termed autonomous robots, and the area that of situated intelligence. It seeks to place human reasoning firmly in the context of 'lower-level' processes such as perception and motor control.

It is possible that this current diversity will in time reveal underlying unifying principles. David Marr suggested that complex information processing problems needed to be understood at several levels: in particular he distinguished between the levels of computation and of implementation. The former deals with the abstract, formal characteristics of a problem, describing the solution in general mathematical terms to which any device whatever must conform. The latter deals with how any particular physical machine, be it made of silicon chips or neurons, carries out that computation. Unity at the computational level can thus coexist with diversity of implementation.

References

Crevier D. (1993) *AI: The Tumultuous History of the Search for Artificial Intelligence*, Basic Books: New York.

Franklin S. (1995) *Artificial Minds*, MIT Press: Cambridge MA.

PAUL DEAN

artificial neural networks *see* neural networks

ascending reticular activating system The ascending reticular activating system is a concept originally proposed by Moruzzi & Magoun in 1949 on the basis of the effects of electrical stimulation of the BRAINSTEM on the cortical ELECTROENCEPHALOGRAM (EEG) in anaesthetized cats. These investigators found that high-frequency stimulation at the core of the RETICULAR FORMATION throughout the brainstem is effective in inducing the activated pattern (so-called desynchronization) of the EEG. Stimulation at the MIDBRAIN level was the most effective. The core region of the reticular formation was thought to be activated by COLLATERALS of specific sensory pathways and send a powerful excitatory drive to the THALAMUS, which in turn activates the CEREBRAL CORTEX. Subsequent studies showed that a LESION of the reticular core does indeed produce chronic EEG inactivation and SOMNOLENCE; the activation of the EEG and behavioural AROUSAL were still possible with strong sensory stimulation, but did not outlast the stimulation. These results provided a new interpretation to the earlier finding by Bremer of continuous EEG inactivation in the CERVEAU ISOLÉ (isolated FOREBRAIN) preparation; this was due to the isolation of the reticular formation from the forebrain, rather than sensory deafferentation as originally interpreted. Theoretically, the work by Moruzzi & Magoun introduced the concept that a 'nonspecific' (see NONSPECIFIC PROJECTIONS) rather than 'specific' sensory system is responsible for EEG

activation. The proposal by Moruzzi & Magoun that the excitatory drive generated in the brainstem core is mediated by the thalamus *en route* to the cortex was later confirmed, and expanded further by Steriade and other investigators using more sophisticated cellular techniques. The seminal studies by Moruzzi & Magoun conceptualized, for the first time, that cortical activation was actively maintained by the tonic activation of brainstem core neurons, and defined the beginning of the modern era of studies on the states of vigilance, stimulating a great deal of research.

Because the anatomy of the reticular formation was poorly understood, the anatomical substrate of the ascending reticular activating system remained an enigma for three decades. It was once thought that the key anatomical feature of the reticular formation was the highly collateralizing axons of so-called isodendritic neurons, but subsequent studies failed to support this idea; cells with such extensive collaterals were the exception rather than the rule. However, the advances in neuroanatomical techniques in the 1980s, in particular TRACT TRACERS and IMMUNOHISTOCHEMISTRY, have delineated the anatomical substrate of the ascending reticular activating system. Interestingly, the sites in the midbrain that were found to be most effective in evoking cortical EEG activation upon stimulation exactly corresponded to an area ventrolateral to the midbrain PERIAQUEDUCTAL GREY where bundles of CHOLINERGIC and MONOAMINERGIC fibres ascend. Thus, it is now commonly held that the reticular activating system is composed of several ascending pathways that use different neurotransmitters and innervate distinct forebrain structures. These pathways include ascending cholinergic, NORADRENERGIC and serotonergic projections as well as reticular projections using unidentified NEUROTRANSMITTERS, possibly GLUTAMATE.

The cholinergic pathway originates from the PEDUNCULOPONTINE TEGMENTAL NUCLEUS and the LATERODORSAL TEGMENTAL NUCLEUS (see also CH1–CH8). These neurons heavily innervate the thalamic nuclei in a topographic manner. The same cholinergic neurons also project to other forebrain structures including the BASAL FOREBRAIN, but their cortical projection is limited to the MEDIAL PREFRONTAL CORTEX. The thalamus, in particular its association nuclei, also receives massive projections from non-cholinergic, probably GLUTAMATERGIC, neurons in the rostral midbrain reticular formation. The noradrenergic pathway arises from the LOCUS COERULEUS, whereas the serotonergic pathway originates in the dorsal and median RAPHE NUCLEI. These monoaminergic pathways reach not only the thalamus but also the cerebral cortex directly. In the thalamus, ACETYLCHOLINE, NORADRENALINE and SEROTONIN block SLEEP SPINDLES and facilitate sensory transmission. Two structures in the forebrain may be regarded as rostral extensions of the ascending reticular activating: the posterior HYPOTHALAMUS containing HISTAMINERGIC neurons innervating the cortex, and the basal forebrain containing cholinergic, GABAERGIC and other neurons innervating the cortex as well as neurons that become selectively active during wakefulness and REM SLEEP (rapid eye movement sleep) or during NON-REM SLEEP.

From both anatomical and functional studies, it is now clear that the neurochemically coded ascending projections with distinct projection patterns can be viewed as the anatomical substrate of the ascending reticular activating system proposed by Moruzzi & Magoun in 1949. The effects of activation of each of these pathways in cortical activation and sensory transmission are being characterized, further defining the role of each component of the system in the mechanisms of EEG and behavioural arousal.

References

Moruzzi G. & Magoun H. W. (1949) Brain stem reticular formation and activation of the EEG. *Electroencephalography and Clinical Neurophysiology* 1: 455–473.
Steriade M. & McCarley R.W. (1990) *Brainstem Control of Wakefulness and Sleep*, Plenum Press: New York.

KAZUE SEMBA

ascorbic acid (ascorbate) A strong anti-oxidant found in high concentrations in nervous tissue. Because it has anti-oxidant properties it can be added to VEHICLE solutions to prevent

OXIDATION of drugs or chemicals. It is also known as vitamin C.

See also: drug ionization

CHARLES D. BLAHA

aseptic technique (from Greek, *a*: not, *sepsis*: putrefaction) Aseptic technique is used in surgical operations and avoids the induction of putrefaction, decay or disease, by the exclusion of microorganisms and other contaminants. It is achieved by heat sterilization of all the equipment to be used in the surgical procedure, by covering the working surfaces with sterile drapes; by covering the subject of the surgical procedure with sterile drapes (except of course at the point of surgical contact); and by the surgeons wearing sterile coverings (masks, gloves, hats, gowns and so on, as required). Though most commonly associated with experimental or therapeutic surgery, aseptic techniques are used elsewhere. For example, 'aseptic' techniques are required when producing microelectronic components.

See also: stereotaxic surgery

asexual Literally, reproduction without sexual activity; see also CLONE.

asomatoagnosia (also spelled *asomatognosia*; *asomatagnosia*) Unawareness of the condition of one's own body, either on both sides, or unilaterally. UNILATERAL asomatoagnosia may involve denial of HEMIPLEGIA.

See also: phantom limb pain; spatial neglect

aspartic acid (aspartate) One of the EXCITATORY AMINO ACIDS; aspartic acid and GLUTAMIC ACID are described as the two major excitatory NEUROTRANSMITTERS in the central nervous system. The concentration of both is relatively high in comparison to other amino acids involved in neurotransmission, such as glycine. However, although a neurotransmitter role for aspartate has been acknowledged, the amount of research on this compared to glutamate has been very small and much remains to be clarified.

See also: amino acid neurotransmitters; drug ionization

Asperger's syndrome A recently introduced diagnosis related to AUTISM. Like autism, it is diagnosed on the basis of social and communicative impairments, with restricted interests and activities. In current diagnosis it is distinguished from autism by intact language and normal INTELLIGENCE QUOTIENT (IQ). These and other possible differentiating features (clumsiness, special interests) remain controversial. Autism and Asperger's syndrome cluster in the same families, and a genetic cause is assumed. The brain regions affected are unknown, although abnormalities of the FRONTAL LOBE and RIGHT HEMISPHERE have been suggested. Epidemiological studies currently suggest a prevalence of 4 per 1000 with a male:female ratio of 4:1.

Reference

Frith U. (ed.) (1991) *Autism and Asperger Syndrome*, Cambridge University Press: Cambridge.

FRANCESCA G. HAPPÉ

aspiration lesion *see* lesion

assembly coding *see* neural assembly

association A link between two events or entities that permits one to activate the other as, for example, when a characteristic odour elicits an image of the place where it was once experienced. (Also, the process of forming such a link.) For philosophers of previous centuries the entities of interest were ideas or states of consciousness. Modern psychology concerns itself largely with the central representations evoked by stimuli. In both cases the aim has been to specify the laws of association, that is, the conditions that must be met for links to be formed and activated.

See also: associative learning; conditioning

GEOFFREY HALL

association cortex The association cortex consists of those parts of the CEREBRAL CORTEX that are neither primary motor nor primary sensory areas (*see* KONIOCORTEX). It constitutes the largest part of the CORTEX in higher mammals, including humans. Association areas are often divided into *unimodal association areas* (integrating different information from within a sensory modality), *polymodal association areas* (integrating information across mod-

alities) and *supramodal association areas* (integrating high order polymodal information). As higher-order integration centres, the association areas receive information from the primary and other areas of the cortex, as well as association nuclei of the THALAMUS. Through these connections, the association cortex processes basic sensations into perception and recognition, and executes skilled movements. Disturbance of these mechanisms by lesion of the association cortex can result in AGNOSIA, APHASIA or APRAXIA.

See also: sensation vs. perception

KAZUE SEMBA

associative agnosia To identify a visual object, what is seen must make contact with previous experience organized in terms of specific episodes and general conceptual knowledge. Associative agnosia refers to impairments of object identification that are demonstrably the outcome of some failure in the mapping of structure to object concepts: what is correctly seen is no longer adequately classified and understood. AGNOSIA may be more severe for objects in particular categories. In addition, the disorder may occur in the auditory or tactile modality, and not in visual perception.

See also: association

DANIEL N. BUB

associative learning As a training procedure, one that involves presenting an organism with a CONTINGENCY between two events (that is, with two events occurring close together in time). An example is the PAIRED ASSOCIATE LEARNING procedure used in studies of human verbal learning in which the subject is presented a list consisting of pairs of words and learns to respond with one when given the other. The basic CONDITIONING procedures used in the study of animal learning similarly involve the co-occurrence of two events. In PAVLOVIAN CONDITIONING the events are both stimuli, as when the sounding of a tone accompanies food delivery. In INSTRUMENTAL CONDITIONING (also called operant conditioning) one event is an action (or response) performed by the animal, as when a lever press results in the delivery of food.

Associative learning also refers to a theoretical interpretation of the outcome of such procedures, an interpretation that supposes that the changes in behaviour they generate are the consequence of the formation of associations or links between the central representations of the events involved. Pavlovian conditioning has been interpreted as resulting in the formation of a STIMULUS–STIMULUS ASSOCIATION (S–S, in this example, a tone–food association). This association allows the first stimulus to activate the representation of the second and thus evoke behaviour (the CONDITIONED REFLEX) appropriate to that stimulus (salivation in this case). In instrumental conditioning associations might be formed between the set of stimuli that constitute the training apparatus and the response that the animal performs (an S–R association); also between the response and the event (food in this case) that this response produces (an R–S association). Experimental evidence supports the conclusion that both these associations can be formed.

The conditioning procedure (in particular the Pavlovian version) has been extensively used in studies directed toward specifying the conditions that are necessary for associations to be formed (the 'laws of association'). In these experiments the conditions of training are varied and the effect on the magnitude of the conditioned response is noted. The size of this response is taken to reflect directly the strength of the S–S association produced by the training. Such experiments have shown that associations are best formed when both the events to be associated are salient and novel and when they are presented close to each other in time and space. But although it is necessary, the contiguous occurrence of the relevant events is not sufficient for association formation to occur. Thus, in Pavlovian conditioning, repeated pairings of the tone with food will not establish a tone–food association if presentations of the food also occur with equal frequency when the tone has not been presented. One interpretation of this effect holds that the association will only be formed when the one stimulus supplies information about the likely occurrence of the other. Again, tone–food pairings have been found to be ineffective if the tone is presented along with some other event, say a light, that has, as a result of previous training, already formed an association with the food (a phenomenon known as BLOCKING: the pre-trained light is said to block learning about the tone). It has been suggested that blocking occurs because the tone supplies no new information, as the food is already predicted by the presentation of the light.

Theorists interested in producing formal models of the associative learning process have been much concerned with effects like those just described. Of the models still current, the most important and influential is that first proposed in 1972 by R.A. Rescorla and A.R. Wagner – the RESCORLA–WAGNER THEORY. The essence of their model is that a stimulus already signalled by some event will lose its effectiveness and thus its ability to enter into new associations. This simple principle allows the model to accommodate the importance of the predictive relationship between the stimuli being associated. It is a principle that has been taken up by others and has gained wide currency among cognitive psychologists whose interest lies in developing connectionist models of learning, perception and language (see CONNECTIONISM).

For many years, theories of associative learning played a dominant role in psychological theorizing generally (indeed, in the guise of connectionism, they may still do so). They have been so influential for two main reasons. First, there is no doubting the central importance of the process of learning in shaping behaviour and associative theory supplies the only well-developed account of a possible mechanism. Second, given what we know about brain structure and function (about neurons and synapses), the associative hypothesis seems, to say the least, very plausible. Although not yet achieved, it seems likely that neuroscientists will soon be able to identify the synapses that are changed when associations are formed and the nature of the changes involved.

See also: Hebbian synapse; learning

GEOFFREY HALL

associative transitivity Transitivity is a property of a relationship between two events (for example, greater than) such that if A is related to B, and B to C, then one may infer that A is related to C. Animals sometimes appear to make such inferences; for example, after training on four simple discriminations, A+ B-, B+ C-, C+ D-, D+ E- (that is, given a choice of A and B, A is reinforced and B is not, etc), animals will choose B over D, even though B and D are equally associated with REINFORCE-MENT. Such performance suggests a non-associative mechanism – perhaps the animals learn A is better than B and so on, and thus infer that B is better than D. But it is possible that, during training, an ASSOCIATION could form between the to-be-discriminated stimuli, specifically between A and B, and D and E. B, associated with the always-reinforced A, might then be preferred over D, associated with the never-reinforced E. Whether this associative mechanism forms the basis of TRANSITIVE INFERENCE in humans is controversial.

CHARLOTTE BONARDI

associative visual agnosia A form of AGNOSIA in which the fully integrated percept of an object is not assigned the correct meaning.

See also: copying and drawing; object agnosia

astereoagnosia An inability to recognize objects by touch, despite other sensory qualities of the objects being recognized. The term is often used more-or-less synonymously with TACTILE AGNOSIA.

astigmatism *see* refractive error

astrocyte *see* glial cells

astrocytic syncytium *see* glial cells

astrocytoma *see* tumour

astroglia The same as astroglia; *see* glial cells

asymmetric synapses *see* synapse

asymmetry Differences between two structures in MORPHOLOGY, or in function in spite of similar morphology. Until recently, twentiethth-century efforts in psychology and neurology have tended to focus on the evidence for asymmetry of function in the two cerebral hemispheres, at the expense of study of somatic preferences (such as HANDEDNESS) and anatomical asymmetries. In Europe in the late

nineteenth century, Karl Wernicke (see WERNICKE'S APHASIA) and his contemporaries helped to popularize the idea that loss of speech related functions tended to follow from damage to the LEFT HEMISPHERE. Very shortly the RIGHT HEMISPHERE became commonly described as the 'minor hemisphere', its role trivialized to such an extent that it was even suggested that its principal function was to hold up the left hemisphere within the skull. The functions which depend more on right-hemispheric mechanisms remained more difficult to describe until well into the twentieth century, when it was established that certain visuospatial functions are compromised more frequently after right-hemisphere damage. For example, patients with damage in the right PARIETAL CORTEX will frequently fail to attend to stimuli on their left side. This symptom, NEGLECT SYNDROME, only occurs rarely (and typically in a less dramatic form) after left-hemisphere lesions. In fact, the occurrence of neglect after right-hemisphere lesions and APHASIA and APRAXIA after left-hemisphere lesions provide the two of the more reliable pieces of evidence for functional asymmetry. It is probably no accident that such disorders involve the inferior parietal lobe in both instances, a region which some anatomists have argued that we do not share with our non-human primate relations. Interest in cerebral asymmetry was revived in the latter part of this century by the pioneering work of Roger Sperry and his colleagues on the so-called SPLIT-BRAIN patients. After the cerebral commissures are cut (commissurotomy – as a treatment for intractable epilepsy) specialized procedures can be used to lateralize sensory input to only one hemisphere; because the information cannot be 'passed on' to the other hemisphere, the limitations of the processing capacities can be deduced by examining the responses of the patient. The majority of dissociations between left- and right-hemisphere skills seen in split-brain patients had been previously demonstrated in neurological patients and alluded to by work on neurologically intact subjects. Nevertheless it was the dramatic way in which asymmetries manifested themselves in split-brain patients that captured the interest of the scientific community as well as the general public. The most obvious behavioural asymmetries have to do with the preferred use of one hand, foot or eye relative to the other. In human samples, the incidence of right-hand preference is typically 90%, and occurs even in the rare populations where there is no obvious cultural bias against left-handedness ('sinistrality' – see SINISTRAL). Less well known behavioural asymmetries are a bias towards right-foot preference (~70–85%) and right-eye preference for tasks which explicitly or implicitly require the use of one eye and not the other (~65–75%). These right-sided preferences are not perfectly related to one another, so it is not completely uncommon for a 'right-hander' to prefer the left foot or the left eye. Nevertheless, the fact that the population-level bias is for right-sided preferences for hand, foot and eye is unlikely to be a coincidence. The right-sided bias might be related to left-hemisphere advantages in the control of movement (although any such model has to be quite complex to account for right-eye preference). Evidence for behavioural asymmetries in non-human primates has been suggested, although the magnitude of the claimed asymmetry is always much smaller than those found in human populations. The recent ascent of imaging techniques such as MAGNETIC RESONANCE IMAGING (MRI) and POSITRON EMISSION TOMOGRAPHY (PET) has generated a renewed interest in functional, as well as anatomical asymmetries in the brain. The list of anatomical asymmetries demonstrated by MRI as well as *post-mortem* examination is growing. To date, the most cited difference is a larger PLANUM TEMPORALE in the left hemisphere relative to the right, although this asymmetry is only present in 65% of brains. HESCHL'S GYRUS, located anterior to the planum temporale; tends to be larger in the right hemisphere than the left (there are often two gyri in the right hemisphere). Because imaging studies like MRI and functional MRI can be performed in large numbers of subjects, studies that try to relate behavioural asymmetries like handedness to anatomical and functional brain asymmetries should do much to unify these three largely independent research domains.

Reference

Springer S.P. & Deutsch G. (1997) *Left Brain, Right Brain*, 5th edn, W.H. Freeman: New York.

DAVID P. CAREY

asymptote In mathematics, an asymptote is a line that approaches a curve but never meets it; asymptotic is the adjectival form or asymptote. In pharmacological studies of, for example, RECEPTOR BINDING, one might find a drug–receptor relationship that could be described as asymptotic – this would imply that 100% binding was never quite achieved. In behavioural studies, one often describes an ASYMPTOTIC BEHAVIOURAL MAXIMUM.

asymptotic behavioural maximum As the size of a behavioural response grows it can either hit a ceiling (followed by abrupt transition to no further growth) or it can gradually approach a limit. The latter case is asymptotic. An application is seen in the RATE–FREQUENCY CURVES. As the pulse frequency of a BRAIN STIMULATION REWARD is increased, behaviour appears to grow and to approach an asymptote. Another application is in the single lever adaptation of the MATCHING LAW where the rate of lever-pressing also grows to an asymptote as the VI schedule (and reinforcements earned) increases (see SCHEDULES OF REINFORCEMENT).

JAMES R. STELLAR

ataxia Poor coordination of movement, often due to cerebellar dysfunction (see CEREBELLUM) or a familial degenerative disorder of the sensory and motor pathways such as FREIDRICH'S ATAXIA. Ataxic movements are inaccurate in positioning, and/or defective in timing and patterning. By far the most common form of ataxia is caused by cerebellar dysfunction. The most common manifestation of this kind of ataxia is disordered finger-to-nose pointing, where an ataxic tremor (or INTENTION TREMOR) is seen during the movement, and tends to increase in magnitude as the target is approached. Additionally, hypermetric errors are often encountered – patients will overshoot target position. Ataxia is invariably worse when the patient is required to make rapid movements. Nevertheless cerebellar ataxia is also revealed in tasks which require manual or ocular tracking of a drifting target. Ataxia of GAIT can be seen in patients with damage to cerebellar structures. The typical pattern in such patients is short steps from a broad base and a tendency to lean forward. Most models of ataxia suggest that a cerebellum plays a role in pre-programming the timing of agonist/antagonist muscle activities before the movement is actually initiated. Abnormal patterns of braking may be consequent to disruption in the pre-programming phase, and lead to movement overshooting, undershooting, and additional abnormal programming of the corrective movements which the ataxic errors make necessary. Additionally, difficulties in processing proprioceptive feedback related to the ongoing movement may be a consequence of cerebellar dysfunction and could contribute to the presence and magnitude of ataxia. Other researchers have suggested that ataxic movements of cerebellar patients could be understood in terms of poor utilization of efference copy (feedforward) signals received from the MOTOR CORTEX. Poor guidance of a limb movement towards a target has been, rather inaccurately, named 'OPTIC ATAXIA' by Rezsö Balint (see BALINT'S SYNDROME). Optic ataxia is a consequence of bilateral or unilateral lesions of the PARIETAL LOBE.

DAVID P. CAREY

atenolol A beta-1 noradrenaline receptor ANTAGONIST; see ADRENOCEPTORS.

atherosclerosis A form of ARTERIOSCLEROSIS (hardening of the arteries) responsible for the large vessel arterial disease that underlies coronary artery and cerebrovascular disease. Atherosclerosis represents the leading cause of death in the UK and the US. Atherosclerotic lesions, consisting initially of LIPID accumulation, and later fibrous change and NECROSIS, develop in the inner arterial walls. The arteries become narrowed, stiffened and weakened. These changes result in reduction in the blood supply to affected areas, which may be sudden and complete if the vessel is occluded, or bursts. Atherosclerosis in the vessels supporting

brain tissue may result in STROKE, or VASCULAR DEMENTIA.

IAN C. REID

athetosis (from Greek, *a*: not, *thetos*: placed) A form of movement disorder, involving non-rhythmic, jerky movements; slower than CHOREA. CHOREOATHETOSIS involves features of both chorea and athetosis.

atmospheric perspective *see* perspective

atom Just as a MOLECULE is the smallest quantity of a substance that retains the properties of that substance, so an atom is the smallest quantity of an ELEMENT possessing the properties of that element – that is, it is the smallest amount of an element able to take part in chemical reactions. Atoms are composed of a NUCLEUS (which has a proton and a neutron) and electrons, circling the nucleus. Protons are positively charged; neutrons are neutral; and electrons have a negative electrical charge. The ATOMIC NUMBER of an element is the same as the number of protons in the nucleus. (Discussion of the phenomena of subatomic particles is not appropriate here; see Campbell, Reece & Mitchell for further detail.) The mass (or weight) of an atom is measured in Daltons, after John Dalton (1766–1844), the eminent British scientists who pioneered atomic theory.

See also: atomic weight; periodic table of the elements

Reference

Campbell N.A., Reece J.B. & Mitchell L.G. (1999) *Biology*, 5th edn, Addison-Wesley: Menlo Park CA.

atomic number *see* atom

atomic weight Literally this is the weight of an ATOM. It is more or less equivalent to the combined weight of the protons and neutrons in an atom (that is, the atomic NUCLEUS) since electrons have next to no mass. The atomic weight alone is rarely of interest to biological psychologists, except in so far as the net weight of all the atoms in a MOLECULE will determine its MOLECULAR WEIGHT.

See also: isotope

atonia Lack or loss of MUSCLE tone; it may occur as part of a normal process (see REM SLEEP) or as part of a muscular disorder (such as MYASTHENIA GRAVIS).

ATP *see* adenosine triphosphate

ATP synthase The enzyme, found in the membranes of MITOCHONDRIA, that manufactures ADENOSINE TRIPHOSPHATE (ATP). The process of doing this is very complex; see Campbell, Reece & Mitchell for a clear exposition of this and of the functions and properties of ATP.

Reference

Campbell N.A., Reece J.B. & Mitchell L.G. (1999) *Biology*, 5th edn, Addison-Wesley: Menlo Park CA.

ATPase An enzyme involved in the breakdown of ADENOSINE TRIPHOSPHATE (ATP).

See also: sodium–potassium pump

atraumatic Not producing trauma; the EAR BARS used on a stereotaxic frame, for example, should be atraumatic (see STEREOTAXIC SURGERY).

atrial natriuretic peptide *see* natriuretic peptides

atrium *see* blood

atrophy (from Greek, *a*: not, *trophe*: food) Atrophy is a term used to indicate degeneration or wasting away; atrophied indicates that something has wasted away or fallen into disuse.

atropine Atropine, an alkaloid, is an ANTAGONIST that blocks the action of ACETYLCHOLINE at MUSCARINIC ACETYLCHOLINE RECEPTORS. This blockade occurs non-selectively at all subtypes of muscarinic receptors. Atropine is also the main content of the naturally occurring anti-muscarinic drugs prepared from belladonna plants. Topically applied to the eye, atropine blocks the action of acetylcholine released from parasympathetic fibres, causing dilation of the pupil. In animal surgery, atropine is often used to reduce mucous secretion. Systemic atropine causes dissociation of the cortical ELECTROENCEPHALOGRAM (EEG) and behaviour in which the cortical EEG shows large slow waves while the animal is behaviourally active.

See also: scopolamine; hyoscine

KAZUE SEMBA

attachment *see* social behaviour

attack *see* aggression

attention Attention is an executive process by which inputs are selected for processing. It describes the means by which humans and animals can identify and process important environmental events in a sustained manner, while ignoring others which are irrelevant. The term is used in a number of different ways, because attention is not a single process. For instance, selective, divided and sustained forms of attention have been identified in humans. SELECTIVE ATTENTION is sometimes also called focused attention. It refers to the ability to detect and analyse a specific portion of the information available to the senses, while ignoring the rest. DIVIDED ATTENTION pertains to the concurrent processing of more than one input. SUSTAINED ATTENTION is required for continuous performance of a task which is not under automatic control. It is sometimes used synonymously with VIGILANCE, although this can be misleading: vigilance is better defined as the constant detection of rare and unpredictable events, which is not something demanded by every continuous performance task.

Many paradigms have been designed to provide a perspective about the way in which people maintain an alert state and detect, orient to and process sensory signals (Posner & Peterson, 1990). These typically involve auditory tasks such as DICHOTIC LISTENING and shadowing, or VISUAL SEARCH tasks. Each can be modified to measure selective or divided attentional processes: in listening/shadowing tasks the subject can be instructed to focus on one or both streams of information; in visual tasks divided attention may be achieved by using a number of salient cue points which require simultaneous monitoring through COVERT ORIENTING. Measurement of shifts in attention are also possible. In cued visual tasks, the increase in response time to a target following an inappropriate cue is a measure of the time required to disengage attention. The

WISCONSIN CARD-SORT TEST provides a way of investigating the attentional importance given to different dimensions of stimuli and the ease with which we shift between them. Sustained attention is typically measured in experiments which involve continuous decisions about target stimuli, or alternatively by testing the resistance of performance to a distraction. Although the data-processing components of each task may be very different, the combination of paradigms can discover whether attentional processes are common to all.

Some attentional paradigms have been successfully modified for animal subjects (Robbins, 1998). For instance, the FIVE-CHOICE SERIAL REACTION TIME TEST measures sustained and divided attention in rats, as they continuously monitor and respond to the presentation of a light in one of five possible locations, for the delivery of a small food reward. Selective attention can also be investigated in this task by including random bursts of white noise amongst the visual stimuli. Paradigms specifically designed to investigate divided attention include those which require monitoring of simultaneously presented visual stimuli, and more recently the performance of concurrently presented conditional discriminations in the auditory and visual domains. The roles of the INTRADIMENSIONAL SHIFT and EXTRADIMENSIONAL SHIFT have been successfully investigated in a modification of the Wisconsin card-sort test for PRIMATES.

Just as attention is not a unitary process, it has been shown that it is not carried out by one particular region of the brain, but by a network of systems which interact with specific stimulus–response processing systems (Posner & Peterson, 1990). Within this network, certain regions have been ascribed specific functions through the use of LESION techniques in animal studies and the development of sophisticated human brain scanning techniques such as POSITRON EMISSION TOMOGRAPHY and MAGNETIC RESONANCE IMAGING. For instance, the SUPERIOR COLLICULUS is likely to have responsibility for movement of visual attention through its involvement in eye movements. The lateral pulvinar of the THALAMUS and the posterior PARIETAL CORTEX have been highlighted as crucial for the engagement and disengagement of attention respectively. The PREFRONTAL CORTEX has been shown to be required for making successful extra-dimensional shifts. In addition, the neurochemistry of attentional processes is beginning to unfold. Forebrain CHOLINERGIC and brainstem NORADRENERGIC systems which innervate the cerebral cortex are thought to be involved in aspects of accuracy, while the brainstem cholinergic, SEROTONERGIC and noradrenergic systems may enhance sensory awareness by their enhancement of the excitability of thalamic relay neurons. The NIGROSTRIATAL DOPAMINE SYSTEM titrates MOTOR READINESS. The discovery that attention can be broken down into distinct neurochemical and neuroanatomical components has supported its investigation within the context of disease states. For instance, the parietal lobes have been linked particularly closely with attentional neglect (see NEGLECT SYNDROME), the frontal lobes have been associated with perseverative deficits in SCHIZOPHRENIA, and attentional deficits in patients with ALZHEIMER'S DEMENTIA have been attributed to a loss of forebrain ACETYLCHOLINE.

See also: attention-deficit disorder

Reference

Posner M.I. & Peterson S.E. (1990) The attention system of the human brain. *Annual Review of Neuroscience* 13: 25–42.

Robbins T.W. (1998) Arousal and attention: psychopharmacological and neuropsychological studies in experimental animals. In *The Attentive Brain*, ed. R. Parasuraman, pp.189–220, MIT Press: Cambridge MA.

WENDY L. INGLIS

attention-deficit disorder Attention-deficit/hyperactivity disorder (AD/HD) is characterized by a triad of symptoms involving persistent age-inappropriate problems of HYPERACTIVITY, inattention and impulsivity. Hyperactivity may be manifested as fidgeting, appearing to be driven by a motor, never sitting quietly and talking excessively. Impulsivity may be manifested as impatience and difficulty in delaying responses, often interrupting others. Inattention may demonstrate as a failing to give attention to detail in work and difficulty in sustaining attention in tasks or play activities.

Epidemiologically AD/HD ranks as, probably, the most common psychiatric disturbance of childhood, affecting an estimated 3–5% of school-age children in Britain, with a greater preponderance of males in clinically referred samples; the sex ratio ranging from 3:1 to 9:1. Non-referred population samples suggest a lower sex ratio of 2:1 to 3:1. The age of onset is usually in toddlerhood with a peak age of onset around 3–4 years of age. Around one half of children with AD/HD in the clinical and general populations are comorbid with oppositional defiant disorder or conduct disorder. There is also a higher prevalence of mood disorders, anxiety disorders, learning disorders and communication disorders in AD/HD children. For most individuals, symptoms of AD/HD usually decrease in adolescence and early adulthood. However, AD/HD is a risk factor for later psychiatric disorder (in particular conduct disorder and adult antisocial personality disorder), SUBSTANCE ABUSE, poor social achievement and poor social adjustment. In addition, academic achievement is impaired in some children with AD/HD. Contributions to the possible causes of AD/HD include both environmental (including psychosocial) and organic (including genetic) risk factors. The psychosocial associations which may be aetiologically important are low socioeconomic status, institutional upbringing and adversity in, or lack of, close personal and family relationships. Genetically, AD/HD appears both familial and moderately heritable. Other suggested aetiological factors include brain dysfunction caused by lead intoxication, food additives, maternal smoking or starvation.

Neuropsychologically, children with AD/HD have impairments on tests of visuospatial functioning, certain MEMORY tests and perform poorly on tests of ATTENTION, showing reduced attention span and problems on tests of sustained, selective and spatial attention. They also demonstrate deficits on tests of EXECUTIVE FUNCTION such as tasks involving problem solving, planning, fluency and cognitive flexibility. Additionally, children with AD/HD may have a lower IQ and poorer reading skills when compared to normal children. Differences in brain structure in AD/HD, as measured by COMPUTERIZED AXIAL TOMOGRAPHY and MAGNETIC RESONANCE IMAGING, show some consonance with the neuropsychological impairments. In AD/HD samples there appear to be abnormalities in the BASAL GANGLIA, CORPUS CALLOSUM, CEREBRAL CORTEX, and the CEREBELLUM. Reduced metabolism and cerebral blood flow in frontal and parietal cortex, and subcortical regions in AD/HD has also been reported. Several theories have been proposed to try and explain the range of impairments seen in AD/HD, such as motoric theories, motivational theories, defects in executive function, a state regulation deficit, dysfunctional LEARNING and abnormal sensitivity to REWARD.

Treatment of AD/HD usually involves stimulant medication such as METHYLPHENIDATE (Ritalin) or dextro-amphetamine (see AMPHETAMINE). They have been used in the treatment of hyperactivity since the late 1950s. Their central nervous system action is to release dopamine and noradrenaline and block their reuptake at the presynaptic terminal. Clinically, treatment improves inattention, reduces motor activity, improves behaviour and, in some children, improves academic performance. Preliminary studies on measurements of brain function during treatment, using BRAIN IMAGING techniques, indicate that methylphenidate appears to increase reduced blood flow to the frontal cortex and basal ganglia and decrease blood flow to the motor cortex and primary sensory cortex.

Treating a child with stimulants may not be the complete solution. Initially it may be a useful means of gaining parental co-operation and is in fact associated with more expressed positive contact from parents and siblings, which could allow for adjunctive psychological treatments to become feasible. Indeed, some hyperactive children appear not to respond to stimulant medication, while side-effects in others necessitate withdrawal. In these cases psychological treatments may also be possible. Examples include behavioural approaches, which are best achieved via school-based programmes; COGNITIVE THERAPY approaches which use self-instruction strategies to enhance self-control and self-regulation; and parental training aimed at improving parental skills and child-behaviour management and reducing stress.

BARBARA J. SAHAKIAN AND MITUL MEHTA

attentional dyslexia *see* acquired dyslexia

attentional set The allocation of ATTENTION to a particular feature or class of features of stimuli. This enables more rapid discrimination of and response to stimuli, as only currently relevant features are selected for further processing and irrelevant features may be rejected.

See also: attentional set-shifting; extradimensional shift; intradimensional shift; mental set

VERITY J. BROWN

attentional set-shifting Discriminating and responding to a STIMULUS based on features of that stimulus results in the formation of an ATTENTIONAL SET, which enhances the efficiency of processing of the relevant features. When the contingencies of discriminating and responding to stimuli change, it may be necessary to abandon the current attentional set and to change, or shift, attention to enable the rapid discrimination of and response to another feature or class of features (see DISENGAGE AND SHIFTING ATTENTION). A class of features or attributes by which stimuli may be classified and discriminated is called a STIMULUS DIMENSION. A dimension might be a physical attribute of a stimulus, such as the colour of a visual object, or it might be a semantic attribute of a stimulus, such as words and non-words. Variations within a stimulus dimension are called exemplars. Thus, yellow is an exemplar of the dimension colour.

See also: extradimensional shift; intradimensional shift

VERITY J. BROWN

atto- Prefix indicating a factor of 10^{-18}, or one million million millionth; see SI UNITS.

attributable risk *see* risk

attribution An attribution is an inference we make about the perceived underlying dispositional characteristics about ourselves or another organism. The subject of our attributions, however, can vary from those aspects of an indi-

vidual's persona such as INTELLIGENCE, humour, or aggressiveness (see AGGRESSION) to the ascription of emotional states (see EMOTION) and intention. Social psychology has largely focused on the latter where intention is considered to be a central component of our system of beliefs about why individuals behave in the way they do and the ascriptions we give regarding causality, responsibility and blame. Attributions can focus on whether behaviour is considered dispositionally or externally based, stable or unstable, global or specific, or controllable or uncontrollable. *Attribution theory* refers to a number of social psychological models which attempt to formalize the psychological processes involved in comparing and weighing available information. The attributions we make, however, are generally regarded to reveal more about the perceiver than the perceived. Attributional research is largely concerned with the consequences of such attributions for our emotions and behaviour.

MALCOLM D. MACLEOD

atypical depression Also known as hysteroid dysphoria is a recognized subtype of DEPRESSION in which the principal SIGNS AND SYMPTOMS are an increase in APPETITE, possibly featuring a craving for CARBOHYDRATE and increased BODY WEIGHT; FATIGUE; a depressed MOOD (which often worsens during the day); and rejection sensitivity (a heightened reactivity to the thoughts and behaviour of others). It is also characterized by resistance to TRICYCLIC ANTIDEPRESSANT therapy. The most common estimate is that some 15 per cent of individuals presenting with depression have this atypical form.

atypical antipsychotic *see* antipsychotic

atypical neuroleptic *see* antipsychotic

audiogenic Literally, produced by sound. Clearly, all sorts of normal actions and reactions are produced by hearing sounds of a wide variety of types. The term AUDIOGENIC therefore tends to be used when there is some particular reason to highlight the role of sound in eliciting a response (for example, audiogenic seizures – see EPILEPSY) or when the behaviour produced by a sound is particularly striking (see STARTLE REFLEX).

audition (from Latin, *audire*: to hear) Audition is synonymous with hearing: it refers to the act of, or the sense of, hearing. (Note that the term audition, meaning a test performance, for instance for a theatrical role, comes for the same Latin root.)

See also: hearing theories

auditory agnosia An agnosia is a failure in obtaining access to stored knowledge or object-specific representation. Auditory agnosia is a specific form of agnosia in which the disturbance in confined to the identification of sounds.

See also: agnosia; object agnosia; tactile agnosia; visual agnosia

auditory aphasia A form of APHASIA in which the main feature is an inability to understand spoken words; it is also known as WORD DEAFNESS.

auditory canal The connecting passage between the outer ear (the PINNA) and the EARDRUM.

auditory cortex The auditory cortex comprises at least half a dozen interconnected and specialized auditory areas in the superior TEMPORAL LOBE that receive specific afferent input at deep layer III and layer IV from the MEDIAL GENICULATE NUCLEUS in the THALAMUS. At least three levels of processing have been distinguished in cat auditory cortex. The primary areas contain a fine-tuned TONOTOPIC REPRESENTATION of the COCHLEA on the contralateral side, whereas the secondary and tertiary areas are broader tuned so that a tonotopic organization is more difficult to demonstrate. In primates the secondary cortical (or belt) areas surround the primary (or core) areas. Besides being tonotopically organized, several neural properties are mapped systematically on the surface of the primary auditory cortex such as sensitivity, frequency-tuning curve bandwidth, capacity to follow periodic changes in sound and sensitivity to binaural or spatial input. In auditory specialized animals such as echolocating bats (see ECHOLOCATION) the auditory cortex contains maps of ecologically valuable echo features such as intensity, echo delay and echo fre-

quency Doppler shift reflecting target size, distance and approach velocity as well as insect wing-beat frequency.

In auditory non-specialists such as the cat (and primates) the primary auditory cortex is specialized in the analysis of broadband, mostly transient, sounds that allows fine timing discrimination important for certain aspects of complex sound (SPEECH PERCEPTION). A LESION in the human primary auditory cortex will abolish consonant–vowel phoneme perception but leave vowel perception or pure tone frequency discrimination intact. The anterior auditory field, also a primary area, appears to prefer temporally structured narrow band sounds with a higher resolution of periodicities but still less than 100–200 Hz. Thus it is doubtful that periodicity pitch (see AUDITORY PERCEPTION) is based on temporal coding in auditory cortex. The secondary or tertiary areas, such as those in the superior temporal gyrus in monkeys, may be specialized for extracting more specific sound features and may be tuned to specific communication calls. Primary auditory cortex analyses sound azimuth based on tonotopic binaural information and is mandatory for the execution of learned sound localization behaviour. A multi-modal tertiary area, the anterior ECTOSYLVIAN SULCUS, shows a modest sensitivity to sound azimuth, improved over that in primary cortex, but without a well defined map of auditory space such as present in the SUPERIOR COLLICULUS.

Reference

Aitkin, L. (1990) *The Auditory Cortex: Structural and Functional Bases of Auditory Perception*, Chapman & Hall: London.

JOS J. EGGERMONT

auditory fusion *see* binaural

auditory meatus (from Latin, *meare*: to go) The term meatus indicates an opening: the auditory meatus is a passageway associated with the AUDITORY SYSTEM. The external auditory meatus (also known as the auditory canal) is a connecting passage between the outer ear (the PINNA) and the EARDRUM; the internal auditory meatus is a passageway through the

TEMPORAL BONE, giving nerves access from the ear to the CENTRAL NERVOUS SYSTEM.

auditory nerve The auditory nerve consists of about 40 000 nerve fibres innervating the INNER HAIR CELLS with about 20 fibres per cell. The nerve fibres run through the petrous bone to trifurcate (split into three) and synapse on cells in each of three specialized subdivisions of the COCHLEAR NUCLEUS. The fibres are myelinated and homogeneous in diameter with a conduction velocity of about 20 m/s. The fibres can be distinguished on basis of spontaneous activity and threshold of activation. Low-threshold fibres have high spontaneous activity and synapse with large contacts on the inner hair cells, higher-threshold fibres have lower spontaneous activity and smaller synaptic endings.

JOS J. EGGERMONT

auditory pathways The auditory pathways begin with the transduction of sound into neural impulses in the COCHLEA. From the cochlea, the COCHLEA NERVE (also known as the AUDITORY NERVE and, with the VESTIBULAR NERVE, one of the principal branches of the VESTIBULOCOCHLEAR NERVE [the eighth cranial nerve]) travels to the COCHLEAR NUCLEUS in the pons via the COCHLEA NERVE GANGLION. The cochlear nerve ganglion contains BIPOLAR NEURONS: one limb receives information from the cochlea; then other limb transmits to the cochlear nucleus. This ganglion is also known as the SPIRAL GANGLION, its shape reflecting that of the cochlea itself. The auditory pathway so far is organized entirely ipsilaterally. At the level of the cochlear nucleus there is crossing of information to enable binaural perception of sound: the anteroventral and posteroventral portions of the cochlear nucleus project ipsilaterally and contralaterally to the SUPERIOR OLIVARY COMPLEX. The dorsal cochlear nucleus projects contralaterally to the INFERIOR COLLICULUS.

From the cochlear nucleus information is transmitted via the TRAPEZOID BODY (a bundle of horizontal fibres that is part of the superior olivary complex) and via the DORSAL ACOUSTIC STRIA and INTERMEDIATE ACOUSTIC STRIA, to the superior olivary complex: the lateral portion of this (the LATERAL SUPERIOR OLIVE) is concerned with the localization of sound in space, while the medial portion (the MEDIAL SUPERIOR OLIVE) is concerned with sound localization. Neurons in the lateral and medial portions of the superior olivary complex, and fibres travelling from the cochlear nucleus that have not made contact with the superior olivary complex at all, then travel via the LATERAL LEMNISCUS to the INFERIOR COLLICULUS. (The lateral lemniscus is made up of fibres from the superior olivary complex and the cochlear nucleus travelling to the inferior colliculus, and it contains some cell bodies in the NUCLEI OF THE LATERAL LEMNISCUS, where some of the auditory fibres SYNAPSE.) The inferior colliculus receives input from the ipsi- and contralateral cochlea, the ispi- and contralateral superior olivary complex, and from both ipsi- and contralateral nuclei of the lateral lemniscus. It projects to the MEDIAL GENICULATE NUCLEUS (or medial geniculate body) in the THALAMUS, which then projects to the AUDITORY CORTEX.

These are the ascending auditory pathways; there are also descending pathways. The superior olivary complex sends axons back to the cochlea via the OLIVOCOCHLEAR BUNDLE, a collection of fibres that travel via the cochlea nerve (which thus has fibres travelling in both directions along it). These axons synapse on the INNER HAIR CELLS, where they use ACETYLCHOLINE as a neurotransmitter (unlike the ascending fibres in the cochlea nerve, which appear to use GLUTAMATE or aspartate [see ASPARTIC ACID] as NEUROTRANSMITTERS).

For further information, see the individual entries for the various structures.

See also: auditory perception; auditory system; hearing theories

auditory perception The extraction, categorization and grouping of sound features that allows the analysis of scenes into well segregated sources are the most important aspects of auditory perception. Hearing comprises a combination of an analysis stage in the COCHLEA and a central stage of synthesis. The analysis stage is characterized by frequency resolution, the capacity to project the components of complex sound on a frequency scale, by nonlinear processing which allows the large dynamic range and generates combination tones, and by lateral suppression providing contrast enhancement in the frequency domain. The ability to hear the myriad of combination tones when two tones are presented simultaneously (see OTOACOUSTIC EMISSIONS) relates to the essential non-linear nature of BASILAR MEMBRANE movement largely caused by the action of the outer hair cells (see HAIR CELLS). Most of the analysis capacities are attributable to cochlear frequency analysis (see AUDITORY TUNING CURVE). For instance the just-noticeable difference (jnd) for frequency is about 0.15% between 500 and 2000 Hz. The jnd for intensity discrimination drops from about 1.5 dB at near threshold levels to about 0.5 dB at levels of 80 dB above threshold. The critical band width, reflecting the perceptual frequency selectivity, is constant at about 150 Hz for frequencies below 1000 Hz and then increases proportional to frequency to become 1500 Hz at 10 kHz.

The synthesis stage allows the perception of LOUDNESS by integrating the total neural activity from the auditory nerve, of TIMBRE by analysing the distribution pattern of neural activity across frequency, and of PITCH by extracting local peaks in that neural distribution. Intensity discrimination, especially of pure tones depends on frequency selectivity. Integrating and comparing across frequency channels, and perceiving changes in the shape of acoustic spectra becomes important. An analysis that takes the profile of the entire ACOUSTIC SPECTRUM into account stresses the importance of, for instance, common rates of amplitude and frequency modulation and constancy of ratios of FORMANT FREQUENCIES. This leads to an emphasis on 'perceptual binding' (see BINDING PROBLEM) of extracted features into a coherent whole based on this covariation of transient changes across frequency and of continuity or slow change in frequency across time. As a result, the separation of an auditory scene in individual sound sources becomes possible.

References

Bregman A.S. (1990) *Auditory Scene Analysis*, MIT Press: Cambridge MA.
Green D.M. (1988) *Profile Analysis. Auditory Intensity Discrimination*, Oxford University Press: New York.

JOS J. EGGERMONT

auditory system The auditory system *en masse* includes all elements from the PINNA through to the AUDITORY CORTEX. The pinna is connected to the AUDITORY CANAL at the end of which is the EARDRUM (the TYMPANIC MEMBRANE). Air pressure here moves this membrane causing movement of the bones on the other side – the OSSICLES. These transmit pressure changes into the COCHLEA, where transduction of these pressure changes into neural signals takes place at the ORGAN OF CORTI (which includes the basilar membrane, HAIR CELLS and the TECTORIAL MEMBRANE). From here the COCHLEA NERVE (a branch of the VESTIBULOCOCHLEAR NERVE, the eighth cranial nerve) carries information away, connecting through the AUDITORY PATHWAYS to the auditory cortex.

See also: auditory perception; ear; hearing theories

auditory tuning curve An auditory tuning curve consists of sound frequency-level combinations that border the receptive field of, for example, an AUDITORY NERVE fibre. The frequency at the lowest sound level of the tuning curve is the characteristic frequency. The ratio of the characteristic frequency to the bandwidth, distance in Hz between the high and low frequency border 10 dB above the level at characteristic frequency, is the quality factor (Q10dB) which ranges from about 1 at low to about 6 at high frequencies. The tuning reflects that of the BASILAR MEMBRANE section under the inner hair cell that the auditory nerve fibre innervates.

JOS J. EGGERMONT

aura (from Latin, *aura*: a breeze) Aura is a term given to the rather unusual sensations that can precede an attack of EPILEPSY.

autism A developmental disorder characterized by impairments in social, imaginative and communicative functions, with restricted repetitive interests and activities. Qualitative impairments are evident by age three, although diagnosis often occurs much later. Since the manifestation of these impairments changes with age, and varies among individuals, autism is sometimes conceptualized as a spectrum. Prevalence is estimated at 4–10 per 10 000, according to the breadth of definition used. Males outnumber females by 3 to 1, and among high-functioning individuals by at least 5 to 1. The disorder is accompanied by general developmental delay/low INTELLIGENCE QUOTIENT (IQ) in perhaps three-quarters of cases, and by EPILEPSY in at least a third. These facts, among others, have argued against the PSYCHOGENIC view of autism as caused by 'refrigerator parenting', an outdated view now abandoned in favour of a biological explanation. Indeed, signs of social peculiarity in parents of children with autism may be results rather than causes of the child's disorder, or may be signs of the 'extended phenotype' of autism, which appears to have a significant genetic component. Concordance rates for MONOZYGOTIC TWINS may be between 30 and 90%, according to the breadth of definition used, compared with a concordance for DIZYGOTIC TWINS of 0–10%. Siblings show a risk of autism at least 50 times that of the normal population. Current research appears to support a multiplicative multilocus model of inheritance. Obstetric complications, which are common in autism, are thought to be the result, rather than cause, of the child's abnormalities.

The brain basis of autism is as yet unclear, with candidate regions including the CEREBELLUM, LIMBIC SYSTEM and FRONTAL LOBE being actively researched. *In vivo* and pathological anatomical studies, biochemical and electrophysiological investigations have provided some suggestive findings, but results have often remained unreplicated, and in many cases show abnormalities unlikely to be either specific or universal to autism. Functional brain imaging investigations have only just begun and may prove useful. At present there is no specific drug treatment for autism but, in the absence of a 'cure', well-informed education and management achieves significant improvements.

More progress has been made in understanding the nature of the cognitive deficits in autism. A challenge here has been to explain why social, communication and imagination deficits should go together (often referred to as WING'S TRIAD, following epidemiological work by Wing and Gould which established this co-occurrence), and why other functions (for instance spatial skills, rote MEMORY) are often intact or even superior in autism. A currently influential hypothesis is that people with autism lack THEORY OF MIND – that is, they are unable to represent mental states (see METAREPRESENTATION), and fail to recognize the thoughts and feelings of those around them. Children with autism fail to show behaviours which require theory of mind (understanding deception, or keeping secrets for example), although other social abilities may be intact (such as attachment to parents). The earliest manifestation of this 'mind-blindness' may be a lack of pretend play, gaze following and joint attention at 18 months. The theory-of-mind account of autism has led to progress in early identification of autism, attempts to teach social insight, and FUNCTIONAL NEUROIMAGING of the regions normally involved in mental state attribution. Some people with autism, especially those with ASPERGER'S SYNDROME, who fall at the able end of the spectrum, do pass tests of theory of mind, though typically they are delayed by many years and appear to have developed alternative strategies for social insight.

Autism is characterized by a range of nonsocial symptoms which defy explanation in terms of theory of mind; motor stereotypies (see STEREOTYPY), obsessive interests, repetitive behaviours, savant skills (see IDIOT SAVANT), markedly uneven IQ sub-test profile, fragmented and anomalous perceptual experiences. Failures of inhibition, and a tendency to perseverate (see PERSEVERATION) as well as difficulties in planning and monitoring behaviour, have led to the suggestion that impaired EXECUTIVE FUNCTION (due perhaps to frontal lobe damage) might explain social and nonsocial handicaps in autism. The only current theory attempting to explain autistic skills and preserved abilities is the notion that people with autism have a different information processing style – referred to as weak 'CENTRAL COHERENCE' – with a processing preference for parts over wholes, and an ability to process information piecemeal independent of context. Research on autism (theory of mind, executive functions and coherence) has had significant influence on current theories of normal cognition.

References

Bailey A., Phillips W. & Rutter M. (1996) Autism: towards an integration of clinical, genetic, neuropsychological, and neurobiological perspectives. *Journal of Child Psychology and Psychiatry* 37: 89–126.

Happé, F. (1994) *Autism: An Introduction to Psychological Theory*, Harvard University Press: Cambridge MA.

FRANCESCA G. HAPPÉ

autobiographical memory Autobiographical memory refers to an individual's personal memories of the events in his or her life. Autobiographical memory, in contrast to SEMANTIC MEMORY, is specific to some earlier time and place. Autobiographical recollection implies mental time travel, that is, the placing of oneself within some previous episode or, alternatively, as an observer of a previous episode. Studies of autobiographical recollections of the remote past document that the general meaning and the general texture of past experiences are remembered accurately. However, it is not uncommon to have confusions about the temporal order of events, to have SOURCE AMNESIA, and to commit errors in recalling specific episodes and events. Finally, autobiographical memory extends back only to about the age of 3½ years to the period of INFANTILE AMNESIA.

See also: episodic memory

LARRY R. SQUIRE

autocatalysis A form of catalysis in which the product of a reaction in turn catalyses the reaction that produced it.

autochthonous (from Greek, *autos*: self, *chthonos*: soil) Something is said to be autochthonous if it is derived from the place in which it is found.

autocrine Paracrine release of a chemical (e.g. NEUROTRANSMITTERS or HORMONES) involves that chemical acting on a cell other than the one which released it. Autocrine release involves a chemical being released in a paracrine-like manner, but acting on the cell that did the releasing.

autografts Transplantation of cells, organs or tissues back into the same individual that has donated those tissues. Cells derived from the donor will not suffer immunological rejection, and autografts avoid the need for IMMUNOSUPPRESSION. Autografts have been used in developmental studies of organization and regeneration in CORTICAL MAPS, for instance after rotation of the barrel fields. Easily accessible peripheral cells (such as fibroblasts) are popular for GENETIC ENGINEERING prior to implantation in the nervous system. Adrenal autografts have been employed in PARKINSON'S DISEASE, but with only limited success.

See also: transplantation

STEPHEN B. DUNNETT

autoimmune disease *see* immune system

autokinetic effect *see* visual direction

automatic action For automatic action, see VOLUNTARY. Automaticity is the adjective that refers to an automatic action.

automatic vs. controlled attention This refers to the proposed distinction between those attentional processes which are thought to draw upon central cognitive resources (controlled attention) and those attentional processes which are thought not to draw upon such resources (AUTOMATIC ATTENTION). This dichotomy also relates to a more general distinction made in cognitive psychology between resource-dependent (controlled) and resource independent (automatic) cognitive processes (Schneider & Shiffrin, 1977). Controlled attentional processing is deemed to be demanding of attention capacity, serial in nature, amenable to conscious control and effortful. By contrast, automatic attentional processing is regarded as demanding little (if any) attentional capacity, being parallel and difficult (if not impossible) to modify or suppress. Controlled and automatic processes may be characterized in operational terms: performance on tasks requiring the allocation of controlled attentional processes should suffer if an individual is required concomitantly to perform another cognitive task, whereas performance on tasks which are mediated by automatic attentional processes should show no such impairment. Unfortunately, the terms controlled and automatic attention are often used more loosely to refer to hypothetical constructs which have not been delineated in an experimental manner.

See also: attention

Reference

Schneider W. & Shiffrin R. M. (1977) Controlled and automatic human information processing: I. Detection, search, and attention. *Psychological Review* 84: 1–66.

JONATHAN K. FOSTER

automatism A feature of EPILEPSY in which consciousness is absent, but muscle tone and posture are retained and simple motor acts can be completed without awareness. The duration of automatism within an epileptic attack can be very variable.

autonomic (from Greek, *autos*: self, *nomos*: law) Self-governing – relating to the actions of the AUTONOMIC NERVOUS SYSTEM.

autonomic nervous system (ANS) A component part of the PERIPHERAL NERVOUS SYSTEM, the ANS was originally considered primarily an effector or motor system, but afferent axons from the VISCERA and central autonomic pathways were also included as elements of the system. The term 'autonomic' was coined by J.N. Langley (1852–1925) at the turn of the twentieth century to reflect the reflex nature and relative independence from conscious control of this component of the nervous system. The ANS exerts largely involuntary control of the activity of viscera, glands and smooth muscle but CONDITIONING experiments and BIOFEEDBACK training demonstrate that limited voluntary control can be achieved over visceral functions. Classically, the ANS consists of two main divisions: the SYMPATHETIC NERVOUS SYSTEM and the PARASYMPATHETIC NERVOUS SYSTEM. A third component known as the ENTERIC NERVOUS SYSTEM is usually considered separately because of its association with the gastrointestinal tract.

Most viscera and glands receive a dual, functionally reciprocal innervation from the sympathetic and parasympathetic divisions of the ANS. The sympathetic nervous system is dominant in situations involving stress (FIGHT-OR-FLIGHT situations) while the parasympathetic system is more active during rest and the conservation and restoration of energy. The two divisions are tonically active and their actions tend to produce opposite effects such that a balance exists between them with the relative dominance of one or the other depending on circumstances. Some organ systems are regulated by only one division, or are regulated by a complementary rather than an antagonistic relationship. The ANS is a highly dynamic, continuously active system which affects virtually every aspect of maintenance of the internal milieu of the body, including adjustments to blood pressure in response to changing POSTURE, THERMOREGULATION, DIGESTION and a constellation of major physiological responses to states of EMOTION and PAIN.

The basic organization of the ANS is a two-neuron chain consisting of a PREGANGLIONIC NEURON in the central nervous system that projects to a POSTGANGLIONIC NEURON in a peripheral autonomic ganglion. The sympathetic or thoracolumbar preganglionic neurons are located in the LATERAL HORN and the intermediomedial nucleus of the thoracic and upper segments of the lumbar SPINAL CORD (T1–L3). They project via ventral roots to peripheral sympathetic ganglia located near the vertebral column (paravertebral and cervical ganglia of the sympathetic trunk) and in neural plexuses of the abdomen (prevertebral sympathetic ganglia). Long unmyelinated postganglionic sympathetic axons then project to the eyes, lacrimal glands, salivary glands, mucous membranes of the head, and to the respiratory, cardiovascular, digestive, urinary and reproductive systems. Sympathetic axons are closely associated with blood vessels which they also innervate, having a vasoconstrictor function. Sympathetic axons in the skin innervate blood vessels, sweat glands and the arrector pili smooth muscle of hair follicles.

Parasympathetic or craniosacral preganglionic neurons are found in the brainstem and sacral spinal cord (S2–S4). Parasympathetic ganglia are found in or near the target organs. Brainstem preganglionic axons leave the brain via four CRANIAL NERVES (third, seventh, ninth and tenth) and project long, myelinated axons to autonomic ganglia in the head. Short, unmyelinated postganglionic axons innervate the eyes, lacrimal glands, salivary glands and mucous membranes. The tenth cranial nerve (the VAGUS NERVE) projects to autonomic ganglia closely associated with the respiratory system, heart, gastrointestinal tract, liver and kidneys.

ACETYLCHOLINE is the neurotransmitter for pre- and postganglionic parasympathetic neurons and for postganglionic sympathetic neurons innervating sweat glands, while NORADRENALINE is the transmitter for all other postganglionic sympathetic neurons. In addition, many neurons of the sympathetic division of the ANS have one or more NEUROPEPTIDES colocalized with their classical neurotransmitters.

Afferent information from the viscera and blood vessels is carried to the spinal cord by axons that travel in autonomic nerves of the viscera, in somatic nerves and in the GLOSSOPHARYNGEAL NERVE and vagus nerve to modulate visceral reflexes and to be relayed to higher levels of the NEURAXIS. Most of the detailed incoming information regarding the state of the viscera is not consciously perceived. Visceral sensations of fullness, motility and pain can be appreciated but not with the precise localization characteristic of somatic sensation. Visceral and somatic pain are among the most powerful activators of the ANS.

Ascending and descending central autonomic neural pathways integrate autonomic, ENDOCRINE and behavioural responses against a background of HOMEOSTATIC and non-homeostatic mechanisms and ongoing MOTIVATION and EMOTION. Central autonomic pathways are characterized by reciprocal connections and redundancy. The NUCLEUS OF THE SOLITARY TRACT and the PARABRACHIAL NUCLEI of the PONS, nuclei that receive afferent visceral information either directly or indirectly from the cranial nerves or spinal cord, are the main ascending waystations of central autonomic pathways. Ascending projections also relay visceral afferent information to the HY-POTHALAMUS, LIMBIC SYSTEM and CEREBRAL CORTEX (insular and prefrontal). Important descending central autonomic pathways arise from the cerebral cortex, AMYGDALA, hypothalamus and periaqueductal GREY MATTER to act upon autonomic centres and preganglionic neurons of the BRAINSTEM and spinal cord.

DAVID A. HOPKINS

autopsy (from Greek, *autos*: self, *opsis*: sight) a *POST MORTEM* examination of a body.

autoradiogram The output of autoradiography; see AUTORADIOGRAPHY.

autoradiography An anatomical technique to localize radiolabelled markers in tissue sections (see RADIOLABEL). Radioisotopes may include ^{3}H, ^{32}P, ^{35}S or ^{125}I. These markers are visualized either by laying X-ray film over histologically processed sections on slides (see HISTOLOGY), or by coating such slides with a photographic emulsion which provides better cellular resolution. Following exposure, the film or slides are developed as in photography, visualizing the labels as dark silver grains. For RECEPTOR BINDING autoradiography, a radioactive label is tagged to a LIGAND of interest. For *IN SITU* HYBRIDIZATION, complementary DNA, RNA or oligonucleotide probes are tagged with a radioisotope.

KAZUE SEMBA

autoreceptor Autoreceptors are the receptors on terminals, soma or dendrites of a NEURON that bind the NEUROTRANSMITTERS released by the same neuron. The function of autoreceptors is best studied in monoamine neurons such as DOPAMINE neurons. Autoreceptors are usually inhibitory, and the activation of autoreceptors at the soma results in HYPERPOLARIZATION , while the activation of autoreceptors at terminals usually results in a decrease in transmitter release. Antagonism at autoreceptors is an effective way of modulating neurotransmission, and autoreceptors are considered to be sites of interest for pharmacological interventions in movement and AFFECTIVE DISORDERS.

See also: heteroceptors

KAZUE SEMBA

autoshaping The approach to or avoidance of a stimulus which, by PAVLOVIAN CONDITIONING, reliably predicts a positive or negative event. For example, pigeons will approach and peck at a disc when it is illuminated (CONDITIONED STIMULUS) just prior to delivery of grain (UNCONDITIONED STIMULUS), but they will avoid the same stimulus if it predicts non-delivery of grain. Autoshaping may be an innate tracking response linked to survival mechanisms, although Pavlovian theory explains it in terms of stimulus substitution: pigeons appear to 'eat' the conditioned stimulus when it predicts food, and 'drink' it when it predicts water.

WENDY L. INGLIS

autosomal chromosome A chromosome which is not a sex (X or Y) chromosome. In DIPLOID organisms, there are two of each autosomal chromosome, and two sex chromosomes.

FIONA M. INGLIS

autosomal dominant/recessive A term describing an ALLELE of a GENE found on an AUTOSOMAL CHROMOSOME. Because there are two of each autosomal chromosome per cell, a dominant allele will mask a recessive allele, so that the dominant characteristic will be observed in the organism. If both alleles are recessive, then the recessive trait will be observed.

FIONA M. INGLIS

autosomal recessive see autosomal dominant/recessive

autosome see cell division

autostereogram see autostereopsis

autostereopsis Any means of presenting the BINOCULAR DISPARITY information for stereoscopic DEPTH PERCEPTION to the viewer without the use of a viewing device such as a stereoscope or image-separating spectacles. The most widespread form of autostereopsis is the lenticular screen of stereoscopic postcards in which two (or more) different images are projected into space for different viewing angles by local refraction at each lenticular cylinder in the screen. A more recent technique is the AUTOSTEREOGRAM, a type of printed image developed by C. W. Tyler from the RANDOM-DOT STEREOGRAM by encoding the information required for both eyes in a single image, from which the binocular disparity information is read out by viewing the image with a small convergence or divergence of the eyes.

Reference

Tyler C.W. (1983) Sensory processing of binocular disparity. In *Vergence Eye Movements: Basic and Clinical Aspects*, ed. C.M. Schor and K.J. Cuiffreda, pp. 199–295, Butterworth: Boston MA.

CHRISTOPHER TYLER

aversive conditioning Aversive conditioning is a CONDITIONING process that involves aversive, as opposed to appetitive stimuli. Aversive conditioning can be employed in a CLASSICAL CONDITIONING paradigm, or an INSTRUMENTAL CONDITIONING paradigm. Aversive instrumental conditioning can include ACTIVE AVOIDANCE, PASSIVE AVOIDANCE or PUNISHMENT procedures.

JOHN D. SALAMONE

aversive stimulus *see* negative reinforcer

avoidance learning *see* active avoidance; animal models of anxiety; passive avoidance

avolition A lack of will, energy and interest; it describes a condition in DEPRESSION and is one of the NEGATIVE SYMPTOMS of SCHIZOPHRENIA.

axial About an axis; so for example, the term axial symptoms would refer to deviations in POSTURE or behaviour about an axis. ROTATION could be described as movement about an axis; similarly, BARREL ROLLING occurs about a rat's long axis.

See also: transplantation

axoaxonic A term describing a synaptic connection between two axons; see SYNAPSE.

axodendritic A term describing a synaptic connection between an axon and a dendrite; see SYNAPSE.

axolemma *see* membrane

axon The axon is the process of a NEURON whose function is to conduct action potentials. Unlike a DENDRITE, a neuron usually has only one axon. Axons can be myelinated (see MYELIN) or unmyelinated, and myelinated axons can conduct action potentials faster than unmyelinated axons due to SALTATORY CONDUCTION which allows action potentials to jump between the NODES OF RANVIER. The axon emerges from either the soma or a PROXIMAL DENDRITE. In humans, the longest axons can approach 1 m in length, as in the cases of MOTOR NEURONS that innervate the foot, or cortical PYRAMIDAL NEURONS that form the CORTICOSPINAL TRACT.

See also: action potential

KAZUE SEMBA

axon guidance The process by which a developing AXON locates its target; see GROWTH CONE; NEURODEVELOPMENT.

axon hillock *see* neuron

axon terminal An axon terminal is the typical presynaptic element of a SYNAPSE; also known as axon bulb, knob or bouton, or (more loosely) a SYNAPTIC TERMINAL.

See also: telodendria

axonal transport *see* axoplasm; cytoskeleton

axoplasm Axoplasm is cytoplasm but contained within an AXON. Axoplasm is not still: transport of various chemicals occurs, often in distinct channels formed within the neuronal CYTOSKELETON. Because there are channels available, axoplasm may be moving from soma to synaptic terminals in one channel and in reverse in another channel within the same axon. This process is known as AXOPLASMIC TRANSPORT.

axoplasmic transport *see* cytoskeleton

axosomatic A term describing a synaptic connection between an axon and a soma; see SYNAPSE.

axotomy Destruction or cutting of an AXON; it can be achieved experimentally by, for example, a KNIFE CUT LESION.

B

B cells *see* immune system

B-HT920 An alpha 2 noradrenaline receptor AGONIST; see ADRENOCEPTORS.

Babinski reflex (Babinski response, Babinski sign) 'Upgoing toe' – normally, stimulation of the sole of the foot produces downward toe-curling, but such stimulation in adult patients with damage in the CORTICOSPINAL TRACT produces upward curling (the same reaction as is produced in children less than 12 months old, in whom the corticospinal tracts are not fully mature).

backpropagation A method of training neural nets to produce correct answers. In SUPERVISED LEARNING, the difference between the output of the net and an externally specified target output, termed the error, is used to adjust the weights on the NETWORK NODES. The DELTA RULE is a procedure for computing the desired change for weights on to nodes in the net's output layer. If the net has one or more hidden layers, the delta rule needs to be generalized: the error signal must be propagated back to the hidden layer so the weights from the input layer can be altered correctly.

PAUL DEAN

backward conditioning A Pavlovian CONDITIONING procedure in which the UNCONDITIONED STIMULUS (US) precedes the CONDITIONED STIMULUS (CS) – the reverse of the sequence in DELAY CONDITIONING. It is sometimes used as a control condition for the assessment of Pavlovian conditioning: it matches subjects for experience of the CS and US but does not usually generate conditioned responding. Backward conditioning is, however, perhaps an unwise control treatment: under some circumstances (for example, when very few pairings are given) it can produce conditioned responding, and with more extended training it can produce CONDITIONED INHIBITION.

See also: trace conditioning

JASPER WARD-ROBINSON

baclofen The most widely used ANTAGONIST at the GABA-B receptor.

bag cell A type of neuron found in APLYSIA. Bag cells contain several NEUROPEPTIDES (known as bag cell peptides) and engage in complex neurosecretory processes during a burst of activity lasting about 20 minutes at the start of egg laying.

Reference

Pulst S.-M., Gusman D. & Mayeri E. (1988) Immunostaining for peptides of the egg-laying hormone / bag cell peptide precursor protein in the head ganglia of *Aplysia*. *Neuroscience* 27: 363–371.

bait shyness A reluctance of an animal to take the bait, usually food. Bait shyness might be the product of FOOD AVERSION LEARNING, although other forms of LEARNING can also be involved, as can SPATIAL MEMORY: food placed in a spatial location associated with NEGATIVE REINFORCEMENT will almost certainly be avoided.

balance The sense of balance is unusual in that there is little or no conscious awareness involved in the detection of imbalance or the correction of it. It is however a critical sense: unless the body is properly balanced, movement cannot occur. The lack of awareness can be considered a mark of the importance of this sense, and of the speed with which it is adjusted. Balance is a principal function of the VESTIBULAR SYSTEM.

See also: vestibular complex

Balint's syndrome A syndrome, first described by Rezsö Balint (1874–1929) in 1909, which follows bilateral damage to the parieto-occipital region of the CEREBRAL CORTEX. Balint's syndrome includes OPTIC ATAXIA (a difficulty in reaching for an object, even though it might be correctly identified and located in space); OCULAR APRAXIA (poor visual scanning in which the patient's eyes will wander off-target); and SIMULTAGNOSIA (a problem detecting more than one object at a time).

See also: ataxia

ballism (also known as ballismus) A form of MOVEMENT DEFICIT in which large, uncontrolled movements of the limbs occurs; see HEMIBALLISMUS.

ballistic (from Greek, *ballein*: to throw) A ballistic movement is one that, once initiated, cannot be interrupted or re-programmed; it is unaffected by feedback. A SACCADE is an example of a ballistic movement.

See also: closed loop, open loop; hemiballismus; servomechanism

band of Gennari *see* striate cortex

barbiturates A group of SEDATIVE drugs with similar chemical structure. The barbiturates comprise a class of compounds that are chemically derived from barbituric acid, which was first synthesized in 1864. All of these compounds (examples of which are PENTOBARBITAL, PHENOBARBITAL and THIOPENTAL) are potent sedative–HYPNOTIC (calming and sleep-inducing) drugs. In medicine these drugs have been used extensively as intravenous general ANAESTHETICS, and also as ANTICONVULSANTS. Considerable differences exist between differ-

ent types of barbiturates (with slightly varying chemical structure) with regard to onset and duration of action. For example, with thiopental the patient may fall asleep within seconds of infusion, and wake up five minutes later. Pentobarbital on the other hand induces sleep within five minutes of administration and has effects which last for up to sixty minutes. Before the development of the BENZODIAZEPINE drugs, barbiturates were also used to treat ANXIETY and INSOMNIA. However, their narrow THERAPEUTIC INDEX renders them quite dangerous, and much safer drugs are now used for these purposes. Barbiturates also have high ABUSE POTENTIAL, and chronic use can result in physical dependence. It is believed that barbiturates increase inhibitory mechanisms of the brain by enhancing NEUROTRANSMISSION at inhibitory GABA RECEPTORS, and generally suppress neuronal excitability.

ANN E. KELLEY

bare nerve ending The same as a FREE NERVE ENDING.

bariatric surgery Surgical interventions for the treatment of OBESITY. Old techniques, such as the insertion of a GASTRIC BALLOON or GASTRIC STAPLING are not favoured any longer, but various forms of intestinal bypass surgery are used to help individuals reduce BODY WEIGHT. The most common is the ROUX-EN-Y GASTRIC BY-PASS. The STOMACH is separated into two portions: the lower part and the upper portion of the small intestine is by-passed, the upper part of the stomach (some 30% of the total volume) being connected directly to the lower portion of the small intestine. Then procedure produces a reduction in food intake and changes in eating patterns. It is a radical inter-vention used only for the most pressing cases.

baroreceptor *see* osmoregulation

barrel cortex The BARREL CORTEX is a region of SOMATOSENSORY CORTEX in mice and rats that contains discrete groups of multicellular units, or barrel cells, each of which receives innervation from a single hair or VIBRISSAE on the contralateral face. Mechanical stimulation of a single whisker leads to local DEPOLARIZATION of the cells within this unit, which can be detected electrophysiologically. Cortical barrels are arranged topographically, resulting in a SOMATOTOPIC map of vibrissal cortical innervation. These barrels are arranged in columns running throughout the depth of the cortex, and thus receive information from, and send impulses to, other cortical and subcortical structures such as the THALAMUS. Cortical barrels are therefore considered computational units which transform vibrissal information and distribute it to various somatosensory processing areas of the brain. Cortical barrels have been studied extensively because of the ease with which single barrels may be excited through whisker stimulation.

See also: cortical columns and hypercolumns

FIONA M. INGLIS

barrel rolling An abnormal behaviour shown by rats, usually as part of range of CONVULSIONS and SEIZURES seen following administration of EXCITOTOXINS. Barrel rolling involves a rat rolling about its long axis (that is, the axis between the nose and tail). Episodes are relatively rare and, when they do occur following excitotoxin administration, never persist for more than approximately 2 hours, during the immediate recovery period.

Barrington's nucleus *see* micturition

basal Towards the base. For instance, the BASAL FOREBRAIN includes tissue in the forebrain towards the base of the brain.

basal cells Cells towards the base (that is, basal) of the olfactory epithelium which can act as STEM CELLS, providing replacement receptor molecules; see OLFACTION.

basal dendrite *see* apical dendrite

basal forebrain The ventral part of the FOREBRAIN. In a narrower definition, it refers to the areas of the ventral forebrain that contain CHOLINERGIC neurons. These areas include the medial septum (see SEPTAL NUCLEI), vertical and horizontal limb nuclei of the DIAGONAL BAND OF BROCA, VENTRAL PALLIDUM, magnocellular PREOPTIC AREA, substantia innominata and NUCLEUS BASALIS OF MEYNERT. Cholinergic neurons are distributed in a continuum across these regions. In a wider definition, the

basal forebrain refers to the entire ventral aspect of the forebrain, including the basal forebrain as above, as well as the ventral STRIATUM, septal nuclei, preoptic areas and anterior HYPOTHALAMUS.

KAZUE SEMBA

basal ganglia The basal ganglia, or basal nuclei, are SUBCORTICAL grey masses lateral to the THALAMUS in the basal parts of CEREBRAL HEMISPHERES. In the strict sense, they include the CORPUS STRIATUM, the CLAUSTRUM and the amygdaloid nuclear complex (see AMYGDALA). However, common usage tends not to group the amygdala with the basal ganglia and instead includes the diencephalic SUBTHALAMIC NUCLEUS and mesencephalic SUBSTANTIA NIGRA within a functional and connectional, rather than a topographical, definition. The corpus striatum is divided traditionally into the CAUDATE NUCLEUS and LENTIFORM NUCLEUS, the latter itself being divided into the medial GLOBUS PALLIDUS (or pallidum/ dorsal pallidum) and a more laterally placed PUTAMEN. This topographical delineation is also misleading. The caudate nucleus and putamen are in fact the same structure, being only separated in primate species by the large size of the INTERNAL CAPSULE, which artificially separates them into two separately named 'nuclei'. The caudate and putamen are often grouped together as the dorsal STRIATUM, to distinguish them from the ventral striatum which is largely comprised of the NUCLEUS ACCUMBENS and underlying OLFACTORY TUBERCLE.

The basal ganglia are interpolated within what is generally referred to as cortico-striato-pallido-thalamo-cortical loop circuitry (see CORTICOSTRIATAL LOOPS). The major AFFERENTS to the basal ganglia are from widespread areas of the CEREBRAL CORTEX and they arrive in the striatum in a topographically ordered pattern. The striatum receives two other major sources of afferents, namely a DOPAMINERGIC input from the midbrain (substantia nigra pars compacta which innervates the dorsal striatum; more medial dopaminergic neurons of the ventral tegmental area which innervate the ventral striatum) and the midline and intralaminar thalamic nuclei (so-called non-specific thalamic nuclei; see THALAMUS). EFFERENTS from the striatum reach various parts of the globus pallidus, which in turn projects to the thalamus (ventral anterior and medial dorsal nuclei) and then back to the FRONTAL and PREFRONTAL CORTEX, hence partially closing a cortico-cortical loop. In fact, discrete areas of the cortex have quite specific connections with sub-regions of the striatum, pallidum, thalamus and frontal lobes and this has been interpreted to indicate the existence of several anatomically segregated cortico-striato-pallido-thalamo-cortical loops with different motor, cognitive and affective functions. Diseases of the basal ganglia are associated with motor disorders and disturbances in cognitive processes. For example PARKINSON'S DISEASE is characterized by degeneration of the midbrain DOPAMINE neurons and hence dopamine depletion of the striatum, giving rise to difficulties in initiating movement (BRADYKINESIA or AKINESIA). Huntington's disease is an inherited disorder associated with degeneration of striatal neurons and is associated with CHOREA (involuntary movements, especially of the limbs) and also with a progressive DEMENTIA.

BARRY J. EVERITT

basal lamina A basal lamina is simply a layer (LAMINA, plural, LAMINAE) at the base (BASAL) of something. It may be a layer of MEMBRANE on an individual CELL or it may be a layer at the base of a structure. The OLFACTORY EPITHELIUM for example is described as having a BASAL LAMINA, i.e. the side of the olfactory epithelium on the inside, furthest from the edge exposed to odorant molecules; see OLFACTION.

basal metabolic rate *see* metabolic rate

base In biology and chemistry, a base is the opposite of an ACID: it is a substance that decreases the hydrogen ION (H^+) content of a solution. This can be achieved by different mechanisms. The principal ones are by dilution: sodium hydroxide (NaOH) for example dissociates in solution into SODIUM ions (Na^+) and hydroxide ions (OH^-). The hydroxide ions can combine with hydrogen ions to form water (H_2O). Alternatively, hydrogen ions can be scavenged. Ammonia (NH_3) for example can attract hydrogen ions in solution, combining

with them to form ammonium ions (NH_4). An alternative name for a base is an ALKALI.

See also: pH

Reference

Campbell N.A., Reece J.B. & Mitchell L.G. (1999) *Biology*, 5th edn, Addison-Wesley: Menlo Park CA.

baseline The phrase ON THE BASELINE relates to STEADY STATE responding. Animals 'responding on the baseline' will show a constant level of performance (the baseline) on small FIXED RATIO SCHEDULES that provide just enough REINFORCEMENT to maintain responding. 'Responding off the baseline' refers to either a decrease or an increase in responding brought about by a stimulus of some sort – for example, drug administration. Removal of the stimulus will lead to a return to responding on the baseline.

basilar artery *see* blood

basilar membrane The human basilar membrane is 35 mm long and located in the inner ear. It distributes sound frequencies via a travelling displacement wave to the HAIR CELLS which activate the AUDITORY NERVE fibres. The basilar membrane has a constant mass per unit length and an exponentially decreasing stiffness from base to apex. It manifests frequency tuning TONOTOPIC REPRESENTATION with high frequencies (20 000 Hz) activating the membrane near the STAPES and lower frequencies also progressively towards the apex (tuned to 200 Hz). Lower frequencies activate similar parts as 200 Hz; however their PITCH is determined by periodicity rather than place of activation.

JOS J. EGGERMONT

basis pedunculi *see* cerebral peduncles

basket cells These are NON-PYRAMIDAL NEURONS, found in the CEREBRAL CORTEX, HIPPOCAMPUS (see HILAR CELLS) and the cerebellum (see CEREBELLUM – ANATOMICAL ORGANIZATION) which function as INTERNEURONS. They are called basket cells (or basket neurons) because they make so many synaptic connections that they appear to surround – to make a basket for – the neurons they make contact with.

See also: stellate cells

basophil *see* immune system

Batani transection *see* cerveau isolé

batswing tremor *see* tremor

Bayesian statistics Bayesian statistics are named after the Reverend Thomas Bayes (1702–1761), a Nonconformist minister who, following his ordination, worked first in London then later in Kent. Bayes' theorem has become a valuable statistical tool. Its importance is in its ability to make probabilistic inferences about the incidence of mutually exclusive, non-repeatable events. The theorem has various expressions, each involving conditional probabilities, written in the form $P(A\backslash B)$, the probability (P) of A given B. It can be expressed, for example, as:

$$P(A\backslash B)*P(B) = P(B\backslash A)*P(A)$$

in which $P(A)$ and $P(B)$ are the unconditional, a priori probabilities of A and B. Bayesian statistics have been widely used in studies concerned with DECISION-MAKING.

beacon homing *see* navigation

Beck depression inventory A common questionnaire (*see* QUESTIONNAIRE STUDIES) for the analysis of DEPRESSION, developed by Aaron T. Beck. It features 21 groups of statements: individuals are asked to isolate the one which most closely describes their feelings over the previous week. For example, Question 1 asks individuals to choose between I do not feel sad (score 0); I feel sad (1); I am sad all the time and I can't snap out of it (2); or I am so sad or unhappy that I can't stand it (3). Higher scores are indicative of depression.

bed nucleus A nucleus (*see* NUCLEUS definition ii) can be called a bed nucleus if it provides support for some other anatomical feature, usually a FIBRE pathway. For example, the BED NUCLEUS OF THE STRIA TERMINALIS has a supporting position with respect to the STRIA TERMINALIS. Similarly, the LATERAL HYPOTHALAMUS has been described as being a bed nucleus for the MEDIAL FOREBRAIN BUNDLE. On the other hand, the ENTOPEDUNCULAR NUCLEUS, even though embedded in the CEREBRAL PEDUNCLES, is not described as a bed nucleus. The bed in bed nucleus refers to support, not embedding.

bed nucleus of the stria terminalis A BED NUCLEUS of the STRIA TERMINALIS known as the bed nucleus of the stria terminalis. It lies below the stria terminalis in its more anterior portion, is relatively large (in the rodent brain) and can be subdivided into a number of discrete sub-nuclei. It has received attention for two reasons recently. First, the anatomical position it occupies has been debated. It was included in early descriptions of the VENTRAL STRIATUM and has more recently been accommodated within the EXTENDED AMYGDALA. Second, it appears to have a function with respect to SEX DIFFERENCES. It is believed to be larger in males than in females. Surprisingly, it has been claimed that in male transsexuals, the bed nucleus of the stria terminalis is smaller than that which is normal for a male, being instead closer to the size of the average female bed nucleus of the stria terminalis.

Reference

Zhou J.N., Hofman M.A., Gooren L.J.G. & Swaab D.F. (1995) A sex difference in the human brain and its relation to trans-sexuality. *Nature* 378: 68–70.

bedwetting *see* nocturnal enuresis

behaviour analysis An approach to understanding behaviour originally based on the OPERANT CONDITIONING approach initiated by B.F. Skinner (1904–1990). Unlike BEHAVIOUR THERAPY, behaviour analysis is based on an understanding of the functional relations into which behaviours enter with the environment. This involves understanding proximal and distal antecedents for behaviour, and the consequences of behaviour. Antecedents may be general setting events – for example the presence of an audience without which a speaker would not deliver a lecture – or specific DISCRIMINATIVE CUES. Consequences which are reinforcing (see REINFORCEMENT) ensure that the behaviour increases in frequency and/ or is maintained in the presence of appropriate antecedents. Consequences which are punishing (see PUNISHMENT) result in a decrease in the frequency of the behaviour and/or the behaviour being at low probability in the presence of specific antecedents.

Behaviour analysis encompasses the experimental analysis of behaviour, which follows closely in the Skinnerian tradition, utilizing strict experimental control, often in laboratory settings using OPERANT CHAMBERS such as the SKINNER BOX. Since the 1970s there has been a decrease in the use of non-human animals, such as rats and pigeons, as experimental subjects, although the hallmark of the field is still its adherence to rigorous control of experimental variables, and the use of specific, single-subject research designs. Behaviour analysis also embraces applied behaviour analysis which involves clinical and other applications in real-world settings. These have included interventions with people with MENTAL RETARDATION, PSYCHOSIS, patients with cancer, head injury and burns, and many other clinical problems. People in industry, sport and the police have used behaviour analysis to improve their efficiency and effectiveness. Education settings, too, have often provided a forum for behaviour analytic interventions. Since the 1980s there has been an increase in community interventions, helping drivers and pedestrians, smokers, televisions viewers and consumers, among others.

Also in the 1980s attention began to be turned to forging relationships with other areas of psychology which had traditionally not been considered the province of behaviour analysis. Building on Skinner's early work behaviour analysts began to explore topics such as PERCEPTION and cognition. Those working in ARTIFICIAL INTELLIGENCE have used computer models to understand human functioning, and behaviour analysts challenged this in exploring the distinction between rule-governed and CONTINGENCY-shaped behaviour. Their argument is that much of human functioning, particularly cognition, is not rule-governed in the way we understand computers to work, but is shaped and selected by the environment just as other biological functions are. This puts behaviour analysis firmly within the sphere of the biological sciences, explaining the operant conditioning process (which is at the basis of behaviour analysis) as an example of variation

and natural selection. In the brain sciences the same approach, together with a rejection of procedural computer models (see PROCEDURAL LEARNING), is to be found in NEURAL DARWINISM.

In the 1990s behaviour analysis began to be described as part of a broader philosophy of contextualism, which is the view that all phenomena can be understood only if one analyses the current circumstances – the context – under which they occur. This does not deny that people have experiences in the past which influence their current behaviour, but somehow these past influences must have an effect upon the current state of the organism. One leading behaviour analyst has described context as 'just another word for contingencies of reinforcement, survival and cultural evolution. Contingencies describe the functional relationships of behaviour to the events in space and time that precede and follow the behaviour, in the lifetime of the individual (reinforcement), in the lifetime of species (survival), or in the lifetime of a cultural group (cultural evolution)' (Hayes, 1987).

Part of the context which must be understood when conducting a behaviour analysis is the physiology of the organism. Although earlier neural modelling based on simple procedural computer models was rejected by behaviour analysts, they have welcomed and embraced CONNECTIONISM and NEURAL NETWORKS models, since these are biologically inspired approaches to learning as opposed to machine (computer) approaches. Behaviour analysts are also interested in using their approach to understand, and even design, communities. Skinner published a highly influential novel in 1948, *Walden Two*, which described a community designed and administered according to behaviourist principles, and since then many have tried to use the approach to help people to achieve more valued lifestyles. Community design of this type is especially relevant in fields such as mental retardation.

Reference

Hayes S.C. (1987) A contextual approach to therapeutic change. In *Psychotherapists in Clinical Practice: Cognitive and Behavioural*

Perspectives, ed. N. Jacobson, Guilford Press: New York.

CHRIS CULLEN

behaviour therapy An approach to maladaptive or unwanted behaviour which is based on CLASSICAL CONDITIONING procedures. The term was initially coined by B. F. Skinner (1904–1990) and Ogden Lindsley in 1954 to describe approaches based on behaviourist learning theory. Its use then became widely promoted by the British psychologist H. J. Eysenck (1916–1997) in the 1960s. Behaviour therapy has followed a path somewhat different to that of BEHAVIOUR ANALYSIS, which is based on OPERANT CONDITIONING.

During its first 20 years behaviour therapy was an approach in opposition to psychoanalysis and psychotherapy, focusing directly on maladaptive behaviour rather than on assumed disease processes, personality structures or unconscious conflict. Treatment goals were defined explicitly and related to observable behaviour which could be easily measured. Behaviour therapists tended to deal with neurotic and emotional disorders (see NEUROSIS), rather than PSYCHOSIS, considering that habits which had been acquired by LEARNING should logically be treated by methods based on learning principles. Examples of problems treated by behaviour therapy are PHOBIA, REACTIVE DISORDERS such as DEPRESSION, OBSESSIVE COMPULSIVE DISORDER, sexual dysfunction, deviant SEXUAL BEHAVIOUR and marital problems. Typical procedures used by early behaviour therapists include the reduction of ANXIETY by relaxation procedures; encouraging people to imitate the therapist in order to learn new behaviours (modelling); flooding, which involves exposing people to their anxiety-evoking situations and instructing them not to escape, or even preventing them from doing so; aversion techniques (which quickly slipped out of favour) which involved exposing a person to circumstances likely to elicit the maladaptive response and then punishing the response, often using electric shock or other noxious stimuli (see AVERSIVE CONDITIONING). Of these, the commonest were probably relaxation procedures, designed to reduce or eliminate the anxiety which often accompanies presenting problems. Also often used were exposure therapies in which the patient would be encouraged to experience the situations which made them anxious. This could be accomplished gradually by procedures such as systematic DESENSITIZATION, or abruptly as in flooding. The confrontation would be either with the real events or stimuli (*in vivo*) or by getting the person to imagine them. In general it was found that the *in vivo* and flooding procedures were more effective.

In the 1970s it became clear that many of these relatively simple and crude behaviour therapy techniques did not, on their own, lead to lasting cures for people, and other psychological approaches and concepts became incorporated into behaviour therapy. One of the pioneers of behaviour therapy, Arnold A. Lazarus (1932–), was among the first to broaden the conceptual basis of behaviour therapy by introducing the notion of multimodal behaviour therapy. He argued that direct intervention across a number of distinct but interrelated modalities is necessary in order to achieve lasting change. These modalities were behaviour, AFFECT, SENSATION, IMAGERY, cognition, interpersonal relationships and medication. This moved behaviour therapy somewhat away from earlier formulations which emphasized the direct treatment of presenting behavioural problems.

A related addition to the behaviour therapy paradigm has been the inclusion of cognitive approaches such as rational emotive therapy, and this led, by the mid 1980s, to the almost universal replacement of standard behaviour therapy procedures in clinical practice initially by cognitive–behavioural therapy and then later by what has become known as COGNITIVE THERAPY. The reason that behaviour therapy has been largely supplanted by cognitive therapy is because of a perception that traditional behaviour therapy did not get to the root of people's problems, but dealt only with their symptoms. One of the originators of behaviour therapy, Joseph Wolpe (1915–1997), has blamed what he describes as the derailment of behaviour therapy on an excessive adherence to exposure therapies which had no real basis in classical conditioning theory, but appeared to be based on the notion that all that was required was that patients should get used to the stimuli which evoked anxiety. However, notwithstanding such calls to return to earlier modes of theory and practice, behaviour therapy has evolved and developed into an approach which has much in common with cognitive therapy and behaviour analysis, adopting a broadened more integrative position, incorporating a wide range of clinical procedures.

CHRIS CULLEN

behavioural assay The use of behaviour to measure physiological or other variables. For example, the degree of DOPAMINE depletion in the STRIATUM following a unilateral 6-HYDROXYDOPAMINE lesion can be measured by the amount of ROTATION an animal displays in response to AMPHETAMINE administration

behavioural checklist A list of categories of behaviour used for scoring the frequency of behaviour over time. There are constraints on behaviour in OPERANT tasks, whether in automatic chambers such as the SKINNER BOX or NINE-HOLE BOX, or in a MAZE. The behaviour of interest (for example, see NOSE POKE VS. LEVER PRESS) is highly predictable, the tasks being arranged to maximize the frequency of that behaviour, in order to record some property of it – choice or latency for example. The measurement of spontaneous behaviour, either in field studies (see ETHOLOGY) or in the laboratory is more complex. Measurement of specific acts such as food intake or liquid consumption is relatively straightforward: one measures for instance the volume of intake, latency to begin, number and duration of bouts. Similarly, certain relatively predictable activities with species-typical features (such as SEXUAL BEHAVIOUR) are straightforward to categorize in terms of the elements that make up that activity. The continuous stream of behaviour an animal emits is more difficult to capture. Behaviour can be recorded on video tape, to avoid missing some important feature, but the scoring of the activity remains problematic. Three different approaches have been used: one is to adopt a system for scoring movement itself, typically in terms of an animal's body position at a series of time points (see ESHKOL–WACHMAN NOTATION).

This is both difficult and rather reductionist (see REDUCTIONISM), scoring behaviour only as movement. An alternative is to measure the temporal patterning of behaviour (see THEME ANALYSIS), an approach that yields considerable information about the patterning of behaviour. However, the most common way for assessing the stream of activity is to measure the frequency with which identified categories of behaviour appear, using a behavioural checklist. This is a simple device, that can be accomplished with either paper and pencil, or by using a computer to record observations. Behaviour is divided into a number of categories (for example, LOCOMOTION, forepaw GROOMING, licking and so on) and behaviour observed for a specific period of time at regular intervals (for example, for 10 seconds every 2 minutes). If an activity occurs, and fits specified criteria (for example, licking for more than 3 seconds) its appearance is recorded. An objective picture of an animal's activity over time is generated and can be statistically analysed. Such an approach has considerable analytic power, though it has been criticized for its reliance on predetermined categorization of behaviour. It has been used for example to examine systematically the different effects of drugs that stimulate activity of DOPAMINE (see Fray *et al.*, 1980; these authors provide a carefully designed behavioural checklist which can be adapted for a variety of uses by modifying the categories of behaviour measured).

See also: Creese–Iversen scale

Reference

Fray P.J., Sahakian B.J., Robbins T.W., Koob G.F. & Iversen S.D. (1980) An observational method for quantifying the behavioural effects of dopamine agonists: contrasting effects of *d*-amphetamine and apomorphine. *Psychopharmacology* 69: 253–259.

VERITY J. BROWN AND PHILIP WINN

behavioural economics General term used to cover the processes animals use to get the most effective return on their time and ENERGY expenditure; for examples, see COST–BENEFIT ANALYSIS; MATCHING LAW; OPTIMAL FORAGING THEORY; SCHEDULES OF REINFORCEMENT; UTILITY.

behavioural inhibition The active suppression of behaviour (as opposed to FORGETTING to do something, or just doing nothing for example).

See also: behavioural inhibition system; cognitive inhibition; response competition; supervisory attentional system

behavioural inhibition system A functional term devised by Jeffrey Gray to describe the operations of a brain system important in the generation of ANXIETY. The function of the system is to inhibit current behaviour and to increase ATTENTION and AROUSAL following presentation of novel stimuli, or stimuli predictive of PUNISHMENT or absence of REWARD. It was suggested to work essentially as a comparator; examining incoming sensory information in relation to expectations, the behavioural inhibition system being activated when a mismatch between expectation and input occurred, or when input suggested some aversive event was likely. The anatomical system mediating this Grey suggested included the SEPTOHIPPOCAMPAL SYSTEM, PAPEZ CIRCUIT, PREFRONTAL CORTEX and CHOLINERGIC and MONOAMINERGIC elements of the ASCENDING RETICULAR ACTIVATING SYSTEM. He also suggested that ANXIOLYTIC drugs, notably the BENZODIAZEPINES and BARBITURATES, had a major action on this system: anxiety was interpreted as overactivation of the behavioural inhibition system, the drugs working to correct this. The ideas Grey presented about the nature of anxiety have had impact (see EMOTION; FIGHT-OR-FLIGHT). The need to interrupt ongoing activity following analysis of fresh sensory data is not in doubt, though the precise way in which this function is achieved by brains remains unclear.

References

Gray J.A. (1982) *The Neuropsychology of Anxiety: An Enquiry into the Functions of the Septohippocampal System*, Oxford University Press: Oxford.
—— (1982) Precis of 'The neuropsychology of anxiety: an enquiry into the functions of the septohippocampal system'. *The Behavioural and Brain Sciences* 5: 469–534.

behavioural neuroscience That part of neuroscience that seeks to understand the relationships between brain systems and the control of behaviour, as opposed to cognitive processes.

behavioural pharmacology *see* psychopharmacology

behavioural silence A term coined by Anthony Dickinson to describe a problem in animal LEARNING: learning is demonstrated by animals through changes in their behaviour. If there is no change in behaviour however, is it correct to assume that no learning has occurred? Evidence from phenomena such as LATENT INHIBITION and LEARNED IRRELEVANCE indicate that animals learn about the world even though they might give no overt indication, at the time, that learning has occurred; see McFarland (1999) for a discussion of this.

References

Dickinson A. (1980) *Contemporary Animal Learning Theory*, Cambridge University Press: Cambridge.
McFarland D. (1999) *Animal Behaviour*, 3rd edn, Longman: Harlow UK.

behavioural state This term refers to the three main states of waking, SLOW-WAVE SLEEP (SWS) and REM SLEEP (rapid eye movement sleep). Each is not a homogeneous state: different behaviours and levels of arousal occur during waking, and in humans, four different stages (depths) of SWS have been identified. Control of behavioural state relies on the interplay between CHOLINERGIC and MONOAMINERGIC neurons in the RETICULAR FORMATION and their interaction with those in the FOREBRAIN, particularly the THALAMUS, HYPOTHALAMUS and CORTEX.

In its most fully developed form, each behavioural state can be differentiated from the other by means of three physiological measures: recordings of the cortical ELECTROENCEPHALOGRAM (EEG), muscular tone as recorded by ELECTROMYOGRAM (EMG) and eye movements recorded by ELECTRO-OCULOGRAM (EOG), although using only the first two of these together is also relatively accurate. The EEG is desynchronized during both waking and REM sleep, but synchronized during SWS (see SYNCHRONY/DESYNCHRONY). Muscle tone is highest during 'active waking', less during 'quiet waking' and SWS, and practically zero in REM sleep. Eye movements can be measured during both waking and REM sleep, although they occur as an involuntary SACCADE during REM sleep. There are also recognizable transition zones between states. For instance, the transition from waking to SWS is marked by a period of drowsiness lasting several minutes, which is depicted by episodic appearance of spindle waves (see SLEEP SPINDLES) and a gradual increase in the amplitude of the EEG. In contrast, the transition from SWS to waking is a sudden change during a period of only a few seconds, incorporating increased frequency and decreased AMPLITUDE of EEG, increased muscle tone and reappearance of voluntary eye movements. The transition from SWS to REM sleep is observed physiologically by 1–2 minutes of sharp PGO WAVES, originating in the PONS and occurring prior to EEG desynchrony and MUSCLE ATONIA.

Behavioural state control was once thought to be a passive process. However, in 1990 Steriade & McCarley proposed a reciprocal interaction model: an active model of behavioural state control, based on mathematical assumptions about two types of neurons, REM-off and REM-on. As REM-off neurons gradually increased their firing, they would activate REM-on neurons by a feed-forward mechanism. The increase in firing of REM-on neurons would precipitate REM sleep and inhibit the REM-off neurons. As activity in the REM-off group subsided, there would be less activation of REM-on neurons and the balance of activity would switch back to REM-off neurons. This model has subsequently been applied to neurons located in the reticular formation, which have state-dependent firing patterns, that is, consistently changing in relation to the behavioural state of the animal. REM-on neurons include the cholinergic neurons in the PEDUNCULOPONTINE TEGMENTAL NUCLEUS and LATERODORSAL TEGMENTAL NUCLEUS, and the GLUTAMATE- and GLYCINE-containing neurons in the medial pontine reticular formation. REM-off neurons include the SEROTONIN neurons in the RAPHE NUCLEI and the NORADRENALINE neurons in the LOCUS COERULEUS. It has been possible to confirm the connections between these nuclei through the technique of TRACT TRACERS. In addition, in most instances, the RECEPTOR subtypes and excitatory or inhibitory relationships which occur between the nuclei have been ascertained by *in vitro* electrophysiological recordings. However, the model is still being developed and modified: one particular point which has not been reconciled with the known anatomy and electrophysiology is that these neuronal groups are all active at once during the waking state.

Although the patterns of EEG, EMG and EOG activity typically measured in each behavioural state are orchestrated by the MESOPONTINE and PONTINE RETICULAR FORMATION neurons, these have crucial interactions with a number of other nuclei to produce such physiological changes. Specifically, control of EEG comes from reticular formation input to the thalamus and cortex, control of muscle tone is through interactions between the pons and alpha-MOTONEURONS, and EOG is modified by pontine interactions with OCULOMOTOR neurons. Important afferent control of these systems also comes from the hypothalamus and SUPERIOR COLLICULUS. For instance, projections from the posterior hypothalamus have been implicated in alertness, and those from the SUPRACHIASMATIC NUCLEUS are likely to be important in entraining the oscillation between behavioural states to the CIRCADIAN RHYTHM; inputs from the superior colliculus play an important role in eye-movement control. There is also likely to be considerable plasticity in these control mechanisms, since it has been shown that patients who are in a PERSISTENT VEGETATIVE STATE still switch between different behavioural states, despite severe damage to the thalamus. In such conditions it would appear that the thalamus is not necessary for behavioural state control, if extrathalamic pathways are intact.

See also: sleep–wake cycle

Reference

Steriade M. & McCarley R.W. (1990) *Brainstem Control of Wakefulness and Sleep*, Plenum Press: New York.

WENDY L. INGLIS

behavioural tolerance Cellular tolerance accounts for TOLERANCE in terms of changed function in cells. In contrast, behavioural tolerance is a form of tolerance that involves behavioural and psychological processes. It has been proposed by Siegel (1989) that part of the effects of drugs is conditioned: the place in which a DRUG is taken, for example, can acquire, by PAVLOVIAN CONDITIONING, effects of its own (see PLACE CONDITIONING). These effects will often involve making the body ready to receive drug. If these preparatory signals are not present, a drug may have a very different effect. It has been suggested that many of the fatalities that result from drug OVERDOSE involve a drug having been administered in a novel environment, where the protective effects of learned responses were not present.

References

Feldman R., Meyer J.S. & Quenzer L.F. (1997) *Principles of Neuropsychopharmacology*, Sinauer Associates: Sunderland MA.
Siegel S. (1989) Pharmacological conditioning and drug effects. In *Psychoactive Drugs: Tolerance and Sensitization*, ed. A.J. Goudie & M.W. Emmett-Oglesby, pp. 115–180, Humana Press: Clifton NJ.

behaviourism Broadly, behaviourism refers to the doctrine that understanding behaviour is fundamental to understanding mental events. Scientific and philosophical forms of behaviourism can be identified. *Scientific behaviourism* has its origins in the work of J.B. Watson (1878–1958) but was given its most vigorous defence by B.F. Skinner (1904–1990). Strict behaviourists argue that behaviour is all that there is to measure: that mental terms and events are of little or no value; and that internal neural events are of no value, in that all behaviour can be described in its terms of actions and the environmental events that precede and follow them. Scientific behaviourism came under attack from cognitive scientists, and in particular from those with an interest in LANGUAGE, a process that behaviourism has great difficulty in accounting for. Behaviourism is still of value in that it generated a series of terms and tools for investigating processes of LEARNING and MEMORY (see for example CONDITIONING and OPERANT CHAMBER), and in its clinical manifestations (see BEHAVIOUR THERAPY). *Philosophical behaviourism* was concerned with the analysis of the meaning of mentalistic expressions; it no longer has impact.

Bell–Magendie law Named after its founders, François Magendie (1783–1855) and Charles Bell (1774–1842), this simply encapsulates the principal that the VENTRAL ROOTS of the SPINAL CORD carry motor information out from the spinal cord to various targets within the body, while the DORSAL ROOTS bring sensory information to the spinal cord from the body.

belladonna alkaloids The most commonly used of these are ATROPINE and SCOPOLAMINE, both MUSCARINIC ACETYLCHOLINE RECEPTOR blockers.

benzedrine Benzedrine is the trade name for the racemic mixture (RACEMATE) of AMPHETAMINE; that is D,L-amphetamine. The slang term 'bennies' refers to benzedrine.

benzodiazepine (BDZ) Any of the group of drugs with ANTICONVULSANT, ANXIOLYTIC, hypnotic and muscle-relaxant properties. They act at the GABA receptor complex type A, where they bind as agonists to a specific benzodiazepine binding site. Here, they facilitate GABAergic inhibitory neurotransmission. Examples of the class include DIAZEPAM (valium) and nitrazepam (mogadon). Benzodiazepines have a variety of indications, including INSOMNIA, termination of SEIZURES, ANXIETY and PANIC disorders. Though very safe drugs, particularly in overdose, there is considerable risk of TOLERANCE and physical and psychological DEPENDENCE.

IAN C. REID

benzodiazepine-induced hyperphagia Drugs that act at the benzodiazepine receptors, as well as having a variety of ANTICONVULSANT, ANXIOLYTIC and hypnotic effects, also affect FEEDING: benzodiazepine-receptor agonists increase food intake while inverse agonists reduce it. The hyperphagic effects appear to be mediated through BRAINSTEM processes, probably at sites within the PARABRACHIAL NUCLEI. Direct MICROINJECTION of the benzodiazepine MIDAZOLAM into the parabrachial nuclei increased food intake but did not produce sedation or changes in gross motor activity, suggesting that the effects of benzodiazepines may be specifically related to some aspect of feeding, rather than a non-specific effect.

Reference

Higgs S. & Cooper S.J. (1996) Hyperphagia induced by direct administration of midazolam into the parabrachial nucleus of the rat. *European Journal of Pharmacology* 313: 1–9.

Berlyne box Equipment used to measure EXPLORATION in rats. It is an OPEN FIELD with a compartment in one wall, normally obscured by a door, that contains a novel object. Once a rat has become familiar with the open field, the compartment is opened, and exploration measured in terms of rats' latency to make contact with the novel object and the amount of time directed to it. This provides a measure of exploration, though one partially confounded by locomotor activity – rats with motor impairments have difficulty showing a preference for novelty in this test, unlike the CARLSON BOX.

Bernstein principle Bernstein was a physiologist working in the Soviet Union whose work became well known in the West with the publication in 1967 of *The Coordination and Regulation of Movements*. Bernstein made many valuable contributions to the study of movement, but became known for suggesting that 'there exist in the central nervous system exact formulae of movements or their engrams and that these formulae or engrams contain in some form of brain trace the whole process of the movement in its entire course in time' (Bernstein, 1967, p. 37). This process he saw as a chaining together of one ENGRAM after another, each concerned with a portion of the total action. These could be chained such that execution of engram A produced activation of engram B, though Bernstein preferred to think of them as not being so slavishly chained. Rather, he preferred the notion that activation of one engram could release several others (a rather more disinhibitory conception). He also believed that while actions could be decomposed, there must be a central representation (a motor image) of the entire action. For a discussion of Bernstein's work, see Jeannerod (1988).

See also: motor control; motor programming; motor system

References

Bernstein N. (1967) *The Coordination and Regulation of Movements*, Pergamon Press: Oxford.

Jeannerod M. (1988) *The Neural and Behavioral Organization of Goal-Directed Movements*, Oxford University Press: Oxford.

beta amyloid protein *see* amyloid

beta blockers Drugs that act as ANTAGONISTS at BETA RECEPTORS (see ADRENOCEPTORS). Beta blockers are often prescribed to suppress activity in the SYMPATHETIC NERVOUS SYSTEM (for example, they can slow HEART RATE and reduce sweating). They are also used in the treatment of such things as POST TRAUMATIC STRESS DISORDER and ANXIETY, but there is little evidence for them having very specific therapeutic actions in these conditions.

beta carboline *see* anxiogenic

beta cells These are the B CELLS of the IMMUNE SYSTEM; see also IMMUNOLOGY; LYMPHATIC SYSTEM; T CELL.

beta conditioning *see* alpha and beta conditioning

beta endorphin *see* endorphins

beta receptor; beta adrenergic *see* adrenoceptors

beta waves *see* electroencephalogram

Betz cells Betz cells, named after Vladimir Betz (1834–1894) who discovered them, are giant (50–80 μm) PYRAMIDAL NEURONS in layer 5 of the primary MOTOR CORTEX. There are about 30 000 Betz cells in the human motor cortex. Their axons contribute to the CORTICOSPINAL TRACT, which contains the axons of about a million neurons.

See also: agranular cortex; cytoarchitecture

bicuculline The most widely used competitive ANTAGONIST (see COMPETITIVE–NONCOMPETITIVE BINDING) at the GABA-A receptor (see GABA RECEPTORS). The GABA-B receptor is discriminated from the GABA-A receptor by virtue of the inability of bicuculline to work there: BACLOFEN is the most common antagonist for the GABA-B receptor.

Bienenstock–Cooper–Munro rule *see* Hebbian synapse

bilateral Affecting or present on two sides: the brain has two hemispheres so, for example, a bilateral LESION of a particular structure would be one that was present in that structure in both hemispheres. A UNILATERAL lesion would be present in that structure in one hemisphere only.

bilingualism Ability to communicate in two languages (in more than two languages, multi-lingualism). A categorical distinction between 'real' bilinguals and non-bilinguals cannot be drawn; rather, there is a continuum from grossly unbalanced to closely balanced mastery of different languages. However, even the most balanced bilinguals differ in how they use their languages – a particular technical vocabulary may be primarily accessible in one language, for instance. The use of more than one dialect (for example, a regional and a standard variant), or of more than one speaking style (such as formal versus informal) draws on the same abilities to select situationally appropriate language.

ANNE CUTLER

binaural Relating to both ears, as opposed to only one (MONAURAL). The term DICHOTIC is also used (see DICHOTIC LISTENING TASK) but in this case different material is presented to each ear, whereas binaural is a word describing normal listening to material using both ears. BINAURAL beat is a periodic elevation of LOUD-NESS accompanying simultaneous presentation of different low frequency tones, one to each ear – it occurs when the peaks of the tones are in synchrony. Similarly, BINAURAL shift is the periodic change in SOUND LOCALIZATION that occurs when two low-frequency sounds are presented – this occurs because of variation in the phase of each sound. BINAURAL fusion is the perception of independent sounds as one single sound (also called AUDITORY FUSION). BINAURAL ratio is the ratio of sound intensity presented to each ear, and BINAURAL summa-

tion is the increase in loudness when a sound is heard through both ears rather than just one.

See also: auditory perception

binding *see* receptor binding

binding affinity *see* affinity

binding problem Processing in neuronal systems is generally accepted to occur in parallel (see PARALLEL VS. SERIAL PROCESSING) and to be distributed (see DISTRIBUTED PROCESSING). A complex visual image, for example, will be processed by many neurons over a wide area of tissue. The question of how the various processes that operate on a single stimulus are reintegrated to form a coherent REPRESENTA-TION is referred to as the binding problem. The idea that single units encode specific complex stimuli is considered implausible. While specific neurons can encode specific stimulus elements (see FEATURE DETECTOR), complex element such as faces (see FACE PERCEPTION) are not coded by individual neurons (see GRANDMOTHER CELL). Explanations for the binding problem are generally sought in various neural coding mechanisms, the synchronization or patterning of neuronal firing for example.

See also: labelled-line theory; neural coding; pattern perception

Reference

Singer W. (1996) Neuronal synchronization: a solution to the binding problem? In *The Mind–Brain Continuum: Sensory Processes*, ed. R. Llinás & P.S. Churchland, pp. 101–130, MIT Press: Cambridge MA.

binding site *see* receptor

binge eating Episodes of over-eating, accompanied by a feeling of loss of control, representing a defining characteristic of BULIMIA NERVOSA and the 'binge eating disorder' of DSM-IV. Binge eating disorder is distinguished from bulimia nervosa in that compensatory mechanisms for increased intake (such as purging and vomiting) do not occur. Binge eating may also occur in atypical forms of DEPRES-SION, and accompany SEASONAL AFFECTIVE DISORDER; and as part of the KLUVER–BUCY SYNDROME or KLEIN–LEVIN SYNDROME. Very rarely, it may occur as a consequence of brain tumours or as an epileptic phenomenon.

IAN C. REID

binocular Pertaining to the use of two eyes. All vertebrates – animals with backbones – have two eyes that provide coordinated visual information about the world to the brain. There are two main arrangements of the two eyes: lateral and frontal. In the lateral placement, there is minimal overlap between the visual fields of about 180° in each eye, which combine to provide 360° coverage of the external world. In the frontal placement, typical of predatory animals and humans, the visual fields of the two eyes overlap, so most of the visual field is binocular. While this arrangement sacrifices coverage to the rear, the binocular overlap provides the advantages of improved SIGNAL-TO-NOISE RATIO from BINOCULAR SUMMATION and depth information by means of BINOCULAR DISPARITY

Reference

Walls, G.L. (1963) *The Vertebrate Eye and its Adaptive Radiations*, Hafner: New York.

CHRISTOPHER TYLER

binocular disparity Relative position in the two eyes. Horizontal disparity is the most direct cue for perceived depth in the third (near–far) dimension. For similar stimuli in each eye, there is a range of positions of one monocular image relative to the other that give the impression of an object nearer or further in EGOCENTRIC distance. The origin for zero disparity is the centre of the FOVEA in each eye. Vertical disparities give no sense of depth directly, but may influence the depth perceived from horizontal disparities. Depth from horizontal disparity is not limited to fused stimuli, and in fact reaches its greatest strength for diplopic (see DIPLOPIA) images.

See also: depth perception

Reference

Howard I.P. & Rogers B.J. (1995) *Binocular Vision and Stereopsis*, Oxford University Press: New York.

CHRISTOPHER TYLER

binocular fusion Combination of images in the two eyes into a single percept. For stimuli that are similar in shape in each eye, there is a range of binocular disparities (see BINOCULAR DISPARITY) over which they appear as a single image midway in position between the positions of the two monocular images. The process by which the two images are combined and shifted is not well understood; the fusion range depends on the size and shape of the binocular images. Outside the range of fusion, when either the horizontal or vertical disparity is too great, the images are seen as diplopic (see DIPLOPIA), the sum of the two monocular views, or in BINOCULAR RIVALRY where dissimilar features overlap.

Reference

Tyler C.W. (1991) The horopter and binocular fusion. In *Vision and Visual Disorders*, vol. 9, *Binocular Vision*, ed. D. Regan, pp. 19–37, Macmillan: New York.

CHRISTOPHER TYLER

binocular rivalry Alternation of the perception of the images in the two eyes. For high-contrast stimuli in each eye that are dissimilar in shape, perception tends to alternate irregularly between the monocular images, with one image being perceptually suppressed while the other dominates. The alternation follows a random pattern that can be described statistically and is generally not under voluntary control. Recent evidence suggests that binocular rivalry is a manifestation of generalized pattern rivalry in the VISUAL CORTEX rather than being based on eye of origin.

Reference

Fox R. (1991) Binocular rivalry. In *Vision and Visual Disorders*, vol. 9, *Binocular Vision*, ed. D. Regan, pp. 93–110, Macmillan: New York.

CHRISTOPHER TYLER

binocular strip A feature of the RETINA: there is an overlap (of approximately 1° in the human eye) along the vertical meridian of the projections of the NASAL and TEMPORAL VISUAL HEMIFIELDS. This part of the retina is therefore in receipt of BINOCULAR information. Some evidence supports the hypothesis that the CORPUS CALLOSUM connections of the primary

VISUAL CORTEX may intervene in some binocular processes such as binocular STEREOPSIS along the mid sagittal plane.

binocular summation The process by which information from the two eyes is combined. Binocular summation is not necessarily limited to linear summation of local contrasts; various combination rules apply in different circumstances, ranging from summing the squares of local contrast to no difference between the binocular and monocular impression (FECHNER'S PARADOX). Recent evidence has revealed that binocular summation may occur between dissimilar images in the same location in the two eyes if they are brief, low contrast or high spatial frequency. Under other conditions, such dissimilar images engender BINOCULAR RIVALRY.

Reference

Howard I.P. & Rogers B.J. (1995) *Binocular Vision and Stereopsis*, Oxford University Press: New York.

CHRISTOPHER TYLER

bioavailability *see* drug administration

biocytin *see* tract tracers

biofeedback Response-contingent stimulation. Biofeedback methods provide subjects with exteroceptive feedback (usually visual or auditory) of variations in some dimension of muscular, visceral or neural activity. The method is based on the (unproven) theory that VOLUNTARY MOTOR CONTROL depends on the integrity of a feedback loop that provides central motor control circuits with information about the activities of to-be-controlled effectors. Activities of deafferented STRIATE MUSCLES as well as those of the VISCERA and the nervous system that are difficult to detect, are resistant to voluntary control. In such cases, biofeedback is thought to facilitate control by augmenting the discriminability of the to-be-controlled activity and thereby enabling the subject to steer the otherwise undetectable and therefore non-voluntary effector activity towards a goal state identified by the feedback stimulus. Most frequently simple binary feedback is used in which a stimulus is presented when the criterion activity occurs and termi-

nates when the activity ceases to meet the criterion. Analog feedback has been used occasionally, for example by linking the position of a meter needle or the volume or pitch of a tone to such dimensions as the time integral of ELECTROMYOGRAM (EMG) activity, the level of diastolic blood pressure or the density of alpha ELECTROENCEPHALOGRAM (EEG) activity. However, it is not clear that analog feedback, which carries more information about effector activity, is more effective than binary feedback.

In the clinical realm, biofeedback is considered to be an 'alternative medicine' treatment and is employed as a means of generating control over a variety of primary disease symptoms. While its effectiveness remains controversial, proponents of the method argue that biofeedback is valuable in treating muscle tension HEADACHE, MIGRAINE headache, Raynaud's disease, ANXIETY, irritable bowel syndrome, incontinence, chronic PAIN and INSOMNIA. Published evidence suggests that the method is most effective in the treatment of disorders that are expressed by a loss of muscular control including tension headache, incontinence and neuromuscular disorders. For other disorders, it is not clear that biofeedback offers therapeutic advantages over relaxation training.

Biofeedback was first popularized by J. Kamiya who published evidence in the early 1960s that when provided with auditory feedback, individuals could increase the prevalence of alpha-wave EEG. Typically, EEG at this frequency (about 10 Hz) is associated with a relaxed attentive state similar to that achieved in meditation. At about the same time that Kamiya's work appeared, H. Kimmel published evidence that the GALVANIC SKIN RESPONSE (GSR) could be influenced by response-contingent REINFORCEMENT. Kimmel's demonstrations were not sufficiently powerful to overturn the received wisdom that autonomically mediated responses were immune to OPERANT CONDITIONING. However by emphasizing response-contingent reinforcement rather than feedback as the defining characteristic of the method, Kimmel cast the biofeedback problem within the more familiar conditioning framework. This stimulated a number of experimental studies that attempted to resolve the question of whether or not autonomically controlled responses were subject to operant conditioning. At the forefront of this experimental effort was a spate of studies that attempted to show that visceral control generated by response-contingent reinforcement was not a reflexive consequence of learned striate muscular control. From the mid 1960s to the early 1970s, a substantial experimental literature evolved on operant conditioning of visceral responses in curarized (see CURARE) animals. This work, which did much to promote the scientific respectability of biofeedback, purported to show that paralysed animals could be trained to produce highly specific visceromotor control. The implication of these demonstrations was that when provided with appropriate feedback, voluntary (or operant) control could be gained over non-voluntary activities. Subsequent work has shown that the phenomena reported in this early literature are not only fragile but of questionable theoretical significance.

Thus, there have been numerous failures to replicate the large effects demonstrated in the early literature. Furthermore, a strong experimental case has been made in support of the proposition that even when paralysed, animals could try to move their striate muscles and thereby generate neural outflow that influenced the visceral organs. Therefore, even if replicable, the curare experiments fail to prove that visceral control in curarized animals is independent of the neural processes that underlie voluntary control or operant conditioning of the striate (voluntary) muscles. Nevertheless, the curare experiments and other basic research that supported the development of biofeedback as a method have stimulated research into the roles of feedback in voluntary motor control and operant conditioning. Through its emphasis on the mediation of operant visceral control, it also refocused attention on the mechanisms in voluntary motor control. Finally biofeedback, which has rested on the idea that the voluntary control of an activity depends on the discriminability of that activity, has spawned research into the ability of individuals to detect variations in their own, mainly visceral, activities.

JASPER BRENER

biogenic amine The term biogenic refers to something that is only derived from living things; an AMINE is a derivative of ammonia in which hydrocarbon radicals have replaced one or more of the hydrogen atoms ammonia possesses. A biogenic amine is therefore simply an amine derived from living things. In practice the term biogenic amine refers to the MONOAMINE neurotransmitters: the CATECHOLAMINES and the INDOLEAMINES.

biological clock A physiological timekeeping mechanism synchronizing organisms' physiology with prominent environmental cycles. A wide variety of rhythmic processes have been observed in the physiology and behaviour of living organisms, with periodicities ranging from milliseconds to years. Some of these periodicities correspond to the periods of the major environmental cycles on the earth and are normally synchronized to them. These include the solar day–night cycle (24.0 h), tidal cycles (~12.4 h), the lunar day cycle (~24.8 h), the monthly lunar cycle (~29.5 days) and the year (365.25 days).

Many of these rhythms have been shown to persist indefinitely with slightly altered periodicity in a variety of organisms housed under artificially constant environmental conditions. The indefinite persistence of these biological rhythms with idiosyncratic periods unrelated to any environmental time cues is the strongest evidence that they are generated by an internal mechanism, called a pacemaker or biological clock, by analogy with a mechanical timekeeping device. Persistent rhythms observed under artificial constant conditions are called FREE RUNNING RHYTHMS, and they are normally synchronized by a process called ENTRAINMENT to cues provided by a corresponding geophysical cycle. The biological rhythms most often studied correspond in period to the solar day. Under constant environmental conditions, however, these rhythms express periods deviating slightly from 24 h, and are therefore called circadian rhythms (from Latin, *circa*: about, *dies*: a day). Such rhythms are found in virtually all eukaryotic organisms (and numerous prokaryotes) and appear to constitute a fundamental temporal organizing framework for most living things. The existence of multiple circadian rhythms and the demonstration of a complex physiological mechanism underlying their expression and environmental synchronization have given rise to the concept of a 'circadian system', by analogy with, for instance, the cardiovascular or gastrointestinal system. The activity of the circadian system serves two major functions. One is to organize the flow of physiological and behavioural events in time. Thus, in humans, particular hormones are secreted at selected times, often in anticipation of the need for them, sleep and waking alternate rhythmically, and aspects of the function of the IMMUNE SYSTEM, circulatory system and nervous system, among others, rise and fall at different times of day. For most of these rhythms, however, the functional significance of their timing is poorly understood: CORTISOL levels, for example, peak just in anticipation of waking, growth hormone rises during sleep, and MELATONIN secretion is initiated in anticipation of the sleep phase. Many believe that the patterns of temporal organization in the physiology of organisms that result from these multiple rhythms are important to normal function and health, and that their deterioration in old age or as a result of pathology can give rise to illness and disability.

The second major function of circadian clocks is to give organisms access to information about local time. By entrainment to local time cues, the physiology of an organism is adapted to local time and the myriad physical and biological events that will occur predictably in that environment. One of the great functional advantages of this process is that organisms can anticipate critical daily challenges or opportunities by appropriate physiological accommodations, rather than dealing with them reactively. Disruptions of the normal relations between internal biological rhythms and external time cues occur during rapid transmeridian flights, giving rise to the disruptions of SLEEP, FEEDING and performance known as JET LAG. Similar disruptions can occur when individuals alter the normal human pattern of nocturnal sleep and daytime work by working at unusual hours, especially when shift work schedules rotate rapidly. The growing prevalence of shift work in industrialized, 24-hour societies is at odds with the natural temporal organization of human physiology and can give rise to serious health and safety concerns. The circadian entrainment mechanism also allows an organism to track seasonal changes in daylength with appropriate physiological and behavioural changes, using the mechanism of photoperiodic time measurement. These changes are pronounced in many species which show seasonal patterns of reproduction, hibernation, migration, weight, coat quality and behaviour. While seasonality is often considered to be vestigial in humans, there are many documented seasonal rhythms in human physiology, and evidence for clinically significant changes in the case of SEASONAL AFFECTIVE DISORDER. Finally, biological clocks give organisms the capacity to measure the passage of time. Thus, the circadian clock not only signals the timing of daily events, but can also be consulted continuously in order to track the passage of time. This phenomenon was first documented in the case of sun-compass orientation in honeybees. In these studies, bees trained to visit a food source at one time of day using the sun as a compass, gave clear evidence that their circadian clock mechanisms allowed them to predict the sun's azimuthal position at any time of day, which could only be accomplished with knowledge of the rate of passage of time.

BENJAMIN RUSAK

biological psychology That part of psychology that seeks biological explanations for psychological phenomena; also known as biopsychology, and more or less synonymous with the term PHYSIOLOGICAL PSYCHOLOGY. Both of these terms incorporate investigations of all biological systems in relation to psychology. CARDIOVASCULAR PSYCHOPHYSIOLOGY for instance could be subsumed under the general term biological psychology. BEHAVIOURAL NEUROSCIENCE, COGNITIVE NEUROSCIENCE and NEUROPSYCHOLOGY are all specifically concerned with the relationships between behaviour, cognition and brain systems.

See also: psychopharmacology; psychophysiology

biological symmetry Biological organisms express an astonishing variety of symmetries, from the precise multi-axial symmetries of single-celled diatoms to the approximate bilateral symmetry of all vertebrate species. Bilateral symmetry is highly associated with directed LOCOMOTION through the environment. The fact that almost all species that move in this way (and most vehicles of human construction) exhibit bilateral symmetry suggests an adaptive value in avoiding navigational bias. That the constraint is not enforced by some genetic template is demonstrated by the violations of symmetry of the internal organs of vertebrates. On the other hand, the extensive variety of symmetries exhibited by invertebrate animals and plants may arise from structural constraints in the microbiology of the genes.

See also: asymmetry; handedness

Reference

Tyler C.W. (1996) Human symmetry perception. In *Human Symmetry Perception and its Computational Analysis*, ed. C.W. Tyler, pp.3–22, VSP Press: Utrecht.

CHRISTOPHER TYLER

biopsy 'Biopsy' pronounced 'bio-sigh' is shorthand for biological psychology. 'Biopsy' pronounced 'biop-sea' is a diagnostic investigation of tissue or fluid taken from a living organism (in contrast to an AUTOPSY, in which examination of dead tissue is made).

biorhythms Three hypothetical rhythms in human physiology for which there is no empirical evidence. This term is sometimes used as a contraction for 'biological rhythms' (see BIOLOGICAL CLOCK), referring to the extensively documented and well-understood CIRCADIAN RHYTHMS that pervade human physiology and other biological systems. This usage leads to great confusion and should be avoided. The concept of three biorhythms (physical, emotional and intellectual cycles with periods of 23, 28 and 33 days), evolved out of numerological musings in the late nineteenth century. These cycles are supposed to be initiated at birth and to express their periodicities stably throughout life. There is no empirical basis for the period lengths attributed to these cycles, although the supposed emotional cycle may have been influenced by the length of the human MENSTRUAL CYCLE. Their beating interactions are supposed to influence each individual's.strength, alertness, MOOD and performance, leading to so-called critical days, and best and worst days for different kinds of athletic and intellectual activities. Periodic interest in biorhythms has been prompted by the appearance of books claiming to predict good days and bad for various activities and, in the modern era, by the development of biorhythms computers.

There are several fatal difficulties with the biorhythms concept. First, there are no empirical data supporting the existence of the three biorhythms. Second, there is no known physiological mechanism that can give rise to them. Third, empirical tests using records of athletic performances and accidents demonstrate that the calculated biorhythms for individuals have no predictive power. Fourth, studies purporting to demonstrate an influence of biorhythms are methodologically flawed and statistically incompetent. Finally, the concept that these rhythms are initiated at birth and progress throughout life with absolutely fixed periodicities is inherently absurd, given our knowledge of how real biological rhythms function. The sales tactics used for biorhythms books and computers include pointing to particular instances in which a calculated 'triple-critical' day for a pilot coincided with a plane crash. These illustrative examples seem to carry more weight with the public than do laboriously calculated statistical demonstrations that plane crashes and car accidents are randomly distributed with respect to the supposed biorhythms of those involved. The concept of biorhythms has more to do with astrology than with biology. By promising effortless predictions of our unknowable futures, astrology and biorhythms both seduce a gullible portion of the population to the profit of purveyors of pseudoscientific nonsense.

BENJAMIN RUSAK

biosynthesis The formation of chemical compounds by ENZYMES; it can be achieved either *IN VIVO* or *IN VITRO*.

biotransformation *see* drug metabolism

biped A biped is an animal that has only two feet on the ground in order to engage in LOCOMOTION; a QUADRUPED has four feet on the ground. Having the upper limbs free for other tasks confers on to the bipedal animal some considerable advantage in such things as, for example, grasping and the development of tool use.

bipolar A general term indicating the presence of two opposite poles; it can describe a variety of things including psychological states (for example BIPOLAR DISORDER) or structures (for example, BIPOLAR NEURON). Unipolar in contrast indicates possession of only one pole (as in UNIPOLAR DEPRESSION, or UNIPOLAR NEURON).

bipolar cells Bipolar cells are INTERNEURONS that link PHOTORECEPTORS (RODS and CONES) to the GANGLION CELLS in the RETINA. Their CELL BODIES are in the inner nuclear layer of the retina, but their processes extend into the outer and inner plexiform layers (see RETINAL CELL LAYERS). Their connectivity gives them a critical position in information flow across the retina. Like ganglion cells, bipolar cells have RECEPTIVE FIELDS that are circular, with a centre and an antagonistic surround: they can be on-centre or off-centre (these terms describing whether or not light applied to the centres turns the cells on or off). A single photoreceptor can simultaneously fire off-centre bipolar cells while inhibiting on-centre cells, a trick achieved through having the same neurotransmitter (GLUTAMATE) released by the photoreceptors produce different effects on the different types of bipolar cell. Further complex synaptic interactions in the inner plexiform layer achieves activation of on-centre or off-centre ganglion cells.

Reference

Kandel E.R., Schwartz J.H. & Jessell T.M. (1991) *Principles of Neural Science*, 3rd edn, Appleton & Lange: East Norwalk CT.

bipolar disorder Mood disorder in which episodes of major DEPRESSION and MANIA occur throughout the course of the illness, as distinct from recurrent episodes of depressive disorder alone (UNIPOLAR DEPRESSION). Classified by some authorities into subtypes: bipolar

I (episodes of major depression and mania) and bipolar II (major depressive episodes alternating with mild mood elevation, not sufficiently severe to be classified as manic – so-called 'HYPOMANIA'). Bipolar disorder is less common than unipolar depression, with a lifetime prevalence of 1%. There is evidence that there is a stronger genetic loading in bipolar disorder than other affective disorders.

IAN C. REID

bipolar electrode *see* electrode

bipolar, multipolar and unipolar neurons MULTIPOLAR NEURONS are the most common type in the CENTRAL NERVOUS SYSTEM: they have a CELL BODY with one AXON and multiple (typically branching) DENDRITES. A UNIPOLAR NEURON has a cell body that gives rise to a single PROCESS (therefore it is unipolar) which divides, one branch of it being the dendrite the other the axon. (These are also known as PSEUDOUNIPOLAR NEURONS, because the process eventually divides into two.) BIPOLAR NEURONS have a cell body that gives rise to one axon and one dendrite (that is, two processes, hence bipolar). Unipolar and bipolar neurons are relatively common in sensory systems: bipolar neurons for example are found in the RETINA, while unipolar neurons are found in SOMATOSENSORY systems.

See also: neuron

bipolar neuron *see* bipolar; multipolar neuron; unipolar neuron

birdsong Birds use a variety of sounds in communication, but the word 'song' is usually restricted to the more lengthy and complex of these. The most notable singers are among the songbirds (Order Passeriformes, Suborder Oscines), some of which have single short and STEREOTYPED phrases, while others may have a repertoire of hundreds of different song types. In most species it is only males in breeding condition that sing, and experimental evidence suggests that song fulfils two different functions: the attraction and stimulation of females and the exclusion of other males from the breeding territory. Females of various species have been found to show solicitation displays when played songs of their own species and, in some cases, song has been shown to stimulate ovarian development. The playing of song from loudspeakers has also been found to repel rival males. Birdsong provides a classic example of how nature and nurture interact during development. Young males isolated from adult song develop very simple songs but, if exposed to singing adults of their own species, will often copy their songs very precisely. Some species will copy from tapes, although in others social interaction is required. There are usually constraints which effectively restrict learning to the young bird's own species. Learning is also often restricted to a SENSITIVE PERIOD early in life, so that males learn as fledglings or as young adults first setting up their territories. Song learning leads to males in an area sharing song phrases, but transmission is not always accurate, so songs often differ from place to place (dialects) and with time (cultural evolution). In some species different song types appear to function in mate attraction and in rival repulsion, but in most all the songs in a repertoire are equivalent to each other in function. Experiments suggest that large song repertoires have evolved by sexual selection: females prefer males with more varied songs and hence it is advantageous for males to develop larger repertoires. Studies of birdsong have given important insights into the neural basis of behaviour. The nuclei involved in learning form a circuit that is different from that involved in production. In canaries, males have repertoires of song phrases that change from year to year. One nucleus, the HIGHER VOCAL CENTRE (HVC) is larger in birds with larger song repertoires, varies in size seasonally in line with singing behaviour and also shows neurogenesis in adulthood.

PETER J. B. SLATER

bisoperol A beta-1 noradrenaline receptor ANTAGONIST; see ADRENOCEPTORS.

blast (from Greek, *blastos*: bud) Blast can appear as a prefix but is more common as a suffix (as in, for example, FIBROBLAST or MYOBLAST); it always indicates that the cells referred to are in DEVELOPMENT.

bleaching (i) Vision: refers to loss of colour in the RETINA produced by exposure to light;

continued absorption of PHOTONS by VISUAL PIGMENTS is responsible for this.

(ii) Histology: refers to the gradual loss of colour from processed sections. FLUORO-CHROMES for example lose the ability to emit light over time – sections that are stored over long periods will lose their resolution as they bleach. Other forms of STAIN can also show bleaching over time.

blepharospasm (from Greek, *blepharon*: eyelid, *spaein*: to convulse) Blepharospasm is a condition in which both the eyelids shows chronic and persistent blinking. The condition is generally known as benign essential BLE-PHAROSPASM, to distinguish it from disorders of blinking that appear as secondary symptoms of other disorders. (It is also to be distinguished from blepharitis, which is an infection of the eyelid.) In the initial stages blepharospasm presents as excessive blinking, but over time this can become so intense that the eyes are to all intents and purposes closed. The spasms disappear during SLEEP and may be controlled by concentration on a particular task. The precise cause of the disorder is not known, but it is believed to be a disorder of BASAL GANGLIA function. (Drugs such as L-DOPA given for the relief of PARKINSON'S DISEASE may initiate blepharospasm as a side-effect – though fortunately one that is alleviated by moderating the dose of L-DOPA.) Misactivation of the fifth (the TRIGEMINAL NERVE) and seventh (the FACIAL NERVE) CRA-NIAL NERVES also occurs. It is treated quite effectively with injections of BOTULINUM TOXIN in very small doses: relief may take up to 2 weeks to develop but will then be present for up to 3 months. However, this is essentially control of the musculature; it prevents expression of the disorder rather than treating the (unknown) core dysfunction in the basal ganglia.

It is not to be confused with HEMIFACIAL SPASM which, although it can initially present as a blepharospasm-like condition, is in fact a more generalized disorder of the facial musculature (but only on one side of the face). It does however form a part of MEIGE SYNDROME (also known as segmental cranial dystonia). In this there is blepharospasm as well as jaw clenching, involuntary mouth opening and tongue extension, which of course also interfere with SPEECH PRODUCTION. Meige syndrome has been found to be associated with the presence of LEWY BODIES in the SUBSTANTIA NIGRA and LOCUS COERULEUS (as they are in Parkinson's disease) and there is evidence of decreased DOPAMINE activity in the STRIATUM.

blind spot The blind spot or OPTIC DISC is the region of the RETINA where the axons of the retinal ganglion cells converge to form the OPTIC NERVE and where they leave the eyeball, accompanied by the blood vessels that form the circulation of the eye. It is located approximately 15° towards the nasal side of the retina and is completely devoid of PHOTORECEPTORS. Visual objects that are imaged in this region cannot be perceived. Under certain circumstances, different geometric shapes imaged on the optic disc can be discriminated because of light scattering into the surrounding retinal regions. This demonstration has been used to critically query the existence of BLINDSIGHT.

DAVID W. HEELEY

blindness The inability to see, caused by damage to the eye or to parts of the VISUAL SYSTEM. It has been defined as a condition in which VISUAL ACUITY is 20/200 (see 6/6 NOTATION); or if the VISUAL FIELD subtends a visual angle of 20° or less.

See also: blindsight; colour blindness; scotoma; spatial neglect

blindsight The non-reflexive residual visual functions that persist in absolute cortically blind visual fields (see CORTICAL BLINDNESS). While visual reflexes like the pupil light reflex can also be elicited in comatose patients who have lost consciousness altogether, the more complex voluntary responses that have been termed 'blindsight' by Weiskrantz and colleagues (1974) are exclusively observed in conscious patients with lesions in the optic radiation and the PRIMARY VISUAL CORTEX. Depending on the extent and location of the LESION, it causes a visual field defect which affects the entire visual field, a HEMIFIELD, a quadrant, or any part of the visual field. The field defect is perimetrically assessed (see PERIMETRY) with respect to extent, location in the visual field and density. The latter differenti-

ates between relative defects where low-level conscious vision can be elicited, and absolute defects where no conscious vision remains. Blindsight is the highest known form of unconscious vision, and reserved for visual functions elicited from absolutely blind fields.

Two types of approaches have been used to uncover blindsight. The first is an indirect approach that demonstrates the responsiveness of the blind field by visually stimulating both the normal and the blind field. The patients are asked to respond to the stimulus they see – that is, the one in the normal field – and their responses are registered as a function of the presence of an additional stimulus presented, unbeknown to the patients, in the field defect. Such an additional stimulus has been shown to lengthen the REACTION TIME and to cause a perceptual completion or alteration of the seen stimulus. The alternative direct approach applies forced-choice guessing paradigms to account for the patient's inability to consciously see stimuli in the blind field. Often, to alert the patient to a stimulus presentation, an acoustic signal is given simultaneously or just before the presentation of a visual stimulus in the blind field. The patient's task is then to guess whether a stimulus has been presented, where it may have been or which one of a small number it was. Stimulus detection, localization by manual pointing or by directing the eyes toward the approximate stimulus position, and discrimination of stimuli differing in orientation, motion, motion direction, flux, intensity or wavelength have been demonstrated in this fashion. Dependent on variables that include retinal position, presentation time, stimulus size, on-and offset characteristics, speed, and adaptation level, the performance of the same patient can be at chance, moderate but statistically significant, or even 100% correct. Compared to sensitivity measured at the corresponding position in the normal field, blindsight sensitivity is reduced by 0.4 to 1.5 log units. In view of the patient's inability to consciously see the stimuli, this residual sensitivity is relatively high. It cannot be explained on the basis of light scattered from the stimulus into the normal visual field because the luminance of stimuli that are presented on the natural BLIND SPOT (optic disc) needs to be 2–3 log units above that required for the normal field. The difference between blindsight and STRAYLIGHT sensitivity is thus in the order of 1.5–2.6 log units.

Although most studies of blindsight have been performed in the last 25 years, the phenomenon of residual visual functions was noted as early as 1905 by Bard. Klüver studied it extensively in cortically blinded monkeys who are now known to show a repertoire of residual visual functions, levels of performance and sensitivity similar to that of patients. In addition, in a signal detection paradigm in which they responded differently to stimulus and no-stimulus (blank) trials, hemianopic monkeys who showed close to perfect detection of supra-threshold stimuli in the affected hemifield, treated these same stimuli like blanks. This result indicates that monkeys too may have blindsight and suffer a loss of conscious vision as a consequence of primary visual cortical destruction. Such destruction, usually of vascular, traumatic or neoplastic (see NEOPLASIA) origin, causes RETROGRADE DE-GENERATION of the dorsal LATERAL GENICU-LATE NUCLEUS and the retinal ganglion cell layer. The large population of ganglion cells that survive the degeneration continue to project to all retino-recipient nuclei. In their turn, these send axons either directly or via other nuclei to the extrastriate visual cortical areas that extend from the OCCIPITAL LOBE into temporal and parietal regions. Indicated by physiological recording in monkeys and FUNC-TIONAL NEUROIMAGING in patients, this residual system remains visually responsive, with the dorsal occipito-parietal areas retaining considerably more activity. Studies of this system and the blind visual functions it mediates are relevant to consciousness research because they may help us understand the difference in the neuronal structures and processes underlying unconscious as opposed to consciously represented vision.

References

Stoerig P. & Cowey A. (1997) Blindsight in man and monkey. *Brain* 120: 101–125.
Weiskrantz, L. (1986) *Blindsight. A Case Study and Implications*, Clarendon Press: Oxford.
Weiskrantz L., Warrington E.K., Sanders M.D. & Marshall J. (1974) Visual capacity in the

hemianopic field following a restricted cortical ablation. *Brain* 97: 709–728.

PETRA STOERIG

blocking (i) *Learning*: The attenuation of PAVLOVIAN CONDITIONING when another previously-trained CONDITIONED STIMULUS (CS) is present during CS UNCONDITIONED STIMULUS (US) pairings. A blocking experiment might involve first training a light as a signal for food. Next, a tone and the light are presented simultaneously and followed by food. Relative to a group receiving a similar treatment, but without the first phase of light-food training, conditioned responding to the tone alone is markedly attenuated. This phenomenon shows that the mere pairing of the tone and the food is insufficient to support LEARNING – the presence of the light makes learning of the tone-food relationship redundant. See also ASSOCIATIVE LEARNING.

(ii) *Pharmacology*: blocking describes the application of an ANTAGONIST to a RECEPTOR (or other appropriate substrate); receptor antagonists are colloquially known as blockers.

(iii) *Histology*: tissue blocking is a term used to describe the cutting of a piece of tissue (such as a brain) accurately through a particular plane (see PLANES OF SECTION) prior to cutting it to obtain repeated SECTIONS. Brain blocking can be done in a STEREOTAXIC FRAME or by using purpose built brain holder with cutting guides.

(iv) *Immunohistochemistry*: a blocking SERUM is applied to tissue prior to the application of primary ANTIBODY to block non-specific binding sites.

(I) JASPER WARD-ROBINSON
AND (II–IV) PHILIP WINN

blood 'Blood' might at first appear an odd topic to be of interest to biological psychologists, but such a first impression would be wrong. Blood is interesting to biological psychologists for three reasons. First, it is critically involved in all bodily processes, including the maintenance of brain function. Second, damage to the brain's blood supply can cause profound neuropsychological impairments (see ANOXIA, CEREBROVASCULAR ACCIDENT, ISCHAE-MIA and STROKE). Third, the bloodstream is a critically important source of sensory information to the brain: the state of the body is very effectively indexed by the composition of blood.

What is blood? Vertebrate blood (which is a form of CONNECTIVE TISSUE) is composed of several types of cells suspended in PLASMA. Some 45% of blood volume is made up of cells, the remainder being fluid: plasma, which is 90% water with various ELECTROLYTES present (these maintain the appropriate OSMOTIC PRESSURE of the blood) and PROTEINS (which have several functions: some transport insoluble LIPIDS, some are ANTIBODIES, and some are involved in blood clotting). There are also many molecules present in the blood that are in transit from one place to another – the bloodstream is a major transport system. The majority of the cells present in the blood are ERYTHROCYTES, which are more colloquially known as red blood cells – the colour comes from the molecule HAEMOGLOBIN, a protein which can carry oxygen. Oxygen transport is the major function of erythrocytes. There are also white blood cells (see LEUKOCYTE): these come in five types: MONOCYTE, NEUTROPHIL, BASOPHIL, EOSINOPHIL and LYMPHOCYTE. All are important components of the IMMUNE SYSTEM. PLATELETS are also present in the blood: these are chips of CYTOPLASM and are important in blood clotting. All of these cells need continually to be replaced: STEM CELLS in bone marrow do this.

What is the function of blood? Single-celled or very simple animals are small enough that chemicals – GLUCOSE and oxygen for example – can diffuse effectively to all the required sites. In larger animals with specialized tissues and organs a transport system is required for moving substances (and heat) around the body. A major function is the transport of oxygen, which is collected by blood in the lungs, while carbon dioxide is expelled from the blood to the air that is exhaled. But there are many other chemicals that are transported through the bloodstream, from their point of RELEASE to target sites elsewhere (see below under *CNS systems for analysing blood*). Blood also has a critical role in maintaining body TEMPERATURE, carrying heat around the body as well as being involved in the mechanisms of body cooling. The function of blood as a transport system is also used very effectively in DRUG ADMINISTRATION. No matter what route of drug administration is chosen, the delivered drug will be transported to sites of active use around the body by the bloodstream.

The cardiovascular system simplified

Right ventricle:	pumps blood to lungs via the pulmonary arteries. In the lungs, capillaries collect oxygen and dispose of carbon dioxide. The pulmonary veins return blood loaded with oxygen to the left atrium. This is the PULMONARY CIRCUIT.
Left atrium:	blood is passed from here to the left ventricle
Left ventricle:	blood is pumped from here, via the AORTA, to the VASCULAR system in the rest of the body. This is the SYSTEMIC CIRCUIT.
Right atrium:	blood, depleted of oxygen which has been taken by the body tissues, returns to the right atrium via the anterior (or superior) vena cava (from the head, neck and arms [forelimbs]) and via the posterior (or inferior) vena cava (from the trunk and legs [hindlimbs]). The right atrium passes blood into the right ventricle, completing the circuit.
Heart beat:	contraction of the heart pumps blood; relaxation allows it to fill with blood. The cardiac cycle is one complete sequence of contraction and relaxation: the contraction is known as a SYSTOLE (giving rise to systolic pressure) and the relaxation is known as the DIASTOLE (diastolic pressure). The rhythm of the beat is controlled by PACEMAKER CELLS in the sinoatrial node (in the wall of the right atrium); heart rate can be measured by the ELECTROCARDIOGRAM (ECG)

The organization of the blood supply. The CARDIOVASCULAR SYSTEM includes the heart, blood vessels and blood itself. The heart is essentially a muscular pump with four chambers: two atria (singular: ATRIUM) and two VENTRICLES, separated by valves ensuring that blood flows in only one direction through the heart: the left side receives blood rich in oxygen, the right side blood that is oxygen-depleted. The ventricles serve as pumps and are therefore composed of thicker MUSCLE walls (made of cardiac muscle). The table on page 111 explains briefly the functions of these atria and ventricles.

Three types of blood vessel are found: CAPILLARY, VEIN and ARTERY. Capillaries are the smallest and are composed of a thin layer of ENDOTHELIUM. Within tissues capillaries form networks known as CAPILLARY beds to facilitate interactions between blood and tissues. Veins and arteries are larger than capillaries and are both made in much the same way: they have three layers of tissue: an outer layer of connective tissue, an intermediate layer of smooth muscle and an inner layer of endothelium. Arteries always carry blood away from the heart (so the blood tends to be oxygen-rich) while veins always carry blood towards the heart (so veins tend to be oxygen-depleted). Of course, arteries do not narrow in a single step to become capillaries but instead narrow gradually. The intermediate portions are ARTERIOLES. Similarly, when blood is flowing away from capillary beds into veins, they pass through VENULES first, venules being wider than capillaries but narrower than veins. Arteries effectively pump blood through the body, having valves present to facilitate this. The flow is regular but discontinuous, reflecting the pumping of the ventricles: this pumping is effectively measured by taking one's pulse. Veins are less actively involved in moving blood, which tends to drain back to the heart rather than being actively pumped. Bodily movement works to keep blood moving in the veins.

Blood flow to the brain. Neurons require a continuous blood supply and the brain has an extensive vascular network supplying all parts (the CEREBRAL VASCULATURE). The blood supply and the brain are separated from direct contact (except at the CIRCUMVENTRICULAR ORGANS) by the BLOOD–BRAIN BARRIER. The importance of the blood supply to the brain is shown by the following: a 1-second interruption of blood flow to the brain is sufficient for all the oxygen present there to be used; a 6-second interruption is sufficient to produce unconsciousness; and interruption of only a few minutes is sufficient to produce neuronal death. Blood is supplied to the brain by two pairs of arteries: the VERTEBRAL ARTERIES and the INTERNAL CAROTID ARTERIES. The vertebral arteries enter the skull at the FORAMEN MAGNUM, giving off branches (the anterior and posterior spinal arteries and the posterior inferior cerebellar artery) before joining to form the BASILAR ARTERY which runs along the MIDLINE on the surface of the PONS, immediately below the brain. The basilar artery divides into the posterior cerebral arteries, anterior inferior cerebellar artery, pontine branches and the superior cerebellar artery. Much of the posterior part of the brain receives its blood supply from the vertebral arteries. The internal carotids enter the skull via the FORAMEN LACERUM and divide at the level of the OPTIC CHIASM into the anterior cerebral arteries. Further branching occurs giving rise to the MIDDLE CEREBRAL ARTERY and striate arteries. It is the anterior parts of the brain that receive their blood supply from the internal carotids. At the base of the brain the carotid and vertebral arteries communicate via the anterior and posterior communicating arteries, which form the CIRCLE OF WILLIS. Blood drains away from the brain via veins, which run into larger veins known as sinuses (singular SINUS) present in the DURA MATER. The superior sagittal sinus and straight sinus join to form the transverse sinus, which flows into the sigmoid sinus which in turn flows into the JUGULAR VEIN, in the neck.

CNS control mechanisms involved in heart rate and blood pressure. HEART RATE can be changed by SYMPATHETIC and PARASYMPATHETIC neurons of the AUTONOMIC NERVOUS SYSTEM. NORADRENALINE released from sympathetic nerve endings increases heart rate by an action on BETA ADRENERGIC receptors. Noradrenaline, again acting at beta receptors, also constricts blood vessels (a process called VASO-

CONSTRICTION) which will increase blood pressure. ACETYLCHOLINE released from para-sympathetic neurons and acting at MUSCARINIC ACETYLCHOLINE RECEPTORS, has the opposite effect: it slows heart rate by an action on cardiac muscle and by changing the function of cardiac pacemaker cells which regulate heart beat. The CENTRAL NERVOUS SYSTEM is also involved in the regulation of blood pressure. BARORECEPTORS detect changes in blood pressure in the carotid artery (which is a major source of blood supply to the brain): these signal via the VAGUS NERVE to the NUCLEUS OF THE SOLITARY TRACT. This connects via a disynaptic pathway to neurons in the rostral ventrolateral MEDULLA and to the motor nucleus of the vagus. Vagal outflow produces a decrease in heart rate. Rostral ventrolateral medulla outflow, via the reticulospinal tract, can effect the heart, but can produce an increase in pressure rather than a decrease. This pathway can also have an action on arterioles to change arterial resistance to blood flow. These medullary sites in brain are therefore able to regulate closely heart rate and blood pressure.

CNS systems for analysing blood. The blood supply to the brain is a very important source of sensory information about the state of the body and there are various systems present in the brain for analysing blood composition and initiating changes on the basis of that monitoring. Such processes are of importance for OSMOREGULATION, ENERGY BALANCE, SEXUAL BEHAVIOUR, responses to STRESS and THERMOREGULATION. For example, detector mechanisms in brain can monitor the amount of water present in the blood and circulating levels of molecules such as ANGIOTENSIN II (important in signalling information about WATER BALANCE); glucose and INSULIN (important in maintaining energy balance and the regulation of FEEDING); CHOLECYSTOKININ (thought to be involved in signalling SATIETY); and various HORMONES involved in stress and sexual behaviour. Brain mechanisms in areas such as the circumventricular organs, PARAVENTRICULAR SYSTEM and HYPOTHALAMUS are especially important for monitoring blood content and temperature.

See also: breathing, neural control of

References

Campbell N.A., Reece J.B. & Mitchell L.G. (1999) *Biology*, 5th edn, Addison-Wesley: Menlo Park CA.

Kandel E.R., Schwartz J.H. & Jessell T.M. (1991) *Principles of Neural Science*, 3rd edn, Appleton & Lange: East Norwalk CT.

blood–brain barrier The blood–brain barrier is exactly what it says: a physical barrier between BLOOD and brain (or more specifically, between PLASMA and brain INTERSTITIAL FLUID). Its importance cannot be overstated: the bloodstream contains very many chemicals: some are required by the brain for effective functioning (such as GLUCOSE) and some act as information signals to the brain (such as HORMONES), but there are many chemicals that are not required by brain (and would be dangerous if present there) and of course DRUGS delivered into the bloodstream deliberately, either for therapeutic or recreational purposes, may or may not be wanted in brain. Those substances that need to be excluded are effectively barred by the blood–brain barrier; those that need access generally have to have that access regulated. (For example, the concentration of glucose in the blood fluctuates dramatically during the day. Brains need to be protected against surging levels of glucose, requiring instead a regulated and controlled flow.) Chemicals that cross the blood–brain barrier typically have a low MOLECULAR WEIGHT and high solubility in LIPIDS, or they cross by virtue of an active transport mechanism. In drug discovery research it is always important to know whether a compound can cross the blood–brain barrier: an agent intended to treat a neurological condition would normally be expected actually to enter brain tissue.

The existence of a barrier was noted first by Paul Ehrlich in the nineteenth century: he injected dye into the bloodstream and noted that it stained all tissues except the brain. The same dye injected into the cerebral VENTRICLES did stain brain tissue, indicating that something normally obstructed the passage of chemicals from blood to brain. The term blood–brain barrier was coined in 1900 by Lewandowski. The blood–brain barrier is formed by complex tight junctions between cells which physically prevent movement of fluids across the membranes. There are a number of places where specialized barriers are formed: (1) the ENDOTHELIUM of blood vessels in brain form tight junctions to prevent fluid escaping from the bloodstream into the brain interstitial fluid. (2) The CHOROID PLEXUS is CONNECTIVE TISSUE found in the VENTRICLES of the brain. It is here that CEREBROSPINAL FLUID (CSF) is formed, this accumulating in the ventricles and flowing out into the extracellular spaces around the NEUROPIL of the brain. A barrier in the choroid plexus epithelium prevents direct exchange of fluids between blood and CSF. (3) The NEUROTHELIUM is a barrier formed in the ARACHNOID MEMBRANE: cells form a barrier on the outside of the arachnoid membrane to prevent blood from vessels in the DURA MATER escaping into brain. (4) There are specialized sites known as the CIRCUMVENTRICULAR ORGANS where exchange between brain and blood can take place. Such sites are critically involved in monitoring the composition of the bloodstream, but nevertheless possess a form of barrier that allows the required communication to take place while preventing non-selective influx of material into brain. This barrier is made of TANYCYTES, specialized ependymal cells.

All of these – blood vessel endothelium, choroid plexus endothelium, neurothelium, tanycytes – show formation of tight junctions to prevent unwanted movement of fluid. Clearly though, blood contains substances such as glucose that need to be extracted by the brain. Specialized transport mechanisms exist to take such substances from the bloodstream and divert them to the required brain sites. ASTROCYTES are involved in this process: they make contact with blood vessels and, using specialized transporter mechanisms, effect passage of required substances into brain in a controlled manner.

blood flow limited access *see* drug administration

blood flow to the brain *see* blood

blood serum *see* serum

blotting There are three types of blotting: all are techniques used in MOLECULAR BIOLOGY to

asses the composition of material. NORTHERN BLOTTING it is used to measure RNA; SOUTHERN BLOTTING is used to measure DNA fragments; WESTERN BLOTTING is used to measure PROTEINS. Southern blotting is named after its inventor; the others are merely named imitatively.

Bmax *see* maximum concentration of available binding sites

body dysmorphic disorder A SOMATOFORM DISORDER in which individuals become overly concerned with defects in their physical appearance; see also BODY IMAGE.

body image Psychological construct of self-evaluation of physical appearance. Body image disturbance is central to EATING DISORDERS and to BODY DYSMORPHIC DISORDER. Three components of body image are generally recognized: a perceptual component which incorporates estimation of body size or shape; an affective component which includes satisfaction, disparagement, and ANXIETY about body size or shape; and a behavioural component which indicates the extent to which individuals might hide their shape or size, or avoid situations in which physical appearance is emphasized. Gender differences in body image satisfaction indicate a significantly greater discontent in women.

See also: anorexia nervosa; bulimia nervosa; obesity

Reference

Thompson J.K. (1990) *Body Image Disturbance*, Pergamon Press: Oxford.

MARION M. HETHERINGTON

body language *see* animal communication

body mass index *see* obesity

body weight It is clear that there are physiological and behavioural processes involved in body weight regulation. For example, if laboratory rats have their food intake restricted and their body weight falls, they will spontaneously begin food HOARDING BEHAVIOUR, regardless of how hungry they are at the time of testing. The level of body weight at which this occurs has been referred to as the defended level of body weight.

In the past, theories have suggested that body weight was closely regulated to a SET POINT (probably in the HYPOTHALAMUS) but evidence for such a theory remains unconvincing. Lesions in parts of the hypothalamus that produce dramatic change in body weight (see VENTROMEDIAL HYPOTHALAMIC SYNDROME; LATERAL HYPOTHALAMIC SYNDROME) have been shown to produce their effects by disrupting multiple processes and do not represent the neural substrates of body weight set points. Moreover, the idea of a single set point is intrinsically unlikely: animals generally have to take advantage of seasonal variation in food intake and as such, body weight must be a flexible construct. Critical to this is the process of fat deposition: body weight is an index total body mass, but changing fat deposition is the most rapid way to affect body weight. Studies of ground squirrels have shown that physiological processes are adjusted to take account of seasonal food availability: the body weight of these animals increases in seasons when food is plentiful. However, if they are maintained in a laboratory on a constant energy intake, their body weight still fluctuates: what is regulated is the proportion of energy intake that is stored as fat. It is ENERGY BALANCE that is important to consider in order to understand body weight regulation.

Energy balance is usually represented as a simple equation: energy intake = energy used + energy stored + excess energy burnt as heat. Body weight can be affected therefore by changing energy intake, use or by thermogenesis. For example, individuals showing the HIGH FAT PHENOTYPE (eating over 44% of their energy as fat) show greater weight gain than low fat consumers (less than 35% energy from fat intake). Similarly, studies of the OB/OB mouse revealed that the failure to use BROWN ADIPOSE TISSUE to engage NON-SHIVERING THERMOGENESIS produced excess fat deposition. Further studies of these genetically obese mice revealed the existence of a protein, LEPTIN, which appears to be released by fat cells and to have an action at several sites in the brain, including the LATERAL HYPOTHALAMUS and the PARAVENTRICULAR NUCLEUS OF THE HYPOTHALAMUS. The actions of leptin appear to trigger a variety of signals which in turn affect processes in the periphery regulating fat deposition. The discovery of leptin has been particularly important because, previously, no clear signal from fat stores to brain that could be involved in the fat regulating component of energy balance had been identified.

It is apparent that there are mechanisms that influence energy balance and the deposition of fat. It is also clear that both humans and animals will voluntarily exceed their energy intake requirements (see SUPERMARKET DIET for example) and that OBESITY is a significant problem in many societies. Evidently, having mechanisms for regulating body weight does not imply that they are going to be used in any strict manner.

See also: eating disorders; feeding; satiety; Zucker rats

References

Cooling J., Barth J. & Blundell J. (1998) The high fat phenotype: is leptin involved in the adaptive response to a high fat (high energy) diet? *International Journal of Obesity* 22: 1132–1135.

Zhang Y., Proenca R., Maffei M., Barone M., Leopold L. & Friedman J.M. (1994) Positional cloning of the mouse obese gene and its human homologue. *Nature* 372: 425–432.

bomb calorimetry *see* calorimeter

bombesin One of the gut–brain PEPTIDES (though oddly enough initially detected in frog skin) bombesin is also found within the CENTRAL NERVOUS SYSTEM of MAMMALS where it is present in both neurons and astrocytes (see ASTROGLIA; NEURONS). It is widely distributed and has three different subclasses of receptors (BB1, BB2 and BB3) (see RECEPTOR). It has been suggested, like CHOLECYSTOKININ, to be involved in the signalling of SATIETY.

bone wax A form of surgical wax used to treat bleeding from bones during surgery. (It is a little-recognized fact that bones contain BLOOD vessels and therefore, if a cut is made along a bone surface during surgery, it bleeds.) Bone wax is not often used now, other, better methods for the control of bleeding being available.

See also: stereotaxic surgery

borderline personality disorder *see* schizotypal personality disorder

borna disease Borna disease is a viral infection: the Bornaviridae are a type of RNA VIRUS, and appear to be relatively new. They cause damage to the CENTRAL NERVOUS SYSTEM without any apparent INFLAMMATION. Of special interest is the fact that borna virus appears to have a particular effect on the HIPPOCAMPUS, inducing loss of the DENTATE GYRUS over a period of a few weeks. Behavioural deficits in LEARNING and MEMORY have been described following this.

Reference

Rubin S.A., Sylves P., Vogel M., Pletnikov M., Moran T.H., Schwartz G.J. & Carbone K.M. (1998) Borna disease virus-induced hippocampal dentate gyrus damage is associated with spatial learning and memory deficits. *Brain Research Bulletin* 48: 23–30.

Boston process approach This refers to the Boston diagnostic aphasia examination, a standard tool for the assessment of APHASIA.

Reference

Goodglass H. & Kaplan E. (1983) *The Assessment of Aphasia and Related Disorders*, 2nd edn, Lea & Febiger: Philadelphia.

botulinum toxin A toxin produced by the bacterium *Clostridium botulinum*: it is occasionally found in processed foods and can be fatal (though more often is not). Neuroscientifically it is of interest because it blocks NEUROTRANSMISSION at the NEUROMUSCULAR JUNCTION: it can be used experimentally in studies of this. Medically it is of value because minute injections direct into the area around the EYE is a recognized treatment for BLEPHAROSPASM.

boundary models Boundary models – the first was developed by Herman & Polivy (1984) to account for FEEDING – are an alternative to strict SET POINT models of HOMEOSTASIS. Rather than use a single set point about which a behaviour must be regulated, the boundaries set upper and lower limits. Deviation of some activity – ENERGY BALANCE, WATER BALANCE or THERMOREGULATION for example – outwith the upper or lower limits triggers metabolic and behavioural changes, but within the limits, control is very flexible.

Reference

Herman C.P. & Polivy, J. (1984) A boundary model for the regulation of eating. In *Eating and its disorders*, ed. A. J. Stunkard and E. Stellar, pp.141–156, Raven Press: New York.

bovine spongiform encephalopathy (BSE) A fatal PRION DISEASE of cattle first diagnosed in Britain in 1986. Cows with BSE behave erratically, become apprehensive and stagger about, hence the term 'mad cow disease'. BSE has been transmitted experimentally by intra-cerebral injection of brain material to cows, mice, monkeys, sheep and pigs and by the oral route to cows, sheep and mice. Between 1986 and 1996 BSE was diagnosed in 160 000 cows in the British Isles and may have infected a further 700 000 cattle, most of which would have been eaten before showing symptoms of disease. It is believed that the epidemic of BSE occurred because the rendering process, by which parts of animal carcasses are processed to make animal feedstuff, was changed in the early 1980s inadvertently allowing the infectious agent of prion disease to escape inactivation. The epidemic probably started because of the rendering of carcasses of sheep affected with SCRAPIE but the main part of the epidemic was caused by the recycling of BSE-infected cattle carcasses into cattle feed. Infection of cattle occurred shortly after birth but the disease was not manifest until animals reached 4–5 years of age. The Ruminant Feed Ban of 1988 prevented the use of ruminant-derived material for ruminant feed and was designed to prevent new cases of BSE but, because of the late age of onset of BSE, the epidemic in Britain did not begin to decline until 1993 and was not expected to be over until at least 1999 despite attempts to destroy the cattle most at risk of developing disease. More than 30 000 cattle which developed BSE were born after the Ruminant Feed Ban. This was initially interpreted as suggesting that the disease could be passed directly from dam to calf but the pattern of the incidence of BSE after the

Ruminant Feed Ban and the Specified Bovine Offals Ban (Part 2), which banned the feeding of specified materials to other farm animals, is more compatible with the possibility that the feed bans were not adequately implemented or enforced in the first instance. Attempts to demonstrate maternal transmission of BSE and other prion diseases have produced equivocal results.

The BSE epidemic affected mainly dairy cows in the British Isles who were fed large amounts of rendered cattle feed. Beef cattle, which are usually suckled and fed mainly on grass, were much less frequently affected. A few animals of several species of antelope kept in British zoos and about 75 domestic cats also developed a spongiform ENCEPHALOPATHY between 1985 and 1995 probably as a result of eating contaminated animal feedstuff. In 1989 the Specified Bovine Offals Ban (Part 1) prohibited the use of bovine brain and spinal cord, which are known to carry high levels of infectivity in affected animals, and other internal organs which might have been infectious, in human food. In March 1996, the British Government acknowledged the possibility that consumption of food made from BSE-affected cattle could have been responsible for the occurrence of 10 cases of a new variant of CREUTZFELDT–JAKOB DISEASE in young people in Britain and banned the use of tissue from any British cattle over 30 months old in human food. At the beginning of 1997 a selective cull was instituted which was intended to destroy about 100 000 cattle which were mainly elderly dairy cows born at the same time and place as cows which developed BSE. It was calculated that this group of cattle would contain the best-targeted proportion of the estimated 7000 cows incubating BSE. The extent of the risk to humans (which could be very small or very large) will not be known for 40 years because of the long incubation time for acquired prion disease in humans. The cost to the British Government in compensation to farmers is estimated to be about £3 billion. The loss of trade and damage to associated industries is incalculable.

References

Tyrrell D.A.J. & Taylor K.C.(1996) Handling the BSE epidemic in Great Britain. In *Prion Diseases*, ed. H.F. Baker & R.M. Ridley, pp. 175–198, Humana Press: Totowa NJ.

Wilesmith J.W.(1996) Bovine spongiform encephalopathy: methods of analysing the epidemic in the United Kingdom. In *Prion Diseases*, ed. H.F. Baker & R.M. Ridley, pp. 155–173, Humana Press: Totowa NJ.

ROSALIND RIDLEY

brachiation (from Latin via Old French, *brace* (modern French *bras*): the arm, arm-power) Brachiation is swinging through the trees, a form of LOCOMOTION practised by certain PRIMATES and by Tarzan of the Apes.

brachium conjunctivum Alternative name for the SUPERIOR CEREBELLAR PEDUNCLE (see CEREBELLUM – ANATOMICAL ORGANIZATION).

brachium pontis Alternative name for the MIDDLE CEREBELLAR PEDUNCLE (see CEREBELLUM – ANATOMICAL ORGANIZATION).

bradykinesia (from Greek, *bradys*: slow, *kinesis*: movement – literally, slowness of movement) Bradykinesia is shown by patients with a variety of conditions, but it is most commonly associated with PARKINSON'S DISEASE.

bradykinin A hormone that causes contraction of MUSCLES and dilation of BLOOD vessels; see KININ.

brain 'Brain' and 'CENTRAL NERVOUS SYSTEM' are not synonyms. The brain is one part of the central nervous system; the other component is the SPINAL CORD. The brains of all VERTEBRATES appear to be built to a common plan (see NEURODEVELOPMENT). Among the MAMMALS there are remarkable similarities between brains across SPECIES, both in structure and functional specialization. It is clear however that two major changes can take place: (1) neurons within a given structure often become complex with, for example, greater ARBORIZATION of their dendrites and more complex patterns of branching in the axons (see DENDRITE; NEURON). While the neurons may fulfil similar functions, a greater complexity evidently can develop in higher species. (2) Structures themselves change in their relative size. For example, the OLFACTORY BULB of a rat is very large compared to the remainder of its brain, whereas in the human, while being much bigger than in the rat, it is relatively small in relation to the remainder of the human brain. The comparison between brains of different species and their relative ENCEPHALIZATION is discussed in NERVOUS SYSTEM.

See also: comparative anatomy; neuroanatomy

brain bank A depository for brains, post mortem. Studies of brain PATHOLOGY rely on a supply of tissue, and it is important that the tissue used is in good condition, having been carefully and appropriately removed and stored. It is also of benefit to have a known life history, with as much information as possible about age, health, medication, socioeconomic status and psychological information (such as scores on any appropriate psychological tests that had been taken). As with any tissue bank, brain banks are expensive to maintain and rely on the willingness of living individuals to agree to donate organs post mortem.

brain cooling *see* transient lesions

brain death Death is not an event but a process in which various systems fail successively and at different times. Brain death is now generally accepted (by the 1976 UK Conference of Medical Royal Colleges and Faculties for example) as the watershed for medico-legal purposes such as organ transplantation or termination of life-support. Criteria for the diagnosis of brain death include absence of pupillary, corneal, vestibulo-ocular and pharyngeal reflexes (see REFLEX), after exclusion of other possible causes (such as drugs, metabolic disturbances or HYPOTHERMIA). A flat ELECTROENCEPHALOGRAM, an imperceptible pulse or the persistence of spinal reflexes are not diagnostically significant.

L. JACOB HERBERG

brain-derived neurotrophic factor *see* nerve growth factor

brain electrical activity mapping Brain electrical activity mapping uses SCALP ELECTRODES and ELECTROENCEPHALOGRAM (EEG) recordings to identify waveforms produced by the brain at different locations and with different frequencies. Statistical techniques can then be used to quantify and map electrical activity in the brain. It has been used to evaluate normal and abnormal brain functioning.

See also: evoked potentials; magnetoencephalography

brain imaging *see* functional neuroimaging

brain injury Injury to the brain can either be focal, in which case pathology is limited to a circumscribed part of the brain, or diffuse, when pathological changes are widespread throughout the brain. In Western society, the most common cause of focal injury is STROKE, which is caused by an interruption of the blood supply to brain tissue. Depending on the location and nature of the interruption, the amount of brain damaged following a stroke can vary enormously. As with all focal injuries, however, the consequences of the damage do not only reflect the amount of tissue that has been destroyed; the location of the damage is equally important. Whereas even a large LESION in some areas of the CEREBRAL CORTEX may have consequences that are barely detectable without special testing, a small lesion in an important subcortical structure such as the THALAMUS may have devastating effects on a wide range of psychological functions. After stroke, the most common cause of focal brain damage is neurosurgery, when brain tissue is removed by the surgeon in an effort to alleviate conditions such as intractable EPILEPSY or brain TUMOUR. Diffuse brain injury has numerous causes, including infection with viruses such as herpes simplex and with prions, such as the one responsible for CREUTZFELDT–JAKOB DISEASE. Among young adults, by far the most common cause of diffuse brain injury is CLOSED HEAD INJURY. Among the elderly, a variety of dementing illnesses, notably ALZHEIMER'S DISEASE, cause progressive and increasingly widespread brain damage. A feature of these progressive diseases is that the accompanying psychological deficits appear at first to be quite restricted (for example, to LONG-TERM MEMORY in the case of early Alzheimer's disease), but become more pervasive as the pathological process produces an increasingly diffuse pattern of damage.

MICHAEL D. RUGG

brain natriuretic peptide *see* natriuretic peptides

brain scan Brain scans provide images of the brain's structure and function. Information about structure (and abnormalities of structure arising from injury or disease) are most commonly obtained by COMPUTERIZED AXIAL TOMOGRAPHY or MAGNETIC RESONANCE IMAGING. Functional information is obtained with POSITRON EMISSION TOMOGRAPHY or other FUNCTIONAL NEUROIMAGING methods.

MICHAEL D. RUGG

brain stimulation reward Literally, any direct stimulation of the brain that has rewarding properties (that is, an animal will seek to repeat the stimulation or seek out conditions or places in the environment where stimulation is likely to recur). In practice, the term brain stimulation reward is often used as a synonym for INTRACRANIAL SELF-STIMULATION.

See also: asymptotic behavioural maximum

brain stimulation studies Studies which use electrical stimulation of the brain (see ELECTRICAL BRAIN STIMULATION). Technically, studies which infuse drugs directly into brain result in brain stimulation but this term typically refers to electrical stimulation.

JAMES R. STELLAR

brain tumour *see* tumour

braincase *see* skull

brainstem (also brain stem) The posterior part of the brain that consists of the MEDULLA, PONS and MIDBRAIN. It is continuous with the SPINAL CORD caudally, and with the DIENCEPHALON rostrally. The brainstem contains numerous sensory and motor pathways which ascend or descend to interconnect the spinal cord and FOREBRAIN. Most sensory and motor pathways are relayed within the brainstem. Brainstem nuclei are involved in life-supporting or homeostatic (see HOMEOSTASIS) functions of the organism such as respiration (see BREATHING, NEURAL CONTROL OF), cardiovascular regulation and control of SLEEP and AROUSAL, as well as in basic sensory and motor functions.

See also: central nervous system

KAZUE SEMBA

brainstem reticular formation *see* reticular formation

brainwashing This is a concept familiar to many but not generally covered in the context of biological psychology. It involves the induction of psychological pressure directed consistently at an individual in order to induce changes in cognitive processing and behaviour. It may be presented in a harsh way, as a form of torture, or in an attempt to induce a false confession (as was the case with Stalinist show-trials) or it may be presented in an apparently open and friendly way, as is the case with pseudo-religious indoctrination. Recovering brainwashed individuals back into normal, free society is a process known as deprogramming.

Brattleboro rats *see* vasopressin

breakdown A rather general term, likely to be used in two main ways in biological psychology: (i) as shorthand for NERVOUS BREAKDOWN; (ii) as a colloquialism for CATABOLISM – the decomposition of molecules (see METABOLISM).

breaking point The point at which an animal will stop responding for reinforcement in a PROGRESSIVE RATIO schedule. In a progressive ratio SCHEDULE OF REINFORCEMENT, the animal must make progressively more fixed ratio responses in order to be rewarded. The breaking point, also termed the break point, is defined as the number of responses (usually lever-presses) in the last completed reinforced ratio performed by the animal, before it ceases responding. The breaking point is thought to be a valid measure of the animal's MOTIVATION for a REWARD, primarily because it is not related to response rate, and it is the subject that determines the number of ratios completed. For example, a hungry animal will have a higher breaking point in lever-pressing for food than a satiated animal (that is, it will continue to respond without immediate reward for much longer). Progressive ratio breaking points have been shown to correlate with the reinforcer magnitude of food, ELECTRICAL BRAIN STIMULATION and DRUG dose.

ANN E. KELLEY

breath Breath is the output of breathing (see BREATHING, NEURAL CONTROL OF). Mammals exhale CARBON DIOXIDE, though many other molecules are carried on the breath. Odorants carried in this way can be detected by a CONSPECIFIC and can carry important information; see SOCIAL TRANSMISSION OF FOOD PREFERENCES.

breathing, neural control of The respiratory system operates in coordination with the CARDIOVASCULAR SYSTEM to regulate OXYGEN, CARBON DIOXIDE and PH levels within all body tissues. In lung-breathing animals, the regulation of blood gases is accomplished by exchange of oxygen for carbon dioxide within blood vessels that course through the lungs. The flow of air into and out of the lung is generated by the periodic contraction and relaxation of muscles innervated by SPINAL CORD MOTONEURONS, and is modulated by the activity of upper airway muscles innervated by cranial motoneurons. The main respiratory pump muscle in mammals is the diaphragm. The intercostal muscles (in the spaces between the ribs) and abdominal muscles also assist in the respiratory act. The rhythmic excitation and inhibition of moto-neurons that control respiratory movements is the result of coordinated central nervous system action.

The respiratory cycle in mammals is divided into three phases, inspiration, post-inspiration and expiration. The synaptic interactions between neurons that are active during each of these respiratory phases generate and modulate the normal pattern of breathing. Neurons within the lower BRAINSTEM (PONS and MEDULLA OBLONGATA) produce spontaneous rhythmic activity even when they are isolated from the remainder of the central nervous system and from peripheral stimuli. This indicates that the basic neural circuitry responsible for producing the respiratory rhythm resides within the pons and medulla oblongata. This neural circuit is commonly referred to as the respiratory network. The respiratory network includes three neuron populations that are named according to their locations in the

brainstem. The dorsal and ventral respiratory groups (DRG and VRG) are located within the dorsal and ventral medulla oblongata, respectively. The pontine respiratory group (PRG) is located in the rostral pons. These respiratory populations contain mixtures of neurons that fire ACTION POTENTIALS during the different phases of the respiratory cycle.

The DRG is located in the NUCLEUS OF THE SOLITARY TRACT (NTS) of the medulla oblongata. The NTS is the main visceral (see VISCERA) sensory nucleus of the brain and utilizes sensory inputs from thoracic and abdominal organs for their negative feedback control. An important sensory mechanism for respiratory control is stretch receptor inputs from the lung. Pulmonary stretch receptors respond to lung inflation and send signals to the respiratory network via VAGUS NERVE projections to NTS that help to terminate inspiration. The NTS also receives chemoreceptor inputs from the carotid body (GLOSSOPHARYNGEAL NERVE) and aortic arch (vagus nerve) that adjust respiratory network function to maintain appropriate levels of blood pH and O_2. The PRG receives sensory inputs regarding lung inflation via projections from NTS and helps to terminate inspiration by projections back to NTS and to the VRG. The combined loss of vagal stretch receptor inputs and lesion of the PRG produces prolonged inspiratory bursts and expiratory pauses (apneustic breathing – see APNOEA). The VRG plays a primary role in respiratory network functions. It contains neurons that generate the respiratory rhythm, and other neurons that transmit the rhythm to respiratory motoneurons in the spinal cord. A portion of the VRG, the pre-Bötzinger complex, is critical for generating the rhythm. The pre-Bözinger complex has a special type of neuron that can produce a rhythmic output even though its inputs do not have a rhythmic pattern. These are called pacemaker neurons. The pacemaker neurons of pre-Bözinger complex are believed to drive the rhythm of the respiratory network. The role of the pacemaker neuron is thought to change during development. In neonatal animals, the respiratory rhythm is dependent on the activity of pacemaker cells and excitatory synaptic connections between neurons of the respiratory network. As the animal matures, the respiratory network develops increased synaptic connections between excitatory and inhibitory neurons and synaptic inhibition assumes a more prominent role in the control of inspiration and the expiratory pause. This may represent a developmental change from a rudimentary, automatic rhythm generating system in the neonate, to a mature system that is more amenable to modulatory influences.

Which of the NEUROTRANSMITTERS is utilized by a neuron is an important indicator of its role within a neuronal circuit. GLUTAMATE is an important neurotransmitter for excitation of respiratory motoneurons during inspiration and is the primary form of excitatory communication between respiratory neurons within the brainstem. Glutamate neurotransmission is required for generation of the respiratory rhythm in the brainstem respiratory network, however, the roles of different classes of glutamate receptor is controversial. The interplay between pacemaker, excitatory, and inhibitory neurons within the respiratory network allows for an extremely wide range of responses to both external and internal cues. With this flexibility, the respiratory pattern is able to respond precisely to varied metabolic demands of the body ranging from deep sleep to heavy exercise, while also allowing for coordination with such behaviours as swallowing, coughing, vomiting, sneezing and phonation.

HOWARD H. ELLENBERGER

bregma A skull landmark (the four-way cross formed by the sutures separating the frontal and parietal bones – see SKULL): important in STEREOTAXIC SURGERY.

brief psychotic disorder *see* schizophreniform disorder

brightfield *see* light microscopy

brightness The term brightness, when used in psychology, refers to the apparent intensity of a visual stimulus. It is not the same thing as the intensity of light, since ambient lighting conditions, contrast and various psychological factors can all affect judgement of brightness. HETEROCHROMATIC BRIGHTNESS MATCHING re-

fers to the judgement of brightness of lights of different colour.

See also: luminance

BRL15572 An agonist at the 5HT1E receptor; see SEROTONIN RECEPTORS.

Broca's aphasia A major clinical syndrome of APHASIA (Goodglass & Kaplan, 1983). A frequently occurring form of NON-FLUENT APHASIA, also known clinically as EXPRESSIVE APHASIA, MOTOR APHASIA, ANTERIOR APHASIA. The primary feature is slow, effortful speech. Melodic intonation tends to be flat or distorted. Some well-learned phrases and conversational stereotypes may be pronounced without error, whereas less familiar words are distorted by PHONETIC disintegration of the sounds that comprise the spoken word. LANGUAGE comprehension is relatively spared although subtle failure to interpret complex or lengthy verbal material may be noted. Some patients classified under the term Broca's aphasia exhibit AGRAMMATISM. The hallmark of this symptom is so-called 'telegraphic' sentence formation in which some or all of the grammatical composition of sentences is omitted or distorted, leaving mainly the content words for sentence composition (for example, 'go store...bread, milk...nothing') to describe a recent outing to the grocery store. Some of these patients demonstrate a similar impairment in the comprehension of grammatical elements of sentences. This particular form of aphasic speech production and comprehension has been the focus of intensive research (see Goodglass, 1993).

The LESION associated with Broca's aphasia encompasses BROCA'S AREA, and may extend posteriorly into the lower portion of the motor strip in the LEFT HEMISPHERE. Because of the close proximity of the lesion to the primary MOTOR CORTEX of the face, hand and arm, patients with Broca's aphasia often exhibit HEMIPLEGIA or hemiparesis. The right side of the body is usually the affected side since aphasia almost always results from a left hemisphere lesion, and hemispheric motor areas control the contralateral side of the body. Purely cortical lesions produce only transient symptoms; chronic Broca's aphasia is associated with lesions extending deep into the periventricular white matter.

References

Goodglass, H. (1993) *Understanding Aphasia*, Academic Press: San Diego.

Goodglass, H. & Kaplan, E. (1983) *The Assessment of Aphasia and Related Disorders*, 2nd edn, Lea & Febiger: Philadelphia.

CHARLOTTE C. MITCHUM

Broca's area An area of the posterior FRONTAL CORTEX named after the French neurologist Paul Broca who, in 1861, described a patient who had a LESION in this area, on the left side of the brain: the patient was unable to speak properly; see BROCA'S APHASIA.

See also: aphasia; arcuate fasciculus; language; Wernicke's area

Brodmann's areas Areas of the human (and to a great extent primate) CEREBRAL CORTEX delineated by Korbinian Brodmann (1868–1918) using stains for Nissl substance to locate cell bodies and for MYELIN to show fibre pathways. Brodmann described about 50 different areas based on cytoarchitectonics (see CYTOARCHITECTURE): for example, area 4 is the PRIMARY MOTOR CORTEX, area 17 the PRIMARY VISUAL CORTEX. More recent research has shown that the organization of the cortex, in particular the association areas, is more complex than Brodmann thought. However, the continued use of the classification system described by Brodmann is testament to his skill and to the power of simple staining techniques allied to careful microscopy.

bromocriptine An ERGOT-derived drug which acts as an AGONIST at DOPAMINE receptors with greater effect at D2 rather than D1 receptors. It is used as an adjunct to L-DOPA in the treatment of PARKINSON'S DISEASE. PERGOLIDE and LISURIDE are similar ergot-derived drugs.

brown adipose tissue Brown adipose tissue (BAT; brown fat) is found in the interscapular, cervical and axillary regions of the body. BAT contains brown adipocytes (see ADIPOSE TISSUE), with large MITOCHONDRIA and is highly vascularized. When activated by the SYMPATHETIC NERVOUS SYSTEM, BAT produces heat through NON-SHIVERING THERMOGENESIS. Increased intracellular levels of fatty acids within BAT serve as fuel for THERMOGENESIS. When these fatty acids are oxidized (see OXIDATION) through the tricarboxylic acid cycle in the mitochondria, heat is produced. Obese animals may have defective brown fat thermogenesis. Thyroid hormones and INSULIN stimulate BAT activity, while GLUCOCORTICOIDS suppress BAT activity. BAT is more important for thermoregulation in small rodents than in humans.

See also: obesity

References

Himms-Hagen, J. (1990) Brown adipose tissue thermogenesis: role in thermoregulation, energy regulation and obesity. In *Thermoregulation: Physiology and Biochemistry*, ed. E. Schönbaum & P. Lomax, pp. 327–414, Pergamon Press: New York.

RICHARD E. BROWN

brown fat *see* brown adipose tissue

Bruce effect The Bruce effect describes the ability of PHEROMONES from a male other than that responsible for impregnation to cause spontaneous termination of a PREGNANCY in mice.

See also: Lee–Boot effect; Vandenbergh effect; Whitten effect

bruxism (from Greek, *brychein*: to gnash – teeth grinding) This can occur as a minor feature of psychological disturbance.

See also: jaw movements

buccal (from Latin, *bucca*: cheek) Buccal is an adjective describing anything that relates to the MOUTH or cheek. The buccal glands secrete saliva.

buffer A buffer is a solution which will work to decrease the ACID or BASE nature of a solution: a buffer can acquire hydrogen ions (H^+) (see ION) when they are present in excess (as is the case with an acid) or can provide them when there are too few (as is the case with a base). A buffered solution leaves the chemical nature of whatever is present unaffected, but changes the acidity of it (either up or down).

See also: pH

Reference

Campbell N.A., Reece J.B. & Mitchell L.G. (1999) *Biology*, 5th edn, Addison-Wesley: Menlo Park CA.

bufotenine N, N - dimethyl - 5 - hydroxytrypta-mine: an hallucinogen related to the neuro-transmitter SEROTONIN and the drugs LYSERGIC ACID DIETHYLAMIDE (LSD) and PSILOCYBIN. At one time it was thought to be present to excess in the brains of patients with SCHIZO-PHRENIA, but this now appears not to be the case.

See also: hallucinogens

bug detector *see* feature detector

bulbar A descriptive term used in respect of the MEDULLA OBLONGATA; it is used synony-mously with the term medullary. So for exam-ple, CORTICOBULBAR fibres are fibres that travel from the CEREBRAL CORTEX to the medulla oblongata.

bulimia nervosa (from Greek, *bous*: ox, *limos*: hunger) Psychiatric disorder involving repeated episodes of BINGE EATING followed by purging. Bulimia nervosa was first defined by Gerald Russell in 1979. However, excessive appetite has been described in the literature as early as 1938. Russell's early observations of the syn-drome were as an ominous variant of ANOR-EXIA NERVOSA establishing a close connection between the two eating disorders. The World Health Organization and the American Psy-chiatric Association agree on the following clinical criteria: repeated episodes of binge eating; evidence of compensatory behaviours such as self-induced vomiting, fasting, abuse of diuretics, laxatives or other purgatives; over-valued ideas about weight and shape. Common to both bulimia nervosa and anorexia nervosa is the intense preoccupation with BODY WEIGHT. Russell named this a morbid fear of becoming FAT and it is this fear which is central to the weight-losing behaviour of anor-exia nervosa and to the purging behaviour of bulimia nervosa. Clinical criteria for bulimia nervosa do not include a weight criterion. Most patients with bulimia nervosa tend to be within normal weight limits, however, those who are 85% of expected would normally meet criteria for anorexia nervosa – bulimic subtype. Eating behaviour (see FEEDING) in bulimia nervosa outside of the binge–purge cycle tends to be highly restrictive and this is reflected in high scores on RESTRAINED EATING. Normal weight status may be maintained in bulimia nervosa despite purgation and dietary restraint, partly as a function of sufficient calories being absorbed during binge episodes coupled with a substantially lowered resting metabolic rate.

Definitions of binge eating focus on both the amount of food consumed and the feelings of loss of control during binge episodes. However, clinical and laboratory reports of binge eating vary enormously (from a few hundred to several thousand kilocalories) and it has been suggested that it is the perception of the food as excessive in combination with lack of control which defines the episode as a binge. Two main subtypes of bulimia nervosa are recognized – the purging and non-purging subtypes. The purging subtype of bulimia nervosa is identified when patients use self-induced vomiting and/or other forms of purga-tion following binge eating episodes, whereas the non-purging subtype is identified when patients rely on starvation and/or excessive exercise. Electrolyte imbalance and severe de-hydration caused by vomiting and abuse of purgatives may lead to cardiac arrhythmias and in some cases to sudden death. Mortality rates at 3% are lower in bulimia nervosa compared to anorexia nervosa.

The incidence of bulimia nervosa is higher than for anorexia nervosa estimated at 11.4 per 100 000 population. Among adolescent and young women the prevalence is at least 1%. Bulimia nervosa, unlike anorexia nervosa where emaciation is apparent, is not easily detected. Signs of bulimia nervosa include dental erosion, calluses on fingers and swelling of the salivary glands. Apart from these signs, there is a high degree of secretiveness about the illness perhaps due to shame, disgust or fear of being discovered. In common with anorexia nervosa, dieting tends to precede the develop-ment of bulimia nervosa. It has been argued that the overeating or COUNTER-REGULATION seen in restrained eaters following consumption of a large food pre-load is a laboratory version of binge eating. However, this comparison has been criticized since counter-regulation fails to meet both criteria of binge eating, that is, loss of control of eating and an objectively large amount of food consumed. Bulimia nervosa is caused by a variety of individual, family and societal factors. It is linked to greater levels of impulse control problems such as substance abuse, stealing and promiscuity. Altered gastrointestinal function may have a significant impact on the perpetuation of disordered eating, since gastric distension, emptying and contractions all have a role in the perception of HUNGER and SATIETY and therefore on subsequent food intake. Bulimics show delayed gastric emptying, blunted CHOLECYSTOKININ release in response to a meal and increased gastric capacity. Therefore, changes in gastrointestinal function may delay satiety and perpetuate overeating. Therapies for bulimia nervosa have developed from those used successfully in DEPRESSION since there is a strong association between eating disorders and AFFECTIVE DISORDERS. In the short term, antidepressants appear to have some success whilst in the longer term, cognitive–behavioural therapy appears to be the most effective treatment of bulimia nervosa.

Bulimia nervosa is characterized by repeated episodes of overeating followed by efforts to get rid of the food. Central to the disorder is a fear of being or becoming fat. Medical consequences in bulimia nervosa are serious and typically derive from electrolyte imbalance. Treatment for bulimia nervosa is successfully achieved using cognitive behavioural therapy.

See also: obesity; body image

MARION M. HETHERINGTON

bungarotoxin Alpha-bungarotoxin is a POLY-PEPTIDE which can bind irreversibly to NICO-TINIC ACETYLCHOLINE RECEPTORS, where it acts as an ANTAGONIST. It has a powerful action at the NEUROMUSCULAR JUNCTION, which it blocks, leading to paralysis and death by asphyxiation. It has been extracted from the venom of the banded krait (*Bungarus multicinctus*), a very dangerous Taiwanese snake.

See also: cone snails; *Naja naja*

burst firing Many neurons in different parts of the CENTRAL NERVOUS SYSTEM display burst firing – the production by an individual neuron of trains of action potentials (see ACTION POTENTIAL) with very short intervals between each spike. It is contrasted to SINGLE SPIKING. Following production of a burst there is usually a quiescent period, followed by further bursts of action potentials. Events within the neuron and the pattern of input to it are influential in determining the pattern of bursting: some neurons are able to show spontaneous burst firing (indicative of an intrinsic mechanism – CALCIUM and POTASSIUM conductance across membranes is often linked to the presence of rhythmic bursting) while in other cases burst firing is linked to sensory stimulation (bursting reflecting altered input to the neuron). There are several instances where burst firing is important. (1) It is a pattern of activity typically shown by injured neurons. (2) In several systems it establishes a rhythmic pattern of firing. For example, in the HEART, burst firing is important in establishing rhythmic muscular activity. In the THALAMUS, two basic modes of action are observed: a burst firing mode, associated with SLEEP and cortical synchrony, and a single spiking mode, associated with the waking state and cortical desynchrony (see SYNCHRONY/DESYNCHRONY). The transition from one state to the other is controlled by input from the CHOLINERGIC, NORADRENERGIC and SEROTONERGIC cell groups in the brainstem RETICULAR FORMA-TION (see for example McCormick & Prince, 1986). In each of these examples the production of rhythmic activity has a clear function: to move muscles or to disable cortical activity during sleep. (3) Burst firing is also seen during the waking state (see BEHAVIOURAL STATE). DOPAMINERGIC neurons in the MIDBRAIN show burst firing in response to sensory input: this phenomenon may be related to the role these neurons have in the coding of REWARD.

See also: oscillations

References

McCormick D.A. & Prince D.A. (1986) Acetylcholine induces burst firing in thalamic reticular neurons by activating a potassium conductance. *Nature* 319: 402–405.

Overton P.G. & Clark D. (1997) Burst firing in midbrain dopaminergic neurones. *Brain Research Reviews* 25: 312–334.

butyrophenones A class of drugs, including HALOPERIDOL, used to treat SCHIZOPHRENIA; see ANTIPSYCHOTIC.

butyrylcholinesterase *see* acetylcholinesterase

C

c. elegans see *caenorhabiditis elegans*

C fibres These are FIBRES involved in the sensation of pain; see A FIBRES (alpha, beta and delta).

c-fos One of the IMMEDIATE EARLY GENES, coding for the protein Fos; note that c-fos (lower case f) is the immediate early gene while Fos (upper case F) is the protein which it codes. Detection of this using IMMUNOHISTO-CHEMISTRY is used as a marker of neuronal activation.

See also: metabolic mapping

c-jun see immediate early genes

C-type natriuretic peptide *see* natriuretic peptides

CA1–CA3 'CA' stands for *cornu ammonis*, the Latin term for AMMON'S HORN. Strictly speaking, Ammon's horn is the HIPPOCAMPUS proper, though in fact the term hippocampus is usually taken to include the DENTATE GYRUS as well. (Terminology relating to the hippocampus is a little tortured: see HIPPOCAMPAL FORMATION.) These areas have a more-or-less identical laminar organization, although CA1 and CA3 are much larger than CA2. The main layer is the stratum oriens, which contains PYRAMIDAL NEURONS (these constituting the vast majority of CA1–CA3 neurons). Below this is a layer of FIBRES called the ALVEUS (see also FIMBRIA). There is also a fibre layer just above CA3 (but not CA1 or CA2) composed of AXONS from the dentate gyrus – this is the stratum lucidum. The stratum radiatum is above the pyramidal cell layer in CA1 and CA2, and above the stratum lucidum in CA3: this layer has fibres that interconnect CA1–CA3, as well as connections with the SCHAFFER COLLATERALS. Above all this is the stratum lacunosum-moleculare, a layer in which there are perforant path fibres from the ENTORHINAL CORTEX, and efferent fibres from the THALAMUS. See HIPPOCAMPUS for a discussion of the connections and functions of CA1–CA3.

RICHARD G. M. MORRIS

cable graft A technique used in clinical practice and experimentally to restore peripheral nerve function. If a nerve is cut it is possible to induce regrowth by placing the cut ends close together. (Indeed, this occurs naturally: a cut at one's finger tip can leave a small patch of tissue without nerve innervation, but regrowth promptly occurs spontaneously.) When the cut ends of a nerve cannot be brought together, sections of nerve can be taken from elsewhere and used to join the cut ends, by providing a channel through which regeneration can occur.

See also: transplantation

cable transmission Term used to describe the transmission of electrical impulses along an unmyelinated AXON. Transmission along myelinated fibres (see MYELIN) is described as SALTATORY – ACTION POTENTIALS 'jump' from one NODE OF RANVIER to the next, a very fast form of transmission. In unmyelinated axons, the electrical signal passively diffuses along the axon in a manner analogous to the passage of electricity along a cable. Signals become weaker with increasing distance, though the degree to which this happens will depend on the characteristics of the axon; see ACTION POTENTIAL.

cachexia Literally, a bad condition; from Greek *kachexia* – *kakos*, bad, *hexis*, condition. It is a term often used to describe the condition of those suffering from wasting disorders such as ANOREXIA NERVOSA.

cadaveric rigidity *see* rigidity

cadherin *see* neural adhesion molecules

caecum *see* digestive system

caenorhabditis elegans (c. elegans) The nematode worm, *Caenorhabditis elegans*, has long been popular with developmental biologists. However, recently it has been presented as a model system for the investigation of the neural basis of LEARNING and MEMORY. C. *elegans* offers the only nervous system for which we have a complete spatio-temporal account of its development, at the level of individual neurons, of which there are only 302, and whose connections are known. In addition, it has been shown that C. *elegans* exhibits many forms of learning, including CLASSICAL CONDITIONING.

MARK A. UNGLESS

cafeteria diet *see* supermarket diet

caffeine This is the most widely used central nervous system STIMULANT, and is present in various beverages including coffee and certain soft drinks. Used at low doses, caffeine enhances alertness and concentration in humans while increasing LOCOMOTION in animals. These effects are thought to be mediated by blockade at ADENOSINE receptors. Adenosine is suggested to be an endogenous SLEEP-promoting factor. At higher doses, caffeine can induce nervousness, irritability, ANXIETY and even CONVULSIONS in humans, most likely due to inhibition of phosphodiesterases. Regular caffeine users may develop caffeine dependence and may experience a WITHDRAWAL syndrome upon reduction of caffeine intake.

KAZUE SEMBA

cage stereotypy *see* stereotypy

calbindin Also referred to as calbindin D28K; *see* calcium-binding proteins

calcarine fissure (from Latin, *calx*: the heel) The term calcarine means 'like a spur'. The calcarine fissure is located in the OCCIPITAL LOBE and runs at right angles to the median longitudinal fissure (see LONGITUDINAL FISSURE) the major fissure along the midline which divides the two hemispheres at the back of the brain. The calcarine fissure is of significance because it is the location of the PRIMARY VISUAL CORTEX.

calcification The deposition of CALCIUM, causing hardening of tissues or the formation of calcium-rich deposits (which can be identified using ALIZARIN RED) within tissues. Calcification is associated with tissue degeneration: following EXCITOTOXIC LESIONS for example, calcium rich deposits often appear around a lesioned area.

calcitonin A hormone released by the THYROID GLAND.

See also: endocrine glands; hormones; hormones – classification

calcitonin gene-related peptide A peptide (see PEPTIDES), it is found to be a NEUROTRANSMITTER in MOTOR NEURONS in the SPINAL CORD and at the NEUROMUSCULAR JUNCTION. At both sites it is co-localized with ACETYLCHOLINE, and simultaneously released (an example of COTRANSMISSION). Calcitonin gene-related peptide has been known for some years, and has been joined recently in a small family of peptide neurotransmitters by CALCITONIN (one of the HORMONES released by the THYROID GLAND), AMYLIN and ADRENOMEDULLIN. A separate RECEPTOR type exists for each of these four, but each appears to have a degree of affinity for all receptors types (that is, calcitonin receptors, CGRP receptors, amylin receptors and adrenomedullin receptors). Calcitonin (or more specifically, salmon calcitonin, as opposed to human calcitonin), CGRP and amylin all appear to bind well in the rat NUCLEUS ACCUMBENS, suggesting CENTRAL NERVOUS SYSTEM actions of these.

calcium An element with a wide variety of functions. It is usually active in its ionic form (see ION). Calcium ions (Ca^{2+}) are plentiful in extracellular fluid, with a concentration around 1 mM, but are present at very low levels intracellularly, at a concentration around 100 nM. This 10 000-fold gradient is maintained by a CALCIUM PUMP that actively transports calcium out of the cell or into internal stores (see ACTIVE TRANSPORT) and by intracellular calcium buffers.

Calcium ions play a major role in NEURO-TRANSMISSION, muscle contraction and as SECOND MESSENGERS. Calcium ions are essential to neurotransmission because they trigger the release of neurotransmitters from SYNAPTIC VESICLES. This is brought about by the entry of calcium into the synaptic terminals through calcium channels that are voltage-dependent. These channels open as a result of DEPOLARIZATION of the terminal with the arrival of an ACTION POTENTIAL. Once inside the terminal, calcium binds to recognition sites on the synaptic vesicles which then permits binding of the vesicle membrane to the presynaptic membrane. This fusion of the two membranes results in opening of the vesicle into the SYNAPTIC CLEFT, or EXOCYTOSIS, and the neurotransmitter is able to diffuse across the cleft to the receptors on the POSTSYNAPTIC membrane. Voltage-gated calcium channels are also present on the dendrites of some neurons, for example in the CEREBELLUM, where they can function to produce action potentials. The time course of calcium-induced action potentials (or calcium spikes) is considerably longer than the sodium-mediated action potential, often resulting in repetitive discharges. Calcium also is able to enter neurons through NMDA RECEPTORS, which are one type of GLUTAMATE receptor. Calcium entering via such channels can act as a second messenger and plays a crucial role in plastic changes such as LONG-TERM POTENTIATION.

Calcium ions also play a critical role in excitation–contraction in muscle. Depolarization is carried along the transverse tubules of the muscle cell and in turn causes the sarcoplasmic reticulum to release calcium ions from its stores. Calcium then blocks the inhibitory interaction between troponin and actin and

allows the sliding filament mechanism between actin and myosin cross bridges to occur, resulting in muscle shortening, or contraction. Following its action, calcium is resequestered in the sarcoplasmic reticulum.

DOUGLAS D. RASMUSSON

calcium channel *see* ion channel

calcium-binding proteins Calcium-binding proteins (more generically known as ANNEXINS) are involved in MOBILIZATION. The principal proteins that bind CALCIUM in the CENTRAL NERVOUS SYSTEM are calbindin-D28k (which is more generally referred to just as CALBINDIN), PARVALBUMIN and CALRETININ. These are not evenly distributed through the central nervous system. As a good example of this, the differential distribution of these has been used to map distinct functional territories within the THALAMUS (see Jones, 1998). CALMODULIN is another calcium-binding protein, but one with a much more widespread distribution: it is found in virtually all nucleated cells (i.e. any CELL with a NUCLEUS) in both animals and plants. There are four BINDING SITES on a calmodulin molecule to which calcium ions (Ca^{2+}) (see ION) can bind. Calmodulin is activated when all four sites are occupied. Together with calcium – in the CALCIUM–CALMODULIN COMPLEX – calmodulin is a regulatory factor in the production of a variety of ENZYMES (such as calcium–calmodulin dependent protein kinase II for instance) and proteins in the CYTOSKELETON (such as FODRIN for example).

References

Jones E.G. (1998) Viewpoint: the core and matrix of thalamic organization. *Neuroscience* 85: 331–345.

calcium–calmodulin complex *see* calcium-binding proteins

calcium/calmodulin dependent protein kinase II A PROTEIN KINASE that acts as a SECOND MESSENGER: it is relatively unusual in that, once activated by increasing CALCIUM concentration, its activity remains elevated even if calcium levels fall. It has to be actively inhibited by ENZYME action. This property has led to suggestions that it might be associated with LONG TERM POTENTIATION, which is known to be a calcium dependent process.

calcium pump The CALCIUM pump is one of several membrane pumps – specialized molecules embedded in a MEMBRANE – that actively pump ions (see ION) across the membrane against the CONCENTRATION GRADIENT. It is an ATPASE-dependent process, working in a manner more or less identical to that of the SODIUM–POTASSIUM PUMP. Management of intracellular calcium concentration is achieved through the action of this pump moving calcium to EXTRACELLULAR spaces; by pumping into the ENDOPLASMIC RETICULUM; and by the use of CALCIUM-BINDING PROTEINS within the CYTOSOL. Accumulation of calcium is fatal to cells – indeed, calcium accumulation within neurons is a principal effect of EXCITOTOXINS.

callosal agenesis Callosal agenesis is a failure to develop properly the CORPUS CALLOSUM. There are a variety of different disorders in which this is known to occur. Neuropsychological deficits associated with callosal agenesis have been reported, though these are not as marked as those that occur when the corpus callosum is surgically severed in adulthood (see SPLIT BRAIN). Moreover, with the introduction of a variety of neuroimaging techniques, such as magnetic resonance imaging and CAT scan (see FUNCTIONAL NEUROIMAGING) it has become clear that there are a number of individuals who have agenesis of the corpus callosum but do not present with psychological impairments. When there are deficits present, they tend to be relatively idiosyncratic and subtle: sensory integration and skilled motor control (tasks involving simultaneous dexterity on both hands for example can present a difficulty), but IQ is generally good. General cognitive performance tends to be within the normal range though rather towards the lower ends of the scales. Evidently, the most interesting aspect of this form of agenesis is the marked differentiation between the failure to develop the corpus callosum properly and the destruction of an established corpus callosum in adulthood (see NEUROPLASTICITY).

Reference

Jeeves M.A. (1990) Agenesis of the corpus

callosum. In *Handbook of Neuropsychology*, vol. 4, ed. F. Boller & J. Grafman J., pp. 99–114, Elsevier: Amsterdam.

calmodulin *see* calcium-binding proteins

calorimeter A calorimeter is a chamber, entirely closed from the outside world, in which one can house an animal and record its body heat. It is used to determine the METABOLIC RATE of small animals – calorimeters for use by large animals (including humans) are used, but less often. Calorimetry is the process of taking such recordings. BOMB CALORIMETRY involves determining the amount of energy present in something by burning it in a sealed unit – a bomb calorimeter – and measuring the heat given off. This is a process occasionally used to determine the energy composition of animal carcasses.

calotte *see* skull

calpain Though referred to singly, strictly this refers not to a single ENZYME but a family of enzymes (the calpains), all activated by CALCIUM and involved in PROTEOLYSIS within CELLS. The actions of calpain have been implicated in many processes to do with changing the structure of SYNAPSE following such diverse events as ISCHAEMIA and LONG TERM POTENTIATION; see FODRIN.

calretinin *see* calcium binding proteins

calvaria *see* skull

Cambridge automated neuropsychological test battery (CANTAB) *see* neuropsychological test battery

camera lucida This describes a technique in MICROSCOPY by which an image from a microscope is projected on to a sheet of paper (using what is known as a drawing tube fitted to the micrscope). Looking through the eyepieces of the microscope, one can then see both the paper (and one's pen or pencil on the paper) and a SECTION on the microscope stage and it is possible to draw accurately what one is looking at. Although the drawings often are aesthetically pleasing, the increasing availability of computerized IMAGE ANALYSIS has reduced the use of camera lucida.

candidate gene analysis Genes influence complex processes, but it is highly likely that the effects of genes on most psychological and behavioural processes (and indeed medical conditions) come about through the action not of single genes but of multiple genes. For example, it is inconceivable that INTELLIGENCE is the product of a single gene: any genetic influence on this will come about through the action of multiple genes. In this regard one refers to QUANTITATIVE TRAIT LOCI: these are genes that have varying degrees of effect in multi-gene processes and systems, each one contributing to the variability in an overall PHENOTYPE. Candidate gene analysis is the general name for the procedure that is used to identify individual genes that contribute to some particular process or condition. It is a procedure increasingly used, though still difficult to apply: the central difficulty lies in determining which genes to investigate as candidates for control of a specific process. For further discussion of this, see Plomin *et al.* 1997.

Reference

Plomin R., DeFries J. C., McClearn G.E. & Rutter M. (1997) *Behavioral Genetics*, 3rd edn, WH Freeman & Co.: New York.

cannabinoids *see* cannabis

cannabis A weed-like plant (*Cannabis sativa*), also known as flowering hemp, which has been used by human societies perhaps as far back as 4000 BC. It is likely that the plant originated somewhere in central Asia, but it is now cultivated in many areas of the world. The hemp plant has been used for many purposes, particularly as a source of fibre for making rope, cloth and paper, and as a medicinal herb. Western interest in the plant developed in the nineteenth century. European physicians expounded the usefulness of hemp as an APPETITE stimulant and ANTICONVULSANT, and also in treating a variety of ills such as migraine and menstrual cramps. In Europe, a French physician named Moreau, after several trips to the Middle East, introduced HASHISH smoking for its PSYCHOACTIVE properties to Parisian literary societies (hashish is a potent form of the drug). It is believed that cultivation and consumption of cannabis in America developed when Mexican labourers introduced the practice of smoking it to the United States in the early twentieth century. In fact, the origin of the term MARIJUANA, which refers to a mixture of dried leaves, stems and flowers from the plant, is derived from the Mexican word *maraguanquo*, 'an intoxicating plant'. Today cannabis is probably the most commonly used illegal psychoactive drug (laws governing its use vary between countries, but in most states or countries it is an illicit drug). In the United States for example, it is estimated that nearly 70 million people have used marijuana at least once, which is a substantial proportion of the adult population. Although cannabis is not considered a highly addictive drug compared with NICOTINE or HEROIN, chronic consumption can lead to motivational and cognitive impairments.

Cannabis contains over 60 compounds known as CANNABINOIDS, concentrated in the resin of the plant. The main psychoactive ingredient is delta-9-TETRAHYDROCANNABINOL, or THC. The concentration of this compound varies with different preparations of the plant. For example, hashish, the concentrated resin, is usually around 10–11% THC, while marijuana leaves contain much lower concentrations. Cannabis is usually smoked, although it is sometimes eaten as well. The study of the cognitive and subjective effects of cannabis has been notoriously difficult, because individuals may have very differing reactions depending on dose, prior experience with the drug, and environmental context. Generally, however, the 'high' is characterized by feelings of well-being and mild EUPHORIA. An initial stimulating effect may be replaced by feelings of tranquillity and dreaminess. Emotional or MOOD changes may occur. Perceptual and sensory changes may be present, but generally these are mild exaggerations of pleasurable experiences, such as enhancement of music or tastes. However, with very high doses of THC, hallucinations and feelings of PARANOIA may occur. A common effect of THC intoxication is 'temporal disintegration' in which the user loses the ability to coordinate information for a goal or purpose, and the sense of time becomes distorted.

For many years little was known about the effects of cannabis on the brain, compared with other psychoactive drugs such as cocaine or heroin. However, in the late 1980s, central binding sites, known as cannabinoid receptors, were localized and characterized, and these receptors eventually cloned. Thus, specific binding sites for THC are localized in certain specific brain regions, such as HIPPOCAMPUS, CEREBRAL CORTEX, BASAL GANGLIA, and CEREBELLUM. Undoubtedly many of the cognitive and motor effects of THC intoxication are due to activation of cannabinoids receptors in these regions. THC has effects on a number of neurotransmitter systems; its many neurochemical actions are inhibition of CHOLINERGIC activity in certain brain areas, and activation of NORADRENALINE and DOPAMINE levels.

ANN E. KELLEY

cannibal *see* carnivore

Cannon–Bard theory of emotions The origins of this neural theory of the emotions are described in a book by Walter B. Cannon (1871–1945) which was written (in 1928) very much as a critical reaction to the JAMES–LANGE THEORY OF THE EMOTIONS. The basic theory was that 'the relays of sensory channels in the thalamus and the evidence that disturbances in that region are all that we need for understanding its relation to the nature of the emotions'. This neural evidence was based in part on cases described by the clinical neurologist Henry Head in which unilateral lesions of the thalamic region produced a marked tendency to react excessively to affective stimuli such as pin-pricks, painful pressure, excessive heat or cold, and even to emotive music, on the damaged side of the body. The affective influences could include conscious states and were thus both 'top-down' as well as 'bottom-up' influences on thalamic processing. Head attributed the former to a release of the THALAMUS from cortical inhibition. Cannon's thalamic theory of the emotions thus postulated that the thalamus added 'feeling-tone' or 'quale' to raw sensation and provided a double output: to the emotional effectors which were responsible for somatic and visceral responses and to portions of the CEREBRAL CORTEX which were

responsible for the perception of emotional experience. He thought that the visceral output was largely undifferentiated and could not therefore provide the substrate of emotional experience. Cannon thus contrasted his account with the James-Lange theory for which he raised five famous objections (see JAMES–LANGE THEORY OF THE EMOTIONS).

Bard (1934) expanded Cannon's thalamic theory further based on his research on the effects of TRANSECTIONS of the brain at various levels on emotional behaviour such as AGGRESSION in the cat. For example, he described the 'sham' rage which occurs when DECEREBRATE cats respond aggressively in the absence of eliciting stimuli. One of the problems with the Cannon–Bard theory is that the thalamus is probably not the major centre for the control of the emotions. For example, it is lesions to the posterior and ventral portions of the HYPOTHALAMUS rather than the thalamus that block the excessive rage that can follow decortication. Therefore, it is probably the latter structures that are released from cortical inhibition rather than the thalamus. Several other lines of work began to cast further doubt on the neurological details of the Cannon–Bard theory. For example, the neurophysiologist Hess found that stimulation of sites in the hypothalamus were more likely to elicit aggressive behaviour in cats than the thalamus and Papez & McLean began to piece together evidence from a variety of sources that eventually implicated in emotion several structures in a distributed neural network of structures now collectively known as the LIMBIC SYSTEM. These structures included the septum, HIPPOCAMPUS, CINGULATE CORTEX, and most notably, the AMYGDALA, which today has become perhaps closest to Cannon's concept of an emotional centre. Nevertheless, something of Cannon's ideas are retained in modern neural theories of emotion. LeDoux for example has described how the CLASSICAL CONDITIONING of FEAR in rats depends upon a transfer of sensory information from the sensory thalamus to the amygdala, and the mediodorsal nucleus of the thalamus, may well have important roles in mediating processing between the amygdala and the ORBITOFRONTAL CORTEX.

References

Bard P. (1934) On emotional expression after decortication, with some remarks on certain theoretical views, parts I and II. *Psychological Review* 41:309–329 and 424–449.

Cannon W. (1928) *Bodily Changes in Pain, Hunger, Fear and Rage: An Account of Recent Researches into the Function of Emotional Excitement*, Appleton-Century: New York.

Grossman S.P. (1967) *A Textbook of Physiological Psychology*, Wiley: New York.

LeDoux, J. (1998) *The Emotional Brain*, Phoenix: London.

TREVOR W. ROBBINS

cannula Small piece of tubing through which either fluid (or another length of tubing) can be passed.

See also: microinjection

CANTAB (Cambridge automated neurological test battery) *see* neuropsychological test battery

Capgras syndrome Delusion, first identified by the French psychiatrist Capgras in the 1920s, that close family members have been replaced by others: despite recognition of an individual's features, there is denial that the person is whom they appear to be; a specific example of the general phenomenon of REDUPLICATION.

See also: delusional misidentification

capillary *see* blood

capsaicin The active ingredient in chilli peppers (the genus *Capsicum* – hence capsaicin). Capsaicin produces a painful burning sensation that is thought to depend on stimulation of nociceptors on C FIBRES and A FIBRES (a-delta fibres). SUBSTANCE P is a neurotransmitter in many pain systems and capsaicin is thought to have an action on substance P neurotransmission: there might be a capsaicin receptor on substance P neurons. Capsaicin has a clinical use, paradoxically in the alleviation of certain forms of pain. Capsaicin is available in a variety of ointment creams and is rubbed on a painful area (a joint or muscle typically). It produces a burning sensation that may counter the original pain and which may lead to inactivation of pain transmission. Many patients however find the treatment worse than the original condition.

Reference

Feldman R., Meyer J.S. & Quenzer L.F. (1997) *Principles of Neuropsychopharmacology*, Sinauer Associates: Sunderland MA.

capsid *see* virus

capsulotomy *see* psychosurgery

carbachol Carbamylcholine chloride: a commonly used analogue of ACETYLCHOLINE, relatively resistant to destruction by acetylcholinest-erase. It acts mainly as a stimulant of MUSCARINIC ACETYLCHOLINE RECEPTORS, though it also has a limited effect at NICOTINIC ACETYLCHOLINE RECEPTORS.

carbamazepine One of the most commonly used ANTICONVULSANT drugs, commercially available as Tegretol. Like PHENYTOIN and SODIUM VALPROATE it is thought to act by inhibition of VOLTAGE-SENSITIVE ION CHANNELS for sodium (Na^+) and possibly calcium (Ca^{2+}) in neuronal membranes. Carbamazepine has also been shown to have effectiveness in treating MANIA and is used for patients who are resistant to the effects of the more common anti-mania treatment, LITHIUM.

Reference

Feldman R.S., Meyer J.S. & Quenzer L.F. (1997) *Principles of Neuropsychopharmacology*, Sinauer Associates: Sunderland MA.

carbohydrate Compounds of carbon, hydrogen and oxygen (with hydrogen and oxygen in the same proportions as in water), carbohydrates are the principal source of ENERGY in food; SUGARS are carbohydrates.

carbon dioxide (CO_2) Carbon dioxide is a by-product of RESPIRATION, carried in the BLOOD and exhaled via the lungs (see BREATHING, NEURAL CONTROL OF). Accumulation of carbon dioxide in the blood is associated with PANIC and with SLEEP APNOEA.

carbon disulphide (carbon disulfide; CS_2) A SEMIOCHEMICAL; see BREATH; SOCIAL TRANSMISSION OF FOOD PREFERENCES.

carbon monoxide (CO) Like NITRIC OXIDE, carbon monoxide is thought to be a novel NEUROTRANSMITTER or neuromodulator in the NERVOUS SYSTEM. It is formed from HEME, which HEME OXYGENASE converts to biliverdin and carbon monoxide (CO). The presence of heme oxygenase has been demonstrated in neural tissue, where it has a distribution different to that of NITRIC OXIDE SYNTHASE, the synthetic enzyne for nitric oxide. There are circumstances though when nitric oxide and carbon monoxide do act as cotransmitters (see COTRANSMISSION). It may function as an intracellular messenger, helping produce CYCLIC GMP. The behavioural or psychological conditions under which it is activated remain uncertain.

Carbon monoxide is poisonous in very high concentrations (usually due to inhalation of EXOGENOUS carbon monoxide). It produces asphyxiation and is often fatal. Patients who survive carbon monoxide poisoning suffer brain damage: lesions in the WHITE MATTER of CEREBRAL CORTEX is often present, as is NEURON loss in diverse structures, including the HIPPOCAMPUS and GLOBUS PALLIDUS. Parkinsonian-like states (see PARKINSON'S DISEASE) can develop, featuring both motor and cognitive disturbances.

carbon paste electrode Chemical probe used in VOLTAMMETRY to detect ELECTROACTIVE substances in solution and whose tip is composed of carbon powder mixed with mineral or silicon oil.

CHARLES D. BLAHA

carbonyl sulphide (carbonyl sulfide; COS) A SEMIOCHEMICAL; see BREATH; SOCIAL TRANSMISSION OF FOOD PREFERENCES.

cardiac muscle see muscles

cardiovascular psychophysiology The subsection of PSYCHOPHYSIOLOGY that examines the effects of psychological processes on the cardiovascular system and, less commonly, vice versa. Most studies in cardiovascular psychophysiology are concerned with the effects of STRESS which can lead to alterations in heart rate, blood pressure, cardiac output, peripheral resistance and blood clotting. In patients with heart disease, stress can lead to disturbances of

heart rhythm and of the blood supply to the heart. The emphasis on stress is because of the possible role of stress in the aetiology of essential hypertension, coronary artery disease and the triggering of myocardial infarction, cerebral STROKE and sudden death in patients with arterial disease.

It is held that tasks that involve active coping (dealing with a demanding stimulus that requires difficult continuous behaviour adjustment, such as a complex video game) leads to increased sympathetic arousal which particularly affects the heart and leads to an increase in cardiac output. This contrasts with tasks requiring passive coping, such as the cold pressor test in which the subject submerges their hand in ice water. These tasks, which do not require effortful behaviour from the subject, are associated with increases in peripheral vasculature resistance, also of sympathetic origin. Both types of tasks lead to increases in blood pressure but the mechanisms are different. It is difficult to determine the autonomic control mechanisms since the heart is under both the sympathetic and parasympathetic control. Blockade studies with beta ADRENERGIC blockade using drugs such as PROPRANOLOL or parasympathetic blockade with ATROPINE can illuminate mechanisms. In addition, studies of heart rate variability using spectral analysis can provide information on the balance between sympathetic and parasympathetic influences on the heart since it is believed that low-frequency variability is primarily sympathetic and higher-frequency variability parasympathetic in origin.

Direct neural effects of the cardiovascular system on psychological process are less easy to demonstrate. It was held for some time that alterations in heart rate affected attentional process through centrally acting feedback from the baroreceptors. This does not appear to be the case but it is likely that baroreceptor activity affects PAIN perception, particularly in people with raised blood pressure. This may relate to the otherwise puzzling finding that raised blood pressure is associated with increased objective but not subjective evidence of stress.

DEREK W. JOHNSTON

cardiovascular system *see* blood

Carlson box A double-sided OPEN FIELD used to investigate EXPLORATION. A large rectangular box is divided into two equal compartments. A rat is confined to one side for 1 hour, becoming familiar with it and leaving its scent there. It is then removed and placed in a start box while the dividing wall separating the two sides of the open field is removed and replaced by another with an opening in the centre at floor level, allowing the rat access from the familiar side to the novel side, which is fresh and clean. The start box gives equal access to both sides once a guillotine door is opened. An experimenter can measure (in a 10-minute test) latency to emerge from the start box; choice of side on which to emerge; and, once the rat is out and the start box closed, time spent on each side of the apparatus, the number of crosses between the two sides, LOCOMOTION and REARING. Exploration is evidenced by a preference for the novel side and increased locomotion and rearing on the novel side compared to familiar. Critically, measures of exploration – side choice and the time spent on the novel side – can be dissociated from locomotion.

See also: Berlyne box

carnivore (from Latin, *carnis*: flesh, *vorare*: to devour) An animal that eats other animals and not plants; a CANNIBAL is a special kind of carnivore that eats other members of its own species.

See also: herbivore; omnivore

case-study approach The use of detailed descriptions of individual humans with neurological or psychiatric SIGNS AND SYMPTOMS to increase our understanding of disordered behaviour or normal brain functioning. Medical science has utilized careful observations of patients to understand and distribute knowledge about disease and mental disorders for hundreds of years. In cognitive and clinical NEUROPSYCHOLOGY, theories about normal brain functioning are developed and tested via the observation and measurement of the responses of patients with neuropsychological disorders, often under carefully controlled experimental conditions. For instance, the case of

H.M. with AMNESIA tells us about MEMORY systems in the normal brain.

JENNI A. OGDEN

castration (from Latin, *castrare*: to castrate) The removal of the reproductive organs: TESTES from a male or the OVARIES from a female. Castration is a surgical procedure used experimentally in studies of SEXUAL BEHAVIOUR, and of the effects of SEX HORMONES on both behaviour and physiology. The loss of sex hormones provided by the testes or ovaries can be examined, and the controlled resupply of missing hormones examined.

Note that castration refers to removal of the organs of reproduction from either males or females: GONADECTOMY which involves, like castration, removal of the GONADS (testes in males, ovaries in females) – is a term that has a more nonsexist ring to it. In general one thinks of castration as a procedure involving males rather than females. In farm animals and race horses it is the males rather than females that are castrated to change their growth (a procedure known as gelding). OVARIECTOMY is the more common term for removal of the ovaries. A further point of association between the use of the term castration and specifically males is the fact that in humans, *castrati* were male singers who had had, as youths, their testes removed to prevent their voices from breaking. Good *castrati* were highly paid and honoured musicians, and in pre-twentieth-century Europe, a large poor family having a son with a fine clear treble voice would count themselves fortunate to have the opportunity to develop a *castrato* who could rescue them from their poverty. Much operatic and religious music written for soprano voice was in fact intended not for women but for *castrati*. Some recordings of the last of the *castrati* exist and are remarkable, the high voice of the singers having a range and power unlike a *falsetto*, a boy or female soprano.

CAT scan; CT scan *see* computerized axial tomography

catabolism; catabolic; catabolite *see* metabolism

catalepsy (from Greek, *kata*: down, *lepsis*: taking) Catalepsy is a state of muscular RIGID-

ITY. It is not a widely used term, though in the past it has been used to describe the immobility present in PARKINSON'S DISEASE. It has been investigated in animals: very large doses of drugs that block dopamine receptors (see D1–D5 DOPAMINE RECEPTORS) induce catalepsy in rats. This was usually measured by placing the rat's forepaws on a raised bar and measuring the time taken for it to step down, or by placing the rat on a grid perpendicular to the laboratory bench and looking again for climb down latency. Cataleptic rats maintain the positions in which they are put. Such studies did not apparently reveal a great deal about the functions of dopamine, or the brain structures it is associated with, and so have been largely abandoned.

See also: cataplexy; catatonia

catalyst A CATALYST is a chemical that is able to exert an effect on physiological processes without itself being changed; catalysis is the process of doing this; to catalyse is to engage in catalysis. An ENZYME can be a catalyst of chemical reactions; for example GLUTAMIC ACID DECARBOXYLASE catalyses the conversion of glutamate to GABA.

cataplexy (from Greek, *kata*: down, *plessein*: strike) Cataplexy (adjective: cataplectic) is a cardinal symptom of NARCOLEPSY in which muscle tone is suddenly lost (ATONIA) as it is during REM SLEEP (rapid eye movement sleep) causing individuals to collapse. It often occurs in combination with a SLEEP ATTACK, though the two states are dissociable. When consciousness is not lost (that is, cataplexy without sleep attack) a distressing condition of waking immobility is produced. Cataplexy is particularly associated with strong EMOTION – intense emotions can trigger an attack. Cataplexy is in effect the opposite of REM WITHOUT ATONIA: cataplexy is the inappropriate presence of atonia during the waking state. REM without atonia is the absence of atonia during REM sleep. The behaviour of animals which 'play dead' in order to avoid predators has also been described as cataplectic, though whether or not this is the same as the condition associated with narcolepsy is uncertain.

See also: sleep paralysis

cataract An operable condition in which the lens of the eye becomes opaque. There is neither pain nor inflammation, but vision is impaired.

See also: amblyopia

catastrophic interference Catastrophic interference occurs when the LEARNING of later items results in severely impaired performance during testing of previously learned items. This extreme form of RETROACTIVE INTERFERENCE can occur in PARALLEL DISTRIBUTED PROCESSING neural network models when sequential training procedures are used. Providing concurrent training trials, giving retraining trials, interleaving trial types during training, encoding 'memories' (see MEMORY; ENGRAM) using only a few units, making the input orthogonal, and giving the network a large amount of prior knowledge through pre-training are all methods that have been shown to reduce catastrophic interference.

HOWARD EICHENBAUM

catatonia (from Greek, *kata*: down, *tonos*: stretching) Catatonia is one of the four types of SCHIZOPHRENIA identified by Kraepelin (1856–1926), the others being paranoid (see PARANOIA) and HEBEPHRENIA. Catatonia involves periods of muscular RIGIDITY and immobility, possibly including the state of 'waxy flexibility' in which patients' limbs can be put in positions which are then maintained. Catatonia is relatively rare, but is of interest in that it highlights the fact that schizophrenia includes motor disturbance as well as the better-known disorders of thought, perception and cognition.

See also: catalepsy; cataplexy

catatonic rigidity *see* rigidity

catch-up saccade *see* pursuit eye movements

catechol-O-methyltransferase *see* dopamine; noradrenaline

catecholamine Catecholamines are the class of MONOAMINE that contain a catechol nucleus and a side chain of ethylamine or one of its derivatives. CATECHOLAMINERGIC is the term used to describe cells – usually neurons – that contain catecholamines. The most important catecholamines are DOPAMINE, NORADRENA-LINE and ADRENALINE, which are small-molecule neurotransmitters. The latter two are also called NOREPINEPHRINE (NE) and EPINEPHRINE, respectively, these being the standard American terms (in contrast to noradrenaline and adrenaline, which are the English terms). The difference in terminology comes from the fact that in the United Kingdom adrenaline was first extracted from the ADRENAL GLAND while almost simultaneously in the United States it was synthesized from kidney tissue (the nephron). The precursor for all catecholamines is TYROSINE, derived from dietary protein. Tyrosine is converted into DOPA, dopamine, noradrenaline, and finally to adrenaline. TYROSINE HYDROXYLASE is the rate-limiting enzyme in this synthetic pathway. The specific enzymes that catalyse each step of this pathway have been used as anatomical markers for neurons that contain dopamine, noradrenaline and adrenaline.

KAZUE SEMBA

catecholaminergic *see* catecholamine

categorical memory Synonymous with SEMANTIC MEMORY.

category-specific agnosia *see* agnosia; prosopagnosia

catheter (from Greek, *kathienai*: to send down) A narrow tube inserted into the body providing access for the infusion or withdrawal of fluids. Catheterization is the process of surgically implanting a catheter.

cathode A negatively charged metallic ELECTRODE toward which cations (see CATION) migrate in an electrolytic cell or tissue medium in which it is placed.

See also: anode

CHARLES D. BLAHA

cation A positively charged ION.

cauda equina *see* spinal cord

caudal At the rear. Caudal is contrasted to ROSTRAL, at the front. The terms rostral and caudal are synonymous with ANTERIOR and POSTERIOR.

caudal cholinergic column, This is an uninterrupted column of CHOLINERGIC neurons stretching from the LOCUS COERULEUS at the most posterior levels to the caudal pole of the SUBSTANTIA NIGRA. It includes the Ch5 and Ch6 cholinergic neurons (see CH1–CH8) in the PEDUNCULOPONTINE TEGMENTAL NUCLEUS and LATERODORSAL TEGMENTAL NUCLEUS. Cholinergic neurons in the SUBPEDUNCULAR TEGMENTAL NUCLEUS bridge between these two structures.

caudate nucleus The caudate nucleus, together with the PUTAMEN, form the dorsal STRIATUM. These two structures should not be thought of as separate and different entities and only appear as such in PRIMATES because of the development and size of the INTERNAL CAPSULE, which projects through an otherwise single nuclear mass, thereby dividing it into the caudate and putamen. Ventrally, both nuclei merge imperceptibly with the core sub-region of the NUCLEUS ACCUMBENS. The caudate and putamen, like the ventral striatum, are primarily distinguishable in terms of the origin of their cortical afferents and efferent projection targets in the GLOBUS PALLIDUS. Thus, the dorsal striatum receives primarily neocortical afferents: the head of the caudate receives inputs from prefrontal cortical areas, while the putamen receives projections mainly from the SENSORIMOTOR CORTEX. By contrast, the nucleus accumbens receives afferents from allocortical structures such as the basolateral AMYGDALA. The caudate and putamen receive a rich dopaminergic innervation from the SUBSTANTIA NIGRA, as well as afferents from the midline and intralaminar thalamic nuclei (see THALAMUS). There is also a substantial SEROTONINERGIC innervation arising in the dorsal raphe nucleus.

The output neurons of the caudate and putamen are the MEDIUM SPINY NEURONS, which make up 95% of the total neuronal mass. They are GABAERGIC and project to the internal and external pallidal segments (see GLOBUS PALLIDUS). At least two major populations of these GABAergic projection neurons have been identified; one also expresses the peptide SUBSTANCE P, is enriched with dopamine-D1 receptors (see D1–D5 DOPAMINE RECEPTORS) and projects mainly to the internal pallidal segment and substantia nigra pars reticulata (the 'direct path'; see CORTICOSTRIATAL LOOPS). The other also expresses the peptide ENKEPHALIN, is enriched in dopamine-D2 receptors and projects to the external pallidal segment ('indirect path'). Other neurons in the dorsal striatum are mainly CHOLINERGIC and peptidergic interneurons, the latter containing somatostatin, neuropeptide Y and the enzyme nitric oxide synthase. The structure of the dorsal striatum is not homogeneous, there being two major and neurochemically distinct compartments, the PATCH-AND-MATRIX ORGANIZATION (or striosomes). The matrix is rich in calbindin immunoreactivity and acetylcholinesterase. The patch compartment is rich in μ-OPIATE RECEPTORS and NEUROTENSIN immunoreactivity but is acetylcholinesterase-poor. Matrix neurons receive their cortical afferents largely from superficial layer 5 pyramidal neurons and project to the pallidum; they are the major contributors to the corticostriato-pallidal circuitry. Patch neurons receive their cortical afferents primarily from deep layer 5 pyramidal neurons and project to the dopaminergic neurons of the substantia nigra pars compacta. The functions of the patch compartment neurons are much less well understood than are the functions of the matrix neurons.

BARRY J. EVERITT

caudate–putamen In the brains of PRIMATES the CAUDATE NUCLEUS and PUTAMEN are separated by the fibres of the INTERNAL CAPSULE. The caudate nucleus and putamen are therefore seen as being two different structures. In brains of species lower in the PHYLOGENETIC SCALE than primates (that is to say, the brains of most mammalian and all other vertebrate species) the caudate nucleus and putamen are not separated but merge one into the other. In these brains the composite structure is therefore known as the caudate–putamen. The functions of this tissue, whether caudate nucleus and putamen, or caudate–putamen, are more or less the same across species.

See also: striatum

causalgia An intense burning PAIN; causalgia is produced by excess activation of EFFERENT fibres in the sympathetic nervous system following an injury to a nerve. It can be treated by giving drugs to block sympathetic nerve activity (that is, drugs that block NORADRENALINE activity).

Cavalieri principle A mathematical principle formulated by Bonaventura Cavalieri (1598–1647) that is fundamental to STEREOLOGY. Estimating the volume of cylinders and regularly shaped objects can be done using formulae based on π – the volume of a cylinder for example is $\pi r^2 l$ (where r is the radius of the cylinder and l its length). Estimating the volume of oddly shaped objects is more difficult. Johannes Kepler (1571–1630) described a method for estimating the volume of wine barrels (*Nova Stereometrica Doliorum Vinariorum* – 'New Measurements of Wine Barrels' [1615]) and Cavalieri refined and developed this procedure (*Geometria Indivisibilibus Continuorum* – 'The Geometry of Indivisibles' [1635]). His 'method of indivisibles' involves taking parallel sections of known thickness through an object, calculating their area and then combining these to give an estimate of total volume.

cavitation Cavitation is the process of tissue collapse, literally producing cave-in of tissue, that can follow destructive insults to the brain.

cell The smallest unit of life. All organisms are composed of cells, tiny compartments limited by a MEMBRANE, in which is contained the full complement of genetic material of the organism. Unicellular organisms such as bacteria and protozoa are composed of one cell which contains all non-nutritional components needed for survival. Multicellular organisms, which include most plants and animals, have cells which are often arranged in tissues or organs, and have specialized functions necessary for survival and reproduction.

Cells can be subdivided into PROKARYOTES, which have no NUCLEUS, and EUKARYOTES, in which a nucleus is present, in which the DNA (deoxyribonucleic acid) is kept separate from other cellular material (see EUKARYOTE). Prokaryotes are bacteria: these have a simple structure, characterized by the presence of a rigid cell wall surrounding the cell membrane. Bacteria have a simple GENOME, and require only basic nutrients to survive. They reproduce by binary fission, in which the cell pinches in two, to form two genetically identical daughter cells. In contrast to the relatively simple structure of prokaryotes, eukaryotic cells are more complex. The DNA is packaged into a number of strands (see CHROMOSOMES), which are confined to the nucleus, providing a greater degree of control over the expression of specific genes. In addition to a nucleus, complex eukaryotes also possess a variety of small specialized structures or ORGANELLES necessary for cell survival. Continuous with the cell nucleus is the ROUGH ENDOPLASMIC RETICULUM, a series of highly convoluted membranous folds to which RIBOSOMES are attached on the cytosolic surface. Ribosomes are catalytic units composed of RIBONUCLEIC ACID (RNA) and proteins, which mediate the translation of messenger RNA into proteins during gene expression. SMOOTH ENDOPLASMIC RETICULUM lacks ribosomes, and is involved in the synthesis of LIPIDS, important for the formation of cell membranes. Proteins synthesized at ribosomes on the rough endoplasmic reticulum enter the endoplasmic reticulum, *en route* to a series of membrane stacks called the GOLGI APPARATUS, where they may be modified before transport to their site of action. Some proteins are synthesized by free ribosomes in the cell CYTOSOL. Proteins made at these sites are released directly into the cell cytosol and act at intracellular sites. Other organelles are important for cell metabolism. Membrane-bound sacs called LYSOSOMES contain enzymes used in intracellular digestion. Similarly, PEROXISOMES contain oxidative enzymes which produce hydrogen peroxide for some cellular functions. Most of the energy used to fuel metabolic processes in eukaryotic cells is produced by the MITOCHONDRIA, which use oxygen obtained during respiration in the production of ADENOSINE TRIPHOSPHATE (ATP). In plant cells, organelles called chloroplasts harness energy from light to produce ATP and to form carbohydrates from carbon dioxide.

While prokaryotic cell sizes and shapes are limited by their cell wall, eukaryotic cell shape is maintained by a CYTOSKELETON, formed from networks of protein FILAMENTS and MICROTUBULES. These structures also allow for intracellular trafficking and motility, and lead to the enormous variety in shape that exists in many cell types in higher organisms. Different shapes underlie the highly specialized functions which cells in higher eukaryotes are required to perform for the survival of the organism. For example, a NEURON is a cell in which the distinguishing feature is the presence of an AXON and DENDRITES, fine elongated processes supported by the cytoskeleton of filaments and microtubules. These features allow neurons to conduct electrical charge, and engage in fast intracellular signalling.

Cells therefore represent complex units of life. While neurons and other eukaryotic cells contain similar basic features, specialization has led to highly defined functions of cells within tissues, which collectively permit the organism to sustain life.

FIONA M. INGLIS

cell assembly *see* neural assembly

cell assembly theory In 1949 Donald Hebb (1904–1985) proposed that SHORT-TERM MEMORY of each experience was represented by neural activity, reverberating in closed loops of initially rudimentarily interconnected neurons, while LONG-TERM MEMORY by structural changes in these neurons' synapses induced if activity was maintained and/or repeated. His proposals regarding the emergence of these cell assemblies had implications for the role early, normally occurring, sensory experiences played in the emergence of the neural circuitry underlying perceptual competencies (for instance, in PATTERN PERCEPTION) and for understanding later conditional and perceptual / cognitive learning. They also set out conditions required to induce MEMORY-related changes – for instance, that the pre- and postsynaptic neurons would be active together, with the presynaptic cell repeatedly taking part in activating the postsynaptic neuron (see HEBB-LIKE RULE; HEBBIAN SYNAPSE; HEBB'S POSTULATE).

RICHARD C. TEES

cell body A cell body (also known as the PERIKARYON, mistakenly, or SOMA) is that portion of a NEURON that contains the NUCLEUS and is the main site of PROTEIN synthesis. The cell body contains a variety of subcellular organelles and gives rise to dendrites and axons.

cell counting (More technically, this is known as HISTOMETRY.) This involves counting the numbers of cells in a given piece of tissue – and of course, in biological psychology, this is typically a count of the numbers of neurons in particular regions of the central nervous system. Cell counting could be undertaken simply in order to calculate the numbers of neurons in a particular structure, but it is more commonly undertaken for any of several reasons: (1) To determine the numbers of neurons of a particular type, identified by a selective visualization procedures (such as IMMUNOHISTOCHEMISTRY, IN SITU HYBRIDIZATION or AUTORADIOGRAPHY, for example). This might involve counting neurons normally present, or the numbers that have survived and developed following TRANSPLANTATION. (2) One might wish to determine the nature of an experimental LESION placed in the central nervous system. In this case, what one is doing is counting the numbers of neurons in control tissue and then making a comparison with the numbers of neurons in the same area in tissue in which a lesion has been made – one is trying to estimate how many neurons are missing from the lesioned brains. (3) One might wish to count the numbers of neurons identified by one form or another of the TRACT TRACERS.

Cell counting used to involve exactly that: either examining tissue sections and counting the numbers of all cells present or using a grid (either in the optical system of the microscope being used or on a monitor screen if the image was being projected) and counting in a given proportion of grid squares and estimating total numbers from the sample counted. In some cases this might be satisfactory, but there are a number of hidden problems. For example, if serial sections are taken (that is, the brain is sectioned and every SECTION is analysed, rather than say, every fifth section) then very probably, cells will be present on more than one section. The degree to which this occurs of course depends on the thickness of the tissue section and the size of the cells: with large cells and thin sections it is certain that most will be represented on a number of sections. Cell counting in such circumstances requires use of the ABERCROMBIE CORRECTION factor. Recent advances in MICROSCOPY and IMAGE ANALYSIS have led to the development of better techniques for cell counting. The method of choice now used is STEREOLOGY.

Reference

West M.J. (1999) Stereological methods for estimating the total number of neurons and synapses: issues of precision and bias. *Trends in Neurosciences* 22: 51–61.

cell culture *see* tissue culture

cell cycle *see* cell division

cell division CELL reproduction occurs in two different ways: MITOSIS and MEIOSIS. Each involves the creation of new cells, but with one critical difference: mitotic cell division produces cells with identical DNA, but meiotic does not – it involves the fusion of GAMETES, creating cells with new DNA profiles.

Mitosis is one part of the CELL CYCLE. During the mitotic phase of the cell cycle (which is further divisible into *prophase*, *prometaphase*, *metaphase*, *anaphase* and *telophase*) two essential steps take place: mitosis itself (the division of the cell NUCLEUS) and *cytokinesis* (the division of the CYTOPLASM). Preparation for these takes place in the second major component of the cell cycle, the *interphase*. The interphase (accounting for some 90% of the cycle) is divisible into three components: G1 (the first gap) (a period of cell growth), the S phase (during which CHROMOSOMES replicate, in preparation for mitosis – each divided cell nucleus must have an exact copy of the GENOME) and finally the G2 phase (second gap, during which further cell growth takes place). Mitosis is regulated by chemical control systems, involving various GROWTH FACTORS external to the cell and a class of kinases known as cyclin-dependent kinases (Cdks) that are found within cells (see KINASE). Mitotic cell division occurs continuously in some cells. Fresh BLOOD cells are, for example, produced in bone marrow throughout an individual's life. Other cells however assume a final form and divide no more: the term POSTMITOTIC indicates a cell that has completed all the mitotic divisions it will go through.

Meiosis involves gametes – sperm and egg cells (see SPERMATOZOA and OVUM). The normal cells of the human body (called SOMATIC CELLS) have 46 chromosomes, arranged in pairs: these are DIPLOID cells, in possession of two sex chromosomes (see X AND Y CHROMOSOMES) and 44 AUTOSOMES (the non-sex chromosomes). The gametes however are HAPLOID, with only half the chromosome set: 22 autosomes plus a single sex chromosome (either an X or a Y chromosome). The combination of male and female gametes produces a diploid ZYGOTE (a fertilized egg) which undergoes mitosis to produce more cells. Like mitosis, meiosis is a complex process involving several stages: interphase I is followed by meiosis I (with prophase, metaphase, anaphase and telophase I) followed by meiosis II (with each subphase repeated). At the start of the first interphase, the diploid cell has homologous pairs of chromosomes. During interphase I these replicate within the cell, yielding a homologous pair of chromosomes, each composed of two sister CHROMATIDS. In meiosis I there is cell division to produce two cells, each with a set of homologous chromosomes: these cells are haploid, each with a pair of identical chromatids. In meiosis II there is a second division to produce four cells, each with only one sister chromatid. These are also haploid, in possession of one chromatid with half the genetic material of the organism. This is what each gamete possesses, and their combination of these into a new zygote during reproduction, one from each parent, is the engine of genetic development. One further process encourages genetic variation. A process known as *crossing over* occurs during meiosis I (in the prophase) when a complex process (mediated by the *synaptonemal complex*) allows homologous parts of two non-sister chromatids to change places. The DNA from two parents can, by this means, be combined on a single chromosome.

See also: evolution; natural selection; reproduction

cell lineage The ancestry of a given CELL: from the ZYGOTE, CELL DIVISION occurs to produce cells in an organism. This can be traced in simple systems (such as CAENORHABDITIS ELEGANS) to produce a cell lineage for each cell.

cell suspension Literally, cells suspended in fluid. When TRANSPLANTATION of neurons into adult brains was begun, solid GRAFTS were used – small sections of tissue taken from a donor and placed into a host brain. However, this approach was replaced by one in which the donor tissue is processed to removed CONNECTIVE TISSUE and other unwanted matter, leaving only neurons in suspension. These can then be injected into a damaged area of host brain.

cellular tolerance Tolerance can develop for different reasons: BEHAVIOURAL TOLERANCE describes mechanisms of tolerance that are behavioural or psychological. Cellular tolerance involves adaptation of function in cells. Given that tolerance develops in the face of administration of a standard amount of DRUG, drug dose cannot be involved in the development of tolerance, and DRUG METABOLISM is unlikely to be involved. Cellular tolerance accounts for tolerance in terms of changes in, for example, RECEPTORS or SECOND MESSENGERS. Cellular tolerance is also known as PHARMACODYNAMIC TOLERANCE.

Reference
Feldman R., Meyer J.S. & Quenzer, L.F. (1997) *Principles of Neuropsychopharmacology*, Sinauer Associates: Sunderland MA.

centi- Prefix indicating a factor of 10^{-2}, or one hundredth; see SI UNITS.

central apnoea Apnoea (failure to breathe) caused by a problem within the CENTRAL NERVOUS SYSTEM, as opposed to that produced by (for example) a DRUG, or *induced apnoea* which is (internationally) brought about under general anaesthesia during surgery.

central canal *see* ventricles

central coherence Central coherence is a term introduced by Uta Frith that describes the use of context in processing sensory information: that is, disparate information which shares a common meaning is held together during processing by the CENTRAL NERVOUS SYSTEM (presumably by some top down pro-

cess – see TOP-DOWN VS. BOTTOM-UP PERCEP-
TUAL/NEURAL PROCESSING). Central coherence
places emphasis on global processing and
integration at the expense of local, detail,
processing. It has been suggested that in AUT-
ISM there is 'weak central coherence' which
Happé has argued can account for the preservation of specific skills in autists (see IDIOT
SAVANT). One test of the hypothesis that there
is weak central coherence in autism is the
EMBEDDED FIGURES TEST. In this, subjects have
to locate one simple object – a triangle for
example – that is embedded within a much
more complex figure (which can either be a
complex but familiar object, or a complex
abstract pattern). Autists perform very well on
this task, while normal subjects, seduced by the
global representation, take much longer to
locate the embedded figure.

See also: attentional set; binding problem;
Gestalt; mental set

References

Frith U. (1989) Autism: Explaining the Enigma, Blackwell Scientific: Oxford.
Happé F. (1999) Autism: cognitive deficit or
cognitive style? Trends in Cognitive Science
3: 216–222.

central dyslexia A group of ACQUIRED READ-
ING DISORDERS – DEEP DYSLEXIA, PHONOLOGI-
CAL DYSLEXIA, SURFACE DYSLEXIA – caused by
impairments to the processing pathways of the
normal READING system.

ELAINE FUNNELL

central executive The central executive is a
component of WORKING MEMORY that lies at
the heart of Alan Baddeley's influential multicomponent model. It is considered the most
sophisticated and most flexible component of
working memory and is implicated in essentially all complex cognitive activities, such as
LANGUAGE comprehension, mental arithmetic
(see MATHEMATICS AND THE BRAIN), and reasoning and DECISION-MAKING. More specifically, the central executive is assumed to be a
limited-capacity attentional system that fulfills
different regulatory functions. For example, it
controls and coordinates the activities of the
more specialized 'slave' systems of working
memory, such as the ARTICULATORY LOOP and

the VISUOSPATIAL SKETCHPAD. It also serves to
regulate the transmission of information between working memory and other parts of the
cognitive system, such as LONG-TERM MEMORY.
These executive functions are assumed to be
fuelled by a limited supply of attentional
resources (see ATTENTION).

Despite its importance in complex cognition,
the central executive is the least understood
component of working memory, and Baddeley
himself once called it the area of 'residual
ignorance'. This situation has been changing
gradually. Theoretically, a model of attentional
control, called the SUPERVISORY ATTENTIONAL
SYSTEM (SAS), has provided a basis for the
conceptual development of the central executive. Empirically, various methodologies have
been devised to study the central executive
functions (see Rabbitt, 1997, for a review of
available methods). At least some of these
methodologies were developed in an attempt
to relate the central executive functions to
those of the FRONTAL LOBE, particularly the
PREFRONTAL CORTEX. Although caution should
be exercised in relating an abstract cognitive
construct like the central executive to a brain
structure, the findings from the neuropsychological studies of frontal-lobe patients (and
other clinical populations that demonstrate so-
called DYSEXECUTIVE SYNDROME) have made
important contributions to the understanding
of the central executive system.

One such contribution from recent neuropsychological studies is that the central executive might not be as unitary a system as it was
once thought to be. The findings from these
studies point to the separability of different
executive functions among patient populations.
Based on such findings (and other experimental
results), Baddeley himself now argues for the
fractionation of the central executive into
different sub-components or independent sub-
processes (see Baddeley, 1996, for an overview
of his recent thinking on this issue). Specifying
what these subcomponents or processes that
comprise the central executive might be is one
of the most important challenges currently
facing working memory research.

See also: Phineas Gage

References

Baddeley A.D. (1996) Exploring the central executive. *Quarterly Journal of Experimental Psychology* 49A: 5–28.

Rabbitt, P. (ed.) (1997) *Methodology of Frontal Executive Function*, Psychology Press: Hove UK.

                                    AKIRA MIYAKE

central grey Synonymous with the PERIAQUEDUCTAL GREY.

central motive state A condition of MOTIVATION or DRIVE which persists independently of extra-neural stimuli. In 1906 Sherrington (1857–1952) introduced the idea of a 'central excitatory state' to refer to the excitability of nerves which persisted for several milliseconds beyond the offset of stimulation. This term extends the concept to more complex behaviours, such as FEEDING and SEXUAL BEHAVIOUR. It is suggested that extra-neural stimulation (HORMONES or external stimuli, for example) activate relevant neural circuits, so increasing their sensitivity to subsequent stimulation.

                                    ERIC M. BOWMAN

central nervous system (CNS) The central nervous system is the integral part of the NERVOUS SYSTEM comprising the brain and the SPINAL CORD. The nerves which emerge from the brain and spinal cord and distribute throughout the body represent the PERIPHERAL NERVOUS SYSTEM. While the peripheral nervous system is primarily concerned with transmitting sensory information about the external and internal milieux to the CNS and conveying motor commands to the effectors such as muscles and glands, the CNS represents a central processing unit that receives such information from the periphery, integrates it, and issues commands for an action or response. The AUTONOMIC NERVOUS SYSTEM, concerned with homeostatic (see HOMEOSTASIS) and ENDOCRINE functions, is a separate functional entity, and is part central and part peripheral.

The brain and spinal cord are protected by cranial bones and spinal vertebra, as well as by MENINGES including the dura mater, arachnoid mater and pia mater. The space between the meninges is filled by the CEREBROSPINAL FLUID, a clear colourless liquid that contains glucose, proteins, lactic acid, urea and electolytes. The cerebrospinal fluid mechanically and chemically protects the brain and spinal cord, and serves as a vehicle for nutrients and waste products. The entire central nervous system is also protected by the BLOOD–BRAIN BARRIER (BBB) against blood-borne toxins.

The spinal cord is the lower part of the CNS, and consists of the GREY MATTER shaped like the letter H at the core, and the WHITE MATTER surrounding the grey matter. The grey matter is comprised of sensory relay neurons and INTERNEURONS in the DORSAL HORN, and MOTOR NEURONS and interneurons in the VENTRAL HORN. Autonomic neurons (see PREGANGLIONIC NERVE) are also present in the lateral horn at all thoracic as well as upper lumbar segments. The white matter represents the columns (or funiculi) which are bundles (tracts) of sensory and motor fibres coursing up and down in the spinal cord. SPINAL NERVES emerge at all levels of the spinal cord. A major function of the spinal cord is to connect the peripheral nervous system with the brain and vice versa, but the spinal cord can also function independently as in reflexes (see REFLEX) which occur in response to specific sensory input from the periphery.

The brain, the upper part of the CNS, can be divided into four parts: the BRAINSTEM, CEREBELLUM, DIENCEPHALON and CEREBRAL HEMISPHERES. The brainstem comprises the MEDULLA, PONS and MIDBRAIN, which are derived from the MYELENCEPHALON, METENCEPHALON, and MESENCEPHALON, respectively. The cerebellum is also derived from the metencephalon. The metencephalon and myelencephalon are collectively referred to as the HINDBRAIN or RHOMBENCEPHALON. The brainstem is concerned with autonomic and homeostatic regulation as well as relay of sensory and motor information. Ten of the twelve CRANIAL NERVES emerge from the brainstem. The cerebellum is attached to the dorsal aspect of the pons via three fibre bundles, and is involved in balance and motor coordination. The diencephalon consists of the THALAMUS and HYPOTHALAMUS. The thalamus is a mass of relay nuclei for all sensory systems except OLFACTION, and the hypothalamus is the master structure for autonomic, homeostatic and endocrine functions. As part of the LIMBIC SYSTEM, the hypothalamus is also involved in species-specific behaviours such as FEEDING, DRINKING and SEXUAL BEHAVIOUR and parental behaviours. The most rostral structures of the brain are the cerebral hemispheres which represent the TELENCEPHALON. The cerebral hemispheres are paired structures that are separated by the longitudinal fissure in the midline, but are also interconnected via commissural fibres (see COMMISSURE) through the CORPUS CALLOSUM. Deep in the cerebral hemispheres are the BASAL GANGLIA and limbic system. The basal ganglia are involved in coordination of movements, whereas the limbic system is involved in emotional and motivational behaviours (see EMOTION; MOTIVATION).

The superficial part of cerebral hemispheres is the CEREBRAL CORTEX, critically important for higher functions including LEARNING and MEMORY and higher sensory functions, such as OBJECT RECOGNITION. These functions reach their highest level of complexity in humans. By comparing brains across different species, what is most striking is the larger proportion of the cerebral cortex in higher mammals. This is in contrast to relatively smooth and thin cortex in lower mammals, or the cortex that is almost non-existent in reptiles or amphibians. Clearly, the process of ENCEPHALIZATION reached its peak in the human brain. Consistent with this, although the human brain weighs about 1400g and comprises only about 2% of total body weight, it consumes about 20% of oxygen in a resting adult. Local blood flow in different parts of the brain varies depending on the nature of mental activity and can be studied by using FUNCTIONAL NEUROIMAGING techniques. These techniques provide an exciting avenue for studying the neurobiological basis of higher psychological functions such as planning, creativity and artistic appreciation that are uniquely human.

KAZUE SEMBA

central pain Pain is normally produced by activation of receptors (see NOCICEPTORS) in the periphery. Central pain is a form of pain that is associated with the CENTRAL NERVOUS SYSTEM directly, there being no external sensory input driving the sensation of pain. It is found following damage in the systems associated with the transmission of pain (see PAIN for a description of these) most notably the THALAMUS. Since the management of chronic pain is a major problem for medicine, surgeons have tried, in extreme cases, making a LESION at various levels of the brain. But even in cases where this has provided an initial relief from pain, it almost inevitably returns, often worse than before. Spontaneous lesions may also generate central pain: STROKE damage in the thalamus may produce this.

central pattern generator MOTOR NEURONS in the SPINAL CORD generate bursts of ACTION POTENTIAL activity after which comes a quiet period of inhibition. This cyclical activity can be produced by networks of spinal cord neurons which are called OSCILLATORS or central pattern generators (CPGs). Central pattern generators in the spinal cord can generate rhythmic LOCOMOTION in the absence of sensory information.

central reading disorder The term central reading disorder can be taken to be synonymous with CENTRAL DYSLEXIA; it is therefore a term that can also be applied to the categories of dyslexia that come under this general heading: see DYSLEXIA for a description of these.

central sensory ending *see* muscle spindle

central sulcus A large SULCUS (also known as the ROLANDIC FISSURE) situated more or less half way between the anterior and posterior poles of the brain. It separates the FRONTAL LOBE from the PARIETAL LOBE. The PRIMARY SOMATOSENSORY CORTEX is located immediately behind the central sulcus (in the area known as the POSTCENTRAL GYRUS) while the primary motor cortex is located immediately in front of it (in an area known as the PRECENTRAL GYRUS).

central tegmental tract A fibre pathway of the HINDBRAIN; see DORSAL NORADRENERGIC BUNDLE; VENTRAL NORADRENERGIC BUNDLE.

centre-surround receptive field *see* lateral inhibition; receptive field; retina

centromere The centromere is the region of the CHROMOSOMES in which the two chromatids are joined.

cephalic reflexes of digestion The cephalic reflexes of digestion are those AUTONOMIC and ENDOCRINE reflexes involved in the metabolism of food that are triggered by sensory contact with food rather than by postingestional mechanisms. They are such things as salivation and INSULIN secretion which prepare the body to receive, digest and absorb food. There are three defining traits: (1) the AFFERENT limb of the REFLEX originates in receptor mechanisms of the head and OROPHARYNX, (2) a relay in the CNS is involved, (3) the EFFERENT limb of the reflex involves autonomic and endocrine processes controlling secretion, absorption and the motility of the gastrointestinal tract. This is a process familiar to us all: for example, the sight and smell of food (1 – the afferent limb) is information processed via the CNS (2 – the CNS relay) that can trigger release of saliva from the salivary glands in the mouth (3 – the efferent limb). It was proposed by Terry Powley that VENTROMEDIAL HYPOTHALAMIC SYNDROME was caused by an exaggeration of the cephalic reflexes of digestion.

See also: cephalic rejection reflex

Reference

Powley T.L. (1977) The ventromedial hypothalamic syndrome, satiety and a cephalic phase hypothesis. *Psychological Review* 84: 89–126.

cephalic rejection reflex A negative form of the CEPHALIC REFLEXES OF DIGESTION, the purpose of which is to avoid ingestion of a noxious substance. Rather than preparing the body to receive food, cephalic rejection reflexes prepare it to reject food.

See also: nausea; vomiting

cephalization *see* nervous system

cerebellar cortex *see* cerebellum – anatomical organization

cerebellar glomeruli *see* cerebellum – anatomical organization; glomerulus

cerebellar hemispheres *see* cerebellum – anatomical organization

cerebellar peduncles The three bundles of FIBRES (superior, middle and inferior) through which cerebellar outflow passes.

See also: brachium conjunctivum; brachium pontis; cerebellum – anatomical organization; inferior cerebellar peduncle; middle cerebellar peduncle; superior cerebellar peduncle

cerebellar rigidity *see* rigidity

cerebellar vermis *see* cerebellum – anatomical organization

cerebellomedullary cistern *see* cisterna magna; ventricles

cerebellum The largest structure of the HINDBRAIN, involved in MOTOR CONTROL and LEARNING. Although its simple neuronal circuitry has made it a popular target of anatomists, neurologists such as Gordon Holmes (1876–1966) have emphasized the motor deficits which follow from cerebellar damage. Holmes described three main signs of cerebellar disease: changes in muscular tone, postural difficulties (see POSTURE) and INTENTION TREMOR. Studies of the cerebellum have therefore focused largely on motor coordination and learning. More recently, there has been a revival of interest in the idea that the cerebellum contributes to some higher-level functions such as LANGUAGE and MEMORY. The cerebellum is typically subdivided into three divisions or lobes. The phylogenetically 'oldest' of these is the FLOCCULONODULAR LOBE (the 'ARCHICEREBELLUM'), largely related to vestibular functions. The anterior lobe (the PALAEOCEREBELLUM) is typically associated with position sense. Damage to these two lobes results in abnormalities in GAIT and decreased muscular tone. The NEOCEREBELLUM (largely synonymous with the posterior lobe) is greatly expanded in species with substantial extents of cerebral cortex. Damage in this lobe can results in ab-normal reaching movements, intention tremor, and so on. The cerebellum receives its inputs via two major systems: the CLIMBING FIBRES and the MOSSY FIBRES. The mossy fibre system is largely concerned with conveying visual information from extrastriate visual cortices and the SUPERIOR COLLICULUS to the cerebellum. The climbing fibre system carries information from many sensory systems, not just vision, and its visual inputs are largely from the pretectal area and the accessory optic system. Some theorists believe that the climbing fibre system detects unexpected sensory stimuli which are not a consequence of the subject's own movements, and as a consequence can serve as 'error detectors', important for recalibration of many sensorimotor systems. The uniformity of cerebellar circuitry implies that similar operations are performed for a number of different sensorimotor activities, including error correction in pursuit eye movements, the vestibulo-ocular reflex, and visually guided limb movements. The cerebellum does not control movements directly; instead it seems to play some sort of regulatory role by inhibiting and disinhibiting motor networks in MOTOR CORTEX, BRAINSTEM premotor networks and the SPINAL CORD. The neocerebellum is massively expanded in man. Given the large connections with many regions of neocortex, some theorists now argue for language and cognitive functions of the cerebellum. Although an attractive hypothesis from the point of view of a physiological psychologist, the evidence for cognitive functions of the cerebellum remains controversial.

See also: ataxia

Reference

Houk J.C., Buckingham J.T. & Barto A.G. (1996) Models of the cerebellum and motor learning. *Behavioural and Brain Sciences* 19: 368–383.

DAVID P. CAREY

cerebellum – anatomical organization The anatomy of the CEREBELLUM is ferociously complex, though quite well understood. It is composed of an outer layer of GREY MATTER (making up the CEREBELLAR CORTEX), an inner core of WHITE MATTER and three pairs of DEEP CEREBELLAR NUCLEI: the FASTIGIAL NUCLEUS, the INTERPOSED NUCLEUS (which divides into the GLOBOSE and EMBOLIFORM NUCLEI) and the DENTATE NUCLEUS. Input to the cerebellum, which makes synaptic contact with both the deep cerebellar nuclei and cortical neurons, comes from the periphery and from many parts of the CENTRAL NERVOUS SYSTEM: there is both

motor and sensory input. The output of the cerebellum all goes through the deep cerebellar nuclei, and the closely related VESTIBULAR NUCLEI in the BRAINSTEM. (The oldest parts of the cerebellum project to the vestibular nuclei: evidently this is a precursor of the deep cerebellar nuclei.) All of the outflow travels in three pathways: known collectively as the CEREBELLAR PEDUNCLES, they are the INFERIOR CEREBELLAR PEDUNCLE (also known as the RESTIFORM BODY), the MIDDLE CEREBELLAR PEDUNCLE (or BRACHIUM PONTIS) and the SUPERIOR CEREBELLAR PEDUNCLE (or BRACHIUM CONJUNCTIVUM).

The cerebellum divides into three lobes, each divided into lobules. The principal lobes are the ANTERIOR LOBE, which is separated by the PRIMARY FISSURE from the POSTERIOR LOBE and, separated by the POSTEROLATERAL FISSURE, the FLOCCULONODULAR LOBE. (These are also known respectively as the PALAEOCEREBELLUM, NEOCEREBELLUM and ARCHICEREBELLUM.) The lobes contain SOMATOTOPIC maps of the entire body, as well as neurons responsive to sensory input. They are organized, one behind the other, on an anterior–posterior axis, and are also divided into three longwise. Running along the centre (that is, down the midline from anterior to posterior) is a strip called the CEREBELLAR VERMIS; the tissues to either side of this are known as the CEREBELLAR HEMISPHERES, one on the right, one on the left. Each area, right and left hemisphere and the vermis, has different connections. These are best described in terms of function, as is outlined in the table on p. 146.

The internal organization of the cerebellum is highly structured (making it of considerable interest to modellers of NEURAL NETWORKS). The cerebellar cortex has three layers: the outer layer is the MOLECULAR LAYER, below which is the PURKINJE CELL layer, below which is the GRANULAR LAYER. The molecular layer is composed of axons from GRANULE CELLS (in the granular layer) which collateralize, sending PARALLEL FIBRES running horizontally through the molecular layer. The dendrites of Purkinje cells (from the layer below) also extend into the molecular layer, interacting with the parallel fibres. Also present in the molecular layer are STELLATE CELLS and BASKET CELLS, which

The functional divisions of the cerebellum and their connections

VESTIBULOCEREBELLUM

Cerebellar component:	flocculonodular lobe
Function:	control of EYE MOVEMENTS; BALANCE
Inputs from:	vestibular nuclei
Outputs to:	vestibular nuclei

SPINOCEREBELLUM

Cerebellar component:	cerebellar vermis and adjacent parts of the right and left hemispheres
Function:	regulation of limb movements by control over descending MOTOR SYSTEM pathways
Inputs from:	spinal cord
Outputs to:	deep cerebellar nuclei (the vermis projects to the fastigial nucleus, the hemispheres to the interposed nucleus)

CEREBROCEREBELLUM

Cerebellar component:	lateral parts of the right and left hemispheres
Function:	planning and initiation of movement (see MOTOR PROGRAMMING)
Inputs from:	PONTINE NUCLEI of the motor system
Outputs to:	deep cerebellar nucleus (dentate nucleus) and from there to the RED NUCLEUS and the MOTOR CORTEX via the THALAMUS

function as inhibitory INTERNEURONS. The Purkinje cell layer contains the impressive Purkinje cells, arranged in a single layer. These are large neurons, with cell bodies 50–80 μm wide and exceptionally extensive dendritic fields that extend into the molecular layer. The axons run down through the white matter to the deep cerebellar nuclei (where they form synapses and use GABA as their neurotransmitter): this is the only output of the cerebellar cortex. The Purkinje cell layer has two main inputs: one from MOSSY FIBRES, the other from CLIMBING FIBRES. These are discriminated both anatomically and electrophysiologically. The mossy fibres come from the granule cell layer (including the CEREBELLAR GLOMERULI) which provide the parallel fibres in the molecular layer, with which Purkinje cell dendrites make contact. Some 200 000 parallel fibres contact each Purkinje cell. The climbing fibres come from outside the cerebellum – from the INFERIOR OLIVE. Axons from the inferior olive come directly through to the Purkinje cells, each fibre making multiple synaptic contacts with approximately ten Purkinje cells. Electro-

physiologically, mossy fibre activation produces very powerful and complex action potentials (see ACTION POTENTIAL) in Purkinje cells. Climbing fibres induce straightforward action potentials. The third layer of the cerebellar cortex is the granular layer, packed with small granule cells and the cerebellar glomeruli, complexes formed by granule cells and mossy fibres. This layer is astonishingly dense: there are more neurons in the human granule cell layer of the cerebellum than there are in the cerebral cortex.

This gives a brief idea of the organization of the cerebellum, introducing the main components and briefly explaining how they interact. However, this is a most complex structure and readers are encouraged to seek further information. The chapter in Kandel, Schwartz & Jessell (1991) is an excellent introduction.

Reference

Kandel E.R., Schwartz J.H. & Jessell T.M. (2000) *Principles of Neural Science*, 4th edn, McGraw-Hill, New York.

cerebral akinetopsia *see* motion blindness

cerebral aqueduct Also known as the AQUE-DUCT OF SYLVIUS; *see* ventricles.

cerebral asymmetry *see* asymmetry; lateralization; paw preference

cerebral blood-flow technique A technique to estimate the rate of blood flow within the brain, using radioactive tracers injected into the bloodstream. Normally, there is a close correlation between cerebral metabolism and the blood flow to a given brain area. In order to measure cerebral blood flow in animals, an inert, radioactive tracer (see RADIOLABEL) is administered, systemically, and its subsequent distribution within the brain measured. Sections of tracer-labelled brain are placed against film, producing a detailed AUTORADIOGRAM, or maps of cerebral blood flow. These techniques allow the effects on cerebral blood flow of various challenges, such as experimental ISCHAEMIA, DRUG ADMINISTRATION, or even cognitive challenge, to be estimated.

See also: cerebral vasculature; stroke

FIONA M. INGLIS

cerebral cortex The cerebral cortex represents the GREY MATTER at the outer surface of the CEREBRAL HEMISPHERES. Evolutionarily, it is the most recent development of the CENTRAL NERVOUS SYSTEM. The human cerebral cortex contains billions of NEURONS and represents the seat of higher psychological functions. As a result of rapid increase in size, the cerebral cortex in higher mammals shows extensive foldings called convolutions. Unfolded, the human cerebral cortex measures about 1600–2500 cm^2 in area. The crest of a fold is called a GYRUS, while a groove that separates gyri is called a SULCUS. Deep sulci are often called FISSURES. The longitudinal fissure separates the two cerebral hemispheres at the midline. Although there are individual differences in detail, certain gyri and sulci are more constant than others, and are used as landmarks. Beneath the cerebral cortex is the WHITE MATTER which consists of descending and ascending fibres, association fibres interconnecting different cortical regions, and commissural fibres connecting the two sides of the hemisphere. The commissural fibres form the CORPUS CALLOSUM.

The cerebral cortex can be divided into four lobes that are named after the bones that cover them: frontal, parietal, occipital and temporal lobes. The central sulcus separates the FRONTAL LOBE from the PARIETAL LOBE. Two important gyri lie anterior and posterior to the central sulcus: the pre-central gyrus, containing the primary motor area, and the post-central gyrus, representing the primary somatosensory area. The parieto-occipital sulcus separates the OCCIPITAL LOBE from the parietal lobe. The TEMPORAL LOBE is located laterally and mostly inferior to the other three lobes, and is separated from the frontal lobe by the lateral fissure. A fifth part of the cortex is the insula (see INSULA CORTEX), which lies deep to the lateral fissure.

The cellular arrangement or CYTOARCHITEC-TURE of the cerebral cortex has been studied by inspecting sections stained for NISSL BODIES and fibres. Most (90%) regions of the cortex have six layers, and as such, represent the ISOCORTEX or NEOCORTEX. The six layers, numbered from 1 to 6 from the surface, have distinct connections. Layer 4 is the input region and is highly developed in the primary sensory areas (see below), whereas layer 5 is the output region that sends information to subcortical structures, and is well developed in the primary motor area. Layers 2 and 3 provide associative connections. In addition to this layering, the neocortex exhibits a vertical radial arrangement of the cells across the thickness of the cortex which is distinct in all the four lobes except for the frontal lobe. In the primary visual area, these columns represent OCULAR DOMINANCE and orientation columns. In contrast to the isocortex, the thickness and density of individual layers in the ALLOCORTEX are so variable that the typical six-layer arrangement is practically obscured. The allocortex includes the archicortex (HIPPOCAMPAL FORMATION and DENTATE GYRUS), and the paleocortex (PYRIFORM CORTEX), which are all part of the LIMBIC SYSTEM. All of these cytoarchitectonic features are used to map the entire cerebral cortex, and the chart of 52 areas described by Brodmann for the human brain is widely used as a reference (see BRODMANN'S AREAS).

The cerebral cortex can be divided into sensory, motor and association areas. Generally, sensory areas are located in posterior regions of the cortex whereas the motor areas occupy the anterior part. The primary somatosensory area is located in the post-central gyrus (Brodmann's areas 1, 2 and 3); the primary visual area (area 17) in the medial surface of the occipital lobe; the primary auditory area (areas 41 and 42) in the superior part of the temporal lobe; the primary gustatory area (area 43) at the base of the postcentral gyrus (see GUSTATION); and the primary olfactory area in the medial aspect of the temporal lobe. The primary motor area (area 4) is located in the precentral gyrus. Adjacent to the base of the precentral gyrus is the motor speech area (area 44), also called BROCA'S AREA. This area is concerned with the production of speech and is usually located on the left side only. Lesions in Broca's area result in APHASIA.

The association areas occupy the largest part of the cortex in the human, and are concerned with higher functions including perception and voluntary motor control as well as cognitive and other intellectual functions. Not all of these cortical functions are bilaterally represented, and LATERALIZATION of functions occurs. For example, language functions are represented mostly in the left hemisphere (in right-handed people), and musical and artistic awareness and spatial and pattern perception are represented predominantly in the right hemisphere. The brain imaging techniques that allow metabolic mapping of the human brain during different mental activities have been rapidly advancing the understanding of neuroanatomical localization of psychological functions in the human brain.

See also: cerebral dominance; association cortex; cortex, sensory; motor cortex

KAZUE SEMBA

cerebral dominance The human brain has a RIGHT HEMISPHERE and a LEFT HEMISPHERE, and each is specialized for some cognitive skills. Cerebral dominance commonly refers to the left hemisphere's LANGUAGE functions. As the right hemisphere is more specialized than the left for some functions (for example SPATIAL MEMORY) the term should be used in

conjunction with a specific ability, and with due regard for the fact that the cerebral dominance is true for most, but not all of the population.

JENNI A. OGDEN

cerebral hemispheres *see* hemisphere; left hemisphere; right hemisphere

cerebral palsy Motor disability occurring as a result of damage to the brain during, shortly before or soon after birth. Common causes include the various complications of pregnancy (such as prematurity, multiple births, difficult deliveries, blood incompatibilities, asphyxia or infection). A few cases are probably genetic. Early symptoms may include involuntary movements or an asymmetrical GAIT, followed by SPASTICITY, ATAXIA, DYSARTHRIA, deafness and squint. Some sufferers are subject to convulsive SEIZURES, and may be mentally retarded. The causative lesions are usually located in the cerebral cortex or white matter, or cerebellum, and their extent determines the severity and nature of disability.

L. JACOB HERBERG

cerebral peduncles 'Peduncle' is derived from Latin, *pedis*, the foot. In plant biology it refers to the stalk of a solitary flower but in biology in general it has come to mean any long thin connection. Cerebral of course refers to the CEREBRUM. The cerebral peduncles lie at the base of the MIDBRAIN and are extensions of the INTERNAL CAPSULE. They carry fibres from the CEREBRAL CORTEX that descend towards the PONS, MEDULLA and SPINAL CORD. The cerebral peduncles are also know by the terms BASIS PEDUNCULI and CRUS CEREBRI.

cerebral vasculature The blood vessels supplying the tissues of the brain. The brain derives most of its energy from OXYGEN and GLUCOSE supplied via the bloodstream. Under normal conditions, cerebral blood flow and energy use are tightly coupled, and the brain must adapt to local alterations in energy requirement by regulating the amount of bloodflow accordingly.

Blood reaches the brain via the carotid and basilar arteries, which surround the brain in a complete arterial circle, known as the CIRCLE

OF WILLIS. This circular arrangement may preserve perfusion to the entire brain in the event that one artery becomes blocked. From this circle arise the anterior, middle and posterior cerebral arteries, which divide into pial arteries. These run over the surface of the brain, and subdivide into short arterioles, which give rise to a high density of capillaries that ultimately supply nerve cells with blood. These capillaries are highly responsive to local changes in potassium ions, resulting in increased blood flow during neuronal activity. Because cerebral blood flow and neuronal activity are inherently linked, studies of cerebral blood flow employing radiolabelled tracers have been used both clinically to estimate disruptions of blood flow in disease or injury, and experimentally to examine the effects of cognition and pharmacological intervention on neuronal activity.

See also: blood–brain barrier; ischaemia; metabolic mapping; stroke

FIONA M. INGLIS

cerebrocerebellum *see* cerebellum – anatomical organization

cerebroside *see* lipids

cerebrospinal fluid (CSF) The fluid surrounding the brain and spinal cord. Cerebrospinal fluid is produced by cells of the CHOROID PLEXUS which secrete it into the cerebral VENTRICLES. CSF circulates through the ventricles and then into the subarachnoid space surrounding the brain. It drains into the bloodstream via the arachnoid villi. Its buoyant effect protects the CENTRAL NERVOUS SYSTEM from damage due to acceleration and deceleration. Excess production or impaired removal of CSF can lead to HYDROCEPHALUS. Metabolic products enter the CSF from the brain. CSF can be analysed for the presence of proteins or cells (for example, lymphocytes and monocytes) that are indicative of various disease states, such as MENINGITIS.

DOUGLAS D. RASMUSSON

cerebrovascular accident *see* stroke

cerebrum (Latin, *cerebrum*: brain) Although technically cerebrum refers to the CEREBRAL HEMISPHERES and those structures immediately associated with them, it is generally used as a synonym for BRAIN.

See also: telencephalon

cerveau isolé A knife cut LESION through the brain that isolates the TELENCEPHALON and DIENCEPHALON from the remainder of it – in effect a PRECOLLICULAR–POSTMAMMILLARY TRANSECTION. It is not a technique that is used any more. Experiments using this in the 1950s described persistent SLEEP in animals following such lesions. Other transections lower in the brain did not however have the same effect, but could produce persistent INSOMNIA (the BATANI TRANSECTION) or leave the SLEEP–WAKE CYCLE unaffected (the ENCÉPHALE ISOLÉ). The idea was presented that the *cerveau isolé* cut the output of the ASCENDING RETICULAR ACTIVATING SYSTEM while the Batani transection, in the PONS, cut the input to the ascending reticular activating system, leaving it permanently 'on' and the animal unable to go to sleep. The *encéphale isolé*, made at the junction of the BRAINSTEM and SPINAL CORD, produced no effect because, in contrast to these other transections, it had no effect on the ascending reticular activating system. These studies were valuable in showing that sleep was an active neural process dependent on brainstem mechanisms. Later studies have concentrated on describing the nature of neural sleep mechanisms in much finer detail, and lesions as gross as these are no longer made.

There is a small note to add about the terms *cerveau isolé* and *encéphale isolé*. The French word *isolé* translates, appropriately here, as 'isolated'. But the terms *encéphale* and *cerveau* can both be translated as 'brain'. The most common French term for brain is *cerveau* though neuroscientists would tend to use *encéphale*. Each major division of the brain, as in English, incorporates this term: MYELENCEPHALON, TELENCEPHALON and so forth. But 'hindbrain' for example would always be translated as *cerveau postérieur* and 'forebrain' as *cerveau antérieur*. Thus, both *cerveau* and *encéphale* can be used to refer to 'brain'. The terms *cerveau isolé* and *encéphale isolé* come from the sleep studies of Bremer (1892–1959), a Belgian neuroscientist. The term *encéphale isolé* is correct, since the transection is made between the spinal cord and the brainstem, leaving the brain intact but isolated. But the term *cerveau isolé* is not strictly correct, since it refers to isolating the forebrain (telencephalon and diencephalon) which is *le cerveau antérieur*. As it stands, *cerveau isolé* really means exactly the same as *encéphale isolé*. Fortunately, there is a general agreement about what the terms actually stand for.

cervical spinal cord *see* spinal cord

Cg1 / 2 / 3 These abbreviations refer to the rat CINGULATE CORTEX, located on the frontal MEDIAL WALL. This nomenclature was introduced by Zilles (1985). Cg1 and Cg2 are thought to be homologous to primate ANTERIOR CINGULATE CORTEX. There is some disagreement about whether Cg3, located ventrally, is part of CINGULATE CORTEX or whether it is the functional equivalent of primate PREFRONTAL CORTEX. The boundaries of cingulate cortex in the rat are still being revised, as additional neurochemical data becomes available. In the STEREOTAXIC ATLAS of Paxinos & Watson, Cg3 is designated PRELIMBIC CORTEX (PrL).

See also: rodent vs. primate prefrontal cortex

References

Paxinos G. & Watson C. (1997) *The Rat Brain in Stereotaxic Coordinates*, compact 3rd edn, Academic Press: San Diego.

Zilles K. (1985) *The Cortex of the Rat: a Stereotaxic Atlas*, Springer-Verlag: Berlin.

VERITY J. BROWN

Ch1–Ch8 The terms Ch1–Ch8 were used by Mesulam to classify the ascending CHOLINERGIC pathways in the central nervous system. Cell group Ch1 was found in the medial septal nucleus (see SEPTAL NUCLEI); Ch2 in the nucleus of the vertical limb of the DIAGONAL BAND OF BROCA; Ch3 in the horizontal limb of the diagonal band of Broca; and Ch4 in the NUCLEUS BASALIS OF MEYNERT (also referred to as the MAGNOCELLULAR BASAL NUCLEUS). Collectively, Ch1–Ch4 are known as the magnocellular basal forebrain nuclei. Ch5 neurons are found in the PEDUNCULOPONTINE TEGMENTAL NUCLEUS, Ch6 in the LATERODORSAL TEGMENTAL NUCLEUS, these are the cholinergic neurons of the PONS. Ch7 are found in the

medial HABENULA and Ch8 in the PARABIGEMINAL NUCLEUS, in the diencephalon and mesencephalon. Populations of cholinergic INTERNEURONS are also found in the CEREBRAL CORTEX, HIPPOCAMPUS and STRIATUM.

Reference

Wainer B.H. & Mesulam M.-M. (1990) Ascending cholinergic pathways in the rat brain. In *Brain Cholinergic Systems*, ed. M. Steriade & D. Biesold, pp. 65–119, Oxford University Press: Oxford.

cerebrovascular accident *see* stroke

change blindness *see* saccadic suppression

characteristic frequency The characteristic frequency is the frequency at the lowest sound level of the AUDITORY TUNING CURVE.

chelating agent Chelating agents are chemicals to which metal ions attach, these ions thereby being removed from any other chemical process in which they were involved (see ION). There are chelating agents with degrees of specificity for particular metal ions. Some chelating agents have significance for biological psychology: DISULFRAM for example is a copper chelator.

chemical messengers A rather broad term indicating chemicals that signal information, which includes NEUROTRANSMITTERS and neuromodulators (see NEUROMODULATION), HORMONES, PHEROMONES, and the various signals of the IMMUNE SYSTEM for example). Typically chemical messengers are released from a CELL and bind to a RECEPTOR on a MEMBRANE that may be proximal to the point of RELEASE or at some distance. However, not all chemical messengers act in this way: for example, some novel neuromodulators such as NITRIC OXIDE diffuse across membranes to affect directly intracellular processes.

chemical neuroanatomy This is a general term used to describe those methods that use chemical means to investigate the structure and development of the nervous system. It allows one to engage in an examination of nervous tissue beyond simple examination of MORPHOLOGY. New techniques for examining tissue are being developed all the time and, consequently, more and more is revealed about the chemical composition and structure of the brain. Although one might imagine NEUROANATOMY to be a rather staid science, it is not: our understanding of the structure and development of the brain is constantly changing and of course, as concepts concerning structure change, so do ideas about brain organization and function.

Analysis can be conducted using standard LIGHT MICROSCOPY, CONFOCAL MICROSCOPY or ELECTRON MICROSCOPY. It includes techniques to map the connections of different parts of the nervous system using TRACT TRACERS; techniques such as HISTOCHEMISTRY, IMMUNOHISTOCHEMISTRY and IN SITU HYBRIDIZATION that allow one to identify cells containing specific chemicals; and techniques (such as METABOLIC MAPPING and FUNCTIONAL NEUROIMAGING) that allow one to examine brain activity. There are also techniques to allow one to identify neurons in specific states – the TUNEL METHOD for example allows one to visualize neurons undergoing apoptosis. DOUBLE LABELLING or even TRIPLE LABELLING allows one to combine different procedures so that, for example, different neuronal elements or the spatial relationships between neurons possessing different types of chemical can be examined.

Reference

Bolam J.P. (1992) *Experimental Neuroanatomy: A Practical Approach*, IRL Press at Oxford University Press: Oxford.

chemical synapse *see* synapse

chemical transmission When synaptic TRANSMISSION was first discovered, the term chemical transmission was used to discriminate chemical from electrical forms of transmission in the CENTRAL NERVOUS SYSTEM (that is to say, synaptic transmission and VOLUME TRANSMISSION, both forms of chemical transmission, from EPHAPTIC TRANSMISSION). It is clear however that the cells of the body communicate in many ways using chemicals: HORMONES and PHEROMONES are chemicals that signal information, while the cells of the IMMUNE SYSTEM have many mechanisms for effecting chemical transmission. The term chemical transmission is evidently now a very broad one: in general, unless conceptual breadth is required, one should specify the form of chemical transmission of interest rather than use this broad term.

See also: neurotransmission

chemically addressed system Synonymous with VOLUME TRANSMISSION: it was coined to indicate a difference between SYNAPTIC TRANSMISSION (which occurs at morphologically specialized synapses) and a system that relied on the chemical specificity of the signal and its type of RECEPTOR, without morphological specialization. HORMONES operate in a chemically addressed manner: they are released into the BLOOD stream and circulate until they find an appropriate receptor to target.

chemoarchitecture Chemoarchitecture is the structure of the NERVOUS SYSTEM as described by CHEMICAL NEUROANATOMY; chemoarchitectonics is the process of describing this.

chemoreceptor Any receptor that converts chemical activity into neural activation. NEUROTRANSMISSION at a SYNAPSE involves chemoreceptors: membrane-bound receptors on neurons that bind neurotransmitter molecules. OLFACTION and taste (see GUSTATION) also involve chemoreceptors to sample molecules present on the tongue or airborne molecules in the nose. But the VISUAL SYSTEM and AUDITORY SYSTEM have receptor mechanisms that transduce not chemical signals but light and sound waves into neural activity.

chemosignals *see* pheromones

Cheyne–Stokes respiration An abnormal pattern of breathing (see BREATHING, NEURAL CONTROL OF) in which there is a gradual increase in the depth of intake followed by a pause (producing APNOEA). Because of its up-and-down pattern it is also known as *tidal respiration*; it is typically seen in COMA following damage to the CENTRAL NERVOUS SYSTEM structures controlling breathing.

chick Chicks are used in LEARNING experiments. They are of interest because, following hatching, they immediately begin learning (see IMPRINTING) and therefore permit study of new learning in the absence of any previous environmental influence.

childhood disintegrative disorder This is a diagnostic category employed by DSM-IV. It is a member of a relatively broad category of PERVASIVE DEVELOPMENTAL DISORDERS which also includes AUTISM, RETT SYNDROME, ASPERGER'S SYNDROME and other developmental disorders. In childhood disintegrative disorder examination looks for such things as: (1) normal early DEVELOPMENT, (2) later loss of skills acquired before the age of 10 (skills include such things as PLAY, social skills, physiological skills such as bladder control and motor skills), (3) communication and socialization disorders. The diagnosis of childhood disintegrative disorder is used if other more specific diagnosis (such as autism) can be made, and other diagnoses (such as SCHIZOPHRENIA) do not better account for the SIGNS AND SYMPTOMS evidenced by the patient.

chimaera (also spelled chimera: the chimaera was a monster in Greek mythology with the head of a lion, body of a goat and tail of a serpent) In contemporary biology chimaera refers to any animal (or indeed plant) that has been created from the genetic material of two different species. Evidently the interest in generating new forms of life by manipulation of GENES and tissues has a considerable history.

chimaeric faces An experimental tool: a chimaeric face is a pictorial or computer-generated representation, the sides of which differ. For example, the right side of a man's face may have been paired with the left side of a woman's face. Asked to fixate a central point, patients who have been commissurotomized (see SPLIT BRAIN) can then either be asked to point or to describe the stimulus. A verbal response will describe the right half of the stimulus, because the LEFT HEMISPHERE, more specialized for LANGUAGE, has input from the right VISUAL FIELD. A motor response will be to the left, the RIGHT HEMISPHERE (with left visual field input) being in control. Patients with SPATIAL NEGLECT also have difficulties with this task.

See also: face perception

chirality (from Greek, *cheir*: hand) Chemicals that can exist in right- or left-handed forms are said to possess chirality (adjective chiral); see ISOMERS.

chloral hydrate Chloral hydrate has been used in animals to induce ANAESTHESIA, and given to patients for the treatment of INSOMNIA. It is not commonly used any more, having been replaced by other drugs, such as BARBITURATES.

chloralose An anaesthetic agent, but one little used in biological psychology: it is an effective and long-lasting anaesthetic, but gives only light ANAESTHESIA, insufficient for procedures such as STEREOTAXIC SURGERY. It has been used in studies of cardiovascular physiology because it does not have a significant effect on AUTONOMIC NERVOUS SYSTEM actions.

Reference

Flecknell P.A. (1987) *Laboratory Animal Anaesthesia*, Academic Press: London.

chlordiazepoxide Commercially known as LIBRIUM, chlordiazepoxide was the first BENZODIAZEPINE drug to be developed.

See also: Valium

chloride (Cl^-) Chlorides are chlorine compounds and are essential for normal neural functioning (see for example ACTION POTENTIAL; CHLORIDE CHANNEL). Chlorine is important in ELECTROLYTE balance in the NERVOUS SYSTEM and elsewhere in the body – it accounts for two-thirds of all negatively charged ions in the BLOOD for example.

See also: ion; periodic table of the elements

chloride channel *see* ion channel

chloroform Non-flammable organic liquid discovered in 1847 and capable of inducing general ANAESTHESIA in animals, but with high toxicity to the liver and cardiovascular depressant effects; virtually never used as an anaesthetic now.

See also: ether; halothane

CHARLES D. BLAHA

chlorpromazine One of the PHENOTHIAZINE drugs, used to treat SCHIZOPHRENIA; see ANTIPSYCHOTIC.

chocolate (from Spanish, *chocolate*, which was derived from Nahuatl (the language of a group of south and central American peoples, including Aztec), *chócolatl*). Chocolate is a paste made from the seeds of *Theobroma cacao* (that is, from cocoa beans) which can be transformed into blocks or other confections. It has been claimed that it is possible to form an ADDICTION to chocolate. Such addiction would reflect the high levels of CAFFEINE found in it; see TEA AND COFFEE for discussion of this.

choice reaction time *see* reaction time

cholecystokinin (CCK) Cholecystokinin was the first of the GUT–BRAIN PEPTIDES to be discovered: it is secreted by the DUODENUM to affect PERISTALSIS and stimulate the activity of the PANCREAS during DIGESTION and is also used as one of the NEUROTRANSMITTERS in the CENTRAL NERVOUS SYSTEM. Cholecystokinin is derived from pre-pro-cholecystokinin, a large POLYPEPTIDE composed of four domains: a 20 amino acid signal PEPTIDE (at the amino [NH₂] terminus; see AMINO ACIDS); a 25 amino acid 'spacer peptide' (cleaved off and discarded during cholecystokinin production); a 58 amino acid domain known as cholecystokinin-58 (CCK-58) , the largest form of cholecystokinin and the part typically detected in tissues; and a C terminal peptide normally discarded during the processing of pre-pro-cholecystokinin. Further processing occurs of CCK-58 to produce cholecystokinin 8 (CCK-8), the active molecule of cholecystokinin that acts as a neurotransmitter in the central nervous system. CCK-8 is found in many parts of the brain. For example, it has a high concentration in the CEREBRAL CORTEX, and is found co-existent with DOPAMINE in the MESOLIMBIC DOPAMINE SYSTEM. It is also present in the BRAINSTEM and SPINAL CORD, in a variety of sensory ganglia, and in the RETINA. Two types of RECEPTOR have been described, CCK1 and CCK2, at which CCK-8 is the most potent LIGAND, with GASTRIN and other CCK fragments (such as CCK-4) also active at them. Both receptors are G PROTEIN coupled.

Cholecystokinin was once thought to function as a signal of SATIETY: it is released from the duodenum during digestion, and it is found in brain. It is questionable whether it does induce feelings of satiation. For example, Ettenberg & Koob (1984) showed that satiety induced by feeding and the 'satiety' induced by administration of CCK had very different effects on INTRACRANIAL SELF-STIMULATION, suggesting that rats did not perceive natural satiety and that induced by CCK to be the same thing.

See also: neurotensin

Reference

Ettenberg A. & Koob G.F. (1984) Different effects of cholecystokinin and satiety on lateral hypothalamic self-stimulation. *Physiology and Behavior* 32: 127–130.

cholera toxin subunit B *see* tract tracers

cholesterol Cholesterol is popularly assumed to be 'a bad thing', but life rarely if ever divides neatly into good things and bad things. Cholesterol is a steroid, the precursor of all STEROID HORMONES, including SEX HORMONES. It is also critically involved in the maintenance of membranes, where it acts to reduce fluidity and maintain stability. It is ubiquitously present in membranes, and as such there are large amounts of cholesterol present in the central nervous system. Clearly, without cholesterol, brain tissue would not operate effectively. However, cholesterol travels in the bloodstream (in particles known as low-density LIPOPROTEINS) and in certain conditions (most notably an inherited condition called hypercholesterolaemia) it can accumulate leading to ATHEROSCLEROSIS. High-density lipoproteins act to reduce cholesterol deposition in blood vessels: exercise increases the ratio of high-density to low-density lipoprotein activity (good) but smoking (see TOBACCO) has the reverse effect (bad). A relationship between dietary cholesterol intake and atherosclerosis is strongly suspected but not proven beyond all doubt.

choline The neurotransmitter acetylcholine is synthesized from ACETYL COENZYME A (acetyl CoA) and choline, a reaction catalysed by the enzyme CHOLINE ACETYLTRANSFERASE. Choline is found in many foodstuffs and is transported across the BLOOD–BRAIN BARRIER by a dedicated carrier mechanism, which may be bi-directional.

choline acetyltransferase (ChAT, CAT) Choline acetyltransferase is the critical synthetic enzyme involved in the production of ACETYL-CHOLINE, catalysing the reaction of ACETYL COENZYME A and CHOLINE. Neurons that contain ChAT are by definition CHOLINERGIC. There are antibodies to ChAT available, allowing IMMUNOHISTOCHEMISTRY to be performed for the determination of cholinergic neuron location. The introduction of this technique was critical in determining the details of cholinergic neuroanatomy in the CNS.

See also: acetylcholinesterase; Ch1–Ch8

cholinergic *see* acetylcholine

cholinergic receptors *see* acetylcholine receptors

cholinoceptive A neuron that is responsive to the neurotransmitter ACETYLCHOLINE is said to be cholinoceptive; a cholinoceptive neuron does not have to be CHOLINERGIC.

cholinomimetic A drug that mimics the actions of the neurotransmitter ACETYLCHOLINE is said to be cholinomimetic.

chorda tympani A branch of the VESTIBULO-COCHLEAR NERVE (the eighth cranial nerve) that carries information from the anterior two-thirds of the TONGUE to the CENTRAL NERVOUS SYSTEM.

See also: gustation

chorea (from Greek, *choreia*: dance) A CHOREA is a rapid involuntary movement; choreiform describes such a movement. Various movements can be described in this way, from the gross motor abnormalities of HUN-TINGTON'S CHOREA, through various types of TIC, to the odd rapid leg movements that many people display while sitting down.

choreoathetosis *see* athetosis

chorion *see* amniotic egg

choroid plexus Connective tissue within the VENTRICLES having a very rich blood supply; CEREBROSPINAL FLUID is produced by the choroid plexuses.

See also: blood–brain barrier

chromaffin cells Cells in the medulla of the ADRENAL GLAND that synthesize and release NORADRENALINE (norepinephrine) and ADRENALINE (epinephrine).

See also: fight-or-flight; stress

chromatid A chromosome consists of a complex of DNA (deoxyribonucleic acid) and PROTEINS (together known as chromatin). During CELL DIVISION, the chromosome duplicates, forming two sister chromatids, each containing a copy of the DNA. These are connected in the middle, in an area called the CENTROMERE.

See also: chromosomes

chromophore *see* spectral sensitivity

chromosome abnormalities There are a number of abnormalities of CHROMOSOMES recognized in humans. Some 4% of all recognized pregnancies involve a foetus with a chromosome abnormality. However, most spontaneously terminate and only some 0.5% of live births involve infants with chromosome abnormalities. A proportion of these will be severe enough to limit life, but infants with a number of recognized conditions do survive and enjoy healthy lives. The majority of the cases of chromosome abnormality involve DOWN SYNDROME or TRISOMY 21, but there are many others: see for example FRAGILE X SYNDROME, KLINEFELTER'S SYNDROME (XXY syndrome), PHENYLKETONURIA, XYY SYNDROME, TURNER'S SYNDROME and TRIPLE X SYNDROME (XXX syndrome)

See also: amniocentesis; X and Y chromosomes

chromosomes Large molecules of DNA (deoxyribonucleic acid) contained within a CELL nucleus, which carry the genetic code necessary for the survival and reproduction of the organism. Bacterial cells have a single chromosome, while in more complex organisms each cell has several chromosomes, which together form the entire genetic code. Chromosomes condense into visible structures during MITOSIS or MEIOSIS (see CELL DIVISION).

See also: chromosome abnormalities

FIONA M. INGLIS

chronic A relatively long-lasting challenge or event, in contrast to a rapid or brief event, which is referred to as acute. For instance, one could measure an acute response to a single injection of a drug or examine the chronic response to long-term drug administration.

chronic fatigue syndrome *see* myalgic encephalitis

chronoamperometry An electrochemistry technique in which short-duration voltage pulses (0.1–1 sec duration) are applied repetitively to an ELECTRODE in solution to measure OXIDATION and/or REDUCTION of ELECTROACTIVE compounds.

CHARLES D. BLAHA

chronobiology The study of temporal aspects of biology. This definition is broad enough to cover virtually any aspect of biology, since all processes occur in a temporal framework. Chronobiology, has, however, been applied mainly to two aspects of one field of study; namely, the analysis of the mechanism of types of BIOLOGICAL CLOCK, and the application of this information to human health.

As a basic science, chronobiology involves the documentation of a variety of physiological and behavioural rhythms in organisms, and the analysis of their underlying mechanisms and functional significance. The rhythms of primary interest are those with periods of 24 hours in the natural world, but other rhythms, with shorter or longer periodicities (see ULTRADIAN RHYTHM; SEASONAL AFFECTIVE DISORDER) are also subjects of interest. This aspect of chronobiology emphasizes the diversity of rhythms that can be measured in essentially all of the body's regulatory systems, their generation by an internal biological clock or multiple clocks (see SUPRACHIASMATIC NUCLEUS), and their synchronization by light and other periodic environmental cycles, a process called ENTRAINMENT.

As an applied science, chronobiology investigates the implications of the pervasive, complex rhythmicity of human physiology for the diagnosis and treatment of disease, and the maintenance of health. A fundamental principle in diagnosis is that single measurements of physiological parameters provide only a sample taken from a temporal stream, the meaning of which depends on the temporal context. Thus, elevated cortisol levels at awakening are normal, while the same levels in the early evening would be abnormally high. The proper unit of measurement for assessing 'normality' for most physiological functions is, therefore, the daily rhythm, not an isolated sample. Assessment of rhythmic patterns may provide more sensitive indices of abnormalities. Chronobiology also emphasizes several important features in treatment of medical conditions. Abnormal conditions are themselves often rhythmic, and should be treated with respect to their temporal characteristics. Thus, asthma or cardiovascular disease may require high drug doses at times of highest risk while lower doses at other times can reduce side-effects. In addition, there is evidence that the timing of pharmacotherapies may alter the effectiveness of treatments for cancer because of different rhythms of sensitivity to toxic drugs in healthy versus cancerous tissues. More generally, the pervasive rhythmicity of animal and human physiology can cause drug treatments of clinical populations (or experimental treatments in a laboratory) to have different, even opposite, effects at different times of day or year.

BENJAMIN RUSAK

chronocoulometry *see* voltammetry

chronological age The actual age, calculated in days, months or years, of an organism; contrasted to MENTAL AGE; see INTELLIGENCE TESTING.

chronotaraxis Disorientation with respect to time; it is a symptom found in certain conditions including, for example, KORSAKOFF'S SYNDROME.

cilia (from Latin, *cilium*: an eyelash; cilia is the plural; the singular is cilium) Cilia are fine hair-like threads present on cells. They have different functions in different locations: for example, they can form the sensory element of certain sensory cells – the hairs on HAIR CELLS for example, or in the olfactory system (see STEREOCHEMICAL THEORY OF ODOUR DISCRIMINATION); they can be used for LOCOMOTION by single-celled animals; they can be used by cells to move fluid within the organs of multicelled animals (ciliated cells in the windpipe move mucus out of the lungs for instance).

ciliary ganglion A GANGLION of the AUTONOMIC NERVOUS SYSTEM: it has input from preganglionic neurons in the EDINGER–WESTPHAL NUCLEUS (via the OCULOMOTOR NERVE). The ciliary ganglion sends out fibres (the axons of postganglionic neurons) that innervate and control the muscles of the pupil of the eye.

See also: cranial nerves; pretectum

ciliary muscle Muscles of the EYE which, via the SUSPENSORY LIGAMENTS, control the LENS.

See also: ciliary ganglion

ciliary neurotrophic factor *see* nerve growth factor

cingulate cortex The cingulate cortex or gyrus is a limbic cortical region located on the medial surface of the CEREBRAL CORTEX deep in the LONGITUDINAL FISSURE immediately above the CORPUS CALLOSUM. Cytoarchitectonically (see CYTOARCHITECTURE), the cingulate cortex represents a type of cortex that is transitional between the ALLOCORTEX and the ISOCORTEX or NEOCORTEX. The major input to the cingulate cortex comes from the anterior thalamic nuclei and its main output is directed to the ENTORHINAL CORTEX. Historically, the cingulate cortex was part of PAPEZ CIRCUIT, and is thought to be involved in expression and experience of EMOTION.

See also: anterior cingulate cortex; limbic system

KAZUE SEMBA

cingulate gyrus *see* cingulate cortex

cingulate motor areas Parts of the CINGULATE CORTEX believed to be involved in motor control; see MOTOR CORTEX.

cingulotomy *see* psychosurgery

cirazoline An alpha-1 noradrenaline receptor AGONIST; see ADRENOCEPTORS.

circadian rhythm (from Latin, *circa*: about, *dies*, a day) A biological rhythm with a period of approximately 24 hours.

See also: biological clock

circannual rhythm A biological rhythm with a period of approximately a year.

See also: biological   clock;   hibernation; migration

circle of Willis *see* blood

circumvallate papillae *see* taste buds

circumventricular organs This is a collective name for a group of structures close to the VENTRICLES of the brain where the BLOOD–BRAIN BARRIER is absent: the principal circumventricular organs are the AREA POSTREMA, ORGANUM VASCULOSUM OF THE LAMINA TERMINALIS and the SUBFORNICAL ORGAN. They are sites at which BLOOD-borne information relating to processes such as OSMOREGULATION and ENERGY BALANCE (indeed any processes requiring information from the blood) can be monitored.

cisterna magna *see* cerebellomedullary cistern; ventricles

citrulline *see* nitric oxide; sodium nitroprusside

CL-316,243 A beta-3 NORADRENALINE receptor AGONIST; see ADRENOCEPTORS.

clade A clade is the name given to any group of animals that are suitable for phylogenetic analysis; the hominoid (Latin name: *Hominoidea*) TAXON – the great apes including humans – is a clade. Cladistics is the method of analysis based upon identification of clades. The value of cladistics is that it permits the history of extinct species, the ancestors of members of the clade, to be derived and some of the characteristics of these extinct species to be inferred. A cladogram is the tree-like representation of the relationships between present and past members of the clade.

See also: evolution; taxonomy

clasp knife rigidity *see* rigidity

class inclusion operations *see* multiple memory systems

classical conditioning Those learning processes where the presentation of two stimuli in TEMPORAL CONTIGUITY leads to the development of an ASSOCIATION between them, such that one stimulus, typically a neutral event, becomes imbued with some of the properties of the other, typically a motivationally salient event (see PAVLOVIAN CONDITIONING). Both the presentation of the two stimuli and the formation of the association between them are entirely independent of the actions of the subject, distinguishing such processes from INSTRUMENTAL CONDITIONING. Classical conditioning typically involves the pairing of an UNCONDITIONED STIMULUS, or US (for example, the delivery of sucrose solution) with a CONDITIONED STIMULUS, or CS (for example, the presentation of a light). Following a number of exposures to the two paired stimuli, presentation of the previously neutral light stimulus (CS) on its own becomes capable of eliciting a range of responses from the subject that were previously elicited only by the sucrose solution (US). These responses could include ORIENTATION and approach to the stimulus, contact and salivation. Such learning has been shaped by evolutionary processes to permit the detection and storage of information about predictive relationships in the environment. Depending on the organization of stimuli in an experiment, a stimulus acting as a CS in one situation may act as a US in another. Thus, the definition of a stimulus as a CS or as a US is relative and is determined by which stimulus elicits the specified response under study. The US will elicit the specified response when presented alone. The CS will only elicit the specified response following a period of training. The pace with which learning (see CONDITIONING) proceeds and the ultimate strength of the association is dependent upon the intrinsic properties of the stimuli involved, the subject's prior experience of the stimuli and the temporal relationship between them. Classical conditioning can occur with both appetitive (see APPETITIVE CONDITIONING) and aversive (see AVERSIVE CONDITIONING) unconditioned stimuli. Conditioning by classical (or Pavlovian) processes plays an important role in the regulation of AUTONOMIC NERVOUS SYSTEM activity and also in the expression of complex behaviours.

See also: autoshaping; discrimination learning;

instrumental conditioning; Rescorla–Wagner theory; stimulus–stimulus association

KEITH MATTHEWS

classification of Dahlström and Fuxe Annica Dahlström and Kjell Fuxe used what was then the novel technique of HISTOFLUORESCENCE to map the location of cells in the central nervous system containing the neurotransmitters NORADRENALINE (A1–A7, A11) and DOPAMINE (A8–10, A12–A15) and SEROTONIN (cell groups B1–B9). The work was magisterial, a landmark in the developing field of CHEMICAL NEUROANATOMY. Cell groups A1–A4 and B1–B4 were found in the MEDULLA OBLONGATA; A5–A7 and B3, B5 and B6 in the PONS; A8–A10 and B7–B9 in the MIDBRAIN and A11 and A12 in the DIENCEPHALON. Cell groups A13–A15 were discovered later. The classification scheme is still used, though perhaps less than previously. The most common terms still used are A9 (the dopamine neurons of the SUBSTANTIA NIGRA pars compacta), A10 (the dopamine neurons of the VENTRAL TEGMENTAL AREA), A6 (the noradrenaline neurons of the LOCUS COERULEUS) and B5–B7 (the median raphe nucleus, caudal dorsal raphe and rostral dorsal raphe; see RAPHE NUCLEI).

Reference

Dahlström A. & Fuxe K. (1964) Evidence for the existence of monoamine-containing neurons in the central nervous system. I. Demonstration of monoamines in the cell bodies of brain stem neurons. *Acta Physiologica Scandinavica* 62, suppl. 232: 3–55.

claustrophobia (from Latin, *claustrum*: an enclosed place, and Greek, *phobos*: fear) A fear of confined spaces. Like its counterpart, AGORAPHOBIA, it is made manifest by typical symptoms of PANIC or PHOBIA: shortness of breath, cardiac palpitations, trembling, dizziness, nausea and choking, numbness, tingling and chest pain; DEPERSONALIZATION and DEREALIZATION are often present also. DSMIV indicates that the change in behaviour brought about by claustrophobia must be sufficient to cause a restriction of the sufferer's daily life.

claustrum The claustrum is composed of a thin sheet of neurons that sits between the CEREBRAL CORTEX and the CAUDATE–PUTAMEN, from which it is separated by the fibres of the EXTERNAL CAPSULE. At the most posterior end it is continuous with nuclei of the AMYGDALA. It has connections with parts of the FRONTAL CORTEX and may be involved in visual ATTENTION. By the strictest criteria, the claustrum can be considered part of the BASAL GANGLIA, though in practice it never is.

climbing fibres *see* cerebellum – anatomical organization

clinical psychology The branch of professional psychology concerned with assessing and assisting individuals with psychological problems. Clinical psychologists are concerned with people at all stages of development from childhood to old age but the majority treat adults of working age and it is the study of this population that has most influenced the development of the profession.

In adults clinical psychologists most commonly treat anxiety-related conditions such as the many varieties of PHOBIA, PANIC attacks and generalized ANXIETY disorders (see PSYCHOPATHOLOGY). They also treat patients with DEPRESSION. In the United Kingdom the usual treatment method is COGNITIVE THERAPY, BEHAVIOUR THERAPY, and BEHAVIOUR ANALYSIS, although in other countries psychodynamic therapies that relate to PSYCHOANALYSIS or various forms of group therapy are widely used. The essential elements of cognitive therapy are that the therapist and patient seek to determine the underlying thoughts and assumptions which are believed to cause the unwanted behaviour or emotion and then alter these cognitions by dialogue, behavioural experiments and the well-established methods of behaviour therapy such as controlled exposure to the anxiety-provoking situation. Randomized clinical trials have shown cognitive therapy is more effective than alternative psychological and pharmacological therapies in the treatment of anxiety conditions and as effective as medication in the long-term treatment of depression. Clinical psychologists also treat patients with severe mental disorders such as SCHIZOPHRENIA, both in mental hospitals and in the community. For sometime the common method of treatment was behaviour modification in which the REINFORCEMENT for

appropriate and inappropriate behaviour was manipulated. Increasingly versions of cognitive therapy are being used in the treatment of PSYCHOSIS or of particularly problematic behaviours in psychotic individuals, such as HALLUCINATION or DELUSION. It is held by some clinical psychologists that diagnostic categories such as schizophrenia are inappropriate and that progress will be made by concentrating psychological theory and treatment on specific disturbed behaviours. When working with children and adolescents clinical psychologists often use versions of cognitive therapy (say in the treatment of EATING DISORDERS) but the focus is often on the family and more family oriented approaches taken. In the elderly there is more emphasis on the possible organic basis of the patient's behaviour but the use of appropriately targeted cognitive therapy is widespread and helpful. Clinical psychologists also get involved in the assessment and rehabilitation of patients with brain injuries. This overlaps with aspects of NEUROPSYCHOLOGY.

DEREK W. JOHNSTON

clitoris A highly sensitive area of erectile tissue and nerve endings at the upper end of the vulva. It consists of the clitoral glans, which contains sensitive nerve endings, the clitoral shaft, which contains spongy erectile tissue, and the protective skin or clitoral hood which covers them. Sensitive to touch, pressure, and temperature, the clitoris becomes engorged with blood during sexual arousal in women, and it functions specifically to relay pleasurable somatosensory stimulation during masturbation or sexual intercourse. Although it is derived embryologically from the same primordial tissue as the glans penis, it does not serve any reproductive or urinary function.

See also: sexual arousal; sexual differentiation

JAMES G. PFAUS

clomipramine An antidepressant drug (one of the TRICYCLICS) that works by blocking the REUPTAKE of SEROTONIN from the SYNAPTIC CLEFT.

See also: depression

clonazepam A benzodiazepine drug, used in the treatment of SOMNAMBULISM and of ANXI-

ETY. Unlike some other benzodiazepines – alprazolam for example – it is of less value in treating PANIC attacks because it has a slow action: clonazepam has relatively low lipid solubility and so has a long-lasting effect, being slowly absorbed and metabolized. Panic attacks, being rapid, need a swifter treatment.

clone A copy, or the act of producing a copy, of a CELL, organism or GENE. Cells derived from the type of CELL DIVISION called MITOSIS or binary fission are genetically identical to the parent cell, and thus can be considered a clone of the parent cell. Some plants can be readily cloned from a single cell: these cells are said to be pluripotent. Complex organisms including animals, which reproduce by sexual REPRODUCTION are more difficult to clone, and as such only a few incidences of cloned animals exist. This has been performed by removing the NUCLEUS from an egg cell, and implanting a nucleus taken from a single cell of another animal. The resulting offspring are genetically identical to (and thus a clone of) the animal from which the implanted nucleus was taken. While cloned cells are genetically identical, they are not necessarily similar in function. Cells in multicellular organisms are organized into tissues each with a specific function. This is achieved by regulating which genes are active within each cell. Copying part of a cell's DNA is also considered cloning. This is often performed by inserting a piece of DNA containing a gene of interest into a PLASMID, which can replicate rapidly in bacterial cultures, producing large numbers of copies of the gene. Cloning enables genes to be expressed in a novel environment such as CELL CULTURE, so that the function of the protein encoded for may be better understood.

FIONA M. INGLIS

clonic *see* tonic–clonic

clonidine Clonidine is an AGONIST at the alpha 2 (and possibly, more specifically, the alpha 2A) noradrenaline receptor; see ADRENOCEPTORS.

clorgyline *see* monoamine oxidase inhibitor

closed head injury Closed head injury refers to brain damage arising from the forces generated when the head is rapidly accelerated or decelerated as a result of trauma – for example, hitting a car windscreen in a traffic accident or striking the ground with the head in a fall. The ensuing BRAIN INJURY has both focal and diffuse components. Focal injuries often include a LESION (in the form of contusion) of the extremities of the brain, notably the frontal and temporal polar regions, and haematomas (blood clots) arising from the rupture of blood vessels. Diffuse injury arises from the stretching and shearing of axons, known as DIFFUSE AXONAL INJURY. Diffuse axonal injury is widespread through the brain, its severity proportional to the strength of the accelerative force generated during the trauma. Long axons, such as those comprising the CORPUS CALLOSUM are particularly at risk.

The immediate effects of a severe closed head injury invariably include a period of unconsciousness (COMA). In the most severe cases, there is no recovery, and the patient remains in a PERSISTENT VEGETATIVE STATE or dies. More commonly, coma is followed by a period of confusion, characterized by an inability to recall or to place events in their proper order (post-traumatic AMNESIA), which is followed in turn by a return to normal CONSCIOUSNESS. The psychological impairments arising from closed head injury can be profound, even in cases where the injury is only moderately severe, and the ensuing periods of coma and post-traumatic injury relatively brief. Typically, patients will suffer from a range of cognitive impairments, including poor MEMORY and concentration, and slowed DECISION-MAKING. These impairments are often accompanied by personality changes, which frequently resemble those that are seen in patients with focal damage to the FRONTAL LOBE. The impairments reflect the combined effects of the focal and diffuse components of the brain damage arising from the injury, which are difficult to separate. Not infrequently, the impairments are of sufficient severity to prevent a patient from returning to employment or leading a normal life.

MICHAEL D. RUGG

closed loop, open loop The term CLOSED LOOP refers to any process in which the output of a system is fed back and alters further output; the term OPEN LOOP refers to a process where feedback from output is not present. BALLISTIC movements such as SACCADE can be referred to as open loop movements, while closed loop movements are those that use sensory feedback to guide the movement in progress (as is the case with a SERVOMECHANISM). The terms can also be used in a more general manner, relating to complex behaviours. The control of FEEDING and DRINKING for example can be thought of as closed loop processes, in which output measures provide feedback to terminate actions. Motor disorders may affect these differentially: in PARKINSON'S DISEASE for example, closed loop movements remain intact while open loop movements are produced only with difficulty.

clozapine An ATYPICAL ANTIPSYCHOTIC drug that, unusually, effects both positive and negative symptoms of SCHIZOPHRENIA and does not induce TARDIVE DYSKINESIA. There is evidence that it affects dopamine receptors (see D1–D5 DOPAMINE RECEPTORS) in the NUCLEUS ACCUMBENS but not those in the CAUDATE–PUTAMEN (consistent with much evidence implicating the nucleus accumbens in schizophrenia) but clozapine has effects on many NEUROTRANSMITTERS other than dopamine. Its clinical use is limited by a variety of unwanted effects, the worst being its toxic effects on bone marrow.

Reference

Feldman R., Meyer J.S. & Quenzer, L.F. (1997) *Principles of Neuropsychopharmacology*, Sinauer Associates: Sunderland MA.

clumsy child syndrome *see* dyspraxia

cluster headache *see* headache

CNQX 6-cyano-7-nitroquinoxaline-2,3-dione (CNQX); 6,7-dinitroquinoxaline-2,3-dione (DNQX) and 6-nitro-sulfamoyl-benzo(f)-quinoxaline-2,3-dione (NBQX) are all competitive antagonists at non-NMDA receptors (see ANTAGONIST; GLUTAMATE RECEPTORS) with rather greater selectivity for AMPA as opposed to kainate (see KAINIC ACID) receptors.

cocaine An alkaloid found in the leaves of the shrub *Erythroxylon coca*, which grows wild and has been cultivated in South America for thousands of years. This stimulant DRUG is commonly used for its psychoactive effects in modern times, but in fact human societies have used it for thousands of years. The custom of chewing the leaves by the native peoples of the Peruvian Andes dates back at least 5000 years. Cocaine was introduced into mainstream Western society in the last two decades of the nineteenth century, in various tonics, patent medicines, and remedies. In 1886, a Georgia pharmacist introduced what was to become the most famous drink of all time, Coca-Cola, which had extract of coca leaves. Cocaine's most famous proponent was Freud, who wrote extensively of its supposed virtues. He believed it could cure MORPHINE and ALCOHOL addiction. Not surprisingly, Freud struggled with a severe addiction to cocaine.

Cocaine induces profound changes in behaviour and psychological state as well as alterations in bodily physiology. It is administered in a variety of ways, but most commonly it is injected intravenously, snorted intranasally, or smoked in its free-base form (CRACK COCAINE). Cocaine activates the SYMPATHETIC NERVOUS SYSTEM. It is a potent vasoconstrictor and increases heart rate and blood pressure. Cocaine also induces changes in MOOD and emotional state. In general cocaine produces feelings of stimulation, well-being, vigour and EUPHORIA. Enhanced alertness, increased sexuality, heightened energy, and deepening of emotions may accompany the cocaine high. In contrast to some drugs, cocaine does not appear to alter perceptual processes or distort reality. It has been said that cocaine and other stimulants produce a neurochemical magnification of the pleasure experienced in most activities. It is clearly these positive properties that attract people to cocaine and underlie its addictive properties (see ADDICTION). However, cocaine can also induce negative emotional states and severe disruptions of behaviour. High doses of stimulants can cause DYSPHORIA and intense ANXIETY, and chronic use can result in hyper-aggressiveness, complete INSOMNIA, irritability, impulsiveness, and PANIC. Cocaine intoxication in extreme cases is characterized by PARANOIA and violent behaviour.

Cocaine is a potently reinforcing drug (see REINFORCEMENT). In fact, of all the drugs that are amenable to SELF-ADMINISTRATION by animals and humans, it may well be the most reinforcing. The cocaine addict will engage in behaviour that entails extraordinary risks to health and social stability. The extreme desire to obtain the drug has been shown in animal studies of cocaine use. Rats and monkeys rapidly acquire self-administration behaviour when given access to intravenous cocaine via a lever-press, and when forced to choose between food or cocaine, will always choose cocaine, even with lethal consequences. In the PROGRESSIVE RATIO paradigm, an animal must make progressively more responses in order to obtain intravenous cocaine reinforcement. It has been shown that a monkey will make up to 6000 presses to obtain one infusion of cocaine. Thus, many animal studies have demonstrated that the rewarding effects produced by cocaine are indeed a powerful motivator of drug-seeking behaviour. Research suggests that cocaine (like amphetamine) is a powerful activator of the brain's central REINFORCEMENT system. Activation of the DOPAMINE system is the primary pharmacological effect. Moreover, release of dopamine in the NUCLEUS ACCUMBENS appears to be directly linked to the rewarding properties of these drugs. Animals that have undergone lesions of the dopamine projection to the nucleus accumbens are not interested in self-administering cocaine or amphetamine. In view of the hypothesis that the nucleus accumbens may be a critical neural substrate for 'natural' rewards (food, sex, and so on), the notion that cocaine amplifies pleasure may actually have a neurochemical basis.

Cocaine addiction reached peak levels in the 1980s, and continues to be a major problem in many societies. Curiously, before the 1980s, cocaine was considered to be a safe, non-addicting stimulant drug. There appeared to be no overt physical symptoms that would constitute a withdrawal syndrome. The spread of crack cocaine in the 1980s changed this perception. Crack (solid, free-base cocaine) was much cheaper than powdered cocaine and became widely available, particularly to the poor. The smoking of the drug leads to a rapid, short-lasting but profound euphoria that is extremely addictive. It rapidly became clear that the criteria for SUBSTANCE DEPENDENCE DISORDER were easily met with cocaine. Compulsive use, loss of control, and a withdrawal syndrome began to be clearly recognized. Cocaine WITHDRAWAL is characterized by several phases. A triphasic abstinence pattern generally follows a cocaine binge. The first phase is termed the crash, which lasts from hours to days. The crash is characterized by a sharp decrease in mood and energy, agitation, anxiety, depression and craving for cocaine. There is an extreme need for sleep, which is usually met by the ingestion of sedatives, alcohol or opiates. The next phase, withdrawal, can last for many weeks and is characterized primarily by an intense dysphoric syndrome. Depression and ANHEDONIA (inability to experience pleasure) contrast with memories of stimulant-induced euphoria and often lead to a repetition of the bingeing cycle. If the user continues to be abstinent, the third phase emerges, extinction. During this phase, normal mood and energy are restored. However, the user may experience occasional cravings for cocaine for months or even years after the last binge. The cravings are usually invoked by stimuli or memories associated with the cocaine experience. A number of different strategies have been tried in treatment programmes, with varying outcomes. Although pharmacological strategies may be useful in achieving initial cocaine abstinence, counselling and intensive psychotherapy are important for long-term success.

Reference

Gawin F. (1991) Cocaine addiction: psychology and neurophysiology. *Science* 251: 1580–1585.

ANN E. KELLEY

cocaine vaccination A novel treatment for ADDICTION to COCAINE that involves the production of ANTIBODY to this drug. When administered to individuals, the antibody binds to cocaine circulating in the BLOOD, rendering it functionally useless. It inhibits SELF ADMINISTRATION of cocaine by experimental animals and might prove to be of value in the treatment of human drug addiction.

Reference

Fox B.S. (1997) Development of a therapeutic vaccine for the treatment of cocaine addition. *Drug and Alcohol Dependence* 48: 153–158.

coccygeal *see* coccyx

coccyx (from Greek, *kokkyx*: cuckoo) The coccyx has a shape that suggested a cuckoo's bill: a triangular bone (actually four smaller bones fused together) at the base of the spine; the term coccygeal describes something belonging to the coccyx; see SPINAL CORD.

cochlea (from Greek, *kokhlos*: land snail) A bony, fluid-filled structure of the inner ear, shaped like a snail. It is divided lengthways into the SCALA VESTIBULI (vestibular stairway), SCALA MEDIA (middle stairway) and SCALA TYMPANI (tympanic stairway). The purpose of the cochlea is to transduce air pressure impacting on the TYMPANIC MEMBRANE into neural signals. Incoming airwaves make the tympanic membrane vibrate. This vibration is transmitted via the OSSICLES onto the OVAL WINDOW, a gap in the cochlea covered by a membrane. Pressure here creates movement in the fluid of the cochlea. (Movement is possible because of the existence of a second membrane, the ROUND WINDOW: were this not present, pressure of the ossicles on the oval window would simply increase pressure within the cochlea rather than fluid movement.) Translation of pressure changes into nerve impulses takes place in the ORGAN OF CORTI, which includes the BASILAR MEMBRANE, HAIR CELLS and TECTORIAL MEMBRANE.

See also: auditory perception; hearing theories; tip link; tonotopic representation

cochlear nerve Also known as the AUDITORY NERVE; with the VESTIBULAR NERVE one of the principal branches of the VESTIBULOCOCHLEAR NERVE (the eighth cranial nerve).

cochlear nerve ganglion *see* auditory pathways

cochlear nucleus The cochlear nucleus is in the PONS, positioned on the outer edge of the CEREBRAL PEDUNCLE. It receives input from the AUDITORY NERVE and is the first point in the central processing of auditory information. It can be divided into different sections. As auditory nerve fibres enter the nucleus they divide to innervate differentially the component sub-nuclei of the cochlear nucleus. This organization allows for TONOTOPIC REPRESENTATION, a feature that is a fundamental property of the nucleus. Projections from the cochlear nucleus travel via three principal pathways: the TRAPEZOID BODY, DORSAL ACOUSTIC STRIA and the INTERMEDIATE ACOUSTIC STRIA; the next step in the auditory processing occurs in the SUPERIOR OLIVARY COMPLEX.

See also: auditory system; hindbrain

codeine An opiate drug with moderate analgesic effects; see HEROIN and MORPHINE.

codon A sequence of three nucleotides of DNA (deoxyribonucleic acid) within a gene, which codes for a specific amino acid in a protein chain. Since there are 64 possible combinations of nucleotides, and only 20 amino acids commonly found in proteins, most amino acids are encoded for by more than one codon. In addition, three codons, named STOP CODONS, are used to signal the end of the protein sequence within a region of DNA.

FIONA M. INGLIS

coenzyme *see* cofactor

coexistence *see* colocalization

cofactor A cofactor is either a COENZYME or an ION required by an ENZYME in order to work properly. Coenzymes are molecules (often produced by vitamins) that bind with apoenzymes (which are always made of protein) to produce a compound that will work as an enzyme. ACETYL COENZYME A (acetyl CoA) is an example of a coenzyme; biotin (also known as vitamin H or coenzyme R) is another.

cognitive enhancers Cognitive enhancers are therapeutic agents aimed at producing improvements in cognitive function and ameliorating or arresting cognitive decline. Their putative action is through higher telencephalic functions of the brain involved in cognitive processes such as LEARNING, MEMORY and

ATTENTION. There have been a large number of candidate cognitive enhancers which include CHOLINERGIC function enhancers, NEUROPEPTIDES, NOOTROPICS, PYROLIDONES, ergot alkaloids, MONOAMINERGIC agents, amino acid regulators, GABAERGIC agents, METHYLXANTHINES and VITAMINS. Examples include the use of METHYLPHENIDATE in the treatment of ATTENTION-DEFICIT DISORDER and cholinergic agents such as TACRINE and NICOTINE which have been reported to ameliorate attention dysfunction in ALZHEIMER'S DEMENTIA.

BARBARA J. SAHAKIAN

cognitive inhibition Cognitive inhibition refers to the active inhibition or suppression of a RESPONSE rather than an inhibitory effect due to the activation of competing or alternative responses. Cognitive inhibition is thought to be the mechanism underlying RETRIEVAL-INDUCED FORGETTING effects. These refer to the ironic phenomenon by which remembering some aspects of an event or items about an individual can cause forgetting of related material. It has been shown to exist for both SEMANTIC and EPISODIC MEMORY, and for visuo-spatial and verbal material. Inhibitory effects arise from a need to overcome INTERFERENCE from competing memories. As RETRIEVAL cues are often insufficiently specified, other related information may compete for retrieval and it is this competition which is thought to trigger inhibitory processes that actively suppress competing items.

See also: response competition; supervisory attentional system

MALCOLM D. MacLEOD

cognitive map A cognitive map is an internal REPRESENTATION of an animal's environment that allows for the reorganization of acquired information so that the organism may be aware of properties of the environment that are beyond its field of perception. An advantage of such a representation is that it allows animals to react to stimuli that are not immediately present to the organism, thereby allowing for greater flexibility and efficiency of behaviour (Poucet, 1993). Two fundamental types of cognitive maps correspond to mental

representations of spatial and temporal information.

See also: hippocampus; spatial mapping

Reference

Poucet B. (1993) Spatial cognitive maps in animals: new hypotheses on their structure and neural mechanisms. *Psychological Review* 100: 163–182.

STANLEY B. FLORESCO

cognitive neuroscience That part of neuroscience that seeks to understand the relationships between brain systems and cognitive processes – LANGUAGE and MEMORY for example.

cognitive overlearning A method of training in which individuals are trained to eliminate a defined, unwanted, behaviour by continuous repetition of an 'I must not ...' statement following production of the unwanted action. Alderman & Ward used this procedure to eliminate perseverative speech patterns in a patient with DYSEXECUTIVE SYNDROME. Following a repetition in speech, the patient spent 1 minute repeating (somewhat paradoxically) 'I must not repeat myself'. This procedure was found to have lasting benefit.

See also: errorless learning; response cost method

Reference

Alderman N. & Ward A. (1991) Behavioural treatment of the dysexecutive syndrome: reduction of repetitive speech using response cost and cognitive overlearning. *Neuropsychological Rehabilitation* 1: 65–80.

cognitive psychology (from Latin, *cognoscere*: to know) Cognition is the act or process of knowing. Cognitive psychology is a programme of study that emerged in the 1950s, pioneered by psychologists such as George Miller and Donald Broadbent (1926–1993). The emergence of cognitive psychology was stimulated by three things. The first was a reaction against BEHAVIOURISM, which was seen as unnecessarily restrictive: its strict emphasis on the analysis of behaviour did not permit investigation of such things as MENTAL REPRESENTATIONS, LANGUAGE or the processes of information handling. The second was the introduction of practical computers, which could be used both to manipulate large amounts of information and provide models of information storage, manipulation and use. The third was the rapid advance of INFORMATION THEORY, which provided mathematical models of information coding and decoding. Cognitive psychology is a term used now to refer to areas of study that include processes of knowing, including sensation and perception (see SENSATION VS. PERCEPTION), ATTENTION and the mechanisms of information handling (including LANGUAGE and MEMORY for example). Cognitive psychology is often contrasted with PHYSIOLOGICAL PSYCHOLOGY but in fact the two are closely related: it is cognitive psychology that supplies the theoretical constructs with which physiological psychologists attempt to understand brain functions. The emergent discipline of COGNITIVE NEUROSCIENCE is the outcome of this happy union.

cognitive restraint The self-imposition of restraint on food intake; more commonly known as RESTRAINED EATING, the term 'cognitive' gives added impact to the fact that the restraint is knowingly and voluntarily applied: it is not a routine physiological process.

cognitive therapy A short-term, focused form of PSYCHOTHERAPY in which the major emphasis is on the examination and modification of the patient's thoughts and beliefs. Initially developed by Aaron Beck as a treatment for DEPRESSION, cognitive therapy is based on the notion that depressed patients make errors in the way that they interpret their current experiences and in the predictions they make about future events.

Cognitive therapy was developed in the 1960s from Beck's clinical work with severely depressed patients. It is defined in terms of the underlying cognitive model rather than in terms of any specific therapeutic techniques that might be used. According to the cognitive model, psychological disorders are characterized by specific patterns of maladaptive thinking. These, in turn, reflect dysfunctional beliefs or schemas (see SCHEMA). Schemas are the basic unspoken rules that we use to live our lives. When core beliefs are maladaptive (for instance, 'If I am not loved I can never be

happy') psychological difficulties often occur. Other treatment approaches such as Rational Emotive Therapy (RET) developed by Ellis, are also based on a cognitive perspective. However, the therapeutic approaches of RET differ from those used in cognitive therapy.

The negative views of the self, the personal world and the future that characterize the depressed person are referred to as the cognitive triad. This is a generalized tendency to interpret the world in a manner that highlights personal shortcomings, limitations of the current environment, and the bleak nature of the future. Specific errors in thinking that might reflect this include selective abstraction, overgeneralization, and all-or-none thinking. Selective abstraction (or selective negative focus) occurs when negative events or implications become the focus of attention at the expense of positive information, which may be ignored or disqualified. For example, a shy young man who finally asks a young female co-worker for coffee feels like a failure when she says no. Overgeneralization is present when the person makes a conclusion based on one small piece of information ('Jane disagreed with me in the meeting. That means she doesn't like me.'), while all-or-none thinking involves creating polarized and extreme consequences from complex and continuous information (such as 'I didn't do well on that test. I'm going to fail this class.').

A typical course of cognitive therapy might involve 10–20 weekly sessions. Treatment sessions are structured and the patient and the therapist work together in a spirit of collaborative empiricism. The therapist plays an active role in the treatment and emphasis is placed on the development of a working alliance. Unlike many other forms of therapy, the patient also provides feedback to the therapist. In cognitive therapy, a major focus is the identification of the patient's automatic thoughts. These are the thoughts that pass through the patient's mind (often without full awareness) and that are believed to be the triggers for dysphoric moods or emotional change. The patient's negative interpretations of events ('I didn't do well in that job interview. I'm never going to get a job. I'm just a loser.') are treated as hypotheses rather than as accurate statements about reality. There is thus a strong empirical tone to the therapy session. Working together, patient and therapist subject the patient's automatic thoughts to a thorough test and evaluate the validity of these thoughts based on positive (evidence for) or negative evidence. This is accomplished through guided discovery whereby the therapist questions the patient in a Socratic manner. The goal is to generate logically based rather than distorted inferences based on the information available and to identify and modify maladaptive schemas. Following the therapy session, the patient is generally given a homework assignment to complete before the next meeting. These assignments are designed to broaden the impact of the therapy. For example, the patient might be asked to work on recognizing automatic thoughts when they occur and to explore the links between these thoughts and mood shifts.

Cognitive therapy has been intensely studied as a treatment for depression and is now an accepted and efficacious form of intervention for this disorder. It has been shown to be as helpful as tricyclic ANTIDEPRESSANTS in several studies. Cognitive therapy can also be used in conjunction with pharmacological treatment. Because of its success as a treatment for depression, cognitive therapy is now being used as a treatment for a variety of other psychiatric and psychological problems. These include ANXIETY disorders, EATING DISORDERS and SUBSTANCE ABUSE, and even SCHIZOPHRENIA. Although specialized techniques are used to treat these different conditions, the conceptualization of the patient's problems within a cognitive framework remains the same.

References
Beck A.T., Rush A.J., Shaw B.F. & Emery G. (1979) *Cognitive Therapy of Depression*, Guilford Press: New York.
Beck J. (1996) *Cognitive Therapy: Basics and Beyond*, Guilford Press: New York.

JILL M. HOOLEY

cognitive–behavioural therapy A structured, flexible, and time-limited form of PSYCHOTHERAPY that is used to treat a broad range of clinical problems. As its name suggests, cognitive–behavioural therapy (CBT) seeks to explore the role of maladaptive cogni-

tions and behaviours in psychological problems and employs a wide variety of techniques to modify these within the context of a short-term (10–20 weeks) treatment.

The historical roots of CBT are in BEHAVIOUR THERAPY and simple models of CONDITIONING. Over time, however, the limitations of these approaches for complex human problems became more and more apparent. The important role of cognitions and emotions began to be recognized and the scope of behaviour therapy was expanded to incorporate more aspects of human experience. Because of this, there is no single or prototypical form of CBT. This flexibility and wide applicability may explain the appeal of CBT to large numbers of therapists and patients. The range of clinical problems that can be treated with CBT includes ANXIETY disorders, DEPRESSION, anger, chronic PAIN, marital problems, and personality disorders. CBT can also be used with children. Although the forms of CBT that are used across disorders vary considerably, some techniques are used quite widely. For example, in self-monitoring the patient is taught to observe and record specific behaviours and to identify the circumstances or contexts that result in increases or decreases in problem behaviours. Graded task assignments, where large goals are broken down into smaller, more manageable sub-tasks are also frequently used. Other forms of intervention in CBT might include diversion, whereby the patient uses physical activity, visualization, or social contact to cope with a specific problem such as anger, anxiety, or depression. These interventions are often combined with more formal cognitive strategies such as cognitive restructuring (see COGNITIVE THERAPY). When we consider that cognitive therapy also includes homework assignments that are often behavioural in nature (a depressed patient might be asked to contact a friend to arrange a pleasurable activity for instance) it becomes apparent that in clinical practice, there are no firm boundaries between cognitive therapy and CBT.

Perhaps the common element in CBT is the emphasis placed on empirical validation. Indeed, the formal measurement of behavioural outcomes is often an integral part of the treatment. Its sound empirical basis and short-term nature may explain why CBT is one of the most accepted and influential treatment approaches in modern psychotherapy.

See also: clinical psychology

JILL M. HOOLEY

cogwheel rigidity *see* rigidity

collagen Produced by fibroblasts, collagen is a protein present in certain types of CONNECTIVE TISSUE. Connective tissue rich in collagen (collagenous fibres) does not stretch far and does not tear easily. There is reckoned to be more collagen present in an animal than any other protein.

collateral sprouting A mechanism used by brains to help overcome damage. If one input to a structure is damaged and lost, other inputs (even in the adult brain) may generate additional axonal terminals – that is they may engage in collateral sprouting.

collaterals Branches in an AXON are called collaterals; neurons that have very branched axons can said to be very collateralized. Collateral help single axons cover a wider area of tissue within a single structure (if they wish to); and allow the axonal process derived from one CELL BODY to transmit to two different structures. The neurons of the ASCENDING RETICULAR ACTIVATING SYSTEM are, for example, very heavily collateralized.

collision test An electrophysiological technique (see ELECTROPHYSIOLOGY), rarely used though very valuable: it is designed to establish whether two structures are connected by a monosynaptic pathway. If one orthodromically stimulates (see ORTHODROMIC ACTIVATION) a neuron one can record (see SINGLE-UNIT ELEC-TROPHYSIOLOGICAL RECORDING) activity that is induced by that orthodromic activation in another structure. However, such recording merely indicates that stimulation of the first structure affects the activity of a second one – it does not establish that the connection is monosynaptic. The collision test is a means for establishing the existence of a monosynaptic pathway: one stimulates orthodromically in one structure and antidromically in another simultaneously. If the structures are monosy-

naptically connected, what one will be doing is to stimulate the same neuron from both ends at the same time, inducing both an antidromic and an orthodromic flow of action potentials. These will cancel each other out. The failure to record the arrival of orthodromically activated action potentials – because they have collided with antidromically activated ones – demonstrates the existence of a monosynaptic connection.

colloidal gold *see* tract tracers

colocalization The existence of two or more NEUROTRANSMITTERS or neuromodulators within the same neuron. When chemical neurotransmission was first identified it was thought that each neuron had only one transmitter. Many people assumed that this was what was meant by DALE'S PRINCIPLE, but that in fact means something rather different. However, it is now clear that many neurons contain more than one neurotransmitter and indeed there are neurons with several: such co-existence implies very sophisticated signalling capabilities. It is even likely that neurons possess the genetic capability to synthesize more neurotransmitters than they express. Interestingly, deafferentation of a neuron can have remarkable effects on neurotransmitter expression: loss of input can cause neurons to reduce expression of some of their neurotransmitters and increase others.

Reference

Persson J.K.E., Lindh B., Elde R., Robertson B., Rivero-Melian C., Eriksonn N.P. & Hokfelt T. (1995) The expression of different cytochemical markers in normal and axotomized dorsal root ganglion cells projection to the nucleus gracilis in the adult rat. *Experimental Brain Research* 105: 331–344.

colostrum *see* lactation

colour agnosia *see* agnosia

colour anomia An ANOMIA for the use of colour names; a selective impairment of colour naming. A rare disorder produced by a cortical LESION in the region of the CALCARINE FISSURE and/or LINGUAL GYRUS of the left TEMPORAL LOBE. The nature and range of deficits is variable. For example, subjects while being unable to name a perceived colour, may still be able to point to a named colour, or may still be able to name the colour of an object from a spoken question (see Davidoff, 1991).

See also: anomic aphasia

Reference

Davidoff J. (1991) *Cognition through Color*, MIT Press: Cambridge MA.

KATHY T. MULLEN

colour blindness A term used to refer to either a total or a partial loss of COLOUR VISION which may be either inherited or acquired. The most common inherited colour vision deficiencies are present from birth and produce a partial loss of colour vision in about 8% of men and under 1% of women. These are forms of DICHROMATIC COLOUR BLINDNESS (PROTANOPIA, DEUTERANOPIA, TRITANOPIA) which arise when one of the three light-absorbing pigments in the cones of the retina is missing, and the milder versions (PROTANOMALY, DEUTERANOMALY, TRITANOMALY) which occur when all three pigments are present but one is anomalous. Much more rarely, colour vision may be absent altogether as a result of an inherited disorder, as in ROD MONOCHROMACY in which all three cone pigments are functionally absent. Acquired colour vision disorders, which onset during the subject's lifetime, have a wide range of causes. They usually produce a relatively mild loss of colour vision, for example due to disease processes or pharmacological agents affecting the retina or optic pathways. These acquired colour vision disorders may affect both red-green and blue-yellow colour OPPONENT PROCESSES, although it is believed that blue-yellow colour vision is more vulnerable when the damage is to the receptoral layers of the retina (KOLLNER'S RULE). A complete loss of colour vision (ACHROMATOPSIA) is very rare and is likely to arise from damage to areas of the temporal lobe of the brain that are specialized for the encoding of colour.

See also: trichromatic theory of colour vision

KATHY T. MULLEN

colour constancy The tendency for the perception of the colour of a surface or object to remain constant despite changes in the spectral content (colour) of the ambient illumination. A property of human and non-human primate COLOUR VISION. The spectral content of the illumination may change greatly, for example, from indoor to outdoor environments. Neural computations, most likely made in the VISUAL CORTEX of the brain, enable these changes to be discounted and the spectral reflectance of the surface or object to be perceived unambiguously. Under extreme conditions colour constancy can fail, and the perceived colour of an object may vary as the spectral conditions of the ambient illumination change.

See also: object constancy; opponent process theory of colour vision; trichromatic theory of colour vision

KATHY T. MULLEN

colour opponent receptive field *see* colour vision; lateral inhibition; receptive field; retina

colour vision A visual sense which informs the organism about the relative spectral composition of light reflected from surfaces and objects in the environment. Among the mammals, the most complex (or trichromatic) colour vision is enjoyed by the Old World primates, although birds, fishes and insects may also possess a highly developed colour sense. For human colour vision, eleven basic colours have been identified from colour-naming experiments, comprising four unique colours (red, green, blue and yellow) (see OPPONENT PROCESS THEORY OF COLOUR VISION), four additional colours (pink, brown, orange and purple), and three 'achromatic' colours (white, grey and black).

See also: colour blindness; colour constancy; cones; dichromatic colour blindness; retina; trichromatic theory of colour vision

KATHY T. MULLEN

coloured noise *see* noise

coma A state of deep and persistent unconsciousness; it is explicitly not a form of deep SLEEP but something pathological. Sleep, especially REM SLEEP, involves significant and widespread neural activity; coma does not. Coma is also discriminated from STUPOR, a state of extreme unconsciousness, but one from which it is possible to rouse individuals by sensory stimulation: patients in coma are not responsive to sensory stimulation. Even REFLEX activation is lost in coma, which is a significant discriminator between this and PERSISTENT VEGETATIVE STATE. Coma is caused by damage or dysfunction in the CENTRAL NERVOUS SYSTEM. These can be divided into three broad groups: the first two are defined by their relationship to the TENTORIUM, a landmark close by the CEREBELLUM: (1) *subtentorial lesions* – that is, any LESION in the BRAINSTEM, typically in the PONS, (2) *supratentorial lesions* – typically damage to the vascular system in and around the MENINGES, (3) disorders of METABOLISM, such as HYPOGLYCAEMIA, which have widespread effects on brain. Coma is rated using any of a variety of neuropsychological instruments: the best-known is the GLASGOW COMA SCALE. For a discussion of the medical and legal issues raised by states such as coma, see PERSISTENT VEGETATIVE STATE.

See also: brain death; consciousness; fainting

Reference

Kandel E.R., Schwartz J.H. & Jessell T.M. (2000) *Principles of Neural Science*, 4th edn, McGraw-Hill: New York.

commensal *see* symbiosis

commissure (from Latin, *commissura*: joining) The term commissure is given to any large bundle of FIBRES that crosses from one cerebral HEMISPHERE to the other, thereby joining them. The largest and best known of the commissures is the CORPUS CALLOSUM. Commissural describes a commissure; and commissurotomy is the act of cutting a commissure (see SPLIT BRAIN).

comorbidity Morbidity relates to disease or illness; comorbidity describes a situation in which an individual meets the criteria for more than one illness. Because the diagnostic criteria (see DSM-IV; ICD 10) for many psychological and psychiatric disorders are relatively flexible, comorbidity occurs more frequently than one might expect with physical disorders. For example, patients with an anxiety disorder may meet the diagnostic criteria for more than one type of anxiety.

comparative anatomy The systematic study of brain structure and organisation in different species, to gain insight into function. A basic and consistent format for the brain has emerged from studies of species as different as reptiles, birds, rodents and PRIMATES. However, the size of different regions in relation to others, and the connectivity between these regions, has informed thinking about the role of different brain areas in specific behaviours.

The BRAINSTEM is recognizable even in the simplest vertebrates, with centres for many simple but important roles within the CENTRAL NERVOUS SYSTEM. The RETICULAR FORMATION is a relatively primitive system of interlacing cells and fibres associated with the motor columns in the brainstem and anterior SPINAL CORD, but becoming more developed in the anterior brainstem and MIDBRAIN. It is important for motor coordination in lower vertebrates in which the motor tracts giving the brain control over activities of the trunk are poorly developed. The reticular formation has developed further in mammals, to promote activation in the higher centres of the THALAMUS and CEREBRAL CORTEX. The degree of development of the CEREBELLUM varies considerably and is roughly correlated with the intricacy of body movements: it is large and elaborately constructed in fish, birds and mammals, but small in reptiles and very poorly developed in amphibia. The brain region which has undergone the greatest evolutionary change is the cerebral cortex. This has been key to the development of 'higher' level behaviours such as complex cognition, including – in the case of man – speech. In lower vertebrates the cortex was the locus of olfactory processing (see OLFACTION), while in tetrapods it became the important centre for correlating sensory signals in general, and in mammals it has become the major centre for associations. Comparative anatomy has highlighted the spectacular evolution of one particular cortical area – the PREFRONTAL CORTEX – in mammals. The prefrontal cortex has increased in size by an average of 3% in cats, 17% in chimps and 29% in humans. In order to accommodate these developments, the cortex is often convoluted to increase its surface area within the confines of the skull. Flattened out, the cortex of the human brain would be more than four times larger in surface area than the cortex of a chimpanzee; the chimp cortex is in turn more than 50 times greater in area than the cortex of a rodent.

Many scientists continue to show an interest in comparative anatomy in order to highlight relationships between the size of a particular structure and its function. So for instance, it has been asked whether animals (such as FOOD-STORING BIRDS) which engage in complex spatial activities have a larger HIPPOCAMPUS (which has been thought to be especially involved in SPATIAL MEMORY) than animals which do not. Such questions highlight the continuing influence of PHRENOLOGY.

WENDY L. INGLIS

comparative psychology The systematic study of behavioural differences across many species. Comparative psychology is the branch of biological science which investigates the development of behavioural differences between animals, the neural mechanisms behind such variations, the function of a particular behaviour, and the evolutionary paths (see EVOLUTION) which have resulted in behavioural variations. Those aspects of comparative psychology which investigate brain mechanisms of behavioural functions have recently developed into the new scientific discipline of BEHAVIOURAL NEUROSCIENCE.

The evolutionary perspective of Charles Darwin (1809–1882) is fundamental to comparative psychology. As part of his Theory of Evolution, Darwin insisted that the rudiments of reasoning should be detectable in most species: 'The difference in mind between man and the higher animals, great as it is, certainly is one of degree and not of kind.' (Darwin 1871, *The Descent of Man*). From Darwin's writings came the idea that humans are one species among many, and therefore that their behaviour may be studied on the same terms and by the same general methods as those of any other animal species. Much early psychology was introspectionist: the measurement of what subjects said they thought about certain events. The move towards a more objective 'behaviourist' approach – which was to become comparative psychology – was led by

John Watson (1878–1958) when he was elected President of the American Psychological Association in 1913. Watson argued that psychology should become the science of behaviour, since scoring and recording actual behaviour was accurate and replicable in ways in which introspective observations were not. The work of two other individuals – Ivan Pavlov (1849–1936) and Sigmund Freud (1856–1939) – also did much to nurture behaviourism. Pavlov argued that physiological methods were required to understand the brain. His studies on conditioning established that animals could be trained to respond in different ways to contrasting external events, demonstrating in an objective way, their ability to make sensory discriminations (see PAVLOVIAN CONDITIONING). Freud's development of the concept of the 'unconscious mind' also played an important role. He was the first to suggest there was an unconscious psychological component to MOTIVATION and cognition, supporting the view that there were likely to be many mental processes which were inaccessible to introspection.

WENDY L. INGLIS

compensatory eye movements A form of SMOOTH EYE MOVEMENT: when the head moves, the eyes can retain FIXATION on a particular point in space by virtue of compensatory eye movements.

competitive antagonists *see* antagonist

competitive binding assay An *in vitro* technique for determining the concentrations of specific molecules in tissue samples. It involves the same procedure as IMMUNOASSAY but rather than determining ANTIBODY–ANTIGEN relationships, it is based on the interaction between PROTEINS – for example, between RECEPTORS and their LIGANDS.

competitive–noncompetitive binding Competitive binding to RECEPTORS involves an AGONIST and an ANTAGONIST competing for access to binding sites. COMPETITIVE ANTAGONISTS for example can be displaced from receptors by increasing the concentration of agonist to compete with them. In noncompetitive binding, this is not the case: no amount of agonist can displace a noncompetitive antagonist.

complement Complement – or more properly, the complement system – is a system of proteins found in blood and involved in the response made by the IMMUNE SYSTEM. Complement proteins are activated directly by ANTIGENS or by the actions of ANTIBODIES on antigens. Complement proteins assist in inflammation; promote phagocytosis; and are themselves involved in the LYSIS of cells.

complementary DNA (cDNA) Deoxyribonycleic acid (DNA) which is made using a template of MESSENGER RNA (mRNA), to produce a complementary piece of DNA. This process is achieved using a viral enzyme called reverse transcriptase and provides a stable copy of the gene which can be used for gene analysis, and determination of the function of the gene in other living systems. cDNA differs from genomic DNA because it contains only exons and no introns, which are removed during mRNA formation (see EXON; INTRON).

See also: clone

FIONA M. INGLIS

complex rearing *see* environmental enrichment

compliance The term compliance used in a clinical setting refers to the willingness (or otherwise) of individuals to maintain a DRUG regime. In order to be properly effective, drugs need in general to be administered systematically to ensure a constant level in the body. Failure to maintain appropriate medication, for whatever reason (for example, wilful avoidance, forgetting or a false belief in recovery from symptoms) can create difficulties. Management of drug regimes to ensure compliance is required in many cases.

compound (i) *Chemistry*: A substance made of two or more elements (see PERIODIC TABLE OF THE ELEMENTS) joined together; a substance produced by the union of two or more separate components. For example, sodium and chloride are elements; sodium chloride – common salt – is a compound.

(ii) *Linguistics*: A unit formed of other separate instances of the same unit; for instance, a word formed from two other words, such as 'mailbox'.

(I) PHILIP WINN; (II) ANNE CUTLER

compound action potential *see* action potential

compulsion Compulsions are repeated actions or thoughts, the activation of which is typically repetitious and not sensibly connected with their apparent purpose. Compulsive handwashing for example is not of any particular value in maintaining cleanliness or avoiding contamination: there is a mismatch between the incidence of the act and its apparent purpose. Compulsions are associated with a variety of disorders, including OBSESSIVE COMPULSIVE DISORDER and AUTISM. Many compulsions appear as *yielding compulsions* when individuals are compelled to engage in some pointless act. There are also *controlling compulsions*, in which the compulsive repetition of some procedure is believed by the individual to prevent some unwanted event or thought occurring. Compulsions can be *cognitive compulsions*, in which repetitious and compulsive thoughts rather than actions are used (usually inappropriately) to achieve a desired outcome.

See also: perseveration; stereotypy

computational neuroscience A form of NEUROSCIENCE that endeavours to understand the nature of CENTRAL NERVOUS SYSTEM computations by analysis of the interactions between individual neurons. It shares many of the interests of COGNITIVE NEUROSCIENCE (in things such as MEMORY for example) but has a focus on the interactions of single neurons or NEURAL ASSEMBLIES rather than on the larger systems that cognitive neuroscience typically has. The generation of testable models concerning neural computations is a central goal.

See also: behavioural neuroscience; neural networks: neuron

computational vision Computational vision refers to an approach to understanding how a VISUAL SYSTEM works. The basic principle behind this approach is that the visual system has the task of computing representations of the scene from optical information. To understand how the visual system achieves this will entail understanding the nature of the scene representations that are required, understanding what the nature of the available optical information is, and how the former can be computed from the latter. Computational vision frequently (although not always) involves a computer simulation or model of the processes.

In 1982, David Marr (1945–1980) in a work published posthumously following his death from leukaemia, distinguished between three levels of analysis in the computational approach: computational theory, algorithm and implementation. The computational theory is concerned with the questions of what is to be computed and from what information. The algorithm is concerned with how those computations are to be carried out. The implementation is concerned with the manner in which the algorithm is expressed in terms of the actual hardware that is used. Thus a computational account of the PRIMAL SKETCH can be framed in these three levels. At the level of the computational theory, it is proposed that the visual system computes the positions on the RETINA of the occluding edges of objects and that this is done by identifying points in the image where luminance changes very rapidly. An algorithm can be proposed that involves calculating the luminance derivative in all directions at each point in the image and then finding places where the resulting function reaches a local maximum. This would be implemented by neurons with a certain type of LATERAL INHIBITION. The key element in the success of this approach is that it forces research to be framed in very specific ways – generally specific enough to allow a computer simulation to be constructed. This means that specific predictions of different models of visual processes can be generated and tested. This approach has proved to be very successful, although it is sometimes seen to be rather divorced from the reality of visual neuroscience. This often arises where the requirements of a computational theory involve a degree of mathematical sophistication that seems to be well beyond the basic precision of neuronal engineering. Unlike many approaches,

it requires that the purposes of vision or any small module of vision be explicitly identified. This will generally involve a relationship between the organism and the environment and is an important step towards understanding the ecological and adaptive aspects of biological vision.

Reference

Marr D. (1982) *Vision*, W.H. Freeman: San Francisco.

ROGER J. WATT

computerized axial tomography (CT, CAT) Computerized axial tomography is a brain imaging technique introduced in the early 1970s. It provides 3-dimensional images of the brain by using a mathematical procedure (tomography) to process information from X-rays of the head taken from many different viewpoints. The introduction of CAT revolutionized clinical practice in neurology and neurosurgery by providing, for the first time, the means accurately to detect and localize brain abnormalities non-invasively.

See also: functional neuroimaging

MICHAEL D. RUGG

concentration gradient Molecules will always move from areas of high concentration to lower concentrations: the difference between the two levels is called a concentration gradient. In practice, concentration gradients typically exist across a membrane, and more particularly, a SEMIPERMEABLE MEMBRANE (see OSMOSIS).

See also: sodium-potassium pump

concentration response curve As the DOSE RESPONSE CURVE and DOSE EFFECT CURVE, but plotting the concentration rather than the dose – concentration being the amount of something present in a solution (represented for example as mg/ml; see SI UNITS), dose being a simple representation of the quantity of a drug or chemical (represented for example in terms of mg).

conceptual nervous system The conceptual nervous system (CNS) was a term used by Donald Hebb (1904–1985) in a classic paper in 1955 to describe the general conceptual framework in which neuroscientific research is carried out. He was making a point similar to that made by Thomas Kuhn in describing the role of the PARADIGM: all scientific research is carried out within a conceptual framework that shapes what is done, how it is done and how data are interpreted.

Reference

Hebb D.O. (1955) Drives and the CNS (conceptual nervous system). *Psychological Review* 62: 243–254.

concordance Concordance is a term used in studies of the genetic basis of traits or conditions. It refers to the percentage of a proband's family who have the same condition as the PROBAND.

Reference

Plomin R., DeFries J.C., McClearn G.E. & Rutter M. (1997) *Behavioral Genetics*, 3rd edn, W.H. Freeman: New York.

concurrent discrimination *see* discrimination

concurrent schedule *see* schedules of reinforcement

concussion (from Latin, *concussus*, derived from *con*: together, *quatere*: to shake) Concussion is a term indicating disturbance or shaking. It has various meanings depending on the context in which it is used, but in neurological terms it refers to a disturbance in brain function, typically following a vigorous blow to the head, which may or may not be associated with a period of unconsciousness. It is associated with two conditions: (1) POST-TRAUMATIC AMNESIA, a loss of memory following trauma, the degree of impairment providing a rough-and-ready index of the degree of brain injury, and (2) POST-CONCUSSION SYNDROME. This is a condition typically associated with the later effects of CLOSED HEAD INJURY and can involve a variety of disturbances. Early signs include such generalized effects as headache, nausea, somnolence and disturbances in the visual system (such as blurred vision). Later signs include continued headache, anxiety, depression, insomnia, fatigue, memory impairments and disorders in vision and auditory perception. These can persist for several weeks or, in some cases, over a year. There is a belief

that while the early symptoms might be related to disturbances in physical processes the later disturbances might be more psychological in origin (as is the case with post-traumatic stress disorder). Repeated concussions can produce more lasting impairments, based on cumulative physical damage to the brain – the so-called PUNCH DRUNK SYNDROME.

See also: amnesia; coma

conditional discrimination The subject is required to discriminate between two or more stimuli or states and, on the basis of the discrimination, select a response. Strictly speaking, it is not the discrimination which is conditional; rather, the response is conditional upon the nature of the discriminated stimulus.

See also: conditioned visual-discrimination task

VERITY J. BROWN

conditional stimulus A stimulus that conditions (or trains) an animal: in a SKINNER BOX there may be lights which can be used as the CONDITIONAL STIMULUS (or DISCRIMINATIVE STIMULI).

See also: classical conditioning; conditioning

conditioned approach Approach towards the location where appetitive unconditioned REWARD is received during the presentation of a CONDITIONED STIMULUS that predicts the delivery of this UNCONDITIONED STIMULUS.

See also: appetitive conditioning

A. SIMON KILLCROSS

conditioned avoidance An response trained by INSTRUMENTAL CONDITIONING that allows PUNISHMENT to be avoided; it is a contrast to CONDITIONED ESCAPE.

conditioned cue preference This is synonymous with CUE CONDITIONING; see PLACE CONDITIONING for discussion of this in relation to CONDITIONED PLACE PREFERENCE.

conditioned emotional response An emotional RESPONSE (such as fear) produced to a previously neutral STIMULUS by CLASSICAL CONDITIONING.

See also: conditioned fear; conditioned suppression; emotion

conditioned escape An response trained by INSTRUMENTAL CONDITIONING that allows ESCAPE from PUNISHMENT; it is a contrast to CONDITIONED AVOIDANCE.

conditioned fear Most fears are not innate but instead are learned through experience. Monkeys in the wild are terrified by snakes whereas monkeys bred in captivity are indifferent to snakes. However, once laboratory raised monkeys see the FEAR reaction of a wild monkey to a snake, they rapidly learn the same fear reaction and display it to the snake thereafter. Hence, primates and many other lower animals readily acquire conditioned fear reactions via associations between formerly neutral stimuli and aversive events. Such a CONDITIONING mechanism is highly adaptive because it allows us to avoid bad things that have happened to us in the past and or things we see others avoid.

Conditioned fear can be studied in the laboratory. For example, when a tone, which initially produces no reaction in a rat, is paired with an aversive stimulus such as a FOOTSHOCK, the tone alone can now elicit a constellation of behaviours (conditioned fear responses) that previously were only produced by the shock (unconditioned fear responses). These might include a change in heart rate and respiration, decreased salivation, stomach ulcers, urination, defecation, increased startle responses, excessive grooming and a cessation of ongoing behaviour called freezing. Behavioural effects produced in animals by this formerly neutral stimulus (now called a CONDITIONED STIMULUS) are similar in many respects to the constellation of behaviours used to diagnose generalized anxiety in humans.

A great deal of evidence indicates that the AMYGDALA plays a crucial role in the expression and acquisition of conditioned fear. Many brain areas to which the amygdala projects mediate specific signs of fear. Electrical stimulation of the amygdala elicits a pattern of behaviours that mimic fear. Lesions of the amygdala block innate and conditioned fear and local infusion of drugs into the amygdala reduces fear in several behavioural tests. People who have an abnormal amygdala do not show normal fear reactions. LONG-TERM POTENTIATION (LTP) in the amygdala may mediate fear conditioning because an NMDA receptor-dependent form of LTP has been observed in the amygdala and local infusion of NMDA antagonists into the amygdala blocks the formation of conditioned fear memories measured with several different tests. The HIPPOCAMPUS may be involved in the memory of the location where a fearful event happened. Projections from the amygdala to various cortical areas probably mediate the conscious experience of fear.

See also: animal models of anxiety; prepulse inhibition

MICHAEL DAVIS

conditioned inhibition In PAVLOVIAN CONDITIONING, conditioned inhibition is a state that is opposite to that produced by excitatory conditioning. For example, if the typical Pavlovian conditioning procedure (that is, FORWARD CONDITIONING) results in a conditional response in a particular direction (such as increased salivation), then inhibitory conditioning results in a response that is in the opposite direction (in this case, decreased salivation). Procedures that produce conditioned inhibition include INDUCTION, NEGATIVE CONTINGENCIES, INHIBITION OF DELAY and conditioned discrimination.

JOHN D. SALAMONE

conditioned place preference *see* place conditioning

conditioned punishment The use of a response-contingent aversive CONDITIONED STIMULUS, rather than an unconditioned aversive event such as mild footshock, to punish an instrumental action.

See also: conditioned reinforcement; instrumental conditioning; punishment

A. SIMON KILLCROSS

conditioned reflex The pattern of behaviour evoked by a CONDITIONED STIMULUS (CS) after PAVLOVIAN CONDITIONING. In this form of training the initially ineffective CS is paired with presentations of some other stimulus (the

UNCONDITIONED STIMULUS, US) that evokes a response (the unconditioned response, UCR). As a result of these pairings the CS itself becomes capable of evoking a response. This conditioned response is often similar, if not identical, to the UCR evoked by the US. Since the UCR is often simple and apparently automatically elicited by the US (that is, it shows the properties of a REFLEX) the version elicited by the CS is also described as a conditioned reflex.

GEOFFREY HALL

conditioned reinforcement The reinforcement brought about by presentation of a neutral environmental stimulus (for instance, a light) when it has previously been paired temporally with a natural REINFORCER (for example, water). Conditioned reinforcement can be made contingent upon the acquisition of an OPERANT, such as LEARNING to respond on a lever to receive the light and water. In this example, water is never presented in the test phase. In this phase, one lever produces the light alone – the conditioned reinforcer – while a second lever does not. Specificity of responding for conditioned reinforcement can be measured by comparing presses on the two levers.

WENDY L. INGLIS

conditioned response see stimulus–reinforcer association

conditioned rotation The phenomenon in which an experimental animal (typically a rat) turns in circles (ROTATION) under the control of a CONDITIONED STIMULUS. It has been described in two circumstances. (1) Thirsty rats are trained by OPERANT CONDITIONING to turn selectively in one direction for water REWARD. The ability to initiate rotation in the CONTRALATERAL direction is abolished by a LESION of the NIGROSTRIATAL DOPAMINE SYSTEM. (2) If rats with unilateral nigrostriatal lesions are tested for drug-induced rotation in a specific environment, that environment will subsequently elicit rotation in the non-drugged animal by associative conditioning.

See also: place conditioning

STEPHEN B. DUNNETT

conditioned stimulus see classical conditioning

conditioned suppression (also known as PAVLOVIAN FEAR) The suppression of an appetitive activity such as licking for water or lever-pressing by an aversive CONDITIONED STIMULUS. A frequently-used measure of CONDITIONED FEAR.

See also: aversive conditioning; fear

A. SIMON KILLCROSS

conditioned visual-discrimination task The subject is required to discriminate between two or more visual stimuli and, on the basis of the discrimination, select a response. The discrimination is conditioned in that it often requires arbitrary associations between the visual stimuli and the subsequent response. These associations must be learned.

See also: conditional discrimination

VERITY J. BROWN

conditioning Sometimes now used as a synonym for LEARNING itself, the term CONDITIONING referred originally to the procedure introduced by I. P. Pavlov (1849–1936) in the early years of the twentieth century for the study of nervous function in animals. In PAVLOVIAN CONDITIONING (also called classical conditioning to distinguish it from other variants of the procedure developed subsequently) animal subjects are given paired presentations of two stimuli, one of which unconditionally evokes a response. As a result of this experience the other stimulus acquires the power to evoke a new response, often (although not invariably) similar in form to that evoked by the stimulus with which it has been paired. Since this newly acquired capacity is conditional upon the animal's having undergone this training, the response has come to be called a conditional (conditioned) response (or reflex) (see CONDITIONED REFLEX) and the entire process gets referred to as conditioning. Pavlov's own view, that the many other forms of learning might be explicable in terms of the basic processes at work in his classical conditioning paradigm, probably contributed to the more liberal use of the term conditioning.

Evidence to show that Pavlov's version of conditioning could not explain all forms even of animal learning came from work conducted in the 1920s by the Polish neurophysiologist J. Konorski (1903–1973). He demonstrated that a dog induced to perform a particular response (for instance, to lift a paw) would come to perform this response with increasing frequency if the response was followed by access to food. In this procedure the critical contingency is between the response and the stimulus (food) that follows it, as distinct from Pavlov's procedure in which the critical CONTINGENCY is between two stimuli. Konorski still used the term conditioning to describe the learning process engaged by his experiments, but called it Type II conditioning to distinguish it from classical Pavlovian conditioning, which he referred to as Type I. The distinction was developed in the United States during the 1930s by B.F. Skinner who similarly pointed out that classical conditioning principles could not explain the increased readiness with which a rat would come to press a lever when that action resulted in the delivery of a food pellet. Skinner christened this form of learning (which is formally identical to that studied by Konorski) OPERANT CONDITIONING, the new term 'operant' being coined to emphasize the fact that the animal must operate upon its environment in order to obtain an effect. (The Pavlovian version was renamed RESPONDENT CONDITIONING.) Operant conditioning is also sometimes referred to as INSTRUMENTAL CONDITIONING, so called because the behaviour of the animal is instrumental in producing an effect.

Since the two types of conditioning procedure are operationally quite distinct (in classical the animal is exposed to a contingency between two stimuli; in operant the contingency is between an action and an outcome) the question arose as to whether they differed in more fundamental ways. One widely canvassed suggestion was that classical conditioning might be effective only in modifying the occurrence of simple REFLEX responses and that the modification of voluntary behaviour depended on operant conditioning processes. The distinction has proved to be untenable, however; there have been demonstrations of

the operant conditioning of involuntary responses and that supposedly voluntary behaviour such as an animal shows in moving around its environment, can be susceptible to classical conditioning. The modern consensus is that both types of conditioning depend on a common ASSOCIATIVE LEARNING process, differing only in the events that enter into association: two stimuli in the case of classical conditioning, a response and a stimulus in the operant case.

Conditioning processes undoubtedly operate outside the animal learning laboratory. It seems likely, for instance that some instances of human PHOBIA are a product of the classical conditioning, of the fortuitous pairing, perhaps early in life, of the feared event with some trauma. And the way in which our everyday behaviour can be shaped by REWARD and PUNISHMENT may be taken to reflect operant conditioning in action. More generally, it has been suggested that the basic associative processes that are revealed in laboratory studies of animal conditioning constitute the underlying mechanism of all (or almost all) instances of individual learning and adaptation in both animals and humans. There is, at present, no convincing evidence to require us either to accept or reject this suggestion.

GEOFFREY HALL

conduction (from Latin, *con*: together, *ducere*: to lead) In biological psychology, conduction typically refers to the passage of an ACTION POTENTIAL along an AXON. In other contexts, it has other meanings.

conduction aphasia A major clinical syndrome of aphasia; a form of FLUENT APHASIA with a predominance of phonemic PARAPHASIAS. The sound transpositions and additions may be confined to nouns and other content words whilst sparing grammatical words. Repetition of words and sentences is poor. Though the symptoms of expressive language impairment may be difficult to discern from WERNICKE'S APHASIA a hallmark of this syndrome is relative preservation of auditory comprehension. Lesions associated with conduction aphasia typically are located in the supramarginal GYRUS of the LEFT HEMISPHERE.

Lesions along the border of the SYLVIAN FISSURE may produce conduction aphasia.

Reference

Goodglass H. & Kaplan E. (1983) *The Assessment of Aphasia and Related Disorders*, 2nd edn, Lea & Febiger: Philadelphia.

CHARLOTTE C. MITCHUM

cone opponency *see* opponent process theory of colour vision

cone opponent *see* dual opponent cells

cone snails A genus of gastropod molluscs, the cone snails posses exceptionally venomous NEUROTOXINS (known as CONOTOXINS) with which they kill fish. Brief consideration of their situation indicates the problem they face: cone snails are relatively small and not particularly agile; fish are a lot quicker and very much more agile. The toxins that the cone snails have evolved therefore need to be exceptionally fast-acting, which indeed they are. Some cone snails appear to wander, capturing small fish at random and poisoning them. Others lie in wait, luring fish with an attractive proboscis, poisoning them and eating them after capture in a stomach that can be extended beyond the snails' body. The most dangerous of the 300 or so known types of cone snail is *Conus geographus*, a 3–5 inch snail that can kill a man.

cones Cone-shaped photoreceptors in the RETINA that are responsible for vision under relatively high (day-time) levels of illumination. Commonly, two or three types of cone exist in the retina, distinguished by the SPECTRAL SENSITIVITY of the light-absorbing PHOTOPIGMENT that they contain.

See also: rods; visual system

KATHY T. MULLEN

confabulation (from Latin, *confabulare*: to talk) To confabulate in the everyday sense is to talk, with an emphasis on the discussion and sharing of confidential information. In psychiatry, however, confabulation refers to the state when a patient, asked to recall a memory, often for an event, will describe things that did not happen, typically mixing various elements, often in a rather unusual manner. There is no attempt at deceit: patients are genuinely recounting their beliefs. Confabulation is a feature of several conditions, including ALZHEIMER'S DEMENTIA, AMNESIC SYNDROME and KORSAKOFF'S SYNDROME, amongst others.

See also: false memory syndrome

configural conditioned stimulus *see* negative patterning

configural discrimination *see* discrimination

configural learning A discrimination problem whose solution necessarily requires subjects to learn about combinations (or configurations) of separable stimuli. One example is the CONDITIONAL DISCRIMINATION: subjects might receive food following the presentation of two compounded conditioned stimuli (CSs), CS1–CS2 and CS3–CS4, but not when these CSs are presented in an alternative configuration, CS1–CS4 and CS3–CS2. Given sufficient training, animals will anticipate food during the reinforced combinations but not during the non-reinforced combinations of the CSs. Notice that none of the CSs uniquely predicts the food.

See also: negative patterning; positive patterning

JASPER WARD-ROBINSON

conflict In biological psychology, conflict generally refers not to AGGRESSION between individuals or groups but to inner struggles. In ETHOLOGY, three types of conflict are identified: *approach–approach*, when an organism has desires to approach two positive reinforcers simultaneously (see POSITIVE REINFORCEMENT); *avoidance–avoidance*, with two stimuli equally to be avoided; and *approach–avoidance*, in which an organism has competing desires to approach and avoid a particular stimulus. Approach–avoidance conflict is the most common, frequently appearing in situations involving courtship. Conflict is often a cause of displacement behaviour, when species typical behaviours will appear out of context. These are assumed to be the product of heightened DRIVE or MOTIVATION triggered by a specific STIMULUS but which cannot be satisfied. (SCHEDULE-INDUCED POLYDIPSIA is thought to be a laboratory analogue of this.)

A CONFLICT TEST test is often used in laboratories in ANIMAL MODELS OF ANXIETY.

conflict test A conflict test is one in which animals are challenged by the presence of both positive and negative reinforcers. GELLER–SEIFTER CONFLICT involves the use of an instrumental conditioning procedure, while VOGEL CONFLICT provides reward or punishment with regard to an animal's unconditioned behaviour.

See also: animal models of anxiety; negative reinforcer; positive reinforcer

confocal microscopy A microscopy technique based on laser illumination of specimens and specialized optics that allow selection and imaging of just that thin plane within a thick object which is in focus, and without blurring by other elements outside the focal plane. Confocal microscopy allows much finer resolution of structure at different planes of focus within 3-dimensional objects (such as cells in a histological section) than can be achieved using conventional microscopy.

See also: histology; image analysis

STEPHEN B. DUNNETT

congener (from Latin, *con*: with, *genus*: type) Literally, of the same type. In biology it generally refers to a member of another species within the same genus.

See also: conspecific; taxonomy

congenital (from Latin, *con*: together, *genitum*: to beget) Something that has been always present – a congenital deformity is one that has been present at least since birth. This term is used in contradistinction to 'inherited' (that is, genetic in origin): a congenital condition is one acquired *in utero*, by infection for example.

congenital hypothyroidism Dysfunction of the THYROID GLAND early in life can lead to various problems with growth and DEVELOPMENT. Individuals with this condition typically have stunted body growth and some degree of facial malformation. More pressingly, there is abnormal NEURODEVELOPMENT: brain size is relatively small and structurally abnormal. The structural abnormality is typically seen as a decreased number of dendrites per neuron and a much diminished number of collaterals on axons. The poor brain development leads to MENTAL RETARDATION. The pejorative term for this condition, CRETINISM, is no longer used.

conjoined feature search *see* feature search

conjugate (from Latin, *con*: together, *jugare*: yoke) A word with many uses; in biochemistry, this means to join molecules together without losing the identity of either one (that is, it is not the formation of a new COMPOUND). For an example, see SAPORIN.

conjugate movement *see* vergence

conjunction search Synonymous with CONJOINED FEATURE SEARCH; see FEATURE SEARCH.

connectionism Connectionism is an approach to developing computer simulations of cognitive processes that attempts to capture the abstract information-processing capabilities of large groups of neurons. Information is represented as distributed patterns of activity over groups of simple, neuron-like processing units. Co-operative and competitive interactions among units are governed by weighted connections between them; these weights are typically learned using an automatic training procedure (see BACKPROPAGATION; HEBB-LIKE RULE) based on experience with environmental inputs and outputs. Connectionist simulations have successfully modelled phenomena in many perceptual, cognitive, and motor domains.

See also: connectionist neuropsychology; distributed processing; neural networks; parallel processing; serial vs. parallel processing models

Reference

McClelland J.L, Rumelhart D.E., and the PDP Research Group (1986) *Parallel Distributed Processing: Explorations in the Microstructure of Cognition*, vol. 2, *Psychological and Biological Models*, MIT Press: Cambridge MA.

DAVID C. PLAUT

connectionist neuropsychology Connectionist neuropsychology is an approach to understanding the cognitive impairments than can arise following BRAIN INJURY by simulating these impairments using connectionist models of cognitive processes (see CONNECTIONISM; NEURAL NETWORKS). A connectionist model is a computer simulation in which information processing takes the form of highly parallel interactions among groups of artificial neurons called units. Weights on connections between units govern how the units interact and are learned through experience. Brain damage can be simulated by removing some of the units in a group, or some of the connections between two groups. The effects of such an artificial LESION is to cause the remaining units to interact in an unusual way, perhaps causing the system as a whole to make incorrect responses to stimuli that the undamaged system processed correctly. An important property of connectionist networks in this regard is that they degrade gracefully with damage; as with patients, performance is typically only partially impaired with partial damage. If the pattern of errors produced by the damaged network agrees with the pattern observed of patients with analogous brain damage, it lends support to claims that the undamaged network represents and processes information in a way similar to how the normal cognitive system operates. Moreover, exploring the relative effectiveness of alternative strategies for retraining the damaged network can help in the design of more effective therapy for the patients.

This approach has been adopted successfully in the study of a wide range of neuropsychological disorders, including VISUAL AGNOSIA, HEMISPATIAL NEGLECT, AMNESIA, APHASIA, DEMENTIA, and SCHIZOPHRENIA. Perhaps the most detailed progress involves modelling selective impairments in reading (see ACQUIRED DYSLEXIA). As an example, consider DEEP DYSLEXIA, which is among the most perplexing of neuropsychological disorders. Its hallmark characteristic is the occurrence of SEMANTIC ERRORS, such as pronouncing the word *river* as *ocean* or *dark* as *night*. Deep dyslexic patients also make visual errors (*scandal* as *sandals*) suggesting a second impairment. However, Hinton & Shallice (1991) demonstrated that the occurrence of semantic errors and their co-occurrence with visual errors is a natural consequence of a single lesion to a connectionist network trained to derive the meanings of written words. In this way, connectionist neuropsychology led to an understanding of the processes of understanding written words,

and the way these can break down when damaged, which would have been difficult to discover within more traditional modular frameworks (see MODULES AND MODULAR ORGANIZATION).

See also: neuropsychology

Reference

Hinton G.E. & Shallice T. (1991) Lesioning an attractor network: investigations of acquired dyslexia. *Psychological Review* 98: 74–95.

DAVID C. PLAUT

connective tissue Connective tissue binds and supports other body tissues. Epithelia have tightly packed cells; connective tissue does not, having few cells embedded in a matrix of FIBRES. It is made of three types of fibres: collagenous fibres (rich in COLLAGEN and providing structural strength), elastic fibres (which give a degree of tension) and reticular fibres (also rich in collagen and proving binding to other structures). The main types of connective tissue are: (1) loose connective tissue (which acts to pack and bind tissues), (2) ADIPOSE tissue, which holds adipose cells (ADIPOCYTES), (3) fibrous connective tissue (which makes tendons that attach MUSCLES to bones), (4) cartilage (which has functions in certain joints and in some other specialized locations – the nasal septum, or between vertebrae in the spine), (5) bon, which is formed from collagen but has a high composition of calcium and other minerals causing it to ossify – to become bone, and (6) BLOOD which has some of the properties of connective tissue; it is essentially a collection of specialized cells supported in plasma. The MENINGES are specialized types of connective tissue.

Reference

Campbell N.A., Reece J.B. & Mitchell L.G. (1999) *Biology*, 5th edn, Addison-Wesley: Menlo Park CA.

conotoxins Conotoxins are the NEUROTOXINS possessed by CONE SNAILS. These are peptide toxins and are found in different classes: omega (ω), alpha (α) and mu (μ) conotoxins act at serial stages of neural activation at the NEUROMUSCULAR JUNCTION to produce exceptionally rapid paralysis and death. Omega conotoxins act at presynaptic sites to prevent calcium entry into neurons and inhibit release of ACETYLCHOLINE; alpha conotoxins act at postsynaptic sites to block acetylcholine RECEPTORS and affect SODIUM CHANNELS in MUSCLE; and mu conotoxins prevent ACTION POTENTIAL formation in muscles.

Reference

Olivera B.M., Grey W.R., Zeikus R., McIntosh J.M., Varga J., Rivier J., de Santos V. & Cruz L.J. (1985) Peptide neurotoxins from fish-hunting cone snails. *Science* 230: 1338–1343.

conscious memory *see* declarative memory

conscious recollection *see* declarative memory

consciousness The state of organisms that enables phenomenal experience and VOLUNTARY behaviour. Commonly, both the graded states of being conscious (as opposed to unconscious) and the content of a conscious experience are called consciousness. Consciousness is lost in COMA, ANAESTHESIA, and dreamless SLEEP, reduced in drowsiness and SOMNOLENCE, and fully present in attentive alertness and hyper-excitation. Loss and disturbance of consciousness can result from multiple causes including lack of oxygen, epileptic seizures, brainstem lesions, and substances like alcohol, barbiturates, ether, and ketamine. Clinically, the degree of disturbance is assessed with the GLASGOW COMA SCALE on the basis of eye opening, motor function, and verbal utterances. The states of consciousness are independent of its particular content: what one is conscious of is irrelevant as long as one is conscious of something. It is therefore not surprising that the degree to which an organism is conscious appears to be mediated by an unspecific neuronal system which involves the brainstem and DIENCEPHALON. In particular, the intralaminar nuclei of the THALAMUS have been suggested to be importantly involved, and were found to have been disproportionately affected in the coma case of Karen Ann Quinlan. This central and phylogenetically old system is present in other animals, as are SLEEP–WAKE CYCLES and REM SLEEP (rapid eye movement sleep) and non-REM phases of sleep which require SEROTONIN and NORADRENALINE release.

In contrast, what an organism can be conscious of once it is in a conscious state depends primarily on its sensory equipment, which in turn depends on the ecological niche in which it evolved. Sensory systems differ widely even among vertebrates, ranging from vision and audition tuned to different parts of the electromagnetic and frequency spectra, to sonar systems and sideline organs. Note that sensory processing *per se* need not be consciously represented and is thus not sufficient to attribute consciousness to an organism. Neuroendocrine and reflexive responses can be elicited from comatose and sleeping subjects and do not require the organism to be conscious. In addition, subjects can be in a conscious state and nevertheless not have a conscious perception in response to sensory stimulation. In normal subjects, paradigms applying subliminal and masked stimulation, or BINAURAL and BINOCULAR RIVALRY, have revealed that unperceived information can exert noticeable influences on the conscious voluntary response. Similarly, in patients with lesions to the central parts of the sensory systems who have lost the conscious representation of stimuli of a particular sensory modality, effects of the unperceived stimuli upon non-reflexive responses have been extensively demonstrated. Examples of such implicit processes come from visual BLINDSIGHT, auditory (deaf hearing), somatosensory (unfeeling touch) and memory domains. Their discovery and description may open empirical avenues to two important questions. The first regards the purpose or function of conscious representations, and can be tackled by studying what is and what is not possible based on sensory information that is demonstrably processed but not consciously represented. The second regards the neuronal substrate mediating conscious representations. What structures are needed? The loss of which structures prevents information from becoming conscious? Are the structures, pathways, neurons, neurotransmitters and neuromodulators that mediate only unconscious sensory processing different from those that mediate conscious perception? Is neocortical participation required for conscious perception? Are all functional sub-divisions of NEOCORTEX equally capable of mediating conscious content?

Neuropsychological data show that different aspects of conscious perception even within a single modality can dissociate following a LESION to different parts of the system. The degree of dissociability is astonishing: MEMORY and LANGUAGE can be lost selectively for narrow groups of objects, object IMAGERY can persist in the absence of OBJECT RECOGNITION, and ALEXIA can occur without AGRAPHIA. The selective loss of pieces of the representation caused by circumscribed lesions demonstrates PARALLEL PROCESSING, but conscious perception also seems to be hierarchically structured. The phenomenal representation of sensory information, for instance as colour or sound, appears prior to the conscious identification of the object having the colour or emitting the sound. In contrast to the unity of experience that many philosophers and psychologists have posited, these findings demonstrate a modularity of the mind. HEMISPHERIC SPECIALIZATION, notably observed in SPLIT BRAIN patients whose CORPUS CALLOSUM has been cut to control epileptic seizures, is a notable feature of this modular organization. LANGUAGE, predominantly represented in one HEMISPHERE, helps in assessing consciousness in both meanings of the term, that of being conscious, and that of being conscious of. Being our major means to exchange and access abstract ideas, it plays a role for the social components of consciousness, and contributes to its contents. Both quality and quantity of content are important for the normal function, disturbances resulting from traumatic life events, from too little input (as in SENSORY DEPRIVATION), and from an overextension of its limited capacity (for example, in certain psychiatric disorders or following sleep deprivation).

See also: binding problem

References

Bogen J.E. (1995) On the neurophysiology of consciousness. I. An overview. *Consciousness and Cognition* 4: 52–62.
Jasper H.H., Descarries L., Castellucci V.F. & Rossignol S. (1998) *Consciousness: At the Frontiers of Neuroscience*, Advances in Neurology 77, Lippincott–Raven: Philadelphia PA.
Marcel A.J. & Bisiach E. (1988) *Consciousness in Contemporary Science*, Oxford University Press: Oxford.
Searle J. (1992) *The Rediscovery of the Mind*, MIT Press: Cambridge MA.
Stoerig P. (1996) Varieties of vision: from sensory processing to conscious recognition. *Trends in Neuroscience* 19: 401–406.

PETRA STOERIG

consensus sequences *see* gene

consolidation The process by which material is established in long term memory. The mechanisms by which it occurs are not clear; see LONG-TERM MEMORY.

conspecific (from Latin, *con*: with, *species*: type or appearance) Conspecific is a term meaning that one organism is of the same species (see TAXONOMY) as another.

See also: congener

constructional apraxia The impairment in assembling elements of a 2- or 3-dimensional whole that occurs even in the absence of a primary motor deficit is referred to as constructional apraxia. Patients may fail to copy drawings (see COPYING AND DRAWING) or even to construct block designs, respecting neither the orientation of objects and their parts nor the spatial relationships between the parts. PARIETAL LOBE damage to either hemisphere is a frequent anatomic correlate of this deficit. It has been argued, however, that the deficit that occurs after LEFT HEMISPHERE damage is one of APRAXIA whereas the deficit that occurs after RIGHT HEMISPHERE damage is one of SPATIAL COGNITION.

MARLENE BEHRMANN

consummatory phase *see* appetitive vs. consummatory phases

content-addressable information Information that is accessed by specifying its *content* rather than its *location*. The MEMORY held by computers is content-addressable; CONNECTIONIST NEUROPSYCHOLOGY operates using content-addressable information.

contention scheduling *see* supervisory attentional system

context-dependent learning A principle of MEMORY which states that recall performance is facilitated when the context in which information is retrieved matches the context in which it was learned. Reinstatement of the ENCODING context at RETRIEVAL is beneficial because the context acts as a retrieval cue. The relative importance of context as a retrieval cue depends on the availability of other, more specific cues in the testing situation. Performance on memory tests that provide few retrieval cues, such as tests of FREE RECALL, benefit the most from reinstatement of encoding context at retrieval, whereas tests of RECOGNITION, in which all items are provided at test, benefit little. Typically, the negative effects of changing context between study and test are not large, however, unless context differences are substantial (such as water vs. land). There is some evidence to suggest that mentally imaging the encoding context can diminish the negative effects of different study and test contexts.

Different aspects of context can influence context-dependent learning. First, context can refer the external environment in which information is learned. For example, exam performance is better when students are tested in the same classroom in which the LEARNING took place, as opposed to a different classroom. Second, context can refer to the internal environment of the individual, such as their physical and/or emotional state. For example, a neutral event learned in one MOOD will be better recalled when in that mood than when in a different mood. Context-dependent learning associated with the internal state of the individual is often referred to as STATE-DEPENDENT LEARNING. These types of environmental context do not alter the meaning of the semantic information, and are therefore generally referred to as extrinsic context. Finally, context that can alter the meaning of item information is referred to as intrinsic context. For example, if the word *jam* was originally learned in the context of *strawberry-jam* it is more likely to be recalled when cued with the context of *strawberry-*, as opposed to *traffic-jam*. Context-dependent learning is one of a class of memory principles that stresses the importance of the relationship between study and test situations.

See also: contextual learning; transfer-appropriate processing

JENNIFER A. MANGELS

contextual conditioned stimulus *see* contextual learning

contextual conditioning Conditioning that occurs to the stimuli constituting the background cues in a learning task (the stimuli providing the experimental chamber, or the animals current state for example) and in the presence of which other events are presented. Some have claimed that contextual cues behave in a qualitatively different way from other types of stimuli, but as yet there is little compelling evidence to support this view. Background cues seem to condition in much the same way as non-background cues.

See also: context-dependent learning

CHARLOTTE BONARDI

contextual learning A term describing a LEARNING procedures in which an UNCONDITIONED STIMULUS (US) is paired with a CONDITIONED STIMULUS (CS) in a specific context. (This CS is therefore known as a CONTEXTUAL CONDITIONED STIMULUS.) Typically, contextual learning involves FEAR conditioning: the US is electric shock, the CS a tone, these being delivered in a specific apparatus. Contextual conditioning is a technique that has been used to detect impairments in the function of the HIPPOCAMPUS, especially in mice genetically modified in ways thought to affect this (see Kiyama *et al.*, 1998). However, it has been suggested (Gerlai, 1998) that contextual learning requires both hippocampal and non-hippocampal mechanisms.

See also: contextual conditioning

References

Gerlai R. (1998) Contextual learning and cue association in fear conditioning in mice: a strain comparison and a lesion study. *Behavioral Brain Research* 95: 191–203.
Kiyama Y., Manabe T., Sakimura K., Kawakami F., Mori H. & Mishina M. (1998)

Increased thresholds for long term potentiation and contextual learning in mice lacking the NMDSA-type glutamate receptor (1 subunit). *Journal of Neuroscience* 18: 6704–6712.

contiguity (from Latin, *contingere*: touching all over) Contiguous things are things that are close together, or occurring next to each other in time. The CONTIGUITY of events is an important consideration in animal LEARNING; see OPERANT. Contiguity is different from CONTINGENCY.

contingency (from Latin, *con*: mutual, *tangere*: to touch) If something is contingent it is dependent on something else happening. It does not mean the same as 'dependent': contingent implies that two events will probably (but not certainly) occur with respect to each other. (The term *contingency plan* captures this: a contingency plan is one that has a probability of being used if certain other things happen.) In animal LEARNING, it is now thought that the statistical correlation – the contingency – between a CONDITIONED STIMULUS and an UNCONDITIONED STIMULUS, (or between a RESPONSE and a REWARD) is important in determining how well animals will learn about the relationships between the two things (see OPERANT). The term non-contingent is used as the opposite of contingent. It is taken to mean that an event – the non-contingent event – is not related to any other event (see, for example, PRIMING).

contingency learning This involves LEARNING that an outcome is contingent upon other events; see CONTINGENCY.

contingent tolerance A form of BEHAVIOURAL TOLERANCE, dependent on learning in which the development of drug TOLERANCE is contingent upon an animal's behavioural experiences. It is a term that derives from the fact that tolerance develops contingent upon the temporal relationships between drug administration and behavioural testing.

Reference

Wolgin D.L. (1989) The role of instrumental learning in behavioural tolerance to drugs. In *Psychoactive Drugs: Tolerance and Sensitization*, ed. A.J. Goudie & M.W. Emmett-Oglesby, pp. 17–114, Humana Press: Clifton NJ.

continuous reinforcement *see* schedules of reinforcement

contour perception Contours (lines and edges) correspond to the boundaries of objects in the field of view, and their visual registration is an essential early stage of shape perception. Neurons in STRIATE CORTEX (AREA VI) with an oriented RECEPTIVE FIELD respond selectively to local sections of a contour. Grouping processes must link these sections together, and can produce SUBJECTIVE CONTOURS even in gaps where no light/dark contour exists in the image; neurons in AREA V2 are known to respond to such contours. Associated neural processes must distinguish the intrinsic boundary which defines an object's shape, from contours occurring where the object is occluded by another (figure–ground segregation).

See also: binding problem; pattern perception

OLIVER J. BRADDICK

contralateral On the opposite side; contrasted to IPSILATERAL, meaning on the same side. These are terms defined in relation to a stimulus or event. For instance, if a LESION was made in only one HEMISPHERE of the brain, that side (whether right or left) would be defined as the ipsilateral side (of the brain and body) while the other (non-lesioned) side would be contralateral to the lesion.

contralateral neglect *see* neglect syndrome

contrast-sensitive receptive field *see* retina

contrast sensitivity Sensitivity to variations in light intensity across the visual field, determined from the THRESHOLD contrast for a SINE WAVE GRATING. (Contrast = $(I_{max} - I_{min}) / (I_{max} + I_{min})$ where I_{max}, I_{min} are the intensities at the peak and trough of the sine wave.) The use of sine waves of different spatial frequencies gives a pure measure of the sensitivity of the VISUAL SYSTEM to contrast at various spatial scales (the contrast sensitivity function). This is greatest at a spatial frequency around 3 cycles/degree. Reduced sensitivity at lower frequencies reflects LATERAL INHIBITION in the RECEPTIVE FIELD of a retinal ganglion cell, which diminishes the neural response from gradual variations of light intensity. At high frequencies sensitivity falls to zero at the limit set by visual ACUITY.

See also: spatial frequency channels

OLIVER J. BRADDICK

contre coup (from French, counterblow) Damage to the side of the brain opposite to an impact point. It is thought to be produced by an impact generating movement of the brain that continues after the head itself has stopped moving: brain tissue opposite the point of contact may come into contact with the SKULL.

See also: closed head injury; meninges

controlled stepping This is a term used to describe the LOCOMOTION at a constant rate displayed by animals engaged in TREADMILL LOCOMOTION.

convergent dissociations *see* multiple memory systems

convergent evolution A term used to describe the EVOLUTION, independently but in parallel, of similar features in different SPECIES. The most common example is that wings are found on birds and bats, but there is no direct relationship between them.

convulsant Any agent that induces CONVULSIONS.

See also: kindling; psychomotor stimulants

convulsions A convulsion is a sudden, quite violent, involuntary contraction of the skeletal MUSCLES. Convulsions are often described as being TONIC or CLONIC. They may be present during epileptic seizures (see EPILEPSY) and are often seen, in rodents, immediately after a LESION has been induced by EXCITOTOXINS (though they do not persist in this case).

coordinate system, stereotaxic During stereotaxic surgery, whether experimental or therapeutic, it is necessary to define a point in the brain using 3-dimensional coordinates – anterior–posterior, medial–lateral and dorsal–ventral. Structures in the brain are identified by their distance from zero reference points. In experimental stereotaxic surgery using animals, the anterior–posterior zero point is typically at BREGMA (a skull landmark) or the INTERAURAL

LINE. The medial–lateral zero point is usually taken as the MIDLINE; and the dorsal–ventral one either skull surface or dura. For humans and the most common experimental animals there are STEREOTAXIC ATLASES available which locate the structures of the brain in these 3-dimensional coordinates.

See also: stereotaxic surgery

coordinate system, visual For a spatial measurement to be made a coordinate system is needed to provide an origin from which locations are calculated and a unit of length. The visual system uses at least three coordinate systems with different origins. First, the retinal image has an origin at the centre of the FOVEA. The relationship between this retinal coordinate system and the location of objects in the scene depends on the direction of the eye. A second origin, the direction straight ahead of the observer, is obtained by combining the retinal coordinate system with the direction of GAZE. Occasionally a third is required, placing the origin at the location of an object in the scene.

ROGER J. WATT

coprolalia (from Greek, *kopros*: dung, *lalia*: talk) Obscene language used repetitively and often in a rather exclamatory way. It has a compulsive and perseverative (see COMPULSION and PERSEVERATION) nature and is a particular feature of TOURETTE'S SYNDROME (though it may occur also in other clinical conditions). One would not usually describe everyday obscene talk as coprolalia: that would be described more appropriately as vulgar.

coprophagia (from Greek, *kopros*: dung, *phagein*: to eat) Eating faecal matter. In humans one would hope never to see this. In rodents (and other species) it is normal: VITAMINS of the B group are synthesized by the microflora of the lower gut, beyond the point in the gastrointestinal tract of maximal absorption. Coprophagia therefore allows rodents the opportunity to capture the vitamins present in their own faecal pellets.

copulation (from Latin, *copulare*: to join together) Copulation in fact refers in general to the joining together of things. Most commonly however it is used to refer to sexual intercourse.

See also: sexual behaviour; social behaviour

copulatory lock During copulation, the PENIS of some male mammals – certain types of dogs and mice for example, but not humans – increases in size to such an extent that it cannot be removed from the female's VAGINA for several minutes.

copying and drawing The ability to copy and draw requires the integration of a number of different cognitive skills such as the visual processing of spatial aspects of the display, the appreciation of form, colour and motion and the possession of sufficiently intact motor abilities to execute the task. Consequently, a deficit to any one of a number of perceptual and motor skills will manifest in impaired copying and drawing. Whereas copying involves the processing of a visually presented stimulus (and hence involves perception), drawing need not and can be done by individuals who are blind. In copying, depending on the severity of the damage, patients with a LESION to the posterior parts of the RIGHT HEMISPHERE may lose the ability to reproduce the overall form of the item, may depict the relationships between elements but not produce the entire design or may even be unable to replicate some of the basic elements in the design. In the case of hemispatial neglect, features on the CONTRALATERAL side may be omitted in copying or drawing whereas those on the IPSILATERAL side may be included. Some patients with right hemisphere damage may depict only details or local aspects of the display whereas in cases with left hemisphere damage, only the global Gestalt of the item may be reproduced without the accompanying details. Patients with APPERCEPTIVE AGNOSIA may not be able to copy even simple geometric displays whereas those with ASSOCIATIVE AG-NOSIA who are able to derive a coherent structural description may be able to copy well but still fail to appreciate the identity of the item being copied. Interestingly, there are several reports of patients who can draw well from memory even though they have profound visual AGNOSIA or object recognition deficits. Damage to motor regions of the LEFT HEMI-

SPHERE disrupt copying or drawing because of a primary motor deficit. Patients with APRAXIA following left hemisphere damage may also be impaired at drawing and copying because of an inability to produce fine skilled motor movements in a well-sequenced and coordinated fashion. The errors produced in copying can be informative; for example, perseverations, rotations, 'closing in' errors and the tendency to write the name of the object rather than to draw or copy its geometric shape are all suggestive of organic pathology. Affective processes or particular MOOD states can also influence copying and drawing although this may be primarily manifest in the emotional content or creativity of the produced item.

MARLENE BEHRMANN

core (nucleus accumbens) *see* nucleus accumbens

cornea The cornea is the centrally situated, transparent portion of the outer tunic of the eye, and is continuous with the white surrounding tissue (the sclera). It comprises six concentric non-vascular layers, and is the main refractive part of the optics of the eyeball.

See also: visual system

DAVID W. HEELEY

Cornelia de Lange syndrome *see* mental retardation

cornu ammonis *see* Ammon's horn; hippocampus

corollary discharge *see* efference copy

coronal section *see* planes of section

corpus callosum The corpus callosum is the largest connecting pathway between the CEREBRAL HEMISPHERES. Estimates of the number of nerve fibres it contains vary from 500 to 800 million. It contains two types of fibres: the larger-diameter mediate sensori-motor coordination, the more numerous small-diameter fibres connect association areas.

For the first half of the twentieth century, the corpus callosum seemed to have no function at all. This stood in sharp contrast to the eighteenth century when some authors believed that this 'callous body' or 'hard part' of the brain was the 'seat of the soul'. By 1941 McCulloch & Garrell concluded that thus far attempts have 'failed to produce any characteristic disorders except, possibly, impairment of co-ordination of the hemispheres in complicated symbolic activity' attributable to lesions of, or even surgical sections of, the corpus callosum. This view was radically revised starting from the classical pioneering studies of Myers & Sperry in the late 1950s, on the INTERHEMISPHERIC TRANSFER of information through the corpus callosum. Fibres originating unilaterally in different regions of the cerebral cortex consistently cross the midline in specific locations. Most of these fibres are found in the corpus callosum. This is true for the interhemispheric fibres of primary motor and somatic sensory cortices, as well as the OCCIPITAL LOBE. At the same time, fibres from certain cortical areas intermingle with fibres coming from other regions. This overlap of callosal trajectories tends to occur between those cortical areas that have contralateral interconnections. A natural corollary of the anatomical studies is that different topographical regions within the FOREBRAIN commissures contain fibres relating to different functional specializations. Somatic sensory motor functions are localized to the central portion of the body of the corpus callosum; the SPLENIUM deals mainly with visual-related functions. Such a view finds support from clinical and experimental evidence indicating that discrete lesions of the forebrain commissures differentially disrupt cortical functions.

The physiological functions of the corpus callosum have been most intensively studied in relation to the VISUAL SYSTEM. Visually responsive cortex in the OCCIPITAL LOBE, TEMPORAL LOBE and PARIETAL LOBE of cat and monkey has been subdivided into several areas, each of which contains a more or less complete and continuous representation of visual space. Whilst the various visual cortical areas receive information chiefly from the contralateral half of the visual field (see VISUAL FIELD) they may in addition, owing to the corpus callosum, be reached by visual information from the ipsilateral hemifield. It has been shown that callosal fibres running between areas 17 and 18 (see BRODMANN'S AREAS) of the two sides are endowed with visual fields on the vertical meridian, and distribute themselves to cortical neurons that are also concerned with the vertical midline of the visual field. Such a pattern of organization appears to apply not only to areas 17 and 18 but to the other visual cortical areas as well. Sperry argued that the visual information carried by the callosal connections and that supplied by the direct input to the cortex are both supplementary, because they make an addition to one another, and complementary, because this mutual addition results in a homogenous whole. The relation of the callosal connections to sensory maps differs for the visual and somesthetic systems. Many physiological studies of the information transmitted between these connections in cats have shown that in the visual modality, of 100 visual receptive fields of the callosal fibres studied, only one lay more than $4°$ from the vertical meridian. In the somesthetic modalities almost 20% of the receptive fields had a distal location on a forepaw. The evidence also supports the hypothesis that the callosal connections of the primary VISUAL CORTEX may intervene in some binocular processes such as binocular STEREOPSIS along the mid sagittal plane, which requires either some overlap along the vertical meridian of the projections from the nasal and temporal hemi-retinae, or a set of interhemispheric connections limited to the vertical meridian representation, or both. Evidence for callosal dependent inhibitory surrounds of excitatory receptive fields lying on the other side of the vertical meridian supports the evidence that callosal influences are compatible only with an uninterrupted visuo-topic representation of the visual space on both sides of the vertical meridian.

Results of extensive studies on patients indicates that in the intact cortex, the corpus callosum exerts a facilitatory, or modulating influence on the neural activity in both hemispheres. Observations of callosotomized patients suggest that callosal section may not only abolish interhemispheric propagation of seizure discharges but may also reduce, or even arrest, abnormal activity in an initial focus. Neurophysiologically almost all callosal fibres are excitatory whilst their functional effects may be either excitatory or inhibitory depending on the nature of the interneurons. It is likely that the normal process of interhemispheric regulation requires a balance between both inhibitory and excitatory influences.

References

Pandya D.N. & Seltzer B. (1986) The topography of commissural fibres. In *Two Hemispheres – One Brain. Functions of the Corpus Callosum*, ed. F. Lepore, M. Ptito & H.H. Jasper, Alan R. Liss: New York.

Sperry R.W. (1964) The great cerebral commissure. *Scientific American* 210: 42–52.

MALCOLM A. JEEVES

corpus striatum The term corpus striatum is not commonly used any longer. It denotes a collection of tissue: the CAUDATE NUCLEUS and the LENTIFORM NUCLEI (these being divided into the GLOBUS PALLIDUS and PUTAMEN). Corpus striatum should not be used as a synonym for STRIATUM, a term which has come to have a rather different usage.

See also: basal ganglia

corresponding retinal points The locations on the two retinae which when stimulated result in the same apparent visual direction in the two eyes.

See also: visual system

DAVID W. HEELEY

Corsi blocks test A neuropsychological test of visuospatial MEMORY for humans: blocks are arranged on a desk. The tester points to a sequence of blocks, which the subject has to reproduce after an interval. The numbers of blocks that a subject can remember (the test having been repeated with increasing numbers of blocks each time) give an indication of their visuospatial memory ability.

cortex From the Latin for bark, the cortex is the outer covering of an organ such as the cerebrum (see CEREBRAL CORTEX), the cerebellum (see CEREBELLAR CORTEX) or organs in the body, such as the ADRENAL GLAND. When neuroscientists use the term cortex without specific reference to a particular structure, it is generally the case that they are referring to the cerebral cortex.

See also: agranular cortex; allocortex; anterior

cingulate cortex; archicortex; association cortex; auditory cortex; barrel cortex (barrel cells); cingulate cortex; cortical layers; cortical development; dorsolateral prefrontal cortex; entorhinal cortex; extrastriate cortex; frontal cortex; gustatory cortex; granular cortex; inferior temporal cortex; infralimbic cortex; insula cortex; isocortex; juxtallocortex; koniocortex; limbic cortex; medial agranular cortex; medial prefrontal cortex; mesocortex; motor cortex; orbitofrontal cortex; neocortex; neocortex ratio; non-primary motor cortex; olfactory cortex; opercular cortex; parahippocampal cortex; paralimbic cortex; parietal cortex; perirhinal cortex; peristriate cortex; piriform cortex; prefrontal cortex; prelimbic cortex; premotor cortex; prestriate cortex; primary motor cortex; primary sensory cortex; primary somatosensory cortex; primary visual cortex; posterior parietal cortex; pyriform cortex; rodent vs. primate prefrontal cortex; secondary somatosensory cortex; sensorimotor cortex; sensory cortex; shoulder cortex; somatosensory cortex; striate cortex; supplementary motor area; supplementary motor cortex; tertiary cortex; ventral orbital cortex; visual cortex; watershed areas of cortex

ERIC M. BOWMAN

cortical blindness A form of BLINDNESS caused by destruction or DENERVATION of the PRIMARY VISUAL CORTEX. Vascular, traumatic, and neoplastic lesions that affect the primary visual cortex (also called STRIATE CORTEX; BRODMANN'S AREA 17; V1) directly or by destroying its afferents, are the most common causes of cortical blindness. As the right visual HEMIFIELDS of both eyes are represented in the LEFT HEMISPHERE, and vice versa, destruction of primary visual cortex in one hemisphere causes a partial cortical blindness restricted to the contralateral visual hemifield, while bilateral destruction causes a complete cortical blindness. The strict TOPOGRAPHY of the representation in V1 accounts for the precise location of the different types of visual field defects that include HEMIANOPIA and QUADRANTANOPIA, with or without MACULAR SPARING, and central, paracentral, or peripheral SCOTOMAS. The extent, position in the field, and density of the defects is assessed with dynamic and/or static PERIMETRY; density refers to the depth or completeness of the visual loss in the defect. While a relative defect allows some residual visual perception, an absolute one is characterized by an absence of all conscious vision. Zones of relative loss often surround absolute scotomata. Even in absolute cortical blindness, unconscious residual visual functions (see BLINDSIGHT) remain.

PETRA STOERIG

cortical blob When stained for the enzyme CYTOCHROME OXIDASE (a marker of neuronal activity) the CEREBRAL CORTEX does not appear uniform, but shows blobs of high activity. In PRIMARY VISUAL CORTEX the response properties of the cells inside the blobs have a circular-surround opponent-colour RECEPTIVE FIELD, whilst those outside (interblob cells) contain orientation selective cells with little colour selectivity. It is believed that the blob and interblob cells may in turn project to differing areas in EXTRASTRIATE CORTEX

ROBERT J. SNOWDEN

cortical colour blindness *see* achromatopsia

cortical column and cortical hypercolumn Many response properties of neurons in the CEREBRAL CORTEX (such as orientation selectivity) show an arrangement such that all cells perpendicular to the cortical surface share the same specificity – this is termed an orientation column. The arrangement of such column is also highly ordered so that neighbouring columns have similar preferences. Hence as one moves tangential to the cortical surface the orientation preference varies slowly and systematically and returns eventually to the orientation preference that one commenced with. This collection of columns that cover all orientations is termed the hypercolumn. Similar arrangements can be found for OCULAR DOMINANCE and directional selectivity in the VISUAL CORTEX.

ROBERT J. SNOWDEN

cortical connection A projection of neurons in the CEREBRAL CORTEX. Cortical connections may be within areas of cortex, between two cortical areas or between areas of cortex and subcortical regions. Cortical neurons are connected locally, making synapses with other neurons within the same CORTICAL COLUMN. Cortical neurons may also give rise to long-

distance projections. Three patterns of long-distance cortico-cortical connection have been distinguished: transcallosal, feedforward and feedback. There are cortical projections to subcortical structures and, in many cases, these connections are bi-directional, such as the feedback connections from cortical areas to the nuclei of the THALAMUS which innervate them.

ERIC M. BOWMAN

cortical deafness Cortical deafness is the impoverished auditory perception resulting from pathology to AUDITORY CORTEX. Depending on the spatial extent and severity of the pathology, the perceptual defect varies from complete unresponsivity to sound, to a putative auditory AGNOSIA in which sounds are detectable but poorly differentiated. In rare instances, the lesion is restricted to the PRIMARY SENSORY CORTEX, and the functional defect is restricted to the perceptual elaboration of brief, closely spaced sounds of the kind required by normal SPEECH PERCEPTION. Cortically deaf listeners are not necessarily aphasic (see APHASIA) but their language processor is deprived of acoustic input.

See also: pure word deafness

DENNIS P. PHILLIPS

cortical development The NEURAL PLATE gives rise to the NEURAL TUBE: the CEREBRAL CORTEX is derived from the walls of the neural tube. It develops in four stages: (1) a VENTRICULAR ZONE appears; (2) the PLEXIFORM PRIMORDIUM (or PREPLATE) develops above this; (3) the INTERMEDIATE ZONE develops between the ventricular zone and preplate; (4) a layered structure emerges, with the ventricular zone at the base, the SUBVENTRICULAR ZONE above this, intermediate zone, SUBPLATE (SUBCORTICAL PLATE), CORTICAL PLATE and marginal zone. Developing neurons move across these layers, guided by RADIAL GLIAL CELLS (a process that has been described as 'riding a glial monorail'). In general the fate of an individual cell is determined late in its lineage, usually around the time of the final MITOSIS. In the developing cerebral cortex neurons retain their original laminar fates when transplanted to a new position just before their last mitosis in the cortex, but change their fates in accordance with this new position if transferred at an earlier stage in their history.

See also: neural migration; neurodevelopment

References

Rosenzweig M.R., Leiman A.L. & Breedlove M.R. (1996) *Biological Psychology*, Sinauer Associates: Sunderland MA.
Uylings H.B.M., Van Eden C.G., Parnavelas J.G. & Kalsbeek A. (1990) The prenatal and postnatal development of rat cerebral cortex. In *The Cerebral Cortex of the Rat*, ed. B. Kolb & R.C. Tees, pp. 35–76, MIT Press: Cambridge MA.

cortical equipotentiality *see* equipotentiality

cortical layers All of the CEREBRAL CORTEX is organized in layers: the NEOCORTEX has six layers, the JUXTALLOCORTEX four or five and the ALLOCORTEX three. The six layers of the neocortex (which makes up about 90% of the cortical mass) have distinct compositions and functions: they are numbered from the outside in. Layer 1 is the outermost layer, immediately below the PIA MATER. It contains relatively few neuronal cell bodies, being made up mostly of GLIAL CELLS and the axons of neurons that run laterally through it. Layers 2 and 3 are associative areas; layer 4 is the input region. Layers 5 and 6 are output layers: layer 5 is the larger, sending output to the BASAL GANGLIA, BRAIN STEM and SPINAL CORD; layer 6 has projections to the THALAMUS. Below layer 6 is WHITE MATTER. Two other important points have to be borne in mind: (1) the thickness of the various layers is different in different parts of the cortex, largely dependent on the function of the particular part of the cortex in question; for example, layer 4 is especially large in sensory areas, layer 5 in motor, (2) the cortical layers are composed of two types of neuron, PYRAMIDAL NEURONS and NON-PYRAMIDAL NEURONS.

See also: agranular cortex; Brodmann's areas; granular cortex

cortical map A representation of functions across a particular area of the CEREBRAL CORTEX; see for example, HOMUNCULUS or AREAS V1–V5 for examples of how functions map onto cortical tissue.

cortical plate *see* cortical development

cortical taste area *see* insula cortex

corticobulbar This describes a direct connection between the CEREBRAL CORTEX and MEDULLA OBLONGATA (see BULBAR).

corticopontine *see* motor system

corticorubral *see* motor system

corticospinal This describes a direct connection between the CEREBRAL CORTEX and SPINAL CORD.

corticospinal tract The corticospinal or pyramidal tract conveys commands for highly skilled voluntary movements from the MOTOR CORTEX to somatic MOTOR NEURONS in the SPINAL CORD that innervate skeletal or voluntary muscles. Most of the fibres cross over to the opposite side in the MEDULLA, so that the motor cortex on one side controls muscles on the opposite side of the body. The crossed fibres descend in the lateral column of the spinal cord, and are referred to as the lateral corticospinal tract. A small minority of the fibres remain uncrossed and descend in the anterior column as the anterior corticospinal tract.

KAZUE SEMBA

corticosteroids A class of HORMONES, including both the GLUCOCORTICOIDS and the MINERALOCORTICOIDS secreted from the ADRENAL GLAND, and the SEX HORMONES (ANDROGENS, ESTROGENS and PROGESTERONE). These sex hormones come into the category of corticosteroids because they are released from the cortex of the adrenal gland (which is of course where the term corticosteroids comes from) but they are more commonly recognized as gonadal steroids – steroids released from the GONADS. Corticosteroids are activated by ADRENOCORTICOTROPIC HORMONE released from the ADENOHYPOPHYSIS; see ENDOCRINE GLANDS; HORMONES – CLASSIFICATION; PREGNANCY; STRESS.

corticosterone A hormone of the GLUCO-CORTICOIDS group.

See also: corticosteroids; endocrine glands; hormones; hormones – classification

corticostriatal *see* motor system

corticostriatal loops Until recently, the STRIA-TUM was seen rather as a funnel for wide-spread neocortical afferents, being a smaller structure than the cortical mantle projecting to it. The striatum appeared to funnel its outflow through the even smaller GLOBUS PALLIDUS to the smaller still motor nuclei of the THALAMUS (ventroanterior and ventrolateral nuclei [VA/VL]) and then to more restricted areas of the FRONTAL CORTEX, including the SUPPLEMENTARY MOTOR AREA. Its functions were seen as predominantly motor and it comprised the major component of what was known as the EXTRAPYRAMIDAL MOTOR SYSTEM. Neuroanatomical data have dramatically altered this view. The fundamental principle of striatal circuitry, namely cortex-to-striatum-to-pallidum-to-thalamus-to-cortex is still appropriate, although striatopallidal outflow also influences a variety of BRAINSTEM structures, such as the PEDUNCULOPONTINE TEGMENTAL NUCLEUS. However, rather than appearing as a funnel, it is now accepted that there exist a series of more or less segregated cortico-striato-pallido-thalamo-cortical loops. The discrete cortical origins and topography of these loops indicates separable functions. For example, the following loops are generally agreed upon: motor loop, oculomotor loop, so-called cognitive loops (at least two) and affective loops (at least two).

Important general points in the organization of these loops are that: (1) the cortical origins are more widespread than the cortical areas of termination of the thalamic projection; (2) quite specific striatal, pallidal and thalamic domains are associated with particular cortical inputs for each loop – hence the notion of segregated loops. For example, the motor loop, which is best understood, originates in the sensory-motor cortex and anterior parietal cortex; it projects in a somatotopic way to the PUTAMEN which in turn projects to discrete portions of the internal pallidal segment/SUBSTANTIA NIGRA pars reticulata and also the external pallidal segment/SUBTHALAMIC NUCLEUS subsidiary loop, all of which retain a somatotopic organization. The outflow from the internal pallidal segment/substantia nigra pars reticulata reaches the ventral anterior and

ventral lateral thalamus, again with somatotopicity preserved and this thalamic nucleus projects back primarily to the supplementary motor area and also to the primary SOMATOSENSORY CORTEX, which is of course itself somatotopically organized. The remarkable feature of this loop circuitry is its precise compartmentalization at each node, leading to the notion of segregated loops. The oculomotor loop involves the FRONTAL EYE FIELDS and supplementary frontal eye fields; the affective loops involve the anterior cingulate cortex and medial orbitofrontal cortex; the cognitive loops involve the dorsolateral and lateral orbital parts of the PREFRONTAL CORTEX. These loops are primarily dependent upon projections to discrete domains of the dorsal striatum, especially the CAUDATE NUCLEUS which in turn, for each loop, projects to specific sub-regions of the globus pallidus and ventral anterior or medial dorsal thalamus. A similar organization has been demonstrated for the ventral striatum, where the cortical origins involve the basolateral AMYGDALA, HIPPOCAMPUS, ANTERIOR CINGULATE CORTEX and PRELIMBIC CORTEX, the striatal node is mainly the NUCLEUS ACCUMBENS and the re-entrant cortical circuitry involves serial relays through the ventral pallidum and DORSOMEDIAL NUCLEUS OF THE THALAMUS, the latter projecting specifically to the prefrontal cortex.

Within this general scheme, there is also considerable fine detail in the organization of the striatum and its outputs and this has helped clarify the way that hypokinetic states arise following the loss of DOPAMINE from the striatum, arising either experimentally or in PARKINSON'S DISEASE. The outflow of the dorsal striatum is now known to be organized in the form of direct and indirect striatal pathways. The direct path consists of projections from the MEDIUM SPINY NEURONS in the striatum to the globus pallidus internal segment (GPi) and the substantia nigra pars reticulata (SNr): these are in essence separate parts of the same structure. They in turn project to the thalamus, SUPERIOR COLLICULUS and pedunculopontine tegmental nucleus. The indirect path consists of projections from striatal medium spiny neurons to the external segment of the globus pallidus (GPe), thence to the subthalamic nucleus (STN) and to the GPi/SNr. Striatal and pallidal neurons are GABAERGIC (that is, they are inhibitory output neurons); the subthalamic nucleus neurons are GLUTAMATERGIC (and therefore excitatory). Thalamic neurons projecting to the cortex and also cortical projections to the striatum are both glutamatergic. It can be seen then that activation of the striatum via excitatory cortical afferents will increase activity in the direct path, so inhibiting GPi/SNr and disinhibiting the excitatory thalamic drive to the cortex. Increasing activity in the indirect path, on the other hand, will disinhibit the STN, increasing the excitatory drive to GPi/SNr, thereby increasing the inhibitory input to the thalamus and so opposing activity in the direct path. However, the NIGROSTRIATAL DOPAMINE SYSTEM powerfully modulates this relationship; dopamine release tends to increase the activity of the direct path, via dopamine D1 receptors (see DI–D5 DOPAMINE RECEPTORS) localized to this population of striatal neurons, but simultaneously also tends to decrease the activity of the indirect path via dopamine D2 receptors localized to this population of striatal neurons. This is the basis of the so-called 'disinhibitory' principle of communication through striatopallidal circuitry and the way that cortical drive to the striatum and its interaction with dopamine reinforces cortical activity subserving movement.

Clearly, it is inappropriate to regard the striatum simply as a motor structure. The striatum has cognitive and affective functions as well, which are dependent upon the specific organization of the segregated corticostriatal loops. While we understand a great deal about the functioning of the motor loop, we know as yet much less about the functions of the other corticostriatal loops, nor how these apparently segregated loops might interact with each other.

BARRY J. EVERITT

corticotectal *see* motor system

corticotropin releasing factor (CRF) This is the same as CORTICOTROPIN RELEASING HORMONE [CRH]). CRF is a HORMONE involved in the control of the release of other hormones (for example adrenocorticotropic hormone

[ACTH]) from the ADENOHYPOPHYSIS (the anterior PITUITARY GLAND). It is found however in a wide variety of places throughout the central nervous system, including the PARAVENTRICULAR NUCLEUS OF THE HYPOTHALAMUS (from where it can control ACTH secretion in the adenohypophysis), the PREOPTIC AREAS, OLFACTORY BULBS, BED NUCLEUS OF THE STRIA TERMINALIS, AMYGDALA (central nucleus), LATERODORSAL TEGMENTAL NUCLEUS, PARABRACHIAL NUCLEI, LOCUS COERULEUS and in other sites in the BRAINSTEM associated with the functions of the AUTONOMIC NERVOUS SYSTEM. There are two different RECEPTOR classes for CRF (CRF$_1$ and CRF$_2$) with the CRF$_2$ receptor being divided further into alpha and beta subtypes: the CRF$_{2\alpha}$ (are found in the brain, CRF$_{2\beta}$ (in other tissues (notably BLOOD and CHOROID PLEXUS). The receptors in the central nervous system are found in a wide variety of sites including CEREBRAL CORTEX, HYPOTHALAMUS, amygdala and SEPTAL NUCLEI, the CRF$_1$ and CRF$_{2\alpha}$ having different distributions. The pattern of distribution of CRF and its receptors indicates clearly that it has NEUROTRANSMITTER functions within the central nervous system in addition to its hormonal actions. It is thought that it is involved in a general coordinating way in responding to stress, mobilizing appropriate processing resources in the central nervous system and physiological responses from peripheral tissues.

corticotropin releasing hormone (CRH) This is the same as CORTICOTROPIN RELEASING FACTOR (CRF).

cortisol A hormone of the GLUCOCORTICOIDS group.

See also: corticosteroids; endocrine glands; hor-mones; hormones – classification

corynanthine An alpha-1 noradrenaline receptor ANTAGONIST; see ADRENOCEPTORS.

cost–benefit analysis A term borrowed from economics, referring to the analysis of market forces. Actions have estimated costs (such as a financial or time investment) and expected outcomes (hopefully, rewards or repayments) and these factors are weighed against each other. Unless the benefits are expected to exceed the costs, the action will be unprofitable and should be rejected. The analysis is often made complex by the fact that the currency of the cost(s) and benefit(s) may not be the same and the exchange rate will vary under different circumstances. In psychology, the concept has been applied in an attempt to understand the processes involved in MOTIVATION. This enterprise has been called behavioural economics.

See also: decision-making

VERITY J. BROWN

cot death *see* sudden infant death syndrome

Cotard syndrome First described by Jules Cotard in 1880, the core of this syndrome is a belief that one is dead. Associated delusions may include the belief that one's body organs are absent or have been turned to stone; that one is immortal; and that one's body is gigantic to a degree way beyond the normal (Cotard described a patient who believed that he could touch the stars) (see DELUSION). It is a rare condition that has been associated with extreme DEPRESSION, though other features are associated with it also, including some of the SIGNS AND SYMPTOMS of SCHIZOPHRENIA. Some studies have associated Cotard syndrome with TEMPORAL LOBE dysfunction, though others have identified FRONTAL and PARIETAL LOBE defects; evidently, its biological basis is obscure.

See also: delusional misidentification

cotransmission An extra dimension in CO-LOCALIZATION: cotransmission is said to occur when two coexistent NEUROTRANSMITTERS are not only present in a NEURON together, but also released simultaneously. An example is the cotransmission of ACETYLCHOLINE and CALCITONIN GENE-RELATED PEPTIDE at the NEUROMUSCULAR JUNCTION.

counter-regulation *see* restrained and unrestrained eating

counterconditioning A conditioning procedure in which the RESPONSE to a STIMULUS is ameliorated or even reversed by associating the stimulus with another UNCONDITIONED STIMULUS that has an opposite effect. For example, the effects of FOOTSHOCK can be reversed by

associating the shock with POSITIVE REINFORCEMENT (food for example).

counterfactual thinking The cognitive process by which people mentally undo an event so that it is envisaged differently and, most often, for the better. Mentally undoing an event may represent an attempt to gain a degree of control over an apparently uncontrollable event. However, where future control is unlikely, counterfactual thinking may contribute to poorer adjustment to traumatic events and may account for the relationship between rumination processes and POST-TRAUMATIC STRESS DISORDER.

MALCOLM D. MacLEOD

courtship *see* animal communication

covariance rule *see* Hebbian synapse

covert attention The allocation of ATTENTION to a location, object or feature of interest, which occurs without overt orientation of the head and/or eyes.

See also: covert orienting; covert recognition; spatial attention

VERITY J. BROWN

covert orienting The movement of SPATIAL ATTENTION to a location of interest. The allocation of attentional resources, being a mental process, is necessarily covert, or unseen. The term covert orienting, however, is used specifically to refer to the allocation of spatial attention when it occurs in the absence of overt orientation of the head and/or eyes.

VERITY J. BROWN

covert recognition The unseen mental process of identification of an object or person. The qualifier, covert, is generally used to refer to the absence of behaviour (that is, an overt response), but it can also refer to RECOGNITION without awareness of the subject.

See also: prosopagnosia

VERITY J. BROWN

CP-93,129 An AGONIST at the $5HT_{1B}$ receptor; see SEROTONIN RECEPTORS.

crack babies *see* drug effects *in utero*

crack cocaine The free base of the alkaloid COCAINE. Cocaine is extracted from the leaves of the coca plant. The initial extraction process results in the alkaloid being converted to cocaine hydrochloride (HCl) salt, which is in crystalline, powdered form. This form is very water soluble and can be administered either orally, intranasally ('snorted'), or injected intravenously. In the 1980s, when the cocaine epidemic was increasing, methods were sought to make cocaine more available, cheaper, and to maximize its psychological effects. Smoking a drug, such as NICOTINE or MARIJUANA, results in greatly increased amounts of the drug getting to the brain, in a rapid amount of time, because the surface area of the lungs is so great. However, cocaine HCl could not be smoked because the active ingredient was destroyed when heated. It was soon discovered that mixing cocaine HCl with some household chemicals such as baking soda, converts cocaine back into its free base. The conversion process results in small lumps of solid, smokable cocaine. These were sold in relatively small amounts, generally enough just for one dose. The availability of crack resulted in a rapid spread of the cocaine epidemic throughout inner-city ghettos and amongst the poor. Although cocaine is the active ingredient in both powdered cocaine and the freebase, because of the intensity of the 'high' that smoking cocaine produces, it is considered much more addictive (see ADDICTION). The rapid, powerful high is very short-lasting and is followed by a 'crash' or depression. Like for cocaine HCl, the main neurochemical mechanism underlying the potent rewarding effects of crack is greatly increased levels of synaptic DOPAMINE.

ANN E. KELLEY

cranial bones *see* skull

cranial cavity *see* skull

cranial nerves The twelve pairs of cranial nerves which originate from the brain are remarkable for their functional diversity. They carry sensory information to the brain from the head and neck, as well as from VISCERA in the neck, thorax and abdomen and are especially significant because of the special senses of smell, vision, taste, hearing and balance. Motor neurons with axons in cranial nerves are responsible for the control of pupil diameter, tear formation, mastication, salivation, swallowing, movements of the facial musculature as well as cardiorespiratory and digestive functions. Collectively, cranial nerves have seven different functional sensory and motor components. These are: the general somatic afferent (GSA), general visceral afferent (GVA), general somatic efferent (GSE), and general visceral efferent (GVE) components that innervate somatic structures (skin and muscle) and viscera (internal organs and glands) and are analogous to the equivalent components found in spinal nerves. In addition, there are three special functional components unique to cranial nerves because of the special senses and structures associated with the branchial (gill) arches. These are the special somatic afferents (SSA) for vision, hearing and balance, the special visceral afferents (SVA) for olfaction and taste, and the special visceral efferents (SVE) for swallowing and phonation.

The following summary emphasizes the major functions and unique features of each cranial nerve. The OLFACTORY NERVE (I; olfaction; SVA) originates in bipolar sensory neurons located in the nasal mucosa of the nasal cavity. Olfactory chemoreceptors are present on the cilia, the distal processes of the bipolar olfactory neurons. The olfactory nerves are made up of numerous bundles of short, unmyelinated axons of the BIPOLAR NEURONS that project centrally to the olfactory bulb. OLFACTION is a very complex sensation and accounts for much of what we experience as taste (see GUSTATION). The OPTIC NERVE (II; vision; SSA) originates in ganglion cells of the RETINA. Optic nerve axons cross entirely or partially depending on the species (50% crossing in humans) at the OPTIC CHIASM and project to the SUPRACHIASMATIC NUCLEUS, LATERAL GENICULATE NUCLEUS, pretectal nucleus and SUPERIOR COLLICULUS. The OCULOMOTOR NERVE (III; eye movements, raising the eyelid, pupillary light reflex, visual accommodation; GSE, GVE) originates in motoneurons of the oculomotor nuclear complex in the MESENCEPHALON and innervates four eye muscles. Preganglionic parasympathetic neurons of the EDINGER–WESTPHAL NUCLEUS also travel in the oculomotor nerve to synapse in the CILIARY GANGLION. The postganglionic axons innervate the pupillary constrictor muscle (part of the iris) and the ciliary muscle. The TROCHLEAR NERVE (IV; superior oblique muscle; GSE) originates from motor neurons of the contralateral trochlear nucleus of the mesencephalon. The trochlear nerve is unusual in that its motor axons decussate completely and it exits dorsally from the BRAINSTEM. The TRIGEMINAL NERVE (V; general sensory for face and head, muscles of mastication, proprioception; GSA, GVE) has three major sensory branches (ophthalmic, maxillary, mandibular) supplying corresponding areas of the face. The central axons of the sensory neurons project to the principal and spinal trigeminal sensory nuclei of the hindbrain and upper cervical spinal cord. Proprioceptive axons for the muscles of mastication originate from the mesencephalic nucleus of the trigeminal nerve. The motor root of the trigeminal nerve originates in the motor trigeminal nucleus in the PONS and innervates the muscles of mastication. The ABDUCENS NERVE (VI; lateral rectus muscle; GSE) originates in motor neurons of the abducens nucleus in the pons. The FACIAL NERVE (VII; muscles of facial expression, stapedius muscle, digastric muscle, stylohyoid muscle, SVE; taste to anterior two-thirds of the tongue, SVA; salivation, tears, GVE) leaves the intracranial region through the internal acoustic meatus to travel in the facial canal in the skull. Special visceral efferent motor neurons for the muscles of facial expression originate in the facial nucleus. Parasympathetic preganglionic neurons are found in the superior salivatory nucleus. The somata of sensory neurons, primarily for taste sensations from the anterior two-thirds of the tongue, are found in the geniculate ganglion of the facial canal. Their distal processes form the chorda tympani nerve. The VESTIBULOCOCHLEAR NERVE (VIII; balance, hearing; SSA) also leaves the skull via the internal acoustic meatus. The vestibular component carries sensory information from specialized receptors in the inner ear to the vestibular complex of the lower pons and upper medulla. The auditory component carries sensory information from hair cells in the cochlea to the cochlear nuclei of the pons. The

GLOSSOPHARYNGEAL NERVE (IX; swallowing, salivation, taste, upper airway sensation, carotid sinus and carotid body pressor and chemoreceptors, SVE, GVE, SVA, GVA, GSA) has a motor component projecting from the nucleus ambiguus to the stylopharyngeus muscle and sensory neurons that transmit baroreceptor and chemoreceptor information from the carotid artery, general sensory input from the oropharynx, and taste from the posterior one-third of the tongue to the nucleus of the tractus solitarius. The VAGUS NERVE (X; swallowing, respiration, secretomotor, cardiomotor, taste, SVE, GVE, GVA, SVA) is widely distributed in the neck, thorax and abdomen. SVE motor neurons innervate muscles of the pharynx, larynx and esophagus. General visceral efferent motor neurons supply secretomotor axons to the stomach, small intestine and pancreas. Cardiomotor neurons project to parasympathetic ganglia on the heart. The ACCESSORY NERVE (XI; swallowing, head and shoulder movements, SVE) has cranial and spinal roots that innervate pharyngeal muscles via branches of the vagus and the sternocleidomastoid and trapezius muscles via the spinal accessory nerve. The HYPOGLOSSAL NERVE (XII; tongue movements; GSE) supplies intrinsic and extrinsic tongue muscles.

DAVID A. HOPKINS

cranium (from Greek, *kranion*: the skull) The cranium is the SKULL; cranial is the adjective used in reference to this.

craving A term used in the fields of MOTIVATION and drug ADDICTION to denote a state of strong desire to obtain a REINFORCEMENT, such as a drug. In clinical psychiatry, the term has been used to described drug craving in addiction (or alcohol in ALCOHOLISM), as well as craving for certain kinds of foods. For example in BULIMIA NERVOSA, patients will often describe uncontrollable cravings for CARBOHYDRATES, FATS and sweet things. In SEASONAL AFFECTIVE DISORDER, carbohydrate craving has been described. In addiction, the term has been used in attempts to understand the motivational or emotional states associated with drug-seeking behaviour. It is believed that increased DRUG CRAVING, even in long-abstinent individuals, is an important factor in relapse to drug use.

See also: priming

ANN E. KELLEY

Creese–Iversen scale A scale developed by Ian Creese and Susan Iversen, used to rate STEREOTYPY (stereotyped behaviour) in rodents. The original scale, modified by later authors to suit their particular purposes, was as shown in the table.

This scale was widely used, and still retains considerable power as a shorthand description of the stereotyped behaviour induced by drugs such as AMPHETAMINE and APOMORPHINE that stimulate activity in DOPAMINE systems. There are though some difficulties with the scale. (1) It is not continuous. Amphetamine given by SYSTEMIC INJECTION has never been shown to induce licking or gnawing in a normal rat, though apomorphine has. Ratings of 5 or 6 therefore are of less value when studying the effects of amphetamine. (2) The ratings are often treated as if they were other than nominal data, but the numbers 0–6 here could be effectively substituted by the letters A through G with no loss of descriptive power. Creese–Iversen data have to be analysed by frequency counts (that is, how many instances of a particular score were there) rather than by taking means or medians. (3) The scale requires one to categorize a behaviour as stereotyped rather than the stereotyped nature of the activity emerging from the description. This is in contrast to what happens when one uses a BEHAVIOURAL CHECKLIST, in which abnormal frequencies of the occurrence of specific acts can lead one to describe a behaviour as stereotyped without prejudging the issue.

References

Creese I. & Iversen S.D. (1975) The pharmacological and anatomical substrates of the amphetamine response in the rat. *Brain Research* 83: 419–436.

Fray P.J., Sahakian B.J., Robbins T.W., Koob G.F. & Iversen S.D. (1980) An observational method for quantifying the behavioural effects of dopamine agonists: contrasting effects of *d*-amphetamine and apomorphine. *Psychopharmacology* 69: 253–259.

crepuscular (from Latin, *crepusculum*: dusky or obscure) Relating to dawn and dusk. A crepuscular animal is one that is most active during twilight.

See also: diurnal; nocturnal

cresyl violet A common histological stain used to show the presence of Nissl substance, which is present in all the cells of the nervous system.

See also: histology

cretinism An obsolete term for CONGENITAL HYPOTHYROIDISM; it should not be used.

Creutzfeldt–Jakob disease (CJD) A fatal neurodegenerative PRION DISEASE of later middle age affecting about 1 person per million population per year world-wide. Symptoms consist of a very rapidly progressive DEMENTIA with some involuntary movements. Neuropathological examination of the brain after death reveals a SPONGIFORM ENCEPHALOPATHY. About 85% of cases of CJD are sporadic in that they occur without any known antecedent events and with no family history. About 15% of cases of human prion disease

The Creese-Iversen scale

0	asleep or stationary
1	active
2	predominantly active but with burst of stereotyped sniffing or rearing
3	stereotyped activity such as sniffing along a fixed path in the cage
4	stereotyped sniffing or rearing maintained in one location
5	stereotyped behaviour in one location with bursts of licking
6	continual gnawing or licking of the cage bars

occur in an AUTOSOMAL DOMINANT pattern in association with mutations in the gene which codes for the prion protein. Different mutations produce slightly different variants of prion disease known as familial CJD, Gerstmann–Straüssler–Scheinker disease, fatal familial INSOMNIA, and atypical prion disease. CJD can also be acquired by contamination with the abnormal form of prion protein from an exogenous source. Contamination during neurosurgery, particularly where DURA MATER grafts made from human MENINGES were used, has caused more than 100 cases and the use of contaminated human pituitary-derived GROWTH HORMONE has been responsible for many cases of CJD. A sporadic case of CJD early in this century is thought to have started the epidemic of about 2550 cases of a prion disease called KURU amongst the Foré people of Papua New Guinea which was spread by ritual cannibalism. The time between contamination and onset of illness in humans ranges from 18 months, following intracerebral contamination with affected brain material, to 4–40 years following oral contamination. It is supposed that a new variant of CJD seen in Britain from 1994 onwards is related to consumption of beef products made from cattle affected with BOVINE SPONGIFORM ENCEPHALOPATHY. It is not possible to predict at present whether many people will be affected by the new variant of CJD. SCRAPIE is not believed to cause CJD in humans.

Reference

Baker H.F. & Ridley, R.M. (1992) The genetics and transmissibility of spongiform encephalopathy. *Neurodegeneration* 1: 3–16.

ROSALIND RIDLEY

crib death *see* sudden infant death syndrome

cribriform plate A bone at the anterior portion of the base of the brain on which the OLFACTORY BULB sits. The sensory neurons of the OLFACTORY EPITHELIUM send their axons through the cribriform plate to synapse on the OLFACTORY GLOMERULI of the MITRAL CELLS, which are in the olfactory bulb immediately above the cribriform plate (see OLFACTION).

critical flicker fusion A task thought to measure AROUSAL or to index in some way overall activity of the CENTRAL NERVOUS SYSTEM. Subjects are shown a flickering light, the frequency of which is slowly increased. Subjects have to report the point at which the flicker disappears and the light instead appears constant. What the critical flicker (that is the highest flicker rate that is perceived as flicker, not constant) is thought to indicate is the maximum number of bits of information that can be centrally processed by the VISUAL SYSTEM, and this is thought to represent overall brain state or arousal. (Note well though that arousal is a difficult concept to investigate and should be treated with care.) It has been used to investigate the effects of different types of DRUG – NICOTINE for example – on brain activity in humans.

Reference

Feldman R., Meyer J.S. & Quenzer L.F. (1997) *Principles of Neuropsychopharmacology*, Sinauer Associates: Sunderland MA.

critical period A biologically determined, specific and fixed period of time, generally early in ONTOGENY, during which some aspect of an organism's neural functioning (and related behavioural competence) is influenced by specific environmental factors. There are constraints on the nature of the environmental input that can modify or influence the organism, and strictly speaking, the beginning, end and length of this window of time are invariant (that is, they cannot be shifted by any developmental circumstances). If the period is missed, the neural circuitry and related competence fail to develop normally, with little or no possibility of later reversal.

See also: sensitive period

RICHARD C. TEES

Crocker–Henderson scale *see* olfactory prism

cross bridges *see* muscles

cross maze *see* plus maze

cross-modal conflict; cross-modal matching; cross-modal transfer Cross-modal tests involve examining stimuli across sensory dimensions. Cross-modal conflict occurs when related information is presented in two sensory dimensions, with slowed or distorted perception resulting; for examples, see McGURK EFFECT and STROOP EFFECT and see also INTERFERENCE. Cross-modal matching is a scaling technique used in sensory psychophysics in which subjects match the intensity of a stimulus in one sensory dimension with the intensity of a stimulus in another dimension. The assignment of arbitrary numerical values to stimulus intensity is of limited value. However, if subjects are asked to rate one stimulus in terms of another – the loudness of a sound gauged by grip force for example – it is possible to derive power functions that allow one to scale stimulus properties with a relatively high degree of accuracy. Cross-modal transfer can be used to examine subjects' ability to relate information across sensory dimensions by having them, for example, touch various sized objects (wood blocks for example) while blindfolded, before attempting to recognize them by sight.

See also: psychophysics

cross-sensitization A drug may be given repeatedly such that SENSITIZATION to it develops. It can then be the case that a second drug also shows sensitization, despite it not having been given before. (One would know that tolerance had developed because a significantly lower amount of the drug than expected would have to be given to produce an effect.) The second drug has shown the effect of cross-sensitization.

See also: cross-tolerance

cross-tolerance A drug may be given repeatedly such that TOLERANCE to it develops. It can then be the case that a second drug also shows tolerance, despite it not having been given before. (One would know that tolerance had developed because a significantly higher amount of the drug than expected would have to be given to produce an effect.) The second drug has shown the effect of cross-tolerance.

See also: cross-sensitization

Reference

Feldman R., Meyer J.S. & Quenzer L.F. (1997) *Principles of Neuropsychopharmacology*, Sinauer Associates: Sunderland MA.

crossed disparity *see* retinal disparity

crus cerebri *see* cerebral peduncles

cryode *see* transient lesions

cryolesion *see* transient lesions

cryopreservation (from Greek, *kryos*: frost) Preserving living cells and vital fluids by freezing; see TRANSPLANTATION.

cryoprotectant *see* fixation

cryostat A cryostat is a MICROTOME enclosed in a temperature-controlled cabinet which can be kept cold.

cue In psychology the term cue refers to any STIMULUS that can guide behaviour or provide information; for examples, see CONDITIONED CUE PREFERENCE; CUE COMBINATION; CUED RECALL; DISCRIMINATIVE CUE; EXTINCTION CUE; PHONEMIC CUEING; REACTION TIME.

cue combination This refers to the process in perception (see SENSATION VS. PERCEPTION) by which individual cues can be combined to give an overall representation of the world, and most especially of depth (see CUE; DEPTH PERCEPTION). Different descriptions of this have been presented, referred to as *weak* or *strong fusion* accounts: weak fusion accounts suggest that individual cues are considered in isolation and then averaged; strong fusion accounts induce that the most probable account is extracted by the CENTRAL NERVOUS SYSTEM. Landy and his colleagues have suggested that neither of these provides the best account and have proposed a *modified weak fusion* account of cue combination in which one cue is able to interact with another to generate information.

References

Landy M.S., Maloney L.T., Johnston E.B. & Young M. (1995) Measurement and modeling of depth cue combination – in defense of weak fusion. *Vision Research* 35: 389–412.

cue conditioning *see* place conditioning

cued choice reaction time *see* reaction time

cued recall Procedure used in humans to examine the ability to RECALL from MEMORY previously encountered items, with RETRIEVAL cues provided. It is a memory task that differs from others such as FREE RECALL and SERIAL RECALL.

See also: declarative memory; episodic memory; explicit memory; recognition; transfer appropriate processing

culture, human Culture as a construct in BIOLOGICAL PSYCHOLOGY might appear to be a rather odd notion. Culture in human terms is difficult precisely to define, but is taken to refer to both the tangible achievements of human societies, as well as the values, attitudes and beliefs that inform those societies. In human societies culture is evidenced by such things as architecture, literature, music and the visual arts. The values that inform such activities are drawn principally from theology and philosophy, including such things as political theory, philosophy of science, moral philosophy and the study of aesthetics. Culture is an inclusive term that collects all of these things together. Problems appear when one begins to compare cultures. Is it possible to describe in the same terms, the cultures of, for instance, Europe or China, with the cultures of the indigenous peoples of Amazonia or New Guinea? Then comes the even more difficult question: do animals other than humans posses cultures? Comparisons of human societies, one with another, do make sense. Though often difficult to describe without seeming patronizing, there are common threads in culture which seem to unite all peoples. But is it possible to describe cultures in other animals without either torturing the definition of culture or reducing human culture to a degree that is both simplistic and demeaning?

It is the notion of 'other animals' that makes the idea of culture of interest to biologists: humans *are* animals, and have been subjected to the pressures of NATURAL SELECTION during the course of EVOLUTION as has every other species. Can the origins of human culture be found in other animals, most notably PRIMATES? The answer appears to be yes, but in order to make this claim it is necessary to use a definition of culture that is, at best, minimalist. Culture defined as *'the non-genetic transmission of habits'* (de Waal, 1999) does exist in chimpanzee societies. Analysis of behaviour patterns in chimpanzee groups at various African sites has revealed quite remarkable variations in behaviours that have been (and, indeed, are being) acquired and transmitted through social groups, establishing patterns of behaviour that are unique to the groups in which they have originated (see Whiten *et al.*, 1999). Indeed, one might go further and predict that in any species that shows SOCIAL BEHAVIOUR and is capable of OBSERVATION LEARNING and the formation of HABITS, forms of culture might be apparent as patterns of behaviour that are acquired and transmitted across generations.

This use of the term culture in biological psychology will remain contentious. So much depends on the definition of culture that is used, and because, in terms of human societies, culture is so difficult precisely to define, it opens the door to those who wish to propose a lowest-common-denominator definition. *The non-genetic transmission of habits* might be sufficient when describing chimpanzee behaviour, but is this really a satisfactory definition to use when describing human societies? Such a definition hardly seems able to account for the development of systematic theologies or philosophies, or the development of rarefied theories of aesthetics, and would be a curious way of describing the achievements of, say, Italian Renaissance artists or the builders of the great Egyptian pyramids. Are these all best described as the non-genetic transmission of habits? Or should the definition of human culture relate not simply to the development of actions that improve biological success (see FITNESS) but to more abstract conceptions to do with the formulation of values and beliefs? Engaging in such arguments about cultural definitions and differences invariably brings the charge from primatologists that the goalposts are being moved to prevent primate culture from being recognized for what it is. There is some justification for primatologists taking this line. Clearly, primate societies do have patterns of behaviour that can be described as forming a culture. But even if one accepts the lowest common denominator definition – *the non-genetic transmission of habits* – as being acceptable in covering culture in all species, there has to be a recognition of the immense gulf between humans and all other animals. To do otherwise is plain silly.

See also: evolutionary psychology; socio-biology

References

de Waal F.B.M. (1999) Cultural primatology comes of age. *Nature* 399: 635–636.
Whiten A., Goodall J., McGrew W.C., Nishida T., Reynolds V., Sugiyama Y., Tutin C.E.G., Wrangham R.W. & Boesch C. (1999) Culture in chimpanzees. *Nature* 399: 682–685.

culture, laboratory science A culture is a collection of cells or microorganisms grown *in vitro* in a laboratory; to culture refers to the process of growing a culture.

See also: tissue culture

cuneate nucleus One of the DORSAL COLUMN NUCLEI OF THE MEDULLA OBLONGATA (the GRACILE NUCLEUS is the other) which receives sensory fibres from the DORSAL FUNICULUS of the SPINAL CORD carrying sensations of fine, discriminative TOUCH and vibration.

cuneate region of the occipital lobe A part of the OCCIPITAL LOBE, on its medial wall (that is within the LONGITUDINAL FISSURE); it is one of the regions of the CEREBRAL CORTEX that, in the RIGHT HEMISPHERE, is larger in females than in males (see SEX DIFFERENCES).

cuneiform nucleus The cuneiform nucleus is a nucleus in the dorsal MIDBRAIN TEGMENTUM located lateral to the central GREY MATTER, ventral to the SUPERIOR COLLICULUS, dorsal to the SUPERIOR CEREBELLAR PEDUNCLE, and dorsal and posterior to the PEDUNCULOPON-TINE TEGMENTAL NUCLEUS. Like other nuclei in the RETICULAR FORMATION, the cuneiform nucleus has extensive ascending and descending projections. Electrical and chemical stimulation of the cuneiform nucleus elicits LOCOMOTION as well as jumping, rearing, and elements of defensive (see DEFENCE) behaviour in cats and rats. It may be part of the so-called MESENCEPHALIC LOCOMOTOR REGION.

KAZUE SEMBA

cupola *see* vestibular system

curare A poison from the tropical plant *Chondrodendron tomentosum*, used by South American Indians to immobilize prey. The active ingredient D-tubocurarine, is an AN-TAGONIST at NICOTINIC ACETYLCHOLINE RECEPTORS, especially at the NEUROMUSCULAR JUNCTION. Curarization – the process of administering curare – is used on occasion in certain clinical procedures in which muscular relaxation is required. Synthetic forms of curare (such as GALLAMINE, PANCURONIUM or DIHYDRO-BETA-ERYTHROIDINE) are used in these clinical conditions. The effects of curare (curarization) can be reversed by administration of ACETYLCHOLINESTERASE inhibitors such as NEOSTIGMINE.

current *see* voltage clamp

current clamp *see* voltage clamp

Cushing's disease The term is properly restricted to those cases of Cushing's syndrome that result from excess secretion of ADRENOCORTICOTROPIC HORMONE (ACTH) by a growth (adenoma) of the anterior PITUITARY GLAND. Excess ACTH leads in turn to overproduction of adrenal CORTICOSTEROIDS. The syndrome may also result from a primary growth in the adrenal gland itself, or from medication. Clinical features include darkening and thinning of the skin, OBESITY especially of the trunk, and muscular wasting, giving the patient an 'orange on matchsticks' appearance. Complications include diabetes, osteoporosis and psychotic DEPRESSION. Treatment may involve surgery or irradiation of the pituitary, or the administration of adrenolytic drugs, such as metyrapone.

L. JACOB HERBERG

cutaneous nerves *see* somatosensory pathways

cutaneous sensation *see* skin; touch

cyclic AMP *see* second messengers

cyclic GMP *see* second messengers

cyclic nucleotide There are two cyclic nucleotides of special interest to neuroscientists: CYCLIC AMP and CYCLIC GMP. These act as SECOND MESSENGERS. The generic term cyclic nucleotide describes a compound that has two properties. First, it is cyclic: it is a closed chain of atoms. If these are all carbon it would be a carbocyclic compound; if carbon and other atoms, it would be a heterocyclic compound. Second, it is a nucleotide: that is, it is a nucleoside with an attached phosphate group (nucleosides being sugar molecules – deoxyribose or ribose – with a purine or pyrimidine base attached). Nucleotides are the individual parts of nucleic acids.

cyclothymic disorder A chronic MOOD disorder with frequent bouts of DEPRESSION and HYPOMANIA. These can be intermixed with periods of normal mood lasting several months. When depressed, cyclothymic patients suffer feelings of inadequacy, becoming socially isolated; they sleep more than usual and become dull. When hypomanic, sufferers have an exaggerated self-esteem and sociability; they tend to INSOMNIA and their previous dullness is replaced by creativity. It is possible to regard a cyclothymic mood disorder as a minor version of the MANIC DEPRESSION.

See also: dysphoria; dysthymic disorder; euphoria

cyproheptadine A drug that is an ANTAGONIST at SEROTONIN RECEPTORS: it has been used as an APPETITE stimulant (see EATING DISORDERS).

cytoarchitecture (from Greek, *kytos*: vessel, and architecture; *cyto-* is a prefix denoting 'CELL'). The measurement of variation in the size and density of cells can be examined (see HISTOLOGY) and these measures used to identify cellular groupings in the brain, thus delineating nuclei by their cytoarchitecture – that is, the cells from which structures are built helps define those structures. Cytoarchitectonics is the process of doing this (see NEUROANATOMY).

cytochrome oxidase Cytochrome oxidase is an enzyme, expression of which can be taken as an index of metabolic activity (see METABOLIC MAPPING). Cytochrome oxidase is found in mitochondria, being involved in the synthesis of ADENOSINE TRIPHOSPHATE (ATP) – remarkably, the reaction involving cytochrome oxidase in ATP formation accounts for more than 90% of oxygen consumption by animals. Cytochrome oxidase activity is in fact the RATE-LIMITING STEP in ATP production. Because of its close association with ATP production, the amount of cytochrome oxidase present in a cell correlates well with the activity of that cell. As such, in brain it can be used as a marker of neuronal activity: more active neurons show a higher degree of cytochrome oxidase activity than inactive neurons. A straightforward histochemical method (see HISTOCHEMISTRY) allows one to visualize cytochrome oxidase in *post mortem* tissue.

Reference

Wong-Riley M.T.T. (1979) Changes in the visual system of monocularly sutured or enucleated cats demonstrable with cytochrome oxidase histochemistry. *Brain Research* 171: 11–28.

cytokine (from Greek, *kytos*: vessel (*cyto-* is a prefix denoting 'CELL') and *kineein*: to move) Cytokines are proteins involved in the actions of the IMMUNE SYSTEM, serving as important signals between cells (and released most notably by helper T CELLS). INTERLEUKIN, INTERFERON, LYMPHOTOXIN and TUMOUR NECROSIS FACTOR are all examples of cytokines.

cytomegalovirus One of any of the family of *Herpes* viruses, including *Herpes simplex* (type I causes cold sores, type II genital sores), *Herpes zoster* (which causes chicken pox) and HERPES ENCEPHALITIS, which infects the CENTRAL NERVOUS SYSTEM. All herpes viruses have a double strand of DNA. The cytomegaloviruses cause cells to swell dramatically.

cytoplasm The term cytoplasm refers to the region between a cell NUCLEUS and the cell MEMBRANE: it consists of CYTOSOL, a semi-liquid fluid in which are suspended various subcellular organelles, such as the ENDOPLASMIC RETICULUM and, in a NEURON, SYNAPTIC VESICLES.

See also: axoplasm; cell

cytoplasmic determinants *see* development

cytosine A nucleotide; see DNA.

cytoskeleton Neurons, like other cells, are not simply formless bags of CYTOPLASM: they have a structure provided by the cytoskeleton – literally, the cell skeleton. The cytoskeletons of neurons have three principal components. MICROFILAMENTS are thin fibres made of two strands of the protein actin. Microfilaments are the most delicate element of the cytoskeleton and are found mostly lining the internal walls of membranes, helping maintain the positions of membrane-bound molecules (receptors, for instance). NEUROFILAMENTS are larger than microfilaments and provide general structural support. MICROTUBULES are hollow tubes formed by thirteen filaments made of the protein TUBULIN. Microtubules are involved in the transport of substances through the AXO-PLASM. Alterations to the neuronal cytoskeleton have been thought to play a part in the process of LONG-TERM POTENTIATION.

cytosol *see* cytoplasm

D

D1–D5 dopamine receptors The different subtypes of DOPAMINE (DA) receptors. Receptors for the neurotransmitter dopamine have several forms, which differ in molecular structure and conformation and in affinities for various dopaminergic drugs. There are two families of DA receptors, the D1 family and the D2 family, named for the two original subtypes characterized. D1 subtypes include D1 and D5 receptors, which are primarily defined by their ability to activate ADENYLATE CYCLASE via a membrane-bound G PROTEIN linked to the receptor. D2-like subtypes include D2, D3, and D4; these subtypes inhibit adenylate cyclase formation via coupling to an inhibitory G protein. Most DA receptors subtypes are found in abundance in regions where dopamine is found, such as the STRIATUM, NUCLEUS ACCUMBENS, and MIDBRAIN. Compounds that are selective agonists or antagonists for various receptor subtypes are useful in elucidating their functions. It is believed that both subtype families are important in dopaminergic transmission.

See also: antipsychotic; dopamine hypothesis of schizophrenia

ANN E. KELLEY

Dale's principle A key concept in neurobiology identified by Dale (1875–1968) was that the metabolic unity of a NEURON extends to all processes, including the release of a common messenger. A generalization of this concept was formulated by Eccles on the basis of his work on the recurrent inhibition of MOTOR NEURONS. Converging Dale's and Eccles's important insights, the modern version of Dale's principle states that a neuron releases the same set of NEUROTRANSMITTERS from all of its axon terminals.

References

Dale C.B.E. (1935) Pharmacology and nerve-endings. *Proceedings of the Royal Society of Medicine* 28: 319–322.
Eccles J.C. (1957) *Physiology of Nerve Cells*, Johns Hopkins University Press: Baltimore.

KAZUE SEMBA

Daltonism *see* dichromatic colour blindness

Dandy's symptom *see* oscillopsia

darkfield *see* light microscopy

data based memory The data based memory system is proposed to encode incoming information about the observer's present environment. It emphasizes facts and events that are usually personal in nature and occur within specific external and internal environmental contexts. The system is concerned only with SHORT-TERM MEMORY or INTERMEDIATE-TERM MEMORY storage. Memories are organized according to their space, time, sensory-perception, response, language, and affect attributes. The data based memory system often works in conjunction with the EXPECTANCY BASED MEMORY system, although these systems are independent of one another.

See also: declarative memory; episodic memory; explicit memory; memory

HOWARD EICHENBAUM

day blindness *see* night blindness

De Groot orientation *see* stereotaxic surgery

dead reckoning A form of NAVIGATION without reference to landmarks: position in space is determined with reference to the time that has been spent travelling and the direction of travel. Such information should be sufficient for navigation, and is used often by humans in piloting aircraft and ships. It would seem to be a complex calculation, but in fact many species (possibly most or even all) are capable of it. Birds can, and indeed one might expect all vertebrates to be able to accomplish dead reckoning, with their ample brains and a need to forage (see FORAGING) for food, often at night, or engage in MIGRATION. However, invertebrates do it: both bees and ants have been shown to be able to do so. This implies that dead reckoning is a computation that can be made by relatively small networks of neurons.

See also: path integration; spatial behaviour

Reference

Pearce J.M. (1997) *Animal Learning and Cognition: An Introduction*, 2nd edn, Psychology Press: Hove UK.

deaf hearing An auditory equivalent to the phenomenon of BLINDSIGHT (see CONSCIOUSNESS).

deafferent To DEAFFERENT a structure is to remove its neuronal inputs (that is, the neurons that are AFFERENT to that structure); deafferentation is the process of doing this; deafferented describes the condition of it having been done. Deafferentation can be achieved by destroying neurons whole or by cutting fibres. For example, if one was to LESION completely a structure, then all the other structures to which the lesioned one normally sends axons to would be (in whole or partially) deafferented. Alternatively, if one made a knife cut lesion just outside a structure, one would sever axons going to that structure without necessarily killing all the neurons to which those axons belonged.

deafness Deafness is the lack of appropriate perceptual or behavioural responsivity to sound that results from pathology to the peripheral or central auditory systems. When the pathology is restricted to the external or middle ears, the hearing loss is termed conductive, reflecting the impoverished conduction of acoustic vibrations to the COCHLEA. When the pathology is restricted to the cochlea, the hearing loss is termed sensorineural, reflecting the impoverished nature of SENSORY TRANSDUCTION, and the impaired transmission of sensory information to the brain. When the pathology lies in the central nervous system, the deafness is usually referred to as central. In all of these cases, the deafness may be more or less severe, depending on the nature or extent of the pathology.

In conductive hearing loss, the essential problem is a failure to deliver appropriate signal amplitudes to the cochlea. Depending on the nature of the pathology (for example, blocked external ear canal, ossicles stiffened by bony adhesions, the middle ear cavity filled with fluids) the impoverished signal amplitudes may be more marked for low or high sound frequencies. In either case, however, since the problem resides in an abnormally low sound amplitude reaching the cochlea, it can often be overcome with appropriate amplification, or by surgical intervention to restore normal sound transmission. In sensorineural or cochlear hearing loss, the essential problem is often pathology to the outer hair cell system (see HEARING THEORIES). In practice, this pathology may reflect predominantly high or low frequencies or the whole frequency range. Pathology of the OUTER HAIR CELLS system at any site results in BASILAR MEMBRANE motion at that site being less sensitive to stimulation, and more broadly tuned to sound frequency than normal. This has two consequences. The first is that the basilar membrane motion to be transduced by the INNER HAIR CELLS has an unusually low amplitude, with the result that the listener has poorer than normal (that is, elevated) sound detection thresholds at the affected frequencies. The second consequence of impaired outer hair cell function is that the ability of the cochlea to execute its normal spectral decomposition is also impaired. This means that there is a poorer than normal mapping of the sound spectrum onto the COCHLEAR NERVE array. The result of this is that fine peaks and valleys in the sound's spectrum are poorly resolved by the cochlea, and so the brain has an impoverished substrate on which to operate. This 'spectral smearing' is exacerbated by the presence of background noise, and can be particularly debilitating to SPEECH PERCEPTION if the hearing loss is in the range required for the discrimination of the consonants. Quite often, sensorineural hearing loss is restricted to relatively high frequencies (such as noise trauma, PRESBYACUSIS). Studies have revealed that normal, low-frequency hearing has inherently poor temporal resolution. Thus, a patient with a high-frequency hearing loss has the disadvantage of pathologically poor spectral resolution at high frequencies, and inherently poor temporal resolution at low ones. Outer hair cell loss is usually permanent. Peripheral amplification can overcome the sensitivity loss of the impaired cochlear transducer, but does not aid the impaired spectral resolution. In some post-lingually deaf patients, it is possible to employ a cochlear implant to bypass the middle ear and transduction process, and to stimulate the surviving cochlear nerve array directly. This device receives the acoustic signal, performs a partial spectral decomposition of it, and then sends appropriate electrical signals to the relevant sectors of the cochlear nerve array.

Central deafness is more complicated and heterogeneous because of the greater structural complexity of the anatomy, the diversity of function ascribed to it, and the individuality of the pathological processes and their loci. Thus, it is quite possible for a human or animal listener to have normal sound detection thresholds, but be poor at SOUND LOCALIZATION. Even in the case of LESION to the cortical auditory system alone (see AUDITORY CORTEX), variations in the size and site of the lesion may produce behavioural consequences as broad as complete unresponsivity to sound (CORTICAL DEAFNESS) or as narrow as a putative PURE WORD DEAFNESS (see Phillips, 1995). Central auditory disorders are difficult to treat medically but, at least in some children, hope may lie in explicit training in the perceptual discriminations that may be the source of higher-level problems (such as delayed language development; see Tallal et al., 1996).

References

Phillips D.P. (1995) Central auditory processing. A view from auditory neuroscience. *American Journal of Otology* 16: 338–352.
Tallal P., Miller S.L., Bedi G., Byma G., Wang X., Nagarajan S.S., Schreiner C., Jenkins W.M. & Merzenich M.M. (1996) Language comprehension in language-learning impaired children improved with acoustically-modified speech. *Science* 271: 81–84.

DENNIS P. PHILLIPS

decarboxylase A decarboxylase is an ENZYME that removes a MOLECULE of CARBON DIOXIDE (CO_2) from a carboxylic group – for example, from one of the AMINO ACIDS, converting it to an amide. The term decarboxylation describes this process. Decarboxylation is a ubiquitous process and account has to be taken of it. For example, when L-DOPA was first used as a treatment for PARKINSON'S DISEASE, large amounts of the drug were found to be required in order to achieve therapeutic benefit. However, it transpired that much of the administered L-DOPA was being decarboxylated in the periphery, before it could get to the CENTRAL NERVOUS SYSTEM. To combat this, a peripheral decarboxylase inhibitor is given.

decerebrate An animal that has had the CEREBRUM removed or made inoperative by disconnection is said to be decerebrate. It is not a procedure often used, being a very crude form of LESION. It is of interest to note though that rats that have been decerebrated are not incapable of action. Decerebration may reveal unexpected abilities of SUBCORTICAL tissue. For example, decerebrate rats eat and drink, and have sufficient skill (see SKILL LEARNING) and MOTIVATION to be able successfully to engage in SEXUAL BEHAVIOUR.

See also: cerveau isolé; decortication

decerebrate rigidity *see* rigidity

deci- Prefix indicating a factor of 10^{-1}, or one tenth; see SI UNITS.

decibel (dB) A unit of physical intensity most commonly applied to sound stimuli though it can also be used to describe the intensity of other physical stimuli, such as light. A bel (named after Alexander Graham Bell, the inventor of the telephone, though abbreviated) represents a tenfold increase in intensity. For example, if one STIMULUS was a million times more intense than another (that is, 10^6 times greater) it would be 6 bel greater. In practice, one uses tenths of bels to make the scale practical, so the standard unit of intensity is not a *bel* but a *decibel*. In AUDITORY PERCEPTION, the threshold of hearing is 0 dB; conversation normally takes place at about 80 dB; and stimuli of around 140 dB cause PAIN.

See also: psychophysics

decision-making In everyday situations, individuals are required to make choices between actions with respect to current behavioural goals, and in the context of information relating to the existing contingencies between particular actions and relevant outcomes. An important project for biological psychology is to specify and describe the neural bases of the psychological processes that allow such choices to be made.

Traditionally, much of the existing research into human-decision making has centred around findings that subjects often make suboptimal choices in comparison to those predicted by normative theories arising out of economic and statistical research, especially in the context of decisions about probabilistic events. For example, seminal work by Tversky and Kahneman demonstrated that subjects' judgements about the probable truth of hypotheses can be inaccurate, relative to Bayesian estimates (see BAYESIAN STATISTICS) because of failure to take full account of the relative frequency of events ('base rates') as well a tendency to focus on information that is either more readily available to the subject, or more consistent with pre-existing prototypes used in the decision-making process (the so-called availability and representiveness heuristics). Other research has shown that the factors which determine the precise strategies used by subjects to arrive at a decision include the number of choices and their attributes, as well as the type and format of material involved in the choice (see Slovic *et al.*, 1988 for review).

The major impetus for research on the neurobiology of decision-making stems from the observation that certain patient popula-tions with neurological or neuropsychiatric conditions, such as those with focal damage to the PREFRONTAL CORTEX, DRUG ABUSE problems, OBSESSIVE COMPULSIVE DISORDER and sociopathic behaviours, often exhibit marked changes in the quality of decision-making in their everyday lives. Of particular interest are those patients who have sustained damage to ventromedial sectors of the prefrontal cortex (VM-PFC) (see MEDIAL PREFRONTAL CORTEX). A classic example is patient EVR (see Damasio, 1994) whose surgery for a tumour left him with a bilateral LESION of this cortical area. Before his operation, EVR was an effective, successful individual in both professional and personal terms. However, after his operation, his behaviour was characterized by a pattern of personally disastrous decisions whose consequences included the failure of his first and subsequent marriages, a series of ill-judged investments and profoundly disrupted interpersonal behaviour. However, his neuropsychological profile showed little sign of gross cognitive decline (as evidenced by a performance IQ of 135 points), and essentially normal performance on instruments known to be sensitive to other aspects of prefrontal dysfunction. Thus, the scientific challenge posed by patients like EVR is to account for their specific inability to make effective choices in social and real-life settings, in the absence of neuropsychological deficits in other functions (such as short-term retention of information in WORKING MEMORY systems, the ability to control mental and motor sets, and basic linguistic competence) widely thought to underpin the complex cognitive operations required to arrive at adaptive, successful decisions.

One possibility is that the real-life decisions which VM-PFC patients find so difficult are characterized by a need to reason about uncertain or poorly understood contingencies between actions and outcomes. In these cases, the available propositional knowledge about the alternative choices and their relative attributes, over which subjects might have been able to deploy a number of cognitive strategies (see above), is insufficient for arriving at a decision and needs to be supplemented by additional, perhaps more implicit, information about the consequences of choices in similar situations encountered in the past. Evidence that VM-PFC patients are not able to use such information to assist their decision-making is seen in the finding that, in a simulated gambling paradigm involving uncertain action–outcome contingencies, VM-PFC patients make choices that earn high REWARD but still higher penalties (resulting in eventual losses) at the expense of choices that earn smaller rewards but still smaller penalties (resulting in eventual gains). Additionally, these risky choices are associated with reduced autonomic responses, suggesting that the basis of this behaviour might be a failure to mark disadvantageous choices with an appropriate somatic marker (see SOMATIC MARKER HYPOTHESIS) that could guide future behaviour.

It is important to emphasize that, at the time of writing, very little is known about the neural basis of decision-making. For example, it is certain that the ventromedial prefrontal cortex is only one station in the wider circuitry mediating the various cognitive processes that underpin decision-making cognition. This circuitry will probably incorporate additional cortical areas (for example, the SOMATOSENSORY CORTEX) as well as those LIMBIC SYSTEM structures (such as the ventral STRIATUM and AMYGDALA) that influence the selection of actions via the provision of reward or emotion-related information. Moreover, precise modulation of this circuitry by the ascending MONOAMINE projections is also likely to be extremely important in the efficiency and quality of decision-making. For instance, extensive clinical evidence indicates that impaired decision-making culminating in violent, impulsive behaviour is associated with reduced levels of SEROTONIN metabolites in the CEREBROSPINAL FLUID of sociopathic individuals. Thus, a full account of the NEUROPSYCHOLOGY of decision-making will need to integrate neuroanatomic and neurochemical information, as well as psychological information about the way subjects reach their decisions.

See also: cost–benefit analysis

References

Damasio A.R. (1994). *Descartes' Error*, Picador: London.

Slovic P., Lichtenstein S. & Fischhoff B. (1988). In *Steven's Handbook of Experimental Psychology*, 2nd edn, ed. Atkinson R.C., Hernnstein R.J., Lindzey G. & Luce R.D., pp. 673–738, Interscience-Wiley: New York.

ROBERT D. ROGERS

declarative memory Capacity for CONSCIOUS RECOLLECTION of past episodes and of knowledge derived from past experience. It includes MEMORY for events distinct in time and space (see EPISODIC MEMORY) and for facts (see SEMANTIC MEMORY). It is distinguished from non-declarative memory capacities (such as PROCEDURAL LEARNING and PRIMING), which are expressed through changes in performance without demanding conscious access to memory content. Declarative memory depends on brain structures that are different from those that support non-declarative memory capacities (see MULTIPLE MEMORY SYSTEMS). Patients with AMNESIA due to medial TEMPORAL LOBE damage (see HIPPOCAMPUS) show impaired declarative but preserved non-declarative memory abilities. Research debates concern whether all aspects of declarative memory (episodic and semantic) depend on the integrity of the medial temporal lobes and to what extent other brain structures (for example, the PREFRONTAL CORTEX) are important.

See also: amnesic syndrome; explicit memory; global amnesia

STEFAN KÖHLER

decortication Decortication is removal of the CEREBRAL CORTEX from both HEMISPHERES; decorticate describes an organism to which this has been done.

See also: *cerveau isolé*; decerebrate; hemi-decortication

decussation As a noun – decussation – this means a crossing of FIBRES, more or less in the shape of an X; as a verb it means similarly to cross – as in 'the OPTIC CHIASM is where the OPTIC NERVE decussates'. It has a Latin root: a *decussis* was a coin worth ten *asses* (*decem asses* shortens to *decussis*) and it was marked with the Roman numeral ten, X.

deep brain stimulation Literally, stimulation of structures relatively deep in the brain. Deep brain stimulation was initially used for the relief of TREMOR in PARKINSON'S DISEASE: ELECTRODE implants were made using STEREO- TAXIC SURGERY under local anaesthesia into the THALAMUS or the SUBTHALAMIC NUCLEUS, structures whose activity is changed in Parkinson's disease – resetting activity in these areas can give symptomatic relief. The electrodes are connected to stimulators implanted beneath the SKIN (typically in the region of the collarbone), patients being able to control the stimulator using hand-held devices. Because deep brain stimulation was initially used for the control of tremor using electrodes in the thalamus, it has been known as TREMOR CONTROL THERAPY or THALAMIC STIMULATION. The same technique has also now been used in the management of other conditions, including STROKE and spinal cord injury. It has also been used for the relief of chronic PAIN, under which guise it has also been referred to as NEURO- AUGMENTATION.

deep cerebellar nuclei *see* cerebellum – anatomical organization

deep dysgraphia *see* agraphia

deep dyslexia An ACQUIRED READING DISORDER in which previously skilled readers can no longer read aloud function words (such as *the*, *when*) and have great difficulty reading abstract words (for instance, *truth*, *skill*). In addition, they are unable to sound-out individual letters or novel letter strings such as *wid* and produce visually similar real words instead (for example, *wid* – *widow*). Concrete words (such as *hospital*, *dog*) and imageable words (for instance, *whisper*, *blue*) are read more successfully. A variety of reading errors occur: semantic errors (for instance, *tiger* read as *lion*); visual errors (*bush* read as *brush*) and visual–semantic errors (*cone* – *cornet*).

Brain lesions tend to be extensive, affecting the cortical and subcortical areas supporting LANGUAGE processing in the dominant (in most cases the left) HEMISPHERE (see LESION). Deep dyslexia is thought to arise when the normal READING system is limited by brain damage to processes which connect written and spoken words directly to a meaning system for concrete and imageable words. If the meaning obtained is not precise, semantic errors occur. Connections in the normal reading system,

which link knowledge of familiar written words to spoken words and allow the pronunciations of novel words to be assembled, have been obliterated by the brain damage. The clinical symptoms of deep dyslexia have been argued to reflect reading processes located in the subdominant hemisphere. Successful therapies for deep dyslexia using lexical strategies and PHONEMIC CUEING have been reported.

See also: central reading disorders; developmental reading disorder; phonological dyslexia; surface dyslexia

Reference

Coltheart M., Patterson K. & Marshall J.C. (eds.) (1987) *Deep Dyslexia*, 2nd edn, Routledge: London.

Funnell E (2000) Deep dyslexia. In *Case Studies in the Neuropsychology of Reading*, ed. E. Funnell, Psychology Press: Hove UK.

ELAINE FUNNELL

deep encoding *see* levels of processing

defence *see* aggression

degeneration In biology this has no moral connotation: degeneration is a process of decay that occurs in systematic stages over time; see for example, NERVE CRUSH; WALLERIAN DEGENERATION. Degeneration might in time be followed by some form of recovery; see RECOVERY OF FUNCTION.

Reference

Kandel E.R., Schwartz J.H. & Jessell T.M. (2000) *Principles of Neural Science*, 4th edn, McGraw-Hill: New York.

Deiter's cells *see* organ of Corti

Deiter's nucleus Also known as the lateral vestibular nucleus; see LOCOMOTION; VESTIBULAR SYSTEM.

delay conditioning A way of scheduling the CONDITIONED STIMULUS and UNCONDITIONED STIMULUS (CS and US) in PAVLOVIAN CONDITIONING in which the US is presented during the final part of the CS presentation (so that both stimuli terminate simultaneously) or when the US occurs immediately on termination of the CS. Delay conditioning is more commonly used than other schedules such as TRACE CONDITIONING and BACKWARD CONDI-

TIONING; this is simply because it typically produces relatively strong conditioned responding.

JASPER WARD-ROBINSON

delayed alternation A behavioural test in which an animal must choose between alternatives, the correct option being determined by the outcome of the preceding trial; specifically the option to be chosen is the one that was incorrect on the previous trial. Thus a monkey might be faced on each trial with two cups side by side; only one cup will contain food and the spatial position of this baited cup will alternate over trials. Imposing a delay between one trial and the next allows the experimenter to determine the interval over which information must be retained. Performance on this task appears to be particularly sensitive to brain damage that involves the FRONTAL LOBE.

GEOFFREY HALL

delayed matching to sample An experimental procedure in which subjects are required on each trial, to respond to a stimulus (that is, the sample) some time after it has been removed (that is, after a delay). Subjects are presented with a number (usually between three and six) of alternative test stimuli and receive POSITIVE REINFORCEMENT if they select one that is identical to the originally presented (sample) stimulus. The procedure is a test of MEMORY in which length of the delay, basic nature of the material (verbal vs. non-verbal for example) and demands of the test and material (for instance the number of alternatives presented during the test phase, as well as the number of stimulus features) can all be manipulated. Delay tests such as this are often used to examine the functions of the PREFRONTAL CORTEX and related structures.

See also: delayed non-matching to sample

RICHARD C. TEES

delayed non-matching to sample An experimental procedure in which a subject is presented on each trial with a sample object and then, after a delay, is presented with a choice between two objects, one identical with the sample, and one a different, unfamiliar object. The subject receives POSITIVE REINFORCEMENT for choosing the non-sample object. In the standard version (which has non-recurring items), brand new objects are used for every trial so that the subject is never confronted with making a choice (match vs. non-match) for an object presented in an earlier trial. Delay tests such as this are often used to examine the functions of the PREFRONTAL CORTEX and related structures.

See also: delayed matching to sample

RICHARD C. TEES

delayed recall Essentially the same as FREE RECALL but with a time delay interposed between presentation of the test material and the memory test.

delayed response A delayed response is, rather obviously, one which is delayed by a given interval. Typically, stimuli are presented and then the subject has to wait for an interval of time before making a response. Delayed response tests are important in assessing MEMORY functions (particularly WORKING MEMORY) and are used as much with experimental animals as with human subjects.

delirium tremens (from Latin, *delirus*: mad, *tremere*: to tremble) A condition associated with excessive alcohol abuse (see ALCOHOLISM) in which vivid and disturbing hallucinations are experienced. It is not a term so much used now; in the past, the term 'DTs' was a commonplace term used to describe the effects of alcoholism.

See also: oneirism

delta rule see backpropagation; neural networks

delta waves see electroencephalogram

delusion (from Latin, *deludere*: to play falsely) In everyday talk, to delude is to deceive or cheat, and a delusion is the process of deluding. More specifically, in psychology a delusion is a false belief, often of a rather improbable nature. Delusions are common in disorders such as SCHIZOPHRENIA.

See also: hallucination; illusions; thought disorder

delusional misidentification As it says, a DELUSION in which there is a misidentification of the true state of things. For example, CAPGRAS SYNDROME involves a belief that one's relatives have been replaced by impostors; COTARD SYNDROME involves a belief that one is dead; and FREGOLI'S SYNDROME involves a belief that other people's bodies have been replaced though their minds remain intact within the changed body.

demented dyslexia *see* hyperlexia

dementia Dementia is a syndrome of progressive global cognitive impairment with MEMORY dysfunction as a prominent feature, accompanied by disorders of LANGUAGE (DYSPHASIA), PRAXIS, and perceptual function (AGNOSIA). Ultimately, memory failure, personality disintegration and behavioural abnormalities may conspire together to completely disable sufferers. The syndrome has many causes, and although generally progressive, some forms of dementia are reversible. These include HYPOTHYROID states, nutritional deficiencies, ALCOHOLISM and abnormal pressure HYDROCEPHALUS. The commonest form of the disorder is ALZHEIMER'S DEMENTIA, followed by the vascular MULTI-INFARCT DEMENTIAS. Other causes include LEWY BODY DEMENTIA, PARKINSON'S DISEASE, and other neurodegenerative disorders such as PICK'S DISEASE, HUNTINGTON'S CHOREA and CREUTZFELDT–JAKOB DISEASE.

IAN C. REID

dementia praecox *see* schizophrenia

demi-syllable A part of a SYLLABLE (see SPEECH PERCEPTION).

demyelination The removal of MYELIN, once formed (in contrast to DYSMYELINATION, which is the failure to form myelin, or UNMYELINATED, which is the natural absence of myelin from axons). Experimentally, there are several ways to remove myelin. Application of ethidium bromide has been used to remove myelin deliberately. EXCITOTOXINS, widely used as agents to destroy neurons, will also demyelinate axons (though spontaneous REMYELINATION occurs: how is not clear). The best known form of spontaneous demyelination is MULTIPLE SCLEROSIS. Neither OLIGODENDROGLIA nor SCHWANN CELLS easily regenerate following damage. When remyelination occurs, it generally requires the recruitment of precursor cells, or cells from another part of the body to invade a damaged area.

References

Brace H., Latimer M. & Winn P. (1997) Neurotoxicity, blood-brain barrier breakdown, demyelination and remyelination associated with NMDA-induced lesions of the rat lateral hypothalamus. *Brain Research Bulletin* 43: 447–455.
Franklin R.J.M., Crang A.J. & Blakemore W.F. (1991) Transplanted type-1 astrocytes facilitate repair of demyelinating lesions by host oligodendrocytes in adult rat spinal cord. *Journal of Neurocytology* 20: 420–430.

dendrite Dendrites are processes of a NEURON whose function is to receive inputs, usually via synapses. After emerging from the SOMA, dendrites taper gradually while dividing into secondary and higher-order branches. The pattern of dendritic branching is unique to each cell population. Dendrites near the soma are called PROXIMAL, while those away from it are called DISTAL. Dendrites often bear protrusions called DENDRITIC SPINES, and certain neurons such as striatal MEDIUM SPINY NEURONS and PURKINJE CELLS have numerous dendritic spines. Although dendrites do not usually release neurotransmitters, certain neurons are known to release neurotransmitters from their dendrites.

See also: axon; synapse

KAZUE SEMBA

dendritic spines *see* medium spiny neurons; dendrite

dendrodendritic A term describing a synaptic connection between two dendrites (see DENDRITE; SYNAPSE).

denervate; denervation; denervated To denervate is to remove the neural input to a structure. This could be removal of a NERVE in the PERIPHERAL NERVOUS SYSTEM, or the removal of neuronal input to a single structure in the CENTRAL NERVOUS SYSTEM; and it could occur by disease, injury or by experimental removal (see LESION).

denopamine A beta-1 noradrenaline receptor AGONIST (see ADRENOCEPTORS).

dense distributed representation *see* neural coding

dental acrylic (dental cement) A quick-curing acrylic cement used to create a HEADCAP that holds securely in position an ELECTRODE or CANNULA implanted into brains. Dental acrylic is not glue – it does not stick directly to the skull surface. SKULL SCREWS are fixed to the skull, the dental acrylic binding around these.

dentate gyrus The dentate gyrus is a U-shaped, inferior region of the HIPPOCAMPAL FORMATION. Its internal region is called the HILUS, and the CA3 (see CA1–CA3) region of the hippocampus extends into the hilus. The dentate gyrus consists of three layers: molecular, granular and polymorphic. Granule cells, located in the granular layer, are the main cell type in the dentate gyrus. They receive excitatory input from the ENTORHINAL CORTEX via the PERFORANT PATH, and send their axons, called MOSSY FIBRES, to activate neurons in the CA3 region of the hippocampus. Mossy fibres contain a high concentration of zinc, but its function is unknown.

KAZUE SEMBA

dentate nucleus *see* cerebellum – anatomical organization

2-deoxyglucose An antimetabolic analogue of GLUCOSE that is taken up by cells but not fully metabolized, thereby accumulating in cells. It is used (1) as a *physiological challenge* to generate eating in experimental animals – its uptake by and accumulation in cells prevents glucose metabolism proceeding properly, leading to an apparent cellular need for energy; and (2) when tagged with a RADIOLABEL, as a tool for *metabolic mapping* studies.

deoxyribonucleic acid *see* DNA

dependence; dependency A state in which an individual is dependent on an external reinforcer, usually a DRUG, for normal functioning. The most common use of the term dependence is in reference to substance dependence, with the word substance denoting either a PSYCHOACTIVE drug or ALCOHOL. The term arose

out of the concept of PHYSICAL DEPENDENCE, which is a state in which an organism needs the presence of a drug in order to maintain physiological HOMEOSTASIS. With physical dependence, if the individual does not take the drug or drink alcohol, a physical WITHDRAWAL SYNDROME can ensue, typified by unpleasant and possible serious physical symptoms. However, the modern definition of dependence has been revised and expanded, and does not require the presence of physical dependence. Rather, the essential feature of substance dependence is a cluster of cognitive, behavioural and physiological symptoms that characterize a maladaptive pattern of substance use. This maladaptive pattern of use leads to clinically significant impairment or distress, and continues in the face of clear knowledge that the behaviour is associated with harmful or dangerous consequences. Dependence is often associated with persistent but unsuccessful efforts to cut down or stop use of the substance, and a great deal of time is spent engaged in activities necessary to obtain or use the substance, or to recover from its effects. Moreover, a further important central feature is a strong, sometimes overpowering desire or compulsion to take the drug (often termed CRAVING or DRUG CRAVING).

The use of 'dependence' as a descriptive construct has gradually replaced the term ADDICTION, particularly in the clinical field. In the early 1980s, the World Health Organization proposed the DEPENDENCE SYNDROME concept, which as noted above, emphasizes the behaviour of the individual in relation to the substance, and also attempts to integrate biological, psychological and social factors contributing to addiction. The terms addiction and drug addict have historically had a negative connotation, with emphasis on failure of will or moral weakness. In contrast, the dependence syndrome concept is meant to underscore the medical model of addiction, in which it is considered as disease or disorder amenable to diagnosis and treatment. It should also be noted that the concept of dependence, as described above, has also been applied to other types of dependent behaviours, such as 'addictions' to sex, television, gambling, food, and exercise. While there may be some overlap in pathological patterns of behaviour, the notion as applied to these situations is controversial and less well studied.

ANN E. KELLEY

dependence syndrome The World Health Organization (WHO) defined, in 1981, the dependence syndrome as 'a cluster of physiological, behavioural, and cognitive phenomena in which the use of a substance or a class of substances takes on a much higher priority for a given individual than other behaviours that once had higher value.'

See also: addiction; state dependency

depersonalization A feeling of being outside one's own body; a symptom of a number of disorders including PANIC, AGORAPHOBIA and SCHIZOPHRENIA.

depolarization A change in the MEMBRANE POTENTIAL of a cell that makes it less negative. In the case of excitable cells, depolarization usually occurs by opening an ION CHANNEL to allow positive charged ions that are abundant outside the cell, such as sodium and calcium (see ION), to flow down their CONCENTRATION GRADIENT into the cell. Depolarization is often called 'excitatory' because it moves neurons closer to their THRESHOLD, thereby making it more likely that an ACTION POTENTIAL will occur.

DOUGLAS D. RASMUSSON

depolarization blockade A condition in which a NEURON becomes depolarized (see DEPOLARIZATION) and remains depolarized. This may be due to massive release of an excitatory neurotransmitter or to an impairment in the normal mechanisms that are responsible for terminating the action of an excitatory transmitter. For example, many muscle paralyzing agents work by blocking the enzyme ACETYLCHOLINESTERASE, which normally breaks down ACETYLCHOLINE, the transmitter at the NEUROMUSCULAR JUNCTION. The excess acetylcholine then keeps the muscle cells in a depolarized state and may result in death.

DOUGLAS D. RASMUSSON

depot injection *see* drug administration

depotentiation The erasure of LONG-TERM POTENTIATION (LTP) at previously potentiated synapses. It is not the same thing as LONG-TERM DEPRESSION (LTD). Depotentiation appears to involve a true reversal of LTP, rather than the superimposition of LTD on LTP; see LONG-TERM DEPRESSION for further discussion.

deprenyl Marketed under the trade name SELEGILINE; a MONOAMINE OXIDASE-B (MAO-B) inhibitor used for the treatment of PARKINSON'S DISEASE, often given in conjunction with L-DOPA.

See also: MPTP

depression Common clinical condition characterized by pathological lowering of MOOD, and inability to experience pleasure (ANHEDONIA). Associated symptoms include SLEEP disturbance with early wakening; poor APPETITE with body weight loss; impaired concentration and memory function; and low or absent sex drive. The disorder tends to be recurrent, and may become chronic. Psychotic symptoms may occur, with auditory HALLUCINATION (taking the form of derogatory voices) and DELUSION (of the nihilistic type). The condition varies widely in severity: mild depressions may go undetected clinically, while rarer, more severe forms of the condition may be lethal, leading to death through SUICIDE or self-neglect. Overall, the condition represents a major public health problem, with one in three of us suffering some degree of depressive disturbance in our lifetime. Depression is encountered in all cultures, and has always been with us – the disorder was described by the Ancient Greeks. There is some evidence that the incidence of the disorder is increasing: the World Health Organization estimates that depression will be the second leading cause of disability and health problems by 2020.

Clinically important depressive disorder is part of a spectrum of affective disorders, which includes DYSTHYMIC DISORDER (a long-standing characteristic predisposition to low mood), UNIPOLAR DEPRESSION (recurrent episodes of pathological low mood) and bipolar depression (MANIC DEPRESSION) where episodes of both low mood and pathological elevation of mood occur recurrently on different occasions. The aetiology of the disorder is complex – there is certainly a marked genetic component (most evident in the form known as manic depression), but social factors and STRESS such as early adverse experience and unpleasant life events are also important. The fact that drugs acting on monoamine systems are effective in depression has led to the idea that SEROTONIN, NORADRENALINE and perhaps DOPAMINE systems may be dysfunctional in depressive disorder. Drugs like PROZAC (fluoxetine) block the REUPTAKE of serotonin by neurons and increase availability of the neurotransmitter. This may lead to the downregulation of presynaptic 5HT1a autoreceptors (see SEROTONIN RECEPTORS) in the cell bodies of the serotonergic neurons in the brainstem with a resultant increase cell firing and increased activity of the system. Other drugs may have similar actions on the noradrenergic system, and some affect both. Experimental depletion of 5HT or blockade of noradrenaline synthesis provokes temporary relapse in treated depressives. Disordered CORTISOL function may play an important role, but it is not clear whether the high levels of cortisol seen in some patients are a cause or an effect of the condition. Recent studies suggest that the expression of a neuroprotective protein, BRAIN-DERIVED NEUROTROPHIC FACTOR, may mediate the effects of stress and antidepressants in a reciprocal manner. FUNCTIONAL NEUROIMAGING studies show functional and structural abnormalities in some depressed patients, with reduced activity in the FRONTAL CORTEX and a reduction in size of the PREFRONTAL CORTEX. Chronic depression may lead to atrophy of the HIPPOCAMPUS, possibly mediated by CORTICOSTEROID dysfunction, with attendant deficits in LEARNING and MEMORY.

Most depression is treated with chemical ANTIDEPRESSANT drugs, such as the serotonin selective reuptake inhibitors (SSRIs), TRICYCLICS or MONOAMINE OXIDASE INHIBITORS. The drugs are highly effective with response rates of 60–70%. Onset of response takes time and is within 3 to 4 weeks of commencing the medication. Psychological therapies, such as COGNITIVE–BEHAVIOURAL THERAPY are also effective. Severe drug resistant depression may be treated with ELECTROCONVULSIVE THERAPY (ECT), which, despite its negative media profile, is safe and highly effective. Rarely, very severe, chronic and intractable disorders may be treated by neurosurgical approaches, as in PSYCHOSURGERY.

IAN C. REID

deprivation To deprive is to dispossess, remove or withhold something. There are a number of ways in which the term is used in biological psychology. These include, for example: (1) maternal deprivation (see MATERNAL SEPARATION/DEPRIVATION) involves examination of the effects of early separation on infant development; (2) SENSORY DEPRIVATION (see SENSORY ENRICHMENT VS. DEAFFERENTATION/DEPRIVATION) involves the with-drawal of sensory stimulation; (3) the most common usage is in food or water deprivation. Animals working in many tests – running in a MAZE or in OPERANT CONDITIONING for example – do so for food or water REINFORCEMENT. In order to increase MOTIVATION, animals will often be maintained on a restricted allowance of food or water in their home cages. An alternative is to motivate performance by presentation of a highly palatable food or fluid. Note that, in the United Kingdom, both food and water deprivation (or more properly, food and water restriction) are procedures licensed by the Home Office. Animals are not allowed to go for 24 hours without food or water. Similar legislation applies elsewhere.

depth perception We have a powerful perceptual experience of a 3-dimensional world, despite receiving only a 2-dimensional visual array on the retina. The view from each eye provides many useful monocular cues about depth: for example texture gradients (see TEXTURE PERCEPTION), SUPERPOSITION, and PERSPECTIVE. The brain can also integrate successive views of the same scene as the head moves from side to side, by use of MOTION PARALLAX: this ability can unmask camouflaged objects like prey. But head movements can be avoided (even better for the predator!) in animals with frontal eyes: here the brain can recover depth from a 2-dimensional image by comparing the two views received through STEREOSCOPIC VISION.

A. DAVID MILNER

depth-of-processing When information is perceived and encoded in MEMORY, the kind of ENCODING that is carried out strongly influences how well the information will later be remembered. Specifically, memory is best when encoding is elaborative and deep; that is, when material is fully processed in terms of its meaning. When encoding is more shallow, for example, if material is processed only in terms of its appearance, then the material will later be remembered less well. Thus, the depth at which material is processed, its depth-of-processing, is an important determinant of how well the material will be remembered.

LARRY R. SQUIRE

derealization A feeling that the world is not real; a symptom of a number of disorders including PANIC, AGORAPHOBIA and SCHIZOPHRENIA.

dermal–epidermal junction *see* skin

dermatome (from Greek, *derma*: skin, *tomos*, section) The SKIN surface can be divided into dermatomes. The dermatomes partially overlap, but each one projects to a particular DORSAL ROOT of the SPINAL CORD, meaning that different parts of the spinal cord are collecting information from different parts of the body. In the upper body the relationship between the spinal cord and dermatomes is fairly straightforward: the CERVICAL SPINAL CORD (at the top) collects information from dermatomes on the back of the head (the face having its own CRANIAL NERVES), neck, shoulders, arms and hands; the THORACIC SPINAL CORD below it collects information from dermatomes around the trunk. But the relationship between the lower body dermatomes and spinal cord is a little more complicated. The hips, front of the legs and upper parts of the feet send information into the dorsal roots of the LUMBAR SPINAL CORD, while the back of the buttocks, backs of the legs, sides and sides of the feet send information to the dorsal roots of the sacral spinal cord. This arrangement appears slightly odd on a BIPED, but reflects quite well the stance of a QUADRUPED: if one bends forwards with one's hand almost touching the floor, the dermatome–spinal cord relationship becomes clearer, sacral spinal cord innervating the most poster-

ior parts of the body, the cervical the most anterior. The size of dermatomes can be examined by touch with a pin prick. In cases of spinal cord damage, the absence of sensation in dermatomes can reveal much about the location of spinal injury.

See also: two-point threshold

dermis *see* skin

desensitization *see* behaviour therapy

desipramine An ANTIDEPRESSANT drug (one of the TRICYCLICS) that works by blocking the REUPTAKE of MONOAMINES from the SYNAPTIC CLEFT: it has a relatively high selectivity for NORADRENALINE reuptake.

See also: depression

desmethylimipramine *see* desipramine

desynchrony *see* synchrony/desynchrony

deuteranomaly *see* colour blindness

deuteranopia *see* dichromatic colour blindness

development The development of a new organism from a single cell, the fertilized egg, is a remarkable feat of nature that has long fascinated biologists and non-biologists alike. During the first 4 weeks of human development the seemingly homogenous egg is transformed into an EMBRYO. As development proceeds further, the primitive elements of all the major body organ systems become precisely organized with respect to each other. By now, the embryo acquires an unmistakably human appearance and is known instead as a FOETUS. Subsequent development builds on this foundation, and largely concerns the growth and elaboration of these structures into the organs proper.

During the earliest stages of development, cells in different regions of the embryo acquire their developmental identity or fate. This involves a number of distinct but nonetheless integrated processes, and many concepts are simply illustrated by considering the development of the limbs. All fingers, for example, are comprised of the same cell types such as bone, cartilage and muscle, but each individual finger has a unique shape and forms in the correct position in the embryonic limb bud. How a finger acquires its individual positional identity is a problem of regional specification or pattern formation. This process controls, and can be distinguished from, cell DIFFERENTIATION, which concerns how precursor cells become restricted in their fates by activating cell type-specific gene expression pathways (see GENE). Pattern formation is directed by MORPHOGENS. These are molecules that impart positional information, such that different embryonic structures are induced to differentiate down specific pathways by different morphogen concentrations. For the limb, a signalling centre on one side of the early limb bud secretes the morphogen, a protein known as SONIC HEDGEHOG (shh), and this diffuses within the bud (see SECRETION and DIFFUSION). As a result, a concentration gradient of shh is established within the bud, with the highest concentration at the site of shh secretion. Distinct digits are then formed as cells differentiate at different positions in the gradient, a little finger appearing at high morphogen concentrations and a thumb at low concentrations. Much of early development, including that of the nervous system, is concerned with such pattern-forming mechanisms. The related concept of MORPHOGENESIS refers to the physical and mechanical events that govern how cells and tissues move in the embryo and mould the final shape of the various organs.

Development also involves a hierarchy of decisions whereby cells become committed to ever more restricted fates, and this involves two major mechanisms. CYTOPLASMIC DETERMINANTS refer to substances localized to specific regions of the egg CYTOPLASM which are then distributed asymmetrically in the dividing embryonic cells to influence their subsequent fates, a strategy seen in the development of invertebrate embryos. By contrast, vertebrate embryos generally use INDUCTION, whereby cells in one region of the embryo are directed by external signals (such as morphogens) produced by cells in other regions. The earliest commitment after fertilization is to a particular germ layer, whether ECTODERM (neural tissue and skin), MESODERM (such as muscle, heart, kidney, liver, blood and bone) or ENDODERM (for example, intestine). Experiments using

amphibian embryos have shown that early mesoderm is induced from tissue that would otherwise make ectoderm, by proteins (such as members of the FIBROBLAST GROWTH FACTOR family and transforming growth factor beta superfamily) emanating from the endoderm.

A critical event after mesoderm induction is GASTRULATION (once defined as a life-event of greater importance than birth, marriage or death). During gastrulation, the mesoderm undergoes a complex series of movements, extending and migrating between the ectoderm and endoderm to generate the definitive positions of the three germ layers. In vertebrates this process is coordinated by a special structure called the organizer (or node) of the PRIMITIVE STREAK, and this is responsible for at least three overlapping activities. It influences subsequent neural development (see NEURODEVELOPMENT) by inducing the overlying ectoderm to form neural tissue (neural induction), and it directs the establishment of the definitive head–tail and dorsal–ventral axes.

One of the most exciting insights of modern developmental biology has come through the study of genes that are responsible for giving body segments their individual identities along the head–tail axis of the fruit fly (Drosophila) embryo, for example distinguishing thoracic, wing-bearing segments from abdominal segments. These HOMEOTIC SELECTOR GENES have their counterparts in vertebrate embryos, and it is striking that their expression patterns and function show a close correspondence in insects and vertebrates (see NEURODEVELOPMENT). Many other genetic signalling pathways that regulate embryonic development have also turned out to be conserved between vertebrates and invertebrates. The differences between organisms presumably lie in the details of the deployment of these pathways, and we are still a long way from understanding how the human brain, in particular, comes to be different from that, say, of a rat.

ROGER J. KEYNES

development of language-specific phonology During the first year of life INFANT SPEECH PERCEPTION becomes attuned to the PHONOLOGY of the environmental language. SPEECH PRODUCTION follows more slowly, but by school age children command production of the PHONETIC contrasts displayed in the language of their environment. Faultless acquisition of more than one language-specific phonology is possible for children, but this ability declines rapidly from the teenage years. For adults, production and PERCEPTION OF SECOND LANGUAGES not acquired in childhood is difficult; in both, the native-language phonology interferes with the learning of a new system, causing 'foreign accent' in production and making perception more effortful.

ANNE CUTLER

developmental aphasia A language-specific learning impairment observed in children. Failure to develop LANGUAGE functions normally can arise from a variety of aetiologies associated generally with mental retardation: chromosomal abnormalities, gestational disorders, metabolic or nutritional disorders, infection, environmental influences, trauma. Use of the term APHASIA is poorly suited for descriptions of developmental language impairment. Aphasia indicates the loss of previously acquired normal language function and therefore applies usually to the adult population. Use of the term aphasia in reference to child language impairment should be reserved for special cases in which normally developing language skills become impaired due to trauma, infection or other aetiology linked to a specific time of onset. Aphasia acquired in childhood generally resolves better than adult-onset aphasia. In young children the brain is capable of reorganizing language in regions of the CEREBRAL CORTEX that would not normally assume language function, including cortical areas of the RIGHT HEMISPHERE. At about the age of puberty the capacity for such reconstitution of language declines and approximates adult levels by late adolescence

Reference

Lennenberg E. (1967) *Biological Foundations of Language*, Wiley: New York.

CHARLOTTE C. MITCHUM

developmental coordination disorder *see* dyspraxia

developmental dyslexia A particular difficulty with learning to read and spell which delays reading development in otherwise able children. DYSLEXIA is diagnosed when the reading level (or READING AGE) of a child is 2 or more years behind the reading level expected for an average child of that chronological age. Dyslexia is a specific difficulty with reading and spelling and is not the result of a general learning difficulty.

Developmental dyslexia has two main forms: DEVELOPMENTAL PHONOLOGICAL DYSLEXIA, and DEVELOPMENTAL SURFACE DYSLEXIA. Children with phonological dyslexia have a limited vocabulary of written words that they recognize by sight. Words with irregular spelling-to-sound correspondences, which do not sound as they are written (for example, *pint*, *yacht*) are read to the same level as words with regular spelling-to-sound correspondences (for example, *mint*, *throng*). Phonetic word-attack skills, which are useful for 'sounding out' unfamiliar words, are deficient and limit the ability to identify unfamiliar written words. Spelling errors tend to be nonphonetic (for instance *daughter* spelled as *duaghter* rather than *dorter*). In contrast, children with developmental surface dyslexia also have a limited sight vocabulary, but have good phonetic word-attack skills. This allows them to sound out regular words more successfully than written words with irregular spelling-sound correspondences. Spelling errors are usually phonetic (for example *ready* spelled as *redee*). Children with deficient PHONIC abilities have been referred to as DISPHONETIC READERS; those with a deficient sight vocabulary, but good phonic skills, as DISEIDETIC READERS.

Current studies of the processing deficits underlying developmental dyslexia note that developmental phonological dyslexia commonly co-occurs with poor auditory–verbal SHORT-TERM MEMORY and with difficulties in repeating spoken words and nonsense words, indicating a basic problem in phonological processing. Such difficulties are thought to be detrimental to the development of skills in phonological awareness, such as segmenting words into sounds, and carrying out rhyming tasks, which are necessary for the development of phonic skills in reading. The processing deficits of surface dyslexia are less well understood. A visual memory disorder, which might hinder memory for the written forms of familiar words, has been suggested but has not been observed in all cases.

Biological causes have been linked to developmental dyslexia. Studies of identical and non-identical twins (see TWIN STUDIES) have indicated a genetic link in cases of developmental phonological dyslexia but not developmental surface dyslexia. AUTOPSY and FUNCTIONAL NEUROIMAGING studies have indicated an underdevelopment of the language areas of the dominant hemisphere, particularly in the area of the PLANUM TEMPORALE of the TEMPORAL LOBE, which forms part of WERNICKE'S AREA. Functional imaging studies of brain activity during reading tasks have also revealed abnormal processing in the these brain areas. Comprehension problems can also cause reading difficulties. In cases of HYPERLEXIA, children with very low intelligence learn to pronounce aloud correctly written words that they then cannot fully understand. Children in the normal intelligence range, but with poor comprehension skills, may also learn to read aloud words to a normal level, but then have difficulties drawing inferences from the text that they have correctly read.

The prognosis for developmental dyslexia is unclear. Difficulties with phonological skills do not always hinder reading development. There are several reported cases of adults with severe deficits in phonological processing who nevertheless have achieved normal levels of oral reading. Little is known about the long-term outcome for children with surface dyslexia. Treatments for developmental dyslexia generally use a variety of methods. Those that report most success have combined training in phonological skills with learning to recognize letters and written words, and with spelling.

References

Ellis A.W. (1993) *Reading, Writing and Dyslexia*, 2nd edn, Lawrence Erlbaum: Hove UK.

Masterson J. (2000) Developmental surface dyslexia. In *Case Studies in the Neuropsychology of Reading*, ed. E. Funnell, Psychology Press: Hove UK.

Snowling M.J. (1987) *Dyslexia. A Cognitive Developmental Perspective*, Blackwell Scientific: Oxford.

ELAINE FUNNELL

developmental phonological dyslexia *see* developmental dyslexia

developmental reading disorder The term DEVELOPMENTAL READING DISORDER can be taken to be synonymous with DEVELOPMENTAL DYSLEXIA; it is therefore a term that can also be applied to the categories of dyslexia that come under this general heading: see DYSLEXIA for a description of these.

developmental surface dyslexia *see* developmental dyslexia

dexamethasone suppression test This is a test for HYPOTHALAMIC-PITUITARY-ADRENAL AXIS function in DEPRESSION. CORTISOL is released from the adrenal cortex, an effect triggered by ACTH, which is released from the PITUITARY GLAND (neurohypophysis) in response to activation by the HYPOTHALAMUS. Cortisol release shows a circadian rhythm: release is high in the morning and low at night. About half of all depressed patients show an abnormality in this: in depression, release of cortisol is generally higher than normal throughout the day, but is markedly higher at night, when it is normally quite low. Dexamethasone is a synthetic glucocorticoid which can inhibit ACTH synthesis, leading to reduced cortisol activation: a poor suppression of cortisol in response to dexamethasone is an indicator of depression. The predictive value of this test for who will respond well to ANTIDEPRESSANT medication is however somewhat ambiguous.

Reference

Feldman R., Meyer J.S. & Quenzer L.F. (1997) *Principles of Neuropsychopharmacology*, Sinauer Associates: Sunderland MA.

dexedrine Dexedrine is the D-ISOMER of AMPHETAMINE: D-amphetamine (or dextroamphetamine): dexedrine is the trade name for it. It is more potent than the L-isomer. The slang name, 'dexys', is of course derived from dexedrine.

dextral (from Latin, *dexter*: right; *dextra*: right hand) Right-handed (see HANDEDNESS) or on the right side (as with an ISOMER).

See also: sinistral

diabetes A condition marked by excessive THIRST and the passage of excessive quantities of dilute urine. There are two distinct diseases: diabetes mellitus (from Greek, *mel*: honey) is a disorder of CARBOHYDRATE metabolism, the patient's urine being rich in unburnt GLUCOSE while diabetes insipidus (from Latin, *insipidus*: weak) is due to impaired kidney function, the urine being unduly dilute.

Diabetes insipidus may result from intrinsic kidney disease (nephrogenic diabetes insipidus) but is more commonly due to a deficiency of VASOPRESSIN (known also as antidiuretic hormone). This is a peptide synthesized in the supraoptic and paraventricular nuclei of the posterior HYPOTHALAMUS, especially in response to increased plasma osmotic pressure or decreased blood volume. The peptide is carried by axonal transport to the posterior PITUITARY GLAND (neurohypophysis) where it enters the bloodstream. On reaching the kidney it serves to increase the concentration of the urine by promoting the resorption of water from the renal filtrate (see OSMOREGULATION). Vasopressin also promotes VASOCONSTRICTION and haemostasis and has been assigned a number of more dubious cognitive functions. In the absence of vasopressin, urine output may exceed 10 litres daily but revert to normal with replacement therapy, administered by injection or intranasal spray.

Diabetes mellitus (or simply, diabetes) is due to deficient production of pancreatic INSULIN, or a defective response to it, associated with retinal, renal, neurological and vascular complications. Raised blood glucose (HYPERGLYCAEMIA) in the fasting subject, and glucose in the urine (glycosuria) are diagnostic. The disease has two forms. The classical young, thin diabetic lacks insulin, commonly as a result of autoimmune destruction of the insulin-secreting pancreatic β-cells. This condition can be controlled by daily replacement therapy. In contrast, diabetes commencing in obese middle-aged patients ('non-insulin-dependent diabetes mellitus', NIDDM) is likely to be due to insulin resistance. Resistance may be hereditary: ethnic groups evolving under conditions of borderline famine may optimize their use of nutriment by putting a metabolic brake on glucose breakdown, and would thus cope poorly with the dietary indulgences of modern society. This may explain the endemic NIDDM and increasing cardiovascular morbidity prevalent in certain immigrant populations. High doses of insulin in these circumstances may be of less benefit than a low-calorie diet. Inadequate management of blood-sugar levels exposes the diabetic patient to episodes of hypo- or hyperglycaemia and predisposes to long-term neurological and circulatory complications. Hypoglycaemia may be associated with transient periods of personality change or confusion, leading to COMA, but can usually be rapidly alleviated, by oral glucose or intravenous injection of a 50% solution.

L. JACOB HERBERG

diacylglycerol (DAG) *see* second messengers

Diagnostic and Statistical Manual of the American Psychiatric Association *see* DSM-IV

diagonal band of Broca The diagonal band of Broca collects AXON fibres from the BASAL FOREBRAIN and the AMYGDALA, courses towards the midline as the horizontal limb, and ascends dorsally into the medial septum as the vertical limb. Mixed with the fibres of the diagonal band of Broca are cell bodies of neurons, referred to as the nuclei of the horizontal and the vertical limbs of the diagonal band of Broca. These nuclei contain numerous CHOLINERGIC neurons that are part of the magnocellular cholinergic cell group in the basal forebrain.

KAZUE SEMBA

dialysate A solution containing the material that passes by diffusion through a dialysis membrane (see MICRODIALYSIS).

CHARLES D. BLAHA

dialysis A filtration process used to separate small from larger molecules in solution by using a SEMIPERMEABLE MEMBRANE.

See also: microdialysis

CHARLES D. BLAHA

diamidino yellow *see* tract tracers

diaschisis A generalized loss of function following a LESION or other form of BRAIN INJURY. It refers to the principle that, in the period immediately following localized damage, there will be a more widespread disruption of function as connections to sites remote from the injury are affected. In time however those remote sites will hopefully resume normal function and lead to an amelioration of the generalized deficit and RECOVERY OF FUNCTION.

diastole *see* blood

diathesis-stress model (from Greek, *dia*: asunder, *tithenai*: to place.) Diathesis refers to the dispositions of the body; the diathesis-stress model is an account of why people develop particular conditions. This model argues that overt biological conditions are an interaction between innate biological predispositions (which may be, for example, physiological or genetic) and life events or environmental stressors. The model has been used to generate hypotheses about various conditions, including SCHIZOPHRENIA.

diazepam *see* valium

dichoptic test A test in which sensory stimuli are presented separately to the right and left eyes, either simultaneously or closely following each other. Such tests have been used to examine LATERALIZATION of function in the brain.

dichotic listening task A non-invasive test of hemispheric LATERALIZATION of function in which subjects hear different material presented to the two ears simultaneously (for instance, one sequence of digits to one ear, and a second presented to the other) and report what they hear. Normal subjects correctly report more verbal material heard by the ear CONTRALATERAL to their dominant hemisphere (usually the LEFT HEMISPHERE) for LANGUAGE. That is, most exhibit a right-ear advantage. In the non-verbal version, subjects are played two different melodies simultaneously and separately to the two ears and are asked to identify the two from a set of four they are subsequently played. In this instance, the left ear

(and RIGHT HEMISPHERE) of most subjects is found to be superior.

RICHARD C. TEES

dichromatic colour blindness An inherited, sex-linked impairment of human COLOUR VISION which results in a reduced range of visible colours. Also called DALTONISM. The deficit is caused by the functional absence of one of the three types of CONES of the RETINA: L cones in PROTANOPIA (so-called 'red' blind), M cones in DEUTERANOPIA (so-called 'green' blind) or S cones in TRITANOPIA (so-called 'blue' blind) (see TRICHROMATIC THEORY OF COLOUR VISION). The most extreme losses occur in protanopia and deuteranopia in which the subject fails to distinguish the colours of red, yellow and green spectral lights. A different range of colours is selectively affected in each disorder, and careful analysis allows the type to be identified. A milder version of the deficiency is more common (PROTANOMALY, DEUTERANOMALY, and TRITANOMALY) in which the associated cone type is anomalous rather than absent and the subject remains trichromatic.

See also: colour blindness; photoreceptors

KATHY T. MULLEN

diencephalic amnesia Permanent failure of LEARNING and MEMORY following damage to structures in the DIENCEPHALON of the brain. Diencephalic amnesia is a variant of the AMNESIC SYNDROME, most commonly encountered clinically as KORSAKOFF'S SYNDROME following vitamin B complex deficiency in the setting of chronic alcohol abuse, though may also follow traumatic brain damage or STROKE. Features are similar to those seen following bi-temporal damage (see AMNESIC SYNDROME), though RETROGRADE AMNESIA is often more extensive, SOURCE AMNESIA more marked and CONFABULATION may occur. These additional features may represent dysfunction of the FRONTAL CORTEX with which diencephalic structures are richly interconnected. The precise diencephalic damage necessary and sufficient to produce amnesia is controversial, but is believed to include the mammillary bodies of

the HYPOTHALAMUS and DORSOMEDIAL NU-
CLEUS OF THE THALAMUS.

IAN C. REID

diencephalon The part of the brain that is
continuous with the MIDBRAIN caudally, and
with the TELENCEPHALON rostrally. The diencephalon consists of four parts: the EPITHALA-
MUS, THALAMUS, HYPOTHALAMUS, and
subthalamus (see SUBTHALAMIC NUCLEUS).
The epithalamus comprises the HABENULA and
PINEAL GLAND. The thalamus contains important relay nuclei for all sensory modalities
except OLFACTION. The hypothalamus is essential for HOMEOSTASIS and MOTIVATION. It also
regulates the release of HORMONES from the
PITUITARY GLAND which is connected with the
hypothalamus via the pituitary stalk. As part of
the BASAL GANGLIA, the subthalamic nuclei are
involved in motor co-ordination.

KAZUE SEMBA

diencephalospinal dopamine system *see*
classification of Dahlström and Fuxe;
dopamine

diestrus *see* oestrus

diet The term diet has two common uses: it
indicates the food that an organism eats – a
balanced diet is one which contains all the
appropriate NUTRIENTS it requires. The second
meaning relates to the restriction of food
intake by humans in order to reduce BODY
WEIGHT (which should properly be referred to
as a weight-reducing diet). It is of interest to
note that there is no SPECIES other than humans that does this.

See also: cognitive restraint

differential display A term used in MOLECU-
LAR BIOLOGY to describe techniques for detecting variation in GENE expression between two
or more CELL populations. The difficulty lies in
measuring gene expression in the first place,
before comparisons can be made.

References

Rushlow W.J., Rajakumar N., Flumerfelt B.A.
& Naus C.C.G. (1999) Characterization of
CArG-binding protein A initially identified
by differential display. *Neuroscience* 94:
637–649.

differential pulse voltammetry A technique
in electrochemistry in which small potential
pulses superimposed on a voltage scan (1–2
minute duration) are applied to an ELECTRODE
to quantify ELECTROACTIVE compounds in solution.

CHARLES D. BLAHA

differential reinforcement of low rates A
schedule of instrumental REINFORCEMENT according to which the animal will receive a
REWARD for making an instrumental response
provided a specified time interval has elapsed
since the previous response. Sometimes referred to as a DIFFERENTIAL REINFORCEMENT
OF OTHER BEHAVIOUR) schedule, because one
way the animal might meet this requirement is
to learn that making responses other than the
target response in the interval between target
responses will help to produce reward.

See also: instrumental conditioning; schedules
of reinforcement

CHARLOTTE BONARDI

**differential reinforcement of other
behaviour** *see* differential reinforcement of
low rates

differentiation The process whereby differences in individuals or tissues are generated.
Animals begin the process of life and growth
with the fusion of sperm and egg (see REPRO-
DUCTION). CELL DIVISION following that produces all the differentiated tissues of
multicelled animals; see DEVELOPMENT; NEU-
RODEVELOPMENT; SEXUAL DIFFERENTIATION.

diffuse *see* focal vs. diffuse

diffuse axonal injury *see* closed head injury

diffuse reflection coefficient (albedo) *see*
luminance

diffusion (i) The movement of a substance
down a CONCENTRATION GRADIENT through a
liquid or gaseous medium. (ii) The scattering of
light rays in MICROSCOPY.

CHARLES D. BLAHA

diffusion limited access *see* drug
administration

digestion Digestion is one of the four stages through which food is processed: these are *ingestion digestion, absorption* and *elimination*. Ingestion is the act of FEEDING; digestion is the process of degrading food components into their MOLECULE constituents for use – molecules small enough to be transported across a cell MEMBRANE have to be generated. CARBOHYDRATES are broken down to simple SUGARS (principally GLUCOSE), FATS to GLYCEROL and FATTY ACIDS, PROTEINS to AMINO ACIDS) and NUCLEIC ACIDS to NUCLEOTIDES. The essential process in this is known as enzymatic hydrolysis – the addition of water to molecules by ENZYME activity, causing them to break down. The third stage, absorption (the absorptive phase) involves cells taking up the molecules presented by digestion; the final stage is elimination, the voiding of waste material.

See also: digestive system; fasting phase; osmoregulation

digestive system All animals need to engage in DIGESTION and are equipped with the means to do so. Animals are in a sense hollow, the ALIMENTARY CANAL (or digestive tract) being a tube that extends from the MOUTH to the anus. The digestive system of MAMMALS contains specialized organs to achieve specific goals. It includes the alimentary canal (MOUTH, PHARYNX, OESOPHAGOUS, STOMACH, SMALL INTESTINE, LARGE INTESTINE, ANUS) and related organs such as the salivary glands, PANCREAS, LIVER and GALLBLADDER. The principal functions of each major section are as follows. (1) MOUTH and pharynx: three main processes occur here: salivary glands secrete saliva to begin digestion of CARBOHYDRATES; a food bolus for swallowing is created; and taste processing occurs (see CEPHALIC REFLEXES OF DIGESTION; GUSTATION). (2) OESOPHAGOUS: this is a passage taking food from the pharynx to the stomach; it transmits a bolus using PERISTALSIS; enzymes in saliva continue to work while the bolus is in transit. (3) STOMACH: this is a large organ capable of storing and releasing food in small quantities such that there is no need to eat constantly. Enzymes begin digestion of PROTEINS: the stomach lining (epithelium) secretes GASTRIC ACID (which is highly acidic [pH 2] to degrade cells)

and PEPSIN (an enzyme that degrades proteins – it is secreted in an inactive form, pepsinogen, which gastric acid converts to pepsin). The stomach is protected from gastric acid by a coating of mucus and constant regeneration of its lining. The stomach mixes food (SMOOTH MUSCLES move it) and the product released at the pyloric sphincter into the small intestine is known as acid chyme. Note that in some mammals there are multiple stomachs – ruminants such as cattle have three stomachs to allow breakdown of complex plant cellulose; other animals (birds for instance) have a crop before the stomach and a gizzard after it to allow for breakdown of foods. Many INVERTEBRATES also have a crop and gizzard. (4) SMALL INTESTINE: this is the principal organ of digestion and the longest part of the human alimentary canal (at 6 metres); the initial 25 cm is known as the DUODENUM, followed by the JEJUNUM and then ILEUM, which connects to the large intestine. In the duodenum, fluids from the pancreas (including ALKALI solutions and enzymes) and the gallbladder (bile – produced in the liver but stored in and released from the gallbladder) are mixed with acid chyme. Enzymes such asCHOLECYSTOKININ, SECRETIN and ENTEROGASTRONES are secreted by the duodenum to affect peristalsis and stimulate the activity of the pancreas. Digestion proceeds in the jejunum and ileum: the lumen of the small intestine and the epithelium (or brush border, so-called because of the microvilli – small finger-like projections – present there) are differentially involved. In the lumen, pancreatic amylases degrade carbohydrates; trypsin and chymotrypsin degrade complex proteins and aminopeptidases and carboxypeptidases break down smaller proteins to amino acids; nucleic acids (DNA and RNA) are broken down by nucleases to NUCLEOTIDES; and FATS are degraded by bile salts and lipases to GLYCEROL, FATTY ACIDS and glycerides (see TRIGLYCERIDES). In the epithelium, disaccharidases degrade DISACCHARIDES to MONOSACCHARIDES; PEPTIDES are degraded to AMINO ACIDS by dipeptidases; nucleotides are reduced to NUCLEOSIDES by nucleotidases and nucleosidases degrade these to even simpler elements. ABSORPTION of NUTRIENTS also occurs: villi and microvilli give the epithelium of the small intestine a huge surface area. Small vessels of the LYMPHATIC SYSTEM (a part known as the lacteal system), BLOOD capillaries and veins transport nutrients away, sometimes by passive diffusion, sometimes with the aid of membrane pumps. The capillaries and veins drain into the hepatic portal vessel, a major blood vessel leading directly to the liver. (5) LARGE INTESTINE: this is also known as the colon: it is connected to the ileum. At this point there is a three-way connection – the CAECUM is also connected. The main component of the caecum is the appendix. Caecum and appendix are involved in cellulose digestion and are relatively small in humans (to the extent that the appendix is removable). The principal purpose of the colon is the reabsorption of water left after digestion in the small intestine. Movement through the colon is relatively slow (12–24 h): the colon terminates at the RECTUM where faecal matter is stored before evacuation via the anus. (The anus and rectum are both sphincters: control over the rectal sphincter is INVOLUNTARY, while control of the anal sphincter is VOLUNTARY.)

digit span task A simple test in which individuals are required to remember strings of digits (see SHORT-TERM MEMORY; WORKING MEMORY).

digital (from Latin, *digitus*: finger or toe) Digit has two meanings: a finger or toe; and the Arabic numerals from 0 to 9. The adjective digital can therefore relate to numbers or to the fingers and toes. For example, digital dexterity refers usually to skilled use of the fingers; digital display will refer to a visual display of numbers.

dihydro-beta-erythroidine A synthetic form of CURARE.

3,4-dihydrodxymandelic acid *see* noradrenaline

3,4-dihydroxyphenylacetaldehyde *see* dopamine

3,4-dihydroxyphenylacetic acid Abbreviated to DOPAC; see DOPAMINE.

3,4-dihydroxyphenylethanolamine *see* noradrenaline

3,4-dihydroxyphenylethylamine The chemical name for DOPAMINE.

3,4-dihydroxyphenylglycoacetaldehyde *see* noradrenaline

3,4-dihydroxyphenylglycol *see* noradrenaline

5,7-dihydroxytryptamine A neurotoxic analogue of SEROTONIN used to destroy selectively serotonin neurons in brain.

See also: 6-hydroxydopamine; neurotoxins

diisopropylfluorophosphate *see* organophosphates

dimorphism (from Greek, *dis*: twice, *morphe*: form) Dimorphism is the possession of two alternative forms. Within biology, the most obvious example is the differentiation of species into male and female forms: SEXUAL DIMORPHISM.

See also: isomer

dinosaur behaviour Since the introduction in 1842 of the term dinosauria (from Greek, *deinos*: terrible, *sauros*: lizard – though they are not lizards) interest in dinosaurs has remained high. In recent years, emphasis has moved away from the straightforward description of the structure of these extinct animals towards an appreciation of how they might have behaved. Books and movies – *Jurassic Park* being the most spectacular example – have established for most people clear images of the behaviour of dinosaurs. Regrettably (and rather obviously) there is little hard evidence about how dinosaurs behaved, though palaeobiologists have been able to make plausible estimates. For example, dinosaur footprints left in rock formations yield considerable information as to the LOCOMOTION, POSTURE and GAIT of specific species of dinosaur (Gatesy *et al.*, 1999). The structure of bones can produce information about the likely MUSCLE formations present on the living animals, which in turn allows predictions to be made about how they might have used those muscles. Bite marks on bones also provide information: teeth marks from adult conspecifics suggest combat within groups, which suggests the presence of SOCIAL BEHAVIOUR. Bite marks from other species can yield information about patterns of attack. The location in which fossils are found can be informative, if it is known what the local environment might have been like when the dinosaurs were alive, and the patterns in which fossilized bones are found is also important. For example, social organization is suggested by finding the remains of a particular species clustered together, while the consistent presence of very small fossilized remains with larger ones could suggest that the smaller species was a parasite. Evidence for nest sites can provide clues to the parenting behaviour of dinosaurs. Increasingly comparison is made between dinosaurs and appropriate living animals, to make inferences about behaviour. This is based on a recognition, probably well-founded, that little has changed in terms of the bare necessities of life between the time of the dinosaurs and now. It seems reasonable to believe that the solutions modern animals have made to particular problems are the same sorts of solutions that extinct animals would have made.

See also: palaeoneurology

References

Crichton M. (1991) *Jurassic Park*, Random House: New York.

Farlow J.O. & Brett-Surman M.K. (1997) *The Complete Dinosaur*, Indiana University Press: Bloomington.

Gatesy S.M., Middleton K.M., Jenkins F.A. Jr & Shubin N.H. (1999) Three-dimensional preservation of foot movements in Triassic theropod dinosaurs. *Nature* 399: 141–144.

diphone Syllables can be further divided into DEMI-SYLLABLES and diphones; see SPEECH PERCEPTION.

diploid Containing two sets of CHROMOSOMES, each containing one full set of GENES. Diploid organisms reproduce sexually, and receive one set of chromosomes from each parent organism.

See also: cell division; haploid

FIONA M. INGLIS

diplopia (from Greek, *diploos*: double, *ops*: eye) Double vision; see BINOCULAR FUSION; RETINAL DISPARITY; STROKE.

dipsogen Any chemical or drug that stimulates DRINKING is called a dipsogen; see ANGIOTENSIN; OSMOREGULATION.

dipsomania (from Greek, *dipsa*: thirst, *mania*: madness) Literally, this term should refer to a deep CRAVING to drink. In practice it refers to a deep craving to drink ALCOHOL and has in the past been sued as a synonym for ALCOHOLISM.

direct agonist *see* agonist

direct and indirect striatal output pathways The principal output stations of the BASAL GANGLIA are the SUBSTANTIA NIGRA pars reticulata and the internal segment of the GLOBUS PALLIDUS (known as the ENTOPEDUNCULAR NUCLEUS in the rat) both of which send inhibitory projection to the THALAMUS and BRAINSTEM (notably the PEDUNCULOPONTINE TEGMENTAL NUCLEUS). The output of the STRIATUM (the largest element of the basal ganglia) to these runs via indirect and direct pathways. The indirect output pathway travels to the internal segment of the globus pallidus via a synaptic relay in the external segment of the globus pallidus (which in the rat is known just as the globus pallidus, the internal segment being the entopeduncular nucleus). The direct output travels, of course, directly from striatum to the internal segment of the globus pallidus. The innervation of the substantia nigra pars reticulata is similarly divided: a direct output arrives from the striatum and an indirect output arrives from the striatum via a relay in the external segment of the globus pallidus.

See also: corticostriatal loops

direct vision A classical problem for understanding visual perception is how distant objects are available to the eyes. Sound and OLFACTION rather obviously come from air which lies between objects and the senses; but before the discovery in the seventeenth century of optical images, especially on the RETINA, how eyes work was simply not understood. Euclid thought of light rays shooting out of the eyes, like fingers touching objects. A medieval notion was that surfaces of objects give off simulacra of themselves, like particles for smell or like rings from a pebble dropped in a pond. Until early this century, some philosophers postulated mysterious entities called 'sense data', existing somehow as intermediaries between objects and eyes. Philosophers like to think of perception as 'direct', making it seem reliable; but this ignores the retinal image, the complexities of the physiology – great variety of illusions. Now – except perhaps for a few psychologists, who are too-literal followers of James J. Gibson – direct accounts have been given up, in favour of explaining perceptions as inferences from neurally signalled coded messages from the senses, read by rich unconscious knowledge to infer the world of objects. This unconscious inference indirect theory was developed towards the end of the nineteenth century, by the German physiologist and physicist Hermann von Helmholtz (1821–1894).

RICHARD L. GREGORY

directional hypokinesia *see* motor neglect

directional selectivity A NEURON is said to show directional selectivity if it responds more strongly to one direction of motion than to others: it is not the same as ORIENTATION SELECTIVE NEURONS. See MOTION PERCEPTION for further information.

disaccharides *see* sugars

disconnection Disconnection refers to the interruption of system of FIBRES connecting structures in the CENTRAL NERVOUS SYSTEM: commissurotomy is an example of a disconnection (see SPLIT BRAIN for a detailed discussion of a disconnecting commissurotomy). A DISCONNECTION SYNDROME is a collection of SIGNS AND SYMPTOMS that appear after disconnection. The term disconnection lesion is often applied to a procedure in experimental animals in which structures rather than fibres are cut. In this instance one identifies two structures that are connected to each other and makes a UNILATERAL lesion in one of them. In the other HEMISPHERE, one makes a LESION in the other structure. Changes in a behaviour indicate that functioning bilateral interconnections between the structures are necessary for its normal expression.

disconnection aphasia Intrahemispheric disconnections can produce aphasic syndromes. These include isolation of the primary language area (TRANSCORTICAL MOTOR APHASIA), and disconnection between WERNICKE'S AREA and the motor-speech execution areas (CONDUCTION APHASIA).

Reference

Goodglass H. (1993) *Understanding Aphasia*, Academic Press: San Diego.

CHARLOTTE C. MITCHUM

disconnection apraxia Inability to produce movements to verbal command (for example, 'Show me how you brush your teeth') with the left hand, while such ability is spared in the right hand. Liepmann was the first to describe this model of APRAXIA, although Norman Geschwind popularized it over 60 years later. The model suggests that motor and premotor cortical systems of the RIGHT HEMISPHERE which control the musculature of the left arm and hand are disconnected from higher-order movement planning systems of the left hemisphere by a frontal LESION which typically involves the CORPUS CALLOSUM.

DAVID P. CAREY

disconnection syndrome Disconnection of the CEREBRAL HEMISPHERES by surgical RESECTION of the fibres of the CORPUS CALLOSUM. A procedure developed as treatment for severe intractable epileptic seizures (see EPILEPSY). Post-surgical commisurotomy patients have been studied (Gazzaniga *et al.*, 1962). Casual observation does not reveal the striking deficits caused by isolation of each cerebral hemisphere. Patients with complete interhemispheric disconnection can verbally describe stimuli that gain access to the language-dominant hemisphere (usually the LEFT HEMISPHERE). For example, an unseen object placed in the left hand of the commisurotomized patient cannot be named because the sensory input is isolated in the right hemisphere and cannot be transferred to the (verbal) left hemisphere. Non-verbal indications of object recognition may be observed (by, for instance, demonstrated use of the object). Once the object is placed in the right hand, it is named easily by the patient. A variety of experimental tests have shown independent function of the cerebral hemisphere (Gazzaniga *et al.*, 1962). Since the environment rarely restricts stimulus input to one cerebral hemisphere, it is not unusual for commisurotomized patients to lead relatively normal lives.

Anterior disconnection syndrome may follow from lesions to the foremost portion of the corpus callosum. Such lesions are associated with infarction of the anterior cerebral artery. Patients demonstrate unilateral APRAXIA of the left hand, and cannot name or otherwise verbalize information about objects held in the left hand. Posterior disconnection syndrome is associated with lesions of the SPLENIUM portion of the corpus callosum. Tumours or infarction of the posterior cerebral artery are common aetiology. Patients may complain of visual disturbances. Functional dissociation between reading impairment (DYSLEXIA) and writing impairment (DYSGRAPHIA) may be associated with some disconnections between the cerebral hemispheres. ALEXIA without AGRAPHIA is attributable to a complex set of lesions that cause dysfunction of the left VISUAL CORTEX in conjunction with a lesion of the posterior corpus callosum which effectively isolates the right visual cortex from the (damaged) left visual cortex. Consequently, both the right and left visual cortices are isolated from the (intact) language area. The intact language areas allow written language production (WRITING) whilst the disconnection of visual stimulus input to the language areas results in failed comprehension of written language (READING). The clinical indication of this complex syndrome is demonstrated by an intact ability to copy or write spontaneously with the striking failure to read what was written.

Reference

Gazzaniga M.S., Bogen J.E. & Sperry R.W. (1962) Some functional effects of sectioning the cerebral commissures in man. *Proceedings of the National Academy of Science* 48: 1765–1769.

CHARLOTTE C. MITCHUM

discrimination In everyday talk this can refer to biased treatment of one individual or group by another individual or group. In experimental psychology it refers to the ability to tell one stimulus from another, regardless of whatever form the stimulus takes. For example, object discrimination involves the discrimination of physically different objects, olfactory discrimination the discrimination of different odours. Clearly, auditory, visual and tactile discriminations can all be made the subjects of DISCRIMINATION LEARNING experiments. The properties of identical stimuli can also be subject to discrimination experiments: for example, DURATION DISCRIMINATION requires measurement of the time over which something occurs while BRIGHTNESS discrimination requires brightness intensity to be discriminated.

Discrimination experiments can involve SERIAL DISCRIMINATION, in which discrimination of a specific target from among a set of possible targets takes place repeatedly. A fresh discrimination is attempted only when this first discrimination has been learnt; a criterion is typically set to define when successful discrimination learning has been achieved - nine out of ten trials with the correct discrimination made for example. In CONCURRENT DISCRIMINATION tasks, several discriminations are attempted simultaneously. (The opposite of this can also be called single discrimination, in which only one discrimination task is presented.) CONFIGURAL DISCRIMINATION involves the discrimination of two different stimuli composed of the same components arranged in different configurations.

See also: drug discrimination; Grice box; Weber's law.

discrimination learning Procedures in which subjects learn to consistently choose a specific stimulus based on prior differential REINFORCEMENT. In an OPERANT CONDITIONING situation, training with differential reinforcement leads to consistent responding (such as a lever press) to one stimulus and not to another. In CLASSICAL CONDITIONING, training leads to elicitation of a CONDITIONED RESPONSE to the presence of a CONDITIONED STIMULUS, but not to an UNCONDITIONED STIMULUS – in a multiple choice discrimination paradigm, stimuli are presented simultaneously and subjects trained with differential positive or negative reinforcement to approach one and avoid others. Other procedures (such as matching to sample) can be employed. Successful discrimination learning is achieved when the rate of correct responding reaches 90% or better over several test days. To evaluate the precise nature of what subjects have learned to discriminate, TRANSFER TESTS are employed.

RICHARD C. TEES

discriminative cue A stimulus cue that signals to an animal that REINFORCEMENT will be available if and when a specific RESPONSE is made.

See also: discrimination; drug discrimination

discriminative stimulus A STIMULUS that allows an animal to respond correctly to another stimulus. For example, a rat could be trained to press a lever on the right side of a SKINNER BOX when a tone was presented and a lever on the left side when a light was presented: this would be a tone–light discrimination.

disease model *see* medical model

disector A procedure used in STEREOLOGY. It is a technique for counting objects within a structure – neurons within a given area of brain tissue for instance. To do this one takes sections of known thickness through an area of tissue: at the simplest level of analysis only two sections are required (hence the name: *di – sector*). The rule for counting objects is straightforward: objects are counted if they are not present on the previous section. In small structures every section can be examined, but in larger structures, sections are taken at intervals and an estimate of the total number of neurons (or whatever else is being counted) made using procedures based on the CAVALIERI PRINCIPLE (that is, one would need to know the distance between sections, thickness of the sections and the numbers of objects counted).

Reference

West M.J. (1999) Stereological methods for estimating the total number of neurons and synapses: issues of precision and bias. *Trends in Neurosciences* 22: 51–61.

diseidetic readers *see* developmental dyslexia

disengage and shifting attention As ATTENTION involves selection of input for processing, there must also be a mechanism by which a current selection is terminated – disengaged –

and attention is realigned or shifted. For example, a commonly used metaphor in visual SELECTIVE ATTENTION is that of an attentional 'spotlight', which scans and alights at different locations within the VISUAL FIELD. This spotlight denotes a region of increased processing efficiency, and can be moved in visual space independently of gaze, (that is, covertly). Work conducted with brain-damaged individuals indicates that COVERT ATTENTION may be broken down into three dissociable components: (1) a disengage process, in which the attentional spotlight is decoupled from a previous region of interest; (2) a shift process, in which the attentional beam moves to another location; and (3) an engage process, in which the attentional spotlight is reapplied to the new region of interest (Posner *et al.*, 1980). The processes of disengaging and shifting attention may be conceptualized independently from the spotlight metaphor (for example, it also applies to ATTENTIONAL SET), but the spotlight analogy represents a useful framework for characterizing these processes.

See also: set shifting

Reference

Posner M.I. Snyder C.R.R. & Davidson B.J. (1980) Attention and the detection of signals. *Journal of Experimental Psychology: General* 109: 160–174.

JONATHAN K. FOSTER

disgust A generally used term to indicate distaste, loathing or disapproval. In biological psychology its use is more restricted, being related principally to FEEDING. In this context disgust is an EMOTION accompanied by specific facial expressions (see FACE PERCEPTION), physiological reactions (NAUSEA and VOMITING) and actions (to create distance from, and removal of, the object of disgust). It is often associated with the ingestion of contaminants (particularly animal waste products) and is not innate – conceptions of disgust develop over the early years of life and are culturally specific. The consumption of invertebrates or certain mammals (dogs for example) is considered very differently across societies. Disgust is a good example of an interaction between physiological, cognitive, emotional and social processes.

See also: eating disorders

Reference

Rozin P. & Fallon A.E. (1987) A perspective on disgust. *Psychological Review* 94: 23–41.

dishabituation Following repeated presentations of a stimulus HABITUATION may occur. If a strong, or motivationally significant, stimulus is now presented, responding is often restored. This restoration of responding is termed DISHABITUATION. For example, a novel noise will elicit a number of responses, including an orienting response. If the noise is presented repeatedly, the orienting response will decline (that is, habituation occurs). If a strong stimulus, such as a shock or a very loud noise, is now presented, it will be observed that responding to the noise is restored (that is, dishabituation has occurred).

MARK A. UNGLESS

disinhibition In neural terms, the removal of an inhibitory stimulus (see INHIBITION) from a NEURON. In behaviour, disinhibition indicates a loss of control. Disinhibition can occur after DRUG use (for example, ALCOHOL consumption can lead to reduced ANXIETY and behavioural disinhibition) and is a common feature of FRONTAL SYNDROME. It is however a difficult construct to use accurately, it being too easy to describe any increase in activity to be a product of disinhibition.

See also: behavioural inhibition system; dysexecutive syndrome

disparate Disparate means unequal or unlike; but in relation to the RETINA there is a more specific meaning; see RETINAL DISPARITY; STEREOPSIS.

disphonetic readers *see* developmental dyslexia

displacement activities *see* ethology; schedule induced polydipsia

display *see* animal communication

dispositional memory The memory system which describes 'dispositions' or habits is also called REFERENCE MEMORY, simple association and TAXON LEARNING. Dispositional memory describes memory for general information about specific items (such as what an 'a' is, what a '2' is). This type of MEMORY is hippocampal-independent, and is usually preserved in amnesic patients. Additionally, this type of memory is very specific and inflexible, which takes it out of the realm of DECLARATIVE MEMORY (or conscious memory). It has been likened to the learning described by traditional CONDITIONING theorists. The associations are less general than those acquired in rule learning, but share the property of hippocampal independence.

HOWARD EICHENBAUM

dissecting aneurysm An aneurysm that causes arterial dissection; see STROKE.

dissociation Spared performance on one task with disrupted performance on a different task in a brain-damaged patient. Such single dissociations cannot prove that the two tasks require independent processes, since differences in difficulty between the tasks could result in failure in one task and not the other. If a second patient is found who shows the reciprocal pattern (disrupted performance on the task the first patient succeeded at and spared performance on the task the first patient failed) then a DOUBLE DISSOCIATION has been uncovered. Double-dissociations provide stronger evidence that the two tasks depend on cognitive processes which are relatively independent in the brain.

DAVID P. CAREY

dissociation constant K_D is the abbreviation given to the dissociation constant, a pharmacological measure of the AFFINITY of a LIGAND for a RECEPTOR. K_A is the abbreviation given to the equilibrium dissociation constant, a measure of the ligand concentration that would occupy half of all the available receptors (see RECEPTOR OCCUPANCY).

dissociative anaesthetics Compounds that produce a form of general ANAESTHESIA but do not necessarily result in complete unconsciousness, and include arylcyclohexylamine compounds, such as KETAMINE and PHENCYLCIDINE, and adjuvant anaesthetics such as

NITROUS OXIDE and diethyl ETHER. Induction of dissociative anaesthesia is characterized by CATALEPSY, CATATONIA, AMNESIA, ANALGESIA, and a particularly strong feeling of dissociation from the environment. Unlike conventional anaesthetics, ketamine-related anaesthetics do not depress activity in the RETICULAR FORMATION in the BRAINSTEM, but act primarily on the CEREBRAL CORTEX and LIMBIC SYSTEM in an excitatory manner similar to other CNS stimulants, such as pentylenetetrazol.

See also: volatile anaesthetics

CHARLES D. BLAHA

dissociative disorders Psychological disorders in which the key symptoms include a disruption in consciousness, memory, identity or perception of the environment, which cannot be accounted for by CLOSED HEAD INJURY or acute or POST-TRAUMATIC STRESS DISORDER. DSM-IV defines dissociative AMNESIA, dissociative FUGUE, dissociative identity disorder, and DEPERSONALIZATION disorder under this heading. The loss of personal identity distinguishes between fugue states and transient amnesic events. Little is know about psychobiological factors in dissociative disorders at present. They would be difficult to detect in any case, since neurological or medical grounds for the state preclude the diagnosis of a dissociative disorder.

DAVID P. CAREY

distal At a distance, in contrast to proximal, close to.

distal dendrite *see* proximal dendrite

distal sensory ending *see* muscle spindle

distress call *see* animal communication

distributed processing Distributed processing involves a large number of separate systems or elements which work together to perform a task more effectively than any one of them could do in isolation. At the level of an individual NEURON, distributed processing refers to the involvement of large numbers of neurons in representing and processing information, as contrasted with a localist (or localizationist) representation which codes specific information by the activity of individual

neurons. At the level of cortical areas, it refers to the coordinated action of multiple brain regions in performing complex cognitive tasks, as contrasted with theories which assign cognitive functions to individual brain regions.

See also: connectionism; cortical equipotentiality; neural networks; parallel processing; parallel vs. serial processing

DAVID C. PLAUT

distributed representations *see* parallel vs. serial processing

disulfram (antabuse) Disulfram is a drug that acts as a copper CHELATING AGENT. This property means that it can affect chemicals in the body that contain copper. One such is the enzyme DOPAMINE BETA HYDROXYLASE, the enzyme involved in the conversion of DOPAMINE to NORADRENALINE. As such, disulfram can be used to inhibit the formation of noradrenaline in neurons. However, its better known medical property probably does not rely on this action. Disulfram is given to patients who have recovered from ALCOHOLISM and who wish to avoid further ALCOHOL ABUSE. Disulfram inhibits (again, by chelation of copper) the activity of the enzyme aldehyde dehyrodgenase, which is involved in the conversion of acetaldehyde to acetate, part of the sequence of alcohol metabolism in the body. Without this enzyme, if alcohol is consumed, levels of acetaldehyde in the body rise and are accompanied by sordid and ghastly effects, including nausea, vomiting and problems with respiration. A single dose of disulfram has effects lasting last for up to 2 weeks, and only a small amount of alcohol is required to trigger the unpleasant consequences. Disulfram therefore helps keep recovered alcoholics away from alcohol by threatening extreme NEGATIVE REINFORCEMENT.

Reference

Feldman R., Meyer J.S. & Quenzer L.F. (1997) *Principles of Neuropsychopharmacology*, Sinauer Associates: Sunderland MA.

disynaptic Having two synapses: a disynaptic pathway involves one NEURON synapsing on another, that one then synapsing on another.

See also: monosynaptic

disynaptic reflex arc *see* reflex arc

diuresis; diuretic From Greek, *dia*, through, and *ouron*, urine: an excess flow of urine; a diuretic is an agent that promotes diuresis.

diurnal (from Latin *diurnalis*: daily, in turn from *dies*: a day) Diurnal animals, in contrast to nocturnal, are awake during the day and sleep at night. Animals often adopt nocturnal habits to avoid predators. Diurnal habits might be maintained by an absence of predation; by a need to detect predators; by a need to maintain body temperature (in ECTOTHERMS; see THERMOREGULATION) or for many other reasons.

See also: crepuscular; nocturnal

divided attention The simultaneous allocation of processing resources to multiple channels of information. This might involve monitoring stimuli in two different sensory modalities, or two sources of inputs within a modality. An example is the monitoring of independent input to each ear simultaneously in the DICHOTIC LISTENING TASK.

See also: attention; selective attention

VERITY J. BROWN

dizocilpine *see* MK801

dizygotic twins Also known as FRATERNAL TWINS, as opposed to IDENTICAL TWINS (MONOZYGOTIC TWINS). Dizygotic twins are the product of two zygotes and always develop each in its own separate CHORION. They can be of different sexes.

See also: twin studies

DNA Deoxyribonucleic acid: the inheritable, chemical substance found in all cells containing genetic codes required to make PROTEINS. DNA is a helical polymer, composed of two strands of NUCLEOTIDES, each joined by a deoxyribose sugar backbone. There are four different nucleotides, or bases, in DNA: adenine, thymine, guanine and cytosine, and the arrangement of these into a specific sequence provides the basis of GENES. Within each strand of DNA, bases are joined in a $5'$–$3'$ manner by a phosphodiester bond, formed between the phosphate group at the $5'$ carbon with the hydroxyl-containing $3'$ carbon of the

next nucleotide. Adjacent strands of DNA are held together by hydrogen bonds formed between bases. Base-pairing is specific, so that adenine will only bond with thymine, and guanine will bond with cytosine. Using one strand of DNA as a template, therefore, a complementary strand may be formed. Strands within a helix are antiparallel: that is the $5'$ end of one strand corresponds to the $3'$ end of the adjacent strand. Replication of DNA before cell division allows genes to be preserved between generations of cells. DNA replication is initiated by the enzyme DNA helicase, which untwists a region of DNA, causing the strands to part in a replication fork. Strands are held apart by single-strand DNA binding proteins, while a small piece of RNA (ribonucleic acid) known as a primer binds to each DNA strand. Pairing of new complementary nucleotides to the $3'$ end of the RNA primer is initiated by another enzyme, DNA polymerase III. Because replication proceeds in a $5'$–$3'$ manner, and the DNA strands are antiparallel, only one complementary strand, the 'leading' strand, will be formed by the continuous addition of nucleotides, as the replication fork progresses along the length of DNA. The other, 'lagging' strand, is formed by synthesis of many short $5'$–$3'$ fragments called Okazaki fragments, each initiated by the addition of an RNA primer, and elongated by DNA polymerase III. RNA primers are excised and replaced with deoxyribose nucleotides by DNA polymerase I, and gaps in the strands are sealed by DNA ligase. In this manner, DNA is replicated to produce two identical molecules, each containing one original strand of DNA. While complementary base-pairing is highly specific, mismatches may occur and must be corrected. Some nucleotides are methylated following replication. If a mismatch is found during replication, the methylated strand of DNA will be preserved and mismatched bases will be replaced in the non-methylated strand. Similarly, irradiation or heat exposure may result in damaged regions of DNA. Enzymes called DNA nucleases remove damaged nucleotides and new bases are added by DNA polymerase I. However, these mechanisms sometimes lead to small alterations in sequences in bases, and consequently an altered gene sequence, or MUTATION. Besides gene sequences, DNA contains large amounts of non-coding sequences, including those which act as recognition sites for enzymes that initiate, enhance or terminate messenger RNA transcription. The precise functions of many regions of DNA are yet to be elucidated.

FIONA M. INGLIS

DNA–DNA hybridization A technique for comparing the DNA of two SPECIES: it has been of interest to biological psychologists in that it has generated the statistic which suggests that there is almost 99% common identity between the DNA of humans and great apes such as gorillas, chimpanzees and bonobos (see PRIMATES). In assessing this it is important to bear in mind two points: first, there is considerable overlap in the DNA of humans with all other vertebrates (possibly as much as 70%). DNA codes for the production of PROTEINS, and there is a huge degree of overlap between species in their physical structure. Second, differences in the human genome have occurred after the divide from the other primates and these may be of considerable functional significance.

References

Chou H.-H., Takematsu H., Diaz S., Iber J., Nickerson E., Wright K.L., Muchmore E.A., Nelson D., Warren S.T. & Varki A. (1998) A mutation in human CMP-sialic acid hydroxylase occurred after the Homo-Pan divergence. *Proceedings of the National Academy of Sciences* 95: 11751–11756.

Sibley C.G. & Ahlquist J.E. (1987) DNA hybridization evidence of hominoid phylogeny: results from an expanded data set. *Journal of Molecular Evolution* 26: 99–121.

DNA fingerprinting The use of a series of enzymes called RESTRICTION ENZYMES, as an aid to DNA analysis, particularly in the area of forensic science. Restriction enzymes cut DNA (deoxyribonucleic acid) at specific, discrete sites along its length. Because DNA from each person is unique, a series of restriction enzymes will cut DNA taken from a person into a set of small fragments, the size of which should be unique to each individual. The fragments can be quantified by GEL ELECTROPHORESIS. If a sample of DNA is obtained at a crime scene, it

can be compared using DNA fingerprinting to a sample taken from a suspect. In the case that two different patterns are produced, then it is likely that the suspect's DNA was not that found at the crime scene.

FIONA M. INGLIS

DNQX *see* CNQX

docking site *see* mobilization

doctrine of specific nerve energies The doctrine of specific nerve energies holds that each sensory nerve, whether visual, auditory or whatever, has its own characteristic quality which informs the organism about the source of the stimulus. Thus it is a theory of neural coding. In 1838 Mueller (1801–1858) theorized that an organism could distinguish between the senses, such as vision and audition, by the different or specific 'energies' these nerves presented to the sensing brain. He based this idea on the fact that however the OPTIC NERVE (for example) is stimulated – by light, or direct stimulation of the eye or optic nerve – the sensation is always visual since the 'visual energy' released would always be the same. However no specific energies were found. But in the same paper he also proposed a contrary and enduring theory that distinctions between the senses depend on the function of the area of the brain to which they project. (Unknown to him, this theory had been proposed by Bell in 1811.) For example, it is beyond doubt that visual sensations depend on activation of a visual part of the brain, and that there is a visual nerve projecting to and activating this area. This is the presently accepted version of the doctrine of specific nerve energies, with the term being a misnomer.

This tradition, that each structure has a different function, was first proposed by Gall. It continued on an implicit level when the unit structure of the brain, the individual NEURON, was discovered. Thus in this theory each individual neuron as well as each nerve is assumed to have a specific function. For example, it is assumed that there are neurons whose activity means 'red' or 'salty' etc. At the neuronal level the doctrine of specific nerve energies is sometimes called the LABELLED-LINE THEORY. Since each neuron is to represent only one stimulus, it is difficult for this theory to account for the fact that individual neurons are usually involved in encoding many different stimuli (see ACROSS-FIBRE PATTERN THEORY). However this theory serves well for some innate mechanisms of unvarying character, such as the escape response of the crayfish which is based on giant motor axons (see MOTOR NEURONS) to the tail; these neurons can be clearly specified or labelled as serving nothing other than escape. The wide range of pheromone-based behaviours, each of which has only one goal, is based on sensory neurons specifically sensitive to that odour, and leading only to that behaviour. Thus these also are specific neurons.

ROBERT P. ERICKSON

dominance Some species of animal form long-lasting social groups. Most commonly, it is thought, this has the biological function of reducing predation risk. The resulting close association of individuals inevitably increases direct, contest competition: for mating, food, and other resources. For any particular pair of individuals, contests often have a consistent outcome, over time and over different types of resource; when this happens, one individual is said to be dominant to the other. Once a dominance relationship is established, the subordinate will often avoid further contests with the dominant, thus reducing risk of injury in aggressive encounters – whose outcome is predictably unlikely to benefit the subordinate itself. (Confusingly, it is sometimes claimed that dominance benefits subordinates, since they can use avoidance to reduce futile aggression – but note that the main resource benefits accrue to the dominant.)

Dominance may be no more than a reflection of relative physical power, weight or weaponry. However, in some species of PRIMATES at least, other factors are involved. Maternal support of offspring generally enables a dependant to win contests with any adult its mother can dominate. In many Old World monkeys, in which females tend to remain in the troop of their birth all their lives, this effect is so prevalent that daughters effectively 'inherit' a rank just below their mother's, and retain it after the mother's death. Among chimpanzees, rank

appears unimportant to females, whereas males invest much energy in status interactions. In male chimpanzees, support from other individuals is often crucial for attaining the highest rank, or ALPHA MALE status. In different populations, this support has been noted to come from kin (an elder brother), from a group of several females, or from a single male. In the latter case, this 'kingmaking' role gives the supporter an opportunity sometimes to switch allegiance between two powerful rivals, thereby gaining personal benefits during the resulting instability.

While dominance relationships may not be transitive, in many species they are (that is, if A beats B, and B beats C, then A beats C). Then, a linear ordering fully describes the dominance structure of the group. This was originally noticed in chickens and called a PECKING ORDER, but is most commonly termed a LINEAR HIERARCHY OF DOMINANCE, often somewhat confusingly shortened to DOMINANCE HIERARCHY. The explanatory value of this concept depends on its generality: where it holds true for several sorts of interaction (mating supplants, monopolization of prime food resources, choice of favoured sleeping sites, and so on) it is a useful and compact description of social relationships. However, this is not always the case. In chimpanzees, for instance, despite the great energy invested by male chimpanzees in competing for rank, dominance rank does not reliably predict access to resources. Access to the most prized food, meat, is a prerogative of older animals, not high-ranking ones; sleeping sites seem to be uncontested; and while the highest-rank male can monopolize matings with any nearby female, females often exercise their own choice, going off temporarily with a male of lower rank when they are fertile.

See also: social behaviour; sociobiology

RICHARD W. BYRNE

dominance hierarchy *see* dominance

dominant allele An allele of a particular gene on one member of an autosomal pair of CHROMOSOMES, which will contribute to the PHENOTYPE of its encoded protein (see PROTEINS), and hence that of the organism, regardless of the form of allele present on the second chromosome. If two co-dominant alleles of a single gene exist, the resultant phenotype will be a mix of the two characteristics encoded for by these alleles.

See also: autosomal chromosome; autosomal dominant; gene; recessive allele

FIONA M. INGLIS

dominant eye The two eyes tend to be asymmetrical in their function. One of the clearest examples of this, and one of the earliest discovered, is in a sighting task where an observer is required to point with a finger at a distant target. Alternate closure of the eyes reveals that when viewed with one of the eyes, the finger and target will remain in alignment, whereas, by definition, this will not be the case with the other eye. The eye that is used for sighting in said to be the 'dominant eye'. Many other tasks also show asymmetries where one eye is favoured or appears to control behaviour, such as conjugate saccadic EYE MOVEMENTS during READING, BINOCULAR RIVALRY, and VISUAL ACUITY. Different estimates of eye dominance do not perfectly correlate, and there are probably many different forms of the phenomenon.

DAVID W. HEELEY

dominant gene *see* dominant allele

domoic acid (domoate) One of the EXCITATORY AMINO ACIDS having actions at the kainate receptor (see GLUTAMATE RECEPTORS). It is rarely used experimentally but is of interest in that it is one of the NEUROTOXINS found in contaminated mussels.

See also: drug ionization

DOPA *see* L-DOPA; dopamine

DOPA decarboxylase *see* aromatic L-amino acid decarboxylase; dopamine

DOPAC Abbreviation for 3,4-dihydroxyphenylacetic acid; see DOPAMINE.

dopamine Dopamine (DA) is a neurotransmitter; neurons that contain dopamine are said to be DOPAMINERGIC. It is one of the CATECHOLAMINE neurotransmitters and therefore a member of the even larger family of MONO-

AMINE neurotransmitters. The full chemical name for dopamine is 3,4-DIHYDROXYPHENYLETHYLAMINE. Dopamine is synthesized from the amino acid L-TYROSINE. The enzyme tyrosine hydroxylase catalyses the conversion of tyrosine to L-DOPA (L-3,4-DIHYDROXYPHENYLALANINE). L-DOPA is then converted by AROMATIC L-AMINO ACID DECARBOXYLASE to dopamine. In dopaminergic neurons, this is as far as the conversion goes, dopamine being transported and packaged for use as a neurotransmitter. However, further conversion of dopamine can produce another catecholamine neurotransmitter, NORADRENALINE. The presence of the enzyme dopamine beta hydroxylase, involved in the conversion of dopamine to noradrenaline, is the principal way to discriminate noradrenaline- from dopamine-containing neurons, dopamine of course being present in all of them. There are multiple receptors for dopamine present in the brain (see D1–D5 DOPAMINE RECEPTORS). The synaptic action of dopamine is terminated in two ways: destruction by enzymes or by reuptake, for which there are specific dopamine transporters. Enzymatic destruction can be achieved by either of two enzymes: MONOAMINE OXIDASE (MAO) or CATECHOL-O-METHYLTRANSFERASE (COMT). (Both MONOAMINE OXIDASE-A and MONOAMINE OXIDASE-B effectively degrade dopamine.) Monoamine oxidase destruction of dopamine leads to formation of the metabolite 3,4-DIHYDROXYPHENYLACETALDEHYDE (DHPA) which ALDEHYDE DEHYDROGENASE further converts to 3,4-DIHYRODXYPHENYLACETICACID(DOPAC).COMT destruction of dopamine leads to production of the metabolite 3-METHOXYTYRAMINE (3-MT) which monoamine oxidase can convert to 3-METHOXY-4-HYDROXYPHENYLACETALDEHYDE (MHPA). DOPAC can be further converted by COMT and MHPA by aldehyde dehydrogenase to produce a final metabolite, HOMOVANILLIC ACID (HVA). Measurement of the metabolites of dopamine (or indeed any other neurochemical) can give important information regarding its synthesis in brain.

Dopamine neurons are found in a variety of places within the brain: the NIGROSTRIATAL DOPAMINE SYSTEM, MESOLIMBIC DOPAMINE SYSTEM and the MESOLIMBICOCORTICAL SYSTEM are the most widely studied, being involved in a variety of psychological process to do with MOTOR CONTROL, cognition and REWARD. Loss of dopamine from the nigrostriatal system gives rise to PARKINSON'S DISEASE, while changes in the dopamine content of the NUCLEUS ACCUMBENS and PREFRONTAL CORTEX have been associated with schizophrenia (see DOPAMINE HYPOTHESIS OF SCHIZOPHRENIA). However, these are just the best known and most often studied dopamine systems. In fact dopamine has a wide variety of functions, indicated by the variety of places in which it is found. Dopamine neurons are also found in all of these places: the DIENCEPHALOSPINAL DOPAMINE SYSTEM projects from the HYPOTHALAMUS to the SPINAL CORD; the PERIVENTRICULAR DOPAMINE SYSTEM projects from the PERIAQUEDUCTAL GREY to the hypothalamus and THALAMUS; the INCERTOHYPOTHALAMIC DOPAMINE SYSTEM is contained within the hypothalamus; the TUBEROHYPOPHYSEAL DOPAMINE SYSTEM projects from the hypothalamus to the PITUITARY GLAND (see also TUBEROINFUNDIBULAR DOPAMINE SYSTEM); the PERIGLOMERULAR DOPAMINE NEURONS are found in the OLFACTORY BULB; and dopamine neurons are also found in the RETINA. (Note that many of these systems also have an 'A' number: the SUBSTANTIA NIGRA pars compacta dopamine neurons are for example the A9 neurons, while those of the VENTRAL TEGMENTAL AREA are the A10 neurons. These relate to the CLASSIFICATION OF DAHLSTRÖM AND FUXE.)

One final note: dopamine has received extensive study since its first description as a neurotransmitter in the 1950s. It is worth considering though the very many tools there are to do this with: there are histological techniques (HISTOFLUORESCENCE and IMMUNOHISTOCHEMISTRY) and biochemical analysis using HIGH-PERFORMANCE LIQUID CHROMATOGRAPHY (HPLC). There are specific lesioning agents, 6-HYDROXYDOPAMINE and MPTP, and a variety of drugs specific for all aspects of dopamine synthesis and degradation, as well as drugs to activate or inactivate receptors, or promote or inhibit dopamine release. Other neurotransmitters have not been nearly so well studied: to what extent is our interest in a given system simply the product of having the tools available with which to study it?

Reference

Feldman R., Meyer J.S. & Quenzer L.F. (1997) *Principles of Neuropsychopharmacology*, Sinauer Associates: Sunderland MA.

dopamine beta hydroxylase *see* dopamine; noradrenaline

dopamine hypothesis of schizophrenia
Theory concerning the aetiology of SCHIZOPHRENIA. The demonstration that effective ANTIPSYCHOTIC drugs have the common property of blocking D2 DOPAMINE receptors led to the idea that hyperactivity of the dopaminergic system may represent the aetiological basis of schizophrenia. However, efforts to demonstrate dopaminergic abnormalities in untreated schizophrenic patients have proved inconclusive, with biochemical, post-mortem, neuroimaging and genetic studies failing consistently to support the hypothesis. The fact that CLOZAPINE, an atypical NEUROLEPTIC, has greater antipsychotic efficacy than traditional neuroleptics, but has less affinity for dopamine receptors further weakens the proposition that schizophrenia is caused by hyperactivity of dopamine. Several reasons have been suggested to account for this. (1) The antipsychotic effects of traditional neuroleptics may be mediated by mechanisms unrelated to the aetiology of schizophrenia. (2) Other (presently unidentified) factors acting in concert with the dopaminergic system may prove to be important. (3) Dopamine activity in the schizophrenic brain may change in different ways in different structures. It has been suggested for example that dopamine activity in the PREFRONTAL CORTEX may be decreased while activity in the NUCLEUS ACCUMBENS is increased, these changes being reciprocally related to each other. The relationship of these changes to the signs and symptoms of schizophrenia remains uncertain, and what causes the changes in the first place is unknown, but such ideas serve to keep the dopamine hypothesis of schizophrenia tantalizingly viable.

Reference

Davis K.L., Kahn R.S., Ko G, & Davidson M. (1991) Dopamine and schizophrenia: a review and reconceptualization. *American Journal of Psychiatry* 148: 1471–1486.

IAN C. REID

dopamine transporter A mechanism for transporting DOPAMINE across a MEMBRANE; see REUPTAKE.

dopaminergic Relating to the neurotransmitter DOPAMINE. For instance, a neuron that synthesizes and releases dopamine is said to be dopaminergic.

dorsal The dorsal surface of the body of a four-legged vertebrate is the top surface (where the SPINAL CORD is). It is contrasted with the VENTRAL surface, the belly, the surface nearest the ground. In two-legged vertebrates such as man the dorsal surface is the back, the ventral surface the front. In terms of brain orientation, dorsal means top (or above), ventral means bottom (or below).

dorsal acoustic stria *see* cochlear nucleus

dorsal bundle *see* dorsal noradrenergic bundle; ventral noradrenergic bundle

dorsal column nuclei of the medulla oblongata These are the GRACILE NUCLEUS and the CUNEATE NUCLEUS.

See also: spinal cord

dorsal column – medial lemniscal system The major ascending pathway for the senses of TOUCH and proprioception (see PROPRIOCEPTORS) for all parts of the body except the head. Primary sensory afferents from touch receptors and proprioceptors enter the spinal cord and ascend in the dorsal columns. Afferents from the feet and legs are medial to those from the hands and arms and synapse in the GRACILE NUCLEUS and CUNEATE NUCLEUS, respectively. These two nuclei are called the dorsal column nuclei. Axons from the second-order neurons in these nuclei cross to the opposite side of the BRAINSTEM and ascend to the THALAMUS in a fibre tract called the MEDIAL LEMNISCUS. Fibres in the medial lemniscus are joined by second-order axons from the trigeminal nuclei which carry similar information for the face and head. Damage to the neurons in the dorsal column-medial lemniscal system produces deficits in fine touch and proprioception.

DOUGLAS D. RASMUSSON

dorsal funiculus *see* spinal cord

dorsal horn A part of the SPINAL CORD: this has dorsal and a VENTRAL HORN and, at thoracic levels, a LATERAL HORN also.

See also: autonomic nervous system

dorsal motor nucleus of the vagus The origin of the motor VAGUS NERVE, in the MEDULLA OBLONGATA. PREGANGLIONIC NEURONS innervate the GASTROINTESTINAL SYSTEM and CARDIOVASCULAR SYSTEM. It receives input from a variety of sites in the central nervous system: several nuclei of the HYPOTHALAMUS (including LATERAL HYPOTHALAMUS and PARAVENTRICULAR NUCLEUS OF THE HYPOTHALAMUS project here).

See also: autonomic nervous system; nucleus of the solitary tract

dorsal noradrenergic bundle The DORSAL NORADRENERGIC BUNDLE (DNAB) and the VENTRAL NORADRENERGIC BUNDLE (VNAB) are the principal NORADRENALINE-containing systems that arise in the PONS and MEDULLA to innervate a variety of FOREBRAIN sites. They are often referred to simply as the dorsal bundle and ventral bundle respectively. Originally described by Ungerstedt (1971), they were initially thought of as being relatively compact, but later studies revealed them to be less so than had been thought.

The ventral bundle arises from the lateral tegmental noradrenaline containing cell groups A1–A5 (see CLASSIFICATION OF DAHLSTRÖM AND FUXE) and is sometimes therefore referred to as the lateral tegmental noradrenergic system. These cell groups lie relatively deep in the brain: cell group A1 for example is close by the AREA POSTREMA and NUCLEUS OF THE SOLITARY TRACT, while A2 lies near the DORSAL MOTOR NUCLEUS OF THE VAGUS. The axons of all of these cell groups collect into the ventral bundle, which passes below the SUPERIOR CEREBELLAR PEDUNCLE before ascending to join the MEDIAL FOREBRAIN BUNDLE. The principal targets of the ventral bundle are subcortical: the largest projections are to the

HYPOTHALAMUS, AMYGDALA and the SEPTAL NUCLEI, though there are other targets, including parts of the THALAMUS and the NUCLEUS ACCUMBENS, and many brainstem targets. Functionally, the ventral bundle has been associated with the transmission of autonomic information and destruction of it is known to lead to deficits in activities such as FEEDING, DRINKING and SEXUAL BEHAVIOUR.

The dorsal bundle arises principally from cell groups A6 and A7. The A6 group is in the LOCUS COERULEUS, while A7 is referred to as being subcoeruleal. The axons of these neurons collect into the dorsal bundle and also pass through and below the superior cerebellar peduncle (though on a course different to that of the ventral bundle). Through the MIDBRAIN they take a course significantly more dorsal to that of the ventral bundle before joining the medial forebrain bundle. Dorsal bundle fibres leave here via a variety of routes (the MAMMILOTHALAMIC TRACT, DIAGONAL BAND OF BROCA, STRIA MEDULLARIS, STRIA TERMINALIS, FORNIX) to innervate sites in the thalamus, amygdala, septal nuclei and nucleus accumbens (as well as brainstem sites) that also receive input from the ventral bundle. However, the principal targets of the dorsal bundle are the HIPPOCAMPUS and CEREBRAL CORTEX which do not receive input from the ventral bundle. Functionally, the dorsal bundle has been associated with ATTENTION and AROUSAL. It is noteworthy in this context that the locus coeruleus has a very strong CARDIOVASCULAR SYSTEM input.

The dorsal and ventral bundles interact with each other and with other nuclei in the ASCENDING RETICULAR ACTIVATING SYSTEM and are involved in discriminably different functions. What remains most remarkable about them however is that such a small number of neurons – only some 2000 in the rat locus coeruleus – should innervate such a wide area of tissue in the central nervous system.

Reference

Ungerstedt U. (1971) Stereotaxic mapping of the monoamine pathways in the rat brain. *Acta Physiologica Scandinavica*, suppl. 367: 1–48.

dorsal noradrenergic bundle; ventral noradrenergic bundle The dorsal noradrenergic bundle is the main ascending fibre bundle arising from the LOCUS COERULEUS. It ascends through the midbrain tegmentum in a position ventrolateral to the PERIAQUEDUCTAL GREY. Upon entering the DIENCEPHALON, the dorsal noradrenergic bundle shifts ventrally and enters the MEDIAL FOREBRAIN BUNDLE, and travels with the latter and its terminal branches into the NEOCORTEX. The dorsal noradrenergic bundle gives off numerous COLLATERALS, providing NORADRENERGIC innervation to virtually all FOREBRAIN and rostral BRAINSTEM structures.

KAZUE SEMBA

dorsal pallidum The terms dorsal and VENTRAL PALLIDUM were introduced in the early 1980s following the conceptual reorganization of CAUDATE–PUTAMEN and NUCLEUS ACCUMBENS (and other structures) into a single (see VENTRAL STRIATUM; DORSAL STRIATUM). The ventral pallidum is the major target for the EFFERENT projections from the ventral striatum while dorsal striatal neurons project to dorsal pallidum. However, while ventral pallidum contains a variety of individual structures, the dorsal pallidum is synonymous with the internal and external segments of the GLOBUS PALLIDUS.

dorsal raphe nucleus *see* raphe nuclei

dorsal root A body of nerves extending from the dorsal portion of the SPINAL CORD. These roots arise bilaterally, at each segment of the spinal cord, from the dorsolateral surface of the cord. They are composed of the axons of SENSORY NEURONS whose cell bodies are found in the DORSAL ROOT GANGLIA. These sensory neurons are PSEUDOUNIPOLAR NEURONS, with cell bodies in the dorsal root ganglia: one branch of the process carries information into the spinal cord, the other branch having collected information from the body.

See also: ventral root

dorsal root ganglion *see* dorsal root

dorsal spatial system *see* dorsal stream

dorsal stream The primary visual area V1 (see AREAS V1–V5), the principal receiving point for information arriving at the CEREBRAL CORTEX from the eye, serves also to distribute different bits of visual information to other areas, both cortical and subcortical. The cortical targets include the secondary visual structures: MIDDLE TEMPORAL REGION (MT or V5), V2, V3, V3A and parts of the PARIETAL LOBE. These areas form the backbone of the dorsal stream, a cluster of areas that begins in area V1 and ends in the posterior parietal complex. The dorsal stream transforms the visual information that guides and controls our actions on a moment-to-moment basis.

See also: visuomotor control

A. DAVID MILNER

dorsal striatopallidal system The dorsal striatopallidal system parallels the VENTRAL STRIATOPALLIDAL SYSTEM (see CORTICOSTRIATAL LOOPS) and is represented by the circuitry that originates in NEOCORTEX, projects to the dorsal striatum (see DORSAL STRIATUM; VENTRAL STRIATUM) and thence to the GLOBUS PALLIDUS, THALAMUS (ventroanterior – ventrolateral nuclei) and back, as re-entrant circuitry, to the CORTEX.

dorsal striatum *see* striatum

dorsal terminal nucleus *see* accessory optic system

dorsolateral funiculus *see* spinal cord

dorsolateral prefrontal cortex The dorsolateral prefrontal cortex in the human brain essentially comprises BRODMANN'S AREAS 9, 46 and 45, from superior to inferior. In non-human primates, two subdivisions of the lateral prefrontal cortex are generally recognized, a dorsal area equivalent to area 9 and the superior part of area 46, and a ventral area comprising the inferior part of area 46 and area 45. In the macaque brain, the dorsolateral prefrontal cortex is usually viewed as the area surrounding the PRINCIPAL SULCUS, but variations in nomenclature of this area of cortex based on cytoarchitectonic distinctions (see CYTOARCHITECTURE) makes it difficult to be categorical about precisely which areas of cortex are included. Generally, it includes areas

9 and 46, but also rostral parts of area 8 (FRONTAL EYE FIELDS). Major afferents to the dorsolateral prefrontal cortex arise in the DORSOMEDIAL NUCLEUS OF THE THALAMUS, but thalamic afferents also arise in the medial pulvinar and ventral anterior nuclei. It receives long association, cortico-cortical, fibres from the posterior and middle SUPERIOR TEMPORAL GYRUS and from the PARIETAL CORTEX. Within the FRONTAL LOBE, afferents arise in the frontal pole (area 10) and the MEDIAL PREFRONTAL CORTEX (area 32). It projects to the SUPPLEMENTARY MOTOR AREA, dorsal premotor cortex and frontal eye field. All these thalamic and cortical connections are reciprocal. This area of the prefrontal cortex is associated with EXECUTIVE FUNCTIONS, including planning, attentional set-shifting and short-term spatial working-memory processes.

See also: cytoarchitecture

BARRY J. EVERITT

dorsomedial nucleus of the hypothalamus A nucleus in the HYPOTHALAMUS with extensive intrahypothalamic connections to the VENTROMEDIAL NUCLEUS OF THE HYPOTHALAMUS, PARAVENTRICULAR NUCLEUS OF THE HYPOTHALAMUS, LATERAL HYPOTHALAMUS, ARCUATE NUCLEUS and others. It is thought to be an important relay in circuitry dealing with FEEDING and BODY WEIGHT regulation, as well as other processes.

Reference

Bernardis L.L. & Bellinger L.L. (1998) The dorsomedial hypothalamic nucleus revisited: 1998 update. *Proceedings of the Society for Experimental Biology and Medicine* 218: 284–306.

dorsomedial nucleus of the thalamus Also known as the medial dorsal nucleus (medialis dorsalis) this is the largest of the medial group of nuclei in the THALAMUS. It lies just lateral to the MASSA INTERMEDIA and can be subdivided into at least three different portions. This nucleus is most notable for its very extensive, reciprocal connections with the PREFRONTAL CORTEX. These connections have a crude topography arranged in medial to lateral strips. Other major connections include inputs from the rostral TEMPORAL LOBE, the AMYGDALA and the BASAL FOREBRAIN. The dorsomedial nucleus is thought to have a general involvement in LEARNING via its frontal interactions. Damage to this nucleus contributes to diencephalic amnesic conditions but is probably not sufficient to cause the amnesia (see DIENCEPHALIC AMNESIA).

JOHN P. AGGLETON

dose dependent The effects of most drugs are dose-dependent; that is, different doses of a DRUG have different effects on whatever is being measured – for example, transmitter release or behaviour. True dose dependency involves showing that there are different effects of different doses of drug, rather than differences between all doses of a drug and a control solution.

See also: dose response curve; EC50; ED50; LD50; Lyon–Robbins hypothesis

dose effect curve The graphic representation of the magnitude of a DRUG effect as a function of the dose of the drug. The dose effect curve, also known as the DOSE RESPONSE CURVE, is an essential feature of well-controlled experiments in pharmacology and PSYCHOPHARMACOLOGY. Although data can be represented in varying ways, the basic curve is a plot of the size or magnitude of the effect on the y-axis and the dose (or concentration) of the compound under study on the x-axis. The ideal dose effect curve has at least three doses of the drug plus VEHICLE, and preferably more. The range of the doses should ideally be quite broad. For example, a common strategy is to test drug doses that vary by log concentrations. It is important to show a relationship between dose and effect in order to clearly demonstrate a specific, physiological effect of the drug. The shape of dose effect curves can vary depending on the pharmacological or neurochemical effects of the drug, as well as the behaviour under study. Most dose effect curves show a positive linear relationship between dose and effect; however, in most systems an asymptote is reached in which further increases in dose will not result in a stronger response. Also common in psychopharmacology are inverted U-shaped dose effect curves. In this case, the maximum effect is reached at a certain dose,

and then decreases with further increases in dose.

See also: dose-dependent; Lyon–Robbins hypothesis; rate–frequency curve; Yerkes-Dodson law

ANN E. KELLEY

dose response curve *see* dose effect curve

Dostoeyevskian epilepsy This is not properly a form of epilepsy at all, but a condition related to it. It is better referred to as interictal syndrome: individuals with this condition show an obsession with work and productivity, and with spiritual matters. It is thought that the Russian novelist Fyodor Mikhailovich Dostoevsky (1821–1881) might have had this condition.

double blind study A study in which neither the subject of the experiment, nor the experimenter controlling it, knows what treatment condition the subject is in. In a study examining the effectiveness of a DRUG on human performance for example, neither the subject nor the experimenter would know whether drug or control was being administered, nor what dose of drug was being given. It is used as a means for controlling possible bias in the results being introduced by experimenter or subject expectations. Such expectations need not be conscious, but may be unconscious biases induced by expectation or observation of the effects of the drug. A SINGLE BLIND STUDY is one in which the experimenter knows what the treatment is but the subject does not. An OPEN STUDY is one in which all participants know what is being done. The terms double blind and single blind relate to experiments in which humans are taking part as subjects. In experiments involving animals there are different considerations. Although animals cannot know or be informed about what treatment they are getting in the way that humans can, they nevertheless can use conditioned (see CONDITIONING) cues to predict events. In experiments involving individual animals receiving both control and test components of an experiment, it is important to make sure that treatment and control conditions are identical and provide no hidden cues. In studies involving experimental animals it is perhaps more important to have the experimenters ignorant of the treatment conditions being used, to prevent observer bias.

See also: placebo

double dissociation This neuropsychology method differentiates two functions that may appear very similar. If symptom A appears in patients with a LESION in area A, but does not appear in patients with a lesion in area B, and symptom B appears in patients with a lesion in area B, but not in patients with a lesion in area A, then symptoms A and B are independent, and should not be categorized together. A single lesion may cause many discrete symptoms if the neural structures underlying them are anatomically close.

See also: dissociation

JENNI A. OGDEN

double labelling Double labelling techniques are anatomical techniques for simultaneous visualization of two markers in tissues, allowing determination of COLOCALIZATION of two markers in the same neurons, or the degree of overlap of two cell populations containing different markers. The markers are tagged to labels that are distinguishable by the colour or other features. Markers may include two RETROGRADE TRACERS, which would allow identification of neurons innervating two targets via branching axons. A retrograde tracer may be combined with an immunohistochemical marker to identify the neurotransmitter in PROJECTION NEURONS. MESSENGER RNA identified with *IN SITU* HYBRIDIZATION techniques may also be used.

See also: histology; immunohistochemistry

KAZUE SEMBA

double opponent process colour cells Also known as DUAL OPPONENT CELLS, these are neurons in the VISUAL SYSTEM, selectively sensitive to colour differences and insensitive to intensity (black/white) differences, which are important for the coding of colour. The RECEPTIVE FIELD of the double opponent neuron has a centre-surround arrangement. The centre is governed by a cone opponent process and the surround has the same opponent process but with inverted sign (see OPPONENT PROCESS

THEORY OF COLOUR VISION). For example, if the centre subtracts the M from the L cone outputs (that is, L–M), the surround will have an M–L cone opponency. These cells were first discovered in the retinas of fish, and later reported in the primate visual cortex, especially the CORTICAL BLOBS of the STRIATE CORTEX.

See also: trichromatic theory of colour vision

KATHY T. MULLEN

down regulation *see* sensitization (receptor)

Down syndrome A chromosomal abnormality that is the commonest cause of MENTAL HANDICAP in children, affecting 1 in 600 live births. Once known as mongolism, Down syndrome is characterized by distinctive morphological features in the development of the face and neck, a shortened stature, immune deficiency, and a developmental heart defect that is the commonest cause of early death, as well as the marked sub-normality. The risk of having a Down syndrome child increases in mothers older than 30 and fathers older than 60. The mental subnormality involves a wide range of social and intellectual functions, and can vary widely in severity. The most severely affected do not acquire the ability to speak, dress or feed themselves, and require total lifelong care, whereas with family support the less affected can develop good language skills, begin to read, maintain good social interactions, and undertake simple work.

Down syndrome is in most cases due to the embryo acquiring an extra copy (trisomy) of chromosome 21 at MEIOSIS (see CHROMOSOMES; CELL DIVISION). In rare cases, the syndrome may also arise from chromosomal translocations in which only a fragment of chromosome 21 is carried in triplicate, implicating the distal part of the long arm of chromosome 21 as the obligate region that determines the syndrome. This segment of the chromosome is associated with genes for SUPEROXIDE DISMUTASE, important in regulating developmental cell death (see APOPTOSIS), and the AMYLOID PRECURSOR PROTEIN implicated in the development of the pathology of Alzheimer's disease. The chromosomal abnormalities can be detected *in utero* by amniocentesis or the newer techniques of chorionic villa sampling, and routine prenatal screening allows the parents, with counselling, to decide whether to terminate the pregnancy.

Until recently, the majority of Down syndrome cases died in childhood and young adulthood, in particular due to the atrioventricular septal heart defect and an impaired immunological response. In the last three decades improved health care has markedly increased the life span of affected individuals, commonly into their 50s. This has revealed an additional burden of an Alzheimer-like dementia with onset at 40–50 years of age, and the same pathology as Alzheimer disease is seen at *post mortem* of senile PLAQUES and NEUROFIBRILLARY TANGLES. Since all affected individuals ultimately develop this pathology and dementia several decades earlier than its occurrence in spontaneous Alzheimer's disease, Down syndrome has become an important source of information for studying the development of Alzheimer-like pathology. It turns out that the first detectable pathological event is the deposition of the β/A4 amyloid protein in the brains in teenage cases. The association of this primary pathology with triplication of a particular chromosome was the critical clue enabling the search for the amyloid precursor protein gene to focus on chromosome 21, leading to its rapid identification and sequencing in 1987.

Trisomy of different chromosomes can be selectively bred in various strains of mice having acrocentric chromosomes by crossbreeding between parents with different Robertsonian translocations. Most trisomies in mice are lethal, as in humans, including trisomy of murine chromosome 16 (syntenic to chromosome 21 in humans) which die *in utero* of a septal heart defect. The murine models have proved useful for detailed analysis of pathology in the development of systems in the brain as well as of peripheral organs. It has been shown that trisomy 16 mouse brain tissues will also develop an Alzheimer-like pathology by transplantation of embryonic cortical donor tissue into the brains of normal host mice.

Reference

Holland A.J. & Oliver C. (1995) Down's syndrome and the link with Alzheimer's disease. *Journal of Neurology, Neurosurgery and Psychiatry* 59: 111–114.

STEPHEN B. DUNNETT

drawing *see* copying and drawing

dreaming Mental activity does not cease at sleep onset. Current scientific evidence suggests instead that it is virtually continuous throughout sleep but that its level of intensity and its formal characteristics change as the brain changes its state with the periodic recurrence of the NON-REM SLEEP and REM SLEEP (rapid eye movement sleep) phases. This entry gives a summary of how the cellular and molecular level changes in the brain which distinguish waking, NREM and REM sleep can be used to account for the concomitant shifts in mental state.

When subjects are aroused from sleep in a laboratory setting or when they awaken spontaneously at home, they give reports of pre-awakening conscious experience that are quite different if their brain state is REM than if it is non-REM. REM sleep dream reports are seven times longer and are far more likely to describe formed sensory perceptions, and vivid visual images than are the reports of NREM dreams which tend to be more thought-like and dull. REM sleep reports are also far more likely to be animated with descriptions of walking, running, playing sports, or even flying. Finally the REM sleep dream scenarios are accompanied by strong emotions such as anxiety, elation, and anger, all of which bear a close relationship to details of the plot. The formal features of dreaming correlate well with changes in the activation level of the brain as measured by the degree of high voltage, slow frequency power in the sleep ELECTROENCEPHALOGRAM. Because the high-voltage slow wave activity of NREM sleep is most intense and prolonged in the first half of the night, reports from awakenings performed then are more likely to show differences from REM reports than are those from the second half of the night. Brain activation is therefore an easily understandable determinant of dream length and visual intensity.

Dreaming may also occur at sleep onset when the brain activation level is just beginning to fall. Sleep onset dreaming is likely to be evanescent and fragmentary with less vivid IMAGERY, less strong emotion and less well-developed story-lines than in REM sleep dreams. Collaborating with the still-high activation level to produce sleep onset dreaming is the rapidly rising threshold to external sensory stimulation. This factor allows internal stimuli to dominate the brain and protects REM sleep brain activation from external sensory influence. If the stimulus level is raised to sufficiently high levels, external information can be incorporated into dream plots but the critical window for such incorporation is narrow and external stimuli more commonly interrupt dreaming by causing awakening. When dreams are interrupted in this way, recall of dreaming is markedly enhanced to levels as high as 95% if the subject is aroused from REM sleep during a cluster of rapid eye movements.

This strong correlation between dreaming and REM sleep with eye movement has encouraged attempts to model the brain basis of dreaming at the cellular and molecular level. The ACTIVATION-SYNTHESIS HYPOTHESIS, first put forward in 1977, ascribed dreaming to activation of the brain in REM sleep by a well-specified pontine BRAINSTEM mechanism. Such distinctive aspects of dream mentation as the vivid visual hallucinations, the constant sense of movement, and the strong emotion were ascribed to internal stimulation of visual, motor and LIMBIC SYSTEM regions of the upper brain by signals of brain stem origins. The bizarreness of dream cognition with its characteristic instability of time, place and person was thought to be due to the chaotic nature of the autoactivation process and to the failure of short-term memory caused by the chemical changes in REM described by the RECIPROCAL INTERACTION MODEL OF BRAIN STATE control first advanced in 1975.

Using microelectrode recording techniques to sample individual cell activity during natural sleep and waking in animal models, it has been possible to show that the neuromodulatory systems of the brainstem behave very differently in waking and REM sleep and the differences help to account for the distinctive psychological features of dreaming, especially the bizarreness and recent memory loss. During waking, cells of the noradrenergic LOCUS COERULEUS and the serotonergic RAPHE NUCLEI are tonically active but in REM they are shut off. This means that the activated brain of REM is demodulated by aminergic neurons so that it cannot – and does not – process information in the same way as it does in waking. Dream bizarreness and dream amnesia are both results of this neuromodulatory effect. Compounding this difference, the pontine cholinergic neurons become reciprocally activated in REM and their intense phasic activity conveys eye movement related information to the visual sensory and motor areas of the brain (accounting for dream hallucinosis) and to the AMYGDALA (accounting for the emotion of dreams).

The specification of these neurochemical differences enables a 3-dimensional state–space model to be constructed which integrates activation level (A), input–output gating (I) with the brain modulatory factor (M). This hybrid psychophysiological construct thus updates both activation synthesis and reciprocal interaction representing the energy (A), information source (I) and processing mode (M) of the brain mind as a single point continuously moving through the state space as a function of the values of A, I and M. According to AIM, dreaming is most likely to occur when activation is high, when the information source shifts from external to internal, and when the neuromodulatory balance shifts from aminergic to cholinergic.

Our natural scepticism about the relevance of animal model data for human psychophysiology has been partially dispelled by recent FUNCTIONAL NEUROIMAGING studies of the human brain which reveal significant regional changes in activation level during REM sleep compared to waking; subjects of these studies all reported dreams after awakening from REM in the scanner. First and foremost is activation of the pontine brainstem, the presumed organizer of the REM sleep brain. Second, is the selective activation of the limbic forebrain and PARALIMBIC CORTEX, the supposed mediator of dream emotion. Third, is the selective inactivation of the dorsal prefrontal cortex, a brain region essential to self-reflective awareness and to executively guided thought, judgement, and action, all functions which are deficient in dreaming.

Unfortunately, imaging techniques do not have the spatial or molecular resolution necessary to confirm the neuromodulatory hypothesis of AIM. But an extensive body of human psychopharmacological data is consonant with the basic assumptions of the model. Drugs which act as aminergic agonists (or REUPTAKE blockers) first suppress REM and REM sleep dreaming. When they are later withdrawn, a marked and unpleasant intensification of dreaming ensues. If those drugs also possess anticholinergic actions, the effects on dreaming are even more pronounced. Finally, and most significantly, human REM sleep dreaming is potentiated by some of the same cholinergic agonist drugs which experimentally enhance REM sleep in animals.

Reference

Kahn D., Pace-Schott E.F. and Hobson J.A. (1997) Consciousness in waking and dreaming: the roles of neuronal oscillation and neuromodulation in determining similarities and differences. *Neuroscience* 78: 13–38.

J. ALLAN HOBSON

dressing apraxia An inability to dress oneself correctly; one of the four principal forms of APRAXIA described by Henry Hecaen (1912–1938).

drinking Drinking is an act controlled by both physiological and psychological factors, and is arguably the most important act that animals engage in. Absence of drinking for more than 24 h produces serious dehydration, which if continued will soon lead to death. There are a variety of physiological mechanisms, closely monitored by the brain, which regulate water balance and trigger the act of drinking – see OSMOREGULATION for discussion of these. As with FEEDING though, there are a variety of non-specific stimuli that trigger drinking, and the composition and taste of fluids on offer is evidently important (see ALCOHOL for example). Note that the terms FEEDING and DRINKING are not as distinct as they might appear. Animals given the opportunity to drink sucrose solutions in high concentrations will consume large amounts, because the taste is very plea-

sant. But in consequence of taking on board a large amount of ENERGY (the sucrose), animals' food intake will fall. The important considerations for animals are ENERGY BALANCE and WATER BALANCE: FEEDING and DRINKING describe behavioural acts that enable proper energy and water balance to be maintained

drive Drive refers to the theoretical construct of a motivational state produced by biological, reproductive or psychological need. As first discussed by psychologists, drive was non-specific in that any unfulfilled need would contribute to a level of generalized activation. Following the work of neuroscientists stimulating or making a LESION in the HYPOTHALAMUS, drive centres were thought to be linked with corresponding satiety centres. Drive is often operationalized by varying the amount of deprivation in behavioural experiments. One mechanism that was hypothesized to control behaviour is DRIVE REDUCTION, in which the organism strives to minimize drive through adaptive responses.

See also: incentive-motivation; motivation;

ERIC M. BOWMAN

drive reduction *see* drive

Drosophila The genus name of fruit flies. *Drosphila melanogaster* has been extensively studied as a model animal. It was first studied by Thomas Hunt Morgan in the early years of the twentieth century. Morgan was the first scientist to associate specific GENES with particular CHROMOSOMES, achieved by experimentation on *Drosophila melanogaster*. It is a species well suited to research in genetics, having only four pairs of chromosomes and, more important perhaps, a 2-week breeding cycle (see Campbell *et al.*, 1999). In biological psychology, research on circadian rhythms (see BIORHYTHMS) has used this fruit fly, associating specific genes with the circadian clock. Research on LEARNING and MEMORY has also employed *Drosophila melanogaster*. Mutant (see MUTATION) strains (with names such as *dunce*, *cabbage*, *turnip*, *rutabaga* or *DDC* – which stands for dopa decarboxylase) have been shown to have specific deficits in learning and memory, and in some cases a mechanism for this has been suggested: for example DDC has a dysfunction in DOPA decarboxylase production, while *rutabaga* has decreased levels of CYCLIC AMP, which of course impairs neural functioning (see Rosenzweig *et al.*, 1996). Use of simpler species such as *Drosophila* (and others such as APLYSIA and CAENORHABDITIS ELEGANS) is providing valuable information about the molecular basis of many processes in NEURODEVELOPMENT as well as in biological psychology.

References

Campbell N.A., Reece J.B. & Mitchell L.G. (1999) *Biology*, 5th edn, Addison-Wesley: Menlo Park CA.

Rosenzweig M.R., Leiman A.L. & Breedlove S.M. (1996) *Biological Psychology*, Sinauer Associates: Sunderland MA.

drug A substance that exerts an effect on a biological system. For the most part, drugs are either derived from living systems (plants for instance) or synthesized in the laboratory. Thousands of different types of drugs exist, which are used for a wide array of purposes ranging from therapeutic to recreational. Drugs that have an effect on the brain and/or behaviour are often termed psychoactive, and are studied in the field of PSYCHOPHARMACOLOGY. Drug effects refer to the changes in the normal biological state that the drug causes. For PSYCHOACTIVE drugs, these changes are usually alterations in behaviour, perception, or subjective feelings. Drugs can, and usually do, have multiple effects; for example, MORPHINE lessens PAIN perception, but also depresses respiratory rate. COCAINE induces EUPHORIA, but also causes changes in heart rate and blood pressure. Drug effects are the result of drug actions, that is, the mechanism by which the drug causes behavioural or physiological effects. Drugs may have multiple actions as well. Although we mostly think of drugs as EXOGENOUS agents, compounds that occur naturally in the body or brain are also synthesized and used as drugs, such as INSULIN, MELATONIN, TRYPTOPHAN, L-DOPA, ADRENALINE and CORTISOL, to name just a few.

ANN E. KELLEY

drug abuse A maladaptive pattern of substance use characterized by significant adverse consequences related to the repeated use of the substance (for instance, ALCOHOL, NICOTINE, COCAINE, HEROIN, CANNABIS). The term is difficult to define precisely because the use of drugs, their adverse consequences, and how society views use of particular drugs varies between and within cultures. Most people, in fact, experiment with psychoactive drugs at some point in their life, and if one includes CAFFEINE, alcohol and nicotine, the majority of people (at least in Western culture) use drugs. Thus a distinction must be made between drug use and abuse. If distress or negative consequences occur in association with drug use, it is generally considered to be drug abuse. Alcohol is a good example of the complexities of defining drug abuse. Alcohol is a legal PSYCHOACTIVE drug in many societies, but also has many restrictions. Thus, drinking a certain amount of alcohol in one's home would not be considered abuse, but drinking the same amount while driving would be defined as abuse (if caught under the influence). Inhaling nicotine into the lungs is not considered abuse in legal terms, while inhaling cannabis is considered abuse. A smoker is generally not called a drug abuser, yet enormous adverse health consequences result from long-term smoking. Thus, many complex legal, physical, psychological and social factors influence the concept of drug abuse.

See also: addiction; alcoholism

ANN E. KELLEY

drug administration Drugs and chemicals are given to experimental animals in different ways and by different routes (and indeed they are given to human volunteer subjects and, therapeutically, to patients). From the point of view of biological psychology there are two main routes via which drugs and chemicals are given: INTRACEREBRAL INJECTION (that is, injection directly into the brain) and SYSTEMIC INJECTION (that is, into any other body system, via one of several different routes). Of course, intracerebral injections can be considered as a particular type of systemic injection. In biological psychology, drugs and chemicals are given for the most part in order to change behaviour or psychological processes – that is, drugs that act on the central nervous system are the main ones used. As such, the major differentiation in

The principal systemic routes of drug administration

intra-cisternal	into a fluid filled space (a general term, rarely used, covering injections into spaces filled with, for example, CEREBROSPINAL FLUID or LYMPH)
intra-dermal (i.d.)	injections into the skin
intra-medullary	into the marrow cavity of long bones (rarely used experimentally: helpful for surgeons treating bone fractures)
intra-muscular (i.m.)	into a muscle
intra-peritoneal (i.p.)	into the abdominal cavity (the peritoneum)
intra-ocular	into the eye
intra-thecal	into the membranes surrounding the SPINAL CORD
intra-tracheal (intubation)	into the windpipe (used to deliver VOLATILE ANAESTHETICS)
intra-venous (i.v.)	into a vein (also, less commonly, INTRA-ARTERIAL, into an artery)
intra-vitreal	into the vitreous humour of the eye
oral administration	by mouth
sub-cutaneous (s.c.)	under the skin
topical	on to the skin
across the skin	transdermal

routes of administration is between those aimed directly at the brain and those that are not.

Intracerebral injections are made by MICRO-INJECTIONS either into brain tissue or into the CEREBROSPINAL FLUID (CSF) contained within the cerebral VENTRICLES (intraventricular or INTRACEREBROVENTRICULAR INJECTIONS). Note that the term intracranial is often used as a synonym for intracerebral: in fact, intracranial refers to injections into the SKULL – the cranium – while intracerebral refers to injections into the brain – the CEREBRUM. Whether into brain tissue or into ventricles, the same techniques are used (see MICROINJECTION). However, injection of a drug or chemical into tissue will let one examine the effect of that drug on that particular tissue, whereas an intraventricular injection allows a drug to diffuse more widely through the brain, without affecting any particular single structure. Of course, the choice of ventricle to inject into will have an effect on drug diffusion: most intraventricular injections are made into the large lateral ventricles in order to maximize drug diffusion. Temporal control over injec-

tions can be achieved using PUSH–PULL PERFUSION or, more commonly, REVERSE MICRO-DIALYSIS.

Systemic administration of drugs or chemicals typically involves injecting, by one means or another, into the bloodstream (see BLOOD). Once in the bloodstream a drug will distribute evenly in blood PLASMA within two or three circulation times (that is, about 1 minute). The drug will remain in plasma if it has a high MOLECULAR WEIGHT similar to other large molecules in the plasma, or if it binds to a plasma protein. If on the other hand the drug does not become bound to protein, and it has a low molecular weight (less than about 1000 daltons) then it will move from the plasma into the fluid in the extracellular spaces: this will take anything from 10 to 60 minutes. Movement of the drug from these extracellular spaces into cells depends on the ability of the drug to penetrate cell membranes. If the drug is lipid-soluble it will gain access quite quickly. If it has low lipid solubility it will either diffuse slowly across membranes, or be excluded altogether. These factors govern what is known as DIFFUSION LIMITED ACCESS. The rate at which drugs concentrate in a particular tissue depend on blood flow to that tissue (BLOOD FLOW LIMITED ACCESS). Clearly, since drugs are being delivered by the bloodstream, the more blood flow to a structure there is the better. Brains are phenomenally well supplied with blood vessels (see VASCULATURE), though of course brains also possess a BLOOD–BRAIN BARRIER which operates to prevent many molecules carried in blood plasma gaining access to the brain. Low-molecular-weight molecules with high lipid solubility cross the blood–brain barrier better than those without these properties. There are also specific transport mechanisms (for example, for glucose) that enable certain molecules to cross the blood brain–barrier (and indeed, to cross cell membranes). The table shows the systemic routes of administration that are used.

BIOAVAILABILITY is a term used to refer to the ability of a drug to reach its targets. Different routes of administration produce varying degrees of bioavailability. Intravenous injections produce very rapid delivery of drugs to target. Subcutaneous injections on the other hand produce a much slower release of drug, which is held up in the tissue and fat beneath the skin. Intramuscular injections produce relatively slow release, though the extent of muscle activity affects drug release. Intraperitoneal injections – the most commonly used in experimental animals – produce degrees of bioavailability between intravenous and subcutaneous. The intratracheal route is used for delivery of volatile anaesthetics: animals are given, under ANAESTHESIA a TRACHEOTOMY and a tube inserted into the windpipe (a procedure called intubation). A mixture of air and volatile anaesthetic can then be delivered directly to the lungs. This would be done if one needed to maintain a constant level of anaesthesia over a long time, something repeated injections of anaesthetics cannot do. It is a rarely used technique: improved face mask design for small-animal surgery has meant that volatile anaesthetics can be delivered without intubation. Oral administration is rarely used in experiments, though if one wished to mimic the oral route of administration used by humans one could administer drugs through an animal's food or water supply. One point of

concern with this route though is the degree to which drugs or chemical will be broken down in the GASTROINTESTINAL SYSTEM. For example, INSULIN cannot be given orally because it would be broken down. Bioavailability can also be restricted by using a DEPOT INJECTION, in which a drug is prepared in a gel which is then implanted, usually subcutaneously. The gel releases the drug only very slowly, at rates that can be measured. Such a procedure avoids having to inject an animal repeatedly. An OSMOTIC MINIPUMP achieves the same end, though with this the outflow of the pump can be targeted at a specific brain site – a means of achieving slow, evenly paced delivery (over several days) of drugs or chemicals to particular intracerebral sites.

It is also worth considering the fact that all these techniques involve drugs *being given* to animals. SELF-ADMINISTRATION techniques (typically, INTRAVENOUS SELF-ADMINISTRATION) involves animals being prepared with catheters which can then be connected to delivery systems that give animals control over drug delivery. Not surprisingly, the effects drugs have can be different depending on whether they are voluntarily or involuntarily administered.

See also: gavage; osmotic minipump; parenteral; slow release

drug clearance This refers to the removal of a DRUG from the body. Once in the body a drug is subject to metabolic change (a process called DRUG METABOLISM, or BIOTRANSFORMATION), the metabolites being eventually excreted. The rate of drug clearance can be determined by measuring the concentration of a drug and its metabolites in the bloodstream. One will be able to measure a maximum concentration of drug in the bloodstream, and after that the concentration of metabolites, which will fall as time goes by. The rate of drug clearance is typically expressed in terms of the HALF-LIFE of the drug.

Reference

Feldman R., Meyer J.S. & Quenzer L.F. (1997) *Principles of Neuropsychopharmacology*, Sinauer Associates: Sunderland MA.

drug craving A term used in the field of drug ADDICTION to denote a state of strong desire to obtain a previously administered drug. The term has been used more extensively in recent years in attempts to define and understand the motivational or emotional states (see MOTIVATION and EMOTION) associated with DRUG-SEEKING BEHAVIOUR. Its use is somewhat controversial, as the concept is very subjective, and it is very difficult to precisely define what is meant by the term. However, it has proved useful as a measure of subjective states in human clinical studies of addiction. For example, in former COCAINE addicts, the subjective measure of CRAVING ('How much do you want the drug, on a scale of 1–10?') is increased by exposure to cocaine-related visual cues or by a small intravenous dose of cocaine. It is believed that increased craving, even in long-abstinent individuals, is an important factor in relapse to drug use. Researchers are interested in developing ANIMAL MODELS of craving in order to better study the neuronal changes associated with this state.

See also: priming

ANN E. KELLEY

drug discrimination A term used to described a behavioural testing paradigm in which animals are taught to discriminate the internal stimulus properties of a DRUG. In this paradigm, the subject is taught to make a particular response (for example, press the right lever) when in one drugged state and to make another (press the left lever) when in the non-drugged state. Thus, the drug itself acts as a DISCRIMINATIVE CUE. With repeated training, animals can make quite accurate assessments of drug and non-drug states. This test is often used to assess the properties, both neurochemical and behavioural, of novel drugs. The novel compound is assessed for its ability to generalize or substitute for the training drug. The procedure can also be useful for evaluating a compound's neurochemical action.

See also: stimulus generalization

ANN E. KELLEY

drug disposition tolerance Tolerance to a drug in which repeated exposure to the DRUG induces biological effects that reduce the amount of drug that reaches active sites, also known as METABOLIC TOLERANCE. Some drugs have the ability to induce effects that alter BIOAVAILABILITY and reduce absorption. For example, sedatives like phenobarbital increase the rate of BIOTRANSFORMATION of the drug by increasing production of metabolizing enzymes. When the drug is repeatedly administered, progressively more enzymes are synthesized that biochemically alter the drug and enhance its rapid elimination. Thus, the biological half-life of the drug is progressively reduced. This is to be contrasted with other forms of tolerance, such as CELLULAR TOLERANCE and BEHAVIOURAL TOLERANCE.

ANN E. KELLEY

drug effects *in utero* Many drugs of abuse (see DRUG ABUSE) taken during PREGNANCY can have effects on the FOETUS during DEVELOPMENT. The placental barrier exists between the circulatory systems of mother and foetus. It protects the foetus from the maternal IMMUNE SYSTEM but many types of MOLECULE do cross from mother to foetus – most are necessary NUTRIENTS, but other agents can cross over (which is why physicians take such care in prescribing therapeutic drugs to pregnant women). Infants rarely if ever come into the world already addicted, but drugs of abuse can have a variety of effects, including induction of the NEONATE NEUROLOGICAL SYNDROME. This syndrome is present within a day of birth and is associated with a variety of signs (including abnormal SLEEP patterning, TREMOR and SEIZURES, FEEDING difficulty and general irritability) and increased risk of other disorders, including SUDDEN INFANT DEATH SYNDROME. It is also important to recognize that, because NEURODEVELOPMENT is not uniform across time, the period in pregnancy during which drugs are taken is often critical.

ALCOHOL, TOBACCO, MARIJUANA, COCAINE and CRACK COCAINE, HEROIN, PCPA and LSD have been associated with various problems including altered MORPHOLOGY (such as low birth weight, often attendant on premature birth, or small head circumference) and behavioural disturbances, initially in sleep and feeding, though other problems may be present, and LEARNING impairments may become apparent later. Probably the most dramatic effects are of alcohol, which causes FOETAL ALCOHOL SYNDROME. Crack cocaine is thought to induce particular problems in so-called CRACK BABIES. One possible mechanism for this is the induction of foetal HYPOXIA, which is associated with a variety of problems in the foetus and PLACENTA during pregnancy. When first identified it was thought that crack babies had a variety of intellectual and behavioural impairments but later research has questioned the severity of the problem. Because heavy drug abuse is often associated with poverty and poor domestic quality, it is difficult to dissociate the effects of the drug *in utero* from the more pervasive effects of deprivation. This is not to say that one should minimize the problems associated with maternal drug abuse, but to indicate that the problems need to be set in a wider context.

drug ionization In solution, a DRUG becomes ionized – that is, it dissociates into its ionic components (see ION). Different terms are sometimes used to indicate drugs in their ionized and non-ionized forms. For example, one refers to GLUTAMIC ACID when it is in a non-ionized form and GLUTAMATE in the ionized form. Similarly, EXCITOTOXINS such as IBOTENIC ACID or KAINIC ACID should be called by these names when not in solution, but IBOTENATE and kainate when in solution.

drug metabolism Drugs are usually metabolized within the body: for a DRUG to be administered, have an effect and then be excreted without change would be very unusual. The metabolism of a drug – also called BIOTRANSFORMATION – occurs in many organs of the body but most of the metabolic processes take place in the liver where various enzymes work to degrade drugs. Elimination of metabolites is achieved by transport to the kidney and excretion in urine.

Reference

Feldman R., Meyer J.S. & Quenzer L.F. (1997) *Principles of Neuropsychopharmacology*, Sinauer Associates: Sunderland MA.

drug patch *see* transdermal drug administration

drug-dependency insomnia Tolerance can develop to sleeping medications (BENZODIAZEPINES for example) leading patients to take ever stronger doses. Eventually patients lose all benefit from the drug and stop using it, leading to a state of INSOMNIA that is perceived to be worse that that originally experienced and for which medication was sought.

See also: sleep disorders

drug-seeking behaviour Behaviours that are directed at bringing an organism into contact with a DRUG that is a REINFORCER. A term used commonly in the ADDICTION field and applied both to humans and animals, drug seeking behaviour is generally thought to be associated with increased MOTIVATION to obtain the drug, and in humans, CRAVING for the drug. In animal experiments, the term drug seeking behaviour is usually used in association with drug SELF-ADMINISTRATION paradigms. Often investigators train the animal to self-administer the drug intravenously and then at a later time period, in the absence of the drug, examine the types and intensity of behaviours that the animal shows when put in an environment where drug was previously available (such as the amount of pressing on a previously rewarded lever). Addiction researchers are particularly interested in the factors that influence reinstatement of drug-seeking behaviour after a period of drug abstinence. STRESS, environmental signals that predict drug REWARD, increased craving, and experiencing an initial dose of the drug (see PRIMING) are all factors that can increase drug-seeking behaviour.

See also: place conditioning

ANN E. KELLEY

DSM-IV The DIAGNOSTIC AND STATISTICAL MANUAL OF THE AMERICAN PSYCHIATRIC ASSOCIATION, 4th edition: a guide to the classification of what might loosely be called mental illness. It is a widely used guide, regularly revised by the American Psychiatric Association to take account of developing knowledge. The main alternative diagnostic aid is the ICD 10. The third edition, and all subsequent editions of DSM, used five axes: axis I, all categories except PERSONALITY DISORDERS; axis II, personality disorders and MENTAL

RETARDATION; axis III, general medical conditions; axis IV, psychosocial and environmental conditions; axis V, current level of adaptive functioning. Rating on each axis is required for diagnosis.

DSP4 DSP4 (N-2-chloroethyl-N-ethyl-2-bromobenzylamine) is a neurotoxin. It is thought to act in a manner similar to 6-HYDROXY-DOPAMINE with the one difference being that it is selective for NORADRENALINE (norepinephrine) neurons rather than targeting those containing a CATECHOLAMINE. It was initially suggested that DSP4 would target selectively noradrenaline containing neurons in the CENTRAL NERVOUS SYSTEM following SYSTEMIC INJECTION but this does not appear to be the case: peripheral nerves containing noradrenaline do appear to be damaged by DSP4. Moreover, it was suggested to have preferential actions on noradrenaline neurons in the LOCUS COERULEUS rather than those located elsewhere in the central nervous system, but this too is doubtful. Nevertheless, if locally applied to specific structures, DSP4 does appear to be an effective agent with which to destroy noradrenaline containing neurons.

See also: neurotoxins

dual centres hypothesis A term used to describe the idea that behaviour can be controlled by reciprocally acting 'centres' in the brain. It is most closely associated with the theory, proposed by Eliot Stellar, that motivated behaviours are controlled by excitatory and inhibitory centres in the HYPOTHALAMUS: the excitatory one switches on an activity (such as FEEDING or DRINKING) while the inhibitory one switches it off. Lesion studies appeared to support this idea (see LATERAL HYPOTHALAMIC SYNDROME; VENTROMEDIAL HYPOTHALAMIC SYNDROME) but the notion of selected centres controlling specific activities has been rejected in favour of more distributed accounts.

Reference
Winn P. (1999) The Physiology of Motivation, by Eliot Stellar. *Brain Research Bulletin* 50: 451–452.

dual opponent cells (double colour-opponent cells) Electrophysiological recordings from cells in the RETINA of fish from the carp family have shown that cells exist that respond in an opposing manner to lights from different ends of the spectrum. For example, the firing rate might increase if the stimulating light was of a long wavelength ('red') and decrease if the light was of a shorter wavelength ('green'). These cells reveal the presence of CONE OPPONENT inputs, in other words mutually antagonistic connections from two different classes of photoreceptors. Very similar behaviour has been shown for cells in the LATERAL GENICULATE NUCLEUS of the optic tract in the rhesus monkey where four types of such opponent cells have been identified, that respond in opposite ways to pairs of the colours blue, yellow, red and green (B+/Y-; B-/Y+; R+/G-; R-/G+). The properties of these cells provide supporting evidence for the OPPONENT PROCESS THEORY OF COLOUR VISION. The properties of some of the cells in cortical area V1 of visual system of the monkey are similar but with the additional property of spatial opponency. The cells are characterized by a RECEPTIVE FIELD comprising a central region and an annular surround. Light falling within the receptive field can influence the firing rate of the cell. Both the centre and surround are colour-opponent, but in a a mutually antagonistic manner. For example, a typical cell might have a central region which has R+/G- colour-opponency with a surround that is R-/G+. Such cells are said to be double colour-opponent. In the monkey V1 cortex (and presumably also in the equivalent region of the human visual cortex – see AREAS V1–V5) such double colour-opponent cells tend to be concentrated in small blobs that are revealed with the histological stain cytochrome oxidase.

DAVID W. HEELEY

dual process theory *see* two-factor learning theory

dualism Theory of the mind as a non-physical thing. According to dualism, although the brain is a physical substance, the mind (or soul) is a non-physical substance, sharing no properties with any physical substance. Minds, on the dualists' hypothesis, can be aware and have experiences, whereas physical substances such as the liver or the brain, cannot. Historically, Plato and Descartes gave substance dualism its most systematic treatment and defence.

Among the problems facing dualism, the most intractable has been the nature of the interaction between the mind and brain. Specifically, the problem is this: how can something with no physical properties whatever causally interact with physical stuff; how can it influence the brain or be influenced by it? Descartes recognized the problem, but hoped an explanation might lie in an interaction between the soul and very fine materials in the PINEAL GLAND, an organ located on the underside of the brain. This proposal was unsatisfactory, however, because even very fine material is still material. No recent proposal has fared any better. With the development of modern science, the interaction problem has become acute, especially because of direct conflict with current physics and the law of conservation of mass-energy. Modern biology also presents dilemmas for dualism. Humans, like other primates, are an evolved species, and brain EVOLUTION appears to hold the key to increased behavioral complexity in non-human animals. In all likelihood, the human brain evolved from earlier hominid brains, and it is known to share much of its organization and chemistry with non-human brains. This suggests that humans' mental capacities to think, feel and so forth have precursors in non-human brains. NEUROSCIENCE, the study of the brain, has failed to reveal any focal structure in the brain that could be the seat of CONSCIOUSNESS, and the pineal gland can be destroyed without any effect on consciousness.

Property dualism tries to avoid some of these problems by dropping the notion of a non-physical substance whilst adopting the hypothesis that the human brain, unlike other physical systems, has the capacity to generate non-physical properties such as feeling PAIN. On this view, mental states emerge from the physical brain, but are not themselves physical. In what sense are they 'non-physical properties'? Adherents say it means the properties cannot be explained in terms of the physical properties of the brain; either they cannot be explained at all or their explanation will require an autonomous science of the mind or perhaps a new physics.

More recent arguments supporting dualism mainly depend on introspective observations concerning how very different are physical properties such as the activity of a neuron, and mental properties such as feeling pain. Like Descartes, some are also convinced that the creative nature of speech (see SPEECH PERCEPTION) and LANGUAGE comprehension implies that mere mechanical devices such as the brain cannot account for language use. Related to this, some philosophers feel that meaningfulness of words and sentences in thought, is evidence that meaning cannot be a physical property.

Several additional reasons motivate dualism, one deriving from the idea of free will, and one from the hope of immortality. Some philosophers consider uncaused choice to be a defining characteristic of humans. Here is the argument: (1) if choice is caused by a mechanism such as the brain, then it is not free; (2) humans do have free will. Therefore: choice and decision-making are independent of physical activity of the brain. Physicalists typically counter this argument by denying the first premise. They suggest that voluntary actions are those that are caused by the agent's desires, reasons and beliefs, and that uncaused choice would be like a random or 'out-of-the-blue' actions. Randomly occurring events would not be the outcome of what the agent really wanted, and hence the agent could not be held responsible for the action. According to this hypothesis, some kinds of causal antecedents of choice involve responsibility, while other conditions, such as having an epileptic seizure or schizophrenic hallucinations, can excuse an agent. Understanding the nature of the causal antecedents, and which do and which do not excuse an agent, is considered to be the joint task of COGNITIVE NEUROSCIENCE and jurisprudence. Belief in an immortal soul that survives the death of the physical body is sometimes a basis for adopting some version of dualism. This belief is a central tenet of many religions, and the apparent conflict between science and religion may be considered resolvable by presuming each to have its autonomous domain of subject matter. Others reject the independence tactic, viewing the conflict to be entirely real, and preferring to try to resolve it, one way or the other.

See also: emergent properties

Reference

Churchland Paul M. (1987) *Matter and Consciousness*, MIT Press: Cambridge MA.

PATRICIA S. CHURCHLAND

duodenum *see* digestive system

duplexity theory (or duplicity theory) Refers to the notion that there may be two mechanisms in vision, one specialized for scotopic conditions (low light levels) which is subserved by the photoreceptors known as RODS, and one specialized for photopic conditions (high light levels) which is subserved by CONES (see SCOTOPIC VS. PHOTOPIC). Intermediate levels, where both rods and cones are active, are known as MESOPIC. Duplexity is often illustrated by the dark-adaptation curve that depicts sensitivity as a function of time in the darkness. The function typically has two branches – an early increase in sensitivity followed by a plateau which is due to cone adaptation, followed by a another increase in sensitivity and plateau that reflects rod mediated thresholds.

ROBERT J. SNOWDEN

dura mater *see* meninges

duration discrimination *see* discrimination

dye *see* stains

dynorphin An opioid peptide; small qualities are found in the brain in localized sites within the BRAINSTEM and BASAL GANGLIA.

dysarthria A deficit in the production of speech. It does not involve APHASIA or any other higher deficit but is a problem caused by failure of the mechanics of SPEECH PRODUCTION.

dyscalculia *see* acalculia

dysexecutive syndrome Dysexecutive syndrome is thought to involve disruption of EXECUTIVE FUNCTIONS. It is a clinical conception that has evolved from what was previously known, rather loosely, as FRONTAL SYNDROME (or frontal lobe syndrome). Patients with FRONTAL LOBE damage show a variety of deficits, including disinhibition of behaviour, the production of inappropriate behaviour, PERSEVERATION and attentional deficits (see ATTENTION). Dysexecutive syndrome is similarly broad and is assessed in various ways: the WISCONSIN CARD-SORTING TASK, the Stroop test (see STROOP EFFECT) and the REITAN TRAIL-MAKING TEST are often used, as is a specific NEUROPSYCHOLOGICAL TEST BATTERY aimed explicitly at dysexecutive syndrome. These usually include simple tests of attention, spatial tasks, tests of planning and SET SHIFTING and temporal judgements (see Wilson *et al.*, 1997).

The term dysexecutive syndrome was introduced by Baddeley in 1986 with the anticipation that the term was only temporary and that it would quickly be superseded by more specific terminologies. This has not happened: dysexecutive syndrome remains a rather vague conception covering many deficits and is not associated with damage to any particular structure. There has been a marked tendency to associate it with the prefrontal cortex, but it is apparent that not all patients with prefrontal damage can be classified as having dysexecutive syndrome while patients without prefrontal damage can show it (see, for example, Robbins *et al.*, 1994). How valuable a term dysexecutive syndrome is remains open to question.

References

Baddeley A. (1986) *Working Memory*, Clarendon Press: Oxford.

Robbins T.W., Owen A.M., Lange K.W., Lees A.J., Leigh P.N., Marsden C.D., Quinn N.P. & Summers B.A. (1994) Cognitive deficits in progressive supranuclear palsy, Parkinson's disease and multiple system atrophy in tests sensitive to frontal lobe dysfunction. *Journal of Neurology, Neurosurgery and Psychiatry* 57: 79–88.

Roberts A.C., Robbins T.W. & Weiskrantz L. (1998) *The Prefrontal Cortex: Executive and Cognitive Functions*, Oxford University Press: Oxford.

Wilson B.A., Evans J.J., Alderman N., Burgess P.W. & Emslie H. (1997) Behavioural assessment of the dysexecutive syndrome. In *Methodology of Frontal and Executive Function*, ed. P. Rabbitt, pp. 239–250, Psychology Press: Hove UK.

dysgenesis A term used to denote diminished development, as opposed to AGENESIS, the complete absence of a structure or region of tissue.

dysgraphia *see* agraphia

dyskinesia A disturbance of movement. The term dyskinesia is usually reserved for the various types of HYPERKINESIA rather than the varieties of AKINESIA. Hyperkinesias include abnormal classes of movements such as chorea (see CHOREA) and ATHETOSIS (non-rhythmic, jerky movements, slower than chorea) and MYOCLONUS. Hyperkinesias are usually consequent to interruptions in pathways from the SUBTHALAMIC NUCLEUS which normally excites GLOBUS PALLIDUS neurons, which in turn inhibit circuits in the ventral THALAMUS. The net result of such a LESION is abnormally increased activity in CORTICOSTRIATAL LOOPS.

See also: basal ganglia; movement deficits

DAVID P. CAREY

dyslexia An acquired or DEVELOPMENTAL READING DISORDER in which some READING is possible. Severe forms of acquired reading disorders are often referred to as ALEXIA. Different categories of dyslexia are identified; these are summarized in the following table. Individual entries for each category are presented.

ELAINE FUNNELL

dysmyelination *see* myelin

dysphagia A difficulty in swallowing, rather than a reduction in food intake. The term APHAGIA is used to refer to the absence (or near absence) of FEEDING; the term HYPOPHAGIA can be used to indicate a reduction (rather than an absence or near absence) in normal food intake.

dysphasia Although the prefix *dys-* (from Greek, meaning bad, ill or abnormal) rather than the prefix *a-* (also from Greek, meaning absence or not) is sometimes used to indicate milder forms of disturbance, dysphasia has been used more or less synonymously with APHASIA. It is a term rarely used.

dysphoria (from Greek, *dysphoria*: affliction) A feeling of uneasiness perhaps best described as the absence of well-being. It is a contrast to EUPHORIA.

dysplasia (from Greek, *dys*: abnormal, *plasis*: moulding) Abnormal growth or development; see, for example, FOETAL ALCOHOL SYNDROME.

dyspraxia From Greek, *dys*, abnormal, and *praxis*, doing: a difficulty in the execution of actions; a milder form of APRAXIA. The term is often encountered with special reference to children: CLUMSY CHILD SYNDROME and DEVELOPMENTAL COORDINATION DISORDER are dyspraxias. These are syndromes, thought to effect boys more than girls and to be caused by slow NEURODEVELOPMENT, that involves clumsiness, poor POSTURE, poor LOCOMOTION and various disorders of coordination (such as catching thrown objects or WRITING difficulties).

dysthymic disorder A chronic condition involving many of the typical signs of

Principal categories of dyslexia

ACQUIRED DYSLEXIA	
i. PERIPHERAL DYSLEXIA	(includes ATTENTIONAL DYSLEXIA, NEGLECT DYSLEXIA and PURE ALEXIA)
ii. CENTRAL DYSLEXIA	(includes DEEP DYSLEXIA, PHONOLOGICAL DYSLEXIA and SURFACE DYSLEXIA)
DEVELOPMENTAL DYSLEXIA	
i. DEVELOPMENTAL PHONOLOGICAL DYSLEXIA	
ii. DEVELOPMENTAL SURFACE DYSLEXIA	

DEPRESSION: ANHEDONIA, SLEEP disturbance, feelings of worthlessness, blunted intellectual capacities and social isolation for example. It is not as extreme as a major depression.

See also: cyclothymic disorder; dysphoria; euphoria

dystonia (from Greek, *dys*: abnormal, *tonos*: tension) A disturbance of the tone of the MUSCLES (which can be either in either direction – slackening or stiffening).

dystrophia (from Greek, *dys*: abnormal, *trophe*: nourishment) A disturbance of nutrition; it is a term that is associated with wasting of the MUSCLES. MUSCULAR DYSTROPHY for example is a condition in which there is a (probably hereditary) abnormality of muscle formation, leading to muscle deterioration.

E

ear The ear is divided into three sections: (1) the external ear includes the PINNA and the AUDITORY CANAL. The pinna – the large flap on the outside of the head – has a function in collecting sound, focusing it, and to some extent filtering it (some sound frequencies are enhanced others dimmed in the pinna). Many animals have muscle systems that can move the pinnae, to aid in sound localization. Some humans can move their ears, others cannot. The auditory canal is the passageway that connects the pinna to the internal machinery of sound transduction. (2) The middle ear: the middle ear includes the TYMPANIC MEMBRANE (the eardrum) and the OSSICLES, a series of small bones. These serve to transduce sound waves into mechanical pressures. In the middle ear there is also the Eustachian tube which connects the middle ear to the throat. It is important in the maintenance of pressure within the ear. (3) The inner ear includes the COCHLEA and the machinery associated with it: the ORGAN OF CORTI, BASILAR MEMBRANE, HAIR CELLS and the TECTORIAL MEMBRANE. The COCHLEAR NERVE connects here.

See also: auditory pathways; auditory perception; hearing theories

ear bar zero *see* stereotaxic surgery

ear bars *see* stereotaxic surgery

eardrum *see* tympanic membrane

eating *see* feeding

eating attitudes test A 40-question test developed to examine the symptoms of ANOREXIA NERVOSA which has been used to examine psychological approach to eating and BODY WEIGHT control in several different populations of subjects.

Reference

Garner D.M. & Garfinkel P.E. (1979) The eating attitudes test: an index of the symptoms of anorexia nervosa. *Psychological Medicine* 9: 273–279.

eating disorders Collective name for psychiatric syndromes involving BODY WEIGHT and eating disorders. Eating disorders might vary from the loss of appetite observed in cancer ANOREXIA to HYPERPHAGIA observed in PRADER–WILLI SYNDROME. However, the term eating disorder is normally restricted to the specific clinical syndromes of ANOREXIA NERVOSA, BULIMIA NERVOSA and BINGE EATING disorder. Central to anorexia and bulimia nervosa is the overvalued idea of becoming or staying slim. To achieve their goal, eating-disordered individuals engage in a range of behaviours from self-starvation and dietary restriction to episodes of overeating followed by compensatory behaviour such as vomiting, fasting or abuse of diuretics and/or laxatives.

The names 'anorexia' and 'bulimia' are problematic since there may be no loss of APPETITE nor excessive appetite as implied by the literal meanings of the terms. The label 'nervosa' closely follows early descriptions of hysteria in women and thus is also problematic since this discourse sought to link mental illness to women's reproductive HORMONES. It is argued that eating disorders are highly specific to women because women in Western societies experience conflict around food. Women are socialized to nurture and nourish others but experience pressure to attain a slender ideal by forsaking such nourishment for themselves. Feminist theories explore the relationship between women's lack of power and low status in our society as critical in the development of eating disorders.

Anorexia nervosa is diagnosed following relative weight loss, loss of menses, fear of being fat despite obvious emaciation and disturbed BODY IMAGE. Bulimia nervosa is diagnosed not on the basis of body weight, but on the loss of control of eating, fear of being fat, and repeated episodes of overeating coupled with attempts to get rid of the energy consumed (vomiting, dieting, excessive intake of laxatives/diuretics, fasting, exercise). Both anorexia and bulimia nervosa are characterized by a pathological fear of fatness, thus the central feature of these disorders is not disordered appetite, but rather overvalued ideas about weight and shape. In contrast to this, binge eating disorder does not share the central feature of a fear of being fat and no attempts are made to compensate for overeating. Rather the suggested diagnosis of binge eating disorder depends upon repeated episodes of binge eating characterised by loss of control and eating an objectively large amount of food in a discrete period; experiencing distress following binge eating; and at least three of the following – rapid eating, eating beyond normal comfort, eating when not hungry, eating alone due to embarrassment and feeling disgust, depression or guilt after overeating. Binge eating disorder may be diagnosed in obese and non-obese (see OBESITY) individuals. However, binge eating disorder is in the early stages of investigation and is at present not a fully recognized eating disorder.

The physiological and behavioural consequences of semi-starvation have been elucidated in a classic studies by Keys and his colleagues who placed young, healthy normal weight men on a diet for 6 months to achieve a 25% loss of body weight. These men developed some of the characteristics of eating disorders. For example, the participants became obsessed with food, some started to collect recipes and to dream about food. Some men binged on food and others reported overwhelming HUNGER sensations. The men became more depressed, lost their ability to concentrate, experienced a reduced SEXUAL AROUSAL and lost interest in their daily activities. Thus, semi-starvation causes changes in cognitive and emotional well-being which may contribute to and exacerbate the development of an eating disorder. Eating disorders are mediated by a variety of predisposing, precipitating and perpetuating events, which might differ considerably from individual to individual. However, predisposing factors (variables which make someone vulnerable to developing an eating disorder) might include societal pressures, family dynamics and eating practices, individual vulnerability and history of individual and family psychiatric illness; precipitating factors (which trigger an eating disorder) might include stress, anxiety, low self-esteem; and perpetuating factors (which maintain the eating disorder) might include semi-starvation resulting from extreme dieting and weight loss; physiological and psychological responses to restriction, bingeing and purging. Multidisciplinary treatment programmes generally include a variety of individual and group psychotherapies, pharmacotherapy, nutritional counselling and psychoeducation. Pharmacological treatments for eating disorders include tricyclic ANTIDEPRESSANTS, ANXIOLYTICS and appetite suppressants (fluoxetine, for example) or appetite enhancers (such as cyproheptadine). Reports suggest that eating disorders are increasing. However, it is difficult to ascertain the degree of increase, given a greater awareness among general practitioners and the general public.

Anorexia and bulimia nervosa are two examples of eating disorders. Both involve an overconcern about weight and shape and behaviours which aim to reduce or maintain body weight. Eating disorders are typically preceded by dieting; however, this is not sufficient on its own to cause eating disorders. A new form of eating disorder named binge eating disorder is currently under investigation. Treatments for eating disorders focus on achieving and maintaining normal weight and rejecting overvalued notions of thinness.

See also: feeding

MARION M. HETHERINGTON

EC50 The effective concentration, 50%; that is, the molar concentration (see MOLARITY) of a substance that produces 50% of the maximum possible response. Such statistics help one decide what concentration of a substance to use in experiments.

See also: ED50; IC50; LD50: TD50; therapeutic index

echoic memory *see* iconic memory

echolalia Repetition of words or phrases produced by someone else; PALILALIA is the repetition of self-generated words of phrases. Echolalia occurs in several disorders, including TOURETTE'S SYNDROME.

echolocation Echolocation is an active form of SOUND LOCALIZATION in which a comparison of an emitted sonic pulse with the echo reflected from a target provides information about the target's location. Thus, the pulse-echo delay provides information about target distance, while a Doppler-shifted echo provides information about the relative velocity of the target. In the auditory cortex of echolocating bats, the computations of these pulse-echo differences take place in specialized territories dedicated to those purposes.

DENNIS P. PHILLIPS

echopraxia Repetition of movements produced by someone else; PALIPRAXIA is the repetition of self-generated movements. Echopraxia occurs in several disorders, including TOURETTE'S SYNDROME.

ecological niche The term ECOLOGICAL NICHE is descriptive of the way in which an organism fits its environment: it is not a location – the word 'habitat' describes this. Ecological niche describes the means by which an organism's survival is maintained: where and what it eats and drinks, how it maintains temperature, the time of day during which it is awake and so on.

ecstasy Ecstasy is the popular name for the drug MDMA (3,4 methylenedioxymethamphetamine). At low doses ecstasy can induce feelings of well-being; at higher doses it is hallucinogenic. Like other amphetamine-related compounds it also has the ability to destroy serotonin-containing neurons (it has neurotoxic properties). Ecstasy has a high ABUSE POTENTIAL and can trigger panic attacks. Its use has also been associated with fatalities, even on very limited exposure.

See also: addiction

Reference

Feldman R., Meyer J.S. & Quenzer L.F. (1997) *Principles of Neuropsychopharmacology.* Sinauer Associates: Sunderland MA.

ECT *see* electroconvulsive therapy

ectoderm The outer one of the three GERM LAYERS present in the developing EMBRYO (the others being MESODERM and ENDODERM), it gives rise to tissues such as neurons and skin (see DEVELOPMENT).

ectohormones *see* pheromones

ectopallium *see* neocortex

ectopic Displaced from the normal position: an ectopic NEURON is one found in an inappropriate structure; in an ectopic PREGNANCY the FOETUS develops outside the UTERUS.

ectosylvian sulcus The SYLVIAN SULCUS is another name for the LATERAL SULCUS, which divides the TEMPORAL LOBE from the FRONTAL LOBE; the prefix ecto- denotes 'outside', thus the ectosylvian sulcus is the tissue on the outside of the Sylvian sulcus. This tissue is involved in SOUND LOCALIZATION (see AUDITORY CORTEX).

ectotherm (poikilotherm) A cold-blooded animal; one that maintains its temperature by absorbing heat from the environment, in contrast to an ENDOTHERM.

ED50 The effective dose, 50%; that is, the dose of a DRUG that produces 50% of the maximum possible response. Such statistics help one decide what drug dose to use in experiments.

See also: EC50; IC50; LD50; TD50; therapeutic index

edema *see* oedema

edge detection Objects are bounded by a physical surface. Where this surface curves away from our line of sight, we see an edge to the object (called an OCCLUDING CONTOUR). Most objects have surfaces that are distinctive from their surrounds, either by being of a different colour and lightness, or by having a different texture. This means that where there is an occluding contour in the scene, there will be a discontinuity of colour, lightness or texture in the optical image formed of the scene. Detecting these discontinuities is termed edge detection. Detecting edges is achieved by finding places in the image where local differences in luminance or texture have high values.

See also: primal sketch

ROGER J. WATT

Edinger–Westphal nucleus A brainstem nucleus involved in OCULOMOTOR control. It contains most of the preganglionic neurons that innervate the CILIARY GANGLION and which make up the OCULOMOTOR NERVE.

See also: pretectum

EEG *see* electroencephalogram

effective stimulus *see* stimulus

effector cells *see* immune system

efference copy This is a copy of a motor output (the signal from the brain's motor centres is termed a COROLLARY DISCHARGE) which is sent to sensory systems in order that sensations caused by the movement are in effect cancelled. For example, movement of the head will change the image on the RETINA: it is important that this change is attributed to the movement of the observer rather than to movement of the external world.

See also: re-afference

efferent (from Latin, *e*: from, *ferre*: carry) Moving away from or outward. Efferent projections (often simply, 'the efferents') of a brain structure are the neurons that project from that structure to another one.

See also: afferent

efferent motor aphasia A major type of APHASIA in the classification scheme of Russian neurologist A.R. Luria (1902–1977). A form of NON-FLUENT APHASIA attributed to an inability to produce sequential kinetic speech movements despite relatively intact production of individual speech sounds.

See also: Broca's aphasia

Reference

Luria A.R. (1970) *Traumatic Aphasia*, Mouton: The Hague.

CHARLOTTE C. MITCHUM

efficacy A pharmacological concept: not every AGONIST has the same effects at RECEPTORS. A high-efficacy agonist can produce a maximal effect while occupying only a small proportion of the receptors available to it. Low efficacy involves poor responding despite high receptor occupancy. RELATIVE EFFICACY of agonists can be determined by measuring the receptor OCCUPANCY required by two different drugs to achieving the same effect.

See also: partial agonist

efflux Efflux is a term used to describe the escape of NEUROTRANSMITTER from NEURONS. It is used more or less synonymously with the terms RELEASE and EMISSION though these two imply an active process (for example, they might depend on ACTION POTENTIALS stimulating NEUROTRANSMISSION) whereas efflux can describe this and the passive release of chemicals from CELLS.

egocentric (from Latin and Greek, *ego*: I) Egocentric means literally self-centred. It is a term familiar to most people, describing someone who is self-centred, psychologically. In studies of animal behaviour, egocentric – again meaning self-centred – refers to an animal's SPATIAL BEHAVIOUR. Position responses are movements made with the body as a reference point, where no external cue is required. These responses are referred to as egocentric. Left/right discriminations are an example of position responses. The opposite of egocentric is ALLOCENTRIC.

egocentric space *see* allocentric space; egocentric space

eicosanoid Eicosanoids are derivatives of ARACHIDONIC ACID; they may function as SECOND

MESSENGERS as well as having other biological functions. PROSTAGLANDIN is probably the best known of the group.

ejaculation The emission of seminal fluid from the urethra. In gonadally-intact males, the seminal fluid contains sperm, thus ejaculation is the mechanism by which sperm exit the male reproductive organs. In humans, ejaculation is typically an extremely pleasurable, involuntary rhythmic sensation, and is nearly always coincident with ORGASM. During masturbation or sexual intercourse, activation of the SYMPATHETIC NERVOUS SYSTEM leads to the ejaculatory response after a requisite amount of sexual stimulation has been achieved. Two disorders, premature ejaculation and inhibited ejaculation, can occur following the administration of certain drugs, or from too much or too little endogenous SEXUAL AROUSAL, respectively.

See also: reproduction; sexual behaviour

JAMES G. PFAUS

Ekman Faces *see* emotion

electrical brain stimulation Low-current pulses applied to small brain regions by an ELECTRODE cause an electron flow that accumulates on the outside of neurons and cause them to fire. Neurons are slightly positively charged on the outside and the accumulating electrons reduce that charge. In an AXON, this reduction of the outside positive charge causes the firing of an ACTION POTENTIAL which travels the length of the axon in both directions and spreads in to all branches of the axon until it reaches a SYNAPTIC TERMINAL, the cell body, or collides with a naturally occurring action potential coming the other way. Some axons are larger than others, which enables them to catch more of the extracellular electron flow and fire earlier. An analogy might be to a sailboat with a bigger sail getting a faster start as the breeze came up over a boat of equal weight and length but with a smaller sail. MYELIN also makes axons more efficient at firing by focusing the extracellular electrons at the NODE OF RANVIER where relatively smaller resistance to electron flow is found. This all assumes negatively charged electrodes in the pulse, but positively charged electrodes can

also fire axons. Positively charged electrodes attract electrons from the brain and fire axons either by next node firing at pulse onset or by adaptation and firing at pulse offset. The next node firing occurs because the electrode draws electrons out of a node of Ranvier close to the electrode which then draws electrons into the axon at neighbouring nodes. This inward flow of electrons at the next node creates the depolarization necessary to fire an action potential. Anodal make firing depends upon a favourable geometry between axonal course and electrode tip. Axons that lie further away from the electrode tip feel the positive current flow more equally at all nodes and will not fire. Axons that are not myelinated cannot concentrate an inward current at the next node and will not fire. The other way that axons fire with positive charge is for their membrane's ionic balance to adapt to charge coming from the electrode. This takes some time (several milliseconds), but when the pulse is suddenly terminated the falling voltage across the membrane triggers an action potential at the electrode tip.

The stimulation effects of positive charge make it difficult to psychophysically match firing frequency of axons to pulse frequency when biphasic stimulation pulses are use or when bipolar electrodes are employed. Thus to preserve simple psychophysical interpretation of the effect produced, the simplest arrangement is to use negatively charged electrodes with short pulses (for instance, 0.1 millisecond). Short pulses will prevent multiple firing of the axon. Short pulses will allow the natural capacitance of the electrode–brain interface to push back all of the electrons between pulses, if the electrode and SKULL SCREW ground are connected together electrically by the stimulator between pulses. This can be accomplished easily by having a switching network on the output stage of the amplifier. Such an arrangement is more important if constant-current amplifiers are used to generate the pulses as they inherently do not provide such between-pulse connections and the electrical charge can summate between pulses resulting in tissue damage. All brain stimulators should check the manufacturer's specifications for compliance with this principle.

See also: intracranial self-stimulation

JAMES R. STELLAR

electrical synapse *see* synapse

electrical transmission *see* electrical synapse; ephaptic transmission; synapse.

electro-oculogram (EOG) Note well: an ELECTRO-OCULOGRAM (EOG) is a recording made by an electro-oculograph. As with the electroencephalograph (EEG), the electro-oculogram measures electrical activity, but in this case it is the electrical activity generated by EYE MOVEMENTS that is recorded. Such recordings are made in many types of study where such activity is a factor of interest, including SLEEP, where movement of the eyes is (obviously) a marked feature of REM SLEEP (rapid eye movement sleep).

See also: electromyogram; polygraph

electroactive A description of MOLECULE whose activity or structure can be changed by passage of electric current; see ELECTROCHEMISTRY.

electrocardiogram *see* blood

electrochemistry Field of analytical chemistry involving the measurement of current signals associated with the OXIDATION and/or REDUCTION of electroactive substances. Several electrochemical methods (for example, CHRONO-AMPEROMETRY, DIFFERENTIAL PULSE VOLTAMMETRY, and RAPID-SCAN VOLTAMMETRY) have been applied *in vivo* to measure changes in extra-cellular concentrations of electro-oxidizable transmitter substances (such as the CATECHOLAMINES, INDOLEAMINES, and their metabolites) involved in synaptic transmission. Electrochemical reactions also play a key role in several cellular events, including electron transport in aerobic respiration and ACTION POTENTIAL conduction.

See also: voltammetry

Reference

Strobel H.A. & Heineman W.R. (eds.) (1989) *Chemical Instrumentation: A Systematic Approach*, Wiley: New York.

CHARLES D. BLAHA

electroconvulsive therapy (ECT) Physical therapy used in psychiatric practice for the treatment of severe mental illness, usually DEPRESSION. ECT was introduced in the 1930s, initially as a treatment for SCHIZOPHRENIA. The procedure has been considerably modified over the years, and presently consists of the electrical induction of an epileptic seizure (see EPILEPSY) in anaesthetized patients, who have been given a muscle relaxant to prevent jerking of the body. The treatment is usually given on a repeated basis, each seizure induction spaced by two to three days. On average, six treatments are given in the course of therapy. The seizure is induced by placing an electrode on each temple, and passing a current of approximately 300 mA. The entire procedure lasts only a few minutes. ECT is highly effective in depressive illness, especially in patients with symptoms of depressive PSYCHOSIS. It is usually reserved for patients who have failed to respond to psychological help or treatment with chemical ANTIDEPRESSANTS, or those for whom the risk of suicide or serious self-neglect requires a rapid treatment response. In the latter situation, ECT may be life-saving. ECT is a remarkably safe treatment, and may be safer than the use of chemical antidepressants in the elderly, physically compromised or pregnant. The principal risks to the patient are similar to those encountered in dental ANAESTHESIA. The main side-effect of ECT is transient MEMORY impairment, with a reversible ANTEROGRADE AMNESIA. RETROGRADE AMNESIA occurs for events just prior to therapy. Because severe depressive illness itself has an impact on memory function, it is difficult to separate the effects of the treatment from the effects of illness. Immediately after treatment, patients may experience an ACUTE CONFUSIONAL STATE and HEADACHE. There is no evidence that ECT causes brain damage of any kind. The mode of action of ECT, like the neurobiology of depression, is poorly understood. ECT modulates monoaminergic neurotransmission in the brain (see MONOAMINE HYPOTHESIS OF DEPRESSION) and has potent ANTICONVULSANT activity, as do some of the drugs used in AFFECTIVE DISORDER (see CARBAMAZEPINE).

See also: cognitive behavioural therapy; cognitive therapy

IAN C. REID

electrode (from Greek, *elektron*: amber, *hodos*: way) A conductor through which electrical current can pass. It is a term used in several contexts in physics and biology – for example, PH is measured usually with a pH electrode. In biological psychology ELECTRODE is most commonly used to describe devices via which one can stimulate tissue with electric current (STIMULATING ELECTRODE) or with which one can measure electrical activity in tissue (RECORDING ELECTRODE).

Electrodes for ELECTROPHYSIOLOGY are used in either a monopolar or bipolar configuration. This applies to both recording and stimulation. MONOPOLAR ELECTRODES are made of single wires. BIPOLAR ELECTRODES usually consist of two wires glued or twisted together, but some are made in a concentric arrangement. With monopolar electrodes, the registered activity indicates the activity of the active electrode in reference to the ground which is electrically inactive. This is achieved through a REFERENCE ELECTRODE: current passes down the stimulating electrode and a second electrode, usually just in the form of SKULL SCREWS fixed in the SKULL conducts the current away. (This arrangement can also be called a skull screw ground.) Monopolar stimulation is usually not recommended because of the spread of current over a large area. Bipolar recording registers the differential activity between the two active electrodes. Similarly, with bipolar stimulation, an electrical current flows between the two electrodes. Stimulating electrodes can also be used to produce ELECTROLYTIC LESIONS: these involve passage of high levels of current down electrodes insulated except at the tip, which produces non-specific chemical reactions at the point of contact with tissue. These destroy tissue non-selectively, leaving a vacancy. It is not a technique routinely employed any longer, more selective LESION techniques being available. In studies involving primates (and often rats also) glass tubes are used to insulate recording and stimulating electrodes. These involve a fine drawn glass tube through which a fine MICROELECTRODE is passed, the tubing then being sealed, leaving only the tip of the electrode (10 μm wide by 20 μm long) exposed. When used in human surgery these are shielded from brain tissue by a metal CANNULA.

In recording studies (see SINGLE UNIT ELECTROPHYSIOLOGICAL RECORDING) the activity of individual neurons, or groups of neurons (called MULTIUNIT RECORDING) is recorded using microelectrodes. These are very fine electrodes used to record activity from single neurons; MACROELECTRODES are bigger and record the activity of populations of neurons. In doing this one can use single electrodes, STEREOTRODES (pairs of electrodes) or MULTITRODES (clusters of electrodes). By comparing activity at more than one electrode it is possible to determine more accurately patterns of activity in neurons. Similarly MOVEABLE ELECTRODES can be used: these are electrodes that can be raised or lowered to record from different locations, rather than being fixed in one position.

Electrodes are also used in ELECTROCHEMISTRY (see also VOLTAMMETRY) and for making ELECTROENCEPHALOGRAM recordings (and see also EVENT-RELATED POTENTIALS). Electrodes for electrochemistry are treated (typically they are CARBON PASTE ELECTRODES) to permit measurement of the OXIDATION and/or REDUCTION of electroactive substances at the electrode surface. For EEG or ERP, SCALP ELECTRODES are used, contact being made with ELECTRODE JELLY.

See also: electrical brain stimulation; microiontophoresis

KAZUE SEMBA AND PHILIP WINN

electrode jelly *see* electroencephalogram

electroencephalogram (EEG) Note well: an ELECTROENCEPHALOGRAM (EEG) is a recording made by an electroencephalograph (colloquially, an EEG machine). When speaking of an EEG one is talking about the recording – the electroencephalogram – made by the machine – the electroencephalograph. The term encephalography refers to the use of the machine – the electroencephalograph. Electroencephalographic is an adjective describing an EEG measure.

EEG is measured using electrodes placed on the scalp (SCALP ELECTRODES), held in place by electrode jelly (which also ensures good contact). It is quite important to have the electrodes placed in consistent positions, as they will measure the massed activity of neurons in regions close to the point of contact. A cap that fits snugly to the head – rather like a bathing cap – with the electrodes pre-fixed in position is often used to maintain consistency of recording placements. EEG measures have been of considerable value in determining brain states in a variety of cases: such measures have diagnostic value in certain pathological conditions, they are widely used in SLEEP research and, in the United States of America, EEG data are used in the legal definition of death (see BRAIN DEATH). Recordings can be made either of spontaneous activity, or of activity in relation to stimulation (these latter being known as EVENT-RELATED POTENTIALS or more colloquially, EVOKED POTENTIALS; see

also P300). With the advent of sophisticated techniques for studying the activity of the living brain (see FUNCTIONAL NEUROIMAGING) the use of the EEG to measure brain activity has been put a little in the shade. However, the EEG retains, for the time being at least, one significant advantage over functional neuroimaging techniques: speed. While it cannot localize events in the brain with anything like the resolution of functional neuroimaging techniques, it can record them with a temporal resolution unmatched by any imaging technique. The use of event-related potentials in combination with functional neuroimaging techniques therefore offers a way to study both *where* (functional neuroimaging) and *when* (event related potentials) brain activity occurs.

Spontaneous activity measured by the EEG can be synchronized (that is, the waveforms measured, reflecting underlying neural activity, is regular and invariant) or desynchronized (that is, the waveforms show variability,

Activity recorded by the EEG

Waking state EEG includes:

alpha waves	Regular, medium frequency waves at 8-12 Hz; synchronized. Produced in the waking state, during quiet rest, when relaxed with little mental activity
beta waves	Irregular, low amplitude, medium to high frequency (13-30 Hz); desynchronized. The typical pattern produced during the waking state; associated with alertness and mental activity; also produced during REM sleep
theta rhythms	Medium amplitude, medium frequency (5-8 Hz). Associated especially with the hippocampus (hippocampal theta) where it has been associated with learning and memory; may also occur during the early stages of slow wave sleep and during REM sleep

Sleep EEG includes:

delta waves	Regular, synchronized waves with high amplitude and low frequency (> 3.5 Hz). Associated with the deepest levels of slow wave sleep
sleep spindles	Short bursts of activity at 12-14 Hz occurring every 2-5 minutes through slow wave sleep. They have been suggested to dampen brain responses to sensory input, permitting an individual to enter deeper sleep stages.
K complexes	Sudden and dramatic waves, appearing approximately once per minute only during stage 2 of slow wave sleep. They occur spontaneously, and in response to sensory events (such as noises)

reflecting the fact that different neurons are differently activated) (see SYNCHRONY/DESYNCHRONY). Different classes of activity (or waveforms as they can be called) are associated with the waking state and sleep. Slow-wave sleep in particular contains many waveforms not present in the waking state, though REM SLEEP shows many similarities with the waking state (hence its alternative name, paradoxical sleep). The various waveforms seen using EEG are listed in the table on page 257.

The state of the body may also be indexed by an ELECTROCARDIOGRAM (ECG) (measuring the activity of the heart), ELECTROMYOGRAM (EMG) (measuring muscle activity) and, ELECTRO-OCULOGRAM (EOG) (measuring eye movements). Research in a sleep laboratory will typically measure EEG, EOG (to indicate the presence of REM sleep) and EMG (to measure the ATONIA that accompanies REM sleep).

See also: polygraph

electroencephalographic afterdischarges Afterdischarges that are recorded using on an ELECTROENCEPHALOGRAM following electrical stimualtion, such as that delivered by KINDLING.

electrolyte Any substance which can be decomposed into electrically charged particles (see ION) is known as an electrolyte. For example, common salt, sodium chloride, breaks down in solution to positively charged SODIUM ions (Na^+) and negatively charged CHLORIDE ions (Cl^-). Because of their electrical properties, electrolytes are critical for neuronal functioning (see ACTION POTENTIAL).

See also: electrostatic pressure

electrolytic lesion *see* lesion

electromyogram (EMG) Note well: an ELECTROMYOGRAM (EMG) is a recording made by an electromyograph. As with the ELECTROENCEPHALOGRAM (EEG), the electromyogram measures electrical activity, but in this case it is the electrical activity generated by MUSCLE activity that is recorded. Such recordings are made in many types of study where muscle activity is a factor of interest, including SLEEP, where ATONIA is a marked feature of REM SLEEP (rapid eye movement sleep).

See also: electro-oculogram; polygraph

electron *see* atom

electron microscopy (EM) This is a form of MICROSCOPY that operates at very much higher level of magnification than either LIGHT MICROSCOPY or CONFOCAL MICROSCOPY, being able to resolve clearly SUBCELLULAR ORGANS with clear resolution at approximately 0.2 nanometers. It works by passing a beam of high-velocity electrons passing through a specimen. The beam that emerges from the specimen is transmitted through lenses and an image can be formed. Electron microscopy is important in assessing the ULTRASTRUCTURE of tissue, but is rarely used for investigation of material in biological psychology experiments.

There are two forms of electron microscopy: transmission EM (TEM) and scanning EM (SEM). In transmission EM the electron beam passes through tissue, allowing one to generate a satisfactory 2-dimensional image. In scanning EM, the electrons behave differently (and more complicatedly) and a three dimensional image can be generated; see FREEZE FRACTURE.

electron transport chain *see* mitochondria; respiration

electrophysiology Literally the study of electrical actions in the CELL and in tissue; in biological psychology this term is typically used to describe studies in which electrical recording of neuronal activity is made.

See also: event related potentials; neurophysiology; single unit electrophysiological recording

electroreceptor A type of RECEPTOR sensitive to changes in electric fields. They are not present in mammalian brain but are specialized receptors used by species that need to be able to detect electrical fields.

electroretinogram (ERG) Note well: an ELECTRORETINOGRAM (EOG) is a recording made by an electroretinograph. As with the ELECTROENCEPHALOGRAM (EEG), the electroretinogram measures electrical activity, but in this case it is the electrical activity generated by the RETINA that is recorded. This is not the same as the ELECTRO-OCULOGRAM.

See also: polygraph

electrostatic pressure Positively charged ions (cations) and negatively charged ions (anions) attract each other but repel their own kind (see ION). Electrostatic pressure is the net result of this ionic attraction or repulsion. Both cations and anions will move away from sites where they exist in high concentrations towards sites where they are in low concentration. Just as OSMOTIC PRESSURE may exist across a SEMI-PERMEABLE MEMBRANE, so there may exist an electrostatic pressure, developed by varying concentrations of anions and cations on either side of a MEMBRANE.

electrotonic Electrotonic conduction is the passive spread of voltage along a neuronal MEMBRANE. The electrotonic gradient is the difference in electronic conduction property between two points on a membrane. The term electrotonic transmission is used to refer to electrical transmission between neurons (EPHAPTIC TRANSMISSION). The electrotonic potential (or RECEPTOR POTENTIAL) is the electronic potential at a given point on a membrane.

electroxidizable A MOLECULE is said to be electroxidizable if it is oxidized (see OXIDATION) by passage of electric current; see ELECTROCHEMISTRY.

element (from Latin, *elementum*: first principle) The word element has many meanings in many different contexts. In chemistry, an element is a substance that cannot be transformed into simpler substances.

See also: atom; periodic table of the elements

elevated mazes Elevated mazes (typically an elevated plus maze – one in the shape of a plus sign) are used to measure ANXIETY-like states in animals. One arm of the maze is enclosed, the other arm open, giving an animal the choice of remaining within a closed area or going out into the open. Apparatus like this is thought to have ethological validity, the pattern of activity on the apparatus reflecting competition between EXPLORATION and AVOIDANCE. Such tests detect well anxiolytic drug action (see BENZODIAZEPINES).

See also: animal models of anxiety

eliminative materialism Materialism is the hypothesis that mental states are states of the physical brain. REDUCTIVE MATERIALISM aims for an explanation of mental functions in terms of neurobiological mechanisms. ELIMINATIVE MATERIALISM is reductive materialism plus the prediction that progress in COGNITIVE NEUROSCIENCE will entail major revisions of psychological categories such as CONSCIOUSNESS, will, belief, and desire. It is predicted that some aspects of the common-sense psychological (FOLK PSYCHOLOGY) may be eliminated altogether, when replaced by a more successful theoretical framework derived from cognitive neuroscience. Despite misconceptions, it does not claim that mental phenomena themselves would be eliminated, but only that how they are categorized, interpreted and understood would be revised.

See also: reductionism

PATRICIA S. CHURCHLAND

ELISA (enzyme-linked immunosorbent assay) An *in vitro* technique for detecting the presence of specific MOLECULES in samples of homogenized tissue, based on the binding of an ANTIBODY to an ANTIGEN. It is a development of the IMMUNOASSAY and RADIOIMMUNOASSAY techniques that involves antibody being coated on specialized reaction tubes.

Reference

Feldman R., Meyer J.S. & Quenzer L.F. (1997) *Principles of Neuropsychopharmacology*, Sinauer Associates: Sunderland MA.

embedded figures test *see* central coherence

embolic stroke A stroke caused by an embolism (see EMBOLUS).

emboliform nucleus *see* cerebellum – anatomical organization

embolus An obstruction in a blood vessel; 'embolism' is a term used to indicate the presence of an embolus (see STROKE).

embryo (from Greek, *en*: in, *bryein*: to swell) An organism in the earliest stages of DEVELOPMENT. During the first 4 weeks of human development the apparently homogenous egg becomes an EMBRYO. Once the principal organs of the body are differentiated and identifiable, even at a rudimentary degree, and the embryo has a human appearance, it is known instead as a FOETUS. The adjective embryonic has a more general (and often imprecise) usage in describing the original stages of things.

emergent properties Something is emergent if it is a function of lower level phenomena and how they are organized. Examples of properties emergent in this sense are being a solid, alive, and a gene (see GENE). In these examples, the macro property does not exist unless the system is organized in a certain way. No single part of a CELL is alive but organized properly, the cell as a whole *is*. Mental phenomena such as feeling PAIN or hoping for a sunny day are emergent with respect to cells in the brain. A more restricted conception of emergence entails that the emergent phenomenon cannot be reduced to or explained in terms of the underlying neural microphenomena.

See also: reductionism

PATRICIA S. CHURCHLAND

emesis *see* vomiting

emission *see* efflux

emotion Emotions are mental states, sometimes described as 'disturbances of mind' that may be associated with certain subjective feelings and characteristic behavioural responses. In experimental psychology, emotions are generally described in terms of three dimensions: the visceral or physiological (including, for instance, AUTONOMIC NERVOUS SYSTEM activity), behavioural (facial expressions, angry postures for example) and the subjective (such things as emotional feelings). Understanding how these three dimensions interact and how they are coordinated is a major aim of research in this area. Related terms to emotion are AFFECT from the older psychological literature and MOOD, terms still commonly used in psychiatry. The distinction between emotions and mood is probably their chronicity: emotions are generally brief experiences of a matter of seconds, whereas moods are much longer lasting.

One of the most enduring questions about the emotions is how many basic forms exist.

Charles Darwin (1809–1882) attempted to classify the basic facial expressions of human emotion as deriving from animal forms. Later, on the basis of cross-cultural studies, Ekman proposed that facial expressions of happiness, surprise, sadness, fear, disgust and contempt are human universals that correspond to the basic emotions. Furthermore, these facial expressions were associated with different patterning of responding in the autonomic system in terms of responses such as blood pressure and skin temperature. However, there is some evidence for rather general or overlapping changes in autonomic reactivity in contrasting emotions if these nevertheless both require behavioural action. There is considerable controversy about when infants develop the capacity to perceive a range of discrete emotions, as distinct from general feelings of contentment and distress. As shown by Bowlby and others, the latter is caused by separation from an attachment figure in unfamiliar circumstances and peaks at about 18 months of age, declining by about 3 years.

The psychological characterization of distinct and shared patterns of emotional response is paralleled by both differentiation and commonality in the neural mechanisms of the emotions. Thus, there is some evidence for discrete regions in control of basic motivational and emotional processes such as particular forms of FEAR or AGGRESSION, together with precise patterns of ENDOCRINE regulation, which may include NEUROPEPTIDES as neuromodulators of specific behavioural responses. The basic behavioural output systems are controlled to some extent by a network of structures termed the LIMBIC SYSTEM, which includes the AMYGDALA, SEPTAL NUCLEI and CINGULATE CORTEX, as well as their interconnecting structures. Theorists such as Jeffrey Gray have attempted to collapse the main emotions into a smaller set of those that are mediated by defined brain systems. For example, according to this scheme, 'frustration' is conceptually related to ANXIETY and is mediated by a brain BEHAVIOURAL INHIBITION SYSTEM that includes the septum and HIPPOCAMPUS. Positive emotions or approach behaviour, by contrast, can be linked to the operation of a general incentive-motivational (see INCENTIVE MOTIVATION) or REWARD system which depends on the functioning of the MESOLIMBIC structures such as the amygdala and NUCLEUS ACCUMBENS. Our understanding of neural mechanisms of the emotions has been enhanced by study of the subjective effects of drugs in human subjects. Many ANTIDEPRESSANTS and ANXIOLYTIC drugs work either directly or indirectly on the ascending monoaminergic neurotransmitter systems (including NORADRENALINE and SEROTONIN, as well as DOPAMINE). Drugs of abuse such as AMPHETAMINE may cause EUPHORIA, presumably by releasing brain dopamine, whereas compounds such as CHOLECYSTOKININ elicit PANIC-like reactions in volunteers. Nevertheless, the subjective effects of these drugs have been shown to depend considerably on the cognitive context in which they are experienced, as postulated in early theories of emotion such as that of Schachter (see JAMES–LANGE THEORY OF THE EMOTIONS).

There have been diverse theories about the causation and functions of emotions, beginning with the James–Lange theory, and its various manifestations, and culminating in more cognitive models emphasizing such factors as appraisal and attribution, and the use of emotions for setting priorities among various goals or as cues to alter goal-directed plans and actions, including social communication (see Oatley & Jenkins 1996 for a review). However, little is known about the cognitive nature and neural basis of these complex mental processes. A key issue is the role of conscious and unconscious emotions. The latter may play an important role in informing conscious DECISION-MAKING. Damasio has recently described how unconscious 'gut feelings' may provide somatic markers for decision-making in normal people that precede a conscious appraisal for making particular choices in a risky situation (see SOMATIC MARKER HYPOTHESIS). However, patients with damage to the ventromedial PREFRONTAL CORTEX apparently lose this capacity and hence continue to make highly risky decisions. It remains possible that the neurochemical basis of the somatic markers corresponds to activity in the central monoamine neurotransmitter systems which innervate the FRONTAL CORTEX. In this way, a

central correlate of William James's postulated visceral reactions underlying emotion may inform complex decision-making at the highest cortical level.

References

Damasio A.R. (1994) *Descartes' Error. Emotion, Reason and the Human Brain*, Putnam Press: New York.

Ekman P. (1981) *Face of Man*, Garland: New York.

Oatley K. & Jenkins J. (1996) *Understanding Emotions*, Blackwell Scientific Publications: Oxford.

TREVOR W. ROBBINS

emotional intelligence An umbrella term that has been applied to a range of learned skills to do with EMOTION. Included under this term are the following qualities: recognizing emotions; coming to terms with the emotions of others; expressing emotions in appropriate ways; regulating and controlling emotions properly; and using emotions appropriately. It is a term that raises intriguing questions about computers: if machines can learn and show intelligent behaviour, can they engage or use affective states?

Reference

Picard R. (1997) *Affective Computing*, MIT Press: Boston MA.

emotional lability questionnaire A questionnaire developed to assess pathological crying and laughing in patients suffering from various forms of brain disorder. Emotional lability has been associated with a variety of conditions, from dysfunction of the FRONTAL LOBE though to TUMOUR damage and DEGENERATION in the BRAINSTEM.

Reference

Newsom-Davis I.C., Abrahams S., Goldstein L.H. & Leigh P.N. (1999) The emotional lability questionnaire: a new measure of emotional lability in amyotrophic lateral sclerosis. *Journal of the Neurological Sciences* 169: 22–25.

emulation Emulation is a form of imitation (see OBSERVATION LEARNING) but is thought to go beyond simple repetition. While imitation can be understood as straightforward copying, emulation involves observing a behaviour and understanding from the specific example seen the deeper principles involved – that is, the *purpose* of the action. In emulating, an organism could therefore use a different form of action to achieve the same goal.

enantiomer An enantiomer is one of a pair of MOLECULES that are mirror-images of each other; every enantiomer is an ISOMER but all isomers need not be enantiomers. Note that the term is derived from the more general one, *enantiomorph* (from Greek, *enantios*: opposite, *morphe*: shape) which describes anything that is one of a mirror-image pair.

encéphale isolé see *cerveau isolé*

encephalitis Inflammatory disease of the brain occurring especially as a direct or delayed reaction to infection, usually by a virus. Inflammation (see IMMUNE SYSTEM) commonly extends to involve the MENINGES and sometimes the SPINAL CORD (as encephalomyelitis), and the acute phase of the illness may mimic the symptoms of MENINGITIS. Encephalitis may also be caused by vaccines (especially rabies and whooping cough vaccines) and by poisons (such as lead). Organisms that commonly give rise to encephalitis are encountered either in epidemics (for instance the viruses for mumps, influenza, whooping cough, glandular fever or measles) or sporadically (the viruses for herpes simplex and herpes zoster, the human immunodeficiency virus and the bacteria for tuberculosis and syphilis). Infections common in the tropics tend to be insect-borne and include various equine encephalitides, Lassa fever and numerous virulent fevers spread by ticks. Trypanosomiasis, or African sleeping sickness, is caused by a parasite spread by the bite of the tsetse fly; it follows a chronic, dementing and eventually fatal course. Most cases of viral encephalitis result from an immunological reaction and develop only about a week after infection. A serious demyelinating condition (see DEMYELINATION), subacute sclerosing panenencephalitis, resembling MULTIPLE SCLEROSIS, may develop many weeks after an attack of measles, but many cases of viral encephalitis are benign and probably pass unnoticed. The pathological changes that develop in the encephalitic brain vary in severity and character and in their anatomical distribution, depending on the identity of the infecting organism. For example, focal invasion of the TEMPORAL LOBE, CEREBRAL CORTEX and LIMBIC SYSTEM by herpes simplex virus may lead to transient behavioural abnormalities, olfactory HALLUCINATION, amnesia, expressive APHASIA and temporal lobe SEIZURES. Delayed post-infective and post-vaccination encephalitides may show a predilection for the BASAL GANGLIA, giving rise to persistent involuntary movements and other signs of extrapyramidal involvement. Specific anti-viral agents are available for treatment in some cases and may improve the prognosis. A separate group of (hitherto) rare encephalitides, including CREUTZFELDT–JAKOB DISEASE, kuru and a human variant of BOVINE SPONGIFORM ENCEPHALOPATHY (BSE), are thought to be caused by invasion of the brain by an abnormal form of protein. The infective agent (abnormal prion protein) lacks DNA or RNA and is thought to replicate by acting as a physical template for its own further production by the host (see PRION DISEASE). The incubation period and clinical course may be extremely prolonged, but the diseases are invariably fatal. There is no effective treatment.

L. JACOB HERBERG

encephalitis lethargica A virus that produces a form of PARKINSON'S DISEASE, known as POST-ENCEPHALITIC PARKINSONISM. Infection leads to an immediate 'sleepy sickness' from which patients may recover. The majority of those infected however go on to develop postencephalitic Parkinson's disease or other neurological disorders. Oliver Sacks in the book *Awakenings* provides a vivid description of this illness, and the recovery, after very many years of untreated Parkinsonism, of a group of patients among the first to be treated with L-DOPA.

Reference

Sacks O. (1976) *Awakenings*, Pelican Books: Harmondsworth UK.

encephalization see nervous system

encephalization quotient see nervous system

encephalomyelitis An acute inflammation of the CENTRAL NERVOUS SYSTEM. There are many forms: BORNA DISEASE for example is an enzootic encephalomyelitis.

encephalon (from Greek, *en*: in, *kephalon*: head) Encephalon is the brain, encephalic, of the brain. It is from this that anatomical terms such as TELENCEPHALON and DIENCEPHALON, and medical terms such as ENCEPHALITIS, are drawn.

encephalopathy Technically this refers to inflammation of the CENTRAL NERVOUS SYSTEM, leading to NEURODEGENERATION. Often however it is used more loosely to refer to any brain disease or disorder.

encoding Encoding is the TRANSDUCTION of material in a different form: neurons encode information, sensory data being transduced into neuronal activity; see LEVELS OF PROCESSING for discussion of DEEP ENCODING and SHALLOW ENCODING.

See also: ensemble coding and population coding; neural coding; neuron

endocannabinoid A chemical naturally found in the body that binds to RECEPTORS for CANNABIS (tetrahydrocannabinol): see ANANDAMIDE.

endocast A cast made of the inside of the SKULL (or indeed other objects); see PALAEONEUROLOGY.

endocrine This term refers to the ENDOCRINE GLANDS and their HORMONES.

endocrine disorder Endocrine organs affecting behaviour include the THYROID GLAND (thyroxin), parathyroid (affecting CALCIUM levels), the OVARIES or TESTES (SEX STEROIDS), pancreatic islets (INSULIN and GLUCAGON), adrenal medulla (ADRENALINE), adrenal cortex (GLUCOCORTICOIDS and MINERALOCORTICOIDS) (see ADRENAL GLAND), posterior pituitary (OXYTOCIN and VASOPRESSIN), and the anterior pituitary (see PITUITARY GLAND). Each endocrine gland is closely regulated by the HYPOTHALAMO-PITUITARY AXIS as well as by intricate feedback systems. This tight control reflects the low tolerances that are permissible: human endocrine function is remarkable in that even small functional drifts, well within what might be thought to be the physiological range, may have profound effects on behaviour or psychological state.

L. JACOB HERBERG

endocrine glands (from Greek, *endon*: within, *krinein*: to separate) The endocrine glands are structures within the body that release HORMONES. They are the so-called 'ductless glands' in contrast to the EXOCRINE GLANDS, which are glands that do have ducts (such as the salivary glands for example). Hormones circulate within the blood stream (see BLOOD) and interact with any structures bearing appropriate receptors. (This is the model for VOLUME TRANSMISSION within the CENTRAL NERVOUS SYSTEM.) The various endocrine glands, their principal hormones and functions are listed in the table on pages 264–266 (adapted from Rosenzweig *et al.* 1996). For the sake of completeness non-endocrine gland hormones are also listed in the table.

See also: fight-or-flight; hormones – classification; menstrual cycle

References
Campbell N.A., Reece J.B. & Mitchell L.G. (1999) *Biology*, 5th edn, Addison-Wesley: Menlo Park CA.
Rosenzweig M.R., Leiman A.L. & Breedlove S.M. (1996) *Biological Psychology*, Sinauer Associates: Sunderland MA.

endocytosis The process whereby a CELL can use a portion of its MEMBRANE to envelope a large MOLECULE or particles of a complex substance and draw it into itself, by cutting of that part of the membrane to form an intracellular VESICLE; PINOCYTOSIS describes this process at SYNAPTIC TERMINALS. Endocytosis is a form of uptake (see REUPTAKE) that does not require specialized molecular machinery embedded in the cell membrane.

See also: exocytosis

endoderm The inner one of the three GERM LAYERS present in the developing EMBRYO (the others being MESODERM and ECTODERM), it gives rise to tissue such as the intestines (see GASTROINTESTINAL SYSTEM).

See also: development

Endocrine glands (and other sites of hormone release) and their functions

Structure	Hormones	Known functions
Endocrine glands include:		
ADRENAL GLAND (adrenal cortex)	corticosteroids including: glucocorticoids (e.g. corticosterone, CORTISOL)	Principally concerned with ENERGY storage and use
	mineralocorticoids (e.g. aldosterone)	Regulation of SODIUM, POTASSIUM activity
	sex hormones	
	androgen	male sexual activity
	estrogen	female sexual activity
	progesterone	female sexual activity
ADRENAL GLAND (adrenal medulla)	adrenaline (epinephrine)	STRESS and AROUSAL
	noradrenaline (norepinephrine)	STRESS and AROUSAL
GASTROINTESTINAL TRACT:		
DUODENUM (mucosa of duodenum)	bombesin	possible role in FEEDING and SATIETY
	cholecystokinin	stimulates gallbladder; satiety signal
	gastric inhibitory peptide	
	gastrin	
	gastrin releasing peptide	
	neurotensin	
	motilin	
	secretin	stimulation of PANCREAS
	somatostatin	
	substance P	
	vasoactive intestinal peptide	
STOMACH	gastrin	stimulation of gastric secretions
GONADS: both female (ovaries) and male (testes) secrete sex hormones:		
OVARIES	estrogens (e.g. ESTRADIOL, ESTRONE)	all involved in female sexual activity
	inhibin	
	progestins (e.g. progesterone)	all involved in female sexual activity and the maintenance of PREGNANCY
	relaxin	secreted near the end of pregnancy
TESTES	androgens (e.g. TESTOSTERONE)	all involved in male sexual activity
	inhibin	

Structure	Hormones	Known functions
PANCREAS	insulin	GLUCOSE storage and use
	glucagon	conversion of GLYCOGEN to glucose
PARATHYROID GLAND	parathyroid hormone	
PITUITARY GLAND: separated into:		
ANTERIOR PITUITARY	adrenocorticotropic hormone	stimulates ADRENAL GLAND
(see also ADENOHYPOPHYSIS)	follicle stimulating hormone	stimulates growth of OVARIES, TESTES
	growth hormone	growth stimulation
	luteinizing hormone	SEX HORMONE stimulation
	melanocyte stimulating hormone	SKIN pigmentation
	prolactin	milk production
	thyroid stimulating hormone	stimulates thyroid gland
POSTERIOR PITUITARY (see also NEUROHYPOPHYSIS)	oxytocin	control of UTERUS; milk production
	vasopressin	OSMOREGULATION
INTERMEDIATE PITUITARY	beta endorphin	see ENDORPHIN
	melanocyte stimulating hormone	skin pigmentation
THYROID GLAND	calcitonin	restricts CALCIUM level in blood
	triiodothyronine (T3)	stimulate METABOLISM
	thyroxine (T4)	stimulate metabolism
THYMUS GLAND	thymosin	
	thymostatin	
	thymoxin	
Non endocrine hormonal release sites include:		
ADIPOSE TISSUE	leptin	Possible role in body weight control
BLOOD	angiotensin II	Produced in the BLOOD; see OSMOREGULATION
BRAIN: Two sites release hormones:		
HYPOTHALAMUS	corticotropin releasing hormone	these are all involved in the control of pituitary hormone release
	gonadotropin releasing hormone	
	growth hormone releasing factor (somatocrinin)	

Structure	Hormones	Known functions
	growth hormone release inhibiting factor (somatostatin)	
	melanocyte stimulating hormone inhibiting factor (possibly dopamine)	
	melanocyte stimulating hormone releasing factor	
	prolactin inhibiting factor (possibly dopamine)	
	prolactin releasing factor	
	thyrotropin releasing hormone	
PINEAL GLAND	melatonin	possible role in CIRCADIAN RHYTHMS
GROWTH FACTORS	epidermal growth factor fibroblast growth factor nerve growth factor somatomedin	All involved in growth; secreted from various cells, not endocrine glands
HEART	atrial natriuretic factor	see OSMOREGULATION
IMMUNE SYSTEM	cytokines (e.g. interferon, interleukin)	Involved in CELL signaling; see IMMUNE SYSTEM
During PREGNANCY, the FOETUS and placenta also release hormones	human chorionic gonadotropin human placental lactogen	maintenance of foetus and placenta

Note: all hormones (and their customary abbreviations) have independent entries which may contain further information about them. The various categories of hormones are also listed under HORMONES: CATEGORIZATION.

endogenous Endogenous means literally generated from within; exogenous means generated from outside. For example, an endogenous neurotransmitter is one found naturally within nervous tissue; if one were to inject, into an animal or patient, neurotransmitter one would be delivering exogenous neurotransmitter.

endogenous depression; exogenous depression Endogenous depression refers to DEPRESSION caused by internal factors, whereas exogenous depression (also known as REACTIVE DEPRESSION) is caused by external forces (such as bereavement for example). The distinction between ENDOGENOUS and EXOGENOUS causes is not easily made, which has led to these terms falling out of favour.

endogenous excitotoxins Excitotoxins occurring naturally in the brain. Their existence has been suggested to account for various forms of damage, most notably that seen in HUNTINGTON'S CHOREA.

See also: kynurenic acid; quinolinic acid

endogenous opiates Enkephalins and ENDORPHINS are NEUROPEPTIDES in the brain which have opiate-like properties. Opiate drugs (see OPIATES) interact with these ENDOGENOUS enkephalin and endorphin systems. It appears then that the brains of mammals have within them NEUROTRANSMITTERS that function as endogenous opiates, and these have been implicated in FEEDING, SOCIAL BEHAVIOUR, STRESS modulation, PAIN transmission, and REINFORCEMENT. Whether activation of one's own enkephalin and endorphin systems (for example by repeated vigorous exercise) can lead to a form of addiction is an open question. Activities that would cause activation of these systems will also have a variety of other effects which might be positively reinforcing.

Reference

Feldman R., Meyer J.S. & Quenzer L.F. (1997) *Principles of Neuropsychopharmacology*, Sinauer Associates: Sunderland MA.

endogenous rhythm A rhythm generated within an organism, unaffected by outside influences (see EXOGENOUS RHYTHM, ZEIT-GEBER). The ENTRAINMENT of endogenous and exogenous rhythms presents the observed OVERT RHYTHM (which may be a rhythm with various periods – CIRCADIAN, CIRCANNUAL, infradian and ULTRADIAN RHYTHMS, for example). The term endogenous rhythm is not commonly used; it is synonymous with FREE RUNNING RHYTHM.

See also: biological clock

endolymph *see* vestibular system

endoneurium *see* nerve

endonuclease Endonucleases mediate the breakdown of DNA (deoxyribonucleic acid) and RNA (ribonucleic acid RNA); see ISCHAE-MIA.

endoplasmic reticulum This may be ROUGH ENDOPLASMIC RETICULUM or SMOOTH ENDO-PLASMIC RETICULUM.

See also: cell; neuron

endorphins Opiate-like neuropeptides found in certain regions of the brain. Endorphins were discovered in 1974, when researchers were attempting to isolate substances in brain extract that bound to the recently discovered opiate receptors. Termed endorphins for '*en-dogenous morphin*e-like' substances, the endorphins comprise a family of peptides derived from the PROOPIOMELANOCORTIN (POMC) gene. The major and most active opioid-like product of this gene (which also synthesizes ACTH) is beta-endorphin. The POMC gene is found in the anterior and intermediate PITUI-TARY GLAND and in the ARCUATE NUCLEUS of

the HYPOTHALAMUS. Endorphin secretion from pituitary is believed to have a neuroendocrine function, while endorphins within the hypotha-lamic neurons (which project to other structures) are presumed to act as NEURO-TRANSMITTERS. The physiological effects of endorphin are very similar to OPIATES. It is believed that endorphins, like other opioid peptides, play a key role in adaptation to STRESS, regulation of PAIN transmission, and many aspects of motivation.

See also: enkephalin

ANN E. KELLEY

endothelin Endothelin is one of the PROTEINS occurring naturally in BLOOD vessels and is involved in regulating their contraction. EXO-GENOUS endothelin can be applied to neural tissue to cause excessive contraction of the blood vessels, thereby generating ISCHAEMIA and consequent NEURODEGENERATION.

endothelium A layer of cells (known as the endothelial cells) lining the inner surface of blood vessels.

See also: blood; blood–brain barrier

endotherm A warm-blooded animal (also known as a homoiotherm); one that maintains its temperature by generating heat internally, in contrast to an ECTOTHERM.

endplate potential *see* neuromuscular junction

energy Energy, from the point of view of biopsychology, concerns several processes re-lated to HUNGER. First, there are energy stores within the body, in the form of calories contained within fat cells or within GLYCOGEN deposits in muscle or liver cells. These energy stores can be called upon for future energy needs. Because there is ample evidence to suggest that BODY WEIGHT and long-term energy stores remain reasonably constant or regulated over the long term, an implication is that the level of these energy stores can be monitored by the brain. A major question has concerned precisely how the brain is able to detect the level of energy stores that are distributed widely over the body. For muscle and liver glycogen, a plausible answer has been that the brain monitors either the level of the chief sugar, GLUCOSE, into which glycogen must be converted before it can be used as an energy source by cells, or else the level of a chemical product that is produced during the metabolism of glucose. An important source of the brain's information about glycogen/glucose stores emanates from chemical detectors within the liver itself, which send projections to the brain via the VAGUS NERVE. It has been more difficult to account for how the brain might monitor the level of energy stores contained in fat cells, since the metabolism of fat does not produce the same chemical signals. However, a substance, LEPTIN, has been reported to be produced by fat cells and to be detected by the brain. Leptin may provide a bloodstream chemical signal to the brain for the long-term regulation of energy stores. Second, energy can refer to the availability of calorie stores for conversion into forms that can be used by either the brain or the rest of the body. Most body cells can metabolize a variety of different chemical forms of energy. The brain, on the other hand, is more limited in its potential sources of energy, partly because of the existence of the BLOOD–BRAIN BARRIER and partly due to the special nature of the NEURON as a cell type. Brain cells typically use only one source of energy: glucose. In cases of extreme starvation, a substitute fuel, KETONE BODIES, may be used by neurons instead. However, in societies where starvation is uncommon it is probable that the vast majority of individuals' brains use glucose as their sole fuel throughout their entire lives. Thus, from the brain's point of view, energy available at the moment concerns availability of glucose itself or of energy stores that can be easily transformed by the liver into glucose. Finally, energy may refer to the actual use of calories by the brain at a given moment. A useful analogy might be the automobile: if energy stores correspond to gasoline (petrol) in the tank, actual use corresponds to the flow of fuel determined by the accelerator pedal. The brain needs to burn glucose constantly in order to supply its unending demand for energy. Interruption of neuronal metabolism of glucose (like blocking the flow of fuel to the engine) by administration of a chemical such as 2-deoxy-D-glucose,

produces an 'energy need' even if there are ample stores of calories (the tank is full). For this reason, administration of 2-deoxy-D-glucose that starves the brain can elicit eating from an animal even if it has already recently eaten.

KENT C. BERRIDGE

energy balance The maintenance of a constant level of ENERGY stores is usually thought to require active regulation by the brain. Calories are continually expended by normal METABOLISM, and even more are lost during exercise. Counterbalancing this loss of energy is food ingestion. The important thing is that over the long term the loss and gain tend to be closely matched, as though they are kept in balance. To do this requires that the brain be able to assess the gain of calories produced by food ingestion, and to keep track of long term energy stores such as FAT deposits in ADIPOSE tissue. A simple equation often presented is:

energy intake = energy used + energy stored

with excess energy burnt as heat.

See also: body weight; brown adipose tissue; feeding; leptin

KENT C. BERRIDGE

engram The physical change in the brain that results from the encoding of an experience. It is often used interchangeably with the term MEMORY TRACE. How are engrams represented at the cellular level? According to the single-neuron hypothesis, each memory in the brain is represented by the firing of only one neuron, such that the memory of your grandmother would be represented by a GRANDMOTHER CELL. However, there are problems with this hypothesis. This would make the brain extremely sensitive to memory loss due to damage. If your grandmother cell died, you would permanently lose your memory for your grandmother unless you saw her again and formed a new representation of her. In addition, if every memory required its own neuron for its representation, an extremely large percentage of the brain would be required just to store memories. Having extremely distinct representations for every memory would make it difficult to generalize across situations. Also, there is little physiological evidence that memories are represented by single cells. While cells that are responsive to particular types of visual stimuli such as faces and 3-dimensional objects have been found in the lateral temporal lobes, single cells that represent particular memories have not been found. The downfall of the single-cell hypothesis has lead researchers to propose that engrams consist of networks of connected cells, or cell assemblies (see CELL ASSEMBLY THEORY) which together represent a memory. In this model, a single neuron can be involved in representing more than one memory. Neuronal connections between engrams and overlapping representations of memories allow the rapid association of related memories. Cellular correlates of memory are reflected in the modulation of cellular firing patterns and in either sustained firing after a LEARNING event, or the ability to reactivate the original neuronal response to a stimulus after the stimulus is no longer present. At the single-cell level, memory encoding can result in changes in the membrane properties that affect ion flow, the growth or retraction of synapses, and changes in presynaptic and postsynaptic neurotransmitter related functions. LONG-TERM POTENTIATION (LTP) and LONG-TERM DEPRESSION (LTD) are thought to play an important role in these cellular memory processes.

Where are engrams located? Research has suggested that there is not a single storehouse for memory in the brain. Karl Lashley (1890–1958) tried to find the location of the memory trace by removing many different sized portions of the cerebral cortex from almost all cortical locations and then giving the lesioned (see LESION) animals memory tests. His results refuted the hypothesis that there is a single or even a few specific memory storehouses in the brain. In addition, while brain stimulation of patients during undergoing neurosurgery has occasionally lead to the vivid recall of memories, these findings are rare and inconsistent, which also suggests that there is not a single storehouse for memory. The inability to find a single memory storehouse has led memory researchers to propose that cortical sensory and motor areas may be involved in the long-term storage of memories. For example, the visual attributes of a memory may be stored in the VISUAL CORTEX, and the olfactory attri-

butes of the same memory may be located in the OLFACTORY CORTEX. The reactivation of a complete memory is hypothesized to occur when cell assemblies in the sensory areas that represent the components of the memory become simultaneously active through synchronous firing. In this model memory is not an entity to be stored, but instead reflects the plasticity within each functional system of the brain.

See also: Hebbian synapse; neural networks

Reference

Lashley K.S. (1950) In search of the engram. *Symposia of the Society for Experimental Biology* 4: 454–482.

HOWARD EICHENBAUM

enkephalin   A type of small neuropeptide found occurring in the nervous system that has actions like those of the OPIATES. In 1975, a year after the discovery of the ENDORPHINS, two opioid pentapeptides (peptide chains of five amino acids) were sequenced: Met-enkephalin (H-Tyr-Gly-Gly-Phe-Met-OH) and leu-enkephalin (H-Tyr-Gly-Gly-Phe-Leu-OH). Since these substances were isolated from the brain, they were termed enkephalin (from Greek, *en*: in, *kephalon*: head). The enkephalin peptides are synthesized from the proenkephalin gene which encodes a 267-amino-acid protein precursor. The enzymatic breakdown of this precursor forms met-enkephalin, leu-enkephalin, and a number of other peptides. Enkephalins are found in many neuronal systems in the brain and SPINAL CORD. It is believed that the distributions of leu-enkephalin and met-enkephalin are identical, although in all areas the levels of met-enkephalin are higher. Examples of areas that have high levels of enkephalins are STRIATUM and GLOBUS PALLIDUS, AMYGDALA, THALAMUS, HYPOTHALAMUS, PERIAQUEDUCTAL GREY region, and the DORSAL HORN of spinal cord. Like other opioid peptides, enkephalins play an important role in many physiological and behavioural functions, such as FEEDING, SOCIAL BEHAVIOUR, STRESS modulation, PAIN transmission, and REINFORCEMENT.

ANN E. KELLEY

ensemble coding and population coding A NEURON is able to code information not only by its individual pattern of FIRING and release of NEUROTRANSMITTERS, but also by communal activation among groups of neurons. Two different types of coding can be identified: population coding involves information (of whatever nature) being represented by the numbers of neurons activated by a stimulus (of whatever sort). In contrast, ensemble coding involves the coding of information by the pattern of activation within a given set of neurons. By analogy, population coding amounts to a vote – the more neurons firing the better – while ensemble coding is better understood in terms of a musical score – the pattern of activity is what generates meaning.

See also: across-fibre pattern theory; neural coding

Reference

Hatsopoulos N.G., Ojakangas C.L., Maynard E.M. & Donoghue J.P. (1998) Detection and identification of ensemble codes in motor cortex. In *Neuronal Ensembles: Strategies for Recording and Decoding*, ed. H. Eichenbaum & J. Davis, pp. 161–175, Wiley: New York.

enteric nervous system The three principal components of the AUTONOMIC NERVOUS SYSTEM are the parasympathetic, sympathetic and enteric divisions. The enteric nervous system innervates the GASTROINTESTINAL TRACT, PANCREAS and gall bladder. Sensory neurons located in these tissues detect muscular and chemical changes and motor neurons are then able to change gut muscular activity, local blood flow and secretory systems. Parasympathetic and sympathetic systems provide external regulation, but the enteric nervous system can function more or less independently and has a critical role in control of gastrointestinal function.

Reference

Kandel E.R., Schwartz J.H. & Jessell T.M. (2000) *Principles of Neural Science*, McGraw-Hill: New York.

enterogastrones *see* digestive system

entopeduncular nucleus The entopeduncular nucleus is an alternative name, in the rat brain, for the medial segment of the GLOBUS PALLIDUS (which is also known as the internal segment of the globus pallidus). It bears this name because it is embedded within the CEREBRAL PEDUNCLES. Some authors use the term entopeduncular nucleus; others have stopped using this term, preferring 'medial segment of the globus pallidus' to maintain consistency with the nomenclature applied to the brains of other species (see STEREOTAXIC ATLAS).

entorhinal cortex The entorhinal cortex provides the major neocortical (see NEOCORTEX) input to the HIPPOCAMPUS. Situated medial to the caudal part of the RHINAL SULCUS, it receives much of its input from the adjacent PERIRHINAL CORTEX and the PARAHIPPOCAMPAL CORTEX, projections from various nuclei of the AMYGDALA, and unimodal input from OLFACTORY CORTEX. Layers II and III (see CORTICAL LAYERS) project to hippocampus and DENTATE GYRUS, while layers IV and V receive projections from area CA1 of the hippocampus and from the subiculum. Often referred to as a 'gateway' to the hippocampal formation, its precise information processing function is unknown. Its importance is highlighted by the observation that it is often the earliest area of the human brain to show pathology in ALZHEIMER'S DEMENTIA.

RICHARD G. M. MORRIS

entrainment Synchronization of a biological rhythm, defined as phase and period control of an endogenously generated biological rhythm by an external cycle. The external cycle is known as a ZEITGEBER (German, 'time giver') and the dominant zeitgeber is the day–night cycle, although some other stimuli are also effective. The use of the term ENTRAINMENT to describe synchronization of daily (CIRCADIAN) RHYTHMS emphasizes that synchrony is not achieved by external cycles directly driving the biological rhythms. Rather, these rhythms are generated endogenously by an autonomous BIOLOGICAL CLOCK, the activity of which is merely synchronized by the external cycle. In the absence of external time cues, circadian rhythms free run (see FREE RUNNING RHYTHM) with periods that differ significantly and idiosyncratically from 24 hours. In the presence of a 24-hour lighting cycle, however, rhythms adopt that periodicity and establish a stable phase relation to the entraining cycle. Phase control is essential: an unstable rhythm expressing a long-term average period of 24 hours, but without adopting a stable phase relation to the lighting cycle, would not meet the definition of entrainment. The conventional model of entrainment depends on the observation that the circadian pacemaker is sensitive to the phase-resetting effects of light at only some phases: light induces delay shifts at one time and advance shifts at another. Entrainment is the result of a daily resetting of the pacemaker by light around dawn and dusk inducing daily advances or delays of the rhythm. The mechanics of this system result in characteristic patterns of entrainment for different combinations of oscillators and zeitgebers. As a rule, a decrease in the period of an oscillator relative to a zeitgeber advances the phase of oscillator entrainment relative to the zeitgeber cycle. Thus, people who entrain spontaneously with early rising and bed times ('larks') can be predicted to have shorter natural free running periods than those who entrain with late rising ('night owls'). Traversing multiple time zones at high speed can lead to transient disruptions of entrainment, experienced as JET LAG. Similarly, the scheduling of work at times incompatible with the typical human pattern of diurnal wakefulness, and the rapid rotation of these shift work schedules, can lead to chronic entrainment disruptions. These are manifest as disorders of SLEEP, waking, digestion and MOOD. Some sleep and biological rhythms disorders occur even in the absence of such stressors. Thus, some visually handicapped people, and others with apparently normal vision, have difficulty entraining normally to day–night cycles.

BENJAMIN RUSAK

entropy In physics, entropy refers to the amount of energy unavailable – energy present but without purpose. It is a measure of disorder in a system. In INFORMATION THEORY, entropy is defined in operational terms as the minimum number of bits of information per symbol required to represent that symbol.

enucleate (from Latin, *e*: from, *nucleus*: a kernel) To enucleate is to remove a NUCLEUS –

in surgery removal of, for example, a BRAIN nucleus, a TUMOUR, or a whole body organ.

enuresis (from Greek, *en*: in, *ouresis*: urination) Inability to inhibit urination; see NOCTURNAL ENURESIS.

enuretic blanket *see* nocturnal enuresis

environmental enrichment A procedure (also called complex rearing) or laboratory environment in which animals are kept in (or given daily experience with) a large complex environment for some period during their lives in which there are additional opportunities to interact with numerous 3-dimensional objects (see SENSORY ENRICHMENT VS. DEAFFERENTATION/DEPRIVATION). While this often happens early in development, some investigators have shown that periods of enrichment also have effects in adult and aged animals (see ISOLATION REARING). While early experiments kept animals in complex environments 24 hours a day, recent findings have shown that 2–3 hours daily enrichment yields virtually all effects of continuous complex rearing and most have adopted the shorter daily exposure. The procedure of regularly changing objects and their locations has a real impact on changes observed, and that also is standard practice.

See also: hypoplasia

Reference

Kemperman G. and Gage F.H. (1999) Experience dependent regulation of adult hippocampal neurogenesis: effects of long-term stimulation and stimulus withdrawal. *Hippocampus* 9:321–332.

RICHARD C. TEES

enzyme A protein that catalyses chemical reactions (typically in the presence of other substances that are necessary for the reaction to occur): see CATALYST. Enzymes are involved in both the synthesis and degradation of chemicals. For example, GLUTAMIC ACID DECARBOXYLASE is an enzyme that catalyses the conversion of glutamate to GABA; ACETYLCHOLINESTERASE is an enzyme involved in the breakdown of acetylcholine.

eosinophil *see* immune system

ependymal cells A layer of cells, also known as the ependyma, lining the inner surface of the ventricles of the brain.

ependymoglial cells These are specialized GLIAL CELLS that are formed from EPENDYMAL CELLS lining the cerebral VENTRICLES. The most commonly encountered in biological psychology are TANYCYTES (important in BLOOD–BRAIN BARRIER function) and MULLER CELLS, specialized glia in the RETINA.

Reference

Kettenmann H. & Ransom B.R. (1995) *Neuroglia*, Oxford University Press: Oxford.

ephaptic transmission Electrical transmission between neurons; see SYNAPSE.

ephedrine A non-selective agonist at NORADRENALINE receptors used in the treatment of asthma and other respiratory disorders. Known to Chinese medicine for over 5000 years – it is derived from the herb *Ephedra vulgaris* – it was in the early nineteenth century a popular medication. A synthetic alternative was developed, AMPHETAMINE. The medical use of amphetamine was very popular for many years until its addictive nature became apparent.

Reference

Feldman R.S., Meyer J.S. & Quenzer L.F. (1997) *Principles of Neuropsychopharmacology*, Sinauer Associates: Sunderland MA.

epibatidine *see* frog skin poison

epidemiology (from Greek, *epi*: among, *demos*: the people) Epidemiology is the study of, strictly speaking, epidemics (which are closely defined in terms of the numbers of individuals affected per head of population). In practice it is used to describe any study into the incidence, prevalence, severity and so forth with which a particular disease or condition appears. For example, it is possible to discuss the epidemiology of a condition such as PARKINSON'S DISEASE without implying in any way that there is an epidemic of this.

epidermal border *see* skin

epidermal growth factor *see* growth factors

epidermis *see* skin

epidural anaesthesia (a word with a made-up modern derivation: partly from Greek, *epi*: among, and partly from Latin *dura mater*: hard mother, the name of part of the MENINGES) Epidural anaesthesia is ANAESTHESIA given to the lowest part of the spinal column. In humans, it is often administered to women during childbirth.

epigenesis (from Greek, *epi*: on or after, *genesis*: formation) Epigenesis is the principle that the DEVELOPMENT of an EMBRYO is a complex and gradual process in which many forces interact and which involves the interaction and organization of many separate parts: embryos are not simply the completed adult form present in miniature. Epigenetics is the study of causal mechanisms in development.

epiglottis *see* mouth

epilepsy A brain disorder characterized by recurrent attacks of altered CONSCIOUSNESS, involuntary motor activity, or disturbed sensory experiences. It occurs sporadically in about 2% of the population but some cases are familial. The most usual form presents first in childhood as bilaterally symmetrical TONIC–CLONIC contractions of the limbs, loss of consciousness and biting of the tongue accompanied by the involuntary passage of urine (see GRAND MAL SEIZURE). However, there are many clinical variants, many different causes, and almost as many attempts at classification. A scheme adopted in 1989 by the International League against Epilepsy defines seizures as Primary (IDIOPATHIC, without known organic cause) or Secondary; and as Generalized (with loss of consciousness) or Partial.

Generalized seizures include infantile spasms, benign neonatal seizures, benign myoclonic seizures, childhood ABSENCE SEIZURES, and the classical convulsive seizures described above. Attacks differ in their clinical and ELECTROENCEPHALOGRAM appearances, the age at which they occur, in prognosis, and with respect to the most effective pharmacotherapy. Some generalized seizures may commence with a brief premonitory sensory AURA, pointing to the presence of an underlying focus; the seizures may also be followed by a POST-ICTAL state marked by HEADACHE, deep SLEEP and MOOD changes. *Partial seizures* are classified according to their site of origin (for example, TEMPORAL LOBE, FRONTAL LOBE, OCCIPITAL LOBE or PARIETAL LOBE), and may occur as simple Jacksonian motor seizures (see JACKSONIAN EPILEPSY), or sensory seizures, or as complex partial seizures – that is, seizures complicated by behavioural AUTOMATISM or mental confusion. Jacksonian seizures commonly point to a focus in the frontal lobes, prominent sensory components suggest a parietal focus, while complex partial seizures, sometimes preceded by an olfactory or gustatory aura, are especially common with temporal lobe (or LIMBIC SYSTEM) foci. Temporal lobe seizures occurring over a period of years are thought by some investigators (but not by others) to be associated with specific alterations in personality, and in some instances to lead to the development of a SCHIZOPHRENIA-like psychosis.

In addition to the above list there is also a ragbag of special conditions, some associated with postinfective or autoimmune ENCEPHALOPATHY, that do not fit easily into any simple scheme. Well-documented case histories have also described seizures elicited specifically and exclusively by music, by computer games, arithmetical tasks, or sexual activity. Isolated epileptiform seizures due to drugs, recent head injury, STROKE, PYREXIA or various metabolic disorders are common but are not, strictly speaking, epilepsy. In STATUS EPILEPTICUS, seizures follow each other in rapid succession without any intervening return of consciousness. Seizures are otherwise terminated probably by an inhibitory neuromodulator such as ADENOSINE ejected by the actively discharging neurons (see NEUROMODULATION).

Various types of *experimental epilepsy* have been evoked in experimental animals by the application of supra-threshold electroconvulsive shock, by KINDLING simulation, by convulsant drugs (such as pentylenetetrazol, pilocarpine, flurothyl), and various GLUTAMATERGIC agonists and GABAERGIC antagonists, or by the intracerebral implantation of long-acting convulsant substances such as tetanus toxin, alumina cream or penicillin. Other methods of eliciting seizures include photic stimulation of predisposed subjects (especially PRIMATES) with stroboscopic lights, and expo-sure to high-frequency sound capable of eliciting audiogenic seizures in susceptible rat strains. Spontaneous recurrent seizures may develop in certain TRANSGENIC or MUTANT mice with genetically abnormal neurotransmission or defective neurotrophins, and in one or two strains of mutant rat.

The causes and pathogenesis of epilepsy are still obscure. Structural changes (aberrant axonal sprouting, possibly leading to the formation of epileptogenic positive feedback circuits) have been detected in the HIPPOCAMPUS of kindled rats, but the significance of these observations is still uncertain. Deficient GABAergic inhibitory tone, or excessive glutamatergic or CHOLINERGIC activity, whether focal or generalized, are obvious possibilities, but are as yet no more than that. Electroencephalographic recordings may serve to corroborate a diagnosis of epilepsy, even during seizure-free intervals, and may sometimes reveal underlying pathology. For example, localized lesions such as tumours may be pinpointed by the presence of an asymmetric focus of slow-wave activity, absence seizures are characterized by distinctive 3-Hz spike-and-wave sequences, while grand mal seizures produce runs of generalized high-voltage spikes. Unfortunately, however, electroencephalographic indications of epilepsy may also be seen in an otherwise completely normal brain. The pharmacological management of epilepsy depends on seizure type. Convulsive seizures respond well to membrane-stabilizing agents (such as CARBAMAZEPINE and PHENYTOIN). These compounds have little effect on pentylenetetrazol seizures in rats but inhibit electroshock-induced seizures, and are believed to act by inhibiting voltage-dependent SODIUM CHANNELS. Absence seizures (PETIT MAL SEIZURE), on the other hand, are best treated with ethosuximide, a compound effective against pentylenetetrazol but not against electroshock-induced seizures, its mechanism of action being quite unknown. Second-line anticonvulsants include various GABAergic agents (for example, valproate, vigabatrin, gabapentin and several BENZODIAZEPINES), some BARBITURATES (for instance PHENOBARBITONE but not PENTOBARBITONE), and some GLUTAMATE antagonists (for example lamotrigine). Temporal lobe seizures tend to be less responsive to pharmacotherapy but are sometimes cured by surgery. Some childhood epilepsies remit spontaneously.

L. JACOB HERBERG

epileptiform Having an appearance like EPILEPSY; typically a description of a SEIZURE or CONVULSIONS, or a related process.

epinephrine Synonymous with ADRENALINE – epinephrine is the term used for this in the United States of America; see NORADRENALINE.

epineurium *see* nerve

epiphenomena (from Greek, *epi*: above) Epiphenomenal events are caused by a system, but exert no causal effects on it – they 'ride above it'. The sound of the heart beating is caused by the heart, but has no causal effects on heart function. Thus the sound is epiphenomenal to the cardiac system. Some dualist (see DUALISM) philosophers hypothesize that mental phenomena are non-physical events that are epiphenomenal relative to the brain. This implies that feelings, desires and so forth cannot influence brain function. Although this view may avoid conflict with the law of conservation of mass-energy, it opens a gap in explaining how decisions yield actions.

PATRICIA S. CHURCHLAND

episodic memory Episodic memory, also called AUTOBIOGRAPHICAL MEMORY is the kind of MEMORY by which individuals can recollect events from their past. Episodic memory has two distinct usages in the psychological literature. First, it refers to autobiographical remembering, to the recollection of an episode that occurred in a particular time and place in the rememberer's past. Second, episodic memory refers to remembering information that was acquired on some particular occasion. For example, one might remember a list of words from an earlier session, or some instructions delivered in an earlier conversation. In this second case, the memory is episodic because the remembered information was presented a single time, not because remembering necessarily re-evokes the circumstances of the learning event itself.

See also: semantic memory

LARRY SQUIRE

episodic vs. semantic amnesia Episodic and semantic amnesia refer to the loss of MEMORY about events and facts, respectively. Events refer to episodes that occurred at a single time and place. Facts refer to accumulated knowledge about the world. When AMNESIA occurs due to brain injury or disease, memory impairment involves both events and facts. There is some loss of memory for events and facts that had been learned about before the onset of amnesia, as well as difficulty learning about new events and facts. Other instances of brain injury, depending on its location, can cause loss of particular kinds of semantic knowledge, for example, aspects of LANGUAGE, the ability to recognize faces (PROSOPAGNOSIA) and the meanings of different kinds of objects (AGNOSIA).

LARRY R. SQUIRE

epithalamus *see* thalamus

epithelial cells A layer of CELLS, also known as the epithelia, lining the outer surface of blood vessels and other tissues.

See also: blood; blood–brain barrier

epitope The portion of an ANTIGEN to which an ANTIBODY binds; see IMMUNE SYSTEM.

EPOR model of sexual excitement A four-stage model of human sexual response proposed by Masters & Johnson in 1966. The model emphasizes a cascade of sexual responses that forms around the build-up and release of sexual excitement: a steep increase in sexual *excitement* (E) during sexual desire and arousal, to a less-steep *plateau* (P) during actual sexual stimulation, to the abrupt release of sexual excitement during *orgasm* (O), and finally to a prolonged period of relaxation known as *resolution* (R). This model applies to the sexual responses of both men and women, although subtle individual differences may exist in the actual response patterns.

See also: orgasm; sexual arousal; sexual behaviour

Reference

Masters, W.H. and Johnson V.E. (1996) *Hu-*

man *Sexual Response*, Little, Brown: Boston, MA.

JAMES G. PFAUS

EPSP/IPSP Abbreviations for excitatory and INHIBITORY POSTSYNAPTIC POTENTIALS respectively. EPSPs hypopolarize a NEURON's membrane and IPSPs hyperpolarize it. Unlike an ACTION POTENTIAL, postsynaptic potentials propagate passively, with the amplitude of the change in voltage dropping sharply as the distance from the SYNAPSE increases. It is thought that the EPSPs, IPSPs and intrinsic oscillatory potentials sum at the AXON HILLOCK to trigger action potentials. Computationally, however, the summing of postsynaptic potentials is not limited to simple excitation and inhibition, as complex non-linear interactions can occur depending on the shape of the neuron's SOMA and dendritic tree (see DENDRITE).

ERIC M. BOWMAN

equilibrium analysis *see* saturation analysis

equilibrium potential *see* Nernst equation

equipotentiality The principle that while sensory input is localized, perception is distributed, involving the entire BRAIN. Theories concerning the LOCALIZATION OF FUNCTION have waxed and waned: in terms of CEREBRAL CORTEX function, it is now accepted that while the posterior cortex contains much that is specific the anterior cortex is less specifically organized. Theories of NEURAL NETWORKS also tend to emphasize the distributed nature of information processing, rather than adopting strict localizationist accounts.

See also: phrenology

equivalence Response equivalence involves making different types of response to achieve an identical goal; it can be considered synonymous with RESPONSE GENERALIZATION. STIMULUS EQUIVALENCE involves a number of stimuli having the ability to elicit a common response; this can be considered synonymous with STIMULUS GENERALIZATION. In vision sciences stimulus equivalence refers to the fact that different sensory impressions can lead to the same perception. We can observe, for example, an object from a variety of different angles and lighting conditions and still recognize it as the same object (*see* METAMERIC MATCH; TRICHROMATIC THEORY OF COLOUR VISION).

erection The filling of the penis or other erectile tissues with blood; also known as TUMESCENCE. Erection typically occurs during periods of SEXUAL AROUSAL, but also occurs involuntarily during REM SLEEP. Erection is driven by activation of the PARASYMPATHETIC NERVOUS SYSTEM, and in particular, by NITRIC OXIDE stimulation of VASOCONSTRICTION. In the penis, blood fills the spongy tissue of the corpora cavernosa and is maintained both by vasoconstriction and contraction of pelvic muscles such as the bulbocavernosus under the base of the penis. Sexual arousal disorders can occur when penile or vaginal blood flow is inhibited by drugs or endogenous factors.

See also: impotence

JAMES G. PFAUS

ergot *see* LSD

ergotamine *see* LSD

ergotism *see* LSD

erotomania The term erotomania describes two conditions: lust in excessive degree; and a belief, typically without foundation, that one is the object of another's strong desire.

errorless discrimination learning *see* errorless learning

errorless learning A form of LEARNING in which subjects are not allowed to make errors, in contrast to learning situations in which subjects engage in trial-and-error procedures, learning from their mistakes. Errorless learning is, at least in certain situations, thought to be more efficient than 'errorful' learning involving trial and error. The first demonstrations were in pigeons, showing what was called errorless discrimination learning. Terrace taught pigeons what is, for them, a difficult discrimination, that between a red key on which they had to peck, and a green key. Pecking on the red key was taught first. Once a good response was established, the key was darkened and presented briefly to the bird while it was not in a position to make effective responses. The key was, over time, gradually changed until it presented as a green key with the same BRIGHTNESS as the red one. Pigeons then allowed access to both keys preferentially pecked the red key. Their ability to make an effective discrimination has been achieved by presentation of the incorrect stimulus, but without allowing pigeons to make a response: they had made no errors in responding. Terrace claimed that pigeons trained in this way displayed less 'emotional' behaviour and learned more efficiently. The technique has been adapted for use with humans, most particularly with children who show MENTAL RETARDATION and with patients in rehabilitation after brain injury. For example, Wilson and her colleagues compared errorless learning with 'errorful' learning in memory impaired individuals using a STEM COMPLETION procedure. In the errorful condition subjects were told that the experimenter was thinking of a five-letter word beginning with (for example) TH. Subjects could make a number of guesses before being told the correct word (THUMB). In the errorless condition subjects were told: 'I am thinking of a five-letter word beginning with TH and the word is THUMB. Please write that down.' Both groups ultimately knew the correct answer: when later challenged to reproduce words that had been learnt, the errorless groups were significantly more successful.

See also: cognitive overlearning; response cost method

References
Terrace H.S. (1963) Discrimination learning with and without 'errors'. *Journal of the Experimental Analysis of Behavior* 6: 1–27.
Wilson B.A., Baddeley A. & Evans J. (1994) Errorless learning in rehabilitation of memory impaired people. *Neuropsychological Rehabilitation* 4: 307–326.

erythrocyte *see* blood

escape *see* aggression; avoidance learning

eserine *see* physostigmine

Eshkol–Wachman notation A movement notation system that permits analysis of behaviour in terms of body parts and their movement. Such notation allows one to de-

scribe the movement itself in abstract terms, rather than describing the movement in terms of its purpose or function. By using a notation scheme such as this psychological terms (such as EXPLORATION) can be dropped in favour of an abstract analytic description of movement.

Reference
Eshkol N. & Wachman A. (1958) *Movement Notation*, Weidenfeld & Nicholson: London.

essential amino acid *see* amino acids

essential fatty acid *see* fatty acids

essential tremor *see* tremor

ester An ESTER is a compound created from ACID and ALCOHOL; an esterase is an ENZYME that degrades an ester. The most important in biological psychology are ACETYLCHOLINESTERASE and BUTYRYLCHOLINESTERASE (also known as pseudocholinesterase.

estradiol *see* estrogens

estrogens (oestrogens) A set of SEX HORMONES including ESTRADIOL and ESTRONE secreted from the ADRENAL GLAND and the OVARIES.

See also: corticosteroids; endocrine glands; estrus; hormones; hormones – classification; menstrual cycle; organization effects of steroid hormones; sex hormones

estrone *see* estrogens

estrous (oestrous) An adjective that pertains to the reproductive cycle of females that display a period of behavioural ESTRUS, as in estrous behaviours, estrous cycles, or estrous secretions. Estrous behaviours are both appetitive responses and consummatory responses that females display during the period of sexual receptivity, usually during the proestrous or estrous phases of the estrous cycle. Estrous secretions are substances found in the vagina, saliva, or as emissions from different glands (for example, the preputial), typically during, but not necessarily limited to, the period of behavioural estrus. Changes in vaginal cell morphology allow the stage of the estrous cycle to be determined.

See also: menstrual cycle; reproduction; sex hormones; sexual behaviour

JAMES G. PFAUS

estrus (oestrus) A noun that defines either the phase of the reproductive ESTROUS cycle during which female sexual behaviour is typically observed, or female sexual behaviour itself, as 'in estrus'. It comes from the Latin word *oestrus*, meaning 'gadfly', and denotes the abrupt change in behaviour when a cycling female goes into HEAT. The estrous cycle is divided into approximately four phases, DIESTRUS, METESTRUS, PROESTRUS, and ESTRUS, each of which correspond to different hormonal and behavioural patterns. For example, in female rodents the estrous cycle is approximately four to five days in length. Dynamic changes in ESTROGEN and PROGESTERONE secretion by the ovaries, and subsequent binding to specific steroid receptors in the brain, are critical for the induction of the cycle and underlie virtually all of the changes in behaviour observed across the cycle. This creates a system in which the behaviour of the female and her neuroendocrine state are tightly linked: her SEXUAL BEHAVIOUR occurs only when she is in an optimal neuroendocrine state to support pregnancy.

The release of FOLLICLE-STIMULATING HORMONE from the PITUITARY GLAND during diestrus signals the growth of the follicle and causes the ovaries to synthesize and secrete 17-b estradiol. As estrogen levels in blood increase progressively during metestrus, estrogen binding in different brain regions (including the PREOPTIC AREA, HYPOTHALAMUS and AMYGDALA) activates intracellular estrogen receptors. Activation of estrogen receptors, in turn, initiates the synthesis of different proteins, such as progesterone receptor, OXYTOCIN receptor, and PREPROENKEPHALIN, and potentiates the release of different neurotransmitters, such as NORADRENALINE. Estrogen activity also promotes the pulsatile release of GONADOTROPHIN-RELEASING HORMONE (GnRH) in the early afternoon of proestrus. GnRH causes the mature follicle to rupture and release the egg, which in turn, transforms the follicle into a corpus luteum, or 'yellow body', which secretes a large amount of progesterone soon

thereafter. Progesterone binds to progestin receptors, most notably in the ventrolateral region of the ventromedial hypothalamus, to facilitate female sexual behaviours. Although estrogen binding in this region potentiates LORDOSIS (the dorsiflexion of the spine consonant with sexual receptivity) activation of progestin receptors in this and other regions (and subsequent protein synthesis induced by such activation) potentiates the full compliment of appetitive and consummatory sexual behaviours in the female, including attractivity, solicitation, proceptivity, and pacing behaviours. Thus, by the evening of proestrus, the female has become sexually excited, aroused, and receptive at a time when the egg she secreted is ready for implantation.

See also: menstrual cycle; reproduction; sex hormones; sexual arousal; sexual differentiation; sexual motivation

JAMES G. PFAUS

ethanol *see* alcohol

ether Highly flammable organic liquid constituting one of the first agents of its kind (*ca.* 1846) capable of inducing general ANAESTHESIA in animals. Virtually never used as an anaesthetic now.

See also: chloroform; dissociative anaesthetics

CHARLES D. BLAHA

ethmoid bone *see* skull

ethology Ethology can be defined only by its approach and not by its content. It was once defined by Tinbergen as 'the objective study of animal behaviour' but this reveals nothing of its nature for the same claim would be made by many other behavioural sciences. Ethology is permanently associated with Konrad Lorenz (1903–1989) and Niko Tinbergen (1907–1988) who, together with Karl von Frisch who first deciphered the dance language of honeybees, shared the 1973 Nobel Prize for Physiology or Medicine. What they achieved during the 1950s and 1960s was the successful re-establishment of behavioural science as a part of biology. The behaviour of animals was to be studied just as any other part of their physical or physiological makeup. In practice this meant that great emphasis was laid on the study of animals in the wild. Both Lorenz and Tinbergen laid great stress on INSTINCT which they regarded as behaviour which had been shaped by NATURAL SELECTION to fit animals to their environment. They saw it as part of a species' inherited characteristics, equivalent to its morphological form.

Given the fact that there was a continuous tradition of field observation and experiment on animal behaviour (for instance by Fabre, Selous, Craig) it may seem hard to justify the attention Lorenz and Tinbergen received. However this is to overlook the atmosphere surrounding animal behaviour studies between the two World Wars. The study of instinct was left to 'amateurs' and largely ignored by biologists. The science of behaviour was totally dominated by American experimental psychology with various behaviourist schools which concentrated almost entirely on LEARNING by rats and pigeons in laboratory settings. So-called 'COMPARATIVE PSYCHOLOGY' had lost its way (see Beach's devastating critique entitled 'The Snark was a Boojum'). Into this rather drab landscape, the ideas of ethology, coming from biologists who were describing the rich panoply of animals in all their diversity, digger-wasps, sticklebacks, jackdaws, geese and ducks, hunting, building nests, fighting and courting in their natural habitats, all came as an intoxicating breath of fresh air. In the 1950s, Lorenz and Tinbergen resumed their collaboration, broken during World War II and rapidly built up school of students, mostly from zoological backgrounds. Much of their early work took a group of related species, gulls, ducks, and worked out in considerable detail the evolution of display behaviour from an ancestral type. It also pioneered the modern study of how displays function as an intra-specific communication system. The key texts setting out the early foundations of ethology are Lorenz's *King Solomon's Ring* (English translation, 1952) – a popular book, but shot through with brilliant insights – and Tinbergen's *The Study of Instinct* (1951).

Concentrating almost entirely upon instinctive behaviour, early ethological theory was rather tightly drawn. Animals inherited hard-wired instinctive systems whereby a series of behaviour patterns, very stereotyped (see STEREOTYPY) in form (aggressive postures, feeding patterns and courtship displays for example) were elicited when the combination of internal and external factors was adequate. The internal factors (see DRIVE) fluctuated with needs (for food, water, warmth and so on) or with levels of HORMONES, as for reproductive behaviour (see REPRODUCTION). The external factors, from the environment or from other animals, were often to be resolved down to particular elements, 'key stimuli' or 'sign stimuli' to which the animal showed inherent responsiveness. A courting male stickleback responds only to the swollen belly of the gravid female; a male robin responds strongly to a tuft of red feathers (key stimulus from a territorial rival) but ignores a whole stuffed robin which lacks any red. Both Lorenz and Tinbergen developed models incorporating interactions between internal and external factors. In particular they tried to explain fluctuating thresholds of response and the results of blocking certain channels of response such that, given high levels of MOTIVATION, thwarted animals sometimes perform apparently irrelevant behaviour – so-called displacement behaviours. Lorenz's model, which became affectionately known as 'PSYCHOHYDRAULICS', used the metaphor of water tanks filling with 'action-specific energy' whose discharge, as instinctive behaviour patterns, was regulated by a spring-loaded value activated by weights – sign stimuli.

Ethology's theoretical framework attracts little attention now, but the influence of its approach has totally pervaded behavioural science. It is now accepted that whatever level of organisation is under scrutiny, explanation is incomplete without knowledge of its place in the life history of the animal subject. In a classic paper Tinbergen (1963) set out four interrelated aims for ethology: to study the function, evolution, causation and development of the behaviour we are studying. These aims have proved as important for psychologists involved in the study of learning or higher cognitive abilities as for zoologists working in the field on the ecological constraints on SOCIAL BEHAVIOUR. The old boundaries between ethology, psychology and physiology have largely broken down as a result. Learning and instinct are no longer seen as alternatives; now we investigate how genetic and environmental influences operate in the development and evolution of all behaviour.

References

Beach F.A. (1950) The Snark was a Boojum. *American Psychologist* 5: 115–124.

Tinbergen N. (1951) *The Study of Instinct*, Oxford University Press: Oxford.

—— (1963) On aims and methods of ethology. *Zeitschrift für Tierpsychologie* 20: 410-433.

AUBREY W. G. MANNING

eukaryote A eukaryote is a CELL in which there is a NUCLEUS present; a prokaryote has no nucleus present. In eukaryotic cells the genetic material is contained in the cell nucleus; in prokaryotic cells it is free in the cytoplasm. Bacteria are prokaryotes; the cells of multicellular organisms are eukaryotic, having DNA packaged into CHROMOSOMES within the cell nucleus.

euphoria A subjective or emotional state of extreme well-being, elation, or positive EMOTION. Although the term can be used to describe any strongly positive natural emotion, in psychiatry it is often used to described the 'high' or rewarding feelings induced by certain drugs of abuse (see DRUG ABUSE). For example, users of STIMULANTS and OPIATES often describe an intense positive feeling or 'rush' following administration of the drug. The term is also used to describe certain features of MOOD disorder, particularly the manic phase of manic-depressive disorder.

See also: dysphoria

ANN E. KELLEY

Eustachian tube *see* ear

euthanization A term (derived from 'euthanasia') used to describe the humane killing of experimental animals.

See also: humane killing

eutherian mammal *see* mammals

euthymic mood Euthymia – euthymic mood – is a tranquil state of 'peace of mind'; contrast this to DYSTHYMIC DISORDER and CYCLOTHYMIC DISORDER.

See also: euphoria; dysphoria

event memory Event memory represents the ability to recall specific events. It is regarded as a form of EPISODIC MEMORY (see MULTIPLE MEMORY SYSTEMS) and its loss is a cardinal feature of TEMPORAL LOBE AMNESIA.

event-related potentials (ERP) Event-related potentials are variations in the voltage of the scalp-recorded ELECTROENCEPHALOGRAM (EEG) time-locked to a discrete event such as the onset of a stimulus or a movement. Because the voltage variations comprising an ERP are very small in relation to other aspects of EEG activity, it is customary to enhance the SIGNAL-TO-NOISE RATIO of ERP waveforms by averaging samples of EEG obtained on multiple (typically, 20–50) experimental trials. ERP waveforms represent the summation of a series of spatially and temporally overlapping components, which arise from the different brain regions activated in response to the event. ERPs are widely employed in the study of sensory, motor and cognitive processing in humans.

Reference

Rugg M.D. & Coles M.G.H. (1995) *The Electrophysiology of Mind*, Oxford University Press: Oxford.

MICHAEL D. RUGG

evoked potentials Evoked potentials is a synonym for EVENT-RELATED POTENTIALS. The term is nowadays largely restricted to brain activity associated with sensory, rather than cognitive or motor, processing.

MICHAEL D. RUGG

evolution In the eighteenth century, when Carolus Linnaeus (1707–1778) systematized the living things into a single classification, he did not question that all living things were individually created by God, to whom he dedicated his work. However, dissatisfaction with this belief – creationism – gradually emerged, and by the mid-nineteenth century there was considerable belief among scientists that species could change or 'evolve' into new ones: evolution. What was missing was a workable hypothesis of how this could take place, a plausible mechanism to produce new organisms that appeared beautifully designed for the lives they led. This need was finally supplied jointly by Darwin and Wallace, the process of adaptation by NATURAL SELECTION; however, not all evolutionary change is adaptive and there is some controversy as to the extent of more neutral mechanisms of change.

Unusually for a scientific theory, there is little alternative to accepting evolution, save for adherence to the doctrine of creationism. The existence of fossil remains of creatures which no longer exist was influential in gaining original acceptance for evolution, but these can also be reconciled with creationism, in two ways. The entire fossil record might have been devised by God as a test of faith. Or, more plausibly, there might have been more than one episode of creation, and extant species reflect only the last of these while fossils give information on previous, imperfect creations. (This account was put forward by the famous French zoologist Cuvier in the eighteenth century.) The pattern in the fossil record, of a series of massive extinction events, gives an impression of empirical support for this view. However, closer examination of post-extinction rock shows some surviving forms after each event, which then radiate out and fill all the vacant ECOLOGICAL NICHES with new species, and change in species also occurs between extinction events.

The strongest reason for treating the theory of evolution as accepted fact, however, is the understanding it gives of the variation among living forms. As Linnaeus discovered, living things are best organized by grouping similar species together, then grouping similar groups – hierarchically – to form ultimately a single, branched tree. This tree structure efficiently describes much of the co-variance in form among living species. Just such a pattern is a prediction of the theory of evolution, since the species most recently diverged from common ancestry will share most features by common descent. Thus a TAXONOMY, rather than in some way reflecting the thought processes of the Creator, as Linnaeus believed, can give a (partial) record of evolutionary history. Each grouping (TAXON), is evidence of an extinct species, ancestral to all the species in the taxon. Evolution can also cause convergence of un-

related species towards similar appearance. This occurs when the form is strongly dictated as a solution to an environmental problem, such as wings for flying. For this reason, it is important to use features unlikely to have evolved more than once, when deriving an appropriate 'evolutionary' or 'phylogenetic' taxonomy. In general, this amounts to preferring for classification the use of complex features, like the vertebral column, rather than simple ones, like green coloration. Molecular structure is normally used now for this purpose, as much of the GENOME appears not to be under active selection and is thus somewhat immune from convergence. In addition, it is important to avoid the error of grouping species by shared possession of primitive features (retained from earlier ancestry), and to use only derived features (evolved in the single ancestor of the taxon) for classification. Taxonomy has not always avoided these pitfalls. The archaic term 'pachyderm' was coined to group 'thick-skinned' animals like rhinoceros and hippopotamus, animals now realized to have converged towards superficially similar appearance. Much more recently, it was realized that the pongid taxon (non-human great apes) was also invalid, since it is based on shared retention of a small brain and various other primitive features. A valid group for phylogenetic analysis, such as the hominoid taxon (great apes including humans), is called a CLADE; the method used is thus often called cladistics. Using a cladistic taxonomy of a group of modern species, the past history of extinct ancestral species can be derived (one per node, in the tree diagram), some of their characteristics can be inferred (those shared by most modern descendants), and the date at which they lived can be estimated (from the amount of subsequent divergence in the structure of their genomes).

RICHARD W. BYRNE

evolutionary psychology For most biological topics (such as anatomy, ecology, genetics, ethology and so on) evolutionary aspects have long been studied and the meaning of the qualifier 'evolutionary' is obvious and uncontroversial. Strangely, this has not been true for psychology, as if psychology were somehow not a part of biology and the brain not a product of EVOLUTION. Partly, this difference reflects the small influence of what little evolutionary study took place within psychology, traditionally termed COMPARATIVE PSYCHOLOGY and handicapped by its laboratory focus, limiting the range of species available for comparison. But in addition it reflects a belief, still current in some branches of the subject, that psychological processes of significance are essentially cultural things, entirely dependent on LANGUAGE and therefore not comparable in any sensible way with animal behaviour. The human brain, on this account, is so flexible that it exerts little constraint on behaviour, which is instead a product of upbringing, society and culture. (Psychologists studying PERCEPTION took an opposite view, to their evident advantage, assuming that perceptual systems would be tightly channelled by genetic constraints and basically similar in related species.)

In recent years, this dogma has become increasingly questioned, and the label evolutionary psychology is both a description of a rapidly developing subject and a banner-headline challenging the orthodoxy of the social sciences (see SOCIOBIOLOGY, which shares both stance and some researchers). Evolutionary psychology contains two complementary methods of study, which address the origins of human traits of different antiquity. ('Trait' is used here in the sense of any behavioural tendency.) Researchers in both schools, however, share a conviction that most psychological processes are strongly affected by a legacy of evolutionary history. Rather than an infinitely flexible product of culture, human behaviour is a product of adaptations for survival by fitness maximization (see NATURAL SELECTION). To understand the origin and nature of evolutionarily 'old' traits, evolutionary psychologists use the comparative method, particularly concentrating on our closest relatives, the PRIMATES. In contrast to the few species studied in laboratories by comparative psychologists, evolutionary psychologists compare a wide range of species living under naturally adaptive conditions. Using a phylogenetic taxonomy (see EVOLUTION), and behavioural data from modern species, behaviour can be reconstructed for a series of ancestral species in the human lineage. On this reconstruction, our shared ancestors with monkeys at 40 million years BP (before the present) already lived in permanent social groups. To reduce the inevitable resource competition this created, they used social manipulation, deception and co-operation, abilities underwritten by a brain twice as large as that of a typical mammal. By 8 million years BP, our shared ancestors with African great apes lived in patrilineal groups, showing stepfather infanticide and homicidal male AGGRESSION towards males of unrelated groups, and probably had some understanding of the intentions of other individuals, and an ability to think non-verbally. These conclusions can be challenged, but they are based on analysis not speculation. To understand human attributes that evolved in the 5 million years since the last shared ancestor with a living ape, a different approach is necessary. Here, evolutionary psychologists use genetical theory to predict which behavioural traits would be adaptive, and then examine modern human behaviour to test these predictions quantitatively (the broad outline of modern behaviour is, of course, often well known in advance). Rapid cultural change since the Neolithic revolution, and especially in industrial societies, means that in many cases observed characteristics will be adaptations to past environments. Some practitioners even assert that all uniquely human behavioural traits are adapted to Palaeolithic hunter–gathering existence, unaffected by modern conditions. This seems unlikely in the face of the inexorability of evolution and the potential for strong selection pressures in elaborate societies (for instance, the genetical impact of polygamy). In addition to insights into human-specific behaviour (for example, the marriage choices of men and women at different ages, universals of sexual attractiveness, pregnancy sickness, female circumcision) quantitative analysis of modern human data has been used to test predictions from the comparative method (for instance, in homicide and risk-taking behaviour by young men, stepfather infanticide, female transfer between groups after puberty).

RICHARD W. BYRNE

evolutionary stable strategy An evolutionary stable strategy is one that cannot be improved upon (provided sufficient individual organisms adopt it). The presence of any mutant GENE will not generate an improvement on this strategy.

ex vivo From the Latin – literally, from life.

excitation Excitation refers to the stimulation of an ACTION POTENTIAL: it is a colloquial way of referring to DEPOLARIZATION and the generation of EXCITATORY POSTSYNAPTIC POTENTIALS (EPSP). INHIBITION refers to the suppression of action potential generation: it is a colloquial way of referring to HYPERPOLARIZATION and the creation of INHIBITORY POSTSYNAPTIC POTENTIALS (IPSP).

excitatory amino acid receptors The two principal EXCITATORY AMINO ACID transmitters are GLUTAMIC ACID and ASPARTIC ACID (glutamate and aspartate – see DRUG IONIZATION) with glutamate being by far the more prominent. The terms excitatory amino acid receptors can be taken as being synonymous with GLUTAMATE RECEPTORS.

excitatory amino acids *see* amino acid neurotransmitters

excitatory postsynaptic potential (EPSP) A DEPOLARIZATION of a NEURON due to input at a SYNAPSE from an excitatory neurotransmitter (see NEUROTRANSMITTERS). EPSPs are local potentials that decay with distance and can summate with other EPSPs and IPSPs that are occurring in the same cell (SPATIAL SUMMATION). They have a slow time course, relative to that of an ACTION POTENTIAL, and therefore show TEMPORAL SUMMATION when repeated inputs occur across the same synapse. Specialized EPSPs, such as at the NEUROMUSCULAR JUNCTION, can be large enough to always lead to an action potential, but in the CENTRAL NERVOUS SYSTEM virtually all EPSPs are too small to reach THRESHOLD without summation.

DOUGLAS D. RASMUSSON

excitotoxic lesion *see* excitotoxins; lesion

excitotoxins Structural analogues of glutamate, which are neurotoxic (see NEUROTOXINS)

when injected into the CENTRAL NERVOUS SYSTEM in appropriate concentrations. They include AMPA, DOMOIC ACID, IBOTENIC ACID, KAINIC ACID, N-methyl-D-aspartate (NMDA), QUINOLINIC ACID and QUISQUALIC ACID – all of which are naturally acidic, but must be titrated to a pH of approximately 7, by adding concentrated sodium hydroxide, an alkali, before they are suitable for injection into the central nervous system. Excitotoxins bind to GLUTAMATE RECEPTORS on neuronal dendrites and excite the neurons to death. Typical histological evidence (see HISTOLOGY) of excitotoxic action includes intense REACTIVE GLIOSIS and neuronal loss in the region of the injection, as seen in sections stained with cresyl violet, and in some cases large calcium deposits around the edges of the lesion, identified with the stain Alizarin red. When excitotoxins were first discovered, they were unique lesion-making tools, because of their ability to make FIBRE-SPARING LESIONS. Other, cruder, lesion-making methodologies included ASPIRATION LESIONS, ELECTROLYTIC LESIONS, KNIFE CUT LESIONS and RADIOFREQUENCY LESIONS.

Kainic acid, AMPA and NMDA have their greatest effects at these particular IONOTROPIC receptors; quinolinic acid has part of its action through NMDA receptors; ibotenic acid activates both NMDA and METABOTROPIC receptors. The exact mechanisms which lead to neuronal death differ according to which receptor is involved. Action of excitotoxins at NMDA receptors leads to massive influx of calcium ions and over-excitation of the neuron; activation at AMPA/kainate receptors involves influx sodium ions; metabotropic receptors initiate second messenger systems such as the INOSITOL phosphate pathway. In all instances, the neurotoxic process itself is relatively fast, and is complete in less than 24 hours. During this period, the animal usually shows signs of SEIZURE activity. In some instances, typically following kainate infusions, evidence has been found of lesions at sites distant from the infusion. The HIPPOCAMPUS is most susceptible to such damage, leading to the hypothesis that it occurs as a result of ANOXIA during seizure activity. Pretreatment with a BENZODIAZEPINE such as DIAZEPAM is an effective means of dampening seizures and reducing the risk of remote damage, without decreasing the excito-toxic action at the site of interest.

Although excitotoxins can make fibre-sparing lesions in the central nervous system, careful histological analyses at different stages post-lesion have shown that the inflammatory response (reactive gliosis) which is part of the excitotoxic process actually leads to breakdown of the BLOOD–BRAIN BARRIER in the injected region. This can result in loss of MYELIN sheaths in lesioned areas which contain diffuse fibre systems. Although initiation of remyelination can be seen after 2–3 weeks, this side-effect has clear implications for studies which involve behavioural testing following an excitotoxic lesion. The size of an excitotoxic lesion is governed by many factors, such as the volume of the infusion, the concentration of the excitotoxic agent and TISSUE TORTUOSITY / receptor profile in the targeted region. Factors specific to a particular excitotoxin may also come into play. For instance, ibotenic acid undergoes enzyme-catalysed decarboxylation to MUSCIMOL *in vivo*, which may act at GABA RECEPTORS to dampen the sensitivity of local neurons to further excitation. This is likely to be the reason why, at well-titrated doses, ibotenate can be used to make small, well-defined lesions. In some instances, ANAESTHETICS such as SODIUM PENTOBARBITONE or CHLORAL HYDRATE, can modify the neurotoxicity of excitotoxins. This is also thought to be related to their action at GABA-A receptors.

An excitotoxin is most effective when neurons of interest in a given region are more susceptible to its toxic effects than others, thereby inducing a relatively selective lesion. Generally, the pattern of damage caused by different excitotoxins is related to the types of glutamate receptors found in the target area, and perhaps even the specific RECEPTOR SUBUNITS which form these receptors. A good example of this is the use of AMPA in the rat BASAL FOREBRAIN, where it can be used to target CHOLINERGIC neurons, if the concentration and volume are titrated correctly. Histochemical and lesion data suggest that this is linked to the high expression of the GluR4 receptor subunit in AMPA receptors in this area. Unfortunately, excitotoxins are never generally more than partially selective neurotoxic agents, and any selectivity which is obtained is critically dependent on the concentration of the infusion. The more recent immunotoxin approach, which uses ribosome-inactivating proteins such as SAPORIN, conjugated to specific receptor antibodies, is a more selective means of making brain lesions.

See also: gliotoxins

WENDY L. INGLIS

executive functions Executive functions are a rather loosely defined set of cognitive functions. The term derives from the CENTRAL EXECUTIVE, a process at the centre of the model of WORKING MEMORY presented and developed by Alan Baddeley and his colleagues. In a lucid discussion of executive functions, Roberts *et al.* (1998, p. 221) identify them as involving 'the optimal scheduling of operation of different components of complex tasks that depend on more dedicated or modular mechanisms (generally mediated by posterior cortical structures). This collection of operations [incorporates] supervisory functions, including for example appropriate inhibitory mechanisms (for example, for selective attention and switching between two or more tasks) and also the monitoring of processes such as retrieval from long term memory and also of performance of intended actions.' There is a degree of consensus in the literature that the term executive function covers processes such as these. There are three debates about it though: first, to what extent is executive function a monolithic construct? Are the separate components in fact independent, and if they are, to what extent can the term executive function be considered valuable? There is a dangerous trend in the literature to use the term rather indiscriminately, which restricts its value considerably. As with the term LIMBIC SYSTEM in NEUROANATOMY, indiscriminate and unspecified usage may debase the concept of executive function to a point where it has no useful meaning at all. Second, are executive functions localizable with the CENTRAL NERVOUS SYSTEM? In many cases executive function appears to be used as a term to describe the functions of the PREFRONTAL CORTEX, but this is a tendency that should be avoided. So, for example, the term

DYSEXECUTIVE SYNDROME has been applied to a condition in which executive functions are impaired following brain damage of one sort or another. Patients with FRONTAL LOBE damage do show dysexecutive syndrome, but it is equally clear that not all patients with frontal damage show it and, moreover, patients with damage outside the frontal lobes can show dysexecutive syndrome. A unique association between the prefrontal cortex and executive functions appears very unlikely.

The third point of discussion concerns two things: the dissociation of executive and non-executive functions and the relationships between executive functions and constructs such as will (see WILLED ACTION) and CONSCIOUSNESS. Both psychologists and philosophers have become embroiled in a debate about the nature of these functions. Rabbitt (1997) identifies the fact that executive functions have much to do with 'novel tasks that require us to formulate a goal, to plan, and to choose between alternative sequences of behaviour to reach this goal, to compare these plans in respect of their relative probabilities of success and their relative efficiency in attaining the chosen goal, to initiate the plan selected and to carry it through, amending it as necessary, until it is successful or until impending failure is recognized' (p3). But Rabbitt notes that complex sequences of actions can be carried out automatically, without obvious 'conscious' control. What distinguishes executive function from non-executive is the degree to which behaviour is controlled automatically. This executive functions appear to relate to conditions in which strategic planning; the initiation of novel behavioural sequences; the active suppression of inappropriate behaviour; allocation of processing resources to more than one task; 'on line' monitoring of performance; and SUSTAINED ATTENTION are all required. Rabbitt distinguishes such processes from automatic functions. These are driven by environmental contingencies and can be thought of as being much the same as HABITS or motor programmes (see MOTOR PROGRAMMING). It is thus conceivable that what starts as an executive function could through repetition become an automatic sequence. The important point to note though is that it is not task complexity

per se that discriminates executive function from non-executive, but such things as novelty and strategic planning. Whether this implies that executive function must be conscious is not clear: some authors imply that there must be a degree of conscious control involved in executive function while others do not. This is a particularly interesting point when considering whether animals other than humans use executive functions. It can be argued, for example, that a laboratory rat, negotiating a complex task such as a RADIAL ARM MAZE for the first time, is in a novel situation and must develop plans and strategies appropriate to its test environment. In humans such processes would be classified as executive, and it is difficult to see why they should not be classified in the same way in a rodent: but are rats and humans conscious in the same way?

See also: supervisory attentional system

References

Rabbitt P. (1997) *Methodology of Frontal and Executive Function*, Psychology Press: Hove UK.
Roberts A.C., Robbins T.W. & Weiskrantz L. (1998) *The Prefrontal Cortex: Executive and Cognitive Functions*, Oxford University Press: Oxford.

exocrine glands (from Greek, *exo*: outside, *krinein*: to separate) The exocrine glands are the so-called duct glands, in contrast to the ductless glands – the ENDOCRINE GLANDS. The best known examples of exocrine glands are the salivary glands.

exocytosis The release of a MOLECULE from within a CELL, involving the fusion of VESICLES with the cell MEMBRANE and expulsion of the vesicle contents into the EXTRACELLULAR space.

See also: endocytosis

exogenous *see* endogenous

exogenous depression *see* endogenous depression

exogenous rhythm Synonymous with ZEITGEBER.

See also: biological clock; endogenous rhythm

exon/intron Regions of GENES involved in the coding and transcription of MESSENGER RNA (mRNA). Exons are regions of genes which code directly for the sequence of AMINO ACIDS in PROTEINS, while introns are large non-coding loops which will be spliced out of mRNA prior to translation into proteins. Introns contain instructional information for their deletion, and what are considered to be long 'junk' sequences, of no obvious function.

FIONA M. INGLIS

expectancy based memory Expectancy based memory is a system that encodes permanent memory representations. It allows for automatic attention (see AUTOMATIC VS. CONTROLLED ATTENTION), IMPLICIT MEMORY activation, elicitation of rules and strategies, and behavioral anticipation. The expectancy or KNOWLEDGE BASED MEMORY system often works in conjunction with the DATA BASED MEMORY system, although these are independent of one another. The system organizes its memories according to their space, time, sensory-perception, response, LANGUAGE, and AFFECT attributes. Interactions between these attributes form scripts, SCHEMA, MOOD and skills.

See also: long-term memory; reference memory; semantic memory

HOWARD EICHENBAUM

experimental design The thoughtful process of planning procedures to determine the causal relationship between two or more variables. The term is also used to refer to an abstract description of the procedures (the experimental variables and the methods by which other variables are controlled) in a scientific study. Several considerations are necessary for good experimental design. Experiments are defined by a set of variables which are manipulated (independent variables) and a set of variables which are measured (dependent variables). Statistical analysis and experimental design should be considered together: a good design is one in which the data (that is to say, the measurement of the dependent variable) can be organized into statistically meaningful results from which the probability of obtaining any observed changes in the dependent variable by chance can be determined. The experimenter will use statistical analysis to assign a prob-ability of the results occurring by chance: if this probability is less than 5% ($p < 0.05$), the result is generally regarded as statistically significant, that is to say that the result is considered as unlikely to have occurred by chance and therefore must be due to the experimental manipulation of the independent variable. Poor experimental design will often result in confounds in the data. For example, it is necessary that, when manipulating one variable, the effects of other variables, not of interest to the experiment, are not unwittingly measured or allowed to affect the result. A Type I error is the erroneous acceptance of the hypothesis that it was the manipulation of the independent variable which influenced the dependent variable. Good experimental design excludes the effects of confounding variables which can cause ambiguity in drawing conclusions regarding the causal relationship between the independent variable and the dependent variable, thereby reducing the likelihood of a Type I error. It is also necessary to avoid a Type II error, which is when the hypothesis is erroneously rejected. Type II errors are most common when the experiment has insufficient power (for example, due to insufficient numbers of observations) or when the manipulation of the independent variable was ineffective. Good design might include another measure to determine the efficacy of the manipulation of the independent variable. Experiments can be distinguished from quasi-experiments, in which all subjects undergo the same procedure but the dependent variable is analysed in terms of different types of subjects. The design of quasi-experiments is less subject to experimenter control, as they do not have experimental manipulations but rather are based on the determination of correlation between observations.

ERIC M. BOWMAN

expert systems *see* artificial intelligence

explant The process of explantation is the growth *in vitro* of tissue taken from an organism; an explant is the term given to what is grown.

See also: tissue culture

explicit memory Form of MEMORY that involves CONSCIOUS RECOLLECTION of prior experiences. It is contrasted with IMPLICIT MEMORY, a non-conscious form of memory. Although the term 'explicit memory' is frequently used synonymously with DECLARATIVE MEMORY, the two terms differ in that the former describes a specific way in which humans can express memory for prior experiences without necessarily implying a distinct underlying memory system in the brain (see MULTIPLE MEMORY SYSTEMS). The term is often used operationally to refer to the class of memory tasks (explicit memory tests) that require conscious recollection of prior experiences, such as FREE RECALL or RECOGNITION.

See also: consciousness; episodic memory

STEFAN KÖHLER

exploration Behaviour that brings an organism into contact with its environment, through which it learns information about the environment. Exploration is a basic instinctive behaviour (see INSTINCT) of many animal species. It is highly adaptive because it provides the organism with information concerning availability of food or other reinforcers, sexual partners, danger, safety, spatial and contextual relationships in the environment. Novelty is a potent stimulus for eliciting exploration. The study of exploratory behaviour has a long history in biological psychology. In 1927, I.P. Pavlov (1849–1936) wrote about the 'investigative reflex'. He wrote that this REFLEX was characterized by the orientation of the appropriate receptor organ towards an external stimulus, bringing about its investigation. Many early theorists considered what factors influenced exploratory behaviour, particularly with regard to approach–avoidance behaviour. It has long been recognized that while novelty stimulates exploration, it can also elicit fear and avoidance. The complexity of these factors makes the study of exploration problematic, particularly with regard to drug effects on exploration.

In the 1950s, several important theoretical developments influenced notions about exploration. DRIVE theory was an important concept at the time, emphasizing that internal drive states, such as HUNGER or THIRST, were the major determinants of behavioural responses. However, many experiments showed that animals would engage in behaviours not associated with any obvious internal drive state, such as SPONTANEOUS ALTERNATION. When given a choice between two arms of a T-MAZE to explore, animals perform non-randomly, consistently alternating between the arms. Animals would learn tasks in order to obtain rewards that did not appear to reduce physiological needs. These phenomena led to the postulate of an exploratory drive (see Montgomery, 1954; Berlyne, 1955). Many other theoretical constructs have influence how psychologists conceptualize exploration, including INCENTIVE MOTIVATION, AROUSAL, and novelty-seeking.

The study of exploratory behaviour and LOCOMOTION in rodents has been an important animal model in PSYCHOPHARMACOLOGY and biological psychology. The brain circuits and NEUROTRANSMITTERS that mediate these behaviours are affected by many classes of PSYCHOACTIVE drugs, such as STIMULANTS, OPIATES, NEUROLEPTICS, and BENZODIAZEPINES. When measuring exploration careful attention must be paid to dissociating true exploratory tendencies from alterations in general motor behaviour. It is generally agreed that the most rigorous way to measure exploration is to use a technique that measures the animal's preference for novelty.

References

Berlyne D.E. (1955) The arousal and satiation of perceptual curiosity in the rat. *Journal of Comparative and Physiological Psychology* 48: 238–246.

Montgomery K.C. (1954) The role of exploratory drive in learning. *Journal of Comparative and Physiological Psychology* 47: 60–64.

ANN E. KELLEY

explosive motor behaviour A form of defence, explosive motor behaviour in rodents involves the immediate production of running at speed away from a stimulus. It is seen after stimulation in the SUPERIOR COLLICULUS and associated structures in the MIDBRAIN, PONS and RETICULAR FORMATION.

expressed emotion Expressed emotion is thought to be one factor in determining the appearance of the SIGNS AND SYMPTOMS of SCHIZOPHRENIA. Research has indicated that the degree of expressed emotion within a family affects the likelihood of relapse in patients who have been discharged to their homes. High expressed emotion (for example, the expression of hostility towards the patient, or emotional over-involvement with the patient) is much more likely to lead to relapse than low expressed emotion. However, the relationships between relapse and expressed emotion remain obscure: do patients' signs and symptoms trigger high levels of expressed emotion or does high expressed emotion trigger them? The role of expressed emotion in generating *de novo* the signs and symptoms of schizophrenia is also unclear.

Reference

Leff J., Kuipers L., Berkowitz R., Vaughn C. & Sturgeon D. (1983) Life events, relatives expressed emotion and maintenance neuroleptics in schizophrenic relapse. *Psychological Medicine* 13: 799–806.

expressive aphasia *see* Broca's aphasia

extended amygdala It has long been known that the centromedial AMYGDALA forms a continuum with the BED NUCLEUS OF THE STRIA TERMINALIS through cell columns distributed along the C-shaped arc of the STRIA TERMINALIS itself. More recently, it has been demonstrated on histochemical and cytoarchitectonic grounds that there is an additional ventral component of this continuum which connects the centromedial amygdala and bed nucleus of the stria terminalis. These cell columns traverse the so-called substantia innominata in the BASAL FOREBRAIN, running between the TEMPORAL LOBE and bed nucleus. Thus, the extension of the centromedial amygdala both alongside the stria terminalis and through the more ventral cell columns in the substantia innominata has been called the 'extended amygdala'. More controversial is the suggestion that this continuum also extends within the shell region of the NUCLEUS ACCUMBENS, the latter being a mixture of striatal and extended amygdala neurons.

See also: cytoarchitecture; histo-chemistry; striatum

BARRY J. EVERITT

extended phenotype Phenotype is an expression of the GENOTYPE and, over time, affects the genotype: certain traits are selected for because they fit an animal better for its environment. But some of the factors that affect the differential survival of a SPECIES are not direct parts of the phenotype – that is, they are not to do with an animal's actual body. For example, a well-constructed nest will help a bird survive. As such the nest can be considered as part of that birds phenotype. Another example, from plant biology, is of a certain type of fungus that grows on ants. The ants pick up the spores, the spores develop in the ant, destroying its nervous system in the process, but of course, while this is going on, the fungus is being effectively distributed around the forest in which it lives. The ant is essential to the fungus: it is in effect part of the fungus' phenotype. EXTENDED PHENOTYPE is a term that allows one to consider more than just the physical characteristics of an animal when attempting to describe how successful phenotypes come to impact the development of a species' gene pool (see GENE).

Reference

Dawkins R. (1982) *The Extended Phenotype*, Oxford University Press: Oxford.

extensor muscles *see* muscles

extensor phase *see* locomotion

external capsule The EXTERNAL CAPSULE, EXTREME CAPSULE and INTERNAL CAPSULE are all fibre pathways that connect the CEREBRAL CORTEX with subcortical structures. The internal capsule is the best known. It can be divided into the anterior limb, genu (the middle portion, which has a bend – *genu* is Latin for knee) and the posterior limb. It carries almost all connections between the THALAMUS and both the STRIATUM and cortex, as well as fibres running from the cortex to the MIDBRAIN and BRAINSTEM. Ascending fibres in the DORSAL COLUMN – MEDIAL LEMNISCAL SYSTEM carrying information from the body travel to the cortex via the internal capsule. The external and extreme capsules also carry information between the cortex and subcortical sites. The three capsules are named by their positions. The internal capsule in the human brain runs between the CAUDATE NUCLEUS and PUTAMEN, closer to the MIDLINE of the brain than either the external or extreme capsules. The external capsule runs on the outside of the putamen, but below the CLAUSTRUM, The extreme capsule lies over the claustrum, immediately below the cortex – it is the most extremely lateral of the capsules.

See also: basal ganglia

Reference

Grossman S.P. (1967) *A Textbook of Physiological Psychology*, Wiley: New York.

external segment of the globus pallidus *see* globus pallidus

externality Degree of influence from salient external (outside the skin) cues to initiate, maintain or terminate behaviour, such as eating; the opposite of INTERNALITY. Initially considered to be responsible for excessive eating found in OBESITY. Early experiments on externality demonstrated a higher level of food intake when external cues were manipulated such as time of day, taste, availability of foods, work necessary to obtain food and proximity of food. The level of externality may be inferred using the external eating sub-scale of the Dutch Eating Behaviour Questionnaire.

Reference

Van Strien T., Frijters J.E.R., Bergers G.P.A. & Defares P.B. (1986) The Dutch Eating Behaviour Questionnaire (DEBQ) for assessment of restrained, emotional and external eating. *International Journal of Eating Disorders* 5: 295–315.

MARION M. HETHERINGTON

exteroceptive *see* interoceptive

extinction (i) *Sensorimotor*: A deficit of visual, auditory or tactile perception most commonly resulting from lateralized parieto-occipital damage. Stimulation presented CONTRALATERAL to the lesioned HEMISPHERE is perceived in isolation, but is not perceived (that is, it is extinguished) when stimulation is presented concurrently IPSILATERAL to the lesioned hemisphere. The same phenomenon has also been referred to as 'INATTENTION', emphasizing the putative role of awareness and ATTENTION in the disorder. Extinction is often classified as part of the neglect syndrome. However, reported cases of neglect without extinction and *vice versa* suggest separable bases for these deficits. See also SIMULTANEOUS EXTINCTION

(ii) *Learning*: Animals are said to be 'responding in extinction' when they continue to respond (for example by lever pressing) for a REINFORCER after it has been discontinued. The response will itself eventually EXTINGUISH.

(iii) *Evolution*: Extinction describes the complete disappearance of a species of animal or plant. Calculating the rate of extinction is difficult to determine, since new species are continually being classified. For example, since 1993, three new species of large mammal have been described in Vietnam.

(I) PATRICIA A. REUTER-LORENZ;
(II, III) PHILIP WINN

extinction cue If a particular STIMULUS is presented during the extinction (see EXTINCTION, definition (ii) learning theory) of a response to a CONDITIONED STIMULUS it can be used subsequently to impede the spontaneous recovery of responding to the conditioned stimulus.

extinguish *see* extinction, definition (ii)

extracellular Outside cells; the extracellular space is the space between cells. The opposite of extracellular is INTRACELLULAR.

extracellular dehydration Loss of water from the extracellular sites; see OSMOREGULATION, PHYSIOLOGICAL CHALLENGE.

extracellular fluid *see* osmoregulation

extracellular matrix The spaces between cells are occupied by fluids (generally known as EXTRACELLULAR or INTERSTITIAL FLUIDS): in the CENTRAL NERVOUS SYSTEM this fluid is CEREBROSPINAL FLUID. However, cells do not just float in this fluid, but are held in place by an extracellular matrix. GLYCOPROTEINS form the bulk of this: COLLAGEN is another important component, held in a network of PROTEOGLYCANS. FIBRONECTINS are a form of glycoprotein that help anchor cells, binding to receptor proteins on cells called INTEGRINS.

See also: neural adhesion molecules

extracellular recording This is an electrophysiological (see ELECTROPHYSIOLOGY) recording of the activity of a NEURON in which the recording ELECTRODE is located outside the cells (that is, it is EXTRACELLULAR). This technique enables neurophysiologists to record the voltage of a neuron: as an ACTION POTENTIAL travels along an AXON it causes local changes in voltage which can be measured by the electrode. Extracellular recording is a form of SINGLE-UNIT ELECTROPHYSIOLOGICAL RECORDING. A more refined technique is INTRACELLULAR RECORDING, in which a single neuron is impaled by a microelectrode, enabling neurophysiologists to measure electrical activity within aneuron. It is a technique for measuring MEMBRANE POTENTIAL and enables examination of the fine details of EPSP/IPSP.

See also: current clamp; neurophysiology; voltage clamp

extradimensional shift Established responding to an exemplar within a STIMULUS DIMENSION, or class of stimulus features, results in the formation of an ATTENTIONAL SET. A change in the contingencies that requires a new pattern of responding is an extra-dimensional shift if the new response is to an exemplar from a different class of stimulus features.

See also: attentional set-shifting; intradimensional shift

VERITY J. BROWN

extrafusal fibre *see* muscle spindle

extraocular muscles The term *extraocular* means, literally, outside the eye, though of course it refers not to anywhere outside the eye, but immediately adjacent to it. The extraocular muscles are three pairs of MUSCLES (the members of each pair working in opposition to each other) that sit outside the eyeball and affect the direction of GAZE: they are the *superior* and *inferior rectus*, the *superior* and *inferior oblique*; and the *lateral* and *medial rectus*.

extraocular nerves The EXTRAOCULAR NERVES are the third (OCULOMOTOR NERVE), fourth (TROCHLEAR NERVE) and sixth (ABDUCENS NERVE) CRANIAL NERVES: they control the EXTRAOCULAR MUSCLES.

extrapyramidal motor system A term not used as much as it once was, the extrapyramidal motor system is that part of the motor system centred on the BASAL GANGLIA rather than the CEREBRAL CORTEX. It was contrasted with the PYRAMIDAL MOTOR SYSTEM, with cell bodies in the PRECENTRAL GYRUS (BRODMANN'S AREAS, number 4) which contained large neurons with a pyramidal shape. These gave rise to the CORTICOSPINAL TRACT (also known as the PYRAMIDAL TRACT), a pathway descending from area 4 of the motor cortex to the SPINAL CORD.

See also: corticostriatal loops; striatum

extrapyramidal side-effects The motor side-effects resembling features of PARKINSON'S DISEASE (such as TREMOR; see TARDIVE DYSKINESIA) caused by ANTIPSYCHOTIC drugs.

extrastriate cortex The STRIATE CORTEX is the PRIMARY VISUAL CORTEX. It is also known as Brodmann area 17 (see BRODMANN'S AREAS) and V1 (see AREAS V1–V5). The area of cortex surrounding V1 is the EXTRASTRIATE CORTEX or PRESTRIATE CORTEX, and contained in the Brodmann areas 18 and 19. It contains numerous other areas (at least 25) that appear to be implicated in visual processing.

extravasation The release of fluids from their appropriate compartments in the body; most commonly it refers to blood loss.

extreme capsule *see* external capsule

eye The receptive organ of the VISUAL SYSTEM; see AQUEOUS HUMOUR; CORNEA; IRIS; LACRIMATION; LENS; OPTIC DISC; PUPIL; RETINA; RETINAL CELL LAYERS; VITREOUS HUMOUR.

eye blink conditioning A form of CONDITIONING requiring minimal movement, used in the study of LEARNING. Rabbits are the typical subjects, because they have a very low spontaneous rate of blinking. It is used with human subjects in conditions where movements need to be kept to a minimum.

See also: conditioned reflex

eye blink reflex A simple REFLEX: movement of objects towards the eyes, or puffs of air directed towards them, produces a blinking reflex.

See also: eye blink conditioning

eye movements Conjugate ocular movements which serve to maintain stability of GAZE. PURSUIT EYE MOVEMENTS and SACCADES are the most extensively studied by psychologists. Pursuit eye movements are driven by slow- to medium-velocity visual targets and can be controlled by the (motion-sensitive) EXTRASTRIATE CORTEX. LESIONS to these regions may temporarily or permanently disrupt smooth pursuit while leaving saccades unaffected. Saccadic eye movements are extremely rapid and are associated with perceptual suppression during the high velocity portion of the movement. Posterior PARIETAL CORTEX and the FRONTAL EYE FIELDS are part of two parallel, semi-independent channels which play a role in voluntary saccades.

See also: eye position; smooth eye movements; smooth following movements; vergence

DAVID P. CAREY

eye position The term eye position refers to the position of the EYE in the ORBITS OF THE EYE, maintained by the EXTRAOCULAR MUSCLES, which both move the eye and counteract rolling motions. In examining the mechanics of eye position, primary, secondary and tertiary positions are identified: *primary position* is defined as the position in which there is no TORSION is evident. (Torsion involves rotation of the eyeball around a front to back axis - either *intorsion* [upper cornea in towards the nose] or *extorsion* [upper cornea towards the temple].) Primary position is usually straight ahead. *Secondary position* is any position achieved by simple horizontal or vertical movement of the eye. *Tertiary positions* are also identified, involving movement through what is known as Listing's plane. LISTING'S LAW indicates that when FIXATION of a point other than one in the primary position occurs, torsion is measured by presuming that it has moved from the initial direction of fixation around an axis perpendicular to it. VESTIBULAR-OCULAR INTERACTIONS are also important in maintaining eye position. For further information, see Davson, 1990.

See also: eye movements

Reference

Davson H (1990) *Physiology of the Eye*, Macmillan Press: London.

F

fa/fa (Fa/Fa) Genes coding for obesity; see ZUCKER RATS.

face agnosia *see* prosopagnosia

face memory Species that depend heavily on social interaction must develop sophisticated MEMORY systems to underpin the need to be able to recognize different individuals and interact with each according to what one knows about them. For humans, the face plays a key role in the recognition of other people. Impairments affecting memory for faces are often found after brain injury affecting the temporal lobes (see TEMPORAL LOBE), and especially the right temporal lobe. These may affect previously stored face memories, as in PROSOPAGNOSIA, or the ability to create new memories, resulting in problems in learning new faces. These findings have been confirmed in FUNCTIONAL NEUROIMAGING studies.

ANDREW W. YOUNG

face perception The interest of the face derives from the range of social signals we get from it – from facial appearance alone we can tell a person's age, sex, whether we know them, and what sort of MOOD they are in. Studies using FUNCTIONAL NEUROIMAGING and neuropsychological techniques show that these different social signals are to some extent dealt with independently by brain regions which have become specialized in dealing with a particular type of information. Generalized perceptual distortions affecting seen faces (METAMORPHOPSIAS) are sometimes found after BRAIN INJURY; faces may then be described as ugly and distorted – often like fish heads. Problems may also affect only one side of the seen face. People with unilateral neglect after RIGHT HEMISPHERE injury often have difficulty in getting information from the left sides of faces (that is, the side falling to their left). This is easily demonstrated with CHIMAERIC FACES, and is sometimes described in a relatively pure form, without other manifestations of unilateral neglect. Other types of selective deficit also occur. A striking example of independent processing of social signals from the face concerns the difference between brain mechanisms used to analyze identity and emotional expression. Neurophysiological studies have found cells responsive to faces in the TEMPORAL LOBE, confirming the importance of the face in species of PRIMATE. Some of these cells respond differentially to the face's identity or its expression; the cells selective for facial expression are mostly located within the SUPERIOR TEMPORAL SULCUS, whereas cells selective for identity tend to be on the INFERIOR TEMPORAL GYRUS. In humans with brain injuries, facial expressions of emotion can be recognized even when there is no overt recognition of the identities of familiar people from their faces (PROSOPAGNOSIA). Conversely, people with brain injuries who show defective comprehension of facial expressions may remain able to recognize identity from the face, forming a DOUBLE DISSOCIATION with the findings from cases of prosopagnosia. In prosopagnosia, the underlying pathology involves lesions affecting ventromedial regions of occipital cortex and temporal cortex; these include the LINGUAL GYRUS, FUSIFORM GYRUS and PARAHIPPOCAMPAL GYRUS, and more anterior parts of the temporal lobes. Functional neuro-imaging studies of normal observers have confirmed the importance of these regions to face perception and FACE MEMORY.

As well as prosopagnosia, there are other types of impairment that can compromise recognition of a face's identity. Some correspond to breakdown at different levels of recognition. Cases of inability to recognize people from their face, voice or name have been described; these seem to reflect loss of SEMANTIC MEMORY for the identities of individuals. There are also reports of problems of name retrieval (ANOMIA), in which familiar people are successfully recognized and appropriate semantic information is accessed, but their names cannot be recalled. These different types of problem fit the view that recognition of others is a multi-stage process. This is consistent with studies of everyday difficulties and errors, which can also reflect breakdown at different levels of recognition. For example: (1) We may completely fail to recognize a familiar face, and mistakenly think that the person is unfamiliar. (2) We may recognize the face as familiar, but be unable to bring to mind any other details about the person, such as her or his occupation or name. (3) We may recognize the face as familiar and remember appropriate semantic information about the person, whilst failing to remember her or his name. Each of these types of everyday face recognition error can also arise after neuropsychological impairment; a brain-injured person will then make her or his characteristic error to many or almost all seen faces.

An interesting feature of neuropsychological problems affecting the recognition of facial expressions of EMOTION is that deficits can compromise the recognition of some emotions more than others. People with AMYGDALA lesions have been found to be poor at recognizing anger and especially fear, with recognition of other basic emotions being less affected. The amygdala is known to be involved in CONDITIONED FEAR and the emotion of FEAR, but it was not immediately obvious that its role would extend to the recognition of fear in others. However, PET and FMRI studies also show amygdala activation when normal perceivers see facial expressions of fear. A plausible hypothesis is that the amygdala is intimately involved in the appraisal of danger in the immediate environment; to which expressions of fear (and anger) by others are a powerful contributory factor. A different pattern of impaired recognition of emotion occurs in people with HUNTINGTON'S CHOREA, for whom recognition of DISGUST is the most affected. Impaired recognition of disgust has also been found for clinically pre-symptomatic people who are carriers of the gene for Huntington's disease. Together with the studies of amygdala damage, these results show double dissociations between impairments affecting the recognition of different basic emotions.

It is clear, then, that face processing impairments reflect damage to a complex underlying system, which can break down in different ways. This point is already well established in other areas, such as LANGUAGE deficits, but it has only been appreciated relatively recently for face perception.

Reference

Ellis A.W. & Young A.W. (1996) *Human Cognitive Neuropsychology: A Textbook with Readings*, Psychology Press: Hove UK.

ANDREW W. YOUNG

facial bones *see* skull

facial masking The description given to the characteristic lack of activity in the MUSCLES in the face present in PARKINSON'S DISEASE.

facial nerve The seventh cranial nerve (see CRANIAL NERVES) composed of motor, sensory and AUTONOMIC fibres. The motor fibres arise in the facial motor nucleus in the rostral MEDULLA and supply superficial facial muscles that are important in facial expression. The sensory fibres are gustatory (see GUSTATION) and innervate TASTE BUDS on the anterior two-thirds of the tongue. These fibres comprise the CHORDA TYMPANI, and their cell bodies are located in the GENICULATE GANGLION in the temporal bone. The autonomic fibres in the facial nerve are involved in the secretion of saliva and tears. Their cell bodies are located in the superior salivatory nucleus in the medulla.

KAZUE SEMBA

facial nucleus The facial nucleus is a point of origin for the FACIAL NERVE (the seventh cranial nerve). It assists in the control of MOTOR NEURONS acting on the muscles of facial expression.

fact memory Fact memory represents the ability to recall specific knowledge without reference to the physical or temporal context in which it was acquired. It refers to the recall of world knowledge (see SEMANTIC MEMORY) rather than the remembrance of a specific event. Studies with amnesic (see AMNESIA) and AGEING patients have demonstrated that fact memory can be dissociated from source memory (see SOURCE AMNESIA). Fact memory is hypothesized to depend on structures in the medial TEMPORAL LOBE.

See also: amnesic syndrome; data based memory; declarative memory; explicit memory; memory

HOWARD EICHENBAUM

fainting More technically known as SYNCOPE, fainting is a transient loss of CONSCIOUSNESS, usually produced by temporarily reduced blood flow to the brain (more severe changes in blood flow – ISCHAEMIA – can produce more severe problems). Vasovagal syncope involves stimulation of the AUTONOMIC NERVOUS SYSTEM and is typically produced by conditions involving PAIN, FEAR and high degrees of EMOTION.

See also: anoxia

false memory syndrome *see* recovered memory

false neurotransmitter A false neurotransmitter is a chemical that is not one of the normal NEUROTRANSMITTERS but which can be taken up by a TERMINAL, packaged into SYNAPTIC VESICLES, and released in response to normal stimulation. PHENYLETHYLAMINE is an example of a false neurotransmitter.

falx cerebelli The FALX CEREBELLI is a fold in the DURA MATER as this follows the geography of the CEREBELLUM: a limb of the falx cerebelli

passes either side of the FORAMEN MAGNUM, producing its sickle shape

falx cerebri (from Latin, *falx*: a sickle) The term falx is a general one, indicating a sickle shape. The FALX CEREBRI is a fold in the DURA MATER (see MENINGES), as the dura mater follows the geography of the brain down into the LONGITUDINAL FISSURE. It is attached to the ethmoid bone (see SKULL) and the TENTORIUM.

familial tremor *see* tremor

fascia dentata Antique term for the DENTATE GYRUS.

fasciculation (from Latin, *fascis*: bundle) Fasciculation has two meanings: (i) it is the term given to rapid contractions of discrete muscle-bundles, detectable in one muscle after another. It is a feature of AMYOTROPHIC LATERAL SCLEROSIS. (ii) It is used to indicate the DEVELOPMENT of bundles of FIBRES in nervous tissue.

fasciculus retroflexus *see* habenula

fast muscle fibres *see* muscles

fast neurotransmission Fast neurotransmission refers to the NEUROTRANSMISSION mediated by the type of RECEPTOR that is directly coupled to an ION CHANNEL. The receptor and an ion channel are both part of a single transmembrane protein in the cell MEMBRANE, representing different domains of the same macromolecule. Fast neurotransmission takes place in the order of a few milliseconds. These types of receptors are called IONOTROPIC, as opposed to METABOTROPIC, and include NICOTINIC ACETYLCHOLINE RECEPTORS, GABA$_A$ RECEPTORS for gamma aminobutyric acid (GABA), 5-HT$_3$ receptors (see SEROTONIN RECEPTORS) for serotonin, and NMDA and non-NMDA GLUTAMATE RECEPTORS.

See also: neurotransmitters; slow neurotransmission; synapse

KAZUE SEMBA

fastigial nucleus *see* cerebellum – anatomical organization

fasting phase During the absorptive phase of DIGESTION, GLUCOSE and other molecules are absorbed by cells. In the FASTING PHASE which follows, when no molecules are being absorbed, glucose concentration must still be maintained, in order for cells to continue working. Glucose is supplied by the breakdown of GLYCOGEN in the LIVER; by the formation of glucose *de novo* from FAT and PROTEINS (GLUCONEOGENESIS); and by having cells metabolize fats rather than glucose.

fat Fat is the major long-term form of ENERGY store. Fat cells contain TRIGLYCERIDES, complex lipid molecules. The ongoing use of lipid molecules as fuel by body cells appears to provide one signal, albeit a relatively mild one, to the brain for HUNGER and SATIETY via the VAGUS NERVE. There has been some controversy as to whether levels of fat are actively regulated, in the sense that the brain monitors them and acts to keep them constant (whether or not their owner wishes this). However, there appears to be reasonable evidence that body fat levels are actively kept constant, at least after adulthood has been attained.

See also: body weight; energy balance; glucose; glycogen; leptin

KENT C. BERRIDGE

fat cell *see* adipose tissue

fatigue Fatigue is the normal sense of tiredness that follows work, either mental or physical. It reduces the ability to respond effectively to stimulation and occurs in all species: rats engaged in very long OPERANT sessions where they are required to emit thousands of lever presses are as likely to show fatigue as is a person engaged in strenuous work. There are pathological syndromes (the so-called CHRONIC FATIGUE SYNDROME) in which fatigue is a major feature.

fatty acids Fat is composed of GLYCEROL and fatty acids, in the proportion of one glycerol molecule to three fatty acid molecules (see TRIGLYCERIDES for further discussion of this). ESSENTIAL FATTY ACIDS are those that organisms cannot synthesize for themselves and which must therefore come from their diets.

fear Fear is a psychological concept that is used to describe the cluster of behaviours that are observed and experienced when a human being faces a threatening situation. If suddenly confronted by a stranger holding a gun to your face, you will realize instantly that you are in danger, that you could be beaten or even killed. Your hands will sweat, your heart will pound and your mouth will feel very dry. You will begin to tremble and feel as if you can't catch your breath. You may feel the hair standing out on the back of your neck and your mind will race, trying to decide whether to hold still, to run, or to try to take the gun out of the assailant's hand. Your sense of smell, sight and hearing will increase and your pupils dilate. Later you will remember this terrible incident over and over again, seeing your assailant's face or the gun in vivid detail. Returning to the location where the incident occurred will revive those awful memories often to the point where you will want to avoid that place forever (see PLACE CONDITIONING). Thus fear is a complex set of reactions which include both the expression and the experience of the emotional event (see EMOTION). Sweaty palms, increased heart rate, altered respiration, hair standing on end, and dilated pupils are part of the expression of fear. The feelings of dread, of potentially being killed, of your heart pounding or the hair standing upright on the back of your neck, are part of the EXPERIENCE of fear. Such reactions depend on the activation of the SYMPATHETIC NERVOUS SYSTEM. Very similar reactions can be seen in animals. If a cat confronts a vicious dog, the cat will assume the familiar 'Halloween posture' with its back arched, hair standing on end, and teeth bared. These expressions of fear can be seen easily and measured objectively. One can presume, based on our own experience, that the cat is experiencing a feeling of fear and a threat to its survival. However, unlike humans, where it is possible to discuss the experience of fear and how it feels, we can only infer that the cat is feeling fearful from looking at the situation and the set of behaviours it displays.

See also: animal models of anxiety; anxiety; conditioned fear

MICHAEL DAVIS

fear-potentiated startle A measure of CONDITIONED FEAR in which the STARTLE REFLEX evoked by a loud noise is enhanced by simultaneous presentation of an AVERSIVE STIMULUS.

See also: animal models of anxiety

SIMON KILLCROSS

feature detector A neuron in a sensory system which responds strongly and selectively to a specific stimulus feature, so that its activity can be taken as a signal that the feature is present. An early example was provided by 'BUG DETECTORS' in the frog RETINA which are active only when a small dark moving object is present in the neuron's RECEPTIVE FIELD. However, it is doubtful how far true feature detectors exist in the mammalian brain; ORIENTATION SELECTIVE NEURONS and other selective neurons in visual cortical areas (see AREAS V1–V5), can probably only convey information by their contribution to a pattern of activity across many different neurons.

See also: cell assembly theory; engram; grandmother cell

OLIVER J. BRADDICK

feature integration framework *see* feature search

feature negative learning *see* feature positive learning

feature positive learning A CONDITIONING technique in which REINFORCEMENT is delivered following presentation of STIMULUS X and stimulus Y, but none is delivered in response to one stimulus on its own. FEATURE NEGATIVE LEARNING involves reinforcement delivery when the individual stimuli are presented, but not when both are present.

feature search The extraction of a specific element from the visual array. The notion of feature search can be related to the FEATURE INTEGRATION FRAMEWORK (see Treisman, 1988), whereby ATTENTION is regarded as the 'glue' which is required to join elementary perceptual features present in the environment. In this framework, feature search is considered to be an automatic, rapid and resource-independent process (see AUTOMATIC VS. CONTROLLED ATTENTION). Phenomenologically, a feature is said to 'pop out' from its background in the visual array; for example, the feature of shading in selecting a filled circle from amongst a background of empty circles. This contrasts with CONJOINED FEATURE SEARCH, in which elements registered in the first feature detection stage are serially conjoined in order to represent more complex feature associations. For example, the features of shading and circularity in selecting a shaded circle from amongst a background of empty circles and filled squares. This conjoined feature stage seems to be resource-dependent and to draw upon effortful or controlled attention.

References

Treisman, A. (1988) Features and objects: the 14th Bartlett memorial lecture. *Quarterly Journal of Experimental Psychology* 40A: 201–237.

JONATHAN K. FOSTER

febrile convulsions The term *febrile* is an adjective that refers to FEVER; FEBRILE CONVULSIONS are CONVULSIONS associated with fever.

Fechner's law A law of PSYCHOPHYSICS formulated in 1860 by Gustav Fechner: the perceived strength of a STIMULUS is a log function of intensity. Mathematically it is expressed as:

$$A = k.\log(I/I_t)$$

where A is perceived strength, I is intensity and I_t the threshold intensity. Like WEBER'S LAW, this formula has held good, though it breaks down when extreme values are used.

Fechner's paradox *see* binocular summation

feeding Feeding is needed for the maintenance of ENERGY BALANCE and requires the integrated activity of many neural and behavioural systems. In order to feed, animals must know about their internal and external environments (when is it time to feed? what is edible, what inedible?), they must be able to search effectively for food (see FORAGING) and be able to activate the MUSCLES necessary to capture it once found (to gather plants or catch and kill other animals) and ingest it. Effective monitoring of internal state is imperative for proper regulation of feeding. Signals indicating both depletion and loss, and repletion and satisfaction are analyzed by the brain. The brain is able to monitor, via analysis of BLOOD composition and receipt of neural input (from the VAGUS NERVE for example) such things as circulating levels of GLUCOSE, activity of HORMONES such as INSULIN and GLUCAGON in the PANCREAS, metabolic activity in the LIVER, gut activity (through CHOLECYSTOKININ concentration for example) and the state of FAT stores (through analysis of LEPTIN concentration). In addition, there are specific mechanisms for the detection of critical diet components such as sodium (see SODIUM APPETITE). The analysis of taste (see GUSTATION) is an important part of feeding: taste serves to give warning of 'badness' or 'goodness' in food and acts as a stimulant to intake. The brain mechanisms involved in this are distributed widely, from, for example, the NUCLEUS OF THE SOLITARY TRACT in the brainstem, the HYPOTHALAMUS in the diencephalon to the FRONTAL CORTEX. Accounts of the neurobiology of feeding have in the past centred on the hypothalamus, which was thought to have specific centres regulating feeding (and other motivated behaviours) but this is seen as over-simplified now (see DUAL CENTRES HYPOTHESIS; LATERAL HYPOTHALAMIC SYNDROME; VENTROMEDIAL HYPOTHALAMIC SYNDROME). Current accounts of the neurobiology of feeding emphasize the distributed nature of its processing.

However, it has to be borne in mind that feeding is not simply a matter of energy regulation and that feeding occurs in response to a wide variety of states and stimuli. In animals it is evident that provision of the SUPERMARKET DIET can lead to excessive intake. This of course can be accounted for by the fact that animals which normally have seasonal variation in food availability should be prepared to overeat when the opportunity presents. But stimuli completely unrelated to nutrition or deprivation, such as TAIL-PINCHING, can also reliably elicit feeding in rats, while in humans it is clear that psychological states of AROUSAL or ANXIETY can trigger feeding (see Slochower, 1983). Evidence such as this points to two conclusions: first, that eating can be triggered by non-specific activation; and second, that in humans at least, LEARNING to attribute (see ATTRIBUTION) the label HUNGER only to appropriate physiological states may be a lot more difficult than is commonly sup-

posed. The most startling evidence of this is presented by Hilde Bruch (1973). She cites (pp.60–61) the developmental history of a grossly obese boy who was fed inappropriately in response to whatever EMOTION he expressed. In consequence he learned that feeding was the appropriate response to a wide variety of psychological and physiological states and ate indiscriminately. Humans generally have mechanisms for monitoring body state and regulating feeding: whether they learn to use them properly is another matter.

See also: digestion; drinking; eating disorders; externality; internality; restrained and unrestrained eating; satiety

References

Bruch H. (1973) *Eating Disorders: Obesity, Anorexia Nervosa and the Person Within*, Basic Books: New York.
Slochower J.A. (1983) *Excessive Eating: The Role of Emotions and Environment*, Humana Sciences Press: New York.

feminine An adjective used to describe any physical or behavioural trait that is typically displayed by females of a given species. Physical or phenotypic traits, such as feminine anatomy (such as the clitoris and vagina, ovaries, cervix, breasts, bone structure) and physiology (for example ESTRUS or the MENSTRUAL CYCLE, ovulation, menopause) are viewed as genetic in nature, being organized perinatally and activated by HORMONES during puberty. Although feminine behavioural traits can also be viewed in this way (for instance, hormonal stimulation of female sexual behaviours) there is little agreement concerning the degree to which feminine behaviours in humans are genetically programmed or learned (see LEARNING).

See also: gender; hormones and cognition; organization effects of steroid hormones; sex differences; sexual behaviour; sexual differentiation

JAMES G. PFAUS

femto- Prefix indicating a factor of 10^{-15}, or one thousand million millionth; see SI UNITS.

fenfluramine Fenfluramine is related to AMPHETAMINE (it is what is known as a substituted amphetamine) and has similar properties.

However, while amphetamine is known principally for its ability to stimulate the RELEASE of DOPAMINE and NORADRENALINE, fenfluramine stimulates the release of SEROTONIN (5-hydroxytryptamine). Like amphetamine, it appears both to stimulate release and block REUPTAKE, but of serotonin rather than the CATECHOLAMINES. It is best known as an APPETITE-suppressant drug, used in experimental animals and also given to humans as part of BODY WEIGHT control programmes (see Blundell & Hill, 1991). The racemate D,L-fenfluramine (available under the trade name 'Pondimin') and the D-isomer, dexfenfluramine ('Redux') are both used clinically in weight-control programmes.

Reference

Blundell J.E. & Hill A.J. (1991) Appetite control by dexfenfluramine in the treatment of obesity. *Reviews in Contemporary Pharmacotherapy* 2:79–92.

fentanyl A narcotic analgesic agent (see ANALGESIA) used as a premedication before surgery (see STEREOTAXIC SURGERY). It provides NEUROLEPTANALGESIA if given in combination with BENZODIAZEPINES such as DIAZEPAM or MIDAZOLAM.

Reference

Flecknell P.A. (1987) *Laboratory Animal Anaesthesia*. Academic Press: London.

festination (from Latin, *festinare*: to hurry) Anything quickened over the normal rate can be described as festination or festinating. Patients with PARKINSON'S DISEASE are described, somewhat paradoxically, as showing festination, or a festinating GAIT. This describes the small shuffling steps they often take, rather than the speed of their actions.

fever *see* immune system

fibre-sparing lesions *see* excitotoxins

fibres (from Latin, *fibra*: a thread or fibre) The term FIBRE of course relates to all sorts of different things. In the context of biological psychology the term is almost always used to mean an AXON, in contrast to the CELL BODY, DENDRITE or SYNAPTIC TERMINALS. A fibre bundle is usually taken to mean a collection of axons running in parallel together (though of

course if one happened to be discussing, for example, MUSCLES and were talking about fibres, one would probably mean MUSCLE FIBRES: context is everything here). The term FIBRE-SPARING LESION relates to a LESION that spares axons but destroys other parts of the NEURON (see EXCITOTOXINS).

See also: connective tissue

fibres en passant *see* fibres of passage

fibres of passage (also known by the French term, *fibres en passant*) This refers to FIBRES that pass through an area without necessarily making synaptic contact with that area. A good example is provided by the relationship between the MEDIAL FOREBRAIN BUNDLE and the LATERAL HYPOTHALAMUS: this bundle passes through the lateral hypothalamus, fibres travelling both anterior to posterior and vice-versa. For the most part these fibres do not make specialized synaptic (see SYNAPSE) contact in the lateral hypothalamus (though there may be VOLUME TRANSMISSION occurring). It is important to recognize that identified structures within the brain are not absolutely solid, forcing fibre pathways to go around them. It is also important, in a more practical sense, to recognize that when one makes a LESION in a given area, one could damage fibres of passage that have nothing to do with the function of the tissue one is trying to damage; for an example of this problem, see LATERAL HYPOTHALAMIC SYNDROME.

fibroblast A fibroblast is a CELL that produces COLLAGEN, a protein that is a basic constituent of CONNECTIVE TISSUE. Some interesting findings were made by Hayflick, who observed that fibroblasts grown in CULTURE will divide to occupy the space available to them in a culture flask. If half of these cells are taken to a new culture flask, they will again divide to cover the available surface. Human fibroblasts can double in number like this about 50 times over a period of up to 9 months, but the process slows and eventually cannot repeat itself. The number of repeats is a function of species lifespan: mouse fibroblasts divide about 15 times; human about 50 and tortoise about 90. The lifespans of these are, in the same order, 3 years, 70 years and 175 years. It has been suggested that this inability continually to reproduce forms a biological basis for AGEING (see also SENILITY). Whatever process is involved appears to be based on the cell NUCLEUS: the nuclei of young and old fibroblasts can be exchanged (using IN VITRO chemical techniques): an old cell with a young nucleus has the properties of a young cell.

fibroblast growth factor One of the GROWTH FACTORS involved early in development, with a variety of functions. It promotes formation of the MESODERM from the ENDODERM (see DEVELOPMENT); and it can stimulate the transformation of CHROMAFFIN CELLS into NEURONS.

fibronectin Fibronectin, secreted by FIBROBLAST cells, is one of the GLYCOPROTEINS and operates as an adhesion molecule; see EXTRACELLULAR MATRIX; GROWTH CONE; NEURAL ADHESION MOLECULES.

fictive locomotion *see* locomotion

field potential A change in the voltage recorded in the CENTRAL NERVOUS SYSTEM reflecting the electrical activity of a large population of neurons or neural elements. The ELECTROENCEPHALOGRAM (EEG) is a measurement of ongoing field potentials in the CEREBRAL CORTEX. Field potentials that are timed to the presentation of a sensory stimulus can be measured in sensory regions of the brain (see EVENT-RELATED POTENTIALS) and can be used to determine how the stimuli are mapped in that region (see MAPS). Field potentials can also be recorded across highly layered regions such as the HIPPOCAMPUS where the AMPLITUDE and shape of the potentials can reflect the synaptic efficiency. Changes in such field potentials have been useful in describing LONG-TERM POTENTIATION and LONG-TERM DEPRESSION.

DOUGLAS D. RASMUSSON

fight-or-flight Unconditioned aggressive or ESCAPE responses that an animal displays when it is exposed to an AVERSIVE STIMULUS. Cannon (1871–1945) introduced the phrase 'fight-or-flight response' in the early 1900s to refer to the physiological reactions that prepare the individual for performing fight or flight. The UNCONDITIONED RESPONSE TO A PUNISHMENT

may be either defensive attacks or attempts to escape. However, fight-or-flight does not depend on the actual punishment delivered but on other stimuli present at the time of punishment. Where effective escape is impossible and there is nothing suitable to ATTACK in the environment, punishing stimuli (such as electric shock) produce unconditioned escape behaviour. However, if a suitable object is present (another animal or small inanimate object for instance) the most likely response is an attack, even though there is no causal relationship between the shock and the object. Given the choice between fight or flight, animals appear to prefer fight. The preference for fight is so great that animals will even work to provide themselves with a suitable stimulus to attack. It is well known that these situations activate the peripheral SYMPATHETIC NERVOUS SYSTEM resulting in AROUSAL, increased heart rate, ADRENAL GLAND release of ADRENALINE, and suppression of digestive activity. However, less is known about central mechanisms underlying these behavioural responses.

Experimental evidence (see Gray, 1987) suggests three separate brain systems that mediate emotional responses: (1) the REWARD system that responds to rewarding (non-punishment) stimuli by activating approach behaviour (positive emotional states); (2) the BEHAVIOURAL INHIBITION SYSTEM that responds to punishing stimuli by suppressing behaviour (passive negative states); and (3) the fight-or-flight system that responds to unconditioned punishment (non-rewards) by activating escape or aggressive behaviour (negative states). The AMYGDALA, HYPOTHALAMUS, and midbrain CENTRAL GREY are thought to be the central components of the fight-or-flight system. The amygdala projects to the medial hypothalamus and then to the central grey to serve as the final fight-or-flight common pathway. The central grey is under inhibitory control from the medial hypothalamus which may be disinhibited by activity from the amygdala. Upon initial exposure to novel stimuli, the behavioural inhibitory system dominates and inhibition of both approach and fight-or-flight is maintained. Attachment of rewarding or punishing significance to these stimuli evokes a change in the medial hypothalamus via the amygdala until either approach or fight-or-flight behaviour dominates.

See also: emotion

Reference

Gray J.A. (1987) *The Psychology of Fear and Stress*, chapters 12–13, Cambridge University Press: Cambridge.

CHARLES D. BLAHA

fighting *see* aggression

filament (from Latin, *filum*: a thread) Filament is a term that can be applied to anything that is thin and threadlike (although of course the degree of thinness will depend on the context: thin in CELL biology is not the same as thin in metalwork necessarily). The CYTOS-KELETON contain various types of filaments, for example.

filopodia *see* growth cone

fimbria The fimbria is a thin band of WHITE MATTER situated laterally in the HIPPOCAMPAL FORMATION. It consists of axons from the PYRAMIDAL NEURONS of the HIPPOCAMPUS and SUBICULUM as well as AFFERENT or incoming fibres to the hippocampal formation. The pyramidal axons initially form the ALVEUS which spreads over the ventricular surface of the hippocampus. The alveus gradually thickens towards the dorsal end of the hippocampus to form the fimbria. The fimbriae from the two sides then merge to form the FORNIX, which projects to the septal region (see SEPTAL NUCLEI) and the HYPOTHALAMUS.

KAZUE SEMBA

final common path The MOTOR NEURONS are the point of convergence of excitatory and inhibitory influences arriving via various routes from different parts of the brain and the periphery. The result of such convergence determines the probability of firing of motor neurons, which in turn controls the degree of muscle contraction (see MUSCLES). Thus, all the influences are funnelled down onto motor neurons which cause the final action, namely, muscle contraction and movement. This integral position of the motor neuron was recognized by Sherrington (1857–1952) when he

coined the term 'final common path' to refer to the motor neuron.

KAZUE SEMBA

finger agnosia The failure to localize and/or identify fingers occurs with approximately equal frequency in patients with RIGHT HEMISPHERE and LEFT HEMISPHERE brain damage and may be associated with many types of damage including diffuse lesions in the posterior PARIETAL LOBE, FRONTAL LOBE and TEMPORAL LOBE. Finger agnosia is not simply attributable to a failure to point to PROXIMAL body parts and patients may fail even on pointing to different fingers on a drawing of a hand. This deficit was originally described as part of the GERSTMANN SYNDROME which includes a combination of finger agnosia, LEFT–RIGHT CONFUSION, ACALCULIA and AGRAPHIA although it may occur in isolation as well.

MARLENE BEHRMANN

finickiness Finickiness in animals refers to a form of food or fluid selection in which palatable foods are overeaten while mildly adulterated foods are rejected. It is typically measured by adding different concentrations of SACCHARIN or QUININE to a standard food or to water. (Saccharin and quinine are used because they have no caloric content: they affect the taste but not nutritional status of food.) Finickiness was a feature of both the VENTROMEDIAL HYPOTHALAMIC SYNDROME and LATERAL HYPOTHALAMIC SYNDROME, as classically described but later studies indicated that it was destruction of neurons outside the HYPOTHALAMUS that produced finickiness.

Reference

Sahakian B.J., Winn P., Robbins T.W., Deeley R.J., Everitt B.J., Dunn L.T., Wallace M. & James W.P.T. (1983) Changes in body weight and food-related behaviour induced by destruction of the ventral or dorsal noradrenergic bundle in the rat. *Neuroscience* 10: 1405–1420.

Fink–Heimer stain *see* Nauta–Gygax stain

firing *see* spike

first-rank symptoms A number of SIGNS AND SYMPTOMS that may be encountered in patients with SCHIZOPHRENIA which were described by

Kurt Schneider (1887–1967) as '*symptoms of the first rank*'. When present, they are considered to be of special value in making a diagnosis of schizophrenia, but they are not specific, nor mandatory, and the diagnosis can be made in their absence. The symptoms are: the experience of thoughts being spoken aloud; third-person auditory hallucinations; auditory hallucinations in the form of a commentary; somatic hallucinations; disorders of possession of thought (that is, thought insertion, withdrawal or broadcasting); delusional perception; passivity experiences (feelings or actions experienced as made or influenced by others).

See also: hallucination

IAN C. REID

fissure *see* gyri and sulci

fistula (from Latin, *fistula*: a pipe) In medicine a fistula can refer to a narrow opening, made by a surgeon. More commonly, it refers to an inserted length of tubing. A GASTRIC FISTULA for example is a tube inserted into the stomach via which stomach fluids can be extracted for analysis, or via which material could be passed into the stomach. The term CATHETER is more or less synonymous.

fitness *see* natural selection

five-choice serial reaction time test A task used to measure the speed and accuracy of ATTENTION, typically in rats. Using a NINE-HOLE BOX, rats are trained to respond with a nose poke in the hole displaying a brief visual stimulus presented at random in any of five locations. The accuracy and latency of responding are measured; error performance – IMPULSIVITY or PERSEVERATION for example – can also yield valuable information.

See also: attention; reaction time

5′–3′ (five-prime–three-prime) In a nucleotide of deoxyribonucleic acid (DNA) or ribonucleic acid (RNA), the carbon atom of each sugar group is numbered 1 to 5, so that the first carbon atom (the one-prime, 1′) atom is that at which the base is attached, and the fifth (five-prime, 5′) is that which contains a phosphate group. Nucleotides are joined together in strands of DNA or RNA by a phosphodiester

bond between the 5′ and 3′ carbon atoms of adjacent bases. Replication of DNA and RNA strands always proceeds in a 5′–3′ manner, so that the 5′ carbon of the incoming nucleotide reacts with the 3′ carbon of the nucleotide at the end of the strand.

See also: antisense

FIONA M. INGLIS

fixation (i) *Vision*: the directing of the EYE such that a particular point in space falls at the centre of the FOVEA; see ACCOMMODATION; FIXATION POINT.

(ii) *Histology*: Fixation (or more appropriately, TISSUE FIXATION) is a procedure that prepares tissue for HISTOLOGY, regardless of how the material is to be visualized (see MICROSCOPY). It is a process that leaves tissue structurally intact but stabilizes PROTEINS, making them insoluble, so that they literally are fixed – they do not move. One is thus able to examine tissue *post-mortem* in as close a state to living as possible. Fixation is typically achieved using an ALDEHYDE solution. FORMALIN is the most commonly used fixative: it is a solution of FORMALDEHYDE gas dissolved in water. 40% formalin is a saturated solution (that is, no more can be dissolved). The most commonly used solution to fix brain tissue is one made up of 10% formalin, this being 10 ml of formalin (at 40%) in 100 ml of solution. The final concentration of formaldehyde in the solution is therefore 4%.

Formaldehyde fixes tissue through the activity of its aldehyde component, which is able to react with the nitrogen present in proteins. Formaldehyde distributes through tissue which is exposed to it very quickly (a matter of minutes) but the protein reaction is much slower (a matter of days). SUCROSE is often added to formaldehyde solutions to act as a CRYOPROTECTANT – it reduces the osmotic (see OSMOSIS) challenge of formaldehyde and prevents shattering of tissue when it is frozen. PARAFORMALDEHYDE is in effect no different to formaldehyde. It is a polymer of formaldehyde which is itself insoluble, but which becomes formaldehyde when added to a BUFFER solution. GLUTARALDEHYDE has two aldehyde groups, which affects its performance as a fixative. It can be used as a fixative for routine material, preserving the ultrastructure of tissue exceptionally well (making it particularly suitable for SECTIONS destined for ELECTRON MICROSCOPY) but it has a negative effect on the quality of material being prepared for IMMUNOHISTOCHEMISTRY (because it affects the numbers of sites at which ANTIBODIES can bind). Mixtures of glutaraldehyde and formaldehyde are often used, combining the advantages of both.

fixation point A visual scene that is to be inspected may often, in laboratory experiments, contain an explicit mark or target to which the observer is instructed to direct their gaze. This fixation point will become imaged on the FOVEOLA, the region of the RETINA with the most acute vision. It is to be noted that even with steady fixation there still exist small EYE MOVEMENTS which prevent the fading of an image that is associated with the perfect stabilization of a visual target.

DAVID W. HEELEY

fixed action pattern A term used in ETHOLOGY to describe a species-specific complex pattern of action, more complex than a REFLEX, often dependent upon the animal's state (of DRIVE for example), and apparently innate rather than the product of LEARNING.

fixed battery A NEUROPSYCHOLOGICAL TEST BATTERY whose contents are fixed: such a battery provides a stable and continuous programme of information which can be used to gauge and compare patients' functions and dysfunctions. The contrast is with tests that are used on an *ad hoc* basis to probe particular problems at particular times. The HALSTEAD–REITAN TEST BATTERY or the LURIA–NEBRASKA NEUROPSYCHOLOGICAL BATTERY are examples of fixed batteries.

fixed interval schedule *see* schedules of reinforcement

fixed ratio schedule *see* schedules of reinforcement

flashbulb memory Flashbulb memory describes a vivid and detailed MEMORY for an event that is typically charged with EMOTION (either positive or negative). The most common example given (at least to individuals of a

certain age) is 'Where were you when you heard of the assassination of President Kennedy?', to which very many individuals can give graphic answers describing a place and the events occurring in it. Some authors have argued that flashbulb memories are supported by special mechanisms; others have suggested instead that the phenomenon of flashbulb memory can be wholly explained using 'ordinary' memory mechanisms; the articles below discuss both sides of this argument.

See also: snapshot memory

References

Cohen N.J., McCloskey M. & Wible C.G. (1988) There is still no case for a flashbulb memory mechanism: reply to Schmidt and Bohannon. *Journal of Experimental Psychology (General)* 117: 336–385.

McCloskey M., Wible C.G.H. & Cohen N.J. (1988) Is there a special flashbulb memory mechanism? *Journal of Experimental Psychology (General)* 117: 171–181.

Schmidt S.R. & Bohannon J.N. III (1988) In defense of flashbulb memory hypothesis: a comment on McCloskey, Wible and Cohen (1988) *Journal of Experimental Psychology (General)* 117: 332–335.

flexor muscles *see* muscles

flexor phase *see* locomotion

flight Flight occurs in many insects and birds and some mammals (bats for instance). Passive flight includes diving (as falcons do) and soaring and gliding (as albatrosses do). In active flight, pectoral muscle contractions generate rhythms in convex-upward shaped wings, resulting in low air pressure on the top of these structures. This produces aerodynamic lift, which in turn provides both weight support and thrust. Wing beats generally produce forward movement, but certain animals can hover or fly backward (for example, hummingbirds). Flight is evolutionary old, being present in certain dinosaurs. Flight may have evolved because it facilitated FORAGING and predator avoidance.

See also: locomotion; migration; navigation;

DONALD M. WILKIE

flinch–jump test *see* analgesia

flip and flop Two alternative variants of the RECEPTOR for AMPA, in which the magnitude of response to GLUTAMATE is markedly different. These two variants are encoded by the same gene for AMPA receptors, but an alternative EXON is used in each case to form the MESSENGER RNA. AMPA receptors which contain flip subunits are much more efficient at passing current than those containing flop subunits. Flip subunits are more prevalent than flop before birth, suggesting a role in SYNAPSE formation in the developing nervous system (see NEURODEVELOPMENT).

FIONA M. INGLIS

flocculonodular lobe *see* cerebellum

flower spray ending *see* muscle spindle

fluent aphasia Part of a clinical dichotomy (vs. NON-FLUENT APHASIA), this is a popular clinical description of aphasia that provides a general characterization of the patient's LANGUAGE disorder based on characteristics of spontaneous SPEECH PRODUCTION. Speech is relatively free-flowing, and easily articulated. Fluent aphasia is associated with LESIONS posterior to the ROLANDIC FISSURE.

See also: anomic aphasia; aphasia; conduction aphasia; transcortical sensory aphasia; Wernicke's aphasia

References

Goodglass H. (1993) *Understanding Aphasia*, Academic Press: San Diego.

CHARLOTTE C. MITCHUM

fluorescence The property of certain substances that allows them to emit light of a greater wavelength than that which they are stimulated by: they glow. Fluorescence can be demonstrated in the nervous system in essentially two ways. (1) A fluorescent marker (a FLUOROCHROME) can be delivered into the nervous system and subsequently detected using fluorescence microscopy. This is the basis for a number of tract tracing techniques (see TRACT TRACERS). (2) Some chemicals in the nervous system will fluoresce if they are treated with FORMALDEHYDE. The discovery that this was the case was very important in allowing for visualization of many MONOAMINE neurotransmitters using the Falck–Hillarp technique

(see CLASSIFICATION OF DAHLSTRÖM AND FUXE). This procedure has largely been overtaken by more modern procedures such as IMMUNOHISTOCHEMISTRY and IN SITU HYBRIDIZATION.

See also: chemical neuroanatomy; histology; microscopy; voltage-sensitive dye recording

fluorescent tracers *see* tract tracers

fluorochrome A fluorochrome is a chemical that emits light (it shows FLUORESCENCE) when light of a specific wavelength is shone on to it; see TRACT TRACERS.

fluorogold A tract tracer, retrogradely transported along an AXON. It labels CYTOPLASM and is especially good in filling dendrites. It also has the virtue of being straightforward to combine with other forms of HISTOCHEMISTRY to achieve DOUBLE LABELLING.

fluoxetine *see* Prozac

fluphenazine A phenothiazine derivative, used to treat SCHIZOPHRENIA; see ANTIPSYCHOTIC.

Flynn effect *see* intelligence

FMRFamide FMRFamide is a neuropeptide transmitter only found in INVERTEBRATES. FMRF is a phonetic anagram: phe-met-arg-phe (phenylalanine, methionine, arginine, phenylalanine) is the amino acid sequence making up this peptide. If one reads out the first letters of phe, met, arg, phe one finds F, M, R, F – and one then calls the peptide *fuh-mur-fuh-mide*.

fMRI The two most important FUNCTIONAL NEUROIMAGING methods are POSITRON EMISSION TOMOGRAPHY (PET) and FUNCTIONAL MAGNETIC RESONANCE IMAGING (fMRI). These both use non-invasive brain imaging methods to localize neural activity in the human brain related to the performance of specific mental functions, and both methods take advantage of the fact that neural activity and blood flow in the normal brain are closely coupled, such that within a few seconds, a change in activity triggers a concomitant change in blood flow. In contrast to PET, fMRI does not measure blood flow directly, but is sensitive to blood oxygenation. The method takes advantage of the remarkable and fortuitous facts that oxy-

and deoxyhaemoglobin have different magnetic susceptibilities, and that the increase in blood flow to an active brain region is greater than that necessary to meet its increased oxygen demand. This means that the blood flowing out of a region is more oxygenated (has a lower concentration of deoxyhaemoglobin) when neural activity in the region is high than when it is low. MRI signals can be made sensitive to the local magnetic variations which covary with the concentration of deoxyhaemoglobin in the blood. Thus MRI can be used to image variations in regional blood oxygenation, and hence, indirectly, regional brain activity. fMRI has a number of advantages as a functional neuroimaging method over PET, and is likely largely to supplant the PET technique within the next few years. Among these advantages are that there is no restriction on the number of observations that can be obtained from a single subject, and that whole-brain images can be acquired in just a few seconds, rather than requiring a minute or so.

See also: functional neuroimaging

MICHAEL D. RUGG

focal ischaemia The process by which the blood flow to a localized region of the brain or other tissue is interrupted. In the brain, focal ischaemia may be the result of head injury, cerebral EMBOLISM or ANEURYSM, and results in death of cerebral tissue, including neurons, GLIAL CELLS and vascular tissue, in the region of ischaemia. Focal ischaemia is often long-lasting, and is characterized by delayed neuronal death in the area of ischaemia and also in brain structures innervated by the ischaemic region. Neurons in the HIPPO-CAMPUS, STRIATUM and CORTEX, which have high densities of GLUTAMATE RECEPTORS, are most at risk of death in focal ischaemia. Occlusion of a specific cerebral artery, such as the middle cerebral artery, provides an animal model of focal ischaemia, and permits studies of functional consequences of ischaemia, and allows effective treatments to be identified. Following focal ischaemia, humans and animals show impairments which are indicative of the localization of the ischaemic INFARCT.

See also: global ischaemia; ischaemia

FIONA M. INGLIS

focal seizure *see* partial seizure

focal vs. diffuse The term FOCAL is derived from the word focus and indicates a high degree of localization. In contrast, DIFFUSE indicates that something is widespread. For examples of the use of these terms, see FOCAL ISCHAEMIA, DIFFUSE AXONAL INJURY.

fodrin Fodrin is one of the PROTEINS that form the CYTOSKELETON. It is of some interest because it has been implicated in the mechanism of LONG-TERM POTENTIATION. The potentiating stimulus driving long-term potentiation has been suggested to increase the entry of CALCIUM into neurons. Calcium influx triggers the action of an ENZYME, CALPAIN, which acts to degrade fodrin, leading to expansion of the neuronal MEMBRANE (the action of fodrin being that of holding it in). Expansion of the surface area of the membrane allows for greater RECEPTOR expression on the membrane, and hence long-term potentiation develops. This is however, only one theory to account for long-term potentiation.

foetal alcohol syndrome A collection of developmental abnormalities caused by embryonic and foetal exposure to ethanol (see ALCOHOL), which readily crosses the PLACENTA after maternal consumption. Foetal alcohol syndrome (FAS) was first described in the medical literature in 1974, and is a leading cause of human mental retardation, with an incidence of about 1 per 1000 live births. The full syndrome is characterized by growth retardation, abnormalities in the head and face (craniofacial abnormalities), defects of the heart and nervous system, and minor joint and limb abnormalities. The type and severity of the various defects may be related to the timing and dosage of maternal ethanol intake and the diagnosis is based on clinical findings and a history of maternal alcohol consumption of more than two drinks per day. Low or moderate intake appears not to be associated with FAS. Typical craniofacial features of the human syndrome range from the well-recognized FAS physiognomy, with a narrow eye opening ('short palpebral fissure') a short nose to upper-lip distance, a thin upper lip and a broad root of the nose, to the more severe frontonasal DYSPLASIA (median cleft face). Structural abnormalities of the CNS include MICROCEPHALY, AGENESIS or underdevelopment of the CORPUS CALLOSUM, enlarged VENTRICLES, underdevelopment of the INFERIOR OLIVES, and a small BRAINSTEM. Up to 90% of affected individuals also have eye defects, often associated with underdevelopment of the OPTIC NERVES, poor VISUAL ACUITY and NYSTAGMUS. The precise cellular and molecular mechanism of action of ethanol in causing abnormal development is unclear. Various biological factors are hypothesized, including maternal/foetal HYPOXIA and formation of FREE RADICALS. In mice, alcohol treatment of pregnant females causes a reduction in the number of myelinated axons (see MYELIN) in the optic nerves, but not peripheral nerves, of young adult offspring, while no differences due to ethanol exposure are detectable during the early postnatal period. This suggests that the effects of ethanol exposure on CNS development can be delayed, although more immediate deleterious effects on developing embryonic and foetal tissues are likely in severe cases. One possible explanation for the craniofacial abnormalities is that ethanol enhances cell death in the population of NEURAL CREST cells (cranial neural crest) that migrates from the developing HINDBRAIN to populate the emerging facial region of the embryo. Little is known about the long-term development and outcome of children with FAS, although in general it appears that in severe cases there is a high rate of persistent psychiatric and cognitive impairment.

ROGER J. KEYNES

foetus (from Latin, *fetus*: offspring; the American spelling, fetus, has therefore remained true to the original form) A developing organism with the principal organs of the body differentiated and identifiable; before this the organism is known as an EMBRYO; see DEVELOPMENT.

foliate papillae *see* taste buds

folic acid (folate) *see* vitamins

folk psychology The term used by many scientists and philosophers to describe normal everyday talk and conceptions of psychological process. Folk psychology is inherently vague and relies on such things as belief, EMOTION and will. ELIMINATIVE MATERIALISM predicts that such talk could be replaced by a description of states couched in terms of the underlying biological processes. What such descriptions would be like – and indeed, whether such descriptions can be provided at all – is a matter of some philosophical debate. In the short term at least it is likely that we will continue to use folk psychology terms such as HUNGER to describe our own states, rather than discussing the concentration of glucose in our blood or the state of our HYPOTHALAMUS.

See also: neurophilosophy

follicle-stimulating hormone (FSH) One of the GONADOTROPHINS.

See also: endocrine glands; estrus; hormones; hormones – classification; menstrual cycle; sex hormones

food-aversion learning If an animal is presented with a food around the same time that it suffers extreme illness or NAUSEA, it will form a strong and persistent aversion to that food. Such striking learning has been observed in a variety of animals, and is likely to be form of LEARNING widely used by animals in their natural environments. Food-aversion learning exhibits certain characteristics, such as relaxed temporal requirements and a clear adaptive significance, which have been taken to suggest that it represents a special form of learning that was uniquely selected during EVOLUTION. Seductive as this notion might be, the issue remains controversial.

MARK A. UNGLESS

food-storing birds Food-storing birds cache food at sites distant from point of capture. Hoarding (see HOARDING BEHAVIOUR) minimizes future food shortages. Costs of storage consist of food loss due to theft, spoilage or failure to retrieve food – FORGETTING where it is. Cache site selection and optimal cache spacing may minimize theft. Food may be cached in areas where robbers are infrequent or cannot gain access to food. By broadly dispersing cache sites – SCATTER HOARDING – food loss is minimized. Behavioural experiments with food-storing birds have shown that MEMORY facilitates cache retrieval. Similar to the case with mammals, lesions of the avian HIPPOCAMPUS result in a reduction in cache recovery.

See also: foraging; optimal foraging theory

DONALD M. WILKIE

footshock A commonly used AVERSIVE STIMULUS for research on aversive or stressful conditions (see STRESS). Electric shocks of various types have been employed to induce a stress response and also to produce aversive CONDITIONING. Footshocks are usually applied by electrification of the grid floor in a test chamber; the shock is delivered when the animal completes the circuit between different poles of the electrified grid. The amount of shock delivered varies substantially depending upon the species. In rats, values of 0.2 – 1.0 mA are often used. It is of interest to note though that, while footshock is generally considered aversive, there have been instances in which animals have been trained to shock themselves, the shock apparently providing POSITIVE REINFORCEMENT. One should not forget that the aversive and rewarding qualities of stimuli are not intrinsic properties, but are perceptions of stimulus quality that can change according to different circumstances.

Reference

Kelleher R.T. and Morse W.H. (1968) Schedules using noxious stimuli. I. Responding maintained with response-produced electric shocks. *Journal of the Experimental Analysis of Behaviour* II: 819–838.

JOHN D. SALAMONE

foraging Activities involved in the location and ingestion of food. Behaviours involved in locating food consist of search, pursuit and capture. Foragers may pursue their prey for long distances or adopt 'sit-and-wait' search. Food may be consumed where it is captured or carried back to a fixed central site for immediate consumption or storage – HOARDING BEHAVIOUR. Many insects, birds and mammals forage in groups while others forage alone. Group foraging may have evolved to minimize predation risk when foraging, to limit intruder access, or to facilitate capture of large prey items thereby maximizing the rate of food energy intake.

See also: food-storing birds; maps; optimal foraging theory

DONALD M. WILKIE

foramen lacerum (from Latin, *foramen*: aperture) The lacerated foramen, at the base of the SKULL adjacent to the OPTIC CHIASM, where the INTERNAL CAROTID ARTERIES (see BLOOD) enter the brain.

foramen magnum (from Latin, *foramen*: aperture) The large opening at the base of the SKULL, where the SPINAL CORD enters the cranial cavity. The vertebral arteries (see BLOOD) also pass through here.

foramen of Magendie *see* meninges; ventricles

foramen of Monro *see* ventricles

foramina of Lushka *see* meninges

forced choice alternation Forced choice alternation is a simple test of SPATIAL MEMORY. It is a simple procedure in which animals are required to alternate choices, having first been forced into one particular choice. For example, in a T MAZE, a barrier can be placed in one arm of the cross bar of the T, such that when an animal comes along the stem of the T to the choice point, it is forced to go one way to collect a simple REWARD. (This has been called the *information run*.) On the next trial the barrier is removed and the animal, on arriving at the choice point has to alternate from the forced choice – that is, to enter the previously blocked arm in order to collect the reward. (This has been called the *test run*.)

See also: spontaneous alternation

forebrain Also known as the PROSENCEPHALON, the forebrain is the most rostral part of the brain. It consists of the CEREBRAL HEMISPHERES (TELENCEPHALON) and the underlying DIENCEPHALON. The superficial part of the cerebral hemispheres represents the CEREBRAL CORTEX. The ventral part of the cerebral hemisphere is composed of the BASAL GANGLIA, including the CAUDATE NUCLEUS, PUTAMEN and GLOBUS PALLIDUS, which are concerned with control of automatic movements. The inner ring of the cerebral hemispheres represents the LIMBIC SYSTEM, which is concerned with emotional behaviours (see EMOTION). The diencephalon consists of the THALAMUS and HYPOTHALAMUS, which are involved in sensory transmission and AUTONOMIC and LIMBIC functions, respectively.

KAZUE SEMBA

forebrain commissures Those commissural systems that are involved in cortical transfer of information in the FOREBRAIN.

See also: anterior commissure; corpus callosum

foreign accent syndrome A rare disorder of speech, first described by Pick in 1919, distinguished by having no impairment in the production of speech or the structure of LANGUAGE: it is the accent in which language is produced that changes. Four principal features have been described: (1) the new accent is considered foreign by the speaker; (2) it is different from the accent adopted before brain injury (though in some cases there is evidence of patients having been exposed to the new accent prior to the onset of the disorder); (3) there will be evidence of structural damage to the brain (though there is no consistent location – cortical and subcortical damage has been reported); and (4) there need be no evidence of the speaker having been fluent in a foreign language.

See also: aphasia; speech production

Reference

Whitaker H. (1982) Levels of impairment in disorders of speech. In *Neuropsychology and Cognition*, vol. 1 (NATO Advanced Study Institute series D, no. 9), ed. R.N. Malatesha & L.C. Hartlage, pp. 168–207, Nijhoff: The Hague.

forgetting Forgetting refers to the inability to recall previously learned information (see LEARNING). There are two major theories of forgetting. According to the first, all learned information is permanently stored in the brain. Inability to RECALL is the result of RETRIEVAL defects but not storage problems. The theory holds that if the person is given the correct retrieval cues, any item can be remembered. On a biological level, this could occur if there was damage to the brain's MEMORY retrieval systems but not the ENGRAM itself. The second major theory of forgetting holds that forgetting occurs as a result of the actual loss of the MEMORY TRACE. When this occurs, the memory can never be reactivated, no matter how good retrieval cues are given. Possible causes of this loss of storage are improper ENCODING, damage, newer memory representations changing the storage of older memories to the point where they can no longer become activated, and loss due to lack of reactivation. It is currently impossible to determine which of these two theories is correct, but both types of processes probably occur. There are many factors that influence the forgetting process. One of the most important factors is time since encoding: newer memories are more susceptible to loss than older ones (see CONSOLIDATION). Rehearsing (see REHEARSAL) information dramatically decreases the likelihood that it will be forgotten. The depth of initial encoding also influences later memory recall. Providing multiple, specific retrieval cues can increase the likelihood that an item will be remembered. Items are also more likely to be remembered if the organism is in the same cognitive state at the time of retrieval as it was during encoding STATE-DEPENDENT LEARNING. The organism's emotional state (see EMOTION) at the time of encoding can also dramatically impact future memory capabilities. In some circumstances traumatic experiences such as rape can cause someone to forget the event, and sometimes they can cause a person to form vivid recollections of certain aspects of the occurrence. Finally, while forgetting may initially seem like a completely undesirable process, the loss of memories can be adaptive. If nothing was ever forgotten, it could become harder to abstract across situations to make generalizations and to form concepts since it would be easy to get lost in the memory of irrelevant details. Forgetting could also allow neurons that had been representing unused information to represent frequently recalled memories more accurately.

See also: amnesia; catastrophic interference;

retrieval induced forgetting; retrograde amnesia; Ribot's law

HOWARD EICHENBAUM

formaldehyde *see* fixation

formalin *see* fixation

formalin test of pain The formalin test of PAIN was developed to model in rodents the pain induced by an acute injury. It involves making a small subcutaneous injection of dilute FORMALIN into the plantar (bottom) surface of one forepaw. A system of rating the behaviours produced by this (including elevation of the treated paw, licking the paw, time spent touching the floor and so on) has been developed to measure the biphasic responses to formalin injection. The fact that responses are biphasic (a short-term response of up to 10 minutes and a longer-term one lasting 40 to 60 minutes) indicates activation of more than one process. This test is self-evidently not pleasant, and is subject to appropriate legislation (by the Home Office in the United Kingdom for example). However, with any test of pain in experimental animals, it has to be borne in mind that pain is not a well-understood phenomenon and that the management of chronic pain in humans and animals is a major challenge to modern medical and veterinary science.

See also: gate control theory of pain

Reference

Abbot F.V., Franklin K.B.J. & Westbrook R.F. (1995) The formalin test: scoring properties of first and second phases of the pain response in rats. *Pain* 60: 91–102.

formant frequencies (from Latin, *formare*: to form) Speech sounds, especially the sounds of vowels, display peaks in spectral energy at particular sound frequencies: these are known as formant frequencies.

See also: auditory perception; speech perception; speech production

formula weight (FW) The weight of a substance without the WATER OF CRYSTALLIZATION; the formula weight plus the water of crystallization gives the MOLECULAR WEIGHT.

fornix A major fibre bundle arising from the HIPPOCAMPUS and SUBICULUM. It contains axons of PYRAMIDAL NEURONS from these regions, as well as afferent or incoming fibres to the HIPPOCAMPAL FORMATION. The body of the fornix travels forward under the CORPUS CALLOSUM, and then separates into two branches of equal size. The precommissural fornix, located anterior to the ANTERIOR COMMISSURE, terminates mainly in the SEPTAL NUCLEI, while the postcommissural fornix courses through the HYPOTHALAMUS to terminate in the MAMMILLARY BODY. The postcommissural fornix primarily contains EFFERENT fibres from the subiculum, rather than the hippocampus.

See also: fimbria; limbic system

KAZUE SEMBA

forskolin A drug that stimulates ADENYLATE CYCLASE activity.

fortification spectra *see* migraine

forward conditioning The standard procedures used in PAVLOVIAN CONDITIONING – the CONDITIONED STIMULUS (CS) precedes the UNCONDITIONED STIMULUS (US) in contrast to BACKWARD CONDITIONING; see CONDITIONED INHIBITION; DELAY CONDITIONING.

Fourier analysis Fourier analysis (or Fourier transformation) is named after Jean Baptiste Joseph Fourier (1768–1830) who derived a proof that all waveforms could be decomposed into individual elements (sine and cosine waves). Fourier analysis can be applied by an experimenter interested in investigating psychophysical phenomena (see PSYCHOPHYSICS) and such decomposition analysis is also performed naturally. For example optic and auditory information is decomposed into elements by the RETINA and COCHLEA respectively.

See also: spatial frequency channels; hearing theories

fourth ventricle *see* ventricles

fovea The central region of the RETINA is the area with the highest density of PHOTORECEPTORS. In humans the region exclusively contains CONES and lacks the RODS associated with scotopic vision (vision at low light levels).

The region is marked by a yellowish pigment that lends the fovea the alternative name of MACULA LUTEA. The cone-rich region contains a pit or 'fovea' which is about 5° in diameter, with a central region (the fovea centralis or FOVEOLA) subtending 1° approximately, containing the smallest diameter photoreceptors in the eye. Behaviourally, the fovea is the area with the highest visual ACUITY and is the region of the retina that an observer turns towards an object in order to inspect it. In normal vision it is the part of the eye that is used for fixation or foveation (see FIXATION POINT).

DAVID W. HEELEY

foveola (fovea centralis) *see* fixation point; fovea

fragile X syndrome A chromosome abnormality in which the X chromosome is, literally, fragile, and can break into two separate parts (see CHROMOSOME ABNORMALITIES; CHROMOSOMES). After DOWN SYNDROME, it is the most frequent chromosome abnormality. It is caused by a single defective gene, possessed by as many as one in 260 women. Estimates suggest that some 1 in 2000 boys and 1 in 4000 girls are affected by it. In both male and female cases, fragile X tends to produce individuals with the following typical features: large underdeveloped ears, long thin faces, broad noses; males also tend to have enlarged testicles. Females may show no outward features of fragile X but their children may still be at risk of inheriting the disorder. More pressing, most males and about one-third of females with fragile X show a degree of MENTAL RETARDATION and other disorders, including AUTISM, which may be quite severe, or may be milder, with limited LANGUAGE and speech difficulties.

See also: X and Y chromosomes

fraternal twins *see* dizygotic twins

free nerve ending A FIBRES and C FIBRES have been thought to terminate in sensory endings known as free nerve endings. These have been suggested to lack organized structure. This is however unlikely to be the case and it is believed that the endings of A and C fibres are in fact more specialized than has previously

been thought: 'free nerve endings' is therefore something of a misnomer.

See also: pain

free radicals A free radical is an atom or MOLECULE which contains an unpaired ELECTRON, rendering it highly reactive. In order to achieve a stable state, a free radical will react with another molecule or atom, resulting in altered state or function of both entities. Free radicals exist both as entities created with a function and as byproducts of reactions. For example, the free radical NITRIC OXIDE is a highly diffusable messenger molecule, found in many tissues throughout the body. However, uncontrolled production of free radicals may lead to pathological alterations in cell function in neurodegenerative conditions such as PARKINSON'S DISEASE.

FIONA M. INGLIS

free recall Procedure used in humans to examine the ability to consciously recollect (see CONSCIOUS RECOLLECTION) information from MEMORY without the aid of specific cues. In a typical set-up, individuals are instructed to memorize a list of items (see LIST LEARNING). Immediately after learning or subsequent to a delay (see DELAYED RECALL), they are asked to generate (that is, to recall) as many items from the list as possible in any order. Free recall differs from other RETRIEVAL tasks, such as CUED RECALL and RECOGNITION, in which additional retrieval cues are provided. It also differs from SERIAL RECALL, a retrieval task that requires recall of previously encountered items in the exact order in which they were presented.

See also: declarative memory; episodic memory; explicit memory

STEFAN KÖHLER

free running rhythm An ENDOGENOUS RHYTHM that expresses a periodicity different from its corresponding environmental cycle under constant conditions. The existence of free running CIRCADIAN RHYTHMS in the physiology and behaviour of most organisms is the strongest evidence that daily rhythms are generated by an internal clock mechanism, and only entrained (see ENTRAINMENT) by external cues. Other biological rhythms that have been demonstrated to free run in some species include tidal and annual rhythms (see BIOLOGICAL CLOCK). The period (length) of a free running rhythm is genetically determined but modifiable by previous experience, especially by the history of entrainment to different lighting patterns.

BENJAMIN RUSAK

freebasing The act of smoking the freebase of a DRUG, usually in reference to freebase COCAINE. Cocaine normally is extracted and produced in its salt, powdered form, cocaine hydrochloride (HCl). However with minor chemical modification it can be converted into its pure, solid freebase form. This form, which is known as CRACK COCAINE is smoked, and results in the drug getting to the brain much faster, and in a much more intense, but short-lasting EUPHORIA ('high'). Other drugs of abuse are also sometimes smoked in the free-base form, such as AMPHETAMINE ('ice') and HEROIN.

ANN E. KELLEY

freeze fracture Literally, freezing tissue and fracturing it. Scanning ELECTRON MICROSCOPY is then used to examine the fractured tissue surface. The point of freeze fracture is that tissue (or indeed anything else) will break under pressure along the line of least resistance – the weakest point. What is produced is an edge that retains the normal 3-dimensional structure, as opposed to cut tissue, which presents a smooth edge. Examination of this edge allows one therefore to understand the geometry of tissue better. Freeze fractured tissue tends to be unstable and does not store well.

freezing see aggression

Fregoli's syndrome A form of DELUSIONAL MISIDENTIFICATION in which patients believe that other people have had their bodies replaced by the bodies of others, though the mind of the original person remains unchanged within the new body: strangers are assumed to contain the minds of other people known to the patient. It is associated with schizophrenia.

See also: Capgras syndrome; delusional misidentification

frequency The term frequency is encountered in everyday talk with reference to the number of times that something repeats or recurs; in PSYCHOPHYSICS, frequency is used to indicate the number of vibrations of cycles per unit time – it typically refers to the intervals between peaks in a waveform.

Friedrich's ataxia see ataxia

frog skin poison Many South and Central American frogs – typically tiny (around 2 cm long) and vividly coloured – have poisons in their SKIN, typically present over all the skin rather than in localized patches. The poisons serve to protect the frogs (as SPECIES) from predation. The skin of many frogs and toads contain chemicals that can cause HALLUCINATIONS, but the skin of poison dart frogs (of which there are many different species) contains a poison that can cause CONVULSIONS, PARALYSIS and eventually death (which is why native peoples have used the skin poisons, carefully collected, to tip darts and arrows used for hunting). The poison is an alkaloid, EPIBATIDINE, which the frogs synthesize from dietary components (see ALKALOIDS). Laboratory analysis has shown that it has an action at NICOTINIC ACETYLCHOLINE RECEPTORS and is a potent analgesic. While epibatidine itself cannot be used therapeutically, derivatives appear likely to be useful analgesic agents.

frontal bone see skull

frontal cortex The CEREBRAL CORTEX is divided into four lobes based on structural landmarks. Thus frontal cortex and the FRONTAL LOBE are the same thing. The term FRONTAL CORTEX has sometimes been used to refer only to granular areas of the frontal lobe (that is, the frontal cortex excluding the MOTOR CORTEX and PREMOTOR CORTEX – see AGRANULAR CORTEX) but such usage is ambiguous and therefore not preferred.

VERITY J. BROWN

frontal eye fields Regions of the FRONTAL CORTEX which, when stimulated electrically, elicit eye movements of the SACCADE type. It is thought that this is the region of the brain that controls voluntary GAZE.

DAVID W. HEELEY

frontal lobe In each HEMISPHERE, the CERE-BRAL CORTEX is divided into four lobes, named after the cranial bones (see SKULL) overlying the cortex. If present in a given species, the CENTRAL SULCUS is the anatomical landmark that defines the posterior extent of the frontal lobe. In species with LISSENCEPHALIC brains, the boundary of frontal cortex must be defined functionally as the boundary between PRIMARY MOTOR CORTEX and PRIMARY SOMATOSENSORY CORTEX.

As with the other lobes of the brain, within the frontal lobes are areas of primary, secondary and association cortex. In the human brain, primary motor cortex is anterior to the central sulcus in the PRECENTRAL GYRUS. Secondary motor cortex (PREMOTOR CORTEX, SUPPLEMENTARY MOTOR CORTEX) occupies the cortex adjacent and rostral to primary motor cortex. The most anterior and the largest portion of the human frontal lobe is higher-order association cortex (PREFRONTAL CORTEX and LIMBIC CORTEX), which can be divided into many functionally distinct sub-regions and includes, for example, BROCA'S AREA. LIMBIC ASSOCIATION CORTEX, which includes ORBITOFRONTAL CORTEX, occupies the ventral and medial aspect of the frontal lobe, but also extends to other cortical lobes, all of which is sometimes referred to collectively as the LIMBIC LOBE. However, as the definition of the four cortical lobes is based on structural landmarks, in contrast to the definition of the limbic lobe, which is based on connectivity and function, it is not, strictly speaking, equivalent to a lobe. There is a hierarchical organization of projections within the frontal lobe, with prefrontal and limbic association areas receiving projections from areas of sensory association cortex in the other lobes. Limbic association cortex projects to prefrontal cortex, which projects to secondary motor cortex, which in turn projects to primary motor cortex.

The frontal lobes control motor output. This is most obviously true of primary motor cortex, which projects directly to the SPINAL CORD (though the bulk of cortical motor output makes synaptic contact with subcortical brain tissue – the BASAL GANGLIA, PONS and MEDULLA for example). It is also true of secondary motor cortex, which is active in response preparation: lesions here impair bimanual co-ordination, response sequencing and other complex motor acts. The functions of the prefrontal cortex are more difficult to define, in part because prefrontal cortex is large and heterogeneous with different functions being associated with different portions of prefrontal cortex. The influence of prefrontal cortex on motor output is perhaps better characterized as response, rather than motor, control. Broca's area is involved in SPEECH PRODUCTION. DORSOLATERAL PREFRONTAL CORTEX is involved in WORKING MEMORY (which may or may not have a spatial component, different areas of prefrontal cortex being implicated accordingly), response planning and response flexibility. Patients with frontal lobe lesions often show disinhibition of responses. Deficits on the WISCONSIN CARD-SORT TEST are typical following damage to prefrontal cortex, characterized by an increase in perseverative responses (see PERSEVERATION). Limbic association cortex is thought to be part of the system wherein information relating to MOTIVATION can influence response output, with damage to orbitofrontal cortex being associated with changes in emotional reactivity and personality (see EMOTION; SOMATIC MARKER HYPOTHESIS). Nevertheless, the definition of the frontal lobe is structural rather than functional and so it is not reasonable to talk about the function of the frontal lobes in anything other than very general terms.

See also: Phineas Gage

VERITY J. BROWN

frontal lobotomy *see* psychosurgery

frontal syndrome A constellation of deficits that occur after damage to the FRONTAL LOBE (especially the PREFRONTAL CORTEX): principal effects are the disinhibition of behaviour; the production of inappropriate behaviour; and PERSEVERATION. Effects such as these are seen after various forms of damage to the frontal lobes, including frontal LOBOTOMY. It is not a generally preferred term however. Terms such as disinhibition can be applied to a very wide range of SIGNS AND SYMPTOMS and as such is not tremendously useful. Moreover, increasing awareness of the anatomical complexity of the frontal lobes and a better ability to specify in close detail what cognitive processes they are involved in has led to better diagnosis. The prefrontal cortex is generally held now to be involved in EXECUTIVE FUNCTIONS, and the term DYSEXECUTIVE SYNDROME is now often used to describe the effects of frontal damage (as well as damage to other parts of the brain).

See also: Phineas Gage

Reference

Ogden J.A. (1996) *Fractured Minds: A Case Study Approach to Clinical Neuropsychology*, Oxford University Press: New York.

fructose (from Latin, *fructus*: fruit) Fruit sugar; a MONOSACCHARIDE sugar. One molecule of fructose combined with one molecule of GLUCOSE makes the DISACCHARIDE sugar SUCROSE.

See also: sugars

fruit fly *see Drosophila*

fugal; petal These are suffixes: *fugal* is from the Latin, *fugere*, to flee; *petal* is from the Latin, *petere*, to seek. They indicate direction: if something is described as fugal it involves movement away, while petal describes movement towards. Thus centrifugal is movement away from the centre, SOMATOFUGAL, movement away from a body. Centripetal is movement towards the centre, SOMATOPETAL movement towards a body.

fugue (from Latin, *fuga*: flight) In music a fugue is a composition in which the principal subject is initiated by one part but then taken up by a second part while the first part switches to accompaniment. In biological psychology, fugue is a form of DISSOCIATIVE DISORDER. Control of the MUSCLES is intact but CONSCIOUSNESS is at best opaque, leading sufferers to wander aimlessly without awareness of what they are doing, where they are, or even who they are. Sufferers are often incoherent during the fugue state (which typically lasts for hours, but may last for days) and typically fail to remember anything of what has hap-

pened to them when they recover. There is disagreement as to whether this condition is associated with EPILEPSY or with other disorders; an older literature associated it with HYSTERIA (though this term is not now generally used).

functional magnetic resonance imaging *see* fMRI

functional mentalism *see* monism

functional neuroimaging Functional neuroimaging refers to the use of non-invasive brain imaging methods to localize neural activity in the human brain related to the engagement of specific mental functions. Such methods have been in use since the late 1980s to investigate the brain regions activated by sensory, motor and cognitive processing in healthy subjects and departures from normal patterns of activation in cases of neurological or psychiatric illness. Functional neuroimaging studies are an important complement to other approaches to understanding brain function, such as the neuropsychological (see NEUROPSYCHOLOGY) investigation of the effects of BRAIN INJURY in humans, and experimental studies of brain function in animals.

The two most important functional neuroimaging methods are POSITRON EMISSION TOMOGRAPHY (PET), which came into use in the mid-1980s, and FUNCTIONAL MAGNETIC RESONANCE IMAGING (fMRI), which was introduced approximately a decade later. Although differing in several important respects the two methods share one important feature, which is that with neither method is neural activity detected directly. Instead, the methods take advantage of the fact that neural activity and blood flow in the normal brain are closely coupled, such that within a few seconds, a change in activity triggers a concomitant change in flow. Thus, if an experimental manipulation has an effect on the net level of neural activity in a given brain region, the effect will be detected as a change in blood flow through that region. It is important to note that changes in the pattern of neural activity in a neural population, rather than in its overall level, will not be accompanied by changes in flow, and thus cannot be detected by PET or fMRI.

The principal goal of functional neuroimaging studies is to identify brain regions in which neural activity is associated selectively with a specific psychological function, such as COLOUR VISION or CONSCIOUS RECOLLECTION, and thereby to identify the regions that support such functions. Typically, this goal is achieved by obtaining functional images during psychological tasks which have been designed to engage the psychological function or functions of interest. An image of the distribution of blood flow or oxygenation obtained during a single experimental task is, however, impossible to interpret, as there is no means of distinguishing between regions in which activity is task-specific, and regions in which it is non-specific. Hence the general experimental strategy in functional neuroimaging studies is to compare images obtained in at least two experimental conditions. In the simplest experimental design, sometimes called the subtraction method, two conditions are employed, a baseline and a task condition. These conditions are designed to make equivalent demands upon sensory and cognitive processes, with the exception of the specific function of experimental interest, which is engaged in the task condition only. Because all other factors are held constant, any differences in the images obtained between the baseline and task conditions can be ascribed to the function of interest. The subtraction method is predicated on a number of key assumptions about the relationship between different cognitive functions which are not always met, and is limited in the range of experimental designs to which it is applicable. More complex experimental designs exist which overcome these problems (see Frith & Friston, 1997).

See also: computerized axial tomography; metabolic mapping

Reference

Frith C.D. & Friston K.J. (1997) Studying brain function with neuroimaging. In *Cognitive Neuroscience*, ed. M.D. Rugg, pp. 169–195, Psychology Press: Hove UK.

MICHAEL D. RUGG

fundamental frequency (Also referred to simply as the FUNDAMENTAL.) The lowest frequency present in a complex sound; see PITCH.

fungiform papillae *see* taste buds

funny bone *see* tingle

fusiform gyrus (from Latin, *fusus*: spindle, *forma*: shape) Fusiform is a general term meaning spindle shaped – fatter in the middle than at either end. The fusiform gyrus is a GYRUS of the ventromedial TEMPORAL LOBE: tissue around here is known to be important in FACE PERCEPTION.

fuzzy logic A means for dealing with the vagueness of the world. Classical logic asserts that objects belong to sets and follow what was called by Aristotle 'the law of the excluded middle' – that is, an object belongs to one set or another, there being no middle ground. A number for example, is either odd or even: there are no degrees of 'oddness' or 'evenness'. Computers deal effectively with classical logic, using precise statements and binary codes. But in the real world, things are more vague than this. Kosko & Isaka (1993) use the example of temperature: air may be cool, just right or warm. A set in classical logic would have to define precisely and exclusively what constituted the set 'warm air'. Fuzzy sets in contrast blend into each other: air may be 20% cool and 80% not cool – fuzziness is the degree to which a condition appears. This is not the same thing as a statement of probability (that is, there is a 20% chance that it will be cool) but a description of the present state: the air *is* 20% cool *and* 80% not cool.

Fuzzy logic is being used increasingly in the development of machines that can control such things as heaters and tumble-driers, using the operators 'if' and 'then'. (For example, *if* the air is too cool *then* set the heater higher, using sliding scales to produce varying degrees of warm and cool.) NEURAL NETWORKS can be used to help fuzzy systems learn rules. In biological psychology, fuzzy logic may prove helpful in a number of ways. For example, they may provide a valuable means for describing how bodies regulate their internal environments. Traditionally, descriptions of FEEDING and DRINKING have relied on biological SET POINTS: if measurement of some body chemical falls below a certain level it will trigger an appropriate corrective action. But measures of ENERGY BALANCE, OSMOREGULATION and TEM-

PERATURE may better be described in fuzzy terms. Rather than suggesting that energy or water intake falls simply into two sets, 'enough' and 'not enough' a fuzzy analysis would enable one to describe degrees of 'enoughness' that might better account for patterns of food and water intake.

See also: homeostasis

Reference

Kosko B. & Isaka S. (1993) Fuzzy logic. *Scientific American* 269: 62–67.

fuzzy set *see* fuzzy logic

G

G protein A family of membrane PROTEINS that play a critical role in transmembrane signalling in the nervous system. G proteins, of which there are several forms, are named for their ability to bind small molecules called GUANINE NUCLEOTIDES, such as GUANINE TRIPHOSPHATE (GTP). In most synaptic transmission, two events occur when an external signal (such as a neurotransmitter or sensory stimulus) has an effect on cellular function. First, the external signal binds to its receptor on the outside of the neuronal membrane. When this occurs, GTP binds to the G protein on the internal surface of the membrane, which is linked to the RECEPTOR, thus making it active. Activation of the G protein regulates the levels of SECOND MESSENGERS, which in turn control the cascade of intracellular events ultimately leading to the cell's physiological response. There are two main types of G proteins: stimulatory G proteins (G_s), which activate transduction and inhibitory G proteins (G_i), which inhibit transduction. The G protein can also be directly coupled to an ION CHANNEL; in this case the activational state of the G protein regulates the permeability of certain ion channels. Although G proteins play many roles in cellular function, among their best known roles is controlling the intracellular levels of the second messenger CYCLIC AMP.

See also: inositol; neurotransmitters

ANN E. KELLEY

GABA (Gamma aminobutyric acid or γ-aminobutyric acid) GABA is the most important of the inhibitory NEUROTRANSMITTERS in the brain (though there are others, including GLYCINE). The term GABAERGIC is used to describe a neuron that contains GABA. About one-third of the synapses in the brain appear to use GABA as their neurotransmitter. It is synthesized from GLUTAMATE, a reaction catalysed by GLUTAMIC ACID DECARBOXYLASE and broken down by GABA aminotransferase to succinic semialdehyde, which is further broken down to SUCCINATE, a reaction catalyzed by succinic semialdehyde dehydrogenase. It is stored in VESICLES prior to release and, following CALCIUM dependent release, there are high affinity REUPTAKE mechanisms to remove it from the synaptic cleft. GABAergic neurons are found virtually in all regions of the CENTRAL NERVOUS SYSTEM, including INTERNEURONS as well as PROJECTION NEURONS such as PURKINJE CELLS in the CEREBELLUM. GABA is found in very few places outside the central nervous system: the PANCREAS has the highest concentration outside the CNS.

KAZUE SEMBA

GABA receptors GABA (gamma aminobutyric acid) RECEPTORS are divided into three classes: A, B and C. The GABA-A receptor is very complex, composed of five subunits, and containing a CHLORIDE channel, estimated to be about 5 nm in diameter. There are multiple BINDING SITES on the GABA-A receptors: sites for GABA obviously exist, but there are also sites for BENZODIAZEPINE drugs, steroids, BARBITURATES and a site biding the drug PICROTOXIN. MUSCIMOL is the most frequently used AGONIST at the GABA-A receptor; BICUCUL-

LINE is the most commonly used ANTAGONIST. Bicuculline is a competitive antagonist (see COMPETITIVE–NONCOMPETITIVE BINDING); picrotoxin is a non-competitive antagonist that blocks the chloride channel. GABA-A receptors are present widely throughout the CENTRAL NERVOUS SYSTEM. GABA-B receptors, which also mediate HYPERPOLARIZATION, were discriminated from GABA-A by their insensitivity to bicuculline. The principal antagonist at these receptors is not this but BACLOFEN. GABA-B receptors appear to exist both pre- and postsynaptically and have a different distribution through the brain compared to GABA-A receptors. GABA-C receptors are less well characterized than either the A or B variants. They mediate potent inhibition when stimulated by GABA and contain a chloride channel. However, these receptors appear not to be affected by benzodiazepines, barbiturates or steroids.

See also: epilepsy; sedative

Reference

Feldman R.S., Meyer J.S. & Quenzer L.F. (1997) *Principles of Neuropsychopharmacology*, Sinauer Associates: Sunderland MA.

GABA transaminase *see* GABA

GABAergic Relating to the neurotransmitter GABA. For instance, a NEURON that synthesizes and releases GABA is said to be GABAergic.

Gage *see* Phineas Gage

gait The regular pattern of walking. Gait has been rigorously investigated by theorists interested in the control of movement, given the precise, reliable nature of the patterns of muscular contraction. Early models suggested that stages of the gait pattern were driven in a feedback manner by the earlier components, such that once the gait sequence was initiated each sub-movement occurred at the correct time because the pattern is effectively a chain of reflexes. These models have been replaced by MOTOR PROGRAMMING theories, which suggest that some central mechanism contains information about the sequencing and timing of the sub-movements required.

See also: locomotion

DAVID P. CAREY

galanin A neuropeptide transmitter: one specific G PROTEIN coupled RECEPTOR type has been identified (GAL1), and galanin has been associated with the control of FAT intake; see G PROTEIN; PARAVENTRICULAR NUCLEUS OF THE HYPOTHALAMUS.

gallamine A synthetic form of CURARE, marketed as Flaxedil.

gallbladder *see* digestive system

Gallyas silver A stain for MYELIN.

See also: chemical neuroanatomy; glial cells

galvanic skin response *see* skin conductance

gametes Cells produced by MEIOSIS (see CELL DIVISION), which are HAPLOID in nature, which are combined in sexual reproduction in order to produce one DIPLOID offspring. In mammals, these cells are sperm and eggs.

FIONA M. INGLIS

gamma aminobutyric acid *see* GABA

gamma motor neuron *see* muscle spindle

ganglion (plural, ganglia) A collection of neurons (see NEURON). Ganglia are found in many places: examples include the BASAL GANGLIA (within the CENTRAL NERVOUS SYSTEM); within the AUTONOMIC NERVOUS SYSTEM; and in invertebrates lacking an organized CNS. In medicine, ganglion also refers to a tumour within a tendon sheath.

ganglion cells These are the output NEURONS of the RETINA. PHOTORECEPTORS (RODS and CONES) in the retina contact the ganglion cells via BIPOLAR CELLS and HORIZONTAL CELLS in the plexiform layer of the retina (see RETINAL CELL LAYERS). In the primate retina there are two types of ganglion cell: M (or Pα) and P (or Pβ). M cells have large RECEPTIVE FIELDS and are responsive to gross features of a stimulus and movement. P cells are smaller and involved in COLOUR VISION. Both types have been implicated in the resolution of fine detail, though P cells appear to be more involved in this than M. The receptive fields of both types of ganglion cell are circular with a centre and an antagonistic surround: they can be on-centre or off-centre (these terms describing whether or not light applied to the centres turns the cells on or off). The on-centre and off-centre neurons send information in parallel along two channels within the OPTIC NERVE. Ganglion cells are always active, increasing their firing slightly to weak illumination and strongly to bright. The ability of these cells to respond to light intensity, and possession of distinctly organized receptive fields, enables them to detect contrast well.

See also: lateral geniculate nucleus

Reference

Kandel E.R., Schwartz J.H. & Jessell T.M. (2000) *Principles of Neural Science*, 4th edn, McGraw-Hill: New York.

ganglioside *see* lipids

gap junction This forms the basis for ELECTRICAL SYNAPSES: membranes on both sides of a gap junction have an ION CHANNEL that permits diffusion of ions directly from one neuron to another. Changes in electrical activity in one neuron, which are of course accompanied by altered ionic activity (see ACTION POTENTIAL) can be communicated to a second neuron across a gap junction.

See also: synapse

gas chromatography Analytical technique similar to HIGH PERFORMANCE LIQUID CHROMATOGRAPHY (HPLC) but which analyses gases rather than liquids.

gastric (from Greek, *gaster*: belly) An adjective indicating association with the STOMACH; see DIGESTIVE SYSTEM.

gastric acid *see* digestive system

gastric balloon Literally, a surgical balloon fitted into the stomach. When inflated it is supposed to generate feelings of SATIETY, and has been used in the management of OBESITY. It is not a technique currently in vogue; see BARIATRIC SURGERY.

gastric by-pass *see* bariatric surgery

gastric distension Literally, stretching of the stomach. It was once thought that the volume of food in the stomach was associated with feelings of HUNGER and SATIETY but this is regarded now as unlikely. Removal of the stomach does not cause dissipation of hunger

sensations. The stomach might be involved in detecting the chemical composition of its contents and this, rather than volume, might be a signal of satiety.

gastric fistula *see* fistula

gastric inhibitory peptide *see* endocrine glands; hormones

gastric stapling A reversible procedure, also known as *gastroplasty*, in which the stomach is reduced (effectively by connecting parts together) by up to 98% of its original size. Individuals who need to lose weight are operated on; following surgery they cannot consume large volumes of food. There are concerns about its safety and effectiveness; a variety of unwanted effects up to and including liver failure have been reported – and in some of the United States of America the procedure is not eligible for support by Medicaid. *Gastric banding* (or *laparoscopic banding*) is a related technique.

See also: bariatric surgery

gastrin *see* endocrine glands; hormones

gastrin releasing peptide *see* endocrine glands; hormones

gastrointestinal system The stomach and intestines; see DIGESTIVE SYSTEM.

gastrulation *see* development

gate-control theory of pain The gate-control theory of Ronald Melzack and Patrick Wall seeks to provide an explanation for the fact that PAIN intensity is not reliably related to the type or intensity of stimulation of the NOCICEPTOR, and that pain can be modified by simultaneous stimulation of other sensory systems and by the psychological state of the perceiver (see ACUPUNCTURE; PLACEBO). The theory is considered in opposition to 'specificity' theory which suggests that pain is felt when a particular class of afferent fibres is activated, and the intensity of pain is proportional to the rate of firing of these fibres. The theory is anatomical rather than abstract and depends on an interpretation of specific features of the known anatomy and physiology of sensory pathways in the SPINAL CORD. The present account outlines the theory as later modified (see Melzack & Wall, 1982) to take account of new anatomical and physiological information. Sensory afferents from the skin and deep tissues have their cell bodies in the DORSAL ROOT GANGLION and project their terminal fibres into the DORSAL HORN of the spinal cord. The dorsal horn of the spinal cord is arranged in six laminae (layers) with lamina 1 the most superficial and lamina 6 the deepest. Laminae 1 and 2 together have a distinctive appearance and are called the SUB-STANTIA GELATINOSA. Nerve fibres are divided into classes according to their size and conduction velocity. Large myelinated fibres are classed as 'A-beta', small myelinated (see MYE-LIN) as 'A-delta', and unmyelinated, which are the most numerous, as 'C'. A-beta fibres carry information about TOUCH but not pain. Pain is associated with activity in A-delta and C fibres, though the majority of A-delta and C fibres do not respond selectively to noxious stimuli. The different classes of fibres terminate in different layers so that the thickest fibres penetrate most deeply, with C fibres and the majority of A-delta fibres terminating in laminae 1 and 2. The large cells that relay incoming sensory information to higher levels of the brain are concentrated in laminae 1 and 5. Melzack & Wall call these 'T' (transmission) cells. The substantia gelatinosa (laminae 1 and 2) also contains many small cells which are stimulated by the sensory afferents and inhibit or excite the relay cells.

According to the theory, pain arises when output of the spinal cord T cells reaches a critical level which enables the T cells to drive a hypothetical 'action system' which generates the behaviour and subjective experience which we call pain. The activity of the T cells is governed by several influences including the activity of large and small afferent fibres, the activity of excitatory and inhibitory substantial gelatinosa cells, and the activity of inhibitory controls that descend in the spinal cord from higher levels of the nervous system. It is proposed that small fibres that respond to noxious stimuli excite T cells and also connect through substantia gelatinosa cells that have excitatory inputs to T cells. The large, fast-conducting fibres can activate T cells but also activate inhibitory interneurons in the substan-tia gelatinosa which damp the firing of T cells. The inhibitory interneurons are also activated by the descending inhibitory controls which can be driven, in a negative feedback loop, by the activity of the T cells themselves. Cognitive processes (that is, higher-level thought processes) activated by fast-conducting fibres are suggested to be able to modify the firing of T cells but the anatomical locus of this action is not specified. Pain, therefore, does not depend on the activation of a specific sensory system but depends on a higher-order process that integrates information from a variety of sensory systems.

The theory has had an extraordinary impact on the field of pain research and has provided a conceptual framework for investigation of a wide variety of phenomena ranging from acupuncture and the influence of MOOD on pain, to the mechanism of action of MORPHINE and drugs that provide ANALGESIA. The clinical impact of the theory is seen in the introduction of TRANSCUTANEOUS electrical nerve stimulation (TENS) as a successful treatment for several chronic pain states, and the introduction of the technique of administering OPIOIDS directly into the space around the spinal cord to control pain (EPIDURAL ANALGESIA). Though many of the tenets on which the theory is based are now widely accepted, the theory has been controversial as a neurological hypothesis. The idea that spinal sensory relay cells are subject to local and descending influences is now universally accepted, but the mechanisms proposed by Melzack & Wall have been disputed. In particular, it has been argued that the theory is incorrect in rejecting the idea that pain is associated with activity in sensory afferents specifically sensitive to noxious stimuli. Also, the proposal that the activity of large afferent fibres inhibits transmission from small afferents in the spinal cord dorsal horn while small fibre activity facilitates it, is not consistently supported by experimental results.

References

Melzack R. & Wall P. (1965) Pain mechanisms: a new theory. *Science* 150: 971–979.
—— (1997) *The Challenge of Pain*, Basic Books: New York.

KEITH B. J. FRANKLIN

gating In biological psychology, a *gate* is a process whose output depends on there being two or more inputs combined appropriately. For example, the term *and gate* is used to indicate a system that is activated only if two independent inputs are present (input one *and* input two). Gating is a term used therefore to describe the interaction of two or more stimuli. It implies that one STIMULUS can block another – as in the GATE-CONTROL THEORY OF PAIN – or that two stimuli interact and modify each other. In this sense it has been suggested that constructs such as DRIVE and INCENTIVE gate each other: higher levels of drive are needed if incentive is low, and vice versa.

Gaussian A Gaussian curve is a smooth mathematical function, of which the bell-shaped curve familiar in distribution statistics is a common example. The Gaussian curve is completely described by just two parameters (the mean and the dispersion). It is often used in visual experiments to taper smoothly the brightness or contrast of patterns employed in psychophysical experiments and displayed on computer-driven display monitors.

DAVID W. HEELEY

gavage (from French, *gaver*: a bird's crop) Gavage is FEEDING by passage of nutrients via a tube inserted into the oesophagous or stomach. It refers also to a procedure for administering other substances, most notably various types of DRUG. While it has the virtue of mimicking the oral route of drug administration typically employed by humans for delivery of therapeutic agents (in so far as the drug is present in the stomach and diffuses into the BLOOD from there) it is not a commonly used technique.

gaze To gaze is to look fixedly at something; direction of gaze is determined by EYE POSITION and maintained by eye movements (see also SACCADE and VERGENCE). The GAZE contingent paradigm is a measure of the duration of perception (see SENSATION VS. PERCEPTION). It works by having a subject read a passage of text: while this is happening letters are altered (computer technology is needed here) and measures are taken of how long it takes the subjects concentration on READING to break.

PSYCHIC PARALYSIS OF GAZE is an alternative name for BALINT'S SYNDROME.

gel electrophoresis A technique for separating and analysing NUCLEIC ACIDS (often DNA, to which ethidium bromide is added to aid visualization) or PROTEINS on the basis of molecular size and electrical charge. The gels are matrices made of agarose or polyacylamide, with channels running through that are the size of the MOLECULE concerned. If an electrical field is applied to the gel (negative pole at the edge where the sample is placed, positive pole on the side opposite) the molecules will migrate across the field (nucleic acids carrying a negative charge). Smaller chain nucleic acids move faster than longer and so they are graded through the gel by size. Previous determination of which nucleic acids are found where in the gel, by use of standards to map their distribution, allows one to determine the content of a sample of material.

See also: blotting; DNA fingerprinting

gelasmus (from Greek, *gelaein*: to laugh) Involuntary hysterical LAUGHTER; see GELASTIC SEIZURE.

gelastic seizure A form of EPILEPSY (also known as *gelastic epilepsy*) in which there is involuntary LAUGHTER (GELASMUS). It is uncertain whether the laughter is produced by simple stimulation of facial motor pathways, or by the content of the AURA associated with the seizure.

Geller–Seifter conflict An instrumental CONFLICT TEST, named after its originators, whereby an instrumental response randomly produces either a REINFORCER that is appetitive or an AVERSIVE STIMULUS such as FOOTSHOCK.

See also: animal models of anxiety; aversive conditioning; instrumental conditioning; Vogel conflict

A. SIMON KILLCROSS

gender (i) *Linguistics*: Mutually exclusive formal grammatical categories into which languages may separate nouns.

(ii) *Biology*: The genetic sex of an individual as female or male, revealed by genotype (that is, XX for females, XY for males, in animals). Gender is often viewed as fixed by genetic factors which stimulate STEROID HORMONES to differentiate the anatomy and physiology of the individual along gender lines during PERINATAL development. This organizational groundwork is then built upon or activated by hormones during puberty: (1) to promote the adult neuroendocrine functions of the gonads (that is, egg production in the ovaries versus spermatogenesis in the testes); (2) to generate secondary sex characteristics (such as growth of facial and body hair, muscle development and deepening of the voice in males; growth of breasts, hip widening and fat deposition in females); and (3) to act on different regions of the brain to promote patterns of release of HORMONES, behaviour or cognitive function that are sexually stereotyped (for example, LORDOSIS in females versus MOUNTING BEHAVIOUR in males). Thus, by adulthood, the gender of most individuals can be recognized by their PHENOTYPE, behavioural patterns or neuroendocrine functions. Gender, as determined by genetic sex, is not always consistent with an individual's gender identity, sex role, or sexual orientation. For example, there are cases in which genetic XY males have had their penises mutilated during postnatal circumcision. Such males are reassigned as females, given appropriate surgery to produce female external genitalia, raised as females in society, and given ESTROGEN and PROGESTERONE during and after PUBERTY to promote and maintain the growth of female secondary sex characteristics. Some of these individuals become the 'other' sex without ever knowing the truth, whereas others do not display a gender identity consistent with the reassignment. Nature also provides genetic mutations that make it difficult to determine gender. Several mutations exist in which chromosomal structure is altered, leading to ambiguous phenotypic traits. Persons can be born with XXY (KLINEFELTER'S SYNDROME), XYY, XXX (TRIPLE-X SYNDROME), XXYY, or XO (TURNER'S SYNDROME) chromosomal structures. Some are born with hermaphroditism, for example, as XX females with CONGENITAL HYPERPLAGIA of the ADRENAL GLAND that has resulted in a partial penis, partial vagina, partial uterus, and malformed ovaries. Some are born as XY males with ANDROGEN INSENSITIVITY SYNDROME that has resulted in external differentiation as a female (although such individuals are sterile). As with cases where the penis has been removed, the sex of these individuals is often reassigned. Such surgical, hormonal and social intervention can create a gender identity consistent with the external gender, but is no guarantee.

See also: feminine; organization effects of steroid hormones; sex differences; sexual differentiation; sexual dimorphism

(I) ANNE CUTLER AND (II) JAMES G. PFAUS

gender identity disorder *see* transsexualism

gender identity disorder of childhood This is a childhood condition, identified by DSM-IV as a persistent and intense desire of a child to belong to the opposite gender. In males it has been colloquially referred to as SISSY BOY SYNDROME, in girls as TOMBOY SYNDROME. Clinically, both conditions go further than what one might expect of normal degrees of boyishness in girls or girlishness in boys. In both instances, examples of gender-appropriate activities are avoided and opposite gender activities are engaged. There is some evidence for physical basis to these conditions, though it is not compelling. However, categorization of gender appropriate behaviour is very heavily loaded with value judgements and care must be taken in dealing with it. Radical therapists dismiss the whole notion of gender identity disorder in childhood, seeing it as an unacceptable form of sex-role stereotyping.

Reference

Davison G.C. & Neale J.M. (2001) *Abnormal Psychology*, 8th edn, Wiley: New York.

gene A linear segment of DEOXYRIBONUCLEIC ACID (DNA) containing a unique series of NUCLEOTIDES, which codes for the sequences of AMINO ACIDS in the PROTEINS required for CELL function. Genes are inherited by successive generations of cells and organisms, and each cell contains a full complement of an organism's genes. The gene has both coding regions, which translate directly into amino acids, and non-coding regions, including sequences used for promoting and enhancing GENE TRANSCRIPTION. When a protein such as an ENZYME is required by the cell, the gene is transcribed in order to produce a messenger ribonucleic acid (MESSENGER RNA) copy, which will be used as a template for building the protein from individual amino acids.

Although each cell in a multicellular organism contains the same genes, these cells use selective sets of genes in order to produce their PHENOTYPE, and therefore control of GENE EXPRESSION is vital to appropriate cellular function. Which genes are expressed as proteins is determined by a series of gene regulatory proteins that bind to specific sequences in the DNA called regulatory regions. These influence the binding of transcription factors and enzymes to a region of the gene called the PROMOTER, and thus influence the initiation of transcription. In a similar manner, gene expression may be up-regulated or down-regulated, depending on the events which occur in the cell, and the consequent requirement for a gene product by the cell at a given time. Variations in sequences close to the gene promoter determine the affinity of transcription factors, and therefore the rate of transcription, providing another degree of control over the rate of gene expression. In every cell, some genes known as HOUSEKEEPING GENES are required to be activated at all times in order to make proteins essential for cell survival. These have highly conserved sequences known as CONSENSUS SEQUENCES, close to the promoter, which greatly enhance the binding of transcription factors, thus ensuring gene expression. Gene expression may be further controlled at the level of mRNA, by a process called RNA EDITING, or ALTERNATIVE SPLICING. For example, during development, different portions of the gene for the NMDA RECEPTOR may be transcribed to form slightly different mRNA molecules, known as SPLICE VARIANTS, each of which produces an NMDA receptor with a different characteristic, such as permeability to CALCIUM ions. Such control of gene expression may underlie many alterations in gene regulation in the developing organism.

While most genes for a specific protein are found in all members of a species, and indeed, many important proteins show a great degree of homology across many species, small variations occur in the precise sequences between individuals. Any different variation of the same gene is called an ALLELE. Such variants are often brought about by random MUTATION involving substitution, loss or addition of one or more nucleotides during DNA replication or repair, and may affect the function of the gene to a greater or lesser extent. Different alleles of the gene for eye colour, for example, may be of little significance to the survival of the species. However, some mutations in structure of a protein or enzyme may alter its function, or prevent it altogether, and this may be highly detrimental to the function of the cell, resulting in disease and possibly death of the individual. Several diseases have been shown to possess a genetic background, including HUNTINGTON'S CHOREA, and familial Alzheimer's disease. The ability to isolate genetic mutations has provided the potential for screening genetic diseases, leading to early detection, and possibly treatment. Strategies such as administration of viral vectors, which aim to replace defective genes, may become viable methods of treating genetic disease (see GENE THERAPY).

FIONA M. INGLIS

gene expression *see* gene

gene knockdown Targeted reduction of a GENE product, or protein. This is commonly achieved through administration of an ANTISENSE OLIGONUCLEOTIDE, a short piece of DEOXYRIBONUCLEIC ACID (DNA) which binds to MESSENGER RNA produced as a result of GENE TRANSCRIPTION. Because the messenger RNA is bound by the antisense oligonucleotide, it cannot be translated into protein, resulting in an artificial downregulation of the protein product of the gene. Gene knockdown is usually transient, lasting for the duration of antisense oligonucleotide administration. Because of the random nature of oligonucleotide binding to mRNA, gene knockdown seldom results in total loss of gene product.

FIONA M. INGLIS

gene knockout The experimental disruption of a specific GENE in an animal, usually a mouse. A knock-out mouse is a TRANSGENIC animal in which a novel piece of DNA is inserted into a specific gene in order to prevent the gene from being transcribed to make protein (see PROTEINS). Often the inserted DNA is a REPORTER GENE, such as the neomycin resistance gene, which has no normal function in the mouse, but can be readily detected in a sample of DNA from the developed mouse. By examining the consequences of gene knockout, the precise function of the gene may be inferred.

FIONA M. INGLIS

gene promoter *see* gene

gene therapy A field of experimental medicine which aims to treat a disease or its symptoms by altering the expression of a GENE, and the subsequent production of PROTEINS. For example, a VIRAL VECTOR may be employed to deliver genes where an essential protein is absent. Alternatively, when a disease is caused by the presence of an abnormal protein, an ANTISENSE OLIGONUCLEOTIDE may be used to bind to specific molecules of MESSENGER RNA (see RNA), preventing production of the protein.

FIONA M. INGLIS

gene transcription *see* gene

gene transfer in the CNS The transfer of novel genes (see GENE) that encode PROTEINS – such as NEUROTRANSMITTERS, RECEPTOR SUBUNITS, ENZYMES, or GROWTH FACTORS – into the nervous system. Three main methodologies are widespread. (1) *Ex vivo* gene transfer: The gene is introduced into cells by a variety of techniques including incorporating the gene into a RETROVIRUS which is then used to infect dividing cells in TISSUE CULTURE. Infected cells can be tested for their inclusion of the gene and for their ability to synthesize and release the gene product. The infected cells are then transferred by TRANSPLANTATION into the host brain. (2) *In vivo* gene transfer: Most viruses only infect dividing cells and so cannot be used to transfer genes into adult neurons. However, various types of virus (for example, adenovirus, adeno-associated virus, and herpes simplex-1) can infect post-mitotic cells (see CELL DIVISION) and so these can be used as vectors to transfer genes into the mature brain by direct inoculation (see VIRAL VECTOR). (3) TRANSGENIC animals: The gene is introduced into the germ line of embryos, and lines of animals carrying the gene are maintained by selective breeding.

Reference

Gage F.H., Kawaja M.D. & Fisher L.J. (1991) Genetically modified cells: applications for intracerebral grafting. *Trends in Neuroscience* 14: 328–333.

STEPHEN B. DUNNETT

general anaesthesia *see* anaesthesia

general paresis of the insane A condition including physical (progressive paralysis) and mental (delusions) dysfunctions that accompanies SYPHILIS. It has historical importance in that it was the first mental disorder to have a physical cause established: syphilitic infection. The fact that a biological cause for a mental dysfunction could be established encouraged late-nineteenth-century scientists to search for biological causes for other mental disorders.

Reference

Davison G.C. & Neale J.M. (1996) *Abnormal Psychology*, 6th edn, Wiley: New York.

generalized anxiety *see* anxiety

generalized seizures Seizures in which the symptoms indicate diffuse brain malfunction, involving both LEFT HEMISPHERE and RIGHT HEMISPHERE. Generalized seizures are often characterized by abrupt loss of CONSCIOUSNESS, with bilateral alterations in motor activity. These motor alterations range in severity, and may consist of several components, either separately or together. For example, TONIC–CLONIC attacks are characterized by extension of muscles of the trunk and limbs (tonic), and rapid muscle jerks (clonic). In contrast, ABSENCE SEIZURE occurs as a momentary lapse in consciousness, motionless staring, and arrest of any ongoing activity. The precise symptoms of generalized seizures indicate the brain areas in which seizure activity is propagated.

FIONA M. INGLIS

genetic engineering *see* gene transfer in the CNS

geniculate ganglion *see* facial nerve

geniculohypothalamic system The HYPOTHA-
LAMUS – in particular the SUPRACHIASMATIC
NUCLEUS – receives information about light
from two sources: the RETINOHYPOTHALAMIC
SYSTEM and the geniculohypothalamic system,
the geniculate nuclei having direct inputs from
the RETINA (see LATERAL GENICULATE NU-
CLEUS). The geniculohypothalamic system originates in the INTERGENICULATE LEAFLET and
uses NEUROPEPTIDE Y as a NEUROTRANSMITTER.

See also: circadian rhythm

**geniculostriate and tectopulvinar visual
pathways** Neurons leaving the eye pass
through the optic tract and terminate in 10
different structures in the brain. Of these the
largest are the SUPERIOR COLLICULUS (sometimes called OPTIC TECTUM, especially in lower
vertebrates), in the MIDBRAIN, and the LATERAL
GENICULATE NUCLEUS (LGN), at the back of
the THALAMUS. The LGN itself has three
subdivisions: layers that contain large or small
neurons (magnocellular vs. parvocellular), and
another group of cells that lie between these
layers (interlaminar neurons). All of these
categories code slightly different features of
the visual world, and indeed they receive their
inputs from different cells in the eye itself.
Neurons in the LGN then send information
(still segregated) up to the primary ('striate')
VISUAL CORTEX, while those in the superior
colliculus pass first to a way-station in the
thalamus (the PULVINAR NUCLEUS) en route to
secondary visual areas in the CEREBRAL COR-
TEX. The LGN receives the kind of high-
resolution visual information that is needed to
tell apart and categorize particular objects, a
CONSPECIFIC vs. another animal, and scenes,
any of which may have learned significance for
the animal. Its separate subdivisions send
information about colour, texture, shape, size
and orientation through a series of processing
stages in the primary and secondary visual
cortex, to the inferior temporal cortex, the
highest level of visual processing in the brain.
This processing route is known as the VENTRAL
STREAM. But the magnocellular input to the
striate cortex is partly also diverted through a
different set of secondary cortical areas – the
DORSAL STREAM – leading ultimately to the
posterior PARIETAL CORTEX). The superior col-

liculus, with other visual structures in the
midbrain, has a much longer evolutionary
history than the LGN. It seems to have evolved
to subserve sensorimotor co-ordination, so as
to allow an animal to detect and ESCAPE from
predators, and to detect and orient towards
prey or other target objects. In higher animals
like PRIMATES, it participates in the visual
guidance of reaching and locomotion, and also
in the control of EYE MOVEMENTS. In achieving
this, it collaborates extensively with visuomotor structures in the dorsal stream. Like the
dorsal stream, its origins in the eye can be
traced back to those that feed the magnocellular LGN layers. The visuomotor role of
the superior colliculus is largely 'hard-wired'
and rule-based, and is unaffected by specific
visual learning (though of course it has to be
honed during early development).

A. DAVID MILNER

genie Genie is a popular acronym, occurring
in many contexts: in neuroscience it usually
refers to a programme based on NEURAL NET-
WORKS for identifying GENE sequences.

genome The total amount of genetic material
– the complete set of CHROMOSOMES and all
the genes they possess – present in each CELL;
see GENE.

genotype The genetic constitution of an individual. Genotype is contrasted with PHENO-
TYPE – the actual observable characteristics,
produced by an interaction between genetic
composition and its modification by experience
and the environment. A genotype is a blueprint; a phenotype is what one actually gets.

genu (from Latin, *genu*: knee) A structure that
has a bend in the shape of a knee can go by the
term genu. For example, the genu of the
CORPUS CALLOSUM is that part of the corpus
callosum at the anterior end where it bends
down and inwards.

geons *see* spatial frequency vs. feature theory

germ layers Three layers of cells (ECTODERM,
MESODERM and ENDODERM) in the developing
EMBRYO that give rise to the tissues of the
body; see DEVELOPMENT.

gerontology (from Greek, *geron*: an old man) The scientific study of the processes and consequences of AGEING.

Gerstmann syndrome A constellation of deficits identified by Josef Gerstmann in the 1930s. It includes AGNOSIA, LEFT-RIGHT CONFUSION, AGRAPHIA and ACALCULIA. Initially it was thought to involve damage in the region of the ANGULAR GYRUS but there is now doubt about the ability to localize these deficits, and indeed it has been argued that the syndrome should not be recognized any longer.

See also: finger agnosia

gestalt The term Gestalt, a German word with no precise translation into English, as a noun indicates a whole object or total configuration. It is a term used to indicate the importance of the whole object rather than the component parts and is neatly encapsulated in the phrase 'the whole is greater than the sum of its parts'. The Gestalt school of psychology (see Wertheimer for a full discussion of this) was important in that it was the first to reject atomism (the examination of parts) in favour of analysis of whole objects, having realized that mental operations work to find whole objects to classify rather than simply describing elements. The VISUAL SYSTEM, for example, although now known to rely on analysis of the component parts of visual stimuli, nevertheless works to produce coherent images of recognizable whole objects.

See also: binding problem

Reference

Wertheimer M. (1987) *A Brief History of Psychology*, 3rd edn, Holt, Rinehart & Winston: New York.

gestation (from Latin, *gestare*: to carry) Gestate is a verb that indicates the carrying in the UTERUS of a FOETUS and EMBRYO; GESTATION is a noun that describes the process of gestating; the *gestation period* is the length of time between conception and birth (a period that varies greatly from SPECIES to species: RATS have a gestation period of only a few weeks; humans have a gestation period of approximately 9 months).

gesture *see* animal communication

Gibsonian perception *see* direct vision

giga- Prefix indicating a factor of 10^9, or one thousand million times; see SI UNITS.

gigantocellular A term indicating an extraordinarily large size of NEURON – larger than MAGNOCELLULAR or PARVOCELLULAR neurons. Gigantocellular neurons are found in parts of the RETICULAR FORMATION.

glabrous skin *see* skin

Glasgow coma scale A scale for the assessment of COMA; it uses three judgements: eye opening (4 points), motor response (6 points) and verbal response (5 points). An overall score is derived simply by adding the score for each element: high scores define normal alertness, scores of 8 or less define acute coma.

Reference

Jennett B. & Teasdale G. (1977) Aspects of coma after severe head injury. *Lancet* 1: 878–881.

Glass pattern A Glass pattern (Glass, 1969) is formed by the superposition of two related patterns. The first is usually an arrangement of randomly placed dots or other similar simple shapes. The second pattern is a transform of the first, such as a radial expansion or a rotation. When the two patterns are combined a strong organization of the dots is seen giving a radial or spiral appearance depending on the transformation used to form the second pattern. Glass patterns are of particular interest to computational theories of vision as the structure that is perceived is thought to be a consequence of the underlying organizational principles of the lower levels of the visual system. Glass patterns have also been used in the study of STEREOSCOPIC VISION.

Reference

Glass L. (1969) Moiré effect from random dots. *Nature* 223: 578–580.

DAVID W. HEELEY

glial cells (from Greek, *glia*: glue) Glial cells are found throughout the nervous system and were initially thought simply to have very limited functions, to be little more than glue, binding neurons in place. Glia cells – or more colloquially, just *glia* – in fact have a variety of functions that are critical to the health and operational well-being of the nervous system. They appear to take no direct part in the computations made by NEURONS: they do not form parts of operational NEURAL NETWORKS and are not involved in neuronal signalling in any direct manner. As such glia are of limited interest to biological psychologists keen to explain the relationships between brain systems, behaviour and psychological processing. However, they are critically involved in the operations of the brain and as such deserve interest. There are four principal classes of glia cell: ASTROCYTES (or ASTROGLIA); MICROGLIA; oligodendrocytes (or OLIGODENDROGLIA); and SCHWANN CELLS. These have different forms, distributions and functions.

Astroglia: there are three main types of astrocyte: *radial astrocytes* (all of which are orientated in a similar plane with respect to the NEURAXIS, and which are found in WHITE MATTER); *fibrous astrocytes* (or non-radial astrocytes, also found in white matter but more diffusely organized); and *protoplasmic astrocytes* (with shorter processes than the other forms and found in GREY MATTER). All astrocytes have a more-or-less star shaped appearance (*astron* is Greek for star; *cyte* is a suffix meaning CELL, taken from the Greek *kytos*, a vessel). The star shape is produced by the processes that spread from the cell body, though the exact form varies dependent on type and location. All astroglia can be detected using IMMUNOHISTOCHEMISTRY for GLIAL FIBRILLARY ACIDIC PROTEIN (GFAP) which marks these cells uniquely. Astroglia are involved in a variety of functions. They make contact with both BLOOD vessels and neurons and appear to be involved in 'trading' between them. It is possible, for example, that astrocytes can form a reservoir for GLUCOSE, accepting it from the blood stream and feeding neurons at the required rate. (This, of course, is consistent with a role for astrocytes in the operation of the BLOOD–BRAIN BARRIER.) Astrocytes also appear to regulate the ionic composition of the central nervous system (CNS). For example, astrocytes form an interconnected network (the so-called ASTROCYTIC SYNCYTIUM) that is able to move potassium ions (K^+) away from sites of high concentra-

tion to sites of low concentration. Astrocytes are also involved in the reuptake of certain neurotransmitters and neurotransmitter metabolites. Astrocytes are critical for the proper chemical operation of the CNS. Pathologically, the most common type of brain TUMOUR forms from astroglia (and is known as an ASTROCYTOMA).

Microglia: these are small glial cells, making up 10–20% of the total population of glia in the nervous system. Three types – or more correctly, *states* – can be identified: *resting* or *ramified microglia*; *activated* or *reactive microglia*; and *phagocytic microglia* (see brain MACROPHAGE). Various other names have been used to characterize microglia, describing their form or function in different states. The transition of microglia from resting to activated to the phagocytic state appears to be regulated by such things as cell death (see APOPTOSIS) and various forms of damage within the brain, which trigger release of substances such as COMPLEMENT and the CYTOKINE group (see IMMUNE SYSTEM; indeed, the microglia can in many ways be considered as part of the immune system). All microglia can be detected using immunohistochemistry for OX-42 (an ANTIBODY for a complement receptor present on microglia).

Oligodendroglia (from Greek, *oligos*: few; *dendron*: tree, *glia*: glue): these are the glial cells that produce MYELIN within the CNS. OLIGODENDROGLIA (or oligodendrocytes as they are also known) come in four basic types, though there appear also to be some transition forms. These are *type I* (spherical cell bodies, many processes: found at many levels of the CNS, often associated with blood vessels or fibre pathways); *type II* (more cuboid than spherical and with fewer processes than type I; only found in white matter); *type III* (three or four processes only: found in the CEREBELLUM, CEREBRAL PEDUNCLES and CEREBELLAR PEDUNCLES, MEDULLA OBLONGATA and SPINAL CORD); and *type IV* (associated with the points of entry of CRANIAL NERVES into the CNS: these oligodendroglia are the most similar to Schwann cells). The function of oligodendroglia is to provide myelin to central nervous system neurons: myelin functions as an electrical insulator of axons, speeding axonal conduction velocities. A single oligodendrocyte will provide myelin for more than one neuron (and one neuron will be myelinated by more than one oligodendrocyte). The processes of myelination involves the processes of oligodendrocytes making contact with an axon and then wrapping around it in a spiral fashion. The process of myelination in humans can take very many years: it is not generally completed until individuals are in their mid-teenage years. Myelin can be visualized in the CNS by various histological techniques (see HISTOLOGY; CHEMICAL NEUROANATOMY) but the most effective is the GALLYAS SILVER stain for myelin.

Schwann cells: the most commonly recognized function of Schwann cells is to provide myelin to neurons in the PERIPHERAL NERVOUS SYSTEM (they are not normally found in the CNS). However, Schwann cells do more than this. All nerve fibres in the peripheral nervous system are sheathed by Schwann cells, whose most basic functions are to provide structural support and to interact with surrounding tissues. Schwann cells are discriminated from oligodendroglia not only by location but also by possession of a basal lamina which serves as a border between the Schwann cell–axon unit and the surrounding CONNECTIVE TISSUE. Peripheral nerve fibres are delicate, yet must travel long distances: the presence of Schwann cells allows the development of effective connective tissue support. In addition to this physical function, Schwann cells can also provide myelin, laying it in sections along axons. Unlike oligodendroglia, a single Schwann cell will provide myelin only along one axon, and only for a particular portion of that axon. (The junctions between myelinated sections are the NODES OF RANVIER; see ACTION POTENTIAL.) Schwann cells do on occasion penetrate the CNS, but only in unusual conditions. They appear to be present in the walls of blood vessels, and if the blood brain–barrier is compromised, Schwann cells can enter the CNS. There are reports of them being engaged in remyelination of CNS neurons following brain damage.

See also: ependymoglial cells; gliotoxins

References

Kettenmann H. & Ransom B.R. (1995) *Neu-*

roglia, Oxford University Press: Oxford. (This is a remarkably thorough and complete account of neuroglia that will answer almost any question about glial cells.)

Kimelberg H.K. & Norenberg M.D. (1989) Astrocytes. *Scientific American* 260: 66–76.

Ransom B.R. & Sontheimer H. (1992) The neurophysiology of glial cells. *Journal of Clinical Neurophysiology* 9: 224–251.

glial fibrillary acidic protein *see* chemical neuroanatomy; glial cells

glial scar *see* reactive gliosis

glioma *see* tumour

gliosis The formation of GLIAL CELLS; see REACTIVE GLIOSIS.

gliotoxins The term gliotoxin has a generic and a specific meaning. Generically, it is a term used to describe any agent that destroys selectively GLIAL CELLS. Ethidium bromide, alpha aminoadipic acid (alpha AAA) and fluorocitrate are all agents that have been used experimentally to destroy glial cells. They have been used to examine, for example, the processes of DEMYELINATIONand REMYELINATION (see Shields *et al.*, 1999) work that hopefully will have important consequences for understanding disorders such as MULTIPLE SCLEROSIS. However, specifically, gliotoxin refers (rather confusingly) to a particular agent: gliotoxin is a fungal toxin that affects plants and animals. Its main properties appear to be suppression of the IMMUNE SYSTEM and destruction of cells (see Richard, 1997).

References

Richard J.L. (1997) Gliotoxin, a mycotoxin associated with cases of avian aspergillosis. *Journal of Natural Toxins* 6: 11–18.

Shields S.A., Gilson J.M., Blakemore W.F. & Franklin R.J.M. (1999) Remyelination occurs as extensively but more slowly in old rats compared to young rats following gliotoxin-induced S+CNS demyelination. *Glia* 28: 77–83.

global amnesia Complete loss or severe impairment of DECLARATIVE MEMORY that is present across all sensory modalities and materials. It usually includes ANTEROGRADE AMNESIA and a variable degree of RETROGRADE AMNESIA. In humans, it contrasts with material-specific amnesia, in which the impairment is selective for specific types of information (for example, verbal). Whereas material-specific amnesia may occurr after unilateral brain damage, global amnesia requires brain damage in both LEFT HEMISPHERE and RIGHT HEMISPHERE. Damage almost always involves the medial TEMPORAL LOBE (see HIPPOCAMPUS) or the DIENCEPHALON. There is a research controversy whether global amnesia in humans affects all aspects of declarative memory or whether it spares SEMANTIC MEMORY.

See also: amnesia; amnesic syndrome; diencephalic amnesia; preserved learning

STEFAN KÖHLER

global aphasia The most severe form of APHASIA. Generally described as a NON-FLUENT APHASIA although speech may be entirely absent. Response to verbal stimuli may be absent or limited to repetitive (and often incorrect) use of familiar words (*okay, yes*), phrases (*here it is*), or phoneme sequences (*tam, tam*). Written LANGUAGE production (WRITING) and comprehension (READING) is similarly severely impaired, hence these patients have no reliable mechanism for communication. Some patients with global aphasia at the onset of symptoms will evolve to lesser-impaired forms of aphasia. Patients with some ability to comprehend and produce speech are clinically described as 'mixed anterior' (a pattern similar to that seen in BROCA'S APHASIA, but with relatively poorer comprehension), or as 'mixed posterior' (a pattern resembling WERNICKE'S APHASIA, but with relatively poorer SPEECH PRODUCTION). Any LESION associated with global aphasia tends to be massive, occupying large regions of cortical tissue in the dominant cerebral HEMISPHERE (usually LEFT HEMISPHERE).

CHARLOTTE C. MITCHUM

global ischaemia Loss of blood flow to the entire brain. Global ischaemia is a characteristic of profoundly reduced blood pressure, most commonly during cardiac arrest. It is usually temporary, and is characterized by widespread damage of NEURONS in the brain. It is modelled in animals by constriction of the carotid and basilar arteries, which provide the brain with blood. Neurons which are most susceptible to ischaemic damage are found in brain regions with high densities of GLUTAMATE RECEPTORS, in particular the HIPPOCAMPUS. Global ischaemia in humans and animals is often followed by cognitive defects, such as impaired SPATIAL MEMORY or OBJECT RECOGNITION tasks.

See also: cerebral vasculature; focal ischaemia; ischaemia

FIONA M. INGLIS

globose nucleus *see* cerebellum – anatomical organization

globus pallidus (Latin, *globus pallidus*: pale globe) This structure forms the medial portion of the LENTIFORM NUCLEUS and comprises an external (lateral) and an internal (medial) segment; PALLIDUM and pallidal are terms used descriptively about the globus pallidus. The internal pallidal segment (known as the ENTOPEDUNCULAR NUCLEUS in the rat brain) is closely related anatomically and functionally to the pars reticulata of the SUBSTANTIA NIGRA. Pallidal neurons contain the neurotransmitter GABA and are larger than the typical striatal MEDIUM SPINY NEURONS, which are the main source of AFFERENT supply to the pallidum. External segment pallidal neurons project to the SUBTHALAMIC NUCLEUS, which in turn projects to the internal pallidal segment/substantia nigra pars reticulata (the 'indirect path' – see DIRECT AND INDIRECT STRIATAL OUTPUT PATHWAYS). Internal pallidal segment neurons (as well as substantia nigra pars reticulata neurons) project primarily to the ventral anterior nucleus of the THALAMUS, but also to the SUPERIOR COLLICULUS and PEDUNCULOPONTINE TEGMENTAL NUCLEUS. These parts of the globus pallidus are generally termed the DORSAL PALLIDUM, emphasizing their connection with the dorsal STRIATUM. There is an equivalent VENTRAL PALLIDUM which receives its afferents primarily from the ventral striatum and projects in turn mainly to the MEDIODORSAL NUCLEUS OF THE THALAMUS.

BARRY J. EVERITT

glomerulus (from Latin, *glomus*: ball of thread) A glomerulus (plural glomeruli) is a cluster of small elements. There are clusters of CAPILLARIES in the kidney known as glomeruli; and the OLFACTORY GLOMERULI are clusters of axons and dendrites; CEREBELLAR GLOMERULI are similar clusters in the cerebellum (see CEREBELLUM – ANATOMICAL ORGANIZATION).

glossopharyngeal nerve The ninth cranial nerve (see CRANIAL NERVES): involved in various processes, including swallowing, taste (see GUSTATION) and sensation in the upper airways.

glottis *see* mouth

glucagon A hormone released from the PANCREAS, having a function opposite to that of INSULIN. Whereas insulin reduces the concentration of GLUCOSE in the BLOOD by enabling cells to capture it, glucagon acts on cells in the LIVER to promote the conversion of stored GLYCOGEN into glucose, thus raising blood glucose concentration. The actions of glucagon are important in making glucose available as circulating levels fall, and in emergency, when additional ENERGY is required (for example, during FIGHT-OR-FLIGHT responses).

glucocorticoids A class of HORMONES, including CORTICOSTERONE and CORTISOL, secreted from the ADRENAL GLAND; with the MINERALOCORTICOIDS, they represent the CORTICOSTEROIDS.

See also: endocrine glands; hormones – classification; immune system; stress

gluconeogenesis The formation of GLUCOSE in the body; see FASTING PHASE.

glucopenia *see* hypoglycaemia

glucoprivation Restriction in the amount of GLUCOSE available (glucose deprivation) and a stimulus to FEEDING; see 2-DEOXYGLUCOSE; PHYSIOLOGICAL CHALLENGE.

glucoreceptors Receptors that detect the presence of GLUCOSE. They are known to be located in the LIVER and in the brain, where they are found in the BRAINSTEM rather than in the DIENCEPHALON (including the HYPOTHALAMUS) or TELENCEPHALON.

Reference
Ritter R.C., Slusser P.G. & Stone S. (1981)

Glucoreceptors controlling feeding and blood glucose: location in the hindbrain. *Science* 213: 452–453.

glucose A monosaccharide, one of the simple SUGARS, contained within many foods, and forming half the constituent of common table sugar, SUCROSE. Glucose is the chief 'common currency' of ENERGY in the body. Many different forms of energy stores (for instance, GLYCOGEN and PROTEINS) can be converted into glucose, and so can be converted into each other via glucose as an intermediate stage. Glucose is also the sole fuel used by most brain neurons, which cannot metabolize most other forms of calories. Glucose is therefore the primary nutrient used by the brain in assessing HUNGER.

See also: carbohydrate; energy balance; fat

KENT C. BERRIDGE

glucose 6-phosphate The first step in the GLYCOLYSIS – the metabolic process by which tissues obtain ENERGY from glucose – is the breakdown of glucose to glucose 6-phosphate, a process catalysed by the enzyme GLUCOSE 6-PHOSPHATASE; see METABOLIC MAPPING for an example of how this process can be used to index neural processing.

glucose 6-phosphatase *see* glucose-6-phosphate; metabolic mapping

glutamate Glutamate (or GLUTAMIC ACID) is an EXCITATORY AMINO ACID, with two isomeric forms: L- and D-glutamic acid. Glutamic and ASPARTIC ACID are the major excitatory NEUROTRANSMITTERS in the CENTRAL NERVOUS SYSTEM. Analogues of glutamic acid such as QUISQUALIC ACID, IBOTENIC ACID, KAINIC ACID and N-methyl-D-aspartate (NMDA) also exhibit marked potency and specificity in the DEPOLARIZATION of neurons. Alongside its role in neurotransmission, glutamate is also involved in intermediary METABOLISM in neural tissue. It is a building block in the synthesis of PROTEINS and PEPTIDES including glutathione, a precursor for the inhibitory neurotransmitter GABA, and plays a role in the detoxification of ammonia in the brain. The diverse roles of glutamate in the central nervous system have led to doubts about its classification as a true neurotransmitter. However, its mechanisms of regulation and release are appropriate for such classification. Glutamate is released from pre-synaptic terminals by depolarization in a cal-cium-dependent manner. After release, glutamate binds to specific postsynaptic recep-tors (see GLUTAMATE RECEPTORS) and induces excitation of the postsynaptic membrane. Glu-tamate transporters pump excess glutamic acid from the extracellular space back into neurons. This reuptake mechanism is important and necessary since glutamate is neurotoxic in high concentrations (see EXCITOTOXINS) and gluta-mate-containing neurons are capable of firing at high frequencies for long periods of time, leading to accumulation of millimolar concen-trations in the SYNAPTIC CLEFT. Some effects of glutamate may be mediated by the novel neurotransmitter nitric oxide: glutamate is a potent stimulator of nitric oxide in the brain and there is evidence that activation of NMDA receptors can regulate nitric oxide neurons. Glutamate has been highlighted as having key roles to play in many normal and pathological brain processes. In the normal brain, it is thought to be critically important for physiolo-gical processes related to LEARNING and MEM-ORY in the HIPPOCAMPUS (see LONG-TERM POTENTIATION), as well as neuroendocrine regulation. It is also thought to play a role in diverse pathophysiological disorders such as HUNTINGTON'S CHOREA, PARKINSON'S DISEASE, ALZHEIMER'S DEMENTIA, AMYOTROPHIC LAT-ERAL SCLEROSIS, EPILEPSY, SCHIZOPHRENIA and STROKE. The importance of these fields means that research is very fast moving, although the roles which glutamate plays are not yet completely understood. One specific research goal is to understand the mechanisms responsible for the massive, uncontrolled re-lease of glutamate in ISCHAEMIA.

See also: drug ionization

WENDY L. INGLIS

glutamate receptors The principal mediators of excitatory synaptic transmission in the vertebrate CENTRAL NERVOUS SYSTEM, also termed EXCITATORY AMINO ACID RECEPTORS. They have been implicated in a wide range of neurophysiological and neuropathological pro-cesses. For instance, they are of fundamental importance in synaptic PLASTICITY, such as

LONG-TERM POTENTIATION and LONG-TERM DEPRESSION. Changes in glutamate systems are also strongly implicated in a variety of pathological conditions including EPILEPSY, ISCHAEMIA and neurodegenerative disorders such as ALZHEIMER'S DEMENTIA and HUNTING-TON'S CHOREA.

Glutamate receptors fall into two broad categories: IONOTROPIC and METABOTROPIC. Activation of ionotropic receptors leads to ION CHANNEL opening; activation of metabotropic glutamate receptors activates cell-signalling pathways (for example PROTEIN KINASE and PHOSPHOLIPASE). Ionotropic glutamate recep-tors can be subdivided into two types – NMDA and non-NMDA receptors – with non-NMDA receptors further subdivided into AMPA and kainate receptors (receptors are all named after their definitive AGONIST). Any SYNAPSE that uses excitatory amino acid transmission may have a combination of ionotropic and metabo-tropic receptor-types available, and these may act synergistically.

The first COMPLEMENTARY DNA encoding a glutamate RECEPTOR SUBUNIT (GluR1) was cloned in 1989. Molecular cloning studies have since identified a number of different subunits which can combine to form a variety of subtypes of ionotropic or metabotropic gluta-mate receptor channels, and IN SITU HYBRIDI-ZATION studies have demonstrated considerable regional variability in the expres-sion of the constituent subunit MESSENGER RNA throughout the brain. NMDA subunits include at least seven alternatively spliced variants of NR1 (or, more cumbersomely, NMDAR1), in addition to four NR2 subunits, NR2A to NR2D; to form a functional NMDA receptor, one of the consituent subunits must be NR1. AMPA receptors are the principal mediators of fast excitatory transmission (see FAST NEURO-TRANSMISSION) and can also be activated by kainic acid. They are constructed from any homomeric or heteromeric combination of two subunits GluR1 to GluR4. In addition, there are at least two types of kainate receptors, which are not activated by AMPA. These are likely to be formed from HIGH AFFINITY kainate subunits such as KA1 and KA2, although these subunits themselves do not appear to form functional homomeric channels. LOW-AFFINITY kainate subunits GluR5 to GluR7 share approximately 40% sequence identity with GluR1 to GluR4. There are at least 8 subtypes of metabotropic glutamate receptor, classified in subgroups according to sequence homology and on their pharmacology and transduction mechanisms when expressed in cell lines. For instance, Group 1 (mGluR1 and mGluR5) are coupled to phospholipase C.

See also: excitotoxins; GABA receptors

WENDY L. INGLIS

glutamatergic Relating to the neurotransmitter GLUTAMATE. For instance, a neuron that synthesizes and releases glutamate is said to be glutamatergic.

glutamic acid *see* glutamate

glutamic acid decarboxylase (GAD; glutamate decarboxylase) Since glutamic acid can also be called glutamate, glutamic acid decarboxylase and glutamate decarboxylase are the same thing; the most common abbreviation is GAD, for glutamic acid decarboxylase. GAD is the essential ENZYME that catalyses the conversion of glutamate to the neurotransmitter GABA. An ANTIBODY is available for GAD, making it a useful marker for neurons able to synthesize GABA.

glutaminase *see* glutamine

glutamine Glutamine is the precursor of the neurotransmitter GLUTAMATE; GLUTAMINASE is the enzyme that catalyses the conversion of glutamine to glutamate (see CATALYST). Curiously, glutamine is synthesized from glutamate, a reaction catalysed by the enzyme GLUTAMINE SYNTHETASE. Why should it be possible to use glutamate to make glutamine, which is then used to make glutamate? The likeliest explanation is that glutamine is stored in NEURONS and glia as an inactive form of glutamate – a reservoir that can be called on if required. It is possible that the conversion of glutamine to glutamate can occur in neurons, though it can certainly occur in astrocytes (see GLIAL CELLS). Astrocytes appear able to transport glutamate across membranes into the neurons they support.

Reference

Feldman R.S., Meyer J.S. & Quenzer L.F. (1997) *Principles of Neuropsychopharmacology*, Sinauer Associates: Sunderland MA.

glutamine synthetase *see* glutamine

glutaraldehyde *see* fixation

glycerol *see* triglycerides

glycine One of the inhibitory AMINO ACIDS; glycine and GABA are described as the two major fast neurotransmitters (see FAST NEUROTRANSMISSION) in the CENTRAL NERVOUS SYSTEM. Glycine is synthesized from SERINE in a reaction catalysed by serine hydroxymethyltransferase. It is stored and used in a manner similar to other AMINO ACID NEUROTRANSMITTERS. It is found principally in the SPINAL CORD and in several brain structures, including the SUBSTANTIA NIGRA (where concentration is high), STRIATUM, RAPHE NUCLEI and various BRAINSTEM structures. Glycine receptors operate in a manner similar to GABA receptors. The well-known poison STRYCHNINE acts at glycine receptors.

glycogen Glycogen is a POLYSACCHARIDE found in MUSCLES and the LIVER. It can be mobilized very rapidly to provide energy to fuel processes such as FIGHT-OR-FLIGHT. (The ENERGY stored as FAT cannot be mobilized quickly.) GLUCAGON, one of the HORMONES liberated from the PANCREAS, promotes the mobilization of glycogen.

See also: insulin

glycolipid *see* lipids

glycolysis The process by which GLUCOSE is broken down by in the CELL to produce ENERGY; also known as the GLYCOLYTIC CYCLE or the Embden–Meyerhof pathway. The other two critical pathways involved in the metabolism of CARBOHYDRATES (of which glucose and the other SUGARS, MONOSACCHARIDES and DISACCHARIDES, are of course members) are the KREBS' CYCLE (also known as the *citric acid cycle*) and the *pentose phosphate pathway*. In physiology, these processes are of the most major significance, since they provide the fuel for cellular processes. In neuroscientific methodology, measurement of glycolysis has been used in METABOLIC MAPPING studies to provide an index of regional brain activity in response to stimulation or challenge.

glycolytic cycle *see* glycolysis

glycoproteins Glycoproteins are conjugated PROTEINS and CARBOHYDRATE. In the brain, glycoproteins act as important ADHESION MOLECULES, providing GROWTH CONE attachments to the local environments.

glycoside The term glycoside refers to any compound derived from a MONOSACCHARIDE; a *glycosidic linkage* is the chemical bond formed between two monosaccharides to make a DISACCHARIDE; see SUGARS.

go/no-go learning An INSTRUMENTAL CONDITIONING paradigm in which the subject must make or withhold a response to cues, rather than approach or avoid them.

IAN C. REID

goal-directed behaviour Literally, behaviour that is directed to achieving a goal of any sort – food, water or anything else. The importance of the term lies in what it does *not* say: it does not use the term MOTIVATION. Some learning theorists (see BEHAVIOURISM) rejected the concept of motivation, arguing that it has the status of an intervening variable, with no effective explanatory power: the mechanisms of LEARNING were sufficient to explain behaviour. Using the term GOAL-DIRECTED BEHAVIOUR therefore allows one to describe certain types of acts without making inferences about the psychological processes underlying them.

Golgi apparatus An organelle, functionally associated with the ENDOPLASMIC RETICULUM in the synthesis and transport of PROTEINS. It is named after the Italian biologist Camillo Golgi (1843–1926).

See also: cell

Golgi method A method for staining neurons (see NEURON) and GLIAL CELLS developed by Camillo Golgi. Only a small number of neurons and glia are actually stained (why only a small proportion is affected is not clear, even now) but it was nevertheless hugely important in allowing the structure of individual neurons

to be described accurately at the end of the nineteenth century.

Golgi tendon organ These, like the GOLGI APPARATUS within the CELL, are named after the man who first described them, Camillo Golgi. Information from MUSCLES – proprioceptive information – is provided principally by two structures: Golgi tendon organs and MUSCLE SPINDLES. Evidently, Golgi tendon organs generate information from tendons, while muscle spindles generate information from muscles. However, while the muscle spindles provide information about muscle *stretching*, the Golgi tendon organs provide information about muscle *contraction*. The Golgi tendon organs are actually attached to both the tendon that connects a muscle to bone and to the muscle itself. They are responsive to shortening of muscle length (as occurs during contraction of the muscle) and generate bursts of ACTION POTENTIAL at a rate proportional to the degree of stretching. That is, the harder a muscle is contracting, the more action potentials will be generated by the Golgi tendon organs.

See also: locomotion

gonadal steroids A class of HORMONES; these are the SEX HORMONES (including ANDROGENS, ESTROGENS and PROGESTERONE) released from the GONADS. Note that these hormones can also be released from the ADRENAL GLAND and so also fall under the category of CORTICOSTEROIDS.

See also: endocrine glands; hormones – classification; pregnancy

gonadectomy Removal of the GONADS; see CASTRATION.

gonadotrophin-releasing hormone One of the HORMONES involved in the control of the release of other hormones from the PITUITARY GLAND.

See also: adenohypophysis; endocrine glands; hormones – classification; neurohypophysis; sex hormones

gonadotrophins The principal gonadotrophins – HORMONES released by the ADENOHYPOPHYSIS that act on the GONADS – are FOLLICLE-

STIMULATING HORMONE and LUTEINIZING HORMONE.

See also: endocrine glands; hormones – classification; menstrual cycle

gonads (from Greek, *gone*: generation) The gonads are the organs that produce sex cells: the TESTES in males and the OVARIES in females; gonadal is the adjectival form of gonad.

gonochorism (from Greek, *gone*: generation, *chorizein*: to separate) Separation into two distinct sexes, male and female; see REPRODUCTION.

goosebumps Also called gooseflesh or goose pimples. An effect observed on hairless SKIN related to PILOERECTION – changing the position of hairs. It is a response to cold: hairs are raised when the environmental temperature is low, in order to trap air which can be warmed to provide an additional insulation; see THERMOREGULATION.

GR113808 An antagonist at the $5HT_4$ receptor; see SEROTONIN RECEPTORS.

gracile nucleus One of the DORSAL COLUMN NUCLEI OF THE MEDULLA OBLONGATA (the CUNEATE NUCLEUS is the other) which receives sensory fibres from the DORSAL FUNICULUS of the SPINAL CORD carrying sensations of fine, discriminative TOUCH and vibration.

graft These terms relate to the TRANSPLANTATION of foreign cells or tissue into host brains, in an effort to restore function after damage.

grammar The grammar of a LANGUAGE is the set of rules controlling the permissible sentences of that language. Grammatical sentences are those which speakers of the language accept as well-formed, ungrammatical sentences are those which they cannot accept. In its widest sense, grammar includes a language's SYNTAX, MORPHOLOGY and PHONOLOGY, and permissible semantic structures. In narrower senses it refers to the permissible sequential structures of words within sentences – that is, syntax plus morphology. Grammars can also be books describing the grammar of particular languages. *Generative grammar* is the notion, proposed by the linguist Noam Chomsky, of grammar as a device for generating all and only the permissible sentences of a language. Transformational grammars – again due to Chomsky – capture the relations between different syntactic forms expressing the same underlying proposition. Thus 'Jack built the house', and 'The house was built by Jack' may be described as having a common underlying structure, with the addition of a passive transformation in generating the second. 'Colourless green ideas sleep furiously' is Chomsky's famous example of a sentence which is syntactically permissible though meaningless; it illustrates the separability of syntax and SEMANTICS. (In certain contexts this sentence is now however highly likely, and thus also illustrates the separability of semantics and frequency of occurrence.) Just as different syntactic forms can express one underlying proposition, so can the same form express more than one meaning: English grammar generates 'Charles is the man I want to succeed' to convey at least five propositions (I want Charles to have success; I want to follow Charles; I need Charles if I am to have success; I want Charles to follow [X]; I need Charles if I am to follow [X]). *Grammatical words* (or function words) are words which primarily perform a syntactic function – such as articles, conjunctions, prepositions, pronouns. They contrast with lexical, or content words: nouns, verbs, adjectives. Languages differ according to whether they largely use independent words for such syntactic functions (as English does), or whether they prefer some other means such as affixes or word order. The degree to which thematic relations of case (for instance, subject, object, instrument), verb mood (for instance, factual, possible) and aspect (for instance, completed, uncompleted) are explicitly represented by the grammar also differ widely across languages. So, again, does preferred order for the basic propositional relations subject, verb, object; across the world's languages all possible orderings may be observed.

References

Borsley R.D. (1991) *Syntactic Theory: A Unified Approach*, Arnold: London.
Hurford J.R. (1994) *Grammar: A Student's*

Guide, Cambridge University Press: Cambridge.

ANNE CUTLER

grand mal seizure Grand mal seizure is one of the GENERALIZED SEIZURES, characterized by widespread changes in the ELECTROENCEPHALOGRAM (EEG) at many sites and loss of CONSCIOUSNESS. Patients will show CONVULSIONS of a TONIC–CLONIC nature. The seizure is followed by a period of confusion, lasting for several minutes, and SLEEP.

See also: epilepsy

grandmother cell A hypothetical construct: the term was coined to highlight the distinction between two different types of coding. Classical ARTIFICIAL INTELLIGENCE theories argue in favour of *symbolic coding*, in which an individual (real or artificial) NEURON codes complex stimuli (such as one's grandmother). CONNECTIONISM however argues that representations of complex stimuli are *distributed* across NEURAL NETWORKS. The term has its origins in the work of Konorski, who used the expression *gnostic units* to refer to the general principle of individual neurons coding complex stimuli. These appear to have mutated into grandmother cells in the early 1970s when Jerry Lettvin, Horace Barlow and Colin Blakemore began to use this term; see Lettvin (1996) for a description of this process.

See also: engram; labelled-line theory; neural coding;

References

Konorski J. (1967) *Integrative Activity of the Brain*, University of Chicago Press: Chicago.
Lettvin J. (1996) Guest editorial: Some reflections on (or by?) grandmother cells. *Perception* 25: 881–886.

granisetron An antagonist at the $5HT_3$ receptor; see SEROTONIN RECEPTORS.

granular cortex The granular cortex refers to those parts of the CEREBRAL CORTEX with an internal GRANULAR LAYER (layer 4 – see CORTICAL LAYERS).

See also: agranular cortex

granular layer *see* cerebellum – anatomical organization; cortical layers

granule cells There is more than one group of granule cells in the brain. One set is in the DENTATE GYRUS: these give rise to MOSSY FIBRES which innervate (see CA1–CA3) in the HIPPOCAMPUS. A second set of granule cells form DENDRODENDRITIC SYNAPSES with MITRAL CELLS in the OLFACTORY BULB and are crucial to the role of the olfactory bulb in olfactory LEARNING (see OLFACTION). A third set are in the CEREBELLUM, where a very great number of granule cells sit beneath the PURKINJE CELLS and emit axons to form the PARALLEL FIBRES of the cerebellum.

granulocyte A granulocyte is a mature granular LEUKOCYTE : there are three types – NEUTROPHIL, EOSINOPHILS and BASOPHILS.

See also: immune system

grapheme (from Greek, *graphema*: something written) A grapheme is the smallest unit of a written LANGUAGE. In English, these are of course the letters of the alphabet; see PHONEME; WRITING.

graphesthesia The ability to recognize symbols (numbers or letters most typically) traced on the SKIN, using only the sensation of TOUCH (the HAPTIC sense) – that is, one does not see the tracing being done, or detect it in any other way. The loss of this ability is of course agraphesthesia.

See also: tactile agnosia

grasp The capture of an object with a manipulandum (typically the hand). Efficient grasping requires scaling the size of the hand opening to the size of the target (grip scaling) as well as rotation of the wrist in two planes in order to position the palmar surface of the hand (when a power grip is required) or the pads of the thumb and index or middle finger (when a precision grip is required). The neural control of grasping in PRIMATES is considered to be relatively independent of the control of the REACHING movement which positions the hand in the appropriate space.

See also: grip

DAVID P. CAREY

Grassman's Laws Grassman's Laws are the laws of colour mixture. Human COLOUR VI-

SION is trichromatic, which is reflection of the fact that in the normal photopic VISUAL SYSTEM there exist three types of CONES each with a different SPECTRAL SENSITIVITY. Consequently if three primary colours are selected so that no single primary can be produced by a mixture of the remaining two (such as red, green and blue) then any other colour drawn from the complete visible spectrum can be matched exactly by a suitable adjustment of the relative proportions of the three primaries:

$$C = \alpha R + \beta G + \gamma B$$

where α, β and γ define the coefficients for the arbitrarily chosen primaries.

See also: opponent process theory of colour vision; trichromatic theory of colour vision

DAVID W. HEELEY

grating acuity The maximum number of lines per degree of visual angle in a pattern comprising alternate dark and light lines that can be reliably distinguished from a uniform grey field. The main limiting factor in grating acuity is the optical characteristics of the eye, and it is closely related to SNELLEN ACUITY (see 6/6 NOTATION).

DAVID W. HEELEY

grey matter and white matter (Note: in general *grey* is used in the UK, *gray* in the USA: both refer to the same thing.) If one slices open the CEREBRAL CORTEX, raw, within it can be seen clearly defined areas of grey and WHITE MATTER. Grey matter is composed principally of CELL BODIES and DENDRITES; white matter is composed of AXONS (FIBRES).

Grice box A piece of equipment in which animals (typically rats) can engage in a DISCRIMINATION experiment. It is named after G. Robert Grice, a psychologist who devoted much time to the investigation of DISCRIMINATION LEARNING. Grice actually used a variety of RUNWAY set-ups and MAZES to investigate discrimination learning, but the apparatus that bears his name can be described as follows. Seen from above, it has the same shape as a conical flask or funnel: the neck forms a start box in which the subject waits behind a door. The body of the box has a more or less

triangular shape: when the animal emerges from the start box it is faced by the end wall (which, in plan view, would be the base of the flask) where there are two objects, one on either side of a dividing wall at right angles to the wall of the box. (There may be doors masking these, though these are not essential.) Each object sits over a food well: moving the correct object reveals a food pellet in the well beneath. Animals have to learn a simple discrimination rule in order consistently to find the food REWARD. Much the same procedure can be accomplished in a Y MAZE, but the distance the animal has to travel is greater. The Grice box affords a speedier way of achieving the same end for visual, tactile and object discriminations. The Y maze however offers other advantages. For example, if olfactory or auditory stimuli are to be discriminated, the Y maze offers the opportunity to separate clearly the two stimuli in a way impossible to achieve in the Grice box.

Reference

Grice G.R. (1948) The acquisition of a visual discrimination habit following response to a single stimulus. *Journal of Experimental Psychology* 38: 633–642.
Osgood C.E. (1953) *Method and Theory in Experimental Psychology*, Oxford University Press: New York. (See this for a contemporaneous account of discrimination learning and the work of Grice and others.)

45° grid test A test of movement: rats are placed on a wire grid angled at 45° to the horizontal with their noses pointing up. The speed and direction with which they return to the level surface are measured. Rats bearing a unilateral 6-HYDROXYDOPAMINE LESION of the NIGROSTRIATAL DOPAMINE SYSTEM show changes in speed and direction of turn.

grip The hand posture used to hold a particular object. The two principle categories of grip are precision and power. A typical precision grip in PRIMATES is used when an object is held in opposition between the index finger and thumb. Precision grip alone allows for movement of a small object relative to the different parts of the hand. In a power grip, all of the fingers and the thumb are used in opposition to the palmar surface of the hand. This type of grip is extremely stable and plays an important role in activities such as non-human primate locomotion. Grip scaling is the process whereby the hand is opened to a degree appropriate to the size of the target.

DAVID P. CAREY

grooming Many species of animals engage in complex grooming which serves to remove irritants, leaving the body clean and in good condition. Grooming can be achieved by an individual acting alone or it can be social, among a CONSPECIFIC group. Many PRIMATES for example groom each other, this activity serving in part to establish the DOMINANCE HIERARCHY and to cement relationships between breeding pairs. Grooming can also occur across species as a form of SYMBIOSIS. For example ox peckers are birds that live symbiotically with large African mammals such as rhinoceroses and water buffalo, eating insects and effectively cleaning their hosts. Grooming in rodents has been closely studied and shows a remarkable degree of organization. Rodents use a variety of identifiable movements which combine to form an overall grooming pattern (see Fentress, 1983).

Reference

Fentress J.C. (1983) Ethological models of hierarchy and patterning of species-specific behavior. In *Handbook of Behavioral Neurobiology*, vol. 6, *Motivation*, ed. E. Satinoff & P. Teitelbaum, pp. 185–234, Plenum Press: New York.

growth cone A growth cone is found at the end of a developing AXON. Projecting from the growth cone are whisker-like filaments called FILOPODIA, (interconnected by membranes called LAMELLIPODIA). The filopodia extend and retract, guiding axons forward as they grow. Axonal growth is actually generated by the growth cone. ADHESION MOLECULES on the growth cone appear to act, in a sense, to drag the axon forward towards targets that are chemically identified.

See also: nerve crush; neuronal migration

growth curve A graph of BODY WEIGHT developed over the course of an animal's lifespan that allows one to track normal DEVEL-

OPMENT. Typically, growth curves show a rapid acceleration early in life, body weight increasing quickly. This tails off to produce a much slower rate of body weight gain over time in mature animals. Growth curves are of value because they provide a standard index of normal development for a population of animals. Having developed a standard growth curve for, say, one's laboratory rats, one can use this in the future to judge the development and health of individual rats, or groups of rats.

growth factors Growth factors do exactly what they say they do: they are factors that promote growth of body tissues. They are PROTEINS or PEPTIDES and their presence is a requirement for growth and DEVELOPMENT. There are a number of growth factors, usually called after the tissues or cells they were first found to operate on: thus EPIDERMAL GROWTH FACTOR works on the epidermis (see SKIN), FIBROBLAST GROWTH FACTOR assists FIBROBLAST growth, NERVE GROWTH FACTOR helps NEURONS grow. SOMATOMEDIN is a liver growth factor. The tendency to name growth factors on the basis of their first discovered function can be misleading, since there are some known to operate in more than one location.

growth hormone Growth hormone is, unsurprisingly, one of the HORMONES involved in growth. It affects many tissues in the body, working to promote normal growth and DEVELOPMENT, both directly and by tropic actions on other systems. Levels are high in children; it is typically secreted to a greater degree during SLEEP than it is during the waking state.

growth hormone release inhibiting hormone (also known as SOMATOSTATIN) One of the HORMONES involved in the control of the release of other hormones from the PITUITARY GLAND.

See also: adenohypophysis; endocrine glands; hormones – classification; neurohypophysis

growth hormone releasing hormone (somatocrinin) A HORMONE involved in the control of the release of other hormones from the PITUITARY GLAND; see ADENOHYPOPHYSIS;

NEUROHYPOPHYSIS; ENDOCRINE GLANDS; HORMONES – CLASSIFICATION.

Guam disease In the 1980s it was recognized that, since the initiation of medical records in 1936, there had been a much higher incidence on Guam than elsewhere of PARKINSON'S DISEASE, ALZHEIMER'S DEMENTIA and MOTOR NEURON DISEASE. It was found that islanders were cooking the seeds of a cycad plant, *Cycas micronesia* which yielded a toxin, B-methylamino-L-alanine. Cell culture methods and animal studies confirmed this as a potent neurotoxin (see NEUROTOXINS), though in the human condition the effect might be considerably delayed (by up to 40 years). This toxin is the same as that found to be causing lathyrism, a disease occurring in Abyssinia, Algeria and India, the signs of which are TREMOR and SPASTICITY.

guanine A nucleotide; see DNA.

guanine nucleotides *see* G protein

guanine triphosphate *see* G protein

guide cannula A small length of (usually) stainless steel tubing implanted into the brain under general ANAESTHESIA using STEREOTAXIC SURGERY. It will be held in place by a HEADCAP and most of the time be plugged with a STYLET (or OBDURATOR) – a pin that fits securely into the guide cannula, filling its entire length. A guide cannula is used, for example, in making a MICROINJECTION or during SINGLE-UNIT RECORDING. It allows an injection CANNULA or MICROELECTRODE to be placed at specific sites in the brains of conscious animals (including humans).

Guillain–Barré syndrome A disorder of the peripheral nerves (see PERIPHERAL NERVES AND SPINAL NERVES), impairing movement. It typically involves respiratory difficulties (possibly requiring assisted ventilation) and affects also the CRANIAL NERVES, leading to PARALYSIS of facial muscles. It is an AUTOIMMUNE DISEASE and can be treated.

See also: motor neuron disease

gustation The sense of taste. Gustation is chemically mediated, receptors on the tongue detecting each of four prototypical tastes:

sweet, sour, bitter and salt. (MONOSODIUM GLUTAMATE, used to enhance flavour, may be a primary taste called UMAMI.) Taste perception begins at TASTE BUDS on the tongue. Taste buds are responsive to specific primary tastes and are differently distributed across the tongue. The tip of the tongue is most sensitive to sweet and salt, the sides to sour, and the back to bitter. Individual taste buds possess 20–50 RECEPTOR cells clustered together and, in order to be tasted, a molecule must be water-soluble and able to bind to one of these receptors. Different prototypical tastes have different actions at receptors: salts operate most simply, sodium ions entering neurons to generate ACTION POTENTIAL. Sourness is detected by hydrogen ions binding to and blocking potassium channels (though the sourness of acids is not only a function of hydrogen concentration). Sweet substances – typically but not only sugars – bind to receptors and activate SECOND MESSENGERS, principally CYCLIC AMP. Bitter substances – quinine for instance – activate INOSITOL TRIPHOSPHATE second messenger systems.

The dendrites of sensory neurons contact taste buds so that information can be sent to the CNS for processing. The action of molecules at receptor sites on the taste buds stimulates activity in these sensory neurons. Several nerves carry information away from the tongue to the CNS: the CHORDA TYMPANI (part of the FACIAL NERVE) carries information from the front of the tongue; the lingual branch of the GLOSSOPHARYNGEAL NERVE carries information from the back; and the VAGUS NERVE carries taste information from the palate and epiglottis. These nerves converge on the NUCLEUS OF THE SOLITARY TRACT from where information is relayed to the THALAMUS (especially the ventral posteromedial nucleus) directly and via the PARABRACHIAL NUCLEI. The thalamus, which is the major relay station for cortical input, sends axons to the primary GUSTATORY CORTEX located in the frontal insular and opercular cortices. This is the principal taste pathway, but fibres conducting gustatory information also reach the AMYGDALA and LATERAL HYPOTHALAMUS. Given that the amygdala is concerned with the ascription of motivational significance to stimuli (that is, deciding whether or not a stimulus is pleasant or aversive) and the lateral hypothalamus performs complex computations involving gustatory and visceral sensations, the representation of gustatory information in these places is not surprising. Perhaps the most curious aspect of the taste pathway however is that taste is not represented bilaterally in the cortex, unlike the other senses.

While taste is carried within these pathways, the nature of the information changes as progress is made through the system. Within the nerves bringing information from the tongue, and in the nucleus of the solitary tract, neurons will respond to any of the prototypical tastes without discriminating between them. As one moves up the system through the thalamus to the cortex, gustatory neurons become increasingly finely tuned: that is, they begin to show selective responding to specific prototypical tastes until, in the gustatory cortex, neurons respond selectively to one prototypical taste only. The perception of complex tastes emerges from an assembly of neurons: it is a function of distributed processing rather than the property of single neurons.

In humans taste has been brought to a state of great refinement. Lovers of fine food and wine for instance are able to discriminate great subtleties of taste. Two points need to be made about this. First, it is clear that taste operates in close conjunction with other senses, particularly olfaction. Vision also has a significant part to play. So, for instance, if one is blindfolded and deprived of olfactory information (by pegging one's nose) it is impossible to discriminate between apples and onions. All of the initial, pre-digestive reactions to food and drink (the CEPHALIC REFLEXES OF DIGESTION) are triggered by receptors in the head and mouth: salivation, GASTRIC ACID and INSULIN secretion are initiated before food has passed into the gullet. It is the sight, smell and taste of food which initiates this cascade. The second point is that taste has a long evolutionary history and an important practical purpose. To survive, animals must ingest parts of the environment, but some things ingested will be wholly or partly poisonous. Sweet and salty substances are in general good, but sourness – acidity – is associated with food which has

gone bad, and bitterness is associated with toxins. Very simple creatures evolved mechanisms of EMESIS (NAUSEA and VOMITING) to deal with this. Moving up the PHYLOGENETIC SCALE however one finds that animals possess ever more complex systems to determine what is toxic and what is not. This is the origin of the taste system.

See also: paraventricular system

gustatory cortex A structure concerned with conscious perception of taste (see GUSTATION). It is located at the base of the POSTCENTRAL GYRUS in the PARIETAL LOBE, corresponding to Brodmann's area 43 (see BRODMANN'S AREAS). The gustatory cortex receives gustatory input from the ventral posteromedial nucleus of the THALAMUS as well as regions of the HYPOTHALAMUS and ventral FOREBRAIN in the LIMBIC SYSTEM. The gustatory cortex lies ventral and rostral to the tongue region of the primary somatosensory area, but appears to have little overlap with it, indicating that taste and somatic senses from the tongue are represented separately.

KAZUE SEMBA

gut–brain peptides A variety of chemical signals regarding HUNGER and SATIETY are sent to the brain from the stomach and intestines. Most of these chemicals are PEPTIDES, related to PROTEINS. Several such as CHOLECYSTOKININ are released into the blood during a meal, as food inside the gastrointestinal tract stimulates their secretion. They may serve to inform the brain that food is currently being digested, and may trigger psychological states of satiety. A MICROINJECTION of cholecystokinin directly into the brain, for example, causes rats to terminate a meal earlier than they ordinarily would, as though the food they ate was extraordinarily satiating. Other peptide molecules, such as NEUROPEPTIDE Y and GALANIN, produce the opposite effect when injected into the brain: they elicit eating from animals that are already sated. However, these eating-eliciting peptides are unlikely to originate from secretion by the gut. Instead, they are produced in the brain itself. This is an important instance of the same molecule being used in two different body locations for two different purposes: the cholecystokinin released by the gut has an action on the brain that is important element in signalling satiety; the cholecystokinin found within the brain acts as a straightforward neuropeptide neurotransmitter and has no specific relationship to FEEDING control

KENT C. BERRIDGE

gyri and sulci The CEREBRAL CORTEX of the human brain is extensively folded – it has a very familiar wrinkled appearance. The cerebral cortex of rodents however is entirely smooth, and other species show varying degrees of gyri and sulci development. The development of extensive folding of the cerebral cortex is an evolutionary strategy for packing more tissue into the limited space available within the skull. (To get an idea of this, think of the cerebral cortex as folded out to a single sheet, which can then be folded into a small space.) Gyri, singular gyrus (from Greek, *gyros*: a circle or ring) are the ridges; sulci, singular sulcus (from Latin, *sulcus*: a furrow) are the grooves. The term FISSURE is used to denote a particularly large sulcus.

gyrus *see* gyri and sulci

H

H.M. Famous neurosurgical case (designated 'H.M.' to preserve patient confidentiality) demonstrating a link between TEMPORAL LOBE function and MEMORY. In 1953, the 23-year-old H.M. underwent bilateral temporal lobectomy in an effort to treat intractable temporal lobe EPILEPSY under the care of neurosurgeon William Scoville. In the operation, the anterior HIPPOCAMPUS, AMYGDALA and UNCUS were removed bilaterally. Although the temporal lobe epilepsy was substantially improved, H.M. was left with a dense, persistent and pure ANTEROGRADE AMNESIA. The patient has been much studied over the years: his inadvertent misfortune laid the groundwork for many studies of the neurology of AMNESIA.

IAN C. REID

H reflex (Hoffman reflex) The H reflex is triggered by electrical stimulation of sensory fibres that travel from MUSCLES to the SPINAL CORD. Consequent activation of muscle is measured on the electromyogram: an *M wave*, produced by direct stimulation of the muscle, and an *H wave*, slower because it involves a synaptic relay in the spinal cord. As stimulus strength is increased, M waves become larger, H waves smaller, ANTIDROMIC activation of motor neurons cancelling out the stimulation evoked from cell bodies in the spinal cord.

habenula The habenula is a major structure in the EPITHALAMUS (see THALAMUS) of the DIENCEPHALON and is closely associated with the LIMBIC SYSTEM. It consists of the medial and lateral sub-nuclei. The input to the habenula comes from FOREBRAIN structures including the SEPTAL NUCLEI, PREOPTIC AREA, anterior thalamic (see THALAMUS) nuclei, and GLOBUS PALLIDUS, via a fibre bundle called the STRIA MEDULLARIS. The output from the habenula is directed to the INTERPEDUNCULAR NUCLEUS, via the habenulointerpeduncular tract or FASCICULUS RETROFLEXUS. Thus, the habenula appears to be a site of convergence of forebrain limbic impulses which are then conveyed to the rostral MIDBRAIN.

KAZUE SEMBA

habits Any persistent pattern of learned behaviour can be referred to as a habit. They are typically thought of as the product of simple stimulus-response conditioning (see INSTRUMENTAL CONDITIONING). Clark Hull (1884–1952) used the expression *habit strength* to indicate the degree of LEARNING that had occurred and *habit family hierarchy* to indicate the different learrned sequences of action that a particular stimulus or situation could elicit. *Habit regression* is a term used to describe the reappearance of a learned sequence of action that had been learned and subsequently abandoned in favour of a later learned sequence.

See also: multiple memory systems

habituation Many stimuli, when presented to an animal for the first time, will elicit a response. Following repeated presentations of such stimuli, responding often declines. This decline in responding is termed HABITUATION. For example, a loud noise will, initially, elicit a startle response. Following repeated presentations of this noise, the startle response will decline and eventually disappear. True examples of habituation are typically thought not to be the result of either sensory adaptation or motor fatigue. Two characteristics, in particular, are often taken as support for this proposal, since they would appear to be uncharacteristic of sensory adaptation or motor fatigue. First, habituation proceeds more rapidly to weak stimuli rather than strong stimuli. Second, presentation of a strong, or motivationally significant, stimulus following habituation will result in restoration of the original response (see DISHABITUATION). Given that habituation is thought to be one of the most simple and primitive forms of LEARNING, it is not surprising that examples of it can be found throughout the animal kingdom. It has been observed, using a variety of stimuli and measuring a variety of responses, in such diverse creatures as leeches, molluscs, insects, birds, and of course mammals, including humans. For example, a snail will rapidly withdraw into its shell following a tap to the surface on which it is placed. Repeated presentations of the stimulus, however, will result in the decline, and eventual abolition, of this withdrawal response. Habituation is certainly an example of learning with which we are all familiar and probably plays a greater role in everyday life than we realise. It is often suggested that the purpose of habituation is to allow animals to ignore, or at least refrain from needlessly responding to, stimuli which do not predict important events. Consequently, it may be a process of considerable adaptive utility, despite its apparent simplicity.

See also: prepulse inhibition

MARK A. UNGLESS

haematoma *see* tumour

haematopoiesis (American spelling: hematopoiesis) (from Greek, *haima*: blood, *poiein*: to make) Haematopoiesis refers to the formation of BLOOD. It is a term that can also be applied to the formation of cells that are derived from blood: a GRANULOCYTE can be spoken of as having haematopoietic origin for example.

haemoglobin (American spelling: hemoglobin) See BLOOD.

haemorrhage (from Greek, *haima*, blood, *rhegnynai*: to burst; American spelling: hemorrhage) Persistent loss of blood from blood vessels; see STROKE.

hair cells There are three rows of OUTER HAIR CELLS (OHC) and one row of INNER HAIR CELLS (IHC) located on the BASILAR MEMBRANE. Ninety-five per cent of AUDITORY NERVE fibres innervates the IHC with up to 20 fibres per IHC. The IHCs are sensory receptors that convert basilar membrane movement into activation of nerve fibres. This process comprises opening of POTASSIUM channels (see ION CHANNEL) in the cilia at the top of the IHC producing a DEPOLARIZATION which allows CALCIUM ions to enter at the base of the IHC and transmitter VESICLES to be released. In contrast, OHCs respond to depolarization by fast length changes that, for low sound levels, provide positive mechanical feedback to the basilar membrane thereby increasing its movement amplitude by up to 100-fold. This permits low-level sounds to depolarize the IHCs. Malfunctioning of OHCs in a given TONOTOPIC REPRESENTATION range increases the hearing threshold by up to 40dB for the corresponding frequencies. OHCs receive an important EFFERENT nerve supply from the brainstem that is affected by the sound level at the same or the other ear. Activation of these nerve fibres causes slow length changes of the OHC which regulate overall movement of the basilar membrane.

See also: cochlea; tip links; vestibular system

JOS J. EGGERMONT

hair follicle *see* skin

hair follicle receptor *see* skin

half-life In pharmacology, half-life refers to the survival of a DRUG once it has been administered to a subject. If one measures the concentration of a drug in the bloodstream one can determine when it achieves a maximal concentration. After this point, the concentration will decline as BIOTRANSFORMATION occurs. The half-life is the time it takes to reduce the concentration of drug by 50%. If the half-life of a drug was 30 minutes one could say that 30 minutes represented one half-life; 60 minutes two half-lives; 90 minutes three half-lives and so on. In terms of radioactive material, half-life refers to the length of time it takes for the radioactivity of a substance to fall by half. In this case however, half-lives may be measured in units of time much longer than minutes.

See also: drug clearance

Reference

Feldman R., Meyer J.S. & Quenzer L.F. (1997) *Principles of Neuropsychopharmacology*, Sinauer Associates: Sunderland MA.

hallucination Abnormality of perception. Defined as a false perception in the absence of a stimulus, which is neither a sensory distortion nor misinterpretation, but which occurs at the same time as real perceptions. Hallucinations may be elementary or complex in form, and may occur in any sensory modality. An elementary visual hallucination may take the form of a flash of light, for example, while a complex auditory hallucination may take the form of a voice or voices. While hallucinations have no diagnostic specificity, there are some recognized associations. Visual hallucinations occur most commonly in organic brain disease, such as DELIRIUM TREMENS, and other forms of ACUTE CONFUSIONAL STATE. Olfactory or gustatory hallucinations are associated with TEMPORAL LOBE EPILEPSY. Auditory hallucinations are often encountered in SCHIZOPHRENIA. Some forms of auditory hallucination are considered FIRST-RANK SYMPTOMS of schizophrenia: hearing one's thoughts aloud, or hearing voices commenting on one's actions. Tactile hallucinations may occur during COCAINE intoxication.

IAN C. REID

hallucinogens A class of PSYCHOACTIVE drugs that have the ability to induce HALLUCINATION (usually visual or auditory). These compounds can be found in different classes of drugs and can have differing chemical structures, but all have the ability to alter perception and thinking. Most are found naturally occurring in plants, and some are synthesized. The most well known hallucinogens are LYSERGIC ACID DIETHYLAMIDE (LSD), PHENCYCLIDINE (PCP), MESCALINE (the active ingredient in the cactus PEYOTE), PSILOCYBIN (found in certain mushrooms). There are many other less well-known hallucinogenic substances found in diverse plants such as ATROPINE (belladonna) in deadly nightshade, jimson in datura, and myristicin in nutmeg. CANNABINOIDS (found in MARIJUANA) are also hallucinogens, but generally are not considered as such since the drug is generally used in sub-hallucinogenic doses. In many native societies, both ancient and modern, hallucinogens have been used in ritual religious ceremonies, presumably to invoke altered mental states associated with spirituality. The precise brain mechanisms underlying hallucinogens are not known, but they generally act to alter SEROTONERGIC, NORADRENERGIC, or CHOLINERGIC systems.

ANN E. KELLEY

Haloperidol (Haldol) *see* antipsychotic

halothane One of the widely used non-flammable VOLATILE ANAESTHETICS administered by flowing oxygenated gases through a chamber promoting vaporization and inhaled by the subject to induce general ANAESTHESIA. It is generally considered a safe anaesthetic, though repeated use on the same subject can induce, in a minority, liver damage known as 'halothane hepatitis'.

CHARLES D. BLAHA

Halstead–Reitan test battery A NEUROPSYCHOLOGICAL TEST BATTERY containing individual tests designed to investigate various psychological processes. It is an established example of a FIXED BATTERY, though the various elements can be used individually to probe specific functions. The sensory tests include the Reitan–Kløve sensory-perceptual examination (a perception of stimuli across different modalities) and the TACTILE form recognition test (a test of shape recognition). The motor tests include finger oscillation, GRIP strength, and tactual performance test all of which are straightforward measures of motor performance in response to simple instructions. The more psychological functions are assessed in various ways: verbal skills are assessed using subtests from the WECHSLER ADULT INTELLIGENCE SCALE, while other components assess spatial and MEMORY functions (see Gaudino *et al.*, 1995; Reitan, 1986).

One of the most widely used components of the battery is the REITAN TRAIL-MAKING TEST. This examines motor speed and visual conceptual and vasomotor tracking. It has two parts, A and B: in trail-making part A, subjects have quickly to draw lines that will interconnect 25 consecutive numbers presented on a page. In trail-making part B, subjects have to draw lines in the same manner, but they must alternate between numbers and letters (see Gaudino *et al.*, 1995 for comparison of parts A and B). This test has been widely used not just as an assessment of motor skill but as a task of planning and EXECUTIVE FUNCTION. Many different patient groups have been assessed with this, including individuals with brain damage and with conditions such as SCHIZO-PHRENIA.

References

Gaudino E.A., Geisler M.W. & Squires N.K. (1995) Construct validity in the trail making test – what makes part B harder? *Journal of Clinical and Experimental Neuropsychology* 17: 529–535.

Reitan R.M. (1986) Theoretical and methodological bases of the Halstead–Reitan neuropsychological test battery. In *Neuropsychological Assessment of Neuropsychiatric Disorders*, ed. I. Grant & K.M. Adams, pp. 3–30, Oxford University Press: New York.

Russell E.W. (1998) In defense of the Halstead Reitan battery. *Archives of Clinical Neuropsychology* 13: 365–381.

hamartoma A growth resembling a NEO-PLASM (see TUMOUR) from which it differs by originating not from inappropriate growths of cells but from incorrect DEVELOPMENT of an organ. It may involve several tissue elements or be an abnormal growth of only one. A hamartoma typically remains at the site of origin and grows at much the same rate as the tissue that spawned it.

handedness Almost 90% of people of every race are right-handed; they use their right hand for most tasks requiring one hand, and their right hand is dominant in tasks requiring both hands. About 95% of these are also right-footed, and two-thirds are right-eyed. Left-handers are less likely to be left-footed and left-eyed. There is little evidence that a consistent population bias for one limb exists outside the human race. Handedness is established by about age 2.

Although evidence suggests that there is some genetic component to handedness, theories disagree on the exact mechanism of this contribution. By far the most popular of the models is the right-shift theory of Marion Annett and her colleagues. The theory suggests that hand preference is a discrete, non-continuous variable, and that the random distribution of hand preference is displaced towards dextrality (right-handedness) in humans. This displacement, according to Annett, is related to the LEFT HEMISPHERE specialization for speech (see SPEECH PERCEPTION; SPEECH PRODUCTION), and the close proximity of regions for hand and speech control in anterior CEREBRAL CORTEX.

See also: asymmetry; corpus callosum;

Reference

Annett M. (1998) Handedness and cerebral dominance: the right shift theory. *Journal of Neuropsychiatry and Clinical Neurosciences* 10:459–469.

JENNI A. OGDEN AND DAVID P. CAREY

haploid Containing a single set of CHROMO-SOMES. In organisms which reproduce sexually, and receive a set of chromosomes from each parent, special cells are created by MEIOSIS (see CELL DIVISION), which contain one set of chromosomes, and are therefore haploid.

FIONA M. INGLIS

haptic Haptic refers to active TOUCH used to purposefully explore objects and the environment. The haptic system incorporates information from cutaneous receptors in the skin with kinaesthetic sensors in muscles, tendons, and joints. KINAESTHESIA integrates hand and finger positions with touch information in a common co-ordinate system. The hand's functional sensitivities are enhanced by the execution of precise motor patterns, called exploratory procedures, which are specialized for extracting specific OBJECT PRIMITIVES (texture, compliance, temperature, size, weight, contour) as well as higher-level functional properties. The haptic system promotes fast, accurate tactile OBJECT RECOGNITION.

See also: grasp; grip; proprioception; soma-esthesis; somatosensory; tactile agnosia; texture perception

Reference

Klatzky R.L. & Lederman S.J. (1993) Toward a computational model of constraint-driven exploration and haptic object identification. *Perception* 22: 597–621.

CATHERINE L. REED

haptic imagery *see* tactile agnosia

harmaline *see* anxiogenic

hashish *see* cannabis

head direction cells These are a type of NEURON that fires when an animal orients its head in a particular direction. Neurons in the anterodorsal THALAMUS, SUBICULUM and MAMMILLARY BODIES (interconnected structures) have this property, which is thought to be of value in the neural computations underlying NAVIGATION.

See also: cognitive map; hippocampus; spatial behaviour; spatial cognition; spatial memory

Reference

Stackman R.W. & Taube J.S. (1998) Firing properties of rat lateral mammillary single units: head direction, head pitch and angular head velocity. *Journal of Neuroscience* 18: 9020–9037.

headache The brain itself is insensitive. The only possible sources of PAIN within the skull are blood vessels, the DURA MATER (see MENINGES), and some of the CRANIAL NERVES. Yet headache is one the most frequent complaints confronting the family medical practitioner. Most cases therefore have an extra-cranial origin, and of these the most common is the so-called TENSION HEADACHE. This condition is thought to be associated with spasm of the muscles of the scalp, triggered in an unknown way by factors such as depression, eye-strain, lack of SLEEP, dietary indiscretion, hangovers and hang-ups. MIGRAINE headaches are quite distinct and are primarily vascular in character: they may be linked to a local disorder of SEROTONIN function, and are usually preceded by transient changes in the underlying CEREBRAL CORTEX. CLUSTER HEADACHE (Horton's cephalalgia) is a distressing variant, with AUTONOMIC involvement. Severe head pain is also a feature of giant-cell arteritis, an auto-immune inflammatory (see INFLAMMATION) condition usually affecting the superficial temporal artery and its branches, and leading to retinal infarction and BLINDNESS unless halted with IMMUNOSUPPRESSANT drugs (see also INFARCT). Pain referred to the head also commonly arises from the teeth, cervical spine, glaucoma, postherpetic and trigeminal NEURALGIA, and inflammation of the nasal sinuses. Intracranial causes of headache include any condition causing mechanical traction or displacement of the dura, blood vessels or cranial nerves. Space-occupying lesions such as tumours, abscesses, cysts and blood clots (haematomata) are obvious examples that usually call for surgery. Sometimes these conditions act indirectly by obstructing the free flow of CEREBROSPINAL FLUID, causing a rise in intracranial pressure and producing HYDROCEPHALUS. Conversely, an abnormally low intracranial pressure following leakage of cerebrospinal fluid after LUMBAR PUNCTURE, is a notorious cause of IATROGENIC headache. Some causes of headache can be recognized by the special character of the pain. The 'mule-kick' headache that follows rupture of an artery in the SUBARACHNOID SPACE is remarkable for its abrupt onset and severity. Recurrent early-morning throbbing headache may signal HYPERTENSION. When in doubt, skull X-ray and other neuroimaging procedures, examination of the cerebrospinal fluid obtained from the spine by diagnostic lumbar puncture, and ophthalmoscopic examination of the RETINA may assist diagnosis. Treatment may be straightforward where a cause is identified, while other cases may obtain symptomatic relief from analgesics (such as paracetamol). Tension headache and psychogenic headache tend to be less responsive to treatment, while the relief of post-concussional headache commonly requires the satisfactory conclusion of legal proceedings.

L. JACOB HERBERG

headcap A construction made from DENTAL ACRYLIC and SKULL SCREWS that sits on an animal's SKULL holding a CANNULA or ELECTRODE securely in place.

health psychology The scientific study of psychological and behavioural processes in health, illness and health care. Much illness in industrialized societies is the direct consequence of health related behaviours such as cigarette smoking (see NICOTINE), excessive ALCOHOL consumption, an inappropriate diet and inadequate exercise. Personality and STRESS may also play a role. Adjustment to illness is clearly psychological and recovery may be determined by adherence to complex medical regimes and a successful interaction with the health care system. A major concern of health psychology is the determinants of health-related behaviours. A number of social cognition models have been proposed to explain the imperfect performance of such behaviours. The theory of planned behaviour is typical and influential. It proposes that the intention to perform a behaviour is a function of the subject's attitude towards the behaviour, the views of others to whom they are exposed (subjective norm), and their belief that they can perform the target behaviour (perceived behavioural control, which is akin to self-efficacy). Such factors explain intention adequately but intention predicts subsequent behaviour poorly. Other models emphasize that people pass through different stages of preparedness to change their behaviour.

It has proved difficult to show that stress is a cause of physical illness in humans although there is excellent supportive evidence in other species, including other PRIMATES. Many aspects of personality have been related to disease, and while the findings are contentious there is support for a link – for example, aspects of hostility are predictive of cardiovascular disease as is DEPRESSION. Studies of patients often examine factors such as coping with illness. An important contrast is drawn between an avoidant coping style which may be helpful in coping with the treatment of acute illness and a vigilant coping style which may be more appropriate for chronic conditions. Patient adherence to treatment regimes is dependent on their understanding of their illness (their illness representations). The belief that one has control of one's own destiny (internal locus of control) also aids recovery. One of the most important findings in this field is that the reporting of SIGNS AND SYMPTOMS is strongly influenced by negative affectivity, the tendency for DYSPHORIA. This has to be allowed for in studies dependent on patient self-report of symptoms. Among the psychological aspects of health care that have been examined are doctor–patient communication, an important determinant of adherence to advice and patient satisfaction. With the advent of evidence-based medicine there is increasing interest in the far-from perfect adherence to treatment guidelines by medical personnel. The cognitive models hitherto applied to patients' behaviour are now being applied to health professions.

DEREK W. JOHNSTON

hearing theories Normal hearing depends on the peripheral and central auditory systems. In the auditory periphery, the PINNA acts as a somewhat directional sound gatherer, and the middle ear OSSICLES conduct the vibrations received by the TYMPANIC MEMBRANE to the COCHLEA, which contains the HAIR CELLS responsible for the transduction of the acoustic pressure waves into neural signals. The cochlea decomposes the incoming stimulus into component frequencies (see FOURIER ANALYSIS). Pressure waves introduced to the cochlear fluids at the OVAL WINDOW are able to vibrate the BASILAR MEMBRANE which partitions the cochlea longitudinally. The basilar membrane is structurally graded so that it can be forced into oscillation at high frequencies near the basal end, and at low frequencies near the apical end. Outer hair cells, arrayed in three rows along the length of the ORGAN OF CORTI, are able actively to enhance basilar membrane motion locally. These two processes have the consequence that basilar membrane motion has a sensitive and fine tuning to tone frequency at each site. This mechanical tuning is directly conferred upon the inner hair cells, which exist as a single longitudinal row in the organ of Corti. The inner hair cells have receptor potentials that are coupled to motion of the basilar membrane; in turn, the receptor potential drives the release of NEUROTRANSMITTERS at the hair cell base, which is the site of contact of the nerve cells that link the hair cells with the auditory processing structures in the BRAIN-STEM.

The foregoing processes have the consequence that the location of vibration along the length of the basilar membrane, and thus the identity of the subset of hair cells and afferent nerves activated, depends on the frequency content of the acoustic stimulus. This is known as the PLACE THEORY. The cochlea can be conceptualized as a linear array of frequency-tuned channels, each functioning relatively independently. The task of any one of these channels is to encode information about the presence, timing and amplitude of stimulus energy at its preferred frequency, and to transmit that information to the brain. For frequencies less than about 3000 Hz, the inner hair cell receptor potential has DEPOLARIZATION and HYPERPOLARIZATION half-periods that are phase-locked to upward and downward motions of the basilar membrane, respectively. Since neurotransmitter release is coupled to hair cell depolarizations, this has the consequence that cochlear nerve fibres are excited by unidirectional elevations of the basilar membrane. Restated, this means that for low frequency sounds, cochlear nerve cells generate a typical ACTION POTENTIAL that is time-locked to oscillations of the basilar membrane at the innervated site and thus to the phase of the stimulus. This constitutes a temporal code for frequency, since the time between spikes will be equal to the stimulus period, or an integral multiple of it. Either by sampling the SPIKE activity of a single such nerve for some duration, or by sampling a number of such nerve cells concurrently, the brain is able to determine the low-frequency spectral content of the sound. This is known as the volley principle.

The central auditory system preserves the place code in the form of a TONOTOPIC REPRESENTATION in each nucleus from the brainstem to the CEREBRAL CORTEX; there is, however, little evidence of phase-locked spike responses for frequencies above 100 Hz, except in the most caudal nuclei. The central auditory pathway has an architecture that shows both PARALLEL PROCESSING and SERIAL PROCESSING. Some brainstem circuits are involved in SOUND LOCALIZATION; others may be involved on processing of a sound's spectral fine structure.

The fact that all such nuclei and circuits are tonotopically organized means that these analyses are performed on a frequency-by-frequency basis. Information from these circuits ultimately reaches the AUDITORY CORTEX. The PRIMARY SENSORY CORTEX, and some adjacent fields, have their own tonotopic representation in the form of strip-like assemblies of neurons tuned to the same preferred frequencies. Overlaying this representation is a patchy mosaic of territories dedicated to elaboration of the processing of other stimulus dimensions initiated in the auditory brainstem. The fidelity of this information sets limits on that available to higher, non-auditory processors (such as ATTENTION and LANGUAGE). In this regard, the auditory cortex on each side of the brain processes spatial information only for the CONTRALATERAL hemifield. It is for this reason that deficits in spatial behavior (attention, sound localization) following a UNILATERAL cerebral LESION are also unilateral, and contralateral to the lesion. By the same token, the strictly temporal fidelity of auditory cortical responses is sufficient to encode the timing of the phonetically important elements of speech

References

Dallos P. (1992) The active cochlea. *Journal of Neuroscience* 12: 4575–4585.

Phillips D.P. (1995) Central auditory processing. A view from auditory neuroscience. *American Journal of Otology* 16: 338–352.

DENNIS P. PHILLIPS

heart An essential organ whose principal function is to pump BLOOD around the body, but important also for OSMOREGULATION. The cardiovascular system is described in the entry BLOOD; and see BREATHING, NEURAL CONTROL OF; ENDOCRINE GLANDS; RESPIRATION.

heart beat *see* blood

heart rate *see* blood

heat (sexual) *see* estrus

heat shock protein Formation of heat shock proteins is induced in neurons (see NEURON) and GLIAL CELLS by a wide variety of stressors (see STRESS) and insults to the CENTRAL NERVOUS SYSTEM, including environmental stressors (such as heat shock) and internal brain events such as the induction of SEIZURES. There are several heat shock proteins, commonly identified by their MOLECULAR WEIGHT. For example, the 70 000 MW heat shock protein (Hsp70) is induced in neurons by stressors; the 27 000 MW heat shock protein (Hsp27) is induced to a greater degree in astrocytes (see ASTROGLIA).

See also: immune system

Hebb's postulate A rule for determining the sign of activity-dependent changes in synaptic efficacy, proposed in 1949 by the psychologist Donald Hebb (1904–1985). Hebb's famous postulate states that: when an axon of cell A is near enough to excite a cell B and repeatedly or persistently takes part in firing it, some growth process or metabolic change takes place in one or both cells such that A's efficiency, as one of the cells firing B, is increased. Hebb proposed his rule in the course of considering how information storage is implemented in a distributed NEURAL ASSEMBLY. The idea has antecedents in the writings of the psychologist William James (1824–1910), who suggested in his 'law of neural habit' that if two regions of the brain were active at the same time each would 'propagate its excitement into the other', and in the work of the neuroanatomists Eugenio Tanzi (1856–1934) and Santiago Ramon y Cajal (1852–1934, winner of the 1906 Nobel Prize for Medicine) who suggested that the SYNAPSE, whose existence as a basic structural entity had been championed by Cajal, was the site of information storage in the brain. Hebb's contribution was to provide a specific rule linking synaptic modification to coincident pre- and postsynaptic activity. The rule is both local and associative. It is local in the sense that the increase in synaptic strength is specific to the synapse linking cells A and B; it is associative in that the activity of cell B is necessarily determined by activity in the whole class of A cells which are afferent to B; thus, a subpopulation of A cells which tend to fire at the same time will generate sufficient postsynaptic activity to satisfy the rule, and the synapses of this subpopulation will accordingly be strengthened. The best-known exemplification of the Hebb rule in the mammalian brain is the phenom-

enon of LONG-TERM POTENTIATION (LTP), in which coincident activity between pre- and postsynaptic cells in the HIPPOCAMPUS leads to a persistent increase in synaptic efficacy. LTP is both associative and input-specific, Hebbian characteristics which derive, at the molecular level, from the voltage-dependent properties of NMDA RECEPTORS. Critics have frequently pointed out that Hebb's rule alone, if unchecked by a mechanism to reduce synaptic efficacy, would lead eventually to a network in which all synapses were saturated at maximum efficiency, and many modifications of Hebb's postulate allowing for activity-dependent synaptic depression have been proposed.

See also: Hebb-like rules; Hebbian synapses; long-term depression

Reference

Hebb D.O. (1949) *The Organization of Behavior*, Wiley: New York.

T. V. P. BLISS

Hebb-like rule A family of rules determining how activity at a SYNAPSE governs changes in synaptic weight in NEURAL NETWORKS. In Hebb's rule (named after Donald Hebb, 1904–1985), which only allows for increases in synaptic strength, changes are proportional to the product of the rate of firing of PRESYNAPTIC and POSTSYNAPTIC neurons. A slightly modified rule, in which the rate of postsynaptic firing is replaced by degree of postsynaptic depolarization, applies to LONG-TERM POTENTIATION (LTP) dependent on NMDA RECEPTORS in the HIPPOCAMPUS. Examples of Hebb-like rules which allow for decreases as well as increases in synaptic strength are the COVARIANCE RULE of Sejnowski, the BIENENSTOCK–COOPER–MUNRO RULE, and the STENT–SINGER RULE.

See also: Hebb's postulate; Hebbian synapse; long-term depression; long-term potentiation

T. V. P. BLISS

Hebbian synapse A SYNAPSE is said to be Hebbian if a period of coincident impulse activity in the neurons linked by the synapse leads to a persistent increase in synaptic efficacy . The existence of such synapses was proposed in 1949 by the Canadian psychologist Donald Hebb (1904–1985) as a mechanism for storing information in neural nets (see HEBB'S POSTULATE; Brown & Chatterji, 1994 provide a contemporary overview). The essential feature of the Hebbian synapse is that its efficacy is controlled by activity in both pre-synaptic and postsynaptic neurons. In that sense, a Hebbian synapse is a coincidence detector. As an illustration of the distinction between synaptic plasticity at Hebbian and non-Hebbian synapses, we may compare LONG-TERM POTENTIATION (LTP) at mossy fibre and Schaffer-commissural synapses in the HIPPOCAMPUS. LTP in mossy fibres is non-Hebbian, since its induction depends only on a period of increased activity in the mossy fibres themselves, and is independent of activity in the target neurons of the CA3 (see CA1–CA3) pyramidal field. In contrast, the synapses made by the axons of these same CA3 cells – the Schaffer-commissural fibres to CA1 pyramidal cells – are the very type of the Hebbian synapse. In these synapses, the induction of LTP requires precisely the ACTION POTENTIAL coincidence in the pre- and postsynaptic neuron postulated by Hebb (Magee & Johnston, 1997). The molecular basis for this property is to be found in the voltage-dependence of the NMDA RECEPTORS (see LONG-TERM POTENTIATION). Note that a typical cortical excitatory synapse does not produce sufficient excitation to fire the postsynaptic cell unaided; thus, the weight of a Hebbian synapse will not change unless there is sufficient coincident input from other excitatory afferents. If these are themselves Hebbian, then changes in synaptic weight will occur associatively; that is, all Hebbian afferents which are simultaneously active will be strengthened.

The performance of NEURAL NETWORKS that contains only Hebbian synapses becomes progressively compromised as the proportion of potentiated synapses increases. At the limit, with all synapses fully potentiated, the network would no longer have any utility as a MNEMONIC device. A number of alternative rules which allow for bi-directional changes in synaptic efficacy, have been postulated to circumvent this problem (see HEBB-LIKE RULE). Four possible conjunction states exist: (1) both

presynaptic and postsynaptic neurons are active (Hebbian conjunction); (2) the postsynaptic cell is active when the presynaptic cell is not; (3) the postsynaptic neuron is active when the presynaptic cell is not, and (4) neither is active. According to the STENT–SINGER RULE, condition (2) leads to LONG-TERM DEPRESSION (LTD) while (3) and (4) are neutral with respect to changes in synaptic weight. A variant of this scheme is the COVARIANCE RULE, due to Sejnowski, in which synaptic weight increases if pre- and postsynaptic activity is positively correlated and decreases if it is negatively correlated. The influential BIENEN-STOCK–COOPER–MUNRO RULE (BCM rule) introduces the further notion of a variable threshold for LTP which is a function of the time-averaged activity in the postsynaptic cell. According to the BCM rule, the change in synaptic weight is determined by the product of activity in the presynaptic neuron and a non-monotonic function, $f(c,<c>)$, whose value is determined both by the activity, c, in the postsynaptic cell, and its time-averaged mean, $<c>$. The polarity of change is determined by the value of f, which for low values of presynaptic activity is negative, but which becomes positive at higher rates of $<c>$, crossing from negative (LTD) to positive (LTP) at a threshold, q, which is itself inversely related to $<c>$. The variable threshold prevents runaway potentiation if high values of $<c>$ are maintained. There is good evidence for bidirectional changes in synaptic weight at synapses in the visual cortex, and in the hippocampus. However, the experimental protocols which induce homosynaptic LTD commonly involve prolonged trains of low-frequency stimulation (see LONG-TERM DEPRESSION). How can this be reconciled with the rules for bidirectional changes in synaptic efficacy discussed above, which emphasize the importance of activity in the postsynaptic cell in determining the direction of change? Present evidence suggests that it is the level of the change in local Ca^{2+} concentration in the postsynaptic cell which determines the direction of change. Synaptic activation alone can produce Ca^{2+} changes which are sufficient to trigger LTD; the association of synaptic activity with postsynaptic firing, leading to BACKPROPAGATION of dendritic action potentials in the postsynaptic cell may produce a non-linear increase in local Ca^{2+} concentration which crosses the threshold for induction of LTP.

The Hebbian synapse has emerged as one of the central concepts in contemporary neuroscience, offering a mechanistic framework for phenomena as diverse as the activity-dependent memory CONSOLIDATION and pruning of synaptic connections (SYNAPTIC PRUNING) in developing sensory systems, and the neural substrate of learning and memory.

See also: artificial intelligence; associative learning

References

Bear M.F., Cooper L.N. & Ebner F.F. (1987) A physiological basis for a theory of synapse modification. *Science* 237: 42–48.

Brown T.H. & Chatterji, S. (1994) Hebbian synaptic plasticity: evolution of the contemporary concept. In *Models of Neural Networks*, vol. 2, ed. E. Domany, J.L. Van Hemmen & K. Schulten, pp. 287–314, Springer-Verlag: New York.

Hebb D.O. (1949) *The Organization of Behavior*, Wiley: New York.

Magee J.C. & Johnston D. (1997) A synaptically controlled, associative signal for Hebbian plasticity in hippocampal neurons. *Science* 275: 209–213.

T. V. P. BLISS

hebephrenia (from Greek, *hebe*: youth, *phren*: mind) An early-onset disorder that formed a category within DEMENTIA PRAECOX, a description used by Emil Kraepelin (1856–1926) but which was later replaced by the term SCHIZOPHRENIA. Hebephrenia included disorders of AFFECT, MOOD and thought. Other categories in dementia praecox included PARANOIA and CATATONIA. These terms remain in use: hebephrenia is a term rarely used now.

hedgehog proteins Hedgehog proteins (hh proteins), coded by hedgehog genes, are important during DEVELOPMENT: they are important in many different structures, not just within the CENTRAL NERVOUS SYSTEM, and are found in species from *DROSOPHILA* through rodents to humans. Their function appears to be to induce the formation of locally appropriate CELL types and to guide their develop-

ment. For example, the DOPAMINERGIC neurons of the SUBSTANTIA NIGRA are stimulated to develop by a particular member of this family of proteins, SONIC HEDGEHOG protein (shh). There is a belief that use of hedgehog proteins might prove valuable in restructuring brains that have been damaged.

See also: neurodevelopment; transplantation

hemangioblastoma *see* tumour

heme Heme is important in several cellular processes, including GENE expression and the transport of PROTEINS: it is present in every type of CELL. Heme is converted by HEME OXYGENASE to CARBON MONOXIDE and biliverdin (a bile pigment).

heme oxygenase There is more than one ISOZYME of heme oxygenase (HO): HO-1 is inducible, activated by a variety of stimuli while HO-2 is a constitutive component of many neurons in BRAIN. Heme oxygenase is important because it is the synthetic enzyme for the novel gaseous neurotransmitter (see NEUROMODULATION) CARBON MONOXIDE. HO-1 is found in discrete sites in brain, identifying those parts of it that can generate carbon monoxide on demand: these include the BRAINSTEM, CEREBELLUM, HYPOTHALAMUS and DENTATE GYRUS. HO-2 is more widely found through the brain.

hemivisual field *see* hemifield

hemiachromatopsia *see* achromatopsia

hemianaesthesia Sensory loss on one side of the body; see STROKE.

hemianopia A lack of vision in one half of the visual field. The dividing line between the intact and blind hemifields is usually (but not always) vertical. There is a partial DECUSSATION of the optic fibres at the OPTIC CHIASM which lies between the eyeball and the LATERAL GENICULATE NUCLEUS. Half of the fibres project to the visual HEMISPHERE of the brain on the same (IPSILATERAL) side, and the other project to the visual hemisphere on the opposite (CONTRALATERAL) side. SECTION of the optic tract above the level of the chiasm therefore will lead to HOMONYMOUS HEMIANOPIA whereby both eyes will be affected, vision being lost in the TEMPORAL VISUAL HEMIFIELD in one eye and the NASAL VISUAL HEMIFIELD in the other. The exact pattern of hemianopia in the two eyes is a critical diagnostic tool for locating the site of a LESION in the visual pathway.

See also: macula sparing

DAVID W. HEELEY

hemiballismus (from Greek, *ballismos*: jumping about) These are uncontrollable writhing and jerky movements on one side of the body, affecting predominantly the limbs. Hemiballismus is seen following damage to the SUBTHALAMIC NUCLEUS, the effect being seen on the side of the body CONTRALATERAL to the LESION.

See also: motor control; movement deficits

DAVID P. CAREY

hemidecortication Hemidecortication is removal of the CEREBRAL CORTEX from one HEMISPHERE only; hemidecorticate describes an organism to which this has been done.

See also: *cerveau isolé*; decerebrate; decortication

hemifacial spasm *see* blepharospasm

hemifield Half of the visual field of the eye. The dividing line is usually vertical as a consequence of the partial crossing of the fibres of the optic tract at the OPTIC CHIASM. Because the dividing line is usually vertical, one typically describes a NASAL VISUAL HEMIFIELD and a TEMPORAL VISUAL HEMIFIELD: the former is that half of the visual field on the side of the eye next to the nose, the latter is the half of the visual field next to the temporal bone (see SKULL) – that is, on the side of the eye furthest from the nose.

DAVID W. HEELEY

hemineglect *see* spatial neglect

hemiparesis Weakness of the muscles on one side of the body, consequent to damage in the CONTRALATERAL side of the brain. HEMIPLEGIA refers to a complete paralysis of the contralateral musculature. Typically, hemiparesis follows some sort of CEREBROVASCULAR ACCIDENT involving the middle cerebral artery.

Recovery from hemiparesis tends to follow a PROXIMAL to DISTAL gradient; the use of the muscles of the upper arm usually precedes recovery of wrist/hand/digit muscle use. Poor control of discrete muscle groups, such as those necessary for individual finger movements, in the contralateral arm/hand is the characteristic feature of the recovering hemiplegic.

See also: motor control; movement deficits

DAVID P. CAREY

hemiplegia Complete paralysis of one side of the body, consequent to CONTRALATERAL brain damage (often a consequence of infarct of the middle cerebral artery). However this term is also often as a synonym for HEMIPARESIS. Hemiplegia is a consequence of a LESION in one of the PYRAMIDAL TRACTS. Typically large lesions in the CEREBRAL CORTEX are necessary, although the tract becomes quite narrow in the INTERNAL CAPSULE where a small infarct can produce a dense hemiplegia. Hemiplegia can be less severe in the contralateral leg than the contralateral face and arm.

See also: corticospinal tract; motor control; movement deficits; paraplegia; spasticity

DAVID P. CAREY

hemispatial neglect *see* spatial neglect

hemisphere One of the two halves of the TELENCEPHALON. Each hemisphere is largely responsible for controlling sensory and motor processes for the opposite side of the body. Psychologists have tended to study functional ASYMMETRY when referring to the hemispheres. The consensus is that (in humans), the LEFT HEMISPHERE plays a critical role in speech (see SPEECH PERCEPTION; SPEECH PRODUCTION) and LANGUAGE functions, and higher-level MOTOR PROGRAMMING and control. There is less agreement on an appropriate label for RIGHT HEMISPHERE specialization, although non-verbal, visuospatial perceptual tasks may rely to some extent on this hemisphere.

See also: aphasia; apraxia; central nervous system; cerebral asymmetry

DAVID P. CAREY

hemispherectomy The surgical removal of one cerebral HEMISPHERE, usually for the treatment of EPILEPSY or cortical TUMOUR (usually a GLIOMA). Patients who have had hemispherectomy are of great theoretical importance for experimental psychology, since they can play a unique role in studies of NEUROPLASTICITY as well as studies of hemispheric function with and without the presence of CEREBRAL CORTEX. For example, such patients have shown some residual abilities to use visual information to guide their movements in the 'bad' visual field (CONTRALATERAL to the hemispherectomy), in spite of no conscious awareness of the presence of a visual stimulus (see BLINDSIGHT).

DAVID P. CAREY

hemispheric specialization *see* lateralization

hemp *see* cannabis

heparin A substance formed naturally in the LIVER and lungs but available also as a prepared compound. It is widely used as an anticoagulant to prevent BLOOD clotting. For example, a heparin solution (heparinized saline) is used to flush the CATHETER used in intra-venous drug SELF-ADMINISTRATION – this prevents blood clotting in the catheter and obstructing it. Similarly, when blood samples are collected from animals for diagnostic purposes, the tubes the blood is collected into will be rinsed with heparin solution to help present clotting.

hepatic Relating to the LIVER or liver function.

herbivore (from Latin, *herba*: herb, *vorare*: to devour) An animal that eats plants and not other animals.

See also: carnivore; omnivore

heredity The process by which characteristics of living CELLS are passed on during replication. The basis of heritability is the genetic code, contained within the DEOXYRIBONUCLEIC ACID (DNA) of all cells. Before cell division, DNA is duplicated and copies of the GENES are inherited by the daughter cells. While most genes are preserved between organisms of the same species, small differences between organisms in the exact structure of DNA lead to variations in gene structure. These differences are manifest in variations in physical characteristics such as eye or hair colour. Organisms which reproduce sexually receive one set of CHROMOSOMES from each parent, each containing half the ALLELES present in each parent. As a result, some allelic variations in gene structure may not be inherited in every offspring. The heritability of psychological traits – the 'NATURE–NURTURE' debate – remains a controversial issue. The relative contribution of genetic, as opposed to environmental factors as determinants of, for example, INTELLIGENCE, is unresolved.

FIONA M. INGLIS

heritability The term heritability refers to the estimation of the degree to which a particular trait or characteristic might be genetically transmitted. The estimation of heritability is a statistical process, and any estimate brings with it a degree of variance. TWIN STUDIES have been used to determine the extent to which traits are heritable, though this method has not been without its critics. Indeed, debates involving heritability – the degree to which INTELLIGENCE is inherited, or the genetic basis of diseases such as SCHIZOPHRENIA – have attracted considerable controversy.

Reference

Plomin R., DeFries J.C., McClearn G.E. & Rutter M. (1997) *Behavioral Genetics*, 3rd edn, W.H. Freeman: New York.

Herman & Polivy restraint scale Test designed to measure the construct of RESTRAINED EATING. The restraint scale was published by C. Peter Herman & Janet Polivy (1980) with 10 items measuring weight fluctuation (four items) and concern for dieting (six items). Restrained eating refers to the degree of chronic dieting. Concern for dieting includes attempts to restrict food intake below a normal or desired limit, and episodes when restraint is abandoned. Therefore, when restrained eaters are given a pre-load of food they consume more than restrained eaters given no pre-load (COUNTER-REGULATION). Subsequent measures of restraint uncouple dietary restriction and tendency to overeat (see Lowe, 1993).

See also: binge eating; eating disorders; obesity

References

Herman C.P. & Polivy J. (1980) Restrained eating. In *Obesity*, ed. A.J. Stunkard, pp. 208–225, W. B Saunders: Philadelphia.

Lowe M.R. (1993) The effects of dieting on eating behaviour: a three-factor model. *Psychological Bulletin*, 114: 100–121.

MARION M. HETHERINGTON

hermaphrodite (from Greek: *Hermaphroditos* was the son of *Hermes* and *Aphrodite* who grew into a single creature with the nymph *Salmacis*) A hermaphrodite is any organism (plant or animal) possessing both male and female reproductive organs; hermaphroditic and hermaphroditism describe this condition. It is not an abnormality: certain species are genuinely hermaphroditic. The term PSEUDO-HERMAPHRODITE (or INTERSEX) describes an individual of a species that divides into male and female who possesses some male and some female characteristics. Such individuals are infertile and, in human cases, raised as females.

See also: gender; reproduction

heroin A semi-synthetic opiate made by adding two acetyl groups to the MORPHINE molecule (see OPIATES). It was first made and promoted by Bayer Laboratories (the same company that makes Bayer aspirin) in 1898. It originally was marketed as a non-addictive substitute for CODEINE. However, as use spread, it soon became apparent that heroin was the most addictive of all the opiates (see ADDICTION). The minor chemical modification makes heroin much more potent than morphine, because it is more lipid-soluble and reaches the brain more quickly and in higher concentrations. Among the opiate addict population, heroin is the drug of choice. It is usually injected into the veins (see INTRAVENOUS SELF-ADMINISTRATION), although it is also injected beneath the skin, which is known as 'skin-popping'. When injected intravenously, heroin is absorbed very rapidly and reaches the brain in a matter of seconds. Subjective accounts by addicts of the heroin high or 'rush' describe a warm flushing of the skin and sensations described in intensity and quality as a 'whole-body ORGASM'. This initial effect lasts for less than 1 minute. TOLERANCE often develops to the EUPHORIA produced by the drug. Heroin can also induce general feelings of well-being, calmness, and a sleepy dream-like state known as 'twilight sleep'. Feelings of ANXIETY, hostility, and AGGRESSION are reduced by heroin. Indeed, in addition to the pleasurable feelings heroin induces, its ability to blunt psychological pain may be an important motivation for using heroin.

Heroin addiction may be associated with a high degree of tolerance and PHYSICAL DEPENDENCE. With repeated use, the dose taken by the user gradually becomes higher. After continued use of fairly high doses, some users can administer doses up to 50 times what would kill a non-tolerant individual. Physical dependence is also classically associated with heroin addiction, and a WITHDRAWAL SYNDROME results in dependent individuals upon cessation of the drug. This syndrome, which varies in intensity depending on the individual and severity of dependence, consists of a number of physiological and psychological symptoms, such as irritability, loss of APPETITE, and TREMOR. At peak intensity, the individual experiences INSOMNIA, violent yawning, excessive tearing and sneezing. Muscle weakness and depression may be pronounced. PILOERECTION resulting in 'goosebumps' gives the skin the appearance of a plucked turkey; hence the expression 'cold turkey' given to signify abrupt withdrawal. Gastrointestinal distress, characterized by cramps and diarrhoea, is also apparent. Gradually, the symptoms subside, although the neuroadaptation that takes place with long-term heroin use may subsist for months or years, and contribute to relapse. The primary treatment for heroin addiction has been pharmacological, with a fair amount of success. Maintenance or substitution therapy has involved substituting an oral synthetic opiate, usually METHADONE, for the intravenous heroin. There are a number of reasons why methadone is preferable to heroin. First, it can be taken orally and thus intravenous injection is avoided. Second, methadone is longer acting than heroin and prevents the onset of withdrawal symptoms for up to 24 hours. Third, little or no euphoria is produced by methadone. Although there is an abstinence syndrome that results from withdrawal from methadone, it is less severe in intensity than withdrawal from heroin. Moreover, methadone seems to block the effects of heroin. Several studies both in the laboratory and in street settings have shown that the heroin addict does not experience the same rush or euphoria if he does take heroin while on methadone, probably because methadone is already occupying the opiate receptors. Since the REINFORCEMENT effects of heroin are diminished and the unpleasant withdrawal state is avoided, methadone therapy is successful in getting users off heroin.

ANN E. KELLEY

herpes encephalitis Infection of the BRAIN by *Herpes simplex* VIRUS. It can lead to damage in the FRONTAL LOBE and TEMPORAL LOBE, producing a LESION that can in some cases be remarkably specific. It often produces an AMNESIC SYNDROME because of damage to structures in the temporal lobe, including the HIPPOCAMPUS.

See also: cytomegalovirus

Heschl's gyrus A cortical gyrus (see GYRI AND SULCI) in the TEMPORAL LOBE that shows, in human brain, ASYMMETRY: it is larger in the right hemisphere than the left.

heterarchy Heterarchy and hierarchy are terms derived from mathematics and linguistics, now applied to NEURAL NETWORKS. A HETERARCHY is a network of nodes (see NETWORK NODES) in which none is permanently uppermost. A HIERARCHY is a network of nodes in which one is uppermost and in which there may be layers of organization.

See also: parallel vs. serial processing; top-down vs. bottom-up perceptual/neural processing

heteroceptor The RECEPTOR on any TERMINAL, SOMA or DENDRITE of a NEURON that binds NEUROTRANSMITTERS released by other neurons. A heteroceptor is contrasted with an AUTORECEPTOR.

heterochromatic brightness matching *see* brightness

heteromer *see* homomer

heterophoria *see* heterotropia

heteropia *see* heterotropia

heterosexual Heterosexual describes sexual attraction, desire or behaviour directed by an individual towards members of the opposite sex.

See also: homosexual

heterosynaptic *see* long-term depression

heterotropia A HETEROTROPIA is a manifest deviation of the optic axis of the eye in the presence of a stimulus – it is a technical term indicating a squint (see STRABISMUS). HETEROPIA is taken to be synonymous with heterotropia. HETEROPHORIA is a deviation of the optic axis when one eye (the non-viewing eye) is covered.

heterozygous In diploid cells, the existence of two different alleles of a particular GENE, often one recessive and one dominant (see DOMINANT ALLELE; RECESSIVE ALLELE), each occurring on one of a pair of AUTOSOMAL CHROMOSOMES.

See also: allele

FIONA M. INGLIS

hibernation A period of dormancy associated with the winter months. Hibernation allows animals to prosper in environments that are fruitful for only part of a year without leaving, in contrast to MIGRATION which involves seasonal transfer between environments. Hibernation occurs annually and is therefore known as a CIRCANNUAL RHYTHM. It is thought that brain mechanisms similar to those controlling circadian rhythms regulate these (see BIOLOGICAL CLOCK). Animals approaching a period of hibernation show changes in their food intake and fat deposition and may engage in HOARDING BEHAVIOUR. Changes in hormonal status and temperature regulation also occur. However, despite the familiarity of hibernation, many key questions remain to be answered fully. Why do some animals in a particular environment hibernate while others do not? Why do animals in environments that seem hospitable nevertheless hibernate? Some species of lemur (the fat-tailed dwarf lemur, *Cheirogaleus medius*) in temperate southern Madagascar hibernate, storing fat in their tails in preparation. What cellular mechanisms regulate the changes in body state? What factors precipitate hibernation? Temperature, and animals' judgement of whether periods of daylight are getting shorter or longer, are thought to be determinants of both hibernation and migration.

See also: aestivation

hierarchy *see* heterarchy

high affinity *see* affinity

high fat phenotype *see* body weight

high-performance liquid chromatography (HPLC) An analytical technique using a liquid mobile phase (carrier) and a stationary phase (column) to separate complex mixtures into individual compounds based on their physiochemical properties. It allows one to determine the chemical content of a solution, for instance the DIALYSATE recovered from the brain using *in vivo* MICRODIALYSIS.

CHARLES D. BLAHA

higher-order conditioning A PAVLOVIAN CONDITIONING procedure in which a previously established CONDITIONED STIMULUS (CS) serves as an UNCONDITIONED STIMULUS (US) in supporting conditioned responding to a new CS. SECOND-ORDER CONDITIONING is a well-established example of higher-order conditioning. Some authors use higher-order conditioning to refer to second-order conditioning; however, the term is more inclusive and can be used to refer to third-order (or more) conditioning, when a third CS is conditioned by its pairing with a second-order conditioned CS.

JASPER WARD-ROBINSON

higher vocal centre *see* birdsong

hilar cells The hilus of the DENTATE GYRUS of the HIPPOCAMPAL FORMATION contains distinct types of INTERNEURONS, including MOSSY CELLS which represent the major cell type. Mossy cells receive numerous synapses (see SYNAPSE) from collateral MOSSY FIBRES of dentate granule cells. Mossy cells are thought to release GLUTAMATE and activate GABAERGIC BASKET CELLS, which in turn directly inhibit

granule cells. Thus, mossy cells are the main component of the RECURRENT INHIBITION circuit that governs the excitability of dentate granule cells. Hilar cells are known to be susceptible to various insults such as neurotoxicity (see NEUROTOXINS) and TRAUMA, and their pathology may be involved in EPILEPSY generated from the TEMPORAL LOBE.

KAZUE SEMBA

hilus *see* dentate gyrus

hindbrain The hindbrain, or RHOMBENCEPHALON, consists of the PONS, CEREBELLUM and MEDULLA OBLONGATA. This term is often encountered in the context of the DEVELOPMENT of the CENTRAL NERVOUS SYSTEM. In contrast, the BRAINSTEM also includes the MESENCEPHALON and DIENCEPHALON. The hindbrain develops from the third of the three primary vesicles of the early embryonic brain. As the brain develops to the five-vesicle stage, the rhombencephalon differentiates into the METENCEPHALON rostrally and MYELENCEPHALON caudally. In the adult brain, the metencephalon includes the cerebellum and pons while the myelencephalon becomes the medulla oblongata.

During development of the hindbrain, the central canal of the embryonic VENTRICULAR SYSTEM enlarges to form the fourth ventricle. In the course of this development, the fourth ventricle opens and expands laterally with the consequence that sensory nuclei of the CRANIAL NERVES of the hindbrain move to a lateral rather than the dorsal position seen in the SPINAL CORD. Similarly, the motor nuclei assume a medial rather than ventral position. This developmental process is a major feature critical to an understanding of the topography and organization of cranial nerve nuclei in the hindbrain. During this process, the roof of the fourth ventricle becomes very thin as it is formed by a layer of ependyma and PIA MATER. The cerebellum eventually expands to lie over and cover the roof of the ventricle in the adult.

Three large fibre tracts, the INFERIOR, MIDDLE and SUPERIOR CEREBELLAR PEDUNCLES attach the cerebellum to the pons. The inferior cerebellar peduncle carries afferent axons from the spinal cord and the INFERIOR OLIVE, the middle cerebellar peduncle carries afferent axons from the pontine nuclei of the pons, and the superior cerebellar peduncle carries efferent axons from the cerebellum to the RED NUCLEUS of the mesencephalon and to the THALAMUS. The fibres of the middle cerebellar peduncle gather on the ventral (anterior) and lateral surface of the PONS, forming a striking white, bridge-like elevation (*pons* is Latin for 'bridge'). The PONTINE NUCLEI, a large collection of neurons giving rise to projections to the contralateral cerebellum, lie deep to the ventral fibres of the middle cerebellar peduncle. The pontine nuclei and their efferent axons occupy roughly half of the pons, while the gray matter dorsal to them forms the PONTINE TEGMENTUM which contains the major cranial nerve nuclei of the pons. The darkly-pigmented ADRENERGIC cells of the LOCUS COERULEUS are found in the dorsal pontine tegmentum. The locus coeruleus has extensive connections with higher levels of the nervous system and has been implicated in many physiological functions related to ATTENTION and EMOTION as well as in the pathophysiology of ANXIETY and DEPRESSION. The COCHLEAR NUCLEUS and VESTIBULAR NUCLEUS are found dorsolaterally while the NUCLEUS ABDUCENS, a motor nucleus, is found medially. The motor TRIGEMINAL NUCLEUS and FACIAL NUCLEUS are located ventrolaterally, consistent with their embryological origin as special visceral efferent neurons which migrate to a ventrolateral position similar to that of the more caudally located special visceral efferent neurons of the NUCLEUS AMBIGUUS in the medulla oblongata. The white matter of the pons is composed of the cerebellar peduncles and longitudinally oriented ascending (for instance, the MEDIAL LEMNISCUS, SPINAL LEMNISCUS, MEDIAL LONGITUDINAL FASCICULUS) and descending (for instance, the CORTICOSPINAL TRACT, medial longitudinal fasciculus) pathways connecting other levels of the NEURAXIS. The medulla oblongata has similarities to the pons in that it contains a large ventrally located precerebellar relay nucleus, the inferior olive, that is closely related both in development and connections to the pontine nuclei. The major medullary somatosensory nuclei are the dorsal column nuclei, which relay information about proprioception and fine touch from the body to the contralateral ventral posterolateral thalamic nucleus, and the spinal trigeminal nucleus, which mediates PAIN and TEMPERATURE sensations from the face and relay it to the contralateral ventral posteromedial nucleus of the thalamus. The NUCLEUS OF THE SOLITARY TRACT relays visceral information to higher levels of the neuraxis. The core of the hindbrain contains the pontine and medullary reticular formations which give rise to widespread ascending and descending projections. Ascending projections, particularly from the pontine reticular formation, are considered to represent part of the anatomical substrate for the ASCENDING RETICULAR ACTIVATING SYSTEM.

DAVID A. HOPKINS

hippocampal commissures In lower species the hippocampal commissure is divisible into dorsal and ventral components, but in PRIMATES, and to an even greater degree in humans, there has been ga progressive reduction in the size of the ventral component, leaving the dorsal hippocampal commissure as a well developed large fibre tract. It travels across the MIDLINE below the SPLENIUM of the CORPUS CALLOSUM and conveys information from the HIPPOCAMPAL FORMATION and TEMPORAL LOBE. It may be important in the seizures associated with EPILEPSY.

Reference

Gloor P., Salanova V., Olivier A. & Quesnay F. (1993) The human dorsal hippocampal commissure. *Brain* 116: 1249–1273.

hippocampal formation The hippocampal formation includes several structures: the DENTATE GYRUS; the HIPPOCAMPUS proper (which also goes by the older name of AMMON'S HORN and includes the three cell groups CA1–CA3); the SUBICULUM and the ENTORHINAL CORTEX. (The subiculum, more properly called the *subicular complex*, is meant here to include the subiculum, PRESUBICULUM and parasubiculum.)

See also: fimbria; fornix; septohippocampal system

Reference

Amaral D.G. & Witter M.P. (1995) Hippocampal formation. In *The Rat Nervous System*, 2nd edn, ed. G. Paxinos, pp. 443–493, Academic Press: London.

hippocampal theta A rhythmical pattern of ELECTROENCEPHALOGRAM (EEG) activity in the HIPPOCAMPUS. Theta, sometimes called RHYTHMIC SLOW ACTIVITY (RSA; Vanderwolf, 1971), occurs at frequencies of 5–12 Hz in rodents and is most prominent during walking, running, swimming and other translational types of movement (involving movements through space). Contrasted with LARGE AMPLITUDE IRREGULAR ACTIVITY (LIA), theta is divisible into a component sensitive to ANTICHOLINERGIC drugs (that occurs during alert immobility in rabbits) and the movement-related component which is sensitive to anaesthetics. Modulated by pacemaker cells in the septum (see SEPTAL NUCLEI) theta is most likely an intrinsic of property of hippocampal cells reflecting activation of specific ION CHANNEL currents. Application of short bursts of high frequency stimulation in a theta-burst manner is very effective in eliciting LONG-TERM POTENTIATION.

Reference

Vanderwolf C.H. (1971) Limbic–diencephalic mechanisms of voluntary movement. *Psychological Review*, 78: 83–113.

RICHARD G. M. MORRIS

hippocampus A major allocortical structure (see ALLOCORTEX) in the medial TEMPORAL LOBE is so named because the interlocking arrangement of GRANULE CELLS in the DENTATE GYRUS and PYRAMIDAL NEURONS of areas CA1 and CA3 (see CA1–CA3) of the hippocampus proper (see AMMON'S HORN) together form the shape of a seahorse whose Latin name is *hippocampus*. Prompted by the observation that patients with brain damage in the medial temporal lobe, including the hippocampus, display AMNESIA (see for example, patient H.M.), it is widely thought to play a critical role in certain types of MEMORY.

The human hippocampus contains approximately 10 million CA1 pyramidal cells (about 30 times more than in the rat brain) and about the same number of CA3 cells. These cells form sheets within an essentially three-layered structure having an intriguing pattern of in-

trinsic circuitry. The hippocampus processes information projected from many regions of the NEOCORTEX, via the ENTORHINAL CORTEX which also serves as one route through which the output of hippocampal processing is fed back to the neocortex. CA3 axons project via the SCHAFFER COLLATERALS to stratum radiatum of area CA1 and to the lateral septal nucleus (see SEPTAL NUCLEI). CA3 receives input from the MOSSY FIBRES of the dentate gyrus and a direct projection of the PERFORANT PATH emanating from layer II of entorhinal cortex. These intrinsic connections are excitatory and have GLUTAMATE NEUROTRANSMITTERS. Excitatory interconnections are modulated by a complex array of inhibitory synapses at DENDRITE, CELL BODY and initial AXON segments, and neuromodulatory input from MIDBRAIN structures involving MONOAMINE and other neurotransmitters. This input reaches the hippocampus via the FORNIX which also provides a route for output from the SUBICULUM to reach the MAMILLARY BODIES and DIENCEPHALON. The hippocampus is also a major site of stress-related CORTICOSTEROID receptors.

Electrophysiological studies have revealed prominent ELECTROENCEPHALOGRAM (EEG) rhythmicity (see HIPPOCAMPAL THETA) and patterns of hippocampal SINGLE-UNIT activity that, in the rodent, reflect some kind of processing of spatial information (see PLACE CELLS). Place cells are pyramidal cells whose firing patterns are influenced by the location of a freely moving (rat or mouse) in a familiar environment, an observation that lies at the root of the COGNITIVE MAP theory of hippocampal function. Other complex cell properties are also observed that probably reflect other contributions to memory processing, including the registration of events. These include activity-dependent changes in synaptic efficacy such as the phenomenon of LONG-TERM POTENTIATION (LTP). LTP is a widely studied model of the synaptic and cellular changes that underlie information storage in the brain, having physiological properties that are ideal for rapid, associatively induced and input-specific changes in synaptic strength. Behavioural studies have provided substantial evidence that an LTP-like mechanism could be involved in

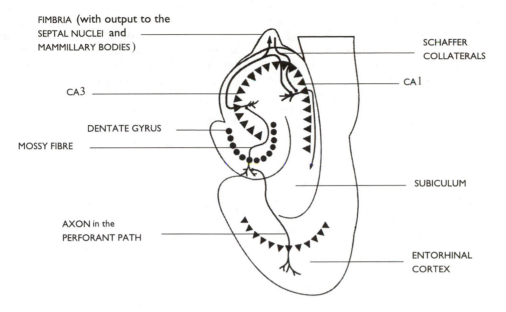

FIMBRIA (with output to the SEPTAL NUCLEI and MAMMILLARY BODIES)

SCHAFFER COLLATERALS

CA3

CA1

DENTATE GYRUS

MOSSY FIBRE

SUBICULUM

AXON in the PERFORANT PATH

ENTORHINAL CORTEX

The Hippocampus

Source: Figure reproduced, with permission, from Carlson, N.R. (1998) *Physiology of Behavior,* 6th edn, Allyn & Bacon: Needham MA.

Notes: In this schematic horizontal section (see PLANES OF SECTION) filled triangles represent the PYRAMIDAL NEURONS of CA1- CA3 and the ENTORHINAL CORTEX. Filled circles represent the NEURONS of the DENTATE GYRUS, which are mainly GRANULE CELLS.

hippocampal-dependent memory; physiological, pharmacological and TRANSGENIC techniques have provided supportive evidence.

There are numerous theories of hippocampal function, most emphasizing its role in some aspect of MEMORY. Prominent amongst these is the proposal that hippocampus is the site of spatial or cognitive maps of the environment used by rodents for NAVIGATION and by PRIMATES (including humans) for organizing the encoding of EPISODIC MEMORY. A LESION of the hippocampal formation in rodents will cause striking impairments of spatial navigation, but will also cause other nonspatial deficits, and certain types of navigation can occur successfully in hippocampal lesioned animals. Another theory is the proposal that the hippocampus plays a critical but time-dependent role in DECLARATIVE MEMORY – the memory for facts and events. This theory is supported by the existence of severe impair-

ments in PROPOSITIONAL or EXPLICIT MEMORY in amnesic patients, including for events that occurred shortly before brain damage, in the absence of any impairment in non-propositional or IMPLICIT MEMORY. However, the claim that this dissociation has been adequately modeled in primates with damage to the hippocampal formation has been undercut by the finding that the integrity of the neighbouring PERIRHINAL CORTEX is critical for RECOGNITION memory. The use of single tasks such as DELAYED NON-MATCHING TO SAMPLE is giving way to the development of new behavioural tasks that point to dissociations within the realm of what has hitherto been considered to be a single unitary process of declarative memory. Other theories of hippocampal function have been developed including the idea that it is critical for the creation of stimulus configurations, for the use of contextual information, for scene memory, and for the flexible use of relational representations. These ideas are a current focus of research.

New insights into the function of the hippocampus are emerging from FUNCTIONAL NEURO-IMAGING work with human subjects using PET and FMRI. These indicate that activation of the human hippocampus and PARAHIPPOCAMPAL GYRUS occur during the recall of navigation through real or virtual environments, supporting the spatial theory. Episodic and declarative memory tasks seem, surprisingly, to activate the PREFRONTAL CORTEX preferentially and to do so differentially on the left or right side of the brain during encoding and recall respectively. However, a developing suspicion is that the hippocampus is metabolically continuously active and so hard to activate differentially using the subtractive methodology widely adopted in imaging work. The hippocampus may therefore play a critical role in some aspect of episodic memory, probably in the more automatic types of encoding that do not depend on intentional or effortful processing characteristic of the FRONTAL LOBE.

Reference

Schacter D.L. and Tulving E. (1994) *Memory Systems 1994*, MIT Press: Cambridge MA.

RICHARD G. M. MORRIS

histamine The neurotransmitter histamine is a BIOGENIC AMINE synthesized from the amino acid histidine by a reaction catalysed by histidine decarboxylase. Neurons that contain histamine are said to be histaminergic. Non-neuronal histamine is released from MAST CELLS during allergic and inflammatory reactions. Neuronal histamine in the CENTRAL NERVOUS SYSTEM originates from a single source, the TUBEROMAMMILLARY NUCLEUS of the posterior HYPOTHALAMUS. The histamine neurons project widely to virtually all regions of the brain and SPINAL CORD. Histamine is implicated in AROUSAL and other functions, and the SEDATIVE) effect of classic ANTIHISTA-MINES (H_1 receptor blockers) is well known. Central HISTAMINE RECEPTORS also appear to mediate actions of certain PSYCHOTROPIC drugs.

KAZUE SEMBA

histamine receptors There appear to be three classes of HISTAMINE receptors in the CENTRAL NERVOUS SYSTEM, designated H_1, H_2 and H_3. H_1 receptors are found in the central nervous system (and on MAST CELLS) and are a target for ANTIHISTAMINE drugs. H_2 receptors predominate in the periphery. H_3 receptors are thought to be a type of AUTORECEPTOR.

histaminergic Relating to the neurotransmitter HISTAMINE.

histochemistry The use of a chemical reaction to generate an insoluble coloured end-product which will demonstrate various tissue elements. Examples of histochemical techniques include NADPH DIAPHORASE to demonstrate the presence of NITRIC OXIDE SYNTHASE; ACETYL-CHOLINESTERASE histochemistry to show the presence of acetylcholinesterase; CYTOCHROME OXIDASE histochemistry to show the presence of cytochrome oxidase. Unlike IMMUNOHISTO-CHEMISTRY, no ANTIBODY–ANTIGEN reactions are required. Simple chemistry is all that is required for histochemistry.

See also: fluorescence

histofluorescence The prefix histo- serves here to indicate fluorescence in histological material; see FLUORESCENCE.

histology Histology is the study of the microscopic structure of biological tissues. It is a subdiscipline of anatomy, and is also called microscopic anatomy. The typical cell types in the brain are NEURONS and glia. Neurons have a SOMA (cell body), dendrites (see DENDRITE) and an AXON. Glial cells, usually smaller than neurons, have a cell body and processes, but no axon. Glial cells are classified into ASTROGLIA, MICROGLIA and OLIGODENDROGLIA, each of which has a distinct MORPHOLOGY. These cells and their cellular elements can be studied with histological staining methods. Histological techniques are also used to examine pathological structures such as various types of TUMOUR, GLIOSIS and AMYLOID deposits in ALZHEIMER'S DEMENTIA. Most histological methods are applicable to all biological tissues, but certain staining methods are specifically developed for neural tissues which contain unique elements. The following summarizes the histological methods that are commonly used for neural tissues.

Certain techniques are used to reveal cell structure. The simplest method is dye staining. Dye is a coloured compound that binds to a substrate in tissues. CRESYL VIOLET stains Nissl substance or RIBOSOMES, thus visualizing the cell bodies of both neurons and glia. Silver methods are used to stain neuronal axons. The GOLGI METHOD stains about 5% of neurons and glia in exquisite detail, including virtually all parts of dendrites and axons. The mechanism of this selectivity is unknown. TIMM STAIN is used to localize heavy metals such as zinc.

A variety of methods are used for staining NEUROACTIVE substances. Histochemical methods are often used to localize known substances such as an ENZYME. These methods take advantage of a chemical reaction that involves the substance of interest and produces a visible reaction product. Enzyme histochemistry is often used for localizing enzymes involved in transmitter functions, including ACETYLCHOLINESTERASE and MONOAMINE OXIDASE. In IMMUNOHISTOCHEMISTRY, ANTIBODIES raised against an ANTIGEN of interest (these are usually PROTEINS or PEPTIDES) are used along with a tag that can be histochemically detected. Monoclonal antibodies, obtained from clones, usually provide superior specificity compared with polyclonal antibodies purified from the whole serum. The presence of MESSENGER RNA of a protein can be detected by using antisense OLIGONUCLEOTIDE probes or COMPLEMENTARY DNA probes that are complementary to the mRNA of interest.

In all of these cases, histological slides can be examined using a standard stereoscopic light microscope or, for greater resolution, CONFOCAL MICROSCOPY. In addition to these, ELECTRON MICROSCOPY is used to examine subcellular elements such as the NUCLEUS, MITOCHONDRIA and ribosomes. The use of electron microscopy is essential for definitive identification of a SYNAPSE.

See also: image analysis; stains; stereology

KAZUE SEMBA

histometry *see* cell counting

histopathology The study of tissue (*histo-*) disease (*-pathology*) as opposed to other forms of the analysis of PATHOLOGY not in tissue but in, for example, urine.

hoarding behaviour The tendency of many arthropod and vertebrate species to accumulate and store valued objects especially items of food in excess of immediate requirements. Hoarding behaviour has attracted scientific interest as an apparent homologue of acquisitive behaviour in man, both normal and pathological, and as a theoretical challenge: how to account for behaviour that is not apparently aimed at the immediate amelioration of a physical or physiological need. The sequestration of food items by birds (see FOOD-STORING BIRDS) and their subsequent faultless retrieval has also offered unique opportunities for the study of animal LEARNING. Clinical manifestations of an innate propensity to hoard may be seen in conditions such as ANOREXIA NERVOSA, commonly associated with inappropriate accumulation of (uneaten) food-stuffs (but see below for the possible role of food deprivation). Hoarding of seemingly worthless objects is also common in elderly patients with early DEMENTIA, and in some instances of OBSESSIVE-COMPULSIVE DISORDER. A more speculative role for a possible hoarding instinct is in the MOTIVATION of activities such as philately and scholarly taxonomy (a notion elaborated by Freud in a somewhat different context). The economic importance of hoarding is exemplified on the one hand by the beneficent labours of the honeybee and on the other by the depredations of rats which may cause much greater losses of warehoused food by hoarding than by eating it. The scientific study of hoarding has focused largely on the laboratory rat. Quantitative studies by C.T. Morgan (1915–1976), Eliot Stellar (1919–1993) and others showed that hoarding of food by male rats occurred only in food-deprived subjects, and depended on nutritional state rather than on the rats' being actually hungry at the time. From this it has since been argued that hoarding is a measure of the extent to which the animal's BODY WEIGHT falls short of its individual genetic norm or SET POINT. Support for this view includes the absence of deprivation-induced hoarding in force-fattened individuals or in ventromedial hypothalamic obesity (see VENTROMEDIAL HYPOTHALAMIC SYNDROME) and, conversely, the persistent, autonomous hoarding produced by ELECTRICAL BRAIN STIMULATION of the LATERAL HYPOTHALAMUS or by corresponding endocrine and neuropharmacological manipulations, and in animals preparing for HIBERNATION. Hoarding patterns in other species sometimes differ from those of the rat and have not been fully accounted for. Hoarding may also be directed to non-food objects, such as nesting materials or water-soaked pledgets of cotton wool (in water-deprived rats). Rats and magpies, like us, will also hoard eye-catching novelties and trinkets for no known reason.

L. JACOB HERBERG

Hodgkin–Huxley equations These are equations derived by Alan Hodgkin and Andrew Huxley who developed the VOLTAGE CLAMP technique, using it to measure activity in the giant axon of the squid nervous system. This work forms the basis of much of what is now known about neuronal MEMBRANE activity. Their work was rewarded by the Nobel Prize for Physiology or Medicine in 1963.

Reference

Kandel E.R., Schwartz J.H. & Jessell T.M. (2000) *Principles of Neural Science*, 4th edn, McGraw-Hill: New York.

hodology (from Greek, *hodos*: a way) The analysis of anatomical structures in relation to their position and connections; a hodological analysis of a particular structure would describe the inputs to and outputs from a structure.

hodophobia (from Greek, *hodos*: a way, *phobos*: fear) A fear of travel.

Hoehn & Yahr scale A classification scheme used to asses the severity of PARKINSON'S DISEASE, described first in 1967. The stages were described by Hoehn & Yahr as follows: Stage I: Unilateral involvement only, usually with minimal or no functional impairment. Stage II: Bilateral or midline involvement, without impairment of balance. Stage III: First sign of impaired righting reflexes. This is evident by unsteadiness as the patient turns or is demonstrated when he is pushed from standing equilibrium with the feet together and eyes closed. Functionally the patient is somewhat restricted in his activities but may have some work potential depending upon the type of employment. Patients are physically capable of leading independent lives, and their disability is mild to moderate. Stage IV: Fully developed, severely disabling disease; the patient is still able to walk and stand unassisted but is markedly incapacitated. Stage V: Confinement to bed or wheelchair unless aided.

The disabilities seen in stage I are TREMOR (unilateral) and RIGIDITY, with possibly some BRADYKINESIA present. In stage II these become worse and FACIAL MASKING might be present. In stage III these become worse, and POSTURE and GAIT are affected. In stage IV these worsen further until in stage V patients are bed-ridden.

Reference

Hoehn M.M. & Yahr M.D. (1967) Parkinsonism: onset progression and mortality. *Neurology* 17: 427–442.

holeboard test A test of EXPLORATION in rodents. A test mostly used for rats and occasionally mice, the holeboard test has traditionally been considered to be a measure of exploratory tendencies of the animal. Although there are variations of this paradigm, the basic test consists of a square or round OPEN FIELD with holes placed in the floor or sides of the apparatus. Since rodents have a strong tendency to explore novel or interesting surroundings by sniffing and nose-poking, this type of environment is conducive to exploratory behaviour. Generally, the dependent measure is the number or frequency of responses in a fixed time period, variously termed 'head-dips', 'nose-pokes', or 'hole visits'. The test is often automated with photocells behind the holes, and further measures can be taken such as length of time spent exploring holes, patterns of exploration, and duration of individual hole visits. The holeboard test has been used extensively in PSYCHOPHARMACOLOGY to test the effects of drugs or lesions on exploratory behaviour, and also as a measure of the response to STRESS if the environment is novel.

ANN E. KELLEY

homeobox genes A GENE family, in which the genes contain a homeobox, a highly conserved sequence of DNA that codes for a protein of approximately 60 AMINO ACIDS, known as a homeodomain protein. These proteins are transcription factors, and are expressed in spatially and temporally distinct patterns in different tissues of an organism during DEVELOPMENT. Studies of GENE KNOCKOUT and MUTATION of these genes indicate that they are important in determining the position and morphological fate of the cells in which they are found. For example, knockout of *Hoxa-1*, one of the *hox* family of homeobox genes, causes delay in closure of the NEURAL TUBE at the level of the HINDBRAIN, and improper position of CRANIAL NERVES, resulting in death of the organism shortly after birth. Knockout of another *hox* gene, *Hoxb-1*, results in failure of migration of MOTOR NEURONS to their proper positions, suggesting that this gene is involved in path-finding of motor neurons to their skeletal targets.

FIONA M. INGLIS

homeostasis (Homoeostasis is an acceptable, though unusual alternative spelling) (from Greek, *homo*: same, *stasis*: stopped, stationary) Homeostasis means, literally, the same state. It describes the observation that living systems tend to maintain constancy. The concept of homeostasis originates with the French physiologist Claude Bernard (1813–1878) but in fact the word homeostasis was coined and first used in 1932 by the American physiologist Walter B. Cannon (1871–1945). It is well established that physiological mechanism, operating at many levels – the individual CELL, systems and whole organisms – tend to maintain a constant state. ENERGY BALANCE, WATER BALANCE, BODY WEIGHT, TEMPERATURE REGULATION are among the basic physiological processes thought to be governed by homeostasis. Brains contain many mechanisms for the detection of change in various physiological measures – for example, the concentration of GLUCOSE in the blood stream, levels of HORMONES, body water content (see OSMOREGULATION) – and there are many effector systems that serve to change physiological processes and behaviour in order to correct imbalances.

Homeostasis is without doubt an important principle, but caveats to it need to be expressed. First, it was once assumed that physiological processes worked by SET POINT mechanisms, with precisely defined levels determined in advance. If a measure deviated above or below this point, corrective processes would take effect to return the system to stability. This would be a very rigid system. A mechanism with upper and lower limits – that is to say an acceptable range of levels rather than a set point value – is more plausible (see Herman & Polivy, 1984 for a description of a boundary model for the regulation of body weight). Second, authors now lay emphasis also on the concept of ALLOSTASIS, which stresses ADAPTATION and flexibility in response to challenge. The role of LEARNING in adapting to changing conditions is emphasized. Clearly, adaptation is of enormous value for either an individual animal or a species to survive. Third, related to this last point, homeostasis is held to be one of the fundamental principles of physiology. Another is NATURAL SELECTION, the engine of EVOLUTION. Natural selection also emphasizes adaptation and FITNESS. It is curious that biology should have two fundamental principles apparently at variance with each other.

See also: boundary model; hypothalamus; neuroadaptation; paraventricular system

Reference

Herman C.P. & Polivy J. (1984) A boundary model for the regulation of eating. In *Eating and its Disorders*, ed. A.J. Stunkard & E. Stellar, pp. 141–156, Raven Press: New York.

homeotherm *see* endotherm

homeothermic blanket A device used during surgery on an animal to maintain its body TEMPERATURE: it is typically an electric blanket, the temperature of which can be adjusted to a desired level. Sensory input from the animal is derived from a thermometer (usually a rectal thermometer) so that if its temperature falls during surgery the blanket is activated until the correct temperature is reached. Maintaining body temperature during surgery is obviously important. Particular care needs to be taken when using certain ANAESTHETICS (such as BARBITURATES) which reduce an animal's ability to maintain proper THERMOREGULATION.

See also: stereotaxic surgery

homeotic selector genes A type of regulatory GENE specifying patterns of DEVELOPMENT; see NEURODEVELOPMENT

hominid A member of the family (see TAXONOMY) Hominidae, which includes modern *Homo sapiens* (modern men and women) and our extinct relatives. (Note though that *Homo sapiens* is often excluded from this: in the same way that once separates man from the animals, one can separate man from the hominids.)

The precise classification of human ancestors is difficult. There appear to be close relationships between *Homo neanderthalensis* (Neanderthal man), *Homo heidelbergiensis*, *Homo erectus* (including Peking man and Java man) and *Homo ergaster*. All of these were bipedal, had a large BRAIN (larger than chimpanzees for instance – see PRIMATES) and engaged to one degree or another in relatively sophisticated activities, including skilled use of stone and other tools. Although usually grouped with these, *Homo habilis* was smaller and in many ways resembled the various classes of australopithecine, of which there might have been as many as 10 different types. These diverged earlier from the evolutionary line of the various *Homo* species and, though they were bipedal, they retained some arboreal climbing ability and had brains hardly bigger than those of chimpanzees. Simple stone tools are associated with *Homo habilis*, and it is likely that australopithecines had similar abilities. Even older, evolutionarily, than these, appears to be *Ardepithecus ramidus*, a species about which little is known but which does appear to predate *Australopithecus*. Whether this is some form of 'missing link' with chimpanzees is an interesting speculation.

More radical speculation concerns the dating of the divergence of various species. MOLECULAR TAXONOMY suggests that *Homo sapiens* diverged from chimpanzees and bonobos about 4.5 million years ago, and from gorillas about 6 million years ago, if the pattern of divergence is calibrated with early ancestors orang utans 12 million years ago. The fossil record however suggests that the divergence of the various *Homo* species and the australopithecines from *Ardepithecus* also occurred about 4.5 million years ago. Clearly, the precise dating of these various divergences is not an exact process, but it can be suggested that the various estimates of dating move one to a position where an argument for including chimpanzees, bonobos and gorillas with hominids could be supported.

One final note: the different forms of *Homo* are often referred to as being different SPECIES. Whether, by strict biological criteria (the presence of two species in a given area without interbreeding, for instance) these are true species is an open question: the more general term 'types' might be preferable to species in this context.

See also: evolution; natural selection

homoiotherm *see* endotherm

homologue *see* homology

homology (from Greek, *homo*: the same) When two or more things are described as showing HOMOLOGY, that is, they are homologous; each one is a HOMOLOGUE (the American spelling of this is *homolog*) of the other. This indicates that they are essentially the same. Anatomical structures in two different species can be described as homologous if they have more-or-less the same position, structure and function; see for example, RODENT VS. PRIMATE PREFRONTAL CORTEX.

homomer The receptors for NEUROTRANSMITTERS are built of subunits (individual building blocks): HOMOMERS are subunits that are the same, HETEROMERS are subunits that differ.

homonymous hemianopia *see* hemianopia

homophones Homophones are words that sound identical but are different in spelling and meaning – *pear* and *pair* for example; see SURFACE DYSLEXIA.

homosexual An individual who prefers exclusive sexual contact with members of the same sex. The terms 'gay' and 'lesbian' are used colloquially to refer to homosexual men and women, respectively. Homosexuality is as old as humanity, and runs the gamut from complete acceptance to complete prohibition in different cultures or during different epochs within a culture. The base rate of homosexuality in human populations is believed to be 10%, although the definition of what constitutes a homosexual is controversial. For example, simply engaging in a homosexual act is not sufficient evidence that the individual is a homosexual or has an exclusive preference for sexual contact with members of the same sex. Likewise, simply being in a heterosexual relationship is no guarantee that an individual has exclusive sexual contact with members of the other sex. Homosexuality is best viewed multidimensionally, in which several factors (such as SEXUAL AROUSAL, sexual activity, self-concept, dominant choice of sex partners, level of exclusivity, sexual history and so on) are considered along converging axes. Homosexuality would thus lie on a multidimensional continuum of sexual or erotic orientation, with individuals being dominantly homosexual, bisexual, or heterosexual.

Until the 1970s, homosexuality was listed as a mental disorder by the American Psychiatric Association. It was taken off the list by a vote in 1974, due to political mobilization by the gay and lesbian community who felt that their lifestyle choice should be respected rather than made the subject of legal hassles, unproven behavioural treatments, and even brain surgery. Recently, the identification of regions in the HYPOTHALAMUS which differ in size between homosexual and heterosexual males has sparked both political and scientific controversy. On one hand, such a discovery suggests that homosexuality has a genetic basis, and therefore should be considered something that an individual cannot help (like being of a particular race or gender) and hence deserving of legal protection. The notion of a genetic basis of homosexuality has also been bolstered by recent findings of an X chromosome-linked domain (see X AND Y CHROMOSOMES) that appears more in homosexual than heterosexual males. On the other hand, the difference in size of these hypothalamic sites or chromosomal regions, if replicable, are merely correlates which do not imply any cause of homosexuality. Indeed, some homosexuals fear that the identification of brain or genetic differences could foster surgical interventions, or lead to the development of genetic probes that will identify whether a FOETUS is 'at risk' for homosexuality.

See also: gender; sexual motivation

JAMES G. PFAUS

homosynaptic *see* long-term depression

homovanillic acid *see* dopamine

homozygous In diploid cells, the presence of the same ALLELE of a GENE in both of a pair of AUTOSOMAL CHROMOSOMES (see DOMINANT ALLELE; RECESSIVE ALLELE).

FIONA M. INGLIS

homunculus (from Latin, the diminutive of *homo*: a man – literally, a little man) In biological psychology it is a term mainly used in respect of a SOMATOSENSORY HOMUNCULUS. That is, it is a picture of a little person with body parts drawn in proportion to their degree of representation in the PRIMARY SOMATOSENSORY CORTEX. The somatosensory homunculus has a disproportionately large head, very large lips, and very large hands, these being the areas of SKIN that are most used in the sense of TOUCH.

Note also that the word homunculus has other meanings; for example, it can be used to refer to a dwarf. More interestingly, it was a term used by Philippus Aureolus Paracelsus (the pseudonym of Theophrastus Bombastus von Hohenheim [1493?–1541]). Paracelsus was a Swiss physician and chemist who is best remembered now for having broken with the ancient belief that disease was caused by imbalance of body fluids (as the Roman physician Galen [129–199?] had indicated) and suggested instead that diseases could be caused by external agents and treated with chemicals (which he attempted to do). Paracelsus, like most scientists of his time, was also interested in the occult and believed it possible to create artificially a tiny man – a homunculus.

See also: motor cortex

horizontal cells Horizontal cells are found in the outer plexiform layer of the RETINA (see RETINAL CELL LAYERS). They interact with the PHOTORECEPTOR cells (RODS and CONES) and with BIPOLAR CELLS. Their interactions with photoreceptors are important in regulating the firing of on- and off-centre surround bipolar cells.

horizontal limb of the diagonal band of Broca *see* diagonal band of Broca

horizontal section *see* planes of section

hormones Hormones are chemical messengers which are synthesized in ENDOCRINE GLANDS, secreted into the circulatory system, and transported through the body in the blood to bind to RECEPTORS on target cells where they exert a specific physiological or biochemical regulatory action. The body has a number of endocrine glands which secrete one or more hormones. The PINEAL GLAND secretes MELATONIN. The posterior PITUITARY GLAND secretes OXYTOCIN and VASOPRESSIN. The anterior pituitary gland secretes GROWTH HORMONE, ADRENOCORTICOTROPIC HORMONE, THYROID-STIMULATING HORMONE, FOLLICLE-STIMULATING HORMONE, LUTEINIZING HORMONE and PROLACTIN. The intermediate pituitary synthesizes MELANOCYTE STIMULATING HORMONE and BETA-ENDORPHIN. There are nine hypopthalamic hormones which regulate the release of pituitary hormones: THYROTROPHIN-RELEASING HORMONE (also known as THYROID-STIMULATING-HORMONE-RELEASING HORMONE), CORTICOTROPIN RELEASING HORMONE, GONADOTROPHIN-RELEASING HORMONE (also known as LUTEINIZING-HORMONE-RELEASING HORMONE), GROWTH-HORMONE-RELEASING HORMONE, GROWTH-HORMONE-RELEASE-INHIBITING HORMONE (also known as SOMATOSTATIN), PROLACTIN-RELEASING FACTOR, PROLACTIN-INHIBITING FACTOR (which in fact may be the neurotransmitter DOPAMINE), MELANOCYTE STIMULATING HORMONE RELEASING FACTOR and MELANOCYTE STIMULATING HORMONE INHIBITING FACTOR (which may also turn out to be dopamine).

The THYROID GLAND produces TRIIODOTHYRONINE (T3), THYROXINE (T4) and CALCITONIN. The PARATHYROID GLANDS produce PARATHYROID HORMONE (PTH). The THYMUS GLAND produces THYMOSIN and THYMOSTATIN. The heart secretes atrial natriuretic factor. ADIPOSE tissue secretes LEPTIN. The mucosa of the GASTROINTESTINAL TRACT secretes over a

dozen peptide hormones, including SECRETIN, GASTRIN and CHOLECYSTOKININ as well as GASTRIC INHIBITORY PEPTIDE, VASOACTIVE INTESTINAL PEPTIDE, SUBSTANCE P, somatostatin, GASTRIN-RELEASING PEPTIDE, BOMBESIN, NEUROTENSIN, and MOTILIN. The endocrine cells of the PANCREAS, the ISLETS OF LANGERHANS, secrete INSULIN and GLUCAGON. The cortex of the ADRENAL GLAND secretes MINERALOCORTICOIDS (ALDOSTERONE), GLUCOCORTICOIDS (CORTISOL and CORTICOSTERONE) and small amounts of the GONADAL STEROIDS (ANDROGENS, ESTROGENS and PROGESTERONE). The adrenal medulla releases ADRENALINE (EPINEPHRINE) and NORADRENALINE (NOREPINEPHRINE). The male GONADS (the testes) produce androgens (TESTOSTERONE) and INHIBIN while the female gonads (the ovaries) produce the estrogens and PROGESTINS and inhibin. When pregnancy occurs, special hormones, including HUMAN CHORIONIC GONADOTROPHIN and HUMAN PLACENTAL LACTOGEN are secreted from the foetal-placental unit and, near the end of pregnancy, the ovary secretes RELAXIN.

Many hormones, however, do not fit the classical definition of a 'true' hormone. PHYTOHORMONES are plant hormones. Some hormones are not synthesized in endocrine glands. ANGIOTENSIN I, for example, is synthesized in the bloodstream. Many hormones of the gastrointestinal tract are not secreted from specific endocrine glands. NEUROHORMONES (oxytocin, vasopressin and the hypothalamic hormones) are produced in neurosecretory cells, which are modified nerve cells. PARAHORMONES, such as histamine and the prostaglandins are hormone-like chemicals which are not produced in endocrine glands, but have all of the other characteristics of a 'true' hormone. GROWTH FACTORS (such as SOMATOMEDIN, NERVE GROWTH FACTOR, EPIDERMAL GROWTH FACTOR and FIBROBLAST GROWTH FACTOR) are hormone-like chemical messengers which are not synthesized in endocrine glands. Likewise, the CYTOKINES (such as INTERFERON γ, and the INTERLEUKINS), which have hormone-like activity, are synthesized by the LYMPHOCYTES, MONOCYTES and MACROPHAGES of the IMMUNE SYSTEM.

The prinicpal chemical categories of hormones

Group	Examples of hormones
amine hormones	adrenaline (epinephrine)
	melatonin
	noradrenaline (norepinephrine)
	thyroid hormones
protein hormones	adrenocorticotropic hormone
	follicle stimulating hormone
	glucagon
	growth hormones
	insulin
	luteinizing hormone
	oxytocin
	prolactin
	thyroid stimulating hormone
	vasopressin (antidiuretic hormone)
	Releasing hormones:
	corticotropin releasing hormone
	gonadotropin releasing hormone
	thyrotropin releasing hormone
	growth hormone releasing factor (somatocrinin)
	growth hormone release inhibiting factor (somatostatin)
steroid hormones	
adrenal	glucocorticoids (e.g. corticosterone, cortisol)
	mineralocorticoids (e.g. aldosterone)
gonadal	androgens (e.g. testosterone)
	estrogens (e.g. estradiol, estrone)
	progestins (e.g. progesterone)

One hormone may be synthesized in a number of glands. Estrogen, for example, is synthesized in the ovaries, testes, adrenal cortex, placenta and by tumour cells. Peptides, such as somatostatin, are called hormones when they are secreted from endocrine glands, and neuropeptides when they are produced by nerve cells in the brain. Some hormones, such as ACTH, are secreted from both endocrine glands and from lymphocytes and other cells of the immune system. Hormones need not be secreted into the bloodstream and transported to their target cells through the circulatory system. Hormones can activate adjacent cells

(PARACRINE action) or even the same cell that releases them (AUTOCRINE action). Neurohormones may be transported by the CEREBROSPINAL FLUID (CSF) as well as by the circulatory system. Although hormones are defined as having a specific action at their target cell, this action may vary according to the type of target cell stimulated. For example, prolactin stimulates the production of milk in the breast; this is an example of a specific hormonal function. Estrogen, on the other hand, can have general effects such as priming cells to respond to other hormones or increasing cell growth. Moreover, some hormones can interact with multiple receptor types such that they have different functions in different target cells. For example, noradrenaline released from the adrenal medulla can bind to either alpha-adrenergic or beta-adrenergic receptors on target cells in the muscles and the physiological action stimulated may differ depending on which receptor was stimulated. On the other hand, many different hormones, no matter what their target cell, induce the same cellular response (for instance, an increase in intracellular CYCLIC AMP production); others may modulate nerve activity by altering the amount of a neurotransmitter synthesized, stored and released from that nerve cell

RICHARD E. BROWN

hormones – classification Hormones can be categorized in many ways – for example, by their location, function or chemical structure. The location of hormones – that is where they are synthesized and stored prior to release – is detailed in the entry ENDOCRINE GLANDS. This also gives details of their function, though this is amplified in the various individual entries for some hormones. The table on p. 363 (adapted from Rosenzweig *et al.,* 1996) presents a categorization of hormones by their chemical groups.

These classes are discriminated by their chemical structure and by their actions. (1) Protein hormones and amine hormones (except thyroid hormones) act at cell surface RECEPTORS (just as NEUROTRANSMITTERS do) with subsequent effects on SECOND MESSENGERS. Steroid hormones in contrast are taken through membranes and exert their effects directly on

intracellular processes. (2) The actions of protein and amine hormones is rapid (just as is the cellular response to neurotransmitters); the response to steroid hormones in contrast is slow.

References

Campbell N.A., Reece J.B. & Mitchell L.G. (1999) *Biology,* 5th edn, Addison-Wesley: Menlo Park CA.
Rosenzweig M.R., Leiman A.L. & Breedlove S.M. (1996) *Biological Psychology,* Sinauer Associates: Sunderland MA.

hormones and cognition Hormone actions in the brain are believed to play an important role in the development and sexual differentiation of certain cognitive abilities. These have been studied to a great extent in humans, especially women, although studies of hormonal function in LEARNING and MEMORY have been conducted largely in rodents. Cognitive abilities in women tend to fluctuate across the MENSTRUAL CYCLE. For example, women perform better on tests of spatial skills during the menstrual phase, when ESTROGEN and PROGESTERONE levels are low, compared to the midluteal phase, when levels of these steroids are high. However, fluctuations in verbal abilities and perceptual speed across the menstrual cycle follow different patterns. Perceptual speed appears greatest during the premenstrual and menstrual phase, whereas verbal abilities are greatest during the midluteal phase. Motor performance also changes across the menstrual cycle with manual speed and coordination being significantly better during the midluteal phase than the premenstrual or menstrual phase. Cerebral LATERALIZATION also changes during the menstrual cycle. The degree of right-ear advantage in tests of dichotic listening diminishes during the menstrual phase, compared to the midluteal phase, suggesting that ASYMMETRY is greatest when circulating levels of estrogen and progesterone are highest. Finally, both visual and olfactory sensitivity (see VISUAL SYSTEM; OLFACTION) seem to be greatest around the time of ovulation. Treatment of postmenopausal women with estrogen increases performance on both verbal and perceptual motor tasks, but does not affect purely spatial tasks.

Learning and memory are also affected by hormones, especially STRESS-related adrenal steroids like the GLUCOCORTICOIDS, anterior PITUITARY GLAND peptide hormones like ADRENOCORTICOTROPIC HORMONE (ACTH), and posterior pituitary peptide hormones like VASOPRESSIN and OXYTOCIN. The adrenal response to stress involves the release of ADRENALINE and CORTICOSTEROIDS (such as CORTICOSTERONE and CORTISOL). In turn, these substances act on the periphery and brain to induce 'FIGHT-OR-FLIGHT' responses, including increased heart rate, glucose metabolism, and awareness of external sensory stimuli. ACTH is released from the anterior pituitary in response to glucocorticoid activation of cells in the HYPOTHALAMUS that release CORTICOTROPIN-RELEASING FACTOR into the pituitary vasculature. Central administration of ACTH to rats potentiates active and PASSIVE AVOIDANCE learning, and prevents AMNESIA (induced by mild HYPOXIA after training). Peripheral injections of vasopressin also enhance learning of avoidance responding, and prevent decay of the memory for several weeks. In contrast, oxytocin seems to enhance FORGETTING, and peripheral or central administrations disrupt active AVOIDANCE LEARNING. Gonadal steroids do not appear to affect learning and memory.

See also: sexual differentiation; sexual dimorphism

JAMES G. PFAUS

horopter The horopter is the locus of points that stimulate CORRESPONDING RETINAL POINTS in the two eyes. If one fixates and converges on a point in space, that point will be foveated (see FOVEA) in the two eyes and will, by definition, have zero RETINAL DISPARITY. There will also be points in space that are not at the fixation point that appear to lie in the same visual direction in the two eyes, and appear to be at the same visual distance as the fixation point. These therefore stimulate corresponding retinal points. The surface that could be plotted through them is known as the horopter. The importance of this for vision is that anything that does not lie on the horopter will not stimulate corresponding retinal points and therefore the two retinal images will be disparate. Retinal disparity is the basis of

stereoscopic vision. Over a limited range of values (which define PANUM'S FUSIONAL AREA) disparities are interpreted by the brain as depth (see DEPTH PERCEPTION). The geometry of the normal viewing situation suggests that the horizontal horopter should be a circle (the VEITH–MULLER CIRCLE). In reality the shape of the horopter depends on fixation distance.

See also: binocular fusion

DAVID W. HEELEY

horseradish peroxidase see tract tracers

hot plate test see analgesia

housekeeping genes see gene

HPLC Abbreviation for HIGH-PERFORMANCE LIQUID CHROMATOGRAPHY.

human chorionic gonadotrophin One of the HORMONES released during PREGNANCY; see ENDOCRINE GLANDS.

human leukocyte antigens see immune system

human placental lactogen One of the HORMONES released during PREGNANCY; see ENDOCRINE GLANDS.

humane killing Animals that have taken part in experiments involving changes to their brains are humanely killed when testing ends to allow experimenters to determine what changes in their brains have been brought about – to measure the size, location and selectivity of any LESION, or determine the placement of an ELECTRODE or CANNULA for example. The most common method is by lethal injection, usually an overdose of BARBITURATES. On occasion rodents will be killed by guillotining, typically when experimenters wish to measure in some way the composition of brain tissue, when administration of drugs could confound results. In the United Kingdom, humane killing is regulated by Schedule 1 of the 1986 Animals (Scientific Procedures) Act and can only be carried out by persons competent to do so. This also specifies which methods of humane killing are appropriate for different species.

See also: animal welfare

humour The term humour has two meanings: (i) it is an antique term describing any body fluids (it derives from Latin, *humor*: moist – and note that the American spelling, humor, is an accurate use of the original Latin term). The adjective humoural (or humoral) is used to describe a body fluid. It is a term that survives in its description of AQUEOUS HUMOUR and VITREOUS HUMOUR, fluids found in the EYE. Ancient wisdom had it that there were four essential body fluids: BLOOD, black bile, yellow bile and phlegm which were associated with different temperaments – respectively, sanguine, melancholic, choleric and phlegmatic. The term melancholic was once used to describe patients who would now be diagnosed as having DEPRESSION. (ii) Humour describes a mental quality – the appreciation of that which has the quality of mirth or levity; see LAUGHTER.

hunger Hunger, like thirst, is a subjective EMOTION: it is an attributional label (see ATTRIBUTION) that humans apply to states they experience. As an expression 'hunger' has value as a predictor of behaviour, but does not necessarily reveal what physiological state a person is in. The predictive value of the term hunger is probabilistic not absolute: ratings of hunger by humans are very variable, both within and between individuals. It is possible that an individual will eat only when a raft of appropriate physiological measures (such as GLUCOSE concentration in the BLOOD for example) indicate that it is necessary to do so, but feeding is clearly triggered by a range of stimuli – conditioned and unconditioned – and emotional states other than these; see FEEDING for further discussion of this.

Huntington's chorea Progressive neurodegenerative disorder characterized by CHOREIFORM (i.e. dance-like; see CHOREA) movements and DEMENTIA. The condition is sometimes associated with PSYCHOSIS and DEPRESSION. The disease is inherited in an autosomal dominant manner (see DOMINANT ALLELE). The disorder was first described by George Huntington in the late nineteenth century: the GENE coding for the disorder (a trinucleotide repeat MUTATION) was discovered in 1993. Accurate diagnostic and predictive genetic testing for the disorder are available. Onset of the disease is usually in the fourth decade of life, though many later-onset, and some juvenile cases have been described. Psychiatric symptoms may occasionally predate the onset of abnormal movements, and occasionally lead to misdiagnosis. The dementing process is usually the last to emerge, with a neuropsychological profile indicating FRONTAL LOBE impairment. Extreme disability requiring institutional care is the usual outcome of the disorder: progressive dementia, severe movement disorder, and occasionally epilepsy make independent self-care impossible. Death usually occurs 10–15 years after onset of symptoms. Pathologically, there is atrophy of CEREBRAL CORTEX with marked frontal involvement, VENTRICULAR ENLARGEMENT, and degeneration of the head of the CAUDATE NUCLEUS and the PUTAMEN of the BASAL GANGLIA. There is no effective treatment for the disorder itself, though the movement disorder and psychotic symptoms may be controlled by the use of NEUROLEPTIC drugs, with MOOD disturbance treated using conventional ANTIDEPRESSANT therapy.

IAN C. REID

hybrid (from Latin, *hibrida*: the issue produced by mating a domestic sow and a wild boar) A hybrid is the product of combining different species or varieties of animal or plant (either individuals or cells). Hybridization and HYBRIDIZE describe the act of producing hybrids.

See also: *in situ* hybridization

hydrocephalus A pathological increase in the volume of CEREBROSPINAL FLUID (CSF) at the expense of brain tissue. In the normal brain, CSF is secreted into the VENTRICULAR SYSTEM by the CHOROID PLEXUS (a vascular excrescence lining the cerebral VENTRICLES), circulates through the ventricular system via the AQUEDUCT OF SYLVIUS and via narrow interconnecting foramina, traverses the length of the SPINAL CORD, and after returning to the SKULL is finally absorbed from the SUBARACHNOID SPACE. In *non-communicating hydrocephalus* circulation of the CSF is obstructed, usually at one or other of the interventricular foramina, with a consequent build-up of intracranial pressure (normally 150–200 mm

H_2O in the recumbent adult), leading to VENTRICULAR ENLARGEMENT and compression of the brain. New-born infants, with soft bone and skull sutures that are not firmly united, may also develop a characteristic enlargement of the skull (MACROCEPHALY). The usual causes of obstruction to the flow of CSF are developmental anomalies, viral or bacterial infection, infestation with parasitic cysts, or a space-occupying LESION such as a TUMOUR or blood clots. Surgery may be curative, but may require the permanent implantation of a tube to bypass the obstruction (Torkildsen's procedure). *Communicating hydrocephalus* is more likely to be seen in adults and results from a mismatch between the rate of formation of CSF (normally 0.3–0.4 ml/min) and its removal. The usual cause is impaired absorption of CSF from the subarachnoid space due to meningeal infection (see MENINGITIS), or the presence of blood following intracranial bleeding. The symptoms of acute onset are the usual signs of raised intracranial pressure: headache, vomiting, constricted pupils, retinal changes, irregular breathing and loss of sphincter control, leading eventually to COMA and death. The condition may be self-limiting, else surgical treatment may require the insertion of a tube to drain the CSF from the skull and into the chest or abdomen. Long-standing untreated hydrocephalus may be associated with MENTAL HANDICAP but in some patients the effects may be surprisingly mild: a celebrated case involved a student of mathematics who more than matched his academic peers at a UK university despite having a cerebral cortex only 1 mm thick.

L. JACOB HERBERG

hydrostatic pressure *see* osmosis

6-hydroxydopamine (6-OHDA) A neurotoxin that selectively damages neurons that contain CATECHOLAMINES as NEUROTRANSMITTERS, including DOPAMINERGIC and NORADRENERGIC neurons. The route of administration determines the population of neurons to be lesioned (see LESION; NEUROTOXINS). Intraperitoneal injections result in chemical 'sympathectomy' which is permanent in neonates but temporary in adults. Systemic injections largely spare central catecholamine neurons because 6-OHDA does not readily cross the BLOOD–BRAIN BARRIER. Selective lesions of central catecholamine neurons can be achieved by injections of the neurotoxin into their target area, or alternatively, in the vicinity of their cell bodies. Such lesions appear to be permanent and there is little evidence for fibre regeneration. The selectivity of 6-OHDA to catecholamine neurons is based on their ability to take up 6-OHDA via selective dopamine or noradrenaline transporters that are present only on catecholamine neurons. The selectivity for dopamine neurons can be achieved by pretreatment with the noradrenaline uptake blocker DESIPRAMINE, which prevents uptake of the neurotoxin into noradrenergic neurons. The mechanism underlying the toxicity of 6-OHDA is not well understood, but is thought to involve the formation of toxic products or by-products during the auto-oxidation process of internalized 6-OHDA. Recent studies have suggested that the formation of neurotoxic free radicals is stimulated by 6-OHDA and that increasing the concentration of certain nerve growth factors in the lesioned area (either by direct injection or by prior gene transfer) can reduce neuronal loss significantly.

Animals with 6-OHDA lesions of the NIGROSTRIATAL DOPAMINE SYSTEM have been used as an animal model of PARKINSON'S DISEASE. Injections of the neurotoxin are made into the STRIATUM, SUBSTANTIA NIGRA or MEDIAL FOREBRAIN BUNDLE. The latter contains nigrostriatal dopamine fibres. Animals with bilateral injections of 6-OHDA show a behavioural syndrome resembling Parkinson's disease, including BRADYKINESIA, ADIPSIA, APHAGIA, decreased exploration and difficulty in initiating motor activity. However, as in Parkinson's disease, the behavioural syndrome and significant reduction in striatal dopamine release occur only when more than 80% of dopamine neurons are damaged due to compensatory mechanisms. Unlike bilaterally lesioned animals, animals with unilateral lesions typically do not show Parkinsonian-like behaviours. They are therefore easier to maintain and more commonly used. One feature of the unilateral lesion model is that it leads to supersensitivity or up-regulation of striatal dopamine receptors on the side of the lesion.

Upon pharmacological stimulation of these receptors, animals shows predictable rotational responses. For example, AMPHETAMINE, which enhances dopamine release, elicits rotation towards the side of the lesion. In contrast, dopamine receptor agonists such as APOMORPHINE elicit contralateral rotation. The mechanism of this rotation is not well understood, but animals with unilateral lesions have been used for screening various compounds to develop effective therapeutic agents for treating Parkinson's disease.

See also: MPTP

KAZUE SEMBA

5-hydroxyindoleacetic acid Metabolite of SEROTONIN routinely measured by HIGH-PERFORMANCE LIQUID CHROMATOGRAPHY and used as an index of serotonin turnover in brain.

5-hydroxytryptamine (5-HT) *see* serotonin

5-hydroxytryptophan Precursor of SEROTONIN, synthesized from L-tryptophan, a reaction catalysed by tryptophan hydroxylase. Amino acid decarboxylase catalyses the formation of serotonin from 5-hydroxytryptophan

hyoid bone *see* skull

hyoscine A cholinomimetic drug, better known as SCOPOLAMINE.

hyper- (from Greek, *hyper*: over) A prefix indicating over, increased or excess. Related prefixes are HYPO- and ISO-. For example, ISOTONIC SALINE (also known as PHYSIOLOGICAL SALINE) is water containing 0.9% sodium chloride (NaCl) (approximately the NaCl composition of seawater). HYPERTONIC SALINE contains more NaCl than this, HYPOTONIC SALINE less.

hyperactivity Simply, an unusually high degree of activity. PSYCHOMOTOR STIMULANT drugs (for example AMPHETAMINE) can induce hyperactivity in both animals and humans. The condition previously known as childhood HYPERACTIVITY is now discussed as ATTENTION-DEFICIT/HYPERACTIVITY DISORDER.

hyperacuity *see* visual acuity

hyperacusia Exceptionally sensitive AUDITORY PERCEPTION.

hyperalgesia Exceptional sensitivity to PAIN.

hypercalcaemia An abnormally high concentration of CALCIUM in the BLOOD.

hypercapnia Excess carbon dioxide in the BLOOD; see BREATHING, NEURAL CONTROL OF; SLEEP APNOEA.

hyperglycaemia (American spelling: hyperglycemia) An excess of GLUCOSE in the BLOOD; it is a condition most commonly encountered in DIABETES.

See also: insulin

hyperinsulinaemia An excess of INSULIN in the BLOOD; this leads to rapid clearance of GLUCOSE from the blood and HYPOGLYCAEMIA, and is a stimulus for FEEDING. It is a principal feature of the VENTROMEDIAL HYPOTHALAMIC SYNDROME.

hyperkinesia *see* dyskinesia

hyperlexia There are two interpretations for the term HYPERLEXIA: (i) in child psychiatry, the acquisition of READING without formal, systematic instruction at an exceptionally early age. This is the more common usage of the term hyperlexia and describes an exceptional ability. (ii) In contrast, hyperlexia has also been used as a term to describe a disability of LANGUAGE in children and in adults: the ability to read out words and spell for example, but without comprehension and without normal SPEECH PRODUCTION abilities. This has also been called DEMENTED DYSLEXIA. This is a condition observed occasionally in adults with DEMENTIA who will read aloud fluently with absolutely no comprehension whatsoever of what is being read.

See also: alexia; dyslexia

hypermetamorphosis A tendency to switch rapidly from one behaviour to another; see KLUVER–BUCY SYNDROME.

hypermetropia Synonym for HYPEROPIA; see REFRACTIVE ERROR.

hypermnesia Hypermnesia is generally regarded as an extreme power of MEMORY. It is also a term used to describe the recovery of memories that were previously inaccessible. This is related to the notion that memories are not simply dispassionate recordings of events but are influenced by a variety of motivational and emotional states, and other psychological processes

See also: Pöetzl effect; recovered memory; retrieval induced forgetting

hyperopia *see* refractive error

hyperorexia Rather antique term indicating over-eating; see BULIMIA NERVOSA; EATING DISORDERS; HYPERPHAGIA.

hyperosmia Exceptional sensitive olfactory ability; see OLFACTION; SMELL; STEREOCHEMICAL THEORY OF ODOUR DISCRIMINATION.

hyperparesthesia Exceptional sensitivity to TOUCH.

hyperphagia Over-eating – the opposite of APHAGIA; see BENZODIAZEPINE-INDUCED HYPERPHAGIA; EATING DISORDERS; VENTROMEDIAL HYPOTHALAMIC SYNDROME.

hyperplagia *see* hyperplasia

hyperplasia (also spelled hyperplagia) The abnormal expansion in size of a tissue due to an increase in the number of cells that comprise it. (The opposite is HYPOPLASIA.) Hyperplasia may result from decreased cell death (APOPTOSIS) and/or enhanced cell division PROLIFERATION, and is distinguished from HYPERTROPHY, where individual cells increase in size, although the two states may coexist. Hyperplasia of a neuronal population may be seen following experimental manipulations during early DEVELOPMENT that increase the number of target cells innervated by that population. It is also seen in the HIPPOCAMPUS of animals reared in an enriched environment (*see* ENVIRONMENTAL ENRICHMENT).

ROGER J. KEYNES

hyperpolarization A change in MEMBRANE potential of a CELL that makes it more negative. In the case of excitable cells, this can be accomplished by opening any ION CHANNEL that is selectively permeable to positive ions (see ION) that are more abundant inside the

cell, such as POTASSIUM, or to negative ions that are more abundant outside the cell, such as CHLORIDE. A hyperpolarizing input is often called 'inhibitory' because it moves the membrane potential away from the neuron's THRESHOLD, thereby making it more difficult for other inputs to excite the cell to threshold.

DOUGLAS D. RASMUSSON

hyperpyrexia Exceptional high body temperature; see THERMOREGULATION.

hyperreflexia The strength of a REFLEX is graded, the degree determined by stimulus strength. Hyperreflexia is a condition in which reflex strength is abnormally exaggerated.

hypersensitive HYPERSENSITIVE and HYPOSENSITIVE are terms commonly encountered in everyday language and are used in the same way in biological psychology: hypersensitivity refers to a state of sensitivity (in whatever domain) that is greater than normal, while hyposensitive is the reverse of this – a lack of sensitivity. The important consideration here is to avoid confusion of these everyday terms with the more specific terms SUPERSENSITIVITY and SENSITIZATION.

See also: sensitization (behavioural); sensitization (drug)

hypersexuality A self-descriptive term: hypersexuality indicates a willingness to engage in any form of SEXUAL BEHAVIOUR. In experimental neuroscience it is a term most commonly encountered when describing the KLUVER–BUCY SYNDROME. In clinical settings, hypersexuality has been described in HUNTINGTON'S CHOREA and after FRONTAL LOBE damage. SEXUAL SEIZURES have also been described, in three types: (1) SEIZURES, shown by EEG recordings to be dependent on PARIETAL LOBE activity, that are accompanied by genital sensations; (2) seizures originating in the sensory cortex producing EROTOMANIA (which can be described therefore as paroxysmal erotomania – see PAROXYSM); and (3) seizures originating in the TEMPORAL LOBE in which hypersexuality of a Kluver–Bucy type appears (though note also that temporal lobe EPILEPSY may be associated with decreased sexual feelings). There is no strong feeling that these effects reflect the organization of some specific sexual control processes: rather they are more likely to be highly idiosyncratic expression of behaviour or emotion following rather generalized brain activation.

hypersomnia Hypersomnia is literally over-SLEEP, a clinical condition recognized by DSM-IV. It is a term reserved for states that are not produced by medication or DRUG use; which are not produced simply by tiredness; which last for more than a month; and which involve sleep at night as well as bouts of sleep during the day; see INSOMNIA.

hyperstriatum ventrale A large structure in the FOREBRAIN of birds, divisible into a number of subnuclei (such as intermediate and medial hyperstriatum ventrale). It is important in IMPRINTING and it is sensitive to the structure of conspecific BIRDSONG. Indeed, the hyperstriatum ventrale pars caudale appears to be critical for the acquisition, perception and production of birdsong and is often now referred to as the HIGHER VOCAL CENTRE (HVC).

hypertension High blood pressure; see BLOOD; HEADACHE; OBESITY; OSMOREGULATION.

hyperthermia Abnormally high body temperature; see THERMOREGULATION.

hyperthyroidism A condition in which the THYROID GLAND is improperly controlled by the HYPOTHALAMO-PITUITARY AXIS leading to excessive release of thyroid HORMONES (see ENDOCRINE GLANDS).

hypertonic *see* isotonic

hypertonic saline *see* isotonic saline

hypertrophy Hypertrophy is literally overgrown, or exceptionally increased in size, whether caused by exaggeration of normal development, disease, experimental manipulation of tissues or processes, or any other cause; the opposite is HYPOTROPHY.

See also: hyperplasia

hypervigilance Hypervigilance is a generally increased state of awareness: it has been reported in accounts of disparate conditions,

from the effects of child abuse through various kinds of PHOBIA to increased sensitivity to physical PAIN.

hypervolaemia Increased BLOOD volume.

hypnagogic This term indicates the beginning of SLEEP.

See also: hypnopompic; narcolepsy

hypnagogic hallucination A vivid, often terrifying, dream-like HALLUCINATION occurring at the onset of SLEEP.

See also: hypnopompic hallucination; narcolepsy; sleep paralysis

hypnopompic (from Greek, *hypnos*: sleep, *pompe*: sending) This term indicates the ending of SLEEP.

See also: hypnagogic; narcolepsy

hypnopompic hallucination A vivid, often terrifying, dream-like HALLUCINATION occurring at the end of SLEEP.

See also: hypnagogic hallucination; narcolepsy

hypnosis (from Greek, *hypnos*: sleep) The origin of hypnosis is generally credited to Franz Mesmer (1734–1815). Mesmer believed in animal magnetism – that all creatures have a universal magnetic fluid, disruption in which could affect psychological state. He affected to cure this by having patients sit in tubs containing iron filings and metal rods, which would enable him to reorganize the animal magnetism in his patients. While appearing ridiculous to modern sensibilities, there is something of interest in this: it is one of the very earliest instances of psychological disturbances being attributed (however oddly) to physical causes. Mesmer's cures have been suggested to have induced a hypnotic state in his patients, which permitted (in some rather unspecified way) therapeutic benefit to be obtained. Indeed, hypnotism – at least stage hypnotism – is still occasionally referred to as mesmerism, and the state of being entranced is known as 'mesmerized'. Hypnotism is still practised in the treatment of certain psychological disorders – Freud used it when he first practised PSYCHOTHERAPY but later abandoned it for other techniques – but it remains unclear what sort of state the hypnotic state is. Is there actually a changed state of CONSCIOUSNESS that can be characterized as hypnotic – a state that is not accounted for by any other SLEEP mechanisms for example? Or is it the case that patients who are hypnotized are not actually in any form of altered consciousness at all but, believing that while hypnotized they are not responsible for their own actions, thoughts or speech, they are freed from inhibitions that would normally prevent them doing, thinking or saying certain things? There is no unambiguous evidence in favour of there being a special hypnotic state of entrancement.

hypnotic sleep Sleep induced by HYPNOTICS.

hypnotics Drugs (such as BARBITURATES, e.g. PENTOBARBITAL, or BENZODIAZEPINES) that induce SLEEP; also known as SEDATIVE–HYPNOTICS, or SEDATIVE–ANXIOLYTIC drugs.

See also: anxiolytic; sedative

hypo- (from Greek *hypo*: under) A prefix indicating under, reduced or less. Related prefixes are HYPO- and ISO-. For example, ISOTONIC SALINE (also known as PHYSIOLOGICAL SALINE) is water containing 0.9% sodium chloride (NaCl) (approximately the NaCl composition of seawater). HYPERTONIC SALINE contains more NaCl than this, HYPOTONIC SALINE less.

hypocalcaemia An abnormally low concentration of CALCIUM in the BLOOD.

hypocretin/orexin This is a PEPTIDE found in the HYPOTHALAMUS. Discovery of this was made simultaneously by two separate research groups: one isolated a peptide from the mammalian hypothalamus which appeared similar to SECRETIN and called it hypocretin. The other group isolated the same peptide and found it could affect FEEDING, so they called it orexin. The term hypocretin/orexin, while clumsy, reflects and credits both discoveries. There are two variants, hypocretin 1/orexin A, and hypocretin 2/orexin B; the former preferentially binds to a RECEPTOR known as hypocretin (orexin) 1 receptors ($Hcrt/OX_1R$) while the latter preferentially binds to hypocretin (orexin) 2 receptors ($Hcrt/OX_2R$). A population of neurons around the PERIFORNICAL HY-POTHALAMUS contain hypocretin/orexin. These have extensive projections to the FOREBRAIN and CEREBRAL CORTEX, and to a variety of sites in the MIDBRAIN and BRAINSTEM. Functionally the hypocretins/orexins have been implicated in the control of both feeding and SLEEP.

References

Kilduff T.S. & Peyron C. (2000) The hypocretin/orexin ligand-receptor system: implications for sleep and sleep disorders. *Trends in Neurosciences* 23: 359–365.

hypofrontality A reduction in activity of the FRONTAL CORTEX, as revealed by FUNCTIONAL NEUROIMAGING studies. The phenomenon has been most extensively studied in SCHIZOPHRENIA, though the finding is not specific to that condition. Hypofrontality may be demonstrated as an ongoing blood flow reduction at rest, or an attenuation of the increase in metabolic activity usually seen when subjects engage in tasks mediated by the frontal cortex (such as the WISCONSIN CARD-SORT TEST).

IAN C. REID

hypoglossal nerve The hypoglossal or twelfth cranial nerve (see CRANIAL NERVES) is a motor nerve innervating the muscles of the tongue. It also contains some sensory (proprioceptive) fibres from tongue muscles. The motor fibres originate in the hypoglossal nucleus in the dorsal MEDULLA. The nerve exits the medulla from its ventral aspect. Damage to the hypoglossal nerve results in difficulty in chewing, swallowing and speaking. There is a loss of movement and muscle tone, as well as ATROPHY of tongue muscles. When the tongue is protruded, it curls towards the side of injury.

KAZUE SEMBA

hypoglycaemia (American spelling: hypoglycemia) An abnormally low level of GLUCOSE in the BLOOD. It is a condition also referred to as GLUCOPENIA.

hypogonadism Abnormal functioning of the GONADS, either in terms of the secretion of gonadal HORMONES or as the production of GAMETES.

hypomania *see* bipolar disorder

hyponatremia An abnormally low concentration of SODIUM in the BLOOD.

hypophagia A reduction (rather than an absence or near absence) in normal food intake; see APHAGIA; DYSPHAGIA; HYPERPHAGIA.

hypophyseal artery *see* adenohypophysis; neurohypophysis

hypophysectomy Literally, cutting of the HYPOPHYSIS – that is, destruction of the PITUITARY GLAND. This can be achieved by cutting the INFUNDIBULUM (the PITUITARY STALK) which connects the pituitary to the HYPOTHALAMUS above it. A cut here causes the pituitary galnd to atrophy.

hypophysis Another name for the PITUITARY GLAND – which divides into the ADENOHYPOPHYSIS (anterior pituitary) and NEUROHYPOPHYSIS (posterior pituitary). Hypophysial and hypophyseal are descriptive of the hypophysis.

hypoplasia Hypoplasia is an under-formation of cells, resulting in abnormal growth (see CELL); the opposite is HYPERPLASIA.

hypopolarization A change in MEMBRANE potential of a CELL that makes it more positive. In the case of excitable cells, this is typically accomplished by opening the ION CHANNEL that is selectively permeable to positive ions (see ION) that are more abundant outside the cell, such as SODIUM. A hypopolarizing input is often called 'excitatory' because it moves the membrane potential toward the neuron's THRESHOLD.

hyposensitive *see* hypersensitive

hyposomnia Hyposomnia would be literally under-SLEEP, though it is a rarely (if ever) used term; instead, see INSOMNIA.

See also: hypersomnia

hypotension Low blood pressure; see BLOOD; HYPERTENSION; OSMOREGULATION.

hypothalamic-pituitary-adrenal axis Descriptive of the hormonal communication that occurs between the HYPOTHALAMUS, PITUITARY GLAND and ADRENAL GLAND.

See also: adenohypophysis; endocrine glands; hormones; hormones – classification; neurohypophysis

hypothalamic-pituitary-gonadal axis Descriptive of the hormonal communication that occurs between the HYPOTHALAMUS, PITUITARY GLAND and GONADS.

See also: adenohypophysis; endocrine glands; hormones; hormones – classification; neurohypophysis; sex hormones

hypothalamo-hypophyseal portal system *see* adenohypophysis; neurohypophysis; pituitary gland

hypothalamo-pituitary axis A general term describing relationships between the HYPOTHALAMUS and the PITUITARY GLAND, and the HORMONE-releasing functions of the NEURONS contained within it; see ADENOHYPOPHYSIS; NEUROHYPOPHYSIS.

hypothalamo-pituitary portal system *see* adenohypophysis; neurohypophysis; pituitary gland

hypothalamus (from Greek, *hypo*: under, *thalamus*: chamber) The hypothalamus is a structure in the DIENCEPHALON, sitting beneath the THALAMUS and is concerned with the control of body processes. It can regulate activity in the PERIPHERAL NERVOUS SYSTEM and controls the release of many HORMONES. It is best known for its role in the control of fundamental activities such as FEEDING, DRINKING, THERMOREGULATION, REPRODUCTION and SEXUAL BEHAVIOUR. It is a nucleated structure: that is, the hypothalamus *en masse* is divided into discrete parts (nuclei) that can be identified using a number of criteria: the nature and density of the NEURONS they contain, the connections they have within and without the hypothalamus, and by their development from embryonic tissue for example.

The division of the hypothalamus into its component nuclei can be systematized, divisions being made both along its anterior–posterior length and longwise, in parallel with the MIDLINE. Four regions are identified along its length: preoptic (the most anterior), anterior hypothalamic, tuberal hypothalamic and mammillary (or posterior hypothalamic) region. Longitudinally, three areas are identified: the periventricular (or midline) zone (the most

Principal divisions of the hypothalamus

	Preoptic	*Anterior hypothalamic*	*Tuberal hypothalamic*	*Mammillary Posterior hypothalamic*
Periventricular (MIDLINE)	Median PREOPTIC N.	Periventricular n.	Periventricular n.	Periventricular n.
		Paraventricular n.	Arcuate n.	Tuberomammillary n.
	Organum vasculosum of the lamina terminalis	Suprachiasmatic n.		
Medial (Core)	Medial PREOPTIC AREA	Anterior HYPOTHALAMIC N.	Dorsomedial n.	Posterior hypothalamic n.
			Ventromedial n.	
	Preoptic nuclei (AV, AD, MPO, PD)			Premammillary n.
				Mammillary bodies
Lateral (Reticular)	Lateral PREOPTIC AREA	Lateral hypothalamus	Lateral hypothalamus	Lateral hypothalamus
	Magnocellular preoptic n.	Supraoptic n.		

Source: Adapted from Simerly (1995)

Notes: AV anteroventral; AD anterodorsal; MPO medial preoptic nucleus; PD posterodorsal; n nucleus

central), the medial (or core) zone and the lateral (or reticular) zone. The nuclei that can be identified within this matrix are listed in the table above; details of the specific functions of individual nuclei are contained in separate entries. The hypothalamus has major connections with: (1) the AUTONOMIC NERVOUS SYSTEM. The NUCLEUS OF THE SOLITARY TRACT and the PARABRACHIAL NUCLEI of the PONS, nuclei that receive afferent visceral information either directly or indirectly from the CRANIAL NERVES or SPINAL CORD, are the sensory nuclei of the autonomic nervous system. These project in turn to the hypothalamus as well as other parts of the LIMBIC SYSTEM and the CEREBRAL CORTEX (INSULA CORTEX and PREFRONTAL CORTEX). Output from the hypothalamus returns to these places and to sites such as the DORSAL MOTOR NUCLEUS OF THE VAGUS, the origin of the efferent limb of the VAGUS NERVE. These connections bring in a wealth of information about the state of the body's tissues. In addition, BLOOD borne information, and information about the body's fluid balance (see OSMOREGULATION) is received via the circumventricular organs. (2) The hypothalamus has extensive neuroendocrine connections, principally by virtue of its relationship with the PITUITARY GLAND: these connections allow the hypothalamus both to monitor hormonal activity in the body and to control the release of HORMONES. The hypothalamus appears also to receive information about the state of the immune system (via the blood) and is able to influence immune system activity (via the activity of hormones it controls). (3) The hypothalamus has sensory information from the external world, as well as the internal milieu. Olfactory input comes from the accessory olfactory system (see OLFACTION) and direct input from the RETINA arrives via the RETINOHYPOTHALAMIC SYSTEM. (4) The hypothalamus has extensive AFFERENT and EFFERENT connections with other structures in the CENTRAL NERVOUS SYSTEM, giving it considerable power in affecting processes such as LEARNING, MEMORY and MOTIVATION.

It has been acknowledged for a long time that the hypothalamus is concerned with HOMEOSTASIS – the maintenance of a stable body state. For many years the prevailing view was that the hypothalamus was divided into discrete drive centres, some acting to turn behaviour on, some to turn it off (see DUAL CENTRES HYPOTHESIS). This is a view that is not generally accepted any longer, though it is still recognized that the hypothalamus is best seen as a coordinating structure: sensory information is received from the body: the autonomic nervous system, hormones, the immune system, sensory systems for monitoring the external environment, and from other parts of the central nervous system. Output is directed towards the goal of bodily maintenance: this is achieved by taking action on the body via hormone release and by the autonomic nervous system and by influencing processes of behavioural selection which in turn will serve to maintain the body. The precise way in which individual hypothalamic nuclei contribute to this is still a matter of active research interest.

See also: arcuate nucleus of the hypothalamus; dorsomedial nucleus of the hypothalamus; lateral hypothalamus; lateral hypothalamic syndrome; paraventricular nucleus of the hypothalamus; periventricular nucleus of the hypothalamus; supraoptic nucleus of the hypothalamus; ventromedial hypothalamic syndrome

References

Altman J. & Bayer S.A. (1986) *The Development of the Rat Hypothalamus. Advances in Embryology and Cell Biology*, vol. 100, Springer-Verlag: Berlin.

Risold P.Y., Thompson R.H. & Swanson L.W. (1997) The structural organization of connections between hypothalamus and cerebral cortex. *Brain Research Reviews* 24: 197–254.

Simerly R.B. (1995) Anatomical substrates of hypothalamic integration. In *The Rat Nervous System*, 2nd edn, ed. G. Paxinos, pp. 353–376, Academic Press: San Diego.

hypothermia Abnormally low body temperature; see THERMOREGULATION.

hypothyroid A deficiency in the production of thyroid hormone.

See also: congenital hypothyroidism; endocrine glands

hypotonic *see* isotonic

hypotonic saline *see* isotonic saline

hypotrophy (from Greek, *hypo*: under, *trophe*: nourishment) Hypotrophy is literally undergrown, or exceptionally reduced in size, whether caused by exaggeration of normal development, disease, experimental manipulation of tissues or processes, or any other cause; the opposite is HYPERTROPHY.

hypovolaemia *see* osmoregulation

hypoxia Hypoxia is a decrease in the level of OXYGEN in the BLOOD or tissues below that which is normal. Anaemic HYPOXIA is caused by a loss of haemoglobin (the oxygen-transporting MOLECULE) form the blood; DIFFUSION hypoxia is caused by a transient decrease in pressure within the lungs (and is rare – it is associated with recovery from ANAESTHESIA); hypoxic HYPOXIA is caused by defective action of the lungs, with a wide variety of possible causes; ischaemic hypoxia (also known as stagnant anoxia) results from reduced blood flow.

See also: anoxia; ischaemia; stroke

hysteria (from Greek, *hystera*: the womb, which was thought by Hippocrates to cause hysteria by wandering about the body) Hysteria is a vague term used to describe disorders where patients complain of symptoms which do not appear to have adequate physical cause. The term is increasingly recognized as unsatisfactory because it has multiple meanings, some of which are pejorative. The designation has been abandoned in DSM-IV and ICD 10 classification systems. Preferred concepts include dissociation syndrome and SOMATIZATION DISORDER.

IAN C. REID

I

iatrogenic (from Greek, *iatros*: physician) Description of a disorder induced by the actions or comments of a physician. See, for example, RECOVERED MEMORY.

ibotenic acid (ibotenate) α-Amino-3-hydroxy-5-isoxazolacetic acid: one of the EXCITOTOXINS, it binds to NMDA and metabotropic GLUTAMATE RECEPTORS and is frequently used to produce a LESION in experimental animals. Ibotenic acid was originally synthesized from the mushrooms *Amanita pantherina* and *Amanita muscaria*.

See also: drug ionization

IC50 The inhibitory concentration 50%; when a substance produces inhibition of a response, the IC50 is the dose or concentration that produces 50% of the maximum inhibition. Such statistics help one decide what concentration of a substance to use in experiments.

See also: EC50; ED50; LD50; TD50; therapeutic index

ICD 10 The *International Statistical Classification of Diseases, Injuries and Causes of Death*, 10th edition. The classification of abnormal behaviour associated with psychological and neurological illness has shown considerable international variation. Efforts have been made to correct this since the end of the nineteenth century. In 1882, in the UK, the Statistical Committee of the Royal Medico-Psychological Association attempted to formulate a classification scheme. In 1886 the Association of Medical Superintendents of American Institutions for the Insane (the forerunner of the American Psychiatric Association) and in 1889, in Paris, the Congress of Mental Science both attempted the same thing. Other congresses and national organizations – and in the United States, state committees – attempted to formulate clear diagnostic guidelines. The World Health Organization added mental illness to the 1939 revision of their *International List of the Causes of Death*. In 1948 this list was revised to become the *International Statistical Classification of Diseases, Injuries and Causes of Death* (ICD). However, despite now running to nine revisions, this classification is still not universally accepted. More commonly used is the American Psychiatric Association's Diagnostic and Statistical Manual (DSM-IV). Any comparison of the incidence of a disorder across international boundaries still has to take account of differing diagnostic criteria, and any attempt to formulate an international standard for diagnosis still has to take account of the fact that certain abnormalities are seen differently by different cultures.

ICI-118,551 A beta-2 noradrenaline receptor ANTAGONIST; see ADRENOCEPTORS.

iconic memory The term ICONIC MEMORY has been used as a synonym for SHORT-TERM MEMORY. More appropriately, it has also been used to indicate a very short-term form of visual memory in which stimulus attributes are preserved but which lasts for only about half a second. The equivalent form of auditory memory is known as ECHOIC MEMORY. (An 'icon' is a form of visual image; an echo is an auditory phenomenon.) Echoic memory is essentially the same as what has been called precategorical acoustic memory.

ictal *see* post-ictal

idazoxan Also known by its development name, RX781094; idazoxan is an ANTAGONIST at alpha 2 noradrenaline receptors (see ADRENOCEPTORS).

ideational apraxia An impairment in the performance of a complex act, but with the individual elements of the act executed correctly; one of the four principal forms of APRAXIA described by Henry Hecaen (1912–1983).

identical twins *see* monozygotic twins

ideomotor action *see* voluntary

ideomotor apraxia An impairment in the execution of single acts, such as waving goodbye; one of the four principal forms of APRAXIA described by Henry Hecaen.

idiopathic (from Greek, *idios*: own, *pathos*: suffering) The term idiopathic is used to describe a condition spontaneously generated by a person for no known reason. Diseases are often referred to as idiopathic. For example, most cases of PARKINSON'S DISEASE are referred to as idiopathic, in contrast to conditions where the symptoms have been produced for a known reason – POST-ENCEPHALITIC PARKINSONISM for example. Idiopathic is therefore a rather grand way of saying 'unknown cause'.

idiot savant An individual showing surprising skill in one area despite low general ability and IQ (see INTELLIGENCE TESTING). Savant skills are typically manifest in one of a narrow range of areas; calculation, music, drawing, MEMORY. Prevalence is approximately 0.06% in mental handicap, and 10% in AUTISM (with a 6:1 ratio of male to female). Research suggests that savant skills are not the product of mere practice or ROTE LEARNING, and reflect implicit (though rarely consciously available) use of extracted rules and regularities. The existence of savant skills has been taken as a challenge to the notion of global intelligence, contributing to interest in the modular organization of the mind.

See also: acalculia; copying and drawing; mathematics and the brain; music and the brain

FRANCESCA HAPPÉ

idiothetic navigation *see* allothetic navigation

IgA; IgD; IgG; IgE; IgM *see* immune system

ileum digestive system

illuminence *see* photometry

illusions We see far more than meets the eyes, though not always correctly, for we experience various phenomena of illusion. Although they are errors, and can be misleading for the physical sciences as well as dangerous in skills such as driving, illusions are useful evidence of how eyes and brains normally work. 'Illusion' is hard to define. Illusions of the senses are departures from physical reality, but what is reality? This is difficult to answer, for we have many descriptions of reality – in science, in art and so on. No doubt all are incomplete, and largely wrong. Certainly physics frequently changes its mind. If we take modern physics' accounts of matter, as atoms and molecules in violent motion with weird effects of quantum mechanics, this is so different from how things appear that we might be tempted to say all perception is illusion. But this is no more helpful than to say that all perceptions are dreams.

We are pushed into thinking that visual and other illusions are departures from quite simple-minded physics – as measured with rulers, protractors, clocks and so on. Illusions include distortions of length, angles and time. There are also phenomena of ghostly fictions, and some figures or objects appear impossible. Others seem to flip from one perception to another, though there is no change at the eyes: they are ambiguous. These are weird and wonderful phenomena, which are central to art and hazards to the physical sciences. They are well worth explaining. It seems useful to try to classify phenomena of illusions, as classifications are important for all science. Chemistry was transformed by the PERIODIC TABLE OF THE ELEMENTS, biology by names of classes of species and varieties (see TAXONOMY). How shall we start for illusions? It is suggestive that illusions of seeing correspond

Causes of visual illusions

Classes	physical causes		cognitive causes	
	Optics	Physiology	Rules	Knowledge
Ambiguities	mist	binocular rivalry	figure-ground	hollow face
Distortions	mirage	café wall	Ponzo	size-weight
Paradoxes	looking glass	rotating spiral	impossible object	Magritte mirror
Fictions	rainbow	afterimages	ghostly shapes	faces in the fire

with errors of LANGUAGE. Appearances of illusions fall into classes which may be named quite naturally from kinds of errors of language: ambiguities, distortions, paradoxes, fictions.

It is intriguing that these apply to vision and to language, for it is more than possible that language grew from pre-human classifications of objects and actions, over many millions of years. This would explain how language developed so rapidly in biological time for early humans – in only tens of thousands of years. Let's compare errors of language with kinds of illusions:

The skeletal Necker cube switches in depth; the upper line of the Ponzo figure looks too long; the Tri-bar looks impossible; the ghostly square (a Kanizsa figure) does not exist.

To discover causes of illusions we need experiments, just as for any science, as well as appropriate explanatory concepts within a general theory or paradigm. Perception starts from what are called bottom-up signals from the eyes and the other senses. After a great deal of signal processing they are 'read' from top-down knowledge of objects, and from general rules (see TOP-DOWN VS. BOTTOM-UP PERCEPTUAL/NEURAL PROCESSING). When these are inappropriate, cognitive illusions occur, though there is nothing wrong with the physiological functioning. (This is rather like 'software' and 'hardware' errors of a computer; though the brain is not very like a digital computer, as it is most probably analogue.) Not all illusions are cognitive in origin. There seem to be four principal kinds of causes of illusions. The first is physical, for vision, optical disturbance between objects and the eyes. The second is physiological disturbance of neural signals, to

and in the brain. The third is extremely different: cognitive errors of reading neural signals in terms of external objects. This occurs in two ways: errors of inappropriate knowledge of objects, and inappropriate general rules (such as depth-perspective applied to the flat surfaces of pictures, and the GESTALT laws of perceptual organisation). When either is inappropriate it can mislead perception, much as for rules and knowledge for thinking. (There are more or less corresponding illusions for the other senses, especially hearing). Here are examples, just one for each kind of visual illusion.

The 'Cafe Wall' distortion occurs with a chess board-like figure, when alternate rows of squares are displaced by half a square width. The rows become long wedges – as the retinal signals are upset by the brightness contrast across each half-square. The Ponzo illusion distortion is very different – perspective convergence of lines in a picture enlarge features that 'should' be more distant.

Distinguishing between objects and spaces between objects ('figure-ground') is the first most basic visual decision: it can be ambiguous. A demonstration of the power of top-down knowledge, here resolving ambiguities, is the hollow face. Though hollow it appears as a normal convex nose-sticking-out face. This is because convex faces are very familiar, and hollow faces extremely unlikely. Knowledge of faces is so strong it overcomes the bottom-up evidence that this face is truly hollow – countering and dominating bottom-up evidence, signalled by the eyes.

The left face is normal; but the right face is a hollow mould. The lighting is the same for both. Through the power of top-down knowledge, the right actually hollow face looks convex, like a normal face.

We always see the present in terms of past experience. We experience cognitive illusions when the past is not appropriate for seeing the present – for survival into the immediate future.

RICHARD L. GREGORY

image (from Latin, *imago*: image) An image is generally conceived of as a REPRESENTATION, and IMAGERY as the product of the imagination. In psychology however it is important to distinguish clearly between different uses of the word 'image'. The term RETINAL IMAGE refers to the pattern of light impinging on the RETINA: this is a physical representation of the visual world on the retina. The term MENTAL IMAGERY refers to a conscious recollection (see CONSCIOUSNESS) of a previous perception in the absence of the physical stimuli that produced that perception (regardless of sensory modality). Images are things that can be discriminated into two different classes: physical representations and non-physical representations (at least in so far as the neural basis of these conscious, 'stimulus free' recollections cannot be specified). It is helpful therefore to use a qualifier before the terms image or imagery to make clear what is meant by their use in any given context.

See also: mental representation; metarepresentation

image analysis Image analysis is a term generally taken to mean the analysis of visual images by computer. Visual images pose special problems for analysis of their content. The human perceptual system is specialized to analyse visual images, in particular distinguish-

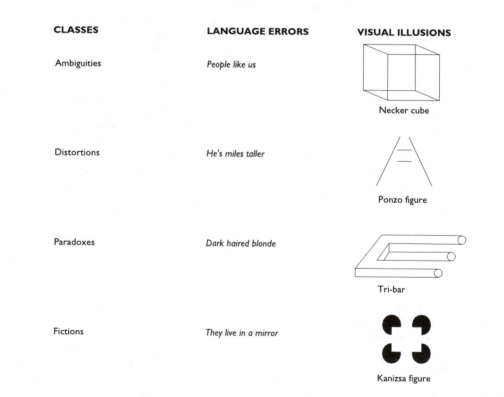

CLASSES	LANGUAGE ERRORS	VISUAL ILLUSIONS
Ambiguities	*People like us*	Necker cube
Distortions	*He's miles taller*	Ponzo figure
Paradoxes	*Dark haired blonde*	Tri-bar
Fictions	*They live in a mirror*	Kanizsa figure

Language errors and illusions of vision

Notes: The skeletal Necker cube switches in depth; the upper line of the Ponzo figure looks too long; the Tri-bar (also known as the Devil's tuning fork) looks impossible; the ghostly square – the Kanizsa figure – does not exist.

ing figures from backgrounds or identifying boundaries or groupings of objects. Nevertheless, image analysis by computers is preferred under conditions such as when there is a large volume of material for analysis (as in the processing of histological specimens – see HISTOLOGY) or when aspects of the image must be quantified objectively. Computers are, in many respects, less good than a human observer. Nevertheless, there are techniques of image analysis which produce consistent results. For example, it is possible to measure the density of pixels of colour and this technique can be used to count histologically-stained neurons (and indeed other cells) or to quantify extent and location of regions of brain activity, as obtained for example from PET (positron emission tomography) scans.

ERIC M. BOWMAN

imagery *see* image

imipramine An ANTIDEPRESSANT drug (one of the TRICYCLICS) that works by blocking the REUPTAKE of MONOAMINES from the SYNAPTIC CLEFT.

See also: depression

imitation learning *see* observation learning

immediate early genes Stimulation of a NEURON leads to activation of SECOND MESSENGERS, which can activate immediate early genes within cells. These encode for PROTEINS called TRANSCRIPTION FACTORS, which enter the NUCLEUS, and bind to the DNA, promoting the expression of the particular GENE involved. The most widely studied immediate early genes are C-FOS and C-JUN, which encode for the proteins Fos and Jun, respectively. These proteins can be measured by IMMUNOHISTOCHEMISTRY, and are found in certain neurons following experimental stimuli such as a LESION, administration of a DRUG, a pathological event such as ISCHAEMIA, or PHYSIOLOGICAL CHALLENGE.

See also: metabolic mapping

FIONA M. INGLIS

immediate memory Immediate memory refers to the ability to RECALL items within seconds after being exposed to them, and it is similar in meaning to the term SHORT-TERM MEMORY. The contents of immediate memory are thought to involve declarative (see DECLARATIVE MEMORY) rather than procedural (see PROCEDURAL MEMORY) information. The capacity of this type of MEMORY system is thought to be 7 plus-or-minus 2 items in normal humans. Some common memory tests that are used to assess immediate memory capabilities are digit span and word list learning. Amnesic (see AMNESIA) patients and animals with damage to the medial TEMPORAL LOBE often have normal immediate memory capabilities but have LONG-TERM MEMORY deficiencies.

HOWARD EICHENBAUM

immobilization Immobilization of course means to render something immovable. In biological psychology it is a term used in two different ways. (i) *Stress*: forced immobilization – the prevention of normal movement – is a means for inducing stress in a rat. Handling a rat is initially stressful to it, but stress responses show HABITUATION as rats become accustomed to the procedure. However, prolonged immobilization of a conscious rat in a restraining device (or by a simple expedient such as taping its legs to a board such that it cannot engage in LOCOMOTION) is stressful. Procedures such as this (which are of course subject to regulation by statutory bodies – the Home Office in the United Kingdom, for example) allow scientists to take measures of the physiological variables affected by stress. It is not a commonly used procedure. (ii) *Chemical activity*: the term immobilize is applied in the following ways: ENZYME immobilization involves fixing an enzyme to a physical substrate such that it is capable of action but incapable of escape from its current location. Other types of CELL (including bacteria) can be immobilized by a physical substrate also. Co-immobilized enzymes are enzymes that have a coordinated action, being physically present together.

immune system The immune system is an essential component of the body's defence against attack. The bodies of MAMMALS have a series of mechanisms to deal with attacks upon them: (1) the body is enclosed in SKIN, a protective (and sensate) layer, and is able to generate secretions (mucous and skin secretions) that protect the body against environmental elements; (2) PHAGOCYTES (principally white blood cells; more properly known as LEUKOCYTES), antimicrobial PROTEINS and INFLAMMATION, all of which act internally and rather non-specifically to protect the body; (3) the immune system, a specific mechanism for dealing with alien cells, based on LYMPHOCYTES and the production of ANTIBODIES. The first of these, skin, is discussed in an entry of its own: the other two are discussed further below. (Note: this discussion is far from complete: the immune system is a highly complex biological process. Readers who wish to understand more about this than can be presented here are referred to Campbell *et al.*, 1999)

Phagocytes (from Greek, *phagein*: to eat, *kytos*: a vessel) are cells that engage in a process called phagocytosis: they are cells that eat other cells. Leukocytes are the principal phagocytes of the body and are present in a variety of types: NEUTROPHILS, MONOCYTES and EOSINOPHILS. (Collectively these are known as GRANULOCYTES – mature leukocytes have a granular appearance.) Most leukocytes (some 65%) are neutrophils, cells which have a short life span and which react to chemical messages emitted by cells invading the body. There are far fewer monocytes, some 5% of the total number of leukocytes. Monocytes leave the blood stream and reside in tissue, where they act as MACROPHAGES. Eosinophils make up less that 2% of the number of leukocytes and are the main defence against parasites, attaching themselves to the cell MEMBRANE of the parasite and using ENZYME action to destroy them. This process, known as lysing (see LYSIS), is not strictly phagocytosis, but is nevertheless a form of destruction. A similar process is adopted by NATURAL KILLER CELLS: these are not leukocytes, but form an important defence against virally infected cells.

These phagocytic cells are all involved in the process of inflammation. This follows the occurrence of a localized TRAUMA – a wound of some sort – which initiates a cascade of events. First, the release of HISTAMINE and PROSTAGLANDINS generates increases in blood flow. Histamine is released by BASOPHILS (a form of leukocyte) and MAST CELLS (in CONNECTIVE TISSUE), while prostaglandins are released by leukocytes. Chemical signals emitted at the site of trauma attract neutrophils and monocytes which phagocytose pathogens. With severe infections – which can generate a sevenfold increase in leukocyte number within hours – FEVER may also develop. Certain leukocytes release PYROGENS which increase body TEMPERATURE: increased temperature facilitates the action of phagocytes and inhibits reproduction of harmful micro-organisms. Microbes are also attacked by proteins in blood SERUM that form the complement system (see COMPLEMENT). Similarly, INTERFERONS are proteins secreted by cells that have had a VIRUS attack. The interferons are of little value to the cells that produce them, but initiate changes in nearby cells to protect them against viral infection. Interferons thus interfere with the spread of infection.

The inflammatory response is a fairly non-specific response to trauma of all sorts. The immune response on the other hand is very much more specific. LYMPHOCYTES – cells of the LYMPHATIC SYSTEM – are central to the immune system and come in two basic types: B CELLS and T CELLS (or B lymphocytes and T lymphocytes: T is for THYMUS GLAND, B is for bone marrow, the points of origin of the two cell types). An ANTIGEN is a molecule that elicits a specific response from lymphocytes: antigens are found on all sorts of things, including viruses and bacteria. The term antigen is an abridged form of the term ANTIBODY generator. B cells produce ANTIBODIES in response to antigens: antigens and antibodies are specifically related (much as a RECEPTOR and LIGAND are) making this a very specific form of defensive mechanism for the body. Indeed, antibodies possess antigen receptors that are, like the receptors of NEUROTRANSMITTERS on a NEURON, membrane-bound proteins. Lymphocytes – T and B cells – have thousands of antigen receptors available with all of the receptors on an individual cell being specialized for a particular antigen. This is an important point: although there are very many lymphocytes circulating in the lymph and blood, an antigen will activate only a small proportion of them – those with the specific receptors for that particular antigen. The primary immune response occurs following combination of an antigen with the receptors on B or T cells. Once this contact has been made, the lymphocyte is stimulated to divide. The division produces EFFECTOR CELLS which continue to fight the antigen, and MEMORY CELLS, in possession of receptors for the activating antigen. Over the subsequent 10–17 days effector B cells (known as PLASMA CELLS) and effector T cells deal with the antigen, eventually clearing it from the body. The secondary immune response is the term given to a second infection by the same antigen. On second presentation, the antigen is dealt with much more quickly. How do the effector cells fight antigens? By the production of antibodies, a group of proteins present in serum known as IMMUNOGLOBULINS (Ig). There are five classes: IgM (the first to appear in response to challenge), IgG (the most abundant), IgA (important in fighting viruses), IgD and IgE (see IGA; IGD; IGE; IGM). Antibodies interface with a small portion of the antigen called the EPITOPE. Antibodies form complexes with antigens, neutralizing them prior to destruction by phagocytosis. Complement is also involved in the elimination of viruses and attacking cells, lysing them. The involvement of complement is triggered by IgM and IgG antibody activity.

During their development in the thymus or bone marrow, lymphocytes are effectively tested for reactivity to body components: clearly one does not want immune cells capable of destroying the host body. (When this does happen it is known as an AUTOIMMUNE DISEASE). Cells with the capacity for autoimmune damage are dealt with by APOPTOSIS, preserving the 'self tolerance' of the body. All the cells in the body are marked by cell surface markers – self-antigens. These are GLYCOPROTEINS (in humans they are called HUMAN LEUKOCYTE ANTIGENS – HLA) and they are coded by a GENE complex known as the MAJOR HISTOCOMPATIBILITY COMPLEX (MHC). There are two classes of these: class I MHC are present on all cells that have nuclei (that is, virtually all cells in the body); class II MHC are found on specialized cells such as macrophages, B cells, activated T cells and cells in the thymus gland. The function of these MHCs is to present antigens to T cells: an infected cell will use the class I MHC to deliver antigen to a cytotoxic T cell (TC); class II MHC molecules are involved in presenting antigens collected by macrophages to helper T cells (TH). The function of the cytotoxic T cell is to destroy invading cells. The helper T cells on the other hand have a signalling role: they release various types of CYTOKINE (such as INTERLEUKIN) which stimualte cytotoxic T cells and B cells. A third type of T cell – suppressor T cells (TS) – appear to be involved in terminating immune response, but their mechanism of action is as yet unclear.

Understanding the immune system, and how it interacts with and affects neural tissue is a developing field – PSYCHONEUROIMMUNOLOGY – of considerable interest. It is evident that brain systems have some degree of control over the immune system via both the AUTONOMIC NERVOUS SYSTEM and neuroendocrine mechanisms controlled by the HYPOTHALAMUS. The immune system appears to provide information to the brain and in return, brain processes help regulate it. Changes in the immune system are associated with several conditions: DEPRESSION and STRESS both suppress immune system activity for example, an action mediated by GLUCOCORTICOIDS and CORTICOTROPIN RELEASING FACTOR: the PARAVENTRICULAR NUCLEUS OF THE HYPOTHALAMUS is critical in regulating activity of these. Why immune responses should be suppressed during stress is not entirely clear. It might be a mechanism temporarily to inhibit the appearance of sickness, to avoid animals subject to predation being identified as weak. On the other hand it might simply be that the energy cost of maintaining the immune system is too high and that all available resources are temporarily shunted to dealing with the more immediate stressor. Moreover, it seems likely that individuals can in fact learn to gain some degree of control over their immune system and, in some sense, 'think themselves better' when ill: this is an area of research actively explored by HEALTH PSYCHOLOGY. The relationship between brain and immune system is also highlighted in other ways as well. For example, brains are privileged sites in which TRANSPLANTATION of neural tissue can take place without the risk of tissue rejection. (Tissue rejection in the rest of the body is a problem caused by the fact that each individual has a unique assembly of different MHC molecules, making it typical for transplanted tissue to be 'rejected' – that is, immunologically fought – by the host.) On the other hand, autoimmune disease such as MULTIPLE SCLEROSIS badly affect nervous tissue. Moreover, STROKE damage within the brain can lead to the irruption into the central nervous system of blood borne cells such as neutrophils that should not normally be there. These can contribute to the process of damage by acting inappropriately within brain. And of course, AIDS can produce dreadful effects on brains, causing AIDS-RELATED DEMENTIA. Understanding the relationships between brains and the immune system is likely to be an important field of research for many years to come.

References

Campbell N.A., Reece J.B. & Mitchell L.G. (1999) *Biology*, 5th edn, Addison-Wesley: Menlo Park CA.

Rosenzweig M.R., Leiman A.L. & Breedlove S.M. (1996) *Biological Psychology*, Sinauer Associates: Sunderland MA.

immunity (from Latin, *in*: not, *munis*: serving; immunity means literally not serving – that is, exempt) It is a term that was in general use before the discovery and characterization of the IMMUNE SYSTEM. In biological terms it has come to refer to protection from infection conferred by the presentation of ANTIBODIES specific to particular ANTIGENS.

immunoassay An *in vitro* technique for detecting the presence of a specific type of MOLECULE in samples of homogenized tissue, based on the binding of an ANTIBODY to an ANTIGEN (see IMMUNE SYSTEM). The technique involves adding known concentrations of antibody to saturating amounts of labelled antigen. In various reaction tubes, different concentrations of unlabelled antigen can be added to this labelled, antigen-saturated solution. Competition between labelled and unlabelled antigen will produce differing amounts of labelled binding with different concentrations of unlabelled antigen present. From the various de-

grees of binding it is possible to estimate the concentration of the molecules of interest.

See also: competitive binding assay; radioimmunoassay

Reference

Feldman R., Meyer J.S. & Quenzer L.F. (1997) *Principles of Neuropsychopharmacology*, Sinauer Associates: Sunderland MA.

immunocytochemistry A term that means, in effect, IMMUNOHISTOCHEMISTRY.

immunofluorescence *see* immunohistochemistry

immunoglobulin *see* immune system; neural adhesion molecules

immunohistochemistry A technique for demonstrating the presence of a specific type of MOLECULE in tissue using antibodies produced specifically for them. ANTIBODIES are produced (or raised, to use the technical term) by sensitizing an animal to a specific molecule (or part of a molecule); that animal will then develop antibodies to that molecule which can be extracted from its BLOOD and purified. The raised antibodies may be polyclonal or MONOCLONAL ANTIBODIES.

In order to do immunohistochemistry one takes sections of tissue and incubates them with a primary antibody. This will produce, within the tissue, ANTIGEN–antibody complexes. These can be visualized in a number of ways. The complex can be tagged with a fluorescent marker (a FLUOROCHROME – a chemical that emits light [fluoresces] when light of a specific wavelength is shone on to it) which can then be detected using a fluorescent microscope. This procedure is known as IMMUNOFLUORESCENCE, and is not commonly used. A more stable visualization technique is to bind diaminobenzidene (DAB) to the antigen–antibody complex using peroxidase. This produces a stable reaction product which is coloured and can be detected using normal light microscopy. It may be the case though that this reaction is difficult to detect. If so, the signal can be increased by the addition of what are essentially further layers of antibody. This is achieved using a secondary antibody which works as follows. If the primary antibody was raised in, for instance, a mouse, an appropriate secondary antibody would be an anti-mouse IGG (IgG being one of the principal types of antibody) raised in another species (goat or sheep for example). This will then bind to the primary antibody, which it will treat as an antigen. Peroxidase–antiperoxidase (PAP) complex to mouse can then be used to bind to the anti-mouse IgG. What this procedure will have done is to increase dramatically the number of sites at which DAB can be bound, but all of the binding is still dependent on the original interaction of the primary antibody with its antigen. This procedure is known as signal amplification: the PAP technique is just one of several that can be used; others include the avidin–biotin complex (ABC) and tyramide signal amplification.

Immunohistochemistry has been an astonishingly successful technique, allowing neuroanatomists to demonstrate the presence in brain of specific molecules. This of course is one of the central techniques of CHEMICAL NEUROANATOMY. An interesting problem that remains is the quantification of immunohistochemically treated material.

See also: histochemistry; *in situ* hybridization; metabolic mapping

immunolesion As a noun, a LESION produced by an IMMUNOTOXIN; as a verb, to make a lesion using an immunotoxin.

immunology Immunology is the study of the IMMUNE SYSTEM.

immunoreaction The outcome of IMMUNOHISTOCHEMISTRY.

immunosuppressant A type of DRUG (or other treatment) given to inhibit the actions of the IMMUNE SYSTEM; important in avoiding the rejection of tissue after tissue TRANSPLANTATION.

See also: myasthenia gravis

immunosuppression The suppression of the immune response (see IMMUNE SYSTEM) which occurs when TOLERANCE develops following repeated exposure to an ANTIGEN; in response to GLUCOCORTICOID hormones (CORTISOL, CORTICOSTERONE), which decrease the number of LYMPHOCYTES in the blood and reduce the

phagocytotic activity of MACROPHAGES and NEUTROPHILS; and by immunosuppressant DRUGS which inhibit T cell activation. X-rays cause immunosuppression by killing lymphocytes. Certain types of VIRUS, such as HIV (AIDS) cause immunosuppression, leaving their hosts open to disease. Parasitoids suppress both the humoral and cellular components of the immune system of their insect hosts by injecting a polydnavirus into them.

RICHARD E. BROWN

immunotoxin An agent for producing a LESION that is made by combining a toxin (often a protein synthesis inhibitor) with a MOLECULE (an ANTIBODY or RECEPTOR BINDING agent) that will be specifically recognized by a cell surface receptor or ANTIGEN. The interaction of the immunotoxin and its binding site on the cell surface enables the toxin to gain access to the internal environment of the cell, leading to its death; see SAPORIN for an example of this.

implant In biological psychology, as a verb, to IMPLANT meanss to introduce material into a subject. For example, one might implant a CANNULA into a rat's brain (see MICROINJECTION), or one might implant foreign cells into a brain structure (see TRANSPLANTATION). As a noun, an IMPLANT is that which has been implanted. For example, the cannula and HEADCAP established to permit intracranial microinjections can be referred to as the implant.

implicit memory Implicit memory refers to non-conscious forms of MEMORY that do not require the explicit, conscious recollection of previously learned facts or episodes. Performance changes as the result of experience, and in this sense deserves the term 'memory', but performance changes without requiring any conscious memory content or even the experience that memory is being used. Examples of implicit memory include the phenomenon of PRIMING, the learning of HABITS, SKILL LEARNING, other examples of PROCEDURAL LEARNING, and CLASSICAL CONDITIONING. In each of these cases, conscious EXPLICIT MEMORY, sometimes called DECLARATIVE MEMORY, may also be acquired, but the explicit memory is often independent of and not relevant to the expression of implicit memory. In other cases, such as complex skill learning, both explicit and implicit memory may be required.

LARRY R. SQUIRE

implicit processes The term implicit indicates that something is present but that there is no awareness of it. Certain forms of MEMORY lack conscious processing and are referred to as IMPLICIT MEMORY. Perceptual processes such as BLINDSIGHT also involve implicit processing. The presence of implicit cognitive and perceptual processes raises important questions concerning the nature of CONSCIOUSNESS.

impotence Failure to gain or maintain an erection, especially during sexual intercourse; also referred to as erectile dysfunction (DSM-IV). It is estimated that over 90% of men experience impotence at least once in their lives. It tends to manifest itself more often in older individuals or in those taking medications that have side-effects which interfere with AUTONOMIC arousal. Impotence can have both organic and psychological causes. Organic impotence is assumed when an individual complaining of erectile dysfunction does not manifest erections during sleep (called NOCTURNAL PENILE TUMESCENCE or NPT), whereas psychogenic impotence is assumed when NPT does occur in such individuals. Impotence is also classified into so-called 'primary' and 'secondary' erectile dysfunction. Primary erectile dysfunction is rare, and is diagnosed when an individual has never been able to achieve an erection sufficient for sexual intercourse. In contrast, secondary erectile dysfunction is diagnosed when an individual has had normal erectile capability in previous sexual relations.

Erectile capacity is rarely 'all-or-none'; loss of erection is usually a matter of degree and is often situational. For example, an individual may experience partial loss of rigidity before or during sexual activity. Some are capable of achieving erection during masturbation but not during sexual intercourse. Some are able to have erections sufficient for sexual intercourse with lovers, but not with their partners, whereas for others the opposite relation is true. More than half of the cases of erectile dysfunction are believed to be caused by disease, prescription medications, or drugs of abuse

(see DRUG ABUSE). Prominent causes of organic erectile dysfunction are DIABETES, ALCOHOLISM, certain neurological disorders such as MULTIPLE SCLEROSIS, and neurological damage from SPINAL CORD injury. Physical injury to the penis, testes, urethra or prostate can also cause impotence, as can low circulating levels of TESTOSTERONE in approximately one-third of hypogonadal men (who may also experience diminished sexual desire). Any drug that interferes with autonomic blood flow can induce organic impotence. Erectile dysfunction is a frequent complaint of men taking medication to treat high blood pressure, and can occur occasionally following other medications (such as ANTIHISTAMINES, pseudoephedrine, and CHOLINERGIC agonists. Short- or long-term use of a variety of illicit drugs, from psychomotor stimulants (such as AMPHETAMINE), to depressants (for example ALCOHOL and BARBITURATES), to sedatives / hypnotics (such as MARIJUANA), to narcotics (for example HEROIN), can interfere with peripheral blood flow, leading to transient or lasting difficulties in achieving or maintaining an erection. Smoking can also cause temporary erectile dysfunction in certain individuals, as it produces mild peripheral VASOCONSTRICTION.

Psychogenic erectile dysfunction can occur in response to a variety of problems that present in everyday life. Such erectile dysfunctions are often temporary, and can occur simply because the individual is tired, stressed or mildly depressed. However, if the momentary inability to gain or maintain an erection is taken too seriously, it can sensitize into an intense FEAR of sexual inadequacy. Such fears produce a kind of feedback inhibition that can sustain erectile and other sexual dysfunctions for a long time.

Treatment of erectile dysfunction has become a billion-dollar industry, and ranges from psychological therapy to pharmacological intervention to surgical implantation of prosthetic hydraulic devices that simulate erection. Psychological treatments are typically broad and attempt to address the many situational variables that may conspire to induce the dysfunction (such as STRESS, emotional and sexual intimacy, fear of inadequacy, drug use and so on). Such treatments are limited to individuals who experience psychogenic impotence, and have their best therapeutic outcome if the individual and his partner can work together. Therapy for organic impotence is just as complicated, and can range from a simple intervention (for example lowering the dosage of the medication with the side-effect) to a more long-term pharmacological treatment. Although pharmacological treatments vary, all have a final common effect of potentiating PARASYMPATHETIC blood flow to the corpora cavernosa, the spongy erectile tissue inside the PENIS. These treatments include oral administration of drugs that stimulate blood flow, such as the NORADRENERGIC antagonists YOHIMBINE and IDAZOXAN, or stimulators of NITRIC OXIDE production, such as nitroglycerine and SODIUM NITROPRUSSIDE. However, taken in high dosages, these drugs can induce PRIAPISM, or painfully distended erectile tissues, and can be dangerous in individuals with high blood pressure. However, some drugs like PROSTAGLANDIN E1 (an EICOSANOID), OXYTOCIN (see NEUROPEPTIDES), or PAPAVERINE (a peripherally active opiate alkaloid) stimulate erection locally following injection into the penis (acting as smooth muscle relaxants and stimulating vasodilation). Many drugs continue to be tested. For example, recent clinical trials with an orally-active stimulator of CYCLIC GMP (VIAGRA) have been promising. Viagra potentiates erection in individuals with organic dysfunction, but only when the individual receives erotic or somatosensory stimulation of the penis (that is, it does not induce priapism). Thus, it could be taken acutely before an anticipated sexual encounter.

See also: ejaculation; erection; sexual arousal

JAMES G. PFAUS

imprinting Learned attachment. Imprinting is particularly widespread in birds. Filial imprinting determines the preferred target for the following response of young birds. Sexual imprinting determines mate preference in birds. Filial imprinting can be reliably produced in the laboratory. Typically, young birds are dark-reared, then they are exposed to a conspicuous object. Several hours or days later, birds are given a preference test. The choice is between the object to which birds were exposed and a novel object. Young birds prefer to approach the object they have seen previously. In sexual imprinting experiments, young birds are cross-fostered with another species. Cross-fostered males exhibit a greater preference for females from the foster species than from their own species. The song of some cross-fostered males (for example, zebra finches) also resembles those of their foster-parent species (see BIRDSONG).

Much of the early research focused on the validity of the definition of imprinting proposed by Konrad Lorenz (1903–1989). Lorenz made four important claims concerning imprinting. (1) Imprinting was confined to a CRITICAL PERIOD early in development. During the critical period, a single exposure to a biologically relevant stimulus activated this process. (2) After the critical period, imprinting was resistant to reversal. (3) Imprinting influenced behaviours that may not be exhibited until later in life (such as SEXUAL BEHAVIOUR). (4) Imprinting differed from other forms of LEARNING such as PAVLOVIAN CONDITIONING and OPERANT CONDITIONING. Imprinting occurs in the absence of any external REINFORCEMENT, is resistant to EXTINCTION and there is a long delay between ACQUISITION and the exhibition of behaviour.

Empirical investigations have extended the original more narrow concept of imprinting proposed by Lorenz. Findings indicate that imprinting is not an all-or-nothing process. Rather, it is characterized by a more gradual diminishment of imprintablity. Hence, the term critical period has been replaced by SENSITIVE PERIOD. Similar to other forms of learning, amount of exposure and the nature of the stimuli used influence sexual imprinting. Under certain conditions, imprinting does appear to be reversible. In general, however, phase specificity and selectivity about the stimuli that are most potent in attaining stable results differentiates imprinting from other types of learning. Neurobiological research on imprinting in birds has shown that the IMHV (intermediate and medial part of the HYPERSTRIATUM VENTRALE) is involved. Damage to the IMHV prior to imprinting prevents the acquisition of preferences. Damage to the area after imprinting, renders the bird amnesic. Following imprinting, changes in POSTSYNAPTIC density and density of postsynaptic receptors are observed. There is a positive correlation between the number of RECEPTOR sites and the degree to which the bird prefers the familiar stimulus at testing. Increase in density could not be attributed to visual stimulation, AROUSAL or locomotor activity but only to how much the chick had learned. Electrophysiological recordings from the left IMHV have shown a positive correlation between neuronal activity and preference tests. Biochemical analysis of TESTOSTERONE levels have shown the influence of hormonal levels on stimulus-dependent effects on imprinting. IMHV is also involved in another type of learning, PASSIVE AVOIDANCE learning. In the passive avoidance task, young birds must learn to recognize the characteristics of particular coloured stimulus and to associate it with an aversive taste. Lesions to the IMHV inhibit successful avoidance learning. Both imprinting and the passive avoidance learning task may require the formation of a representation of a specific visual object. Individual stimulus recognition may then be the common characteristic that is critical for the involvement of the IMHV in both types of learning.

Further research has revealed other developmental processes besides filial and sexual imprinting in birds. These include the development of host preferences in parasitic species and the establishment of preference for food, habitat and locality. In addition, imprinting occurs in other animals besides birds. Imprinting to olfactory stimuli plays a crucial role in spawning MIGRATION of salmonoids such as the Pacific salmon. After hatching, juvenile fish mature in their natal fresh water streams. At about 18 months of age the fish undergo morphological changes called MOLTIFICATION that prepares them for life in salt water. At this time the fish also imprint to the olfactory bouquet of their natal streams. The hormone THYROXINE seems to be involved in both moltification and home stream odour imprinting. The salmon then swim downstream to the ocean where there live for 1–4 years before migrating back to their natal stream to spawn and die. During this return migration the salmon appear to swim up a concentration gradient of home steam odours. Imprinting may have an adaptive benefit for any organism characterized by rapid ontogenetic development and by early dispersal of young. The time course of the sensitive phase also appears to have a selective advantage. It is geared to the age requirement when information is needed for the first time and capitalizes on the opportunity to acquire that information under favourable learning conditions.

See also: ethology

DONALD M. WILKIE

impulsivity The result of a failure of response INHIBITION. Impulse control disorder is the DSM-IV term for any condition in humans in which individuals act on impulse; exhibitionism or compulsive gambling fall into this category. Impulsivity (impulsiveness) is also a feature of ATTENTION-DEFICIT DISORDER.

VERITY J. BROWN

in situ **hybridization** A technique for examining gene presence and activity in tissue. When a GENE is activated, MESSENGER RNA (mRNA) is produced, and sent to the CYTOPLASM for protein formation (see PROTEINS). *In situ* hybridization employs ANTISENSE OLIGONUCLEOTIDES as a probe for gene activity. These oligonucleotides have a sequence complementary to that of the mRNA under investigation and will hybridize with the mRNA. Thin sections of tissue are incubated with the antisense oligonucleotide: the amount of oligonucleotide hybridized to the mRNA in the sections is determined by techniques such as AUTORADIOGRAPHY, or IMMUNOHISTOCHEMISTRY. The presence of the hybridization product implies the activity of the gene.

See also: chemical neuroanatomy; histology

FIONA M. INGLIS

in utero Latin term meaning, literally, in the womb (that is, the UTERUS).

in vitro (from Latin, *vitrum*: glass) Literally, in glass; that is, in a test tube, beaker, dish or in fact anything other than in a living organism. The opposite is IN VIVO.

in vivo (from Latin, *vivus*: alive) Literally, in a live organism, as opposed to *in vitro*, in glass.

inadequate stimulus *see* adequate stimulus

inattention *see* extinction, definition 1

incentive A reason to perform an action. In selecting a RESPONSE, an organism performs a COST–BENEFIT ANALYSIS. Incentives are a critical part of this equation, as both positive incentives (REWARD) and negative incentives (avoidance of PUNISHMENT) represent the expected benefits. Hull's DRIVE REDUCTION theory of MOTIVATION holds that the incentive for all action is the elimination and avoidance of discomfort. Incentives may be tangible and external to the organism, as in the acquisition of food, a sexual partner or warmth, or they may be internal in the sense of interpretations of tangible events, as in the fulfilment of curiosity or feeling of safety.

See also: incentive motivation; reinforcement

VERITY J. BROWN

incentive motivation Incentive motivation is contrasted with PRIMARY MOTIVATION. DRIVE is often thought of as a force that produces behavioural change: it refers to the theoretical construct of a motivational state produced by biological, reproductive or psychological need. Food or water deprivation, for example, create drive states. MOTIVATION produced by a drive state is referred to as primary motivation; on the other hand, motivation produced by the presence of a STIMULUS (such as food or water) in the absence of primary motivation, is referred to as incentive motivation. Primary motivation and incentive motivation are not independent: they gate each other. The incentive motivational properties of stimuli depend in part on the state of primary motivation. In crude and simple terms, one will, if sufficiently food deprived, eat things that one would not in other circumstances wish to while, in contrast, if one is not food deprived, the incentive motivational properties of a food stimulus need to be relatively high in order to generate eating.

incertohypothalamic dopamine system *see* classification of Dahlström and Fuxe; dopamine

incidental learning Incidental learning is that which happens with neither INTENTION nor

MOTIVATION; in contrast intentional learning is that which occurs in a directed manner.

See also: latent learning; observation learning

incisor bar *see* stereotaxic surgery

inclusive fitness *see* sociobiology

incus *see* ossicles

indirect agonist *see* agonist

individual fitness *see* sociobiology

indoleamine Indoleamines are monoamines that are based on a five member ring including nitrogen, joined to a benzene ring. The most important member of this class of NEUROTRANSMITTERS is without doubt SEROTONIN (5-hydroxytryptamine). MELATONIN is another biologically significant indoleamine.

See also: catecholamine

inducible NOS *see* nitric oxide

induction (i) *Learning* theory: I.P. Pavlov (1849–1936) observed that presenting an inhibiting CONDITIONED STIMULUS immediately prior to a positive one increased the power of the second one: he called this positive induction. Negative induction is the reverse – the effect of a an excitatory stimulus before a negative one increases the effect of the negative one.
(ii) *Philosophy*: unlike deduction, the method of induction reasons from specific instances to general cases. Deduction has more power, but inductive reasoning is more common.

infant reflexes Newborn human infants show various types of STRETCH REFLEX, mainly used for controlling POSTURE and head movements. Vestibular reflexes and sensory reflexes develop after birth and reflexes important for the control of LOCOMOTION follow. These reflex movements gradually give way to controlled voluntary movements. The presence or absence of infant reflexes are important in gauging developmental progress.

See also: Moro reflex; rooting reflex

infant speech perception Speakers of all languages begin life with identical LANGUAGE processing systems, but attune to the PHONOLOGY of the environmental language during their first year. Early in that year infants discriminate many PHONETIC contrasts, but by mid-year they begin to acquire the relevant environmental phonological categories; at about 10 months they are, like adult listeners, inattentive to contrasts not used in the phonology of the environmental language. PERCEPTION OF SECOND LANGUAGES in later life is not helped by this efficient early specialization.

Reference

Goodman J.C. & and Nusbaum H.C. (eds.) (1994) *The Development of Speech Perception*, MIT Press: Cambridge MA.

ANNE CUTLER

infanticide *see* aggression

infantile amnesia There are at least two effects associated with infantile FORGETTING. First, memories of events that have occurred infancy are often either difficult or impossible to retrieve when tested in adulthood. Second, forgetting over intervals of a few seconds or minutes itself is much more rapid in infancy than it is later. The argument has been advanced that the mode and perhaps place of coding of memories changes with the dramatic changes in neuronal growth with MATURATION between the time LEARNING occurs in infancy and the time of testing. Hence, the original neural changes associated with those infantile memories are obscured and irretrievable. As for rapid forgetting, evidence is available that the NEONATE has not fully developed a neural substrate for one of the memory systems which is responsible for constructing a stable representation of event context.

See also: engram

RICHARD C. TEES

infarct (from Latin, *in*: in, *farctus*, from *farcire*: to fill, cram) An infarct (or infarction) is a section of tissue, isolated and dying following cessation of its blood supply.

inferior In an anatomical sense, the terms inferior and superior refer to above (superior) and below (inferior) – they are to do with relative position, rather than being judgements of quality. So for example, the SUPERIOR

COLLICULUS is placed above the INFERIOR COLLICULUS in the brain.

inferior cerebellar peduncle A large fibre tract carrying information from the INFERIOR OLIVE and SPINAL CORD to the CEREBELLUM; see HINDBRAIN.

inferior colliculus The inferior colliculus in the MIDBRAIN is receiving direct input from the IPSILATERAL dorsal division of the COCHLEAR NUCLEUS and from the CONTRALATERAL and ipsilateral nuclei of the LATERAL LEMNISCUS. It is a mandatory way station of the auditory pathway to the MEDIAL GENICULATE BODY. The central nucleus of the inferior colliculus is tonotopically organized (see TONOTOPIC REPRESENTATION) and specifies auditory spatial maps in the SUPERIOR COLLICULUS from BINAURAL information it receives from the BRAINSTEM. It likely provides temporal processing relevant for PITCH perception. The external nucleus of the inferior colliculus is the origin of the extra lemniscal pathway to the THALAMUS and CEREBRAL CORTEX.

See also: auditory perception

JOS J. EGGERMONT

inferior nasal concha *see* skull

inferior olivary complex The inferior olivary complex of the rat brain is divisible into three subnuclei, all with complex further subdivisions: the medial accessory olive (abbreviated IO), the dorsal accessory olivary nucleus (IOD) and the principal olive (IOPr). They receive SOMATOSENSORY input from the SPINAL CORD, TRIGEMINAL NUCLEUS and DORSAL COLUMN NUCLEI OF THE MEDULLA OBLONGATA and optic input from the SUPERIOR COLLICULUS. The output of the inferior olivary complex is directed via CLIMBING FIBRES to the CEREBELLUM. The inferior olivary complex has a role in cerebellar function, though it is not wholly clear what that role is. One suggestion is that it provides a pattern of rhythmic firing which serves as a timing mechanism for the co-ordination of actions.

inferior olive *see* inferior olivary complex

inferior parietal lobule The PARIETAL LOBE in PRIMATES is conventionally divided into two parts on the dorsolateral surface of the CERE-BRAL HEMISPHERES, the INFERIOR and SUPER-IOR PARIETAL LOBULES (IPL and SPL), separated by the deep INTRAPARIETAL SULCUS. There is controversy over whether this division is homologous in man and monkey. The anatomist Brodmann thought not (see BROD-MANN'S AREAS). He numbered the IPL as area 7 in the monkey, but placed area 7 right along-side area 5 in the SPL in the human brain. The IPL in humans he distinguished as areas 39 and 40, numbers he did not use in his parcelation of the monkey cortex.

A. DAVID MILNER

inferior temporal cortex It has been known since the work of Klüver & Bucy in the mid-1930s that the TEMPORAL LOBE of PRIMATES, and not just the OCCIPITAL LOBE at the back of the brain, is an important part of the VISUAL SYSTEM. Their experiments showed that bilat-eral damage to the temporal lobe caused visual AGNOSIA (among other things): specifically a failure to recognize food or food-associated shapes through the sense of vision. In the 1950s, the work of Mishkin narrowed down the critical region to the inferior part of the temporal lobe. Damage to this area (sometimes called AREA TE) reliably causes profound fail-ures to learn about and recognize objects visually. It also causes difficulties in distin-guishing colours, and in recognizing objects when seen in different orientations. We now know that neurons in the inferior temporal cortex (ITC) have highly complex visual prop-erties, responding only to specific shapes and colours, or even to the sight of particular static or moving body parts such as faces or arms, or whole bodies. Visual processing in ITC seems designed for the animal to recognize or cate-gorize objects irrespective of the particular viewpoint or illumination conditions of the moment. In general this will be the most useful way to store visual memories. Thus ITC may be considered the highest level of visual proces-sing in the brain, and anatomically it constitu-tes the endpoint of the VENTRAL STREAM. It is intimately associated with brain structures concerned with the formation and retrieval of MEMORY, including the HIPPOCAMPUS. We now know that there is a similar area in the human

brain, which has been discovered using FUNC-TIONAL NEUROIMAGING techniques. It is lo-cated on the underside of the brain, at the junction between the occipital and temporal lobes, apparently somewhat further back than in the monkey. It is the principal region where activity is found to increase when people are viewing real pictures of objects rather than scrambled pictures. In agreement with this, APPERCEPTIVE AGNOSIA results in humans from damage in the occipito-temporal region, pre-sumably damaging the human equivalent of ITC or disconnecting it from visual cortical input areas. The DISCONNECTION can be quite selective, affecting only colours or only objects, or even only places or faces. Or it can affect various combinations of these visual cate-gories. The human ITC is asymmetrically dis-posed in the brain, with the right cerebral hemisphere playing the greater role. Indeed some agnosic patients have brain damage restricted entirely to the right side of the brain.

See also: Klüver–Bucy syndrome; prosopag-nosia

A. DAVID MILNER

inferior temporal gyrus The TEMPORAL LOBE has three principal gyri (see GYRI AND SULCI) clearly visible on its outer surface: the inferior, middle and superior temporal gyri (the inferior being most ventral, the superior most dorsal); see FACE PERCEPTION.

inferotemporal cortex A term used synony-mously with INFERIOR TEMPORAL CORTEX (or AREA TE).

inflammation *see* immune system

information theory Information theory (or *communication theory*) is a subtle and abstract mathematical theory concerned with the trans-mission of information, first developed by Claude Shannon. He was concerned with information transmission in electronic engi-neering, with the emphasis firmly on the process of transmission itself, rather than analysis of the content of what was being transmitted. 'Information' here relates to the coding and discriminability of stimuli without consideration of the validity of the code in rela-tion to that which is being coded. Information theory lies behind the major expansion in communication capacity that occurred in the second half of the twentieth century: increased telephone communication, the internet (your modem – a device classified by how many kilobytes of information per second [kbps] it can process – is quintessentially a information theory device), information storage on CD-ROM are all examples of developments reliant on information theory. It is moreover a theory that has impacted on other disciplines. Philosophers became interested in it, less for its 'transmission' features than for its use in developing an understanding of how arbitrary stimuli (the 'bits' of information) gain meaning. Linguists have an interest in it, since information theory demonstrates that many elements of LANGUAGE are actually unnecessary for the communication of meaning. So for example 'mny lmnts of lang r actlly unncsry for communtn of meang' is an intelligible signal: it omits predictable elements, the resolution of uncertainty being the essential problem in communication.

In biological psychology, information theory has had an impact on the way in which theorists approach the BRAIN. Information theorists worked with model systems that typically included an information source; a mechanism for transmitting information; a communicable signal (which would interact with noise emanating from other sources); a received signal (a product of the transmitted signal and noise); a receiver and a decoder. Shannon described this as a *source – encoder – channel – decoder – destination* model though such systems are essentially three-step processes: source coding, channel transmission and destination decoding. Clearly, brains are devices that receive information which is derived from a source, comes through various channels and which requires decoding. Information theory provides mathematical tools with which to analyse neural activity, in order to understand how information is processed and represented in brain.

See also: artificial intelligence; entropy; neural networks

References

Presentation made by Lucent Technologies

(Bell Labs Innovations) *50 years of Information Theory* at http://www.lucent.com/informationtheory/.

Shannon C.E. (1948) A mathematical theory of communication. *Bell System Technical Journal* 27: 379–423 and 623–656.

infradian rhythm A biological rhythm with a period more than 24 hours (the prefix infra-indicating a low frequency).

See also: biological clock; circannual rhythm; overt rhythm

infralimbic cortex An area of FRONTAL CORTEX of the RAT, located on the medial wall. In the STEREOTAXIC ATLAS of Paxinos & Watson infralimbic cortex is found on coronal sections between 3.2 mm to 2.2 mm anterior to BREGMA, located ventral to PRELIMBIC CORTEX. There is some disagreement whether infralimbic cortex is to be regarded as part of rat PREFRONTAL CORTEX. Thalamic input is from the extreme medial portion of the DORSOMEDIAL NUCLEUS OF THE THALAMUS, with the main thalamic input from the PARAVENTRICULAR NUCLEUS OF THE THALAMUS. Furthermore, infralimbic cortex is thinner, with a less distinct laminar structure, than other areas of putative rodent prefrontal cortex. On the other hand, infralimbic cortex, in common with prelimbic cortex, does have DOPAMINERGIC input from the MIDBRAIN. There is also no consensus on the function of infralimbic cortex of the rat. This is due to several factors, including the difficulty of making selective a LESION and the paucity of sensitive behavioural tasks by which areas of frontal cortex can be functionally dissociated.

Reference

Paxinos G. & Watson C. (1997) *The Rat Brain in Stereotaxic Coordinates*, compact 3rd edn, Academic Press: San Diego CA.

VERITY J. BROWN

infraorbital (from Latin, *infra*: below) Infra is a prefix meaning below: infraorbital refers to tissue below the ORBITS OF THE EYE.

infundibulum Also known as the PITUITARY STALK; see ADENOHYPOPHYSIS; PITUITARY GLAND.

infusion An INFUSION involves delivering fluid to a particular site; PERFUSION involves bathing an area, typically delivering and recovering fluid. Either term can refer to the delivery of fluid into a receptacle or into an organism. For example, injections (see DRUG ADMINISTRATION) are typically infusions, whereas drug delivery by MICRODIALYSIS or PUSH–PULL PERFUSION involves perfusion. In addition the term perfusion is used colloquially to mean TRANSCARDIAL PERFUSION.

inhibin One of the HORMONES secreted from the OVARY and TESTES.

See also: endocrine glands; hormones; hormones – classification

inhibition (i) *Neurophysiology*: see EXCITATION. (ii) *Behaviour*: see BEHAVIOURAL INHIBITION; BEHAVIOURAL INHIBITION SYSTEM; COGNITIVE INHIBITION; RESPONSE COMPETITION; SUPERVISORY ATTENTIONAL SYSTEM.

inhibition of delay Classical CONDITIONING typically involves pairing an UNCONDITIONED STIMULUS (US – for example, the delivery of sucrose solution) with a CONDITIONED STIMULUS (CS – for example, the presentation of a light). The term inhibition of delay refers to the prevention of responding in the period preceding presentation of the unconditioned stimulus. During CONDITIONING, shorter delays are typically used at first, though these can be lengthened as conditioning proceeds.

inhibitory amino acids *see* amino acid neurotransmitters

inhibitory postsynaptic potential (IPSP) A HYPERPOLARIZATION of a NEURON evoked by input at a SYNAPSE by an inhibitory neurotransmitter. IPSPs are local potentials that decay with distance and can summate with other IPSPs and ESPSs (EXCITATORY POSTSYNAPTIC POTENTIAL) that are occurring in the same cell. They have a slow time course (tens or hundreds of milliseconds) and therefore show TEMPORAL SUMMATION when repeated inputs occur at the same synapse. They are called inhibitory because they move the membrane potential away from the neuron's

THRESHOLD, making it less likely for the neuron to produce an ACTION POTENTIAL.

DOUGLAS D. RASMUSSON

inner hair cells *see* hair cells

innervate To INNERVATE means to send an AXON to and make contact with; innervation describes this. So for example, one can say that the SUBSTANTIA NIGRA innervates the CAUDATE–PUTAMEN. RE-INNERVATION describes the regrowth of axons into an area following some form of damage or LESION.

innervation ratio This is concerned with MOTOR UNITS. The ratio of the axons of MOTOR NEURONS to MUSCLE FIBRES: a low ratio indicates a dense innervation and is characteristic of the innervation of muscles involved in fine motor control.

inositol A molecule that is the basic component of many LIPIDS found in many types of neuronal and non-neuronal MEMBRANE. Inositol lipids are the molecular backbone of phosphoinositide-derived SECOND MESSENGERS, which play a key role in intracellular signalling (transforming external signals into specific cellular events). In this pathway, inositol is transformed into phosphotidylinositol (PI), and subsequently into other polyphosphoinositides such as phosphatidylinositol-4-monphosphate (PIP) and phosphatidylinositol 4,5-biphosphate (PIP2). Two breakdown products of PIP2, inositol 1,4,5-triphosphate (IP3) and diacylglycerol (DAG). IP3 and DAG stimulate the activity of intracellular CALCIUM and PROTEIN KINASE C (PKC), respectively.

ANN E. KELLEY

inositol triphosphate *see* second messengers

insertional plaque *see* tip links

insomnia Difficulty with the initiation and maintenance of SLEEP is so common a problem as to be considered normal when it is situational, short-lived, and followed by refreshing compensatory sleep. From an evolutionary point of view, it is clear that adaptation to such environmental uncertainties as temperature fluctuation and the threat of predation often require the temporary postponement of sleep. In modern life the social equivalents of such environmental uncertainties are the ANXI-ETY and STRESS of urban life both of which cause AROUSAL which counteracts sleep.

When stress and anxiety become chronic, sleep may become so disrupted as to constitute a functionally significant disability, warranting symptomatic treatment by psychotherapy, behavioural manipulation (see COGNITIVE–BEHAVIOURAL THERAPY) or medication with SEDATIVES. But before any of these treatments is instituted, a thorough medical investigation, including special inquiry about specific sleep disorders, should be undertaken. This is because almost any medical or psychiatric disease may present with, or be complicated by, nonspecific insomnia and these underlying specific conditions must be recognized and treated first. In the case of such specific sleep disorders as sleep APNOEA which can present as the excessive daytime sleep that insomniacs may complain of, treatment with sedatives is actually contraindicated because it may be harmful. And when insomnia is symptomatic, treatment of the underlying cause relieves the symptoms without recourse to sedatives.

Most normal individuals are able to fall asleep within 5–10 minutes with occasional increases in sleep latency to 30 minutes. Depending on the subject's age, sleep is then maintained for 6–8 hours with one to three brief interruptions. In evaluating deviations from these norms, it should be recognized that (1) sleep, like all other biological variables, is extremely variable in that normal people may need as few as 4 or as many as 10 hours of sleep to feel rested; (2) that insomniacs often grossly exaggerate their sleeplessness (see PSEUD-INSOMNIA); and (3) that the dynamic response to sleep deprivation protects the insomniac from harm due to sleep loss itself. Chronically anxious individuals typically complain of difficulty falling asleep while depressed subjects more typically go to sleep promptly only to awaken early in the morning (see DEPRESSION). For anxiety insomnia the treatment of choice is relaxation and sleep hygiene training and this naturalistic approach should be vigorously pursued before turning to sedative medication. There is, as yet, no physiological sedative and all of the available medications incur some risk with the frequently prescribed BENZODIAZE-

PINES being particularly problematic. If the insomnia is due to a major affective disorder the medications of choice are the TRICYCLIC ANTIDEPRESSANTS or amine reuptake blockers rather than sedatives. Understanding insomnia in anxiety and depression is helped by recognizing the dynamics of sleep–wake neurophysiology. Waking is mediated by the AMINERGIC modulatory systems of the subcortical brain which energize the THALAMUS and CEREBRAL CORTEX. These systems are brought further into play by the anxiety and stress of real and imagined threats to an individual's security. When so exaggerated, the aminergic systems oppose the CHOLINERGIC modulation of sleep and thus impair both deep NON-REM SLEEP and REM SLEEP preventing the profound physical and psychic restoration conferred by those sleep phases. The result is an unhealthy interaction which traps the patient in an endless cycle of anxious days and restless nights until the process can be reversed by the interventions discussed below.

Because of the discrepancy between the subjective experience and objective signs of insomnia and because of the difficulty managing such cases, the evaluation of a patient's complaint should begin with an alliance-building inquiry into the patient's lifestyle. This investigative process is abetted by scrupulous sleep charting with notation of other significant behaviours such as the time of getting up in the mornings, daily activity and exercise, exercise, food, and DRUG intake. Bed partners or family member collaborators are particularly helpful allies, and should be recruited early in the evaluation period. They are in an ideal position to inform the clinician about the objective signs of sleep disorder, to assure compliance with diagnostic or treatment programs, and to evaluate the efficacy of interventions. Sleep laboratory studies have their place in the ruling out of specific sleep disorders and in reassuring the patient that his symptom, while upsetting, is not indicative of organic disease but the sleep laboratory is not an end in itself and is no substitute for a sound behavioural approach. The strongest antidotes to insomnia are a positive mental attitude and a vigorous physical activity pattern, two attributes that are notoriously difficult to inculcate in chronically anxious insomniac people. Before prescribing drugs it is also critical to restrict the intake of CAFFEINE, a potent opponent of sleep that is often taken in excess by anxious insomniacs to counteract sleepiness and improve mood. NICOTINE, taken via cigarette smoking, is another problematic stimulant chemical which is easily available and difficult to withdraw from anxious subjects especially if they have become functionally disabled. Finally, ALCOHOL must not be used as a sedative because of its propensity to interrupt sleep later in the night when the ALDEHYDE products of its hepatic degradation are produced after sleep onset. Recent evidence indicates that chronic insomnia is best treated by behavioural means. When carefully screened subjects are seen in groups led by therapists well-versed in sleep hygiene and relaxation response training techniques, significant improvement in symptoms can be obtained in 95% of the patients within eight weeks.

J. ALLAN HOBSON

instinct Instinct can be conceptualized as a form of behaviour that is innate, elicited by internal or external stimuli – responses triggered by what early ethnologists called sign stimuli. For example, during breeding male three-spined sticklebacks have red bellies. A red stimulus, however crudely related to the shape of the fish, will elicit AGGRESSION in other males. Such sign stimuli were hypothesized to trigger *innate releasing mechanisms* to generate action. Instinct is however a difficult concept. Some activities certainly appear to be pre-programmed (SUCKLING for example) but it is also clear that neonatal organisms are capable of LEARNING: IMPRINTING for example occurs very rapidly after birth. The extent to which complex activities are truly instinctive as opposed to learned is difficult to determine.

See also: critical period; sensitive period

instrumental choice avoidance Performance of one particular instrumental response rather than another in order to avoid presentation, or cause termination, of an aversive event such as mild FOOTSHOCK.

See also: active avoidance; animal models of anxiety; aversive conditioning; passive avoidance

A. SIMON KILLCROSS

instrumental conditioning Those learning processes where an action or response emitted from an organism's behavioural repertoire becomes associated with a specific outcome that leads, in turn, to a change in the rate of production of the action or response that elicited the outcome. Where the frequency, or the probability, of an action is increased, the outcome is deemed a positive reinforcer (see POSITIVE REINFORCEMENT). That is, there is a positive CONTINGENCY between a behavioural response (see OPERANT) and an appetitive-reinforcing stimulus (see APPETITIVE REINFORCEMENT). Where the frequency, or the probability, of an action is decreased, the outcome is deemed a negative reinforcer (see NEGATIVE REINFORCEMENT). That is, there is a negative contingency between a behavioural response and an appetitive–reinforcing stimulus. A special category of negative reinforcer is that of PUNISHMENT, where outcomes are considered to have unpleasant consequences and lead to avoidance. That is, there is a positive contingency between a behavioural response and an aversive (or punishing) reinforcing stimulus (see AVERSIVE CONDITIONING). Whereas stimulus organizations that lead to CLASSICAL CONDITIONING or PAVLOVIAN CONDITIONING occur independent of an organism's actions, instrumental conditioning processes are entirely reliant upon an organism's actions leading to environmental change. As a general rule, the behavioural effects of instrumental conditioning increase in magnitude with increases in the quantity and quality of the reinforcer. Rapidity of acquisition of instrumental conditioning is also influenced by the temporal CONTIGUITY of the action and outcome and also by the action–outcome contingency. That is, instrumental conditioning is most favoured where the action immediately precedes the outcome and where each action leads to the outcome. The capacity for instrumental learning has been shaped by evolutionary processes to permit the prediction of events and causal relationships in the environment. Such learning is crucial for the development of optimal adaptation to the environment and to maximise reproductive resources. Instrumental conditioning can be supported by a broad range of SCHEDULES OF REINFORCEMENT . These schedules dictate how an action-outcome association is learned and maintained. They also dictate how rapidly learning can be reversed (see EXTINCTION). Where a lack of control over the delivery of reinforcement is imposed in an experiment (a loss of action-outcome contingency), the behavioural consequences have been termed LEARNED HELPLESSNESS, a putative model of DEPRESSION.

See also: differential reinforcement of low rates; habits; partial reinforcement; stimulus–reinforcer association; unconditioned behaviour; yoked control

KEITH MATTHEWS

insula cortex The insula cortex lies deep in the floor of the LATERAL SULCUS, being surrounded by a circular sulcus and hidden from view on the lateral aspect of the HEMISPHERE because it is overlapped by the growth of adjacent neocortical areas of the FRONTAL, PARIETAL and TEMPORAL LOBES (the so-called 'OPERCULA OF THE INSULA' – see OPERCULAR CORTEX). Functionally, the rostral insula and adjoining opercular part of the inferior frontal gyrus represent the CORTICAL TASTE AREA and receives its input from the ventral posteromedial nucleus of the THALAMUS.

See also: gustation; neocortex

BARRY J. EVERITT

insulin A hormone secreted by the PANCREATIC BETA CELLS within the ISLETS OF LANGERHANS in the PANCREAS. A polypeptide (see PROTEINS) with an approximate molecular weight of 35 000, this hormone is essential for the uptake of GLUCOSE into all cells and for regulating normal blood sugar (glucose) levels. Insulin release is stimulated by the ingestion of CARBOHYDRATE and FAT, in order to aid in the metabolism of the substances. In diabetics, no insulin is produced or there is insulin resistance, and thus blood sugar levels and metabolism must be controlled with injected insulin or blood-sugar-lowering drugs, depending on the type of DIABETES. There are also insulin receptors in the brain, which in addition to

regulating glucose uptake may play a role in long-term metabolic signalling.

See also: feeding; hunger; satiety

ANN E. KELLEY

insulin-like growth factor *see* insulin receptors

insulin receptors Insulin is released from the PANCREAS and circulates in the BLOOD stream: many cells in many organs posses receptors for it. Insulin appears to cross the BLOOD–BRAIN BARRIER only with difficulty, but there are nevertheless receptors for it within the CENTRAL NERVOUS SYSTEM. These are part of a family of receptors that bind insulin and INSULIN-LIKE GROWTH FACTORS I and II (IGF-I and IGF-II). These receptors are unevenly distributed in brain, being most heavily concentrated in the CEREBRAL CORTEX, CEREBELLUM and HIPPOCAMPUS, with binding present also in other areas, including OLFACTORY BULB and HYPOTHALAMUS. Activity at these receptors have been associated with changed metabolic activity and growth. In CELL CULTURES, insulin and the insulin-like growth factors promote NEURITE growth and cell survival. They also act on GLIAL CELLS: the insulin-like growth factors can promote MYELIN formation by OLIGODENDROGLIA and GLUCOSE utilization in ASTROCYTES. In the past there has been speculation that circulating insulin, acting on the brain, might be important in BODY WEIGHT regulation. Whether circulating insulin provides a key signal for body weight or FEEDING regulation remains unclear.

integrative agnosia This subcategory of VISUAL AGNOSIA falls between the ASSOCIATIVE AGNOSIA and APPERCEPTIVE AGNOSIA, and can be characterized as an intact ability visually to perceive object *parts* but an impairment in the ability to integrate those parts into *whole* objects. Patients with integrative agnosia have usually sustained a (BILATERAL) LESION of the occipital cortex. To illustrate, patient M.H. with integrative agnosia (see Ogden, 1993), can copy complex line drawings accurately but has no idea what he is copying (see COPYING AND DRAWING). When shown an object he cannot recognize it but can describe it element by element: that is, when shown a key M.H.

described it as 'a circle; there is a long thin piece off one side; it is smooth on the top but seems to have a jagged edge on the bottom'. He attempts to guess (usually incorrectly) what the object is from his own description, but on picking up the key, he recognizes it instantly. His good ability to visually perceive simple elements is demonstrated by his accuracy in picking out triangles with curved lines from triangles with straight lines, and discriminating circles, squares, rectangles and other shapes. Patients with integrative agnosia also suffer from PROSOPAGNOSIA (the inability to recognize familiar faces) or ALEXIA (the inability to read). One hypothesis is that patients with integrative agnosia will also suffer prosopagnosia when the right occipital lesion is more extensive than the left, because their underlying problem is an impairment in the representation of complex parts (and a face is composed of complex parts). If the occipital lesion on the left is larger than that on the right, the patient will have alexia along with the agnosia because the underlying impairment is to the representation of numerous parts (and a word is composed of numerous parts or letters). Patients who suffer either prosopagnosia or alexia but do not have visual agnosia are considered to have milder impairments of the appropriate underlying representational system. That is, visual agnosia is a more severe impairment than either alexia or prosopagnosia. Published cases of visual agnosics support this in that they also suffer from alexia and/or prosopagnosia. There are, however. many cases of patients who have alexia or prosopagnosia without visual agnosia.

Reference

Ogden J.A. (1993) Visual object agnosia, prosopagnosia, achromatopsia, loss of visual imagery, and autobiographical amnesia following recovery from cortical blindness: Case M.H. *Neuropsychologia* 31: 571–589.

JENNI A. OGDEN

integrin *see* neural adhesion molecules

intellectual impairment *see* mental retardation

intelligence Cognitive ability. The fundamental attribute underlying alternative definitions is cognitive or information-processing ability in general or thinking ability in particular. Intelligence is the most thoroughly researched of the individual differences that have been identified by psychologists, and a survey of researchers has revealed a high degree of consensus that its major components are verbal intelligence, problem-solving ability, and practical intelligence.

Intelligence cannot be observed directly but can be inferred from observable behaviour. A person's intelligence is usually expressed as an IQ (intelligence quotient) score. Techniques of INTELLIGENCE TESTING include standardization of IQ tests to ensure that the average IQ score for all age groups is 100, although cognitive ability increases from early childhood up to about 18 years of age. Cross-sectional studies have shown that, on average, people in their 30s achieve significantly lower IQ scores than people in their 20s, and that every older age group achieves a lower average score than the immediately younger group, but this is not due entirely or even mainly to age-related decline in intelligence. Although individual performance on IQ tests does tend to decline slightly from about 60 years of age, especially on test items requiring perceptual or motor speed, the gross differences between age groups from 20 years of age onwards are due mainly to a cohort effect. Each successive generation achieves a higher average IQ score than its predecessor, resulting in an average increase of approximately 3 points per decade. This phenomenon, called the FLYNN EFFECT after the New Zealand psychologist James Flynn who first drew attention to it in 1984, has been occurring since intelligence tests were first introduced. It has been found in the United States, the United Kingdom, Belgium, Canada, France, New Zealand, the Netherlands, Norway and Japan, and although the effect is large and well documented, its cause remains obscure.

Controversy has raged throughout the history of psychology over the relative contributions of heredity and environment to intelligence. The HERITABILITY of intelligence has been estimated by three main methods. First, TWIN STUDIES have focused on MONOZYGOTIC TWINS separated soon after birth and raised in separate homes. Because they share all their genes in common, differences between their IQs are attributable entirely to environmental factors and, provided that their separate home environments are no more similar than chance, any correlations between their IQs must be due to genetic factors. Although several independent twin studies have been published, they provide inconclusive evidence regarding the heritability of intelligence, largely because only one study claimed to have established that the twins were raised in truly uncorrelated environments, and that study, by Sir Cyril Burt (1883–1971), is now known to be untrustworthy and almost certainly fraudulent. Second, kinship studies have compared correlations between the IQs of people of varying degrees of genetic relatedness and have generally yielded estimates of heritability between 30% and 60%, but the mathematical models used to derive these estimates require a number of controversial assumptions. Third, adoption studies have focused on the correlations between the IQs of children raised in adoptive homes and the IQs of their natural parents or their adoptive parents or siblings, but these studies have been vitiated by methodological problems and have yielded mutually contradictory heritability estimates.

Race differences in intelligence have been hotly debated for over a century by psychologists and lay people. The point at issue is the interpretation of data on racial differences in IQ scores, such as evidence showing that, on average, black Americans score about 15 points below white Americans on IQ tests, and that people of West Indian descent in Britain score between 5 and 13 points below indigenous white people. During the late 1960s and early 1970s, evidence regarding the heritability of intelligence was deployed in support of the argument that these differences are probably due mainly to genetic differences between the black and white races, but it was later shown that an average difference between groups can be entirely due to environmental factors even if the heritability within each group is 100%, and consequently heritability values, which in any event are not clearly established, are largely irrelevant. Racial admixture studies have capitalized on the fact that black Americans have varying amounts of white ancestry, and correlations between percentage of white ancestry and IQ have turned out to be close to zero, suggesting that race differences are not genetic in origin. In racial crossing studies, IQs have been examined in black, white and mixed-race children all living together in the same residential homes, or in the same white adoptive families, or in other unusual circumstances ensuring broadly similar environments, and under these conditions race differences in intelligence have tended to disappear, suggesting once again that they are due mainly or entirely to environmental rather than genetic factors.

ANDREW M. COLMAN

intelligence quotient (IQ) *see* intelligence testing

intelligence testing The construction and use of instruments for measuring INTELLIGENCE. The first attempt to measure intelligence scientifically was made by Francis Galton (1822–1911) in 1884 using tests of sensory discrimination and reaction time, but the tests turned out not to correlate with one another or with measures of scholastic performance. In 1905 Alfred Binet (1857–1911) and Théodore Simon (1873–1961) devised a test to detect and classify mentally retarded children in France. It was translated and introduced into the United States in 1916 as the STANFORD-BINET SCALE, which became the prototype of most subsequent tests of intelligence and the foundation of modern intelligence testing.

The Binet–Simon scale was designed to measure children's ability to follow instructions, exercise judgement, and solve reasoning problems. Relying on the fact that cognitive ability generally increases as children grow older, Binet & Simon selected 54 items according to how well they discriminated in practice between children of different ages. This led to the establishment of test norms and the introduction of the concept of mental age. For example, if a child passed just those items that average 6-year-olds in the standardization sample could pass, the child was said to be functioning at a mental age of 6 years. The German psychologist William Stern (1871–1938) pointed out in 1912 that MENTAL AGE (MA) indicates intelligence only in relation to actual or CHRONOLOGICAL AGE (CA), and he introduced the concept of the INTELLIGENCE QUOTIENT, which he defined as the ratio MA/CA. The American psychologist Lewis Terman (1877–1956) later introduced the abbreviation IQ (intelligence quotient) and suggested multiplying Stern's ratio by 100 to convert it to a percentage, yielding the familiar formula IQ = MA/CA × 100, according to which an IQ of 100 is average by definition.

Although Terman's formula continues to appear in elementary textbooks, it is no longer used in psychometric practice. It was first abandoned by the American psychometrician David Wechsler (1896–1981) in 1939, largely because it leads to absurdities when applied to adults. Cognitive ability stops increasing around 18 years of age, yet a 40-year-old who performs at the level of an average 20-year-old could be said to have an IQ of 20/40 × 100 = 50, suggestive of severe mental retardation. To avoid the problems of the old formula, Wechsler introduced a purely statistical definition of IQ according to which IQ is a normally distributed variable with a mean or average of 100 and a standard deviation (a statistical measure of variability) of 15, and test scores are converted to this scale. Because of the known properties of the normal distribution, this means that 68% of IQ scores fall between 85 and 115, 95% between 70 and 130, and so on. This statistical definition of IQ has been generally adopted by test constructors since World War II.

A revised form of the Stanford–Binet scale is still used by researchers and educational psychologists. There are three different Wechsler scales for use with different age groups: the WECHSLER ADULT INTELLIGENCE SCALE (WAIS), the Wechsler Intelligence Scale for Children, and the Wechsler Pre-school and Primary Scale of Intelligence. Each of these scales has to be administered individually by a trained tester, and each yields separate scores for verbal IQ, performance IQ, and full-scale IQ. The British Ability Scales, first published in 1979, are a set of 23 tests designed to measure a wide diversity of mental abilities, yielding separate scores for visual IQ, verbal IQ and general IQ. RAVEN'S PROGRESSIVE MATRICES, first published in 1938 and revised several times since then, is a non-verbal test designed to measure abstract reasoning ability through the use of geometric diagrams. There are many other intelligence tests in common use, including various multiple-choice tests that can be administered to large groups of respondents at the same time. Interest has been growing since the late 1980s in biological measures of intelligence based on EVENT-RELATED POTENTIALS and in processing speed as a possible basis for intelligence, as first suggested by Galton.

Scores on different IQ tests correlate highly with one another, partly because a new test is not considered valid unless it correlates with existing tests. The most impressive finding to emerge from decades of research into intelligence is that different tests and subtests correlate with one another no matter how different they are in content. Most contemporary psychologists interpret this fact as evidence for a single common factor, which was labelled g (for general intelligence) by the British psychologist Charles Spearman (1863–1945) in 1927. A rival interpretation, first suggested by the American psychologist Louis Leon Thurstone (1887–1955) in 1938, focuses on the fact that the correlations are not perfect and that certain types of test items usually correlate more highly with one another than with other types. Thurstone believed that these clusters indicate the existence of seven independent primary mental abilities, which he labelled number, word fluency, verbal meaning, memory, reasoning, spatial perception, and perceptual speed.

ANDREW M. COLMAN

intention In everyday language, intention means to have a conscious aim, purpose or design to one's actions. There is clearly a good deal of philosophical (and indeed legal) debate over the term intention and its relationship to concepts such as free will. Philosophers have identified acting with intention as including the action; desires and beliefs appropriate to that action; and a relation between the action and the belief that in some sense is explanatory. *Walking to Fisher and Donaldson's to buy a pastry* is an example of this: there is action (walking), there is belief (that Fisher and Donaldson's sells pastries) and the belief explains the action. The concept of INTENTION-

ALITY is also important in a philosophical sense, over and above its everyday use. Intentionality is used to describe properties of certain mental states in which reference is made to something else. It is identifiable by a quality of 'aboutness'. The mental states of *hope* or *desire* for example have a quality of aboutness – one hopes for things, one desires things.

In biological psychology the term intention is fraught with difficulty when applied to the behaviour of animals. There is transparently a sense in which the behaviour of animals has intention, in so far as it has *purpose*: animals emit actions which will produce predictable outcomes. It is also clear that appropriate actions can be produced in a given situation, indicating that a *selection process* has occurred. But whether one can infer from *purpose* and *selection* that an animal has a mental state in which intention is represented is very far from clear. In some ways the debate about this can be characterized as one between *cognitive* types of explanation, in which mental states are used to explain behaviour (see COGNITIVE PSYCHOLOGY, and behaviourist explanations (see BEHAVIOURISM) in which the mechanisms of learning are thought sufficient to explain the actions, without recourse to (unknowable and hypothetical) mental states in animals (or, indeed, for strict behaviourists, humans). Others have adopted what has become known as an INTENTIONAL STANCE in which mentalistic explanations are used but, as it were, without prejudice: they are used in effect as shorthand because they provide explanations that are manageable, when other types of explanation would not be. This hardly seems satisfactory, but as long as the mental states of animals remain unclear to human observers, questions about intention in animals are not likely to be resolved.

See also: executive functions; consciousness; mentalism; supervisory attentional system

intention tremor *see* tremor

intentional learning *see* incidental learning

intentional stance *see* intention

intentionality *see* intention

inter-ictal syndrome *see* Dostoeyevskian epilepsy

interaural line *see* stereotaxic surgery

intercalated discs *see* muscles

interference The reduction in performance that occurs when a critical task-relevant process or REPRESENTATION is disrupted or displaced by another of a similar type. Interference can also refer to the underlying processes responsible for this disruption or displacement. Interference between processes can occur when tasks compete for processing resources that are too limited to support both tasks simultaneously (see ATTENTION). The degree of interference between tasks can be used as a technique for determining whether these tasks involve similar processes (as in, for example, the selective interference paradigm). Interference between representations is a major determinant of FORGETTING in both SHORT-TERM MEMORY (see also WORKING MEMORY) and LONG-TERM MEMORY. The degree of interference between representations is determined by similarity. Items that are conceptually or perceptually similar (though not identical) are more likely to interfere with each other than items that are dissimilar. Three subtypes of interference in memory are RETROACTIVE INTERFERENCE, or forgetting resulting from activities occurring after information is learned (but before retention is tested); PROACTIVE INTERFERENCE, or forgetting of information resulting from activities occurring before LEARNING; and REPRODUCTIVE INTERFERENCE, which is the term given to the inability to reproduce previously learned material caused by learning other material.

In long-term memory, the likelihood that interference will occur in a retroactive or proactive direction is largely determined by the relative strengths of the competing memory traces (see ENGRAM). For example, after one has moved to a new residence, memory for the phone number of one's previous residence can interfere with memory for the new phone number (proactive interference). Once the new phone number is well learned, however, it can interfere with the ability to remember the phone number from the previous residence (retroactive interference). Damage to the PRE-

FRONTAL CORTEX renders an individual more susceptible to interference on many tasks. Any LESION in the FRONTAL LOBE can lead to increased distractibility, susceptibility to proactive interference, and PERSEVERATION to previously rewarded responses, as on a DELAYED ALTERNATION task or WISCONSIN CARD-SORT TEST. The increased susceptibility to interference of patients with frontal-lobe lesions has been interpreted as an impairment in inhibiting information that is not (or no longer) task-relevant (see Dempster [1992] for a developmental perspective on the role of the frontal lobes in inhibitory control).

See also: cross-modal conflict; delayed matching to sample; delayed response; dorsolateral pre-frontal cortex; inhibition; latent inhibition

References

Dempster F.N. (1992) The rise and fall of the inhibitory mechanism: toward a unified theory of cognitive development and aging. Developmental Review 12: 45–75.

JENNIFER A. MANGELS

interferon see cytokine; immune system

intergeniculate leaflet see geniculo-hypothalamic system; massa intermedia; suprachiasmatic nucleus;

interhemispheric fibre pathways see anterior commissure; commissure; corpus callosum; interhemispheric transfer; massa intermedia

interhemispheric fissure see longitudinal fissure

interhemispheric transfer Literally the transfer of information from one CEREBRAL HEMISPHERE to the other, via INTERHEMISPHERIC FIBRE PATHWAYS (the cerebral COMMISSURES). It is possible to present information to one hemisphere only and then determine whether the other hemisphere has access to it.

See also: corpus callosum; lateralization; split brain; Wada test

interleukin see cytokine; immune system

intermediate acoustic stria see cochlear nucleus

intermediate lobe of the pituitary see adenohypophysis

intermediate reticular nucleus see medullary reticular formation

intermediate-term memory Intermediate-term memory refers to the ability to recall items minutes to days after initial exposure. It is the time period of recall between the few seconds of remembrance mediated by IMMEDIATE MEMORY, and the permanent storage of LONG-TERM MEMORY. Items in intermediate-term memory are still being consolidated (see CONSOLIDATION) although they are not subject to as much INTERFERENCE as immediate memories are. Animal research has suggested that PROTEIN KINASE activity may be very important for memory storage processes during the intermediate-term memory time frame.

intermediate zone see cortical development

See also: short-term memory; working memory

HOWARD EICHENBAUM

intermittent explosive disorder The DSM-IV characterizes intermittent explosive disorder as involving episodes of uncontrolled AGGRESSION directed against persons or property. It is relatively poorly characterized and has been associated with other conditions, from BIPOLAR DISORDER through ANXIETY to specific cases of organic brain damage – it has been observed following removal of a TUMOUR from the CENTRAL NERVOUS SYSTEM. It has been treated with a variety of drugs including CARBAMAZEPINE and SELECTIVE SEROTONIN REUPTAKE INHIBITORS.

intermittent schedule see schedules of reinforcement

internal capsule see external capsule

internal carotid artery see blood

internal genitalia In females, the internal genitalia are the OVARIES, oviducts, UTERUS, cervix and (possibly) the upper VAGINA; and for males, the epididymis, vas deferens and seminal vesicles are the internal genitalia.

See also: gonads; Müllerian internal genitalia; sexual differentiation

internal segment of the globus pallidus see globus pallidus

internality Degree of influence from internal (under the skin) cues to initiate, maintain or terminate behaviour such as eating; the polar opposite to EXTERNALITY. In relation to ingestion, internal cues might include dry mouth, gastric contractions (stomach rumbling or emptiness), dizziness, weakness linked to low blood sugar. Internality is not measured directly but rather inferred from various subjective and objective measures. Measures of INTEROCEPTIVE awareness on the Eating Disorders Inventory (Garner *et al.*, 1983) indicate to what extent individuals accurately identify and respond to emotional states, HUNGER and SATIETY cues.

Reference

Garner D.M., Olmstead M.P. & Polivy J.P. (1983) Development and validation of a multidimensional eating disorder inventory for anorexia nervosa and bulimia. *International Journal of Eating Disorders* 2: 15–34.

MARION M. HETHERINGTON

interneurons Interneurons are a type of NEURON whose AXONS are confined to the anatomical NUCLEUS or region that contains their SOMATA (cell bodies) (see AXON; SOMA). The type of neuron sending axons to distant locations is called PROJECTION NEURON. Typically, interneurons have well developed DENDRITES but, as expected, short axons. The main function of interneurons is to integrate information from various afferents and convey it to projection neurons. In this role, interneurons are often referred to as LOCAL CIRCUIT NEURONS. Many interneurons are inhibitory, providing recurrent inhibition to principal neurons as in RENSHAW CELLS or enhancing SIGNAL-TO-NOISE RATIO as occurs in LATERAL INHIBITION in sensory systems.

KAZUE SEMBA

interoceptive (from *interior* plus *receptor*, Interoceptive refers to the detection of stimuli from within the body (signals transmitted through the BLOOD or the AUTONOMIC NERVOUS SYSTEM for example) whereas EXTEROCEPTIVE (from *exterior* plus *receptor*) relates to the detection of stimuli in the external world (through the VISUAL SYSTEM or OLFACTION for example).

interocular 'From one eye to the other'. An example is INTEROCULAR TRANSFER of ADAPTA-

TION (stimulation of one eye can lead to measurable perceptual effects when the partner eye is tested monocularly).

DAVID W. HEELEY

interocular transfer The assessment of the extent to which visual knowledge or a visuomotor skill learned by a subject exclusively with one eye is evident when the subject is asked to utilize that information or demonstrate the skill solely guided by the other eye – that is, when the sensory input arrives centrally by way of a different AFFERENT pathway. Assessment has been used, for example, to test whether a history of BINOCULAR perceptual experience was necessary to show complete interocular transfer of learned pattern discriminations, and to assess whether normal or SPLIT BRAIN subjects could combine specific information received by each HEMISPHERE separately to solve perceptual or cognitive tasks.

See also: pattern perception

RICHARD C. TEES

interpeduncular nucleus A nucleus that lies along the midline, between the right and left VENTRAL TEGMENTAL AREA OF TSAI. (Properly, the term VENTRAL TEGMENTAL AREA should include all of the structures at the base of the MIDBRAIN TEGMENTUM, including the interpeduncular nucleus, but common usage does not do this: the term ventral tegmental area is taken to be synonymous with the ventral tegmental area of Tsai.) Little is known about the interpeduncular nucleus. It sits equidistant from the CEREBRAL PEDUNCLES in each HEMISPHERE, behind the MAMMILLARY BODIES and in front of the most anterior parts of the RAPHE NUCLEI. The interpeduncular nucleus receives output from the HABENULA and projects to the dorsal tegmentum, among other places. Its function is unclear. A rather old literature, based on ELECTROLYTIC LESIONS, suggests it might have a role in certain forms of LEARNING. It is a structure in need of reassessment.

interposed nucleus *see* cerebellum – anatomical organization

interposition *see* superposition

intersex *see* hermaphrodite

interstimulus interval The length of time between the termination of one STIMULUS and the beginning of the next (typically in an experiment using an OPERANT CHAMBER). The duration of the interstimulus interval has an effect on the rate of LEARNING.

interstitial fluid *see* osmoregulation

intertrial interval The interval of time between one TRIAL and the next: it can be imposed by an experimenter (as in, for example, DELAYED ALTERNATION) or it can reflect the performance of a subject. For example, the interval between collecting REINFORCEMENT and resuming lever pressing increases with a higher FIXED RATIO SCHEDULE in PROGRESSIVE RATIO tests.

interval schedule *see* schedules of reinforcement

interval timing *see* timing

intra-arterial injection *see* drug administration

intracellular Inside cells; the intracellular space is the space inside cells. The opposite of intracellular is EXTRACELLULAR.

intracellular dehydration Loss of water from within cells; see OSMOREGULATION; PHYSIOLOGICAL CHALLENGE.

intracellular fluid *see* osmoregulation

intracellular recording *see* extracellular recording

intracerebral injection Direct injection of a DRUG or chemicals into the BRAIN.

See also: drug administration; intracranial injection; microinjection

intracerebroventricular injection Direct injection of a DRUG or chemicals into the cerebral VENTRICLES; also called INTRAVENTRICULAR INJECTIONS; see DRUG ADMINISTRATION.

intracisternal injection *see* drug administration

intracranial injection To be precise, this refers to direct injection of a DRUG or chemicals into the SKULL. However, it is generally used to refer to injections into the BRAIN. INTRACEREBRAL INJECTION is the more correct term for this.

See also: drug administration; microinjection

intracranial self-administration *see* self-administration

intracranial self-stimulation (ICSS) Weak electrical currents applied to the tip of an ELECTRODE placed at a number of specific locations in the brain leads to a strong reinforcing effect that supports OPERANT self-stimulation behaviour. This phenomenon was discovered by James Olds (1922–1976) in the laboratory of Donald Hebb (1904–1985) at McGill University, and resulted in a first paper published in 1954 with Peter Milner. Although purring by cats in response to electrical brain stimulation was noted earlier in a 1949 monograph by the Nobel Prize winner W.R. Hess (1881–1973) the Olds & Milner paper started this exciting field within psychobiology. That field continues on a smaller scale today. Early excitement was based on the apparent high degree of strength of the REINFORCEMENT effect and concomitant new reports that same year of feeding and other motivational centres in the HYPOTHALAMUS, leading to speculation that understanding of reinforcement process in the brain was imminent.

A dramatic change in the field occurred when complexities emerged about behavioural measurement (for instance, the separation of reinforcement and motor debilitating effects associated with certain DRUG or brain LESION effects). Resulting contradictory or confusing findings which deflated some of the initial enthusiasm. However, about the same time, now 20 years after the initial discovery, a new group in the self-stimulation field emerged utilizing a psychophysical approach. Such an approach is possible in rats due to the high degree of stimulus control and the lack of satiation effects in self-stimulation. Like vision researchers, self-stimulation psychophysicists gathered much data on how the quantitative variations in one parameter of the reinforcing stimulation burst (for example, frequency of square-wave pulses) trade off with systematic changes in another parameter (such as cathodal current intensity) to achieve the same behavioural level (that is, threshold). These 'trade-off' functions as they became known within the psychophysical field led to two important developments. First, in the late 1970s they led to methods for the isolation of reinforcing effects on self-stimulation behaviour from contaminating motor effects when some manipulation is made (the delivery of a drug or brain lesion for example). This reinforcement-specific measure is usually accomplished by finding the behavioural threshold of one aspect of a brain stimulation parameter and noting that the drug raises or lowers threshold (decreases or increases the brain stimulation reinforcement effect). While several threshold methods are in use today, one such method that was developed directly from the psychophysics is the RATE FREQUENCY CURVE method. This method employs the half-maximal behavioural point as its threshold and has served as the basis for a many studies of drug or brain lesion effects. For a potential drug of abuse, enhancement of the brain stimulation reinforcement effect (reduced threshold) is highly related to the ability of that drug to support self-administration in animals and therefore addiction in humans.

The second major development associated with self-stimulation psychophysics is the better defining of aspects of the brain structure underlying the self-stimulation reinforcement process itself. For example, studies in the late 1970s and 1980s led to the assertion that the reinforcement effect of medial forebrain bundle stimulation was carried by medium-size, myelinated axons (see MYELIN)and that these axons carried ACTION POTENTIAL activity in the caudal direction. These findings led to the conclusion that self-stimulation does not directly (but may indirectly) activate the ascending MESO-LIMBIC DOPAMINE SYSTEMS which are composed of small unmyelinated neurons. Prior to these findings, it had been widely assumed that the dopamine or NORADRENALINE neurons were directly activated as they travel though many of the brain areas which support self-stimulation behaviour. Today, this work continues utilizing a variety of biological techniques (such as electrophysiology, brain lesions, C-FOS expression; see IMMEDIATE EARLY GENES) to identify at least some of the neuronal cell bodies whose axons are activated in the

medial forebrain bundle and whose action potentials begin the self-stimulation reinforcement process. Self-stimulation can be obtained from a variety of brain structures, principally in the medial forebrain bundle as it passes through the hypothalamus and its extensions into the BRAINSTEM and FOREBRAIN (to structures such as the FRONTAL CORTEX, NUCLEUS ACCUMBENS and AMYGDALA). Self-stimulation has been reported in the CEREBELLUM, CAUDATE NUCLEUS, and other brain structures not classically associated with the medial forebrain bundle. Self-stimulation has been obtained in a variety of species ranging from alligators to humans. While most commonly studied in intact adult rats, self-stimulation has been obtained from day 3 infant rats and from adult rats with complete removal of the forebrain above the hypothalamus (with hypothalamic electrode). The lateral hypothalamus and medial forebrain bundle remain the best studied places and are the sites which generate the most robust self-stimulation behaviour. It is highly likely that the reinforcement effects from widely different brain sites, animals, or preparations differ substantially in the circuits employed or in the nature of the reinforcement effect that is generated. Indeed, early papers cautioned against assuming that lower rates of response from a septal (see SEPTAL NUCLEI) site automatically meant that the reinforcement was greater at the comparison site (such as the hypothalamus) which supported more rapid lever pressing. While dopamine neurotransmission remains a focus of much thinking about how reinforcement effects from many sources are organized in the brain, it is far from clear that this is the only mechanism by which reinforcement processes work. Finally, ELECTRICAL BRAIN STIMULATION activates neurons indiscriminate of their function, so that any REWARD or reinforcement effect generated in a self-stimulation situation is likely to be accompanied by other physiological and psychological effects (such as aversive side-effects). These side effects must be taken into account before adequate theories of reinforcement related mechanisms or behavioural effects can be generated.

JAMES R. STELLAR

intradermal injection *see* drug administration

intradimensional shift Established responding to an exemplar within a STIMULUS DIMENSION, or class of stimulus features, results in the formation of an ATTENTIONAL SET. A change in the contingencies that requires responding to a different exemplar is an intradimensional shift if the new exemplar is from the same class of stimulus features as the previous exemplar.

See also: attentional set-shifting; extradimensional shift

VERITY J. BROWN

intrafusal fibre *see* muscle spindle

intrahemispheric pathways Fibre pathways that remain within one HEMISPHERE.

intralaminar nuclei *see* thalamus

intramedullary injection *see* drug administration

intramuscular injection *see* drug administration

intraocular injection *see* drug administration

intraparietal sulcus A sulcus within the PARIETAL LOBE; see INFERIOR PARIETAL LOBULE; PARIETAL CORTEX.

intraperitoneal injection *see* drug administration

intrathecal injection *see* drug administration

intratracheal injection *see* drug administration

intrauterine Within the UTERUS or womb.

intravascular fluid *see* osmoregulation

intravenous injection *see* drug administration

intravenous self-administration (IVSA) *see* self-administration

intraventricular injection Direct injection of drugs or chemicals into the cerebral VENTRICLES; also called INTRACEREBROVENTRICULAR INJECTIONS; see DRUG ADMINISTRATION

intravitreal injection Effectively an INTRAOCULAR INJECTION, into the VITREOUS HUMOUR of the eye; see DRUG ADMINISTRATION.

intrinsic neuron A neuron whose elements are contained within a given anatomical unit. It is not quite synonymous with INTERNEURON: a neuron could be intrinsic to the BASAL GANGLIA for example yet project from one structure to another within this.

intromission (from Latin, *intro*: inward, *mittere*: to send) *Intromission* is the noun, *intromit* the verb: in general use intromission refers to any insertion, as the etymology implies. In biology, intromission refers to a component of SEXUAL BEHAVIOUR: the insertion of the PENIS into the VAGINA. In a single sexual interaction, a male rat will typically intromit several times before finally ejaculating.

intron *see* exon

intubation *see* drug administration

invalid cue *see* Posner effect

inverse agonist *see* agonist

invertebrates Any of the animals without a vertebral column (i.e. a backbone composed of individual vertebrae); not one of the VERTEBRATES.

involuntary *see* voluntary

involuntary nervous system An alternative name for the AUTONOMIC NERVOUS SYSTEM.

ion A molecule or ATOM that is electrically charged, having either gained or lost electrons. A CATION has a positive charge, an ANION has a negative charge. In solution many substances break down into their component parts: common salt – sodium chloride (NaCl) – for example breaks down in water into positively charged sodium ions (Na^+) and negatively charged chloride ions (Cl^-). The relative balance of positively and negatively charged ions on either side of a neuronal MEMBRANE determines the RESTING POTENTIAL of a NEURON. The movement of ions across the membrane is critical for ACTION POTENTIAL generation. Movement of ions across a membrane can be a RECEPTOR-mediated process, occurring via the receptor-regulated ION CHANNEL system, or a process mediated by specialized transport mechanisms such as the SODIUM–POTASSIUM PUMP and the CALCIUM PUMP.

ion channel Ion channels are water-filled pores in the cell MEMBRANE through which ions (see ION) can move into or out of cells depending on the MEMBRANE POTENTIAL or the action of NEUROTRANSMITTERS. They occur in three states: resting, open and closed. Because the movement of ions generates a CURRENT and membrane potential changes, ion channels have a fundamental role in controlling neuronal excitability. An ion channel has selective permeability to different ions including SODIUM (Na^+), CALCIUM (Ca^{2+}), POTASSIUM (K^+). Such currents can be measured from a small patch of neuronal membrane containing one or a few ion channels. This technique, called single channel recording, represents a significant technical advance in modern neurobiology.

KAZUE SEMBA

ionotropic Receptors that are directly coupled to the ION CHANNEL within a single macromolecular complex in the cell MEMBRANE are referred to as ionotropic receptors. Ionotropic receptors, thus, directly gate their ion channels, allowing the flow of selected ions (see ION) (Na^+), CALCIUM (Ca^{2+}), POTASSIUM (K^+) and CHLORIDE (Cl^-). In contrast, METABOTROPIC receptors gate ion channels indirectly via SECOND MESSENGERS. An ionotropic receptor is composed of several subunits, and their combination determines the properties of the receptor. Examples of ionotropic receptors are NICOTINIC ACETYLCHOLINE RECEPTORS, NMDA and NON-NMDA RECEPTORS and GABA-A RECEPTORS.

See also: fast neurotransmission; glutamate receptors

KAZUE SEMBA

iproniazid A drug that can block the actions of MONOAMINE OXIDASE. Iproniazid was in use in the 1950s in the treatment of tuberculosis. It was found to have an independent effect on MOOD and consequently was tested for ANTIDEPRESSANT activity, which it was found to have. Subsequently it was found to achieve this effect by virtue of monoamine oxidase inhibition. It is no longer in clinical use but has a venerable position in PSYCHOPHARMACOLOGY.

ipsapirone An agonist at the $5HT_{1A}$ receptor; see SEROTONIN RECEPTORS.

ipsilateral *see* contralateral

IPSP *see* EPSP/IPSP

IQ *see* intelligence testing

iris A coloured circle of MUSCLES surrounding the PUPIL of the EYE, the contraction or relaxation of which controls iris diameter.

iron (Fe) Iron is an important MINERAL and a major component of haemoglobin in the BLOOD and important in ENERGY metabolism; there is some evidence in favour of there being a SPECIFIC APPETITE for iron; see MALNUTRITION.

irreversible antagonist *see* antagonist

irreversible binding *see* receptor binding

ischaemia A loss of BLOOD flow to a tissue or organ. The brain derives most of its energy from the oxidative metabolism of GLUCOSE: both glucose and OXYGEN are supplied to the brain by an extensive CEREBRAL VASCULATURE. When the blood supply is compromised, ischaemia leads to a series of events, culminating in neuronal death. Ischaemia can occur globally, usually due to cardiac arrest, or focally, for example due to the blockage of an isolated cerebral vessel, or STROKE. GLOBAL ISCHAEMIA and FOCAL ISCHAEMIA are different in both the scale of damage done, and the region in which the damage occurs. Global ischaemia due to temporary cardiac arrest is usually short-lived and fully reversible, and results in neuronal damage throughout the brain. In contrast, focal ischaemia is often long-lasting, and involves death of neurons and other cerebral tissue, such as EPITHELIAL CELLS in the cerebral capillaries, in a localized region known as the INFARCT. In addition, neuronal death is often seen spreading in a rim around the infarct, known as the penumbra, and in remote brain structures which are innervated by the region of infarct. A feature of both focal and global ischaemia is that much neuronal death occurs some time later than the initial insult. This observation suggests that mechanisms secondary to the ischaemic insult are responsible for this delayed neuronal death.

In both global and focal ischaemia, there is a hierarchy within neurons in susceptibility to ischaemic damage. Neurons most at risk from ischaemic damage are in regions of brain which have high densities of GLUTAMATE RECEPTORS, and include STRIATUM, CORTEX and HIPPOCAMPUS. Ischaemia is associated with elevated extracellular GLUTAMATE levels, and antagonists to both AMPA and NMDA receptors are found to prevent delayed neuronal death in animal models of ischaemia. This suggests that glutamate acts as an excitotoxin (see EXCITO-TOXINS) in ischaemia, and that NMDA and AMPA antagonists may be useful in clinical treatment of ischaemia.

Without the supply of oxygen and glucose, neurons quickly become depleted in ADENO-SINE TRIPHOSPHATE (ATP), and are unable to fuel normal cellular reactions. An immediate consequence is the loss of function of the SODIUM–POTASSIUM PUMP, an ion pump which maintains the negative membrane potential through active uptake of potassium ions and extrusion of sodium ions. The consequent increase in extracellular potassium concentrations results in bursts of DEPOLARIZATION in neurons, followed by electrical silence. Cell depolarization leads to release of large amounts of neurotransmitter, including gluta-mate. Most glutamate released during normal neuronal firing is rapidly taken up by GLIAL CELLS, where it may be metabolized to GLUTA-MINE, and exported to neurons for resynthesis of glutamate. During ischaemia, however, there is a lack of ATP to fuel uptake mechanisms in glial cells, and so the action of glutamate on neurons is prolonged. Activation of glutamate receptors during normal neuronal firing leads to an influx of CALCIUM ions through NMDA receptors, and some calcium-permeable AMPA receptors. Antagonists of calcium channels are protective against ischaemic damage in animal models, indicating that calcium influx in ischaemic tissue, probably through glutamate receptors, causes neuronal death. In normal cells, cytosolic calcium concentrations are tightly controlled by sequestration into ENDO-PLASMIC RETICULUM and MITOCHONDRIA, through an ATP-dependent sodium-calcium pump. Small increases in cytosolic calcium concentrations affect many cellular reactions.

Calcium is required for initiation of phospha-tase and KINASE action, regulating the activity of cellular enzymes, receptors, SECOND MES-SENGERS and GENE expression. Other enzymes which act to break down cell components are also calcium-dependent. For example, increases in calcium concentration result in stimulation of proteases, which break down proteins, and ENDONUCLEASES, which mediate the break-down of DNA and RNA, the genetic material of the cell. Calcium also stimulates the production of FREE RADICALS, including production of NIT-RIC OXIDE through stimulation of nitric oxide synthase. Free radicals, being highly reactive, are potentially destructive, and can mediate breakdown of membranes and nuclear mate-rial. All of these mechanisms may be initiated by prolonged exposure of a neuron to high extracellular glutamate levels during ischaemia, and each may over a duration lead to the death of the cell, through disruption of its enzymatic processes, loss of control of gene expression, and breakdown of PROTEINS, membranes and genetic material, vital for survival of the cell.

The consequences of cerebral ischaemia may be death, or severe cognitive impairment, the exact symptoms of which vary depending on the location of the ischaemic damage. Thus, the observation that most neuronal death occurs hours after the initial insult is important in treating patients with ischaemia. This delay may represent a window of opportunity, often referred to as the therapeutic window during which drugs such as glutamate antagonists may be used to prevent delayed neuronal death as a result of ischaemia.

FIONA M. INGLIS

islets of Langerhans *see* insulin

iso- (from Greek, *isos*: equal) A prefix indicat-ing equal or the same. Related prefixes are HYPO- and HYPER-. See ISOTONIC SALINE for an example of the usage of these prefixes.

isocortex An alternative name for the NEO-CORTEX.

isodendritic core A part of the RETICULAR FORMATION, in which the DENDRITE structure identifies three types of NEURON. *Isodendritic neurons* are symmetrical with long dendrites extending equally in all directions, to adjacent cell groups and into fibre systems. These are the most common type of reticular formation neuron. *Idiodendritic neurons* have dendrites retained within the host structure. *Allodendritic neurons* are different to both iso- and idiodendritic neurons and have specialized functions. As with all neurons of the reticular formation, the CELL BODY and dendritic field have an organization best seen in coronal sections (see PLANES OF SECTION) and have axons (see AXON) that travel in the CENTRAL TEGMENTAL TRACT (if ascending) or RETICULOSPINAL TRACT (if descending).

isolation rearing A laboratory environment in which animals are housed alone for some time. This manipulation was created to assess whether or not certain kinds of social or sensory experience normally available during some stage (usually early) in development play a role in subsequent (usually adult) neural or behavioural functioning. Assessments of specific behavioural consequences (on adult social competence for instance) and/or neural effects (for example on dendritic branching of cortical neurons) need to be made in respect to other comparison animals (also randomly) assigned to be raised together (see ENVIRONMENTAL ENRICHMENT, and SENSORY ENRICHMENT VS. DEAFFERENTATION/DEPRIVATION). Inevitably, while social experiences may be the focus of investigation, the sensory experience (whether tactual, auditory, visual or whatever) of these animals is also reduced relative to those of animals raised together and the term impoverished rearing is often used synonymously.

See also: social behaviour; social isolation

RICHARD C. TEES

isomer (from Greek, *isos*: equal, *meros*: part) Certain chemicals can exist in two different forms, called isomers. This property arises when there is an asymmetry in the structure of a MOLECULE. Because of this asymmetry, any other components of the molecule attached to the asymmetric component will be biased in one direction or another. The bias may be to the right (the D-isomer) or to the left (the L-isomer): 'D' stands for *dextrorotatory* (rotating to the right, or clockwise), 'L' stands for *levorotatory* (rotating to the left, or anti-

clockwise). It is important to note that isomeric forms of a molecule have essentially the same properties, though there may be important differences. For example, AMINO ACIDS exist in isomeric forms. In this case, the isomerism comes from the fact that one of the carbon atoms, to which a side chain bonds, is asymmetric. Physiologically, L-amino acids are more important than the D- form. For instance, only L-amino acids are incorporated into PROTEINS. AMPHETAMINE is another example of an isomerized chemical. D-amphetamine is more potent that L-amphetamine, and a RACEMATE form also exists.

Reference

Feldman R., Meyer J.S. & Quenzer L.F. (1997) *Principles of Neuropsychopharmacology*, Sinauer Associates: Sunderland MA.

isoproteronol A non-selective beta NORADRENALINE receptor AGONIST; see ADRENORECEPTORS.

isotonic ISOTONIC describes a solution of equal OSMOTIC PRESSURE to INTRACELLULAR FLUIDS: bathing a CELL with an isotonic solution produces no net flux of water across the cell MEMBRANE. HYPERTONIC: more concentrated than isotonic: bathing a cell with a hypertonic solution will cause water to move out of that cell. HYPOTONIC: less concentrated than isotonic: bathing a cell with a hypotonic solution will cause water to move into that cell.

See also: isotonic saline; osmoregulation

isotonic saline Saline is simply salt solution: isotonic saline refers to 0.9% saline: that is, water containing 0.9% sodium chloride (NaCl). (This is bought commercially or made by adding 9 g NaCl to 100 ml water: a percentage solution refers to the number of grams of a substance in 100 ml of solution.) This concentration of saline will not affect normal animal cells. That is, it will not draw water out of them, or cause them to take on more water. Isotonic saline, also known as PHYSIOLOGICAL SALINE, is very commonly used as a VEHICLE for DRUG solutions. HYPERTONIC SALINE is a saline solution containing more than 0.9% NaCl, HYPOTONIC SALINE is a saline solution containing less than 0.9%. 5% Hypertonic saline is given to animals as a PHYSIO-

LOGICAL CHALLENGE: it makes them drink by generating INTRACELLULAR DEHYDRATION.

See also: osmoregulation

isotope Isotopes are variants of the same ELEMENT. Every ATOM of a particular element contains the same number of protons, but some have more neutrons (and therefore weigh more; see ATOMIC WEIGHT). Isotopes are very common in nature: most elements of biological importance have several isotopes. For example, carbon always has 6 protons, but can have 6, 7 or 8 neutrons. While these all have different atomic weights they are nevertheless isotopes of each other. Isotopes can be stable or radioactive: stable isotopes are those whose atomic nuclei remain stable: they have a number of protons and neutrons and retain those numbers. A radioactive isotope (or RADIOISOTOPE) is one in which the atomic nucleus decays, releasing protons and energy and, because protons are lost, turning the element from one thing to another. There is a received style for presenting elements that indicates their nuclear composition: carbon-12 has a total of 12 neutrons and protons. Since all forms of carbon have 6 protons, it follows that carbon-12 (or ^{12}C, or $^{12}_{6}C$) has 6 neutrons. Carbon-13, by the same arithmetic, has 7 neutrons, carbon-14 has 8. Carbon-12 and carbon-13 are stable; carbon-14 is radioactive and decays over time to form nitrogen. Radioisotopes are useful in a variety of neuroscientific procedures: see for example, AUTORADIOGRAPHY; FUNCTIONAL NEUROIMAGING; RADIOIMMUNOASSAY; RADIOLABEL.

isozyme An isozyme is one of an ENZYME group whose members have similar functional properties but slightly different physical characteristics: for example, there are different isozymes of ACETYLCHOLINESTERASE and HEME OXYGENASE.

isthmus (from Greek, *isthmos*, a derivative of *ienai*: to go) This term generally refers to a narrow land bridge between two larger land masses. In anatomy it has had two uses, neither well defined or common: (i) Swanson notes that the term ISTHMUS was used (but is no longer) to refer to a region between the ventricles of the MIDBRAIN and HINDBRAIN during NEURODEVELOPMENT. (ii) Grossman uses the term to refer to that part of the CINGULATE GYRUS that communicates with the hippocampal gyrus.

Reference

Grossman S.P. (1967) *A Textbook of Physiological Psychology*, 1st corrected printing, Wiley: New York.

Swanson L.W. (1992) *Brain Maps: Structure of the Rat Brain*, Elsevier: Amsterdam.

J

Jacksonian epilepsy (Jacksonian seizures) A form of EPILEPSY first described by the remarkable nineteenth-century English neurologist John Hughlings-Jackson (1835–1911). It is a form of epilepsy which begins with a convulsion in a part of the body and spreads until the sufferer becomes 'a clotted mass of spasm'. Involvement of the FRONTAL LOBE is also indicated.

Reference

Critchley M. and Critchley E.A. (1999) *John Hughlings Jackson: Father of English Neurology*, Oxford University Press: Oxford. (For review of this, see *Times Literary Supplement*, March 5 1999, No. 5005, p.36.)

James–Lange theory of the emotions The common-sense or FOLK PSYCHOLOGY view that conscious emotional experience causes emotional responses was rejected by William James (1824–1910) in 1884. He turned around this causal sequence, based on what was known then from clinical case histories, introspection and a burgeoning interest in brain function. Thus, fleeing from danger is not caused by FEAR; the fear is a consequence of the running away. Following the perception of the EMOTION-eliciting event by the sensory portions of the CEREBRAL CORTEX, motor and SOMATIC responses are produced by stimulation of the appropriate output areas and descending projections, partly based on learned (see LEARNING) associations, as well as innate dispositions. Then it is the perception of the feedback from these responses, at the cortical level, that forms the raw substrate of emotional experience. It is important to note that James did not postulate a specific brain centre for the emotions. The neurologist Carl G. Lange (1834–1900) published, apparently independently, a similar version of James's theory in 1885. The theory is thus generally referred to as the James–Lange theory of the emotions, although there are subtle differences between the two formulations. Lange for example did not refer to a mechanism by which feedback from the VISCERA is perceived and emphasizes the expression of emotion via somatic channels, thus laying the foundations for modern psychosomatic medicine.

The James–Lange theory is of only historical interest today. It was criticized strongly by Cannon (see CANNON–BARD THEORY OF THE EMOTIONS) on five major grounds. (1) Total separation of the viscera from the CENTRAL NERVOUS SYSTEM did not eliminate emotional behaviour; note, for example, the lack of effect of sympathectomy on fear avoidance responses in dogs. (2) The same visceral changes occur in different emotional states, even polar opposites such as joy and sadness. (3) The viscera are relatively insensitive. (4) Visceral changes are too slow to be the origin of emotional feelings. (5) Artificial production of visceral changes found in emotion does not actually lead to emotional experience. Cannon proposed instead his own neurological theory of the emotions, which came to be known as the Cannon–Bard theory.

It appears, however, that Cannon's critique was somewhat of an overkill. His criticism about the slowness of visceral responses being unsuitable substrates for emotional experience is countered to some extent by learning in which such autonomic feedback can be conditioned to readily perceived external stimuli. The apparent difficulties of emotional differentiation are also largely overturned by the discoveries of Ekman and others about the patterning of emotional responses (see EMOTION). The James-Lange theory was rescued to some extent by a modified theory proposed by Stanley Schachter which posited emotion to be a joint product of two factors, visceral feedback and its cognitive interpretation. Schachter referred to the (now considered controversial) evidence that paraplegic patients (see PARAPLEGIA) continued to express emotional responses and yet appeared to have reduced emotional feelings when questioned on the nature of their post-operative subjective experience. The hypothesis was that the subjects had previously learned emotional behavioural responses appropriate to particular situations, but had lost the capacity to experience their visceral consequences as a consequence of the LESION to their SPINAL CORD. The subjective intensity of the emotions was inversely related to the level of the spinal cord lesion, with the greatest effects being evident at the lowest levels of TRANSECTION (which correspondingly prevented greater levels of autonomic feedback). He also performed an important experiment (Schachter & Singer, 1962) in which volunteers unknowingly receiving ADRENALINE in different conditions were either unaware or misinformed of the effects of the drug. The intensity of emotions was greatest in such conditions – that is, where subjects were less able to predict or rationalize its effects and accordingly more prone to hypothesize about their possible origin. The results supported the view that emotional experience was the joint product of intensity of visceral responses and the cognitive context in which they are experienced.

Modern applications of the James–Lange–Schachter theory are to be found in the phenomenological and pharmacological study of ANXIETY. It is now evident that PANIC attacks and other forms of somatic anxiety arise largely from a tendency to misinterpret bodily feelings, and this has become a central factor in the cognitive treatment of anxiety (see COGNITIVE THERAPY; COGNITIVE–BEHAVIOURAL THERAPY). It is also apparent that certain somatic forms of anxiety may be treated with any DRUG that produces a reversible blockade of sympathetic activity by acting as NORADRENERGIC beta receptor antagonist, such as propranolol. However, of equivalent theoretical weight is the lack of efficacy of such compounds in many forms of neurotic anxiety, although they may objectively ameliorate the visceral manifestations of anxiety. These disorders often yield to treatment with BENZODIAZEPINES such as Librium or Valium, despite their reduced efficacy at reducing sympathetic activation.

References

Robbins T.W. (1988) Emotion and conditioning. In *Psychology for Medicine*, ed. T.W. Robbins & P.J. Cooper, pp. 190–240, E. Arnold: London.

Schachter S. (1966) The interaction of cognitive and physiological determinants of emotional states. In *Anxiety and Behavior*, ed. S. Spielberger, pp. 193–224, Academic Press: Orlando.

TREVOR W. ROBBINS

jargon aphasia One of five APHASIA types described in the taxonomy of Wepman & Jones (1961). The speech of these patients is rendered meaningless by the excessive use of unintelligible sequences of sounds. Speech generally follows normal patterns of intonation and PITCH, and obeys rules of sound combination (consonant/vowel patterns mimic what normally is permissible for real words). Although the preservation of speech melody and normal use of word boundaries can initially deceive the listener, this striking pattern of aphasic speech is detectable clinically.

See also: paraphasia; speech perception; speech production

Reference

Wepman J. & Jones J. (1961) *Studies in Aphasia: An Approach to Testing. The Language Modalities Test for Aphasia*, Education–Industry Service: Chicago.

CHARLOTTE C. MITCHUM

jaw movements Researchers in PSYCHOPHAR-
MACOLOGY have identified a number of different jaw movement responses that can be
induced by various pharmacological or neurochemical conditions. Administration of a CHO-
LINOMIMETIC or depletion of DOPAMINE has
been reported to produced tremulous jaw
movements. These are defined as rapid and
repetitive bursts of jaw movements that resemble chewing but are not directed at any
particular stimulus. These movements are
called tremulous because they are characterized
by some degree of periodicity, with a frequency
in the Parkinsonian tremor range (see PARKIN-
SON'S DISEASE). They also have been called
VACUOUS JAW MOVEMENTS, with the term
vacuous connoting the non-directed quality of
the movement. Two older terms, PURPOSELESS
CHEWING and VACUOUS CHEWING, also are
used in the literature to describe similar types
of drug induced jaw movement. The clinical
significance of these movements is not clear,
and it has been suggested that the movements
may be related to DYSTONIA, DYSKINESIA or
Parkinsonian tremor.

JOHN D. SALAMONE

jejunum *see* digestive system

jet lag Disturbances of physiology and behaviour caused by the rapid transit of multiple
time zones. The term implies that high-speed
transportation via jet aircraft results in a
mismatch between the ENDOGENOUS body time
of the traveller and local time at the destination. The 'lag' in adjustment to local time
results from the inertia of an endogenous
BIOLOGICAL CLOCK system which is set to local
time at the place of origin, and can only
gradually be resynchronized or entrained (see
ENTRAINMENT) to local time cues at the destination. The symptoms of jet lag include disturbances in SLEEP, alertness, and digestion,
and poor mental and physical performance.
These symptoms can be understood as the
result of the attempt to function in synchrony
with local schedules – sleeping at night, eating
meals at the usual clock times and working or
competing in sporting events during the day –
even though the internal circadian clock mechanisms that regulate these functions are still
entrained to a schedule that may be displaced

by up to 12 hours from local time. Thus, the
jet-lag sufferer may attempt to sleep while his
or her body is becoming aroused, attempt to
eat when the regulators of feeding are effectively shut down, and try to work while
neuroendocrine mechanisms are preparing for
sleep. If an individual is exposed to several
local ZEITGEBER cycles, including especially the
day–night cycle, the circadian clock mechanism
shifts gradually toward local time and the
symptoms of jet lag abate. Many factors
probably affect the rate of re-entrainment, but
requiring a day of adjustment for each time
zone traversed is a rough guide. Jet lag may be
exacerbated by repeated shifts without intervening stable periods of entrainment, especially
when combined with irregular work and sleep
schedules. This pattern is characteristic of
international flight crews on aircraft, who
may suffer from severe and possibly dangerous
disruptions of temporal organization. Jet lag
has much in common with the disorders
suffered by those working night shifts or on
rotating shift-work schedules. Changing work
shifts may be somewhat like crossing multiple
time zones in terms of work schedule, sleeping
time and meals, but exposure to local zeitgebers may be only partially altered, further
complicating physiological adjustment. Treatments for jet lag that have had some success
include appropriately timed doses of the
PINEAL GLAND hormone MELATONIN, timed
exposure to light pulses, and exercise, all of
which are known from animal and human
research to shift the circadian clock mechanism.

See also: circadian rhythm

BENJAMIN RUSAK

jiggle plate A device for measuring TREMOR in
animals. A base plate is mounted on ball
bearings such that it 'jiggles'. Fixed to the plate
is a pointed plumb bob that hangs in a socket.
When bob and socket make contact an electric
circuit is completed: the number of times this
happens is recorded to give an index of tremor
in an animal housed in a box on the base plate.

jimpy mutant mouse Mice with inherited
disorders of MYELIN formation; QUAKING and

SHIVERER MUTANT MICE also have myelin formation disorders.

joint attention The ability to share a focus of ATTENTION with another, such as by showing or pointing to an object, which indicates an appreciation of another's independent mental state.

See also: theory of mind

VERITY J. BROWN

jugular foramen *see* vagus nerve

jugular ganglion The VAGUS NERVE has two sensory ganglia (see GANGLION): the JUGULAR GANGLION (superior) is one and the NODOSE GANGLION (inferior) the other. The jugular ganglion contains general somatic afferent neurons that innervate the DURA MATER (see MENINGES) and SKIN of the EAR and external acoustic meatus.

jugular vein *see* blood

juxtallocortex The juxtallocortex is older than the NEOCORTEX but younger than the ALLO-CORTEX (with which it is often combined in the rather vague term LIMBIC CORTEX). Whereas the allocortex has three cell layers (see CORTI-CAL LAYERS), the juxtallocortex can have four to five (which of course still fails to meet the criteria for neocortex: possession of six cell layers). Included in the juxtallocortex are the CINGULATE CORTEX, OPERCULAR CORTEX and parts of the FRONTAL CORTEX that fail to meet the criteria for inclusion in the neocortex. Older literature might refer to the juxtallocortex as the MESOCORTEX or PALAEOPALLIUM.

K

K complex The K complex is a high-amplitude slow wave pattern (> 0.5 seconds in duration) consisting of an initial sharp negative component and subsequent slower positive component. It occurs during SLOW-WAVE SLEEP either spontaneously or evoked by sensory stimuli, particularly sounds. Evident during stage 2 sleep, the K complex is often accompanied by a SLEEP SPINDLE (12–14 Hz) riding on the trailing positive component. During this stage, K complexes occur about 1–3 times per minute. They most likely occur during stages 3–4 of slow-wave sleep as well, but are not evident on the background of high-amplitude delta waves (1–4 Hz). They may be the manifestation of the 'slow oscillation' (< 1 Hz) that occurs through slow-wave sleep and upon which the other delta and spindle waves ride.

See also: electroencephalogram; sleep

BARBARA E. JONES

kainic acid (kainate) 2-Carboxy-4-(1-methylethenyl)-3-pyrrolidinacetic acid: one of the EXCITOTOXINS, frequently used for LESION production in experimental animals, and the definitive AGONIST at a class of GLUTAMATE RECEPTORS. Kainate was the first excitotoxin used but is less frequently employed now because its extraordinarily high potency tends to produce lesions larger than required.

See also: drug ionization

kairomones *see* pheromones

Kallman's syndrome An ENDOCRINE DISORDER featuring deficiency of gonadotropic hormones (principally FOLLICLE-STIMULATING HORMONE and LUTEINIZING HORMONE). It involves HYPOGONADISM, reduced stature and ANOSMIA. It is treatable by appropriate REPLACEMENT THERAPY.

Kamin's effect Also called the BLOCKING effect, this phenomenon of CLASSICAL CONDITIONING, first described by Leon Kamin, refers to the situation in which an already established association between a CONDITIONED STIMULUS (CS) and UNCONDITIONED STIMULUS (US) prevents the formation of a CONDITIONED RESPONSE (CR) to another CS presented in combination with the first CS. The defining experiments used a CONDITIONED EMOTIONAL RESPONSE paradigm in which a CS is paired with a foot shock US and the strength of the classical conditioning tested by presenting the CS while the subject is working on an OPERANT task for food reward. The CONDITIONED FEAR reaction (CR) induced by the classical conditioning causes the CS to be able to suppress operant responding for food. In the blocking demonstration, two phases of classical condition exist. In the first phase, one type of CS (for example, a tone stimulus) is paired with shock until it gains the ASYMPTOTIC BEHAVIOURAL MAXIMUM ability to suppress operant responding for food. Then, in phase two, further training is given with a combination of this CS and another CS (for example, a light). If the second CS (the light in this case) is presented during operant responding for food, a weaker fear reaction is noticed compared to a control experiment where only phase two is given – that is, the combination CS stimuli (light and tone) is used without phase one pre-training on one of the stimuli. The idea behind blocking is that the second stimulus is redundant and subjects are less likely to learn a classical conditioned association if the new information is not useful to predicting the occurrence of the US. Kamin went even further to suggest that for conditioning to work, the CS has to be unexpected and even surprising to the subject, but also (of course) predictive of the US.

See also: Rescorla–Wagner theory

JAMES R. STELLAR

kanamycin *see* ototoxic drugs

Kennard principle The formulation that it is easier to recovery from brain damage earlier in life than it is later. However, many factors can affect the psychological and neural responses to brain damage and it is growing more clear that this is by no means an absolute principle, correct in all circumstances; see RECOVERY OF FUNCTION.

kenophobia (from Greek, *kenos*: empty, *phobos*: fear) A FEAR of empty spaces.

ketamine An arylcycloalkylamine related to PHENCYCLIDINE and utilized to induce ANAESTHESIA and ANALGESIA and characterized by feelings of detachment from the environment.

See also: dissociative anaesthetics

CHARLES D. BLAHA

ketanserin An antagonist at the $5HT_{2A}$ receptor; see SEROTONIN RECEPTORS.

ketone bodies *see* energy

kidney *see* osmoregulation

kilo- Prefix indicating a factor of 10^3, or one thousand times; see SI UNITS.

kin selection *see* sociobiology

kinaesthesia The sense of body position in space, achieved through detecting the positions of the MUSCLES, tendons and joints and incorporating this with HAPTIC information and information from the VESTIBULAR SYSTEM.

kinase A kinase is an ENZYME that catalyses the PHOSPHORYLATION (that is, the transfer of a phosphate group) of its substrate by a reaction involving ADENOSINE TRIPHOSPHATE (ATP). There are many types, usually differentiated by a specific term: for example, a PROTEIN KINASE is a kinase involved in phosphorylation of PROTEINS.

kindling Graham Goddard coined this term for his fortuitous discovery that an electrical stimulus (see ELECTRICAL BRAIN STIMULATION) delivered to the brain at daily intervals may at first have no overt behavioural effect but eventually cause TONIC–CLONIC epileptiform SEIZURES (see EPILEPSY) at almost every trial. Hundreds of studies later the underlying mechanisms remain enigmatic as ever, apart from some well-established basic principles. For example, the electrodes must be suitably positioned in the AMYGDALA, HIPPOCAMPUS, FRONTAL CORTEX or anterior HYPOTHALAMUS but not in the BRAINSTEM; the electrical stimuli must be strong enough to evoke local AFTERDISCHARGES (see ELECTROENCEPHALOGRAM), and interstimulus intervals usually have to exceed 30 minutes. All the usual experimental species are susceptible, and electrical stimulation may be substituted for by MICROINJECTION of CONVULSANT agents such as PICROTOXIN or kainate.

In the rat, kindled seizures usually evolve through RACINE'S FIVE STAGES: respectively facial twitching, head movement, forelimb clonus, clonus plus rearing on hind legs, rearing plus falling. The resulting kindled status is virtually permanent, and is generalized to other potential kindling sites (but the progress of kindling is disrupted if an additional site is kindled concurrently). The neural substrate is unknown. Structural changes – apart from seizure-induced cell loss – are minimal (but see below); biochemical changes are often reported but seldom replicated. The temporal and electrophysiological paramenters of kindling do not match those of LONG TERM POTENTIATION and the two phenomena are probably not analogous. The pharmacology of kindling resembles that of epilepsy, and kindled rats have been useful in the assay and development of ANTICONVULSANT drugs. But there are significant differences, including the inhibition of kindling (but not established seizures) by noradrenergic alpha-2 receptor antagonists (see

NORADRENALINE RECEPTORS), by NERVE GROWTH FACTOR antagonists and by protein synthesis blockers (see PROTEINS). Kindling is similarly affected in MUTANT or TRANSGENIC strains that mimic the effects of these pharmacological manipulations.

Kindling has long been thought to offer a possible model for plastic neural changes that underlie normal DEVELOPMENT and LEARNING. Specific staining has since shown that the progress of kindling is accompanied by SPROUTING of ZINC-laden nerve processes extending from hippocampal PYRAMIDAL NEURONS in the HIPPOCAMPUS; treatments which prevent this sprouting (such as an ANTAGONIST of nerve growth factor) serve also to retard kindling and to impair learning. Another significant role for kindling may be in the development of seizures after repeated cycles of exposure to and withdrawal from certain types of DRUG OF ABUSE. Thus the unravelling of the kindling phenomenon may be an important step linking the learning process to clearly discernible changes in brain structure.

Reference

Cain D.P. (1996) Kindling and the amygdala. In *The Amygdala: Neurobiological Aspects of Emotion, Memory and Mental Dysfunction*, ed. J.P. Aggleton, pp. 539–560, Wiley-Liss: New York.

L. JACOB HERBERG

kinematics *see* kinetic

kineme An individual movement with communicative properties that is the non-verbal communication (see ANIMAL COMMUNICATION) equivalent of a MORPHEME in LANGUAGE.

See also: kinetic

kinesics *see* kinetic

kinetic (from Greek, *kineein*: to move) As an adjective, KINETIC refers to motion. KINETICS is the scientific study of the actions of forces in producing motion: kinetic energy is the energy that a body possesses by virtue of its motion. KINEMATICS is the science of action without reference to force. KINESICS is the scientific study of communication through the movement of body parts.

kinetic tremor *see* tremor

kinin A hormone found in plants that promotes CELL DIVISION; kinin also refers to a group of polypeptides that all cause dilation of BLOOD vessels and contraction of SMOOTH MUSCLE.

See also: bradykinin; cholecystokinin; tachykinin

Kleine–Levin syndrome A rare condition seen mostly in young men who become subject to repeated episodes of overeating, hypersexuality, irritability and confusion, followed by a period of deep sleep that may last a day or two – or, with interruptions, for several weeks. The cause is quite unknown. A resemblance to the effects of a TUMOUR of the DIENCEPHALON in man or a LESION in the ventromedial HYPOTHALAMUS of rodents (see VENTROMEDIAL HYPOTHALAMIC SYNDROME) may be no more than coincidental. Reports of abnormal neurotransmitter levels have not been confirmed. The condition may remit spontaneously. The reported efficacy of treatment with LITHIUM suggests a possible aetiological kinship with MANIC DEPRESSION.

L. JACOB HERBERG

Klinefelter's syndrome A relatively common genetic disorder of males (1 in 700 live births) caused by the presence of one or more extra X CHROMOSOMES (represented schematically as 47,XXY or 48,XXXY and so on). Disability due to the condition may be relatively mild because of the tendency for supernumerary X chromosomes to be genetically inactivated, as in normal female development. Abnormalities shown by affected individuals include underdeveloped testes (eunuchoidism), infertility, enlarged breasts, and some degree of MENTAL HANDICAP. A mosaic variant of the syndrome affects only a random sample of the body's cells, and its effects are correspondingly milder.

L. JACOB HERBERG

Klüver–Bucy syndrome A bizarre array of behavioural changes sometimes observed after bilateral TEMPORAL LOBE damage. Components of the syndrome are: (1) VISUAL AGNOSIA; (2) a loss of emotional reactivity; (3) ORALITY – a tendency to examine objects with the mouth; (4) HYPERMETAMORPHOSIS – a tendency to switch rapidly from one behaviour to another; (5) HYPERSEXUALITY; (6) abnormal dietary changes. These changes are consistently observed following bilateral removal of the temporal lobes in monkeys (Klüver & Bucy, 1939) but are only occasionally reported in humans. Many of the changes, notably the loss of emotional reactivity, result from the loss of connections between the CEREBRAL CORTEX and AMYGDALA.

See also: emotion

Reference

Klüver H. & Bucy P.C. (1939) Preliminary analysis of functions of the temporal lobes in monkeys. *Archives of Neurology and Psychiatry* 42: 979–1000.

JOHN P. AGGLETON

knee jerk *see* stretch reflex

knife cut lesion *see* lesion

knowledge based memory Knowledge based memory involves the recall of factual information about the world that has been accumulated over one's lifetime. It is a LONG-TERM MEMORY system that can operate in the absence of incoming information. The term is closely related to EXPECTANCY BASED MEMORY and SEMANTIC MEMORY.

See also: memory

HOWARD EICHENBAUM

Kohonen network *see* neural networks

Kölliker–Fuse nucleus *see* parabrachial nuclei

Kollner's rule *see* colour blindness

koniocortex (from Greek, *konis*: dust, and Latin *cortex*: bark) Koniocortex is characterized as having a prominent granular layer (layer 4 – see CORTICAL LAYERS). The PRIMARY SENSORY CORTEX is characterized in this way, regardless of sensory modality, and is thus often referred to as the koniocortex.

Korsakoff's amnesia *see* Korsakoff's syndrome

Korsakoff's psychosis *see* Korsakoff's syndrome

Korsakoff's syndrome A syndrome characterized by degeneration of brain tissue and most notable for severe deficiencies in MEMORY and LEARNING. It is closely associated with significant degree of ALCOHOL ABUSE, which leads to deficiency of VITAMINS; it is the loss of THIAMINE (vitamin B1) which leads to brain damage, by virtue of interruption of GLUCOSE metabolism.

The naming of Korsakoff's syndrome is a little confusing. Sergei Korsakoff (1853–1900) – whose name is often spelt Korsakov – described in 1887 a syndrome involving memory loss resulting from a variety of causes (including blood poisoning, typhus, tuberculosis, diabetes mellitus [see DIABETES], LEAD POISONING and ERGOTISM) though by far and away the most common cause was ALCOHOLISM. This has been variously known as Korsakoff's syndrome, Korsakoff's psychosis and Korsakoff's amnesia. In 1881 Carl Wernicke (1848–1904) had described related psychological changes in patients (one with alcoholism, the other poisoned by sulphuric acid), describing what became known as WERNICKE'S SYNDROME. Another eminent neurologist, Gudden, made a connection between the two, effectively creating what became known as WERNICKE–KORSAKOFF SYNDROME. This term is often used to describe the features of Korsakoff's syndrome though Wernicke's syndrome differs: Korsakoff's syndrome has AMNESIA as the central feature, whereas Wernicke's syndrome includes a general cognitive dysfunction and motor problems, including DYSPHAGIA and DYSARTHRIA, and disturbances of EYE MOVEMENTS and GAIT. The features of Wernicke's syndrome may precede those of 'true' Korsakoff's syndrome (see WERNICKE–KORSAKOFF SYNDROME).

The psychological disturbance in Korsakoff's syndrome is characterized by both ANTEROGRADE AMNESIA and RETROGRADE AMNESIA, CHRONOTARAXIS and CONFABULATION. In addition, patients will present with SIGNS AND SYMPTOMS characteristic of excessive alcohol use: visual disturbance, motor dysfunction, dry SKIN and loss of hair, altered sensation in the extremities may all be present. Brain damage in the DORSOMEDIAL NUCLEUS OF THE THALAMUS and in the MAMMILLARY BODIES (to which the dorsomedial nucleus of the thalamus are connected via the MAMMILOTHALAMIC TRACT) is thought to be critical in the production of the deficits. Neural damage is thought to be induced by a form of MALNUTRITION induced by excessive alcohol intake. Levels of thiamine (vitamin B1) are severely depleted. This loss creates a difficulty in metabolizing glucose, which in turn leads to neural dysfunction and cell death. Why neuronal loss should be restricted and not widespread is uncertain, though studies with animals have made it clear that thiamine deficiency does have consequential neurotoxic effects. The incidence of Korsakoff's syndrome varies depending on alcohol consumption: rates above 2% of the population showing Korsakoff's syndrome are unusual but not unknown. Treatment for both Wernicke's and Korsakoff's syndromes can be attempted by eliminating alcohol intake and offering thiamine replacement in the diet.

See also: diencephalic amnesia

Krause's end bulbs *see* skin

Krebs' cycle *see* respiration

kuru From a local word meaning 'trembles', kuru is a PRION DISEASE present amongst the Foré people of Papua New Guinea which was spread by ritual cannibalism; see CREUTZFELDT–JAKOB DISEASE.

kynurenic acid (kynurenate) 4-Hydroxyquinoline-2-carboxylic acid: a metabolite of TRYPTOPHAN; a broad-spectrum ANTAGONIST at GLUTAMATE RECEPTORS. It is closely related to QUINOLINIC ACID. Just as it has been suggested that quinolinate might be classed as one of the ENDOGENOUS EXCITOTOXINS, kynurenate has been proposed to be a natural antagonist of this. If this were to be the case, damage would result from an imbalance of kynurenate and quinolinate.

See also: drug ionization

L

L-3,4-dihydroxyphenylalanine The full chemical name for L-DOPA.

L-DOPA Abbreviation for L-3,4-dihydroxyphenylalanine, the direct biochemical precursor for DOPAMINE (see NEUROTRANSMITTERS). In the biosynthetic pathway for CATECHOLAMINE synthesis (dopamine, NORADRENALINE and ADRENALINE), the amino acids TYROSINE and phenylalanine are converted to L-DOPA by the enzyme TYROSINE HYDROXYLASE. L-DOPA is then converted to dopamine by the enzyme DOPA DECARBOXYLASE. In the dopamine-containing neurons of the brain, the dopamine is packaged into VESICLES and serves as the neurotransmitter for that neuron. In noradrenaline-containing neurons, the dopamine is further transformed into noradrenaline. Thus, L-DOPA serves as a precursor for both dopamine and noradrenaline. L-DOPA is best known for its role as the principle pharmacotherapeutic treatment for PARKINSON'S DISEASE, offering relief from symptoms by temporarily increasing levels of dopamine, thus improving motor function. Such treatment is known as a REPLACEMENT THERAPY because it seeks to replace chemicals absent from the diseased brain. L-DOPA is taken orally by patients in combination with a peripheral decarboxylase inhibitor to prevent the L-DOPA being degraded in the gut. (When it was first introduced into clinical practice, very large doses were given because it was not realized how much L-DOPA was being broken down before it reached the brain – see Sacks, 1976.)

Reference

Sacks O. (1976) *Awakenings*, revised edition, Pelican Books: Harmondsworth.

ANN E. KELLEY

lab chow The standard feed given to laboratory animals is always known as lab chow. Specific forms of lab chow are available for different species, often in different forms for growing animals and adults. It is typically in pellet form and contains a balance of all the nutrients required for the maintenance of good health.

labelled-line theory The labelled-line coding theory posits that the meaning of activity in a given NEURON (line) is unequivocally labelled in its meaning: for instance, it codes the sensation of red, sour, or 1000 Hz. Structures such as the kidneys, heart and peripheral nerves have clear, unique functions. But individual neurons each seem to be involved in many functions. A 'red' neuron will respond to many wavelengths, and a 'sour' neuron will respond to taste stimuli other than sour. However this theory accounts well for some stereotyped stimulus–response relationships (see DOCTRINE OF SPECIFIC NERVE ENERGIES). This theory is a small version of the modular coding of more complex events; on both scales the problems of limited information capacity and the BINDING together of various aspects of an event are demonstrated. See the ACROSS-FIBRE PATTERN THEORY for a different orientation to neural coding.

See also: binding problem; engram; grandmother cell

ROBERT P. ERICKSON

labyrinth *see* vestibular labyrinth

lac z A GENE that codes for beta galactosidase (see LACTOSE) and which is often used as a REPORTER GENE in gene transfer experiments.

lacrimal bone skull

lacrimation (Also spelled lacrimation) The production of tears, from the lacrimal gland, in the corner of the EYE (adjacent to the NASAL BONE; see SKULL). Control of lacrimation is achieved by the AUTONOMIC NERVOUS SYSTEM and by innervation from the FACIAL NERVE. Functionally, the production of tears is essential for movement in the ORBITS OF THE EYE and for oxygenation of the CORNEA. In mammals that spend time in the sea (such as otters), lacrimation can help rinse salt water away. Humans are the only SPECIES known to produce excess fluid from the lacrimal gland in response to EMOTION. There is no clear explanation of this phenomenon.

lactation (from Greek, *galaktos*: milk, via Latin, *lactis*: milk) The production of milk by mothers for the nourishment of their offspring. The milk secreted by human mothers (and other mammals) changes composition over time: the initial secretions (for a week) is COLOSTRUM, which contains VITAMINS, milk fat (see LIPIDS), LACTOSE, PROTEINS, MINERALS and IMMUNOGLOBULINS (IgG; see IMMUNE SYSTEM) in different concentrations to the mature milk that is produced after three weeks (the period between colostrum and mature milk production being a transitional phase). Milk production is under the control of various HORMONES: during PREGNANCY; ESTROGEN, PROGESTERONE and CORTICOSTEROIDS are involved in preparing tissues to produce and secrete milk. In late pregnancy, levels of STEROID HORMONES and PROLACTIN levels are high in preparation for active lactation. After birth, steroid, estrogen and progesterone levels fall, but prolactin levels remain high in order to maintain lactation.

See also: suckling

Reference

Johnson M. & Everitt B, (1980) *Essential Reproduction*, Blackwell Scientific Publications: Oxford.

lactose A sugar; a DISACCHARIDE (see SUGARS) also known as milk sugar since it is found in milk. During digestion it is broken down into GLUCOSE and galactose by the ENZYME beta galactosidase. The gene that codes for this is LAC Z.

lambda A skull landmark (the three way cross, shaped like the Greek letter lambda, Λ, formed by the SUTURE junction separating the occipital and parietal bones – see SKULL): important in STEREOTAXIC SURGERY.

Lambertian sources *see* luminance

lamellipodia *see* growth cone

lamina (from Latin, *lamina*: a thin plate) Lamina (plural laminae) is a term used to describe a layer. Neurons (see NEURON) in certain structures are often arranged in layers, often called laminae (for example REXED'S LAMINAE in the SPINAL CORD). Layered structures are said to be laminated.

laminin Laminin is one of the GLYCOPROTEINS that operates as an ADHESION MOLECULE.

See also: growth cone; neural adhesion molecules

landmark task A task used to discriminate perceptual and motor difficulties in SPATIAL NEGLECT. Subjects are presented with a line that has been bisected with another line, perpendicular to it (see LINE BISECTION). They are required to indicate, either verbally or by pointing, the end of the line closest to the transection. Patients with spatial neglect typically indicate the end of the line at the left (their lesion being in the right hemisphere).

See also: parietal cortex

References

Harvey M., Milner A.D. & Roberts R.C. (1995) An investigation of hemispatial neglect using the landmark task. *Brain and Cognition* 21: 59–78.

Bisiach E., Ricci R., Lualdi M. & Colombo M.R. (1998) Perceptual and response bias in unilateral neglect: two modified versions of the Milner landmark task. *Brain and Cognition* 37: 369–386.

language The human faculty of communication; or, a system of spoken communication particular to a community. 'Man has an instinctive tendency to speak', wrote Charles Darwin (1809–1882) in *The Descent of Man*. Human beings acquire language from their environment without explicit instruction being necessary; and although unimpaired individuals will naturally acquire spoken language, SIGN LANGUAGE can also be acquired via environmental exposure. A human being who is exposed to no linguistic input at all in childhood will however fail to acquire normal linguistic competence; in particular, the individual's command of GRAMMAR will be impaired. Language is species-specific (see ACQUISITION OF LANGUAGE BY NON-HUMAN PRIMATES), and is supported by specialized language areas of the brain, especially in the FRONTAL LOBE and TEMPORAL LOBE of the LEFT HEMISPHERE (BROCA'S AREAS, WERNICKE'S AREAS); damage to these areas results in APHASIA.

The particular linguistic system acquired by a developing human will be that of the environment, not of the individual's progenitors: a child of English-speaking parents adopted as an infant by Eskimos will acquire perfect Inuktitut, not English. In childhood, more than one language can be acquired easily (see BILINGUALISM), but languages acquired after childhood will rarely be acquired to full competence, especially in their phonological system (see DEVELOPMENT OF LANGUAGE-SPECIFIC PHONOLOGY).

Eastern African hominids dated by archaeologists at about 100 000 years ago display the lower larynx and larger pharynx characteristic of modern humans, and may have been the first of our ancestors capable of wide-ranging vocal communication. There are currently around 5000 distinct languages in the world, most of which can be grouped into 30 or so language families. English is a member of the West Germanic branch of the Indo-European family, which includes most of the languages of Europe, parts of the Near East, and the Indian subcontinent. It is hard to define what counts as a distinct language versus a dialect; such distinctions are more often drawn for political rather than linguistic reasons. Norwegian and Danish are thus termed separate languages although they are largely mutually intelligible, while Alabama English and Newcastle-upon-Tyne English, or Neapolitan versus Genoan Italian, each pair of which may fail the mutual intelligibility test, are held to be, respectively, dialects of English and Italian. The most important properties of natural language are: (1) the encoding of meaning via sound is arbitrary: with only extremely rare exceptions, the form of language is independent of the meaning it signifies. ('Language' is no more transparent of its meaning than 'Sprache' or 'langue'.) (2) Language is compositional: sentences, words, syllables, phonemes are all composed of elements which can be combined in other ways to make other sentences and so on. (3) Language is systematic and rule-governed. Rules of grammar apply to the order of words within sentences, rules of MORPHOLOGY to the order of morphemes within words, rules of phonology to the order of phonemes within syllables, and so on. In English, *man bites dog* is a possible sentence, but *bites dog man* is impossible; *un-November-y* is a possible word coinage, but *y-November-un* is not; *slomp* is a possible syllable but *lsopm*, *oslmp* and *pmlso* are not. (4) Language is creative; most sentences that a language user speaks, hears (and reads or writes) are novel, at least to that person. Further, because the grammars of natural languages allow recursive operation, every language user is in principle capable of producing an infinite number of different sentences.

The language faculty in humans is not simply dependent upon general cognitive abilities; retarded individuals, with for example WILLIAMS SYNDROME, may have unimpaired linguistic competence, while the condition known as SPECIFIC LANGUAGE IMPAIRMENT is just that – mental impairment which is specific to the use of language, while other cognitive abilities are in principle intact. Language may be encoded in secondary representations such as WRITING. In contrast to the development of spoken language in childhood, the use of such cultural forms of representing language – that is, reading and writing – can only be learned via explicit instruction. Written language, which serves to transmit meaning in the absence of personal contact between the producer and the comprehender, differs from spoken language in many ways: it tends to be more formal, and more elaborate (sentences with several subordinate clauses, and parentheses, such as this one, are more likely to occur in written than in spoken language); it tends to contain fewer contextually bound expressions such as *here* and *this* than spoken language; and in many orthographies writing provides a structural system of punctuation with no direct parallel in speech. Disorders of reading and writing due to developmental impairment or brain injury may also exist independently of other areas of linguistic competence (see ALEXIA, DYSLEXIA, AGRAPHIA, DYSGRAPHIA).

References

Crystal D. (1997) *The Cambridge Encyclopaedia of Language*, 2nd edn, Cambridge University Press: Cambridge.

Pinker S. (1994) *The Language Instinct*, Penguin: London.

ANNE CUTLER

large amplitude irregular activity *see* hippocampal theta

large intestine *see* digestive system

laryngeal Relating to the LARYNX; see MOUTH.

larynx *see* mouth

latent inhibition Latent inhibition (LI) occurs when the repeated non-reinforced presentation of a stimulus retards the subsequent CONDITIONING to that stimulus (Lubow, 1989). Therefore, a latent inhibition experiment typically has two main stages. The first stage pre-exposes the to-be-conditioned stimulus (CS) and the second examines the effects of this pre-exposure on conditioning to the CS. The typical LI effect is that the pre-exposed group show retarded conditioning to the CS, by comparison with a control group that has not received pre-exposures. This means that impairments in LI are expressed by superior conditioning in the non-pre-exposed control group. Impaired latent inhibition is shown when the pre-exposed group do not show retarded conditioning, that is, their performance is significantly *better* than usual (see

Robbins *et al.*, 1993 for idealized data). This is a convenient outcome when studying the effects of neural manipulations such as a DRUG or LESION because it rules out non-specific deficits produced by the neural manipulations such as sensory loss or lack of MOTIVATION in explaining the results.

A simple interpretation of the latent inhibition phenomenon is that it results from an inability to screen out irrelevant stimuli (in this case, the pre-exposed CS). A prominent theory of LI refers to learned inattention as a mediating intervening variable (Lubow, 1989). Several groups have capitalized on this hypothesis to advance latent inhibition as a model for attentional dysfunction in SCHIZOPHRENIA (see Gray *et al.*, 1991). Central to their theorizing is the finding that systemic treatment with rats with AMPHETAMINE reduces latent inhibition, whereas similar treatment with an ANTAGONIST at the dopamine receptor (see DI–D5 DOPAMINE RECEPTORS) such as HALOPERIDOL enhances it. These effects are related to other results which implicate HIPPOCAMPUS–ventral STRIATUM circuitry in the mediation of latent inhibition (see Gray *et al.*, 1991 for a review). However, there is some contradictory evidence – notably manipulations which enhance ventral striatal dopamine function such as intra-accumbens infusions of amphetamine do not appear to affect it (for example, see Killcross & Robbins, 1993). It is beyond the present scope to consider in much more detail this controversy. There is also currently much theoretical debate about the exact interpretation of LI, and explanations other than those considering solely attentional, as distinct from associative, factors need further investigation (see Hall, 1991).

References

Gray J.A., Feldon J., Rawlins J.N.P., Hemsley D.R. & Smith A.D. (1991) The neuropsychology of schizophrenia. *Behavioural and Brain Sciences* 14:1–84.

Hall, G. (1991) *Perceptual and Associative Learning*, Oxford University Press: New York.

Killcross A.S. & Robbins T.W. (1993) Differential effects of intra-accumbens amphetamine and systemic amphetamine on latent inhibition, using an on-baseline, within-subject conditioned suppression paradigm. *Psychopharmacology* 110: 479–489.

Lubow, R.E. (1989) *Latent Inhibition and Conditioned Attention Theory*, Cambridge University Press: Cambridge.

Robbins T.W., Muir J.L., Killcross A.S. & Pretsell D. (1993) Methods for assessing attention and stimulus control in the rat. In *Behavioural Neuroscience: A Practical Approach*, vol. 1, ed. A. Sahgal, pp. 13–47, IRL Press: Oxford.

TREVOR W. ROBBINS

latent learning One kind of learning, is that which results from practice, experience or observation, without the necessity of INCENTIVE MOTIVATION. The term latent learning emerged in the 1930s when Tolman (1886–1959) showed that fully satiated animals allowed to explore a specific environment (a maze for example) would (when later motivated) learn to traverse that environment more rapidly than controls, who had not had the previous, non-reinforced exposure. Hence, some latent learning took place during exposure, specifically related to the details of observed environment, whose influence was not revealed until later testing. In contemporary theories of LEARNING and REINFORCEMENT its acceptance as a form of PROCEDURAL LEARNING or PERCEPTUAL LEARNING and its role in the development of such things as spatial knowledge are relatively well established.

RICHARD C. TEES

lateral Away from the middle, in contrast to MEDIAL, which is toward the middle.

lateral fissure The fissure (see GYRI AND SULCI) that separates the TEMPORAL LOBE from the FRONTAL LOBE and PARIETAL LOBE above it; it is alternatively known as the LATERAL SULCUS, SYLVIAN SULCUS or SYLVIAN FISSURE. It is one of the principal landmarks on the outside of the brain.

lateral geniculate nucleus A nucleus of the THALAMUS devoted to vision, the lateral geniculate nucleus (LGN) relays information from retinal ganglion cells to the PRIMARY VISUAL CORTEX. The nucleus contains six layers, three of which receive input from each eye. Each layer contains a RETINOTOPIC map of one half of the VISUAL FIELD, the left LGN representing the right visual hemifield, and vice versa. Each layer contains relay cells, which project to the visual cortex, and local inhibitory INTERNEURONS. In primates, the two ventral layers (the MAGNOCELLULAR layers) contain large cells that receive their input from the large M-type retinal ganglion cells. The four dorsal layers (the PARVOCELLULAR layers) contain relatively small cells that receive their input from the small P cells of the RETINA. The RECEPTIVE FIELD of LGN relay cells largely reflects the properties of their retinal inputs. All are roughly circularly symmetric, and many have a centre surround organization. ON-centre/OFF-surround cells are excited by increased illumination of the receptive field centre and by decreased illumination of the receptive field surround. OFF-centre/ON-surround cells respond oppositely. Cells in the parvocellular layers have small receptive fields and so represent the visual image with high resolution. They are often colour-selective, with centre and surround regions of the receptive field being most sensitive to different wavelengths of light, for example, red and green, or blue and yellow. Magnocellular cells are much less sensitive to colour than parvocellular cells and have much larger receptive fields. They are, however, more sensitive than parvocellular cells to rapidly changing stimuli such as flickering or moving objects. In addition they may receive stronger input from RODS than do parvocellular cells, and so may be important for night or scotopic vision. Finally, magnocellular cells are more sensitive than parvocellular cells to very small changes in illumination and so are more sensitive to faint (low-contrast) image features. In line with these properties, lesions of the parvocellular layers result in a reduction of VISUAL ACUITY and loss of colour vision. Lesions of the magnocellular layers leave acuity and colour sensitivity intact, but reduce sensitivity to motion. Magno- and parvocellular relay cells project to different layers of the visual cortex (4ca and 4cb), and so the form and colour pathway is kept separate from the motion pathway at several further stages of vision processing. The LGN receives what are thought to be modulatory

synaptic inputs from the RETICULAR FORMA-
TION of the BRAINSTEM. Electrical activation of
these inputs alters the responsiveness of geniculate neurons, and so the likely function of
these inputs is to modulate geniculate function
during changes in attentional state, but the
exact function of these inputs is not well-
understood.

See also: colour vision; visual system

DAVID L. FERSTER

lateral horn A part of the SPINAL CORD: this
has a DORSAL HORN and VENTRAL HORN and,
at thoracic levels, a lateral horn containing
PREGANGLIONIC NEURONS of the SYMPATHETIC
NERVOUS SYSTEM.

See also: autonomic nervous system

lateral hypothalamic syndrome (LH syndrome) Bilateral electrolytic lesions (see LE-
SION) of the lateral area of the
HYPOTHALAMUS produce a characteristic syndrome, first described in 1951 by Anand &
Brobeck, characterized initially by profound
APHAGIA, ADIPSIA and loss of BODY WEIGHT.
However, Teitelbaum & Epstein (1962)
showed that rats recover through an orderly
sequence of stages and are able to maintain
themselves eventually on normal lab chow and
water. In recovery though they continue to
have problems: for example, their MOTIVATION
to work on SCHEDULES OF REINFORCEMENT is
lowered, they fail to respond properly to a
PHYSIOLOGICAL CHALLENGE that normally stimulates eating and drinking and they fail to
show appropriate PRANDIAL DRINKING. They
are also show FINICKINESS in response to
adulteration of their food or water. The LH
syndrome was an integral part of Stellar's DUAL
CENTRES HYPOTHESIS: it appeared to provide
evidence of a brain centre that normally
stimulated feeding. Later theories emphasized
other features, such as the regulation of body
weight, but no account satisfactorily explained
all the signs within one conceptual framework.
In the later 1960s and early 1970s work on the
LH syndrome changed direction for two reasons. First, Valenstein and his colleagues
showed that the eating which followed electrical stimulation of the lateral hypothalamus
was non-specific – if the food was removed,

stimulated rats would more on to another
activity. Second, Ungerstedt showed that 6-
HYDROXYDOPAMINE lesions of the fibres of the
NIGROSTRIATAL DOPAMINE SYSTEM, which travel through the LATERAL HYPOTHALAMUS,
could produce aphagia, adipsia and loss of
body weight without damage to the lateral
hypothalamus. Such lesions also produced a
marked AKINESIA and loss of reactivity to
sensory stimuli, features which also appeared
following lateral hypothalamic lesions. That
the LH syndrome was dissociable was confirmed by studies using EXCITOTOXINS, which
destroyed the lateral hypothalamus but spared
DOPAMINE fibres. Such lesions affect food and
water intake, but to nothing like the degree
that bilateral electrolytic lesions (or nigrostriatal lesions) do. That the lateral hypothalamus
has a role in the control of feeding is supported
by these excitotoxic lesion studies (and electrophysiological experiments indicating that neurons show SENSORY SPECIFIC SATIETY); see
Winn (1995) for a review of this. However,
the LH syndrome, as defined by bilateral
electrolytic lesions is of little academic interest
any more. As with the VENTROMEDIAL HY-
POTHALAMIC SYNDROME, it persists principally
in the continuing popular, but erroneous, belief
that feeding and drinking are controlled by
'brain centres'.

References

Anand B.K. & Brobeck J.R. (1951) Hypothalamic control of food intake in rats and
cats. *Yale Journal of Biological Medicine*
24: 123–140.
Teitelbaum P. & Epstein A.N. (1962) The
lateral hypothalamic syndrome: recovery of
feeding and drinking after lateral hypothalamic lesions. *Psychological Review* 69:
74–80.
Winn P. (1995) The lateral hypothalamus and
motivated behavior: an old syndrome reassessed and a new perspective gained. *Current
Directions in Psychological Science* 4:
182–187.

lateral hypothalamus A long rather diffuse
area running the entire anterior–posterior
length of the HYPOTHALAMUS. The term 'lateral hypothalamic area' has been sometimes
used, indicating that the lateral hypothalamus
is an area lacking precise definition. Indeed, it

does not have the clearly defined structure of nuclei in the midline and core areas of the hypothalamus, and in many ways can be considered as not being part of the hypothalamus. It does not, for example, derive from the same PRIMORDIUM as the remainder of the hypothalamus, developing before all other areas. It is crossed by the many fibre systems of the medial forebrain bundle, for which the lateral hypothalamus appears to serve as a BED NUCLEUS. It has reciprocal connections with many areas of the brain, including the PREFRONTAL CORTEX, NUCLEUS ACCUMBENS, THALAMUS, HIPPOCAMPUS, AMYGDALA and several nuclei in the BRAINSTEM, including the LOCUS COERULEUS, RAPHE NUCLEI and PEDUNCULOPONTINE TEGMENTAL NUCLEUS. It also has connections with the AUTONOMIC NERVOUS SYSTEM via the MEDULLARY RETICULAR FORMATION and DORSAL MOTOR NUCLEUS OF THE VAGUS. It has been implicated in many functions, including FEEDING, DRINKING and SEXUAL BEHAVIOUR. Once thought of as a HUNGER centre (see DUAL CENTRES HYPOTHESIS; LATERAL HYPOTHALAMIC SYNDROME) it is still thought to have a role in the regulation of MOTIVATION, though that role appears more subtle than once thought.

Reference

Winn P (1995) The lateral hypothalamus and motivated behavior: an old syndrome reassessed and a new perspective gained. *Current Directions in Psychological Science* 4:182–187.

lateral inhibition A feature of RECEPTIVE FIELD organization in SENSORY NEURONS (and in other neural systems) whereby signals from a RECEPTOR in one region can be inhibited by those from surrounding regions. This causes the neuron to be strongly activated by contrast (difference between nearby regions) but only weakly by uniform stimulation, giving an efficient sensory code which emphasizes significant stimuli. Lateral inhibition has been most studied in the eyes of arthropods (for example *LIMULUS*) and in mammalian retinal ganglion cells (see RETINAL CELL LAYERS) but it is also an important feature in AUDITORY PERCEPTION and somatosensation.

See also: contrast sensitivity; pattern perception; retina

OLIVER J. BRADDICK

lateral lemniscus (from Greek, *lemniskos*: a ribbon or bandage) A pathway of FIBRES made up of axons (see AXON) coming from the SUPERIOR OLIVARY COMPLEX and the COCHLEAR NUCLEUS and travelling to the INFERIOR COLLICULUS. It also contains cell bodies in the NUCLEI OF THE LATERAL LEMNISCUS, where some of the auditory fibres SYNAPSE.

See also: auditory pathways; dorsal column – medial lemniscal system

lateral line *see* vestibular system

lateral preoptic area *see* preoptic area

lateral reticular area *see* medullary reticular formation

lateral reticular nucleus *see* medullary reticular formation

lateral septum *see* septal nuclei

lateral sulcus *see* lateral fissure

lateral superior olive *see* auditory pathways; sound localization; superior olivary complex

lateral tegmental tract A fibre pathway of the HINDBRAIN; see DORSAL NORADRENERGIC BUNDLE; VENTRAL NORADRENERGIC BUNDLE.

lateral terminal nucleus *see* accessory optic system

lateral ventricles *see* ventricles

laterality *see* lateralization

lateralization In general terms this refers to placing to one side any structure or function in a living organism. The term is usually applied to brain functions mediated asymmetrically by either the left or right cerebral HEMISPHERE, and is closely aligned to the terms CEREBRAL DOMINANCE and HEMISPHERIC SPECIALIZATION; for example, speech functions can be said to be lateralized to the left hemisphere, or the left hemisphere is dominant or specialized for speech functions. In 1861, Broca demonstrated the laterality of cerebral functions when he reported that speech was impaired by damage to BROCA'S AREA, in the left FRONTAL

LOBE. Since then other functions, including speech comprehension (see SPEECH PERCEPTION; SPEECH PRODUCTION), READING, WRITING, calculation (see ACALCULIA, MATHEMATICS AND THE BRAIN), verbal memory (see MEMORY), generating images (see VISUAL SYSTEM), and purposeful skilled movements (see APRAXIA) have been shown to be lateralized to the left hemisphere. Functions lateralized more to the RIGHT HEMISPHERE include SPATIAL COGNITION, music perception (see MUSIC AND THE BRAIN), emotional expression (see EMOTION), non-verbal memory (see MEMORY), and FACE PERCEPTION. Generally, LANGUAGE functions are more lateralized to the LEFT HEMISPHERE than functions are lateralized to the right hemisphere. About 30% of left-handers and 4% of right-handers have speech lateralized to the right hemisphere, although it is less certain whether functions normally lateralized to the right are mediated by the left hemisphere in these people. A number of methods have been developed in order to measure lateralization of human brain functions. The most common approach is to assess patients with lesions restricted to one hemisphere to discover what they cannot do. A second approach is to study patients who have undergone a commissurotomy (see COMMISSURE), where the CORPUS CALLOSUM connecting the two hemispheres is cut to reduce otherwise untreatable generalized SEIZURES. The patient's behaviour is generally unaffected by the DISCONNECTION of the two hemispheres, but psychologists can project stimuli to one half of the brain and by recording the patient's response can isolate functions lateralized to one hemisphere. Methods where sensory stimuli are restricted to one hemisphere can also be used in normal subjects (see DICHOTIC LISTENING TEST, DICHOPTIC TEST). Other methods allowing the study of lateralization include assessing patients who have had a WADA TEST or undergone a HEMISPHERECTOMY. Why lateralization occurs is unknown, but theories include the possibility that left and right hemisphere functions are incompatible and keeping them separate ensures optimal performance, or that the neural space taken up in the left hemisphere by language results in other cognitive functions being relegated to the right hemisphere.

See also: asymmetry; handedness

JENNI A. OGDEN

laterodorsal tegmental nucleus (LDTg) A nucleus embedded in the central grey, perhaps in some ways best considered as a caudal extension of the PEDUNCULOPONTINE TEGMENTAL NUCLEUS. It is best known as the site of the Ch6 CHOLINERGIC neurons (see CH1–CH8) which, with the Ch5 neurons of the pedunculopontine tegmental nucleus, provide the largest cholinergic input to the THALAMUS. Together, the Ch5 and Ch6 neurons, constitute the CAUDAL CHOLINERGIC COLUMN, an uninterrupted column of cholinergic neurons stretching from the LOCUS COERULEUS at the most posterior levels to the caudal pole of the SUBSTANTIA NIGRA. These neurons are thought to form part of the ASCENDING RETICULAR ACTIVATING SYSTEM and to have a role in SLEEP. The difficulty in dealing with laterodorsal tegmental nucleus technically has limited the growth of knowledge about its function. There are no agents with which to make a selective LESION of central cholinergic neurons, and the position of the laterodorsal tegmental nucleus in the central grey adjacent to the CEREBRAL AQUEDUCT makes it very difficult to approach surgically.

laudanum see morphine

laughter Spontaneous laughter as a response to stimuli that can be generically described as comical has not been widely investigated. Rather obviously, there is an inherent difficulty in examining the neuroscience of HUMOUR and comedy, and the responses to it: what is found to be funny does not easily generalize across individuals, or even within a single individual. What is comical in one context may not be in another (and indeed may be, in other contexts, irritating, offensive or embarrassing). However, laughter can be both voluntary (that is, a response to amusing stimulation) or it can be involuntary – that is to say, not under the control of an individual and apparently unrelated to any type of stimulation. The following types of studies into laughter have been conducted. (1) Certain conditions – including HAMARTOMA in the HYPOTHALAMUS and NEURINOMA in the TROCHLEAR NERVE – have been shown to produce GELASTIC SEIZURE. GELAS-MUS is a condition of involuntary hysterical laughter, and has nothing to do with the appreciation of humour. It is a condition often associated with a variety of other pathological signs. (2) Laughter is an emotional response (see EMOTION) and has been used as an index of emotional dysfunction (measured using questionnaires such as the EMOTIONAL LABI-LITY QUESTIONNAIRE). For example, following STROKE or degenerative disorders, emotions may become more labile than normal, and may appear at inappropriate times. Inappropriate emotion is a recognized feature of damage to the frontal lobes (see FRONTAL SYNDROME) but has also been found to follow damage in other, deeper, parts of the brain. For example, patients with AMYOTROPHIC LATERAL SCLERO-SIS have been shown to produce both laughter and crying inappropriately (see for example, McCullagh *et al.*, 1999). (3) The normal appreciation of humour and control of voluntary laughter has been examined using FUNC-TIONAL NEUROIMAGING. Relatively little research has been done, though there is a suggestion that the frontal lobes are involved (Shammi & Stuss, 1999). Given that the appreciation of humour involves quite complex cognitive and social processes it is not surprising perhaps that frontal systems should be involved. Whether there is any possibility of characterizing any part of the brain as being uniquely involved in recognizing 'funny' as opposed to being involved in cognitive processes such as WORD RECOGNITION, WORKING MEMORY, OBJECT RECOGNITION, METAREPRE-SENTATION and so on – processes required to interpret and understand the cognitive and emotional states of ourselves and others – is very far from clear. (4) Some speculation has occurred as to the origin of laughter and humour. Ramachandran (1998) has suggested that it might be possible to account for laughter and humour as derivatives of our past as social PRIMATES, and that they serve as signals of threat, or the removal of threat. (5) Do animals laugh? There has been speculation (in the popular press) that rats laugh. The basis of the speculation is the observation of Panksepp and his colleagues (see Knutson *et al.*, 1998) that rats engaged in PLAY emit high frequency

ultrasonic VOCALIZATIONS. Moreover, exposure to environments in which play has taken place induces more vocalization than exposure to a novel arena, and young rats appear to emit more of these vocalizations than older ones. Of course, the mental states of animals are not accessible to us (only their behaviour is) and as such one cannot know if rats are laughing in a manner that could be considered analogous to human voluntary laughter.

See also: tickle

References

Knutson B., Burgdorf J. & Panksepp J. (1998) Anticipation of play elicits high-frequency ultrasonic vocalizations in young rats. *Journal of Comparative Psychology* 112: 65–73.

McCullagh S., Moore M., Gawel M. & Feinstein A. (1999) Pathological laughing and crying in amyotrophic lateral sclerosis: an association with prefrontal cognitive dysfunction. *Journal of the Neurological Sciences* 169: 43–48.

Ramachandran V.S. (1999) The neurology and evolution of humour, laughter, and smiling: the false alarm theory. *Medical Hypotheses* 51: 351–354.

Shammi P. & Stuss D.T. (1999) Humor appreciation: a role of the right frontal lobe. *Brain* 122: 657–666.

law of effect Very few descriptive principles of psychology are called a 'law'. The law of effect has achieved such status as it has become the very foundation of OPERANT psychology and therefore of modern behavioural study of RE-WARD and ADDICTION – particularly to drugs of abuse (see DRUG ABUSE) – in animal psychobiology. The law of effect was coined by E.L. Thorndike (1874–1949) in 1898 and concerned the ability of certain stimuli, to which he referred as 'satisfiers' (we would call them reinforcers) to increase the frequency of behaviours which produced them. Skipping nearly half a century, Skinner used this basic idea in his concept of REINFORCEMENT where a specific stimulus strengthens an operant behaviour that produces that stimulus. Skinner's use has been incorporated into modern psychobiology. Thus the law of effect is used every time a researcher tests the PLACE CONDITIONING, drug SELF-ADMINISTRATION, or any other operant behaviour that is designed to produce a stimulus or an expectation of it, no matter how simple. To most psychobiologists, no more is needed. However, other aspects of Thorndike's thinking, such as 'stamping in' of stimulus–response connections, or the effects of 'annoyers' (as opposed to satsifiers) had a part to play in early studies of LEARNING.

JAMES R. STELLAR

law of mass action The law of mass action relates to RECEPTOR BINDING. Feldman, Meyer & Quenzer express it as 'the drug and free receptors must combine to form an active complex which leads to a cellular response in proportion to the fraction of receptors occupied' (p. 13). That is, there are a number of RECEPTOR sites to be bound and there are a number of molecules of the LIGAND waiting to bind. The interaction between these is dynamic, with ligand and receptor binding and unbinding continuously, until the ligand is cleared away (see DRUG CLEARANCE). At any given moment, the effect of the binding on cellular activity will be in proportion to the numbers of receptors bound.

Reference

Feldman R., Meyer J.S. & Quenzer L.F. (1997) *Principles of Neuropsychopharmacology*, Sinauer Associates: Sunderland MA.

law of specific energies *see* doctrine of specific nerve energies

lazy eye Colloquial term for AMBLYOPIA.

LD50 The lethal dose, 50%; that is, the dose of a DRUG that kills 50% of the animals tested. The LD50 has been used in the safety testing of commercial products. It is no longer widely used and is never used in experimental studies.

See also: EC50; IC50; ED50; TD50; therapeutic index

lead pipe rigidity *see* rigidity

lead poisoning Lead poisoning, now increasingly rare, has been a noted cause of MENTAL RETARDATION. Generally the SIGNS AND SYMPTOMS of mental retardation would present first. The involvement of lead as an aetiological factor is evidenced by the presence of punctate basophilia (tiny blue grains) in the red BLOOD cells. Lead in the environment has been a notable pollutant, but is now much reduced. The elimination of lead from petrol (gasoline) and from paint has been of significant benefit in this regard.

learned appetite *see* malnutrition

learned helplessness A theory concerning the aetiology of DEPRESSION that suggests that uncontrollable aversive events generate a sense of helplessness from which the SIGNS AND SYMPTOMS of depression develop. The theory was developed by Seligman on the basis of experiments with dogs. Experiments were performed in which dogs worked in yoked conditions (see YOKED CONTROL). Both animals experienced identical conditions: both had levers present in their cages, and both received electric shocks. However, only one animal had control over this: if this animal pressed the lever, the shock was turned off for both dogs. The dog that experienced shocks but had control over their termination remained fit and healthy. The dog that received exactly the same treatment but had no control over it became distressed and then passive and, in later parts of the experiment, had difficulty in acquiring appropriate AVOIDANCE LEARNING. It is this condition that was termed learned helplessness. Later studies showed that this condition was seen in rats and other species, could be ameliorated by ANTIDEPRESSANT treatment and that, behaviourally at least, the condition appeared to fulfill DSM-IV criteria for at least some types of depression.

Some experiments involving humans failed to reproduce these effects and some even showed that situations involving 'helplessness' could improve rather than detract from performance. In humans, ATTRIBUTION plays an important role in determining how situations are perceived. In the face of aversive events, the attributions made by individuals – the degree to which they will accept blame – are important considerations in determining whether or not depression will follow. *Attributional helplessness* reformulates the models developed by Seligman and his colleagues to suggest that a tendency to attribute aversive events to stable and global inadequacies in themselves is a precursor of depression.

Reference

Seligman M.E.P. (1975) Depression and learned helplessness. In *The Psychology of Depression: Contemporary Theory and Research*, ed. R.J. Friedman & M.M. Katz, pp. 83–125. Winston-Wiley: Washington DC.

learned irrelevance An effect seen with CLASSICAL CONDITIONING: an animal LEARNING that a CONDITIONED STIMULUS is irrelevant to another stimulus will ignore it when the events are paired. If the conditioned stimulus is then subsequently used to signal a different UNCONDITIONED STIMULUS, learning will be unimpaired, and even improved. It is an example of the effects of experience on learning.

See also: Kamin's effect; latent inhibition

Reference

Pearce J.M. (1997) *Animal Learning and Cognition*, 2nd edn, Psychology Press: Hove UK.

learning The process whereby an organism interacts with its environment and becomes changed by the experience so that its subsequent behaviour is modified. It will be noted that this definition encompasses a wider range of phenomena than those that would usually be considered as instances of learning by the layperson. For the latter, the term is restricted for the most part to the processes involved in the explicit ACQUISITION of new information (as when a new academic subject is mastered) or of a new skill (as in learning to read or to drive a car). These are clearly instances of learning in terms of the definition just offered, but so is the following. If you leave the room in which you now are and return to it an hour later, your behaviour on returning will be different, because of what you have experienced here on the present visit and also because of what you experienced in the intervening hour. The ways in which your behaviour is changed may not be very dramatic – perhaps you will simply be better able to find this book on the shelf and will want to look up a different entry because of something asked of you while you were away – but these behavioural changes none the less constitute examples of learning in terms of our definition. It is because they have generally adopted this wider interpretation of the concept that psychologists have historically devoted so much effort to the study of the learning process: the way in which behaviour is modified by interaction with the environment is a central topic of psychology.

It is normal to distinguish different types of learning and many different categorizations have been offered. Sometimes distinctions are drawn for immediate practical reasons – for some purposes it may be useful to distinguish motor skill learning from other forms of learning. For other purposes we might want to identify a separate category of rewarded learning as distinct from that generated by the attempt to avoid aversive events; and so on. Such descriptive classifications are not problematic but attempts to distinguish different types of learning that differ at a more fundamental level (for instance, in terms of the mechanisms that underlie them) have provoked considerable debate. Thus, for example, some theorists have maintained that PAVLOVIAN CONDITIONING and INSTRUMENTAL CONDITIONING involve quite different processes, whereas other have emphasized what they take to be important similarities between the two. (The modern consensus is that both should be viewed as versions of ASSOCIATIVE LEARNING, differing principally only in the nature of the events that enter into association.) Again, some have wanted to make a distinction between learning based on the cumulative effect of a series of training trials (as when a rat slowly acquires the behaviour of pressing a lever to obtain food) from behaviour patterns that are suddenly acquired (as when an ape in a flash of 'insight' piles boxes together to get to an item of food otherwise out of reach). But others have pointed out that the behaviour of the ape can be shown to depend on its having had, earlier in its life, protracted experience of manipulating objects such as boxes and of the consequences of these actions and to this extent the ape's behaviour too is a product of the cumulative effect of a series of (informal) training trials.

The distinction that seems most likely to survive is that between associative and non-associative learning. The former depends on the animal having experience of paired events and the change in behaviour produced by this experience is the consequence of the formation of some link between the central representations of these events. (Pavlovian conditioning constitutes the paradigm case.) There are, however, a number of examples of learning in which the animal is exposed not to a pairing but to just a single event, thus precluding any simple explanation in terms of the associative mechanism. Examples include HABITUATION (the waning of the unconditioned response initially evoked by a stimulus as a consequence of repeated presentations of that stimulus); IMPRINTING (the acquisition by a young animal of filial responses to a conspicuous object experienced early in life); PERCEPTUAL LEARNING (enhancement of the discriminability of a stimulus as a result of exposure to that stimulus). It should be noted, however, that these instances are defined solely by exclusion (that is, simply as not being associative) and thus there is no guarantee that all are products of a common underlying mechanism. Closer examination could reveal that a distinctively different learning process operates in each case.

GEOFFREY HALL

learning curve A graph plotting degree of success on a task against time or the number of trials (see TRIAL): one expects improvement over time, the rate of improvement reflecting an interaction between task difficulty and subject aptitude.

learning difficulty *see* mental retardation

learning disability *see* mental retardation

learning set In an attempt to evaluate one aspect of the proposition that subjects can learn a new problem faster if they have experiences with other problems of the same type, a number of procedures, paradigm or tasks, most notably the learning set task, have been developed. In the classic version of this learning set task, subjects are presented with two different and unfamiliar stimulus objects on a trial. The choice of one (S+) is paired with positive REINFORCEMENT while the choice of the other (S−) is not. The same objects are used as S+ and S− for a total of six trials, which constitutes one DISCRIMINATION problem. Another two new unfamiliar objects serve as S+ and S− for the subsequent six trials of the second discrimination problem,

then another two objects for the third and so on. (Usually, objects used in one problem never reappear in later discrimination problems.) Harlow (1905–1981) was the first to use this kind of task to demonstrate that animals can learn more in a discrimination task than which stimulus dimension they should attend to – that is, they could 'learn to learn'. The improvement in the rate of learning observed in normal adult members of several species tested across the many different discrimination problems reflected the development of a learning set. Performance for extensively tested and retested subjects is close to 100% on trials 2–6 in each of the discrimination problems they are tested on. The subjects respond as thought they are aware that if a stimulus choice is correct on first trial, that the same object is correct for all six trials of each problem. If their stimulus choice on the first trial is incorrect, then the other stimulus will be correct on the remaining five trials in the same way they learn the left-right position of the objects is irrelevant. Thus, on the basis of whether they are reinforced on each first trial on a problem, they adopt a WIN–STAY, LOSE–SHIFT strategy for the remaining trials and problems. Acquisition of a learning set can also demonstrated in other experimental test circumstances (such as in repeated discrimination reversal, single or double alternation tasks).

See also: learning

RICHARD C. TEES

lectin *see* tract tracers

Lee–Boot effect The name give to the observation that female animals housed together show a slower than normal (or even stopped) MENSTRUAL CYCLE, an effect caused by the presence of specific PHEROMONES.

See also: Bruce effect; Vandenbergh effect; Whitten effect

left hemisphere The left hemisphere of the human brain looks very like a mirror image of the right hemisphere, and in terms of gross anatomy, and primary sensory and motor functions it also parallels the right hemisphere. It differs, however, from the right hemisphere with respect to the higher cognitive functions it mediates. Most obviously it is specialized for LANGUAGE functions, but is also better able to perform many other functions that are dependent upon or associated with purposeful actions, sequencing or generative abilities.

Both cerebral hemispheres can be divided into four lobes; the FRONTAL LOBE, PARIETAL LOBE, TEMPORAL LOBE, and OCCIPITAL LOBE. The cerebellar hemispheres at the base of the cerebral hemispheres are concerned mainly with motor coordination, muscle tone, and balance. Each side of the body is mapped topographically onto areas of PRIMARY MOTOR CORTEX and PRIMARY SENSORY CORTEX in the opposite cerebral hemisphere. Thus if a LESION is placed in the thumb area of the left motor cortex, the right thumb would be paralysed, or if the lesion was in the left thumb area of the sensory cortex, the right thumb would feel numb. Primary cortex in the left temporal lobe receives auditory information, mainly (but not entirely) from the right ear, and primary cortex in the left occipital lobe receives visual information from the right visual field. Adjacent to the areas of primary cortex lie zones of secondary or ASSOCIATION CORTEX. The neurons in these zones receive information from the primary cortices and integrate it into meaningful wholes. Thus the ability to perceive what one is touching (parietal), hearing (temporal) or seeing (occipital) may be impaired when these zones are damaged. Where the association cortices of the parietal, temporal and occipital lobes meet is an area called the TERTIARY CORTEX. Here information from the different lobes is integrated, and damage to this zone can lead to complex, cross-modal higher cognitive impairments (such as an inability to write to dictation). Another large area of tertiary cortex lies at the very front of the frontal lobes; this is called the PREFRONTAL CORTEX. This area mediates executive functions such as strategic planning, problem solving, abstract thinking, and the ability to behave appropriately, and there appears to be little LATERALIZATION of these functions.

While the two hemispheres share some higher functions, each is specialized to a greater or lesser degree for many abilities. For example, the medial left temporal lobe (the HIPPOCAMPUS) is more adept at learning new

verbal material like word lists, and the right hippocampus is better at learning new patterns and tunes (non-verbal material). The main difference between the two hemispheres is the left hemisphere's specialization for language functions. The right hemisphere has no functions that are as clearly specialized as these. Damage to BROCA'S AREA in the third frontal gyrus, and WERNICKE'S AREA in the left posterior superior temporal lobe, result in expressive and receptive APHASIA respectively. Other types of aphasia and acquired reading, WRITING and SPELLING impairments result from damage to other areas of left-hemispheric cortex and connecting fibre tracts. Interestingly, deaf people fluent in SIGN LANGUAGE also become aphasic in the same way as normal speakers following the same sorts of left-hemispheric damage. The ability to talk has lead to the idea that the left brain is the conscious, self-aware brain, although there is evidence from experiments on SPLIT BRAIN patients that the mute right brain is also self-aware and conscious; but must express this non-verbally.

Performing purposeful actions (PRAXIS) is the other primary specialization of the left brain. Disorders of praxis, i.e. the various types of APRAXIA, are usually caused by damage to the left parietal cortex. For example, the patient may not be able to demonstrate the use of a toothbrush (with either hand), may be unable to copy actions performed by someone else, or may even be unable to blow a kiss. One explanation for apraxia is that the left parietal lobe contains the movement formulas for the execution of skilled movements. Damage to this area or its connections to the motor strip of the frontal lobe can result in apraxia. Damage to the CORPUS CALLOSUM, the fibre tract connecting the hemispheres, can also result in apraxia for movements attempted by the left hand. This may be because the right-hemispheric MOTOR STRIP controlling the left hand is disconnected from the movement formulas in the left hemisphere. Finally, there is some evidence that the left brain is the 'happy brain' and the right brain the 'depressed brain', as some patients with large left-hemispheric lesions become severely depressed (because their intact right hemisphere takes over their EMOTION). Of course, becoming aphasic may be sufficient to cause depression, and the happy behaviour of some patients with right-hemispheric lesions may be associated with other symptoms of unawareness related to right-hemispheric damage.

JENNI A. OGDEN

left–right confusion This is also known as RIGHT–LEFT CONFUSION; and the term disorientation can be used instead of confusion. During normal development most children learn to differentiate right and left, both in external space and in terms of the bilateral organization of their own bodies. A deficit in discrimination can take several forms – it can present as a straightforward inability to tell left from right or, more complicatedly, an inability to recognize right–left mirror images. Difficulties in INTERHEMISPHERIC TRANSFER might underlie these problems. Left–right confusion features in a number of syndromes, including GERSTMANN SYNDROME and TURNER'S SYNDROME. There is some evidence from clinical studies that damage to the left PARIETAL LOBE might be involved, though brain damage is not thought likely to lie behind the simpler forms of right–left confusion.

lemniscus *see* dorsal column – medial lemniscal system; lateral lemniscus

lens The crystalline lens of the EYE is the secondary refractive component of the visual apparatus, the main one being the CORNEA. In man, the shape of the lens capsule can be altered by muscular effort (ACCOMMODATION) and this provides a means by which the optical power of the eye and hence its focal length may be adjusted to suit a range of viewing distances. This ability is lost through ageing leading to an almost total lack of accommodative power (PRESBYOPIA).

DAVID W. HEELEY

lentiform nuclei (from Latin, *lens*, *lentis*: a lentil) Lentiform is a term used to describe anything that has the shape of a lentil or lens. The lentiform nuclei include the GLOBUS PALLIDUS and PUTAMEN.

See also: basal ganglia; corpus striatum

leptin Leptin is a PROTEIN secreted from FAT CELLS and the PLACENTA which has actions to control FEEDING, BASAL METABOLIC RATE and some reproductive functions (principally to do with the placenta). Leptin release from fat cells is stimulated by such things as GLUCOCORTI-COIDS and agents that act at beta ADRENOCEP-TORS. Leptin circulating in the blood has access to specific RECEPTORS in the CENTRAL NERVOUS SYSTEM (most likely in the HYPOTHALAMUS, but possibly in other structures as well) and binding of leptin to these receptors affects, directly or indirectly, the release of a variety of peptides, including NEUROPEPTIDE Y and GALANIN – secretion of both of these is reduced. These actions lead to changes in peripheral tissues: both GLUCOSE and INSULIN levels in the blood are decreased. Lack of leptin, as occurs in the OB/OB MOUSE and ZUCKER RAT for example, leads to increased food intake, and low ENERGY expenditure, which of course promotes OBESITY.

Lesch–Nyhan syndrome A rare neurological disorder, affecting only males. First described over 30 years ago, this X-chromosome-linked recessive disease (see X AND Y CHROMOSOMES) is characterized by severe mental retardation, spasticity, CHOREOATHETOSIS, and compulsive self-mutilation. It is caused by an inherited deficiency in the levels of an enzyme important for PURINE metabolism called hypoxanthine-guanosine phosphoribosyl transferase (HPRT or HGPRT). The lack of this enzyme results in overproduction of uric acid. The HPRT gene has been isolated on the long arm of the X chromosome, and its structure characterized. While a great deal of research has been done on the genetic basis of the disorder, the precise neuropathological basis of the severe behavioural and neurological symptoms is not known. There is also a marked depletion of DOPAMINE in the BASAL GANGLIA associated with the disorder. Thus it is hypothesized that disruptions in neurotransmitter functions within basal ganglia and other brain regions are responsible for the symptoms.

ANN E. KELLEY

lesion Lesion is used both as a noun and as a verb to describe damage done to the central nervous system (a lesion) and the process of making it (to lesion). Lesions may be present in patient groups or may be inflicted deliberately on experimental animals. Lesioning is one of the main techniques used experimentally to investigate brain–behaviour relationships, the rationale being that if a selected piece of brain tissue is removed, subsequent behavioural changes (compared to non-lesioned subjects) will reveal something about the normal function of the lost tissue. Lesions have revealed much about brain function, but caution has to be used in assessing their effects. For instance, the absence of a particular function does not necessarily imply that, normally, lesioned tissue exclusively mediates that function.

Experimental lesions are made in several ways. Fibre pathways can be interrupted by a KNIFE CUT LESION. This involves insertion of a microknife which can be moved to sever fibre pathways. Tissue at the surface of the brain can be destroyed by an ASPIRATION LESION (which sucks tissue away) or by SPRITZING (dusting NEUROTOXINS onto the brain). Within the brain, lesions can be made by passing electric current via an electrode, insulated except at the tip (ELECTROLYTIC LESIONS or RADIOFREQUENCY LESIONS). All these techniques are relatively non-selective in terms of tissue destruction. Greater selectivity can be achieved using chemical neurotoxins. EXCITO-TOXINS destroy neurons but spare fibre systems, while GLIOTOXINS destroy GLIAL CELLS rather than neurons. However, often the goal of experimental lesioning is to produce as selective a lesion as possible, which means targeting chemically identified neurons. 6-HY-DROXYDOPAMINE (6OHDA) acts only on CAT-CHOLAMINE neurons and 5,7-DIHYDROXYTRYP-TAMINE (5,7DHT) acts only on SEROTONIN neurons. Other than these though there are no neurotoxins selective for particular neurochemical systems. One way round this difficulty is to raise an ANTIBODY selective for a molecule which uniquely identifies a population of neurons and which can be internalised (taken inside a neuron). If the antibody is tagged with a neurotoxin (such as SAPORIN) normally excluded from the inside of the neuron, it can provide entry for the toxin into the neuron. This technique has been used successfully but is still in development.

In order to relate behavioural change to damage done, it is critical to have as accurate an understanding as possible of the damage present in the central nervous system. Lesions must be verified therefore by HISTOLOGY, measurement of brain neurochemistry, or some form of FUNCTIONAL NEUROIMAGING.

See also: ablation; conotoxins; endogenous excitotoxins; Huntington's chorea; ischaemia; transient lesions; tumour

lethal dose 50 *see* LD50

letter-by-letter alexia *see* letter-by-letter reading

letter-by-letter reading An ACQUIRED READ-ING DISORDER in which words are identified letter-by-letter rather than as complete forms. Also known as PURE ALEXIA.

ELAINE FUNNELL

leucine An amino acid; see TRACT TRACERS.

leucotomy *see* psychosurgery

leukaemia A cancerous disorder of tissue responsible for the formation of white blood cells. Some cases may result from exposure to chemicals, radiation or viruses. Acute and chronic forms of leukaemia differ in their clinical course according to the type of cell series affected; for example, acute lymphoblastic leukaemia predominates in children and is rapidly fatal but may be curable with IMMU-NOSUPPRESSANT anti-cancer drugs. Acute and chronic myeloid leukaemia affects LEUKOCYTES of the polymorphonuclear series (NEUTRO-PHILS, EOSINOPHILS and BASOPHILS) originating in the bone marrow and spleen, and response to treatment is less favourable.

L. JACOB HERBERG

leukocyte A white blood cell; found in the BLOOD and an important component of the IMMUNE SYSTEM.

leupeptin A protease inhibitor (that is it inhibits the actions of any ENZYME that degrade proteins) which has been used to interfere with the development of LONG-TERM POTENTIATION. It has fairly non-specific effects though and has not, consequently, been widely used. However, see Morris *et al.* (1987) for an interesting example of its use in biological psychology.

Reference

Morris R.G.M., Hagan J.J., Nadel L., Jensen J., Baudry M. & Lynch G.S. (1987) Spatial learning in the rat – impairment induced by the thiol proteinase inhibitor, leupeptin, and an analysis of [3H] glutamate receptor binding in relation to learning. *Behavioral and Neural Biology* 47: 333–345.

level skull *see* stereotaxic surgery

levels of processing A theoretical framework in human cognitive psychology that states that the type of processing that is applied to information when it is registered (see ENCODING) determines how well this information can later be consciously recollected (see CONSCIOUS RECOLLECTION). It is assumed that incoming stimuli can be processed at different levels of analysis, with deeper levels reflecting more meaningful processing (see SEMANTIC). If stimuli are processed in terms of their meaning (DEEP ENCODING), they will be remembered better in EXPLICIT MEMORY tests than if they are processed in terms of their physical appearance (SHALLOW ENCODING). Evidence from FUNCTIONAL NEUROIMAGING studies suggests that deep encoding engages left PREFRONTAL CORTEX regions more strongly than shallow encoding does.

See also: declarative memory; engram; episodic memory

STEFAN KÖHLER

lever press *see* nose poke vs. lever press

Lewy bodies These bodies, named by Frederic H. Lewy (1885–1950) a German neurologist working in the USA, are found within the brain in certain pathological conditions. They are found within the CYTOPLASM of neurons and are particularly associated with PARKINSON'S DISEASE, for which they are considered a pathological marker. They have been considered as a potential cause of Parkinson's disease, but this is thought to be unlikely: they are more probably an index of neuronal degeneration rather than a cause of it. In this condition they accumulate in several parts of the BRAINSTEM, most particularly in the SUBSTANTIA

NIGRA. They also appear in the brains of patients with ALZHEIMER'S DEMENTIA and in a condition known as LEWY BODY DEMENTIA. The principal component of Lewy bodies appears to be alpha SYNUCLEIN.

Lewy body dementia This is a form of senile DEMENTIA (it is also known as SENILE DEMENTIA of the Lewy body type) in which there are extensive deposits of LEWY BODIES. Features of this disorder include motor deficits reminiscent of those seen in PARKINSON'S DISEASE; a rather variable cognitive impairment (which resembles that seen in ALZHEIMER'S DEMENTIA) and features such as HALLUCINATION more commonly associated with conditions such as SCHIZOPHRENIA. Patients are very sensitive to ANTIPSYCHOTIC medication, so some care is need in diagnosis of Lewy body dementia. The disorder has only been classified relatively recently, but evidence is accumulating that loss of ACETYLCHOLINE from the CEREBRAL CORTEX and HIPPOCAMPUS is a significant feature (as it is in Alzheimer's disease).

Reference

Perry R., McKeith I. & Perry E. (1997) Lewy body-dementia – clinical, pathological and neurochemical interconnections. *Journal of Neural Transmission* (Supplement) 51: 95–109.

lexical decision task In this task, subjects are asked to discriminate real words (spoken or written) from nonsense words, saying 'yes' to *mate*, for example, but 'no' to *mave*. The measures of interest are the accuracy and speed with which subjects can accept different types of words (varying in word frequency or part of speech or semantic class for example) and reject different types of non-words (for instance, varying in degree of phonological or orthographic similarity to real words). This task is often used in studies of SEMANTIC PRIMING, where the speed of accepting a target word is facilitated by a preceding semantically related prime word (the response 'yes' to *nurse* is faster if the word *doctor* has just been heard or seen). Lexical decision has been considered a relatively pure measure of access to the internal lexicon, though it is now clear that many different factors/sources of information may influence lexical decision responses.

ELAINE FUNNELL AND KARALYN E. PATTERSON

lexicon (mental lexicon) The MEMORY store containing the pairing of word form and meaning for all vocabulary items a person knows. These may be single WORDS, or compound words (*look up*; *hot dog*), or fixed phrases (*good heavens*; *break the ice*), or stems (*hench-*), or affixes (*un-*, *-able*). The content of the lexicon differs across languages, some languages having mostly stand-alone words, others mostly stems and affixes. The size of an educated adult's lexicon has been estimated at over 150 000 entries. Access of the lexicon in WORD RECOGNITION involves mapping a word form (spoken or written) onto its meaning; in SPEECH PRODUCTION meanings are activated first, word forms later.

See also: language

ANNE CUTLER

libido *see* sexual behaviour

librium *see* chlordiazepoxide

lick suppression Obviously, lick suppression is the cessation of licking. It is used as a measure in many studies where the ability of a STIMULUS to prevent behaviour needs to be measured: studies involving CONDITIONING of FEAR for example often use lick suppression to measure the extent to which a fear inducing stimulus can inhibit activity that would otherwise proceed (because the lick would be directed to collecting a POSITIVE REINFORCER).

lidocaine Lidocaine is a LOCAL ANAESTHETIC, related to PROCAINE and indeed to COCAINE (which has local anaesthetic properties). Lidocaine has also been used successfully to make TRANSIENT LESIONS in the CENTRAL NERVOUS SYSTEM.

lie detection It is assumed that when individuals are about to lie, and when they are in the act of lying, physiological changes take place. These are AROUSAL-like changes mediated by the AUTONOMIC NERVOUS SYSTEM. Measurement of such things as changes in SKIN CONDUCTANCE and brain electrical activity using a POLYGRAPH is thought to enable scientists to discriminate when lies are being told, a procedure familiar from countless movies and television programmes. It is not as accurate as might be hoped, and is not therefore in routine use. It has more technically been called interrogative polygraphy.

ligand (from Latin, *ligare*: to bind) Strictly, any chemical that forms a complex with another; in practice, a chemical that binds to a RECEPTOR molecule. Any DRUG that binds to a receptor, whether an AGONIST or ANTAGONIST, can be described as a ligand. NEUROTRANSMITTERS can be described as the natural ligands for specific types of receptor.

ligand-gated ion channels *see* voltage-sensitive ion channels

ligature (from Latin, *ligare*: to bind) A LIGATURE is a binding; to *ligate* is the verb and *ligation* refers to the act of making a ligature. Although ligature can refer to any form of binding, in medicine it refers generally to a small, surgically applied binding, often made with the intention of closing off a VESSEL of some sort. For example, ligation of the VAS DEFERENS is the principal feature of a VASECTOMY (see TESTES).

light microscopy In light microscopy, tissue SECTIONS are examined under a microscope with either an artificial light source or natural light; it is routine microscopy as generally conceived. The term BRIGHTFIELD indicates light coming through the condenser of the microscope which is focused on the object under study on the microscope stage. In contrast, the term DARKFIELD indicates that a special condenser is being used which directs light that is oblique to the objective through which material is being examined. This allows one to examine a CELL against a dark background. FLUORESCENCE microscopy requires incident light – light directed down onto the material under study. The resulting fluorescence of the material is returned though the objectives and is seen.

See also: confocal microscopy; electron microscopy; histology

light therapy The presentation of bright light for periods every day to simulate sunshine, used in SEASONAL AFFECTIVE DISORDER.

Likert scale *see* questionnaire studies

limbic This is a term often used as an adjective to describe either BRAIN structures or functions. Of course, it relates to the LIMBIC SYSTEM: member structures are described as 'limbic', and the functions of those structures are described as 'limbic'. However, 'limbic system' as an anatomical construct has attracted criticism (see the references below) because it has become a rather imprecise term. To describe functions as limbic amounts very often to little more than a vague acknowledgement that an action has something to do with EMOTION. Limbic is not a particularly helpful term to use and should probably be avoided, other than when used in a clearly defined manner.

References

Blessing W.W. (1997*a*) Inadequate framework for understanding bodily homeostasis. *Trends in Neuroscience* 20: 235–239. [This article was then the subject of a short debate in the literature; the letters below followed this one.]

Spyer K.M. & Herbert J. (1997) Do we need a limbic system? *Trends in Neuroscience* 20: 508–509.

Blessing W.W. (1997*b*) Reply. *Trends in Neuroscience* 20: 509.

limbic cortex A rather vague term, more or less synonymous with the terms ALLOCORTEX and JUXTALLOCORTEX combined. In practice, limbic cortex can be defined as those parts of the CEREBRAL CORTEX included in the LIMBIC SYSTEM.

limbic system (from Latin, *limbus*: border) The limbic system consists of a ring of structures that line the inner border of the cerebral hemispheres, as well as the diencephalic (see DIENCEPHALON) structures closely associated with them. These include the PARAHIPPOCAMPAL GYRUS, CINGULATE CORTEX, SUBCALLOSAL GYRUS, HIPPOCAMPUS, AMYGDALA, MAMMILLARY BODIES of the HYPOTHALAMUS, and anterior thalamic (see THALAMUS) nuclei. Other structures that are often included in the limbic system are the entire hypothalamus, the SEPTAL NUCLEI and the HABENULA. The limbic system governs emotional aspects of behaviour, memory, and pleasure and pain.

The concept of the limbic system derives from the term *grand lobe limbique* that was used by Paul Broca (1824–1880) in 1878 to refer to the inner cortical structures. He did not discuss its function. In 1937, James Papez (1883–1958) proposed that a closed neuronal circuit through these structures underlies the expression of emotion. This circuit, known as PAPEZ CIRCUIT, starts with the hippocampus, and is relayed through the mammillary body, anterior thalamic nuclei, and cingulate cortex, and back to the hippocampus. In 1937, Klüver & Bucy reported that bilateral damage to the temporal lobes (see TEMPORAL LOBE), including the hippocampus and amygdala, produces dramatic changes in emotional behaviour in monkeys (see KLÜVER–BUCY SYNDROME). In the 1950s, Paul MacLean suggested the term limbic system which refers to all of the structures mentioned as well as the hypothalamus, septal nuclei, NUCLEUS ACCUMBENS, and ORBITOFRONTAL CORTEX. McLean also suggested that the limbic system represents a phylogenetically old part of the brain. These early studies provided the basis for studying the neurobiological basis of EMOTION.

Although the general scheme of the limbic pathways conceived by the early investigators was validated by modern anatomical studies, many corrections were also made in the details, and many connections have been added to the old scheme. The major input to the hippocampus is now known to come from the ENTORHINAL CORTEX via the PERFORANT PATH, not from the cingulate cortex, which instead projects to the SUBICULUM. Because the entorhinal cortex receives input from the adjacent ASSOCIATION CORTEX in the temporal lobe, it provides a link between the NEOCORTEX and the limbic system. The projection to the mammillary body via the FORNIX has been found to arise in the subiculum, and not in the hippocampus as originally thought. The mammillothalamic tract has been confirmed, but the anterior thalamic nuclei have been found to project to the subiculum, rather than to the hippocampus proper. The subiculum in turn projects to the entorhinal cortex, the origin of the perforant path to the hippocampus. The subiculum also has reciprocal connections with association areas of the neocortex. Thus, like the entorhinal cortex, the subiculum is an important link between the neocortex and the limbic system.

The only major output of the hippocampus, originating from its PYRAMIDAL NEURONS, is directed to the lateral septum. Different hippocampal regions map in an orderly way onto the lateral septum, and from there onto the hypothalamus. These topographic (see TOPOGRAPHY) or orderly projections may have a role in mediating the expression of different classes of goal-oriented behaviour. The lateral septum also projects to the medial septum, which in turn projects back to the hippocampus through CHOLINERGIC and GABAERGIC pathways. These pathways are important in the generation of the HIPPOCAMPAL THETA waves, a characteristic rhythmical activity of the hippocampal ELECTROENCEPHALOGRAM in animals. The amygdala consists of three regions, the corticomedial nuclei which receive massive olfactory input, the basolateral nuclei which are interconnected with certain neocortical regions, and the central nucleus which projects directly to the hypothalamus and certain autonomic nuclei in the BRAINSTEM. The amygdala and the hippocampal formation are also interconnected. Thus, the limbic system may be viewed as an interconnected network interfacing between the neocortex and the hypothalamus, thus functionally associating MOTIVATION and EMOTION with cognitive functions.

The scope and the function of the limbic system have expanded considerably since its original conception. Much of what is now recognized as the limbic system was originally known as the RHINENCEPHALON or 'smell brain'. However, the early studies had already made it clear that the limbic system governs not only OLFACTION, but also emotional behaviour. Furthermore, more recent studies have convincingly shown that some parts of the limbic system are involved in cognitive functions which are not traditionally associated with the limbic system. For example, the amygdala, while having a role in olfaction

through its extensive olfactory input, is involved in memory associated with emotion. Similarly, the hippocampal formation is clearly involved not only in olfaction and emotion, but also in LEARNING and MEMORY. These advances in our understanding of the function of limbic structures have made the term limbic system somewhat less useful than it was in the past. As suggested by several authors, most recently Blessing, time may have come to abandon the term 'limbic system'.

KAZUE SEMBA

limbic system-associated membrane protein That a typical MEMBRANE possesses PROTEINS – NEURAL ADHESION MOLECULES – which can serve as signals during NEURODEVELOPMENT is well known. These have the potential to identify particular anatomical units or systems. Levitt and his colleagues identified LIMBIC SYSTEM ASSOCIATED-MEMBRANE PROTEIN, one of the GLYCOPROTEINS of 64–68 000 molecular weight that appears to identify selectively neurons in LIMBIC SYSTEM structures and in structures receiving projections from this. Identification of molecules such as this might provide a basis for identification of the limbic system, an entity whose composition has not been without controversy.

Reference

Côté P.-Y., Levitt P. & Parent A. (1995) Distribution of limbic system-associated membrane protein immunoreactivity in primate basal ganglia. *Neuroscience* 69: 71–81.

limbic–motor interface The location, or network of locations, in the brain where information from the LIMBIC SYSTEM (that is, information concerned with EMOTION and MOTIVATION) gains access to the motor system, in order that desires and goals can influence behavioural output. The ventral STRIATUM has been considered as the anatomical area most likely to fulfil this role: it is appropriately connected, receiving direct input from many components of the limbic system, thus privy to motivational information, whilst also having privileged access to the motor system. Indeed, the term LIMBIC–MOTOR INTERFACE was used by Mogenson (1931–1991) to describe the functions of the ventral striatum (see Mogenson, 1980). However, the anatomical location has not been unequivocally established (see Winn, 1997) and therefore this term, notwithstanding the anatomical implications of 'limbic', is more usefully used with reference to the psychological processes rather than anatomical structures or systems. Motivational information can affect motor output in different kinds of ways. An alternative approach to asking the anatomical question concerning the structures wherein limbic and motor information may converge, is to define the psychological functions of the limbic-motor interface and to consider the neural basis of these functions. It is likely that in the future, this approach will lead to the identification of a network of areas which compromise the limbic-motor interface. The selection of responses is based upon intention, goals and drive. Without an interface of limbic and motor systems, the organism would be unable to select responses appropriately and might be unable to translate a CENTRAL MOTIVE STATE to action. Thus, firstly, limbic information needs to access the systems determining response choice. A second aspect of motor behaviour which is modulated by motivation is the strength (or vigour) of a response. Thus, limbic information needs access to the systems governing response vigour. Finally, on the basis of changing conditions, there is an interruption of ongoing behaviour, either to switch to a new response or simply to cease the current response. The persistence of a response is an aspect of response control with implications for both response choice and vigour: in the absence of competing responses or diminishing desire, the response will persist, but responses will also persist longer when the initial drive is greater and therefore persistence might also be correlated with response vigour. In the absence of limbic information influencing the motor system, responses will terminate or persist without relevance to motivation.

References

Mogenson G.J., Jones D.L. and Yim C.Y. (1980) From motivation to action: functional interface between the limbic system and motor system. *Progress in Neurobiology* 14: 69–97.

Winn P., Brown V.J. and Inglis W.L. (1997) On the relationship between the striatum and

the pedunculopontine tegmental nucleus. *Critical Reviews in Neurobiology* 11: 241–261.

VERITY J. BROWN

limen *see* threshold

Limulus An arthropod – a crab of the king crab genus – that has been used extensively in experiments examining LATERAL INHIBITION.

line bisection A simple task used to examine patients with SPATIAL NEGLECT: individuals are asked simply presented with a line drawn on a sheet of paper and asked to place a line at 90° to this, as near as they can to the exact halfway point along it. Normal subjects make a reasonably accurate guess at this. Patients with spatial neglect, not attending to one side of space, will consistently place their line off to one side.

See also: landmark task

linear hierarchy of dominance *see* dominance

linear perspective *see* perspective

lingual Pertaining to the TONGUE; for example, the lingual part of the GLOSSOPHARYNGEAL NERVE deals with the tongue.

lingual gyrus A major gyrus (see GYRI AND SULCI) of the TEMPORAL LOBE that is an important part of the VISUAL SYSTEM.

See also: colour anomia; face perception

lipase An enzyme that degrades LIPIDS.

lipids Lipids are molecules that have the properties of FAT. Neuronal membranes are composed of lipids known as PHOSPHOLIPIDS (because they contain phosphates). Other lipids in neural tissue are the CEREBROSIDES, found in MYELIN. Cerebrosides are members of the lipid classes GLYCOLIPIDS (because they contain one of the SUGARS) and SPHINGOLIPIDS (because they contain sphingosine). GANGLIOSIDES are lipids found in neuronal membranes. PROTEOLIPIDS have a protein component. Disruption of lipid synthesis, structure or activity can lead to dysfunction of neuronal membranes, which of course can lead to profound disturbance of function.

Reference

Feldman R.S., Meyer J.S. & Quenzer L.F. (1997) *Principles of Neuropsychopharmacology*, Sinauer Associates: Sunderland MA.

lipid bilayer membrane The MEMBRANE of a NEURON is composed of PROTEINS and LIPIDS. Such a membrane is often referred to as a LIPID BILAYER MEMBRANE, being composed of two layers of lipids. The lipids are each made of three components: a hydrophilic head (it repels water), a GLYCEROL spine and two tails of FATTY ACIDS. On each side of the membrane, a hydrophilic head faces outwards; the tails interlock centrally. RECEPTOR molecules and other forms of TRANSPORT process are embedded in this lipid bilayer.

lipid solubility Neuronal membranes are composed of LIPIDS. Any DRUG that is highly lipid soluble will have better access through membranes therefore. Lipid solubility is a property of a drug that can be tested for, giving an indication of the likely degree to which it will penetrate brain tissues.

Reference

Feldman R.S., Meyer J.S. & Quenzer L.F. (1997) *Principles of Neuropsychopharmacology*, Sinauer Associates: Sunderland MA.

lipoprivation Restriction in the amount of FAT available (fat deprivation); a stimulus to FEEDING.

lipoprotein A lipoprotein is a conjugated LIPID and PROTEIN. They are found in BLOOD where they transport CHOLESTEROL.

liposome (from Greek, *lipos*: fat, *soma*: body) A globule of any of the LIPIDS found in the CYTOPLASM of a CELL.

liposuction (from Greek, *lipos*: fat, and English, suction) The removal of fat by surgically withdrawing it using of negative pressure. It is a radical treatment for the reduction of BODY WEIGHT.

Lissauer's tract Lissauer's tract (also known as *Lissauer's fasciculus* in older literature) is found in the SPINAL CORD. Its typical AXON has its CELL BODY in the SUBSTANTIA GELATINOSA and projects topographically to neighbouring segments of the spinal cord. It has functions related to PROPRIOCEPTION.

lissencephalic (from Greek, *lissos*: smooth, *enkephalon*: brain) Having a smooth CEREBRAL CORTEX, without GYRI AND SULCI. The human brain is most definitely not lissencephalic; the RAT brain most definitely is.

list learning Procedure for MEMORY testing that requires the acquisition of a group of items which form a list – for instance, words in humans; object-reward associations in non-human animals.

See also: discrimination learning; free recall; learning

STEFAN KÖHLER

Lister hooded rats *see* rat

Listing's law *see* eye position

lisuride An ergot-derived drug which acts as an AGONIST at DOPAMINE receptors with greater effect at D2 rather than D1 receptors. It is used as an adjunct to L-DOPA in the treatment of PARKINSON'S DISEASE. BROMO-CRIPTINE and PERGOLIDE are similar ergot-derived drugs.

lithium (Li) Alkaline metal element, used as carbonate or citrate salt in the treatment of AFFECTIVE DISORDER. Principal indications include the prevention of MOOD swings in MANIC DEPRESSION, prophylaxis of recurrent UNIPOLAR DEPRESSION and as an ADJUVANT in the treatment of poorly responsive DEPRESSION. As the drug is potentially toxic, regular blood tests are required to ensure that the amount of lithium in the blood is sufficient to be effective but below toxic levels (range: 0.5–1.0 mmol/litre). Lithium appears to exert its therapeutic effect by acting on SECOND MESSENGERS in the central nervous system.

IAN C. REID

lithium chloride (LiCl) A salt of LITHIUM not used in the treatment of AFFECTIVE DISORDER (as other lithium salts are). In biological psychology lithium chloride is injected into experimental animals after exposure to a novel food or fluid in order to produce a state of NAUSEA as part of FOOD-AVERSION LEARNING tests.

liver A lobed structure that sits immediately below the ribcage with many vital functions. It is the largest single internal organ in the mammalian body and has critical functions, mostly to do with BLOOD. Blood comes to and from the liver from the intestine, spleen, gall bladder, pancreas and stomach via the *hepatic portal vein* and the *hepatic artery* (HEPATIC is the adjective meaning pertaining to the liver). The liver has many functions relating to the synthesis of PROTEINS for PLASMA; detoxification of the blood (removal of DRUG metabolites for example); and storage. It is an important site for the storage of certain VITAMINS (the human liver contains sufficient vitamin B12 to last for 12–36 months) and GLYCOGEN, a POLYSACCHARIDE found in MUSCLES and the liver. It is important because it can be mobilized very rapidly to provide energy to fuel processes such as FIGHT-OR-FLIGHT. (The ENERGY stored as FAT cannot be mobilized quickly.) The pancreatic enzyme GLUCAGON promotes the mobilization of glycogen. The liver is under neural control of the VAGUS NERVE, as well as the SPLANCHNIC NERVE and PHRENIC NERVE. The vagus nerve also carries sensory information back to the central nervous system. OSMORECEPTORS, GLUCORECEPTORS and mechanisms for detecting the ION (e.g. SODIUM) balance in the blood are all present in the liver and all capable of relaying information to the central nervous system. Similarly, structures in the BRAINSTEM and HYPOTHALAMUS are involved in the regulation of liver function. The state of the liver appears to be a critical determinant of behaviour, especially of FEEDING. Glucose applied to the liver in experimental conditions promotes strong firing in the vagus, while infusion of glucose into the hepatic portal vein inhibits it. Several authors have speculated that the liver has a greater degree of control over feeding than does the brain.

lobe A lobe is a division of tissue or an organ: in biological psychology the term lobes is generally taken to mean the four principal lobes of the BRAIN: FRONTAL LOBE, PARIETAL LOBE, OCCIPITAL LOBE and TEMPORAL LOBE.

lobectomy The surgical removal of a lobe from the BRAIN, usually the TEMPORAL LOBE (for the control of EPILEPSY) or frontal tissue; see PSYCHOSURGERY.

lobotomy Casual term for early psychosurgical procedure destroying the frontal lobes (see FRONTAL LOBE) in an effort to treat psychiatric disorder.

See also: leucotomy; psychosurgery

IAN C. REID

local anaesthetic A drug that induces a lack of sensation when applied locally to a relatively small region. Typically, local anaesthetics block nerve conduction in the affected region, thus reducing or blocking transmission of PAIN signals to the brain. Local anaesthetics are extremely useful and are used extensively in many minor surgical procedures, dentistry, ophthalmic and nasal surgery. They are also used in spinal and epidural anaesthesia. In this case they are injected into the appropriate region of the spinal column, usually in combination with other drugs, and induce blockade of nerve conduction in a large body area. Commonly used drugs of this type include LIDOCAINE, PROCAINE, and COCAINE.

ANN E. KELLEY

local circuit neuron *see* interneurons

local enhancement *see* stimulus enhancement

local representation *see* neural coding

local signs *see* retinal local signs

locale memory *see* memory

localization of function The degree to which psychological or behavioural functions are localized within the brain remains a matter of some controversy. Much of the thinking about this has been dominated by PHRENOLOGY. Phrenologists believed that different areas of the brain controlled different functions and that the larger an area was, the more the function it controlled would be developed. They measured the size of different regions of the skull in the belief that this would provide a representation of the volume of brain tissue below. This methodological approach is now clearly discredited, but the underlying theory persists and twentieth-century theorists used and developed similar lines of argument. For example, it was thought for many years that states such as HUNGER, THIRST and SEXUAL AROUSAL were controlled by specific drive centres in the HYPOTHALAMUS (see DUAL CENTRES HYPOTHESIS). However, recent thinking about DISTRIBUTED PROCESSING and NEURAL NETWORKS has created a climate in which it is much less clear how psychological processes could be localized to particular brain centres.

What is important when considering localization of function in the brain is the nature of the function under study. Clearly the brain is not a uniform mass of cells: some neurons have properties that others do not. The magnocellular neurons of PARAVENTRICULAR NUCLEUS OF THE HYPOTHALAMUS and the SUPRAOPTIC NUCLEUS OF THE HYPOTHALAMUS are the only ones in the central nervous system that synthesize and release VASOPRESSIN into the bloodstream in response to dehydration, a function unambiguously tied to these neurons. At a rather more psychological level, it is evident that different parts of the visual cortex (see AREAS V1–V5) have different functions and that damage in different parts of it will produce different visual deficits. But MEMORY is a process that seems to be less clearly localized, though it is associated with specific neural processes (see LONG-TERM POTENTIATION; HEBBIAN SYNAPSE). Skinner thought that the relationship between memory and the brain was best understood as being the same as that between a battery and electricity: no matter how a battery might be cut up, the electricity will not be found. It is a property of the battery rather than a localizable function. One might conclude therefore that some processes are localized to specific neurons; some are localized to particular brain systems; and some are the properties of distributed networks of neurons.

One further point is worth considering. Sensory processes; learning and memory, and the organization of motor systems are things achieved by all of the VERTEBRATES and a great many INVERTEBRATES. These seem to be fundamental neural properties. In humans at least, one has also to consider emotions. States such as hunger or thirst do not have the same status as visual perception or learning. Hunger and thirst are types of EMOTION, interpretations of

bodily states that we learn to make for ourselves. It has been argued that emotions are critical for decision-making (see SOMATIC MARKER HYPOTHESIS) but it can also be argued that emotions are not intrinsic brain properties. As Ryle (1949) suggested, they are things for which diagnoses are required rather than things required for making diagnoses. How emotions localize to brain systems is a complex issue.

See also: attributions; equipotentiality; equivalence; redundancy; dualism

References

Damasio A.R. (1994) *Descartes' Error: Emotion, Reason and the Human Brain*, Putnam Press: New York.

Farah M.J. (1994) Neuropsychological inference with an interactive brain: a critique of the 'locality' assumption. *Behavioural and Brain Sciences* 17: 43–104.

Ryle G. (1949) *The Concept of Mind*, Hutchinson: London.

localization of sound *see* sound localization

locomotion Most forms of locomotion in VERTEBRATES are rhythmic, involving repeated cycles of movements of the body and/or the limbs. (An exception is BRACHIATION – the swinging through trees practised by certain PRIMATES.) During behaviours like WALKING, RUNNING, SWIMMING and FLIGHT, locomotor movements are produced by coordinated contractions of ANTAGONISTIC MUSCLE pairs. Rhythmic locomotion comprises two phases of movement: the POWER STROKE (when thrust is generated against the environment) and the RETURN STROKE (when reverse thrust is minimized). In swimming vertebrates, like fish and amphibian tadpoles, the segmented myotomal muscles on opposite sides of the body act as antagonists to bend the body to the left and right sides. Each side of the body acts alternately as the power and the return stroke. For limbed vertebrates, muscles controlling the joints of each limb are also arranged as antagonists that are active in alternation during locomotion. Most limb muscles are associated with either the FLEXOR PHASE (return stroke) or the EXTENSOR PHASE (power stroke) of the movement cycle. The power stroke, when the limb is generating thrust against the substrate, is also called the STANCE PHASE; when the limb is flexed, moving forwards above the substrate in preparation for the next power stroke, it is said to be in the SWING PHASE.

During each cycle of locomotion spinal MOTOR NEURONS discharge an ACTION POTENTIAL burst followed by a quiescent period when they are inhibited from firing. This cyclical bursting activity can be produced by a network of spinal cord neurons, often called an OSCILLATOR or CENTRAL PATTERN GENERATOR (CPG). Spinal CPGs can generate rhythmic locomotor activity in the absence of both sensory information (following deafferentation) and descending signals from the brain (following SPINALIZATION). The sequence of rhythmic discharge in motor neurons generated after deafferentation and spinalization is called FICTIVE LOCOMOTION. The synaptic input to motor neurons during locomotion consists of periods of excitation (caused by excitatory postsynaptic potentials; see EPSP/IPSP) leading to action potential bursts, separated by periods of inhibition (caused by inhibitory postsynaptic potentials; see EPSP/IPSP) when motor neurons are prevented from firing. In a wide range of vertebrates the excitation results mainly from activation of GLUTAMATE RECEPTORS. Two types of glutamate receptor are activated: NMDA and non-NMDA (kainate/AMPA) receptors. In some vertebrates a component of the excitation during locomotion is known to result from central cholinergic connections between spinal motor neurons. Vertebrate motor neurons use the transmitter ACETYLCHOLINE (ACh) at the NEUROMUSCULAR JUNCTION to elicit muscle contraction. The intrinsic membrane properties of motor neurons may also contribute to rhythm generation: in several animals motor neurons oscillate between two voltage levels (one near RESTING POTENTIAL and the other near action potential THRESHOLD) following activation of NMDA-type glutamate receptors. These non-linear responses occur independently of, but may sum with, the synaptic drive during locomotion. They rely upon the unusual properties of the NMDA receptor type of ION CHANNEL which allows CALCIUM entry into neurons and

which is voltage-dependent in the presence of MAGNESIUM ions.

The inhibition that occurs between motor bursts (called mid-cycle or RECIPROCAL INHIBITION) is coincident with activity in antagonistic motor neurons. The inhibition hyperpolarizes the membrane potential of motor neurons and reduces their input resistance to prevent action potentials. During reciprocal inhibition, chloride ion channels open to allow the influx of negatively charged chloride ions into motor neurons. The channels are associated with membrane bound receptors for the inhibitory amino acid GLYCINE and they are opened when spinal inhibitory INTERNEURONS release glycine onto motor neurons. Reciprocal inhibition during locomotion can be blocked by the glycine receptor antagonist, strychnine. The mid-cycle inhibition helps to ensure that antagonists are active in alternation.

Although spinal CPGs can operate without sensory information, feedback resulting from locomotor movements is important for adjusting the timing and intensity of motor neuron activity. Proprioceptive feedback (see PROPRIOCEPTION feedback) (also called REAFFERENCE) arises from sense organs that are activated by the movements that occur during locomotion. Two important sources of sensory feedback to spinal CPGs are the MUSCLE SPINDLE and GOLGI TENDON ORGAN that generate information about muscle length and tension, respectively. They generate information that encodes both limb position (for instance, joint angle) and the amount of load over the body. Proprioceptors are important in determining the timing of transitions between the two phases of movement. Golgi tendon organs generate positive feedback during the stance phase (power stroke), while muscle spindle activity increases towards the end of stance to terminate stance and trigger swing. The rhythmic signals from proprioceptive afferents can entrain the central motor program (see MOTOR PROGRAMMING): for example, during TREADMILL LOCOMOTION the feedback that is generated causes walking speed to match that imposed by the treadmill.

Sensory information changes if unexpected motor errors occur (for example, when an unexpected obstacle is encountered). This activates EXTEROCEPTIVE afferents that elicit corrective reflexes. The form of the reflex can depend upon the phase of the movement cycle in which the sensory input occurs (called PHASE-DEPENDENT REFLEXES). In cats, for example, tactile stimulation of the dorsal surface of the paw elicits limb flexion if the stimulus coincides with the stance (flexion) phase, but limb extension is evoked if the same stimulus occurs when the limb is on the ground during the stance phase.

Spinal CPGs are also influenced by systems of neurons in higher brain centres, especially those of the BRAINSTEM. Populations of brainstem neurons that influence locomotion form discrete clusters called nuclei. Brainstem nuclei interact with spinal CPGs in three ways: (1) initiation of locomotion; (2) fast adjustments to locomotion; and (3) slow modulation of locomotor intensity and frequency. Locomotor activity can be initiated following electrical stimulation of the so-called MESENCEPHALIC LOCOMOTOR REGION which might initiate locomotion by activating reticulospinal neurons. Once in progress, locomotion can be altered by activation of fast descending pathways. These pathways derive from particular brainstem nuclei and act on specific phases of the movement cycle. For example, DEITER'S NUCLEUS gives rise to the VESTIBULOSPINAL TRACT and is thought to regulate ipsilateral extensor activity; the RETICULAR FORMATION and the RED NUCLEUS give rise to the RETICULOSPINAL TRACT and the RUBROSPINAL TRACT and are thought to act on the flexion phase of the movement cycle. The intensity and duration of motor bursts during locomotion can also be modulated by descending brainstem pathways such as those from the LOCUS COERULEUS and the RAPHE NUCLEI. Most is known about the raphe nuclei whose neurons are predominantly SEROTONERGIC. Serotonin affects many aspects of CPG function but the main effect is to increase the intensity and duration of motor bursts in each cycle of locomotion.

There is considerable interest in the neural mechanisms of locomotion, both in their own right and for functional reasons. The analysis of gait, posture and the pattern of running and walking is, for instance, of considerable value to professional athletes and to physiotherapists developing rehabilitation programmes for patients who have suffered injuries. In psychopharmacological studies of animals, locomotion is often examined to determine whether or not a treatment of some sort – typically drug administration – has a generalized effect on behaviour. It is assumed (not always correctly) that if a drug has stimulant properties it will, in the absence of anything more interesting for the recipient to do, generate locomotion. For instance, AMPHETAMINE will increase selectively responding on a lever associated with CONDITIONED REINFORCEMENT (as opposed to a non-reinforced lever) but the doses of amphetamine that have this effect will also stimulate locomotion, if there is nothing else for the animal to do. Locomotion can thus be seen in this example as a 'default activity' in which an animal will engage if there is nothing more interesting to do. These actions of amphetamine have been associated not with brainstem mechanisms but with activation of dopamine systems in the NUCLEUS ACCUMBENS. Stimulation of the HIPPOCAMPUS can also elicit a strong locomotor response. There has been some debate in the literature about whether the locomotion stimulated from the nucleus accumbens and hippocampus is merely activation or EXPLORATION.

The measurement of locomotion in laboratory animals can be done in several ways. The simplest way is to count the numbers of times an animal crosses floor markers. If an arena is divided on the floor into quadrants, the numbers of crosses from one quadrant to another can be counted, either by direct observation or from video recordings. Rather more sophisticated are cages equipped with photocell beams that detect and register movement without an animals being aware of the recording. Hinged floor plates which activate microswitches are occasionally used to give similar output, though movement of the floor can distract an animal. Exploration can be measured in a BERLYNE BOX, CARLSON BOX or HOLEBOARD TEST. OPEN FIELD locomotion can also be measured. In these, animals will typically restrict their movements to the perimeter until they have became accustomed to the environment. Movement into the centre of an open field can therefore be used experimentally to measure degrees of NEOPHOBIA or ANXIETY.

References

Robbins T.W. (1997) A critique of the methods available for the measurement of spontaneous locomotor activity, in *Handbook of Psychopharmacology, vol. 7, Principles of Behavioral Pharmacology*, eds Iversen L.L., Iversen S.D. & Snyder S.H., pp.37–82, Plenum Press: New York.

Sillar K.T. (1994) Synaptic specificity: development of locomotor rhythmicity. *Current Opinion in Neurobiology* 4:101–107.

KEITH T. SILLAR

locus coeruleus (from Latin, *locus*: place, *coeruleus*: sky blue) The locus coeruleus, so named after its slightly bluish colour in fresh human brain sections, is located in the dorsal PONS and contains about 12 000 neurons on each side in humans. This small collection of neurons is, astonishingly, the major source of NORADRENALINE in most structures in the CENTRAL NERVOUS SYSTEM. While their projections are topographically (see TOPOGRAPHY) organized, many locus coeruleus neurons innervate more than one target, sometimes widely separated structures such as the CEREBRAL CORTEX and CEREBELLUM. The locus coeruleus is implicated in the modulation of sensory, motor and autonomic functions, as well as AROUSAL and ATTENTION.

See also: ascending reticular activating system; dorsal noradrenergic bundle; reticular formation; sleep; ventral noradrenergic bundle

KAZUE SEMBA

locus of rise *see* rate frequency curve

long-term amnesia The inability to form new long-term memories. This falls under a more general classification of memory deficits called ANTEROGRADE AMNESIA, which indicates the inability to form new long-term memories. This is distinct from RETROGRADE AMNESIA, which is the inability to recall memories formed prior to the onset of amnesia (memory for past events). Long-term amnesia spares many realms of cognition. PRIMING, skills, and the LEARNING of HABITS are intact in long-term amnesiac patients. Additionally, long-term amnesia does not cause WORKING MEMORY or SHORT-TERM MEMORY deficits.

HOWARD EICHENBAUM

long-term depression Long-term depression (LTD) is an activity-dependent form of synaptic plasticity, the counterpart to LONG-TERM POTENTIATION (LTP). LTD can be HOMOSYNAPTIC (in which the activated synapses themselves are depressed) or HETEROSYNAPTIC (in which depression in one set of synapses is induced by activity in a neighbouring set). There are persuasive theoretical reasons for postulating the existence of a mechanism for reversing LTP, in order to avoid the loss of plasticity which would occur if LTP were to become saturated. On the other hand, this argument does not demand the existence of LTD, since LTP itself decays naturally over a period of days. Be that as it may, while there were sporadic reports of both homosynaptic and heterosynaptic LTD in the hippocampal (see HIPPOCAMPUS) literature following the first description of LTP in 1973, it was not until the publication of a reliable protocol for the experimental induction of homosynaptic LTD by Dudek & Bear (1992) that the phenomenon became accessible to routine experimental investigation. The induction protocol for producing LTP in young animals requires a long train of low-frequency stimuli, typically 900 stimuli at 1 Hz; in the adult animal, a modification of this protocol consisting of repetitive pairs of pulses, is more effective. Like LTP, LTD is input-specific; whether it is also associative has not been established, although in most (but not all) studies, its induction has been found to be dependent on NMDA RECEPTORS. Induction of LTD is also blocked by protein phosphatase inhibitors.

Long-term depression in naive, unpotentiated synapses should be distinguished from a related phenomenon, DEPOTENTIATION or erasure of LTP at potentiated synapses: the same stimulus protocols which induce LTD will also reduce a previously potentiated response to baseline levels. Is depotentiation simply LTD superimposed on LTP, or is it rather a true reversal of LTP? The following observation suggests the latter: if LTP is first saturated by delivering repeated episodes of tetanic stimulation, and depotentiation is then induced with a low-frequency train, synaptic efficacy can once again be increased by tetanic stimulation (see

TETANUS), indicating that LTP is no longer saturated, and must have been reversed. There is evidence that the degree of tetanus-induced calcium increase in the postsynaptic cell determines whether LTP or LTD is produced. Both LTP and LTD have been implicated in the activity-dependent mechanisms which control and refine the mapping and segregation of axons in the developing visual system.

See also: Hebb's postulate; Hebb-like rule; Hebbian synapse

Reference

Dudek S.M. & Bear M.F. (1992) Homosynaptic long-term depression and effects of N-methyl-D-aspartate receptor blockade. *Proceedings of the National Academy of Science USA* 89: 4363–4367.

T. V. P. BLISS

long-term memory Permanent or lasting memories for objects, facts, personal experiences, and other events. The amount of time between the original learning experience and the permanent establishment of long-term memory can range from seconds to years. Long-term memory consists of several different types of memory, typically separated into DECLARATIVE MEMORY, or EXPLICIT MEMORY, versus non-declarative, procedural, or IMPLICIT MEMORY.

Uncertainty surrounds the issue of when long-term memory begins and when its final CONSOLIDATION ends. Several issues must be taken into consideration, including species, experimental tools for assessing memory (biochemical, physiological, behavioural), and whether one is looking at FORGETTING after LEARNING or RETROGRADE memory loss after some sort of brain insult (see RETROGRADE AMNESIA). For example, biochemical and physiological studies of facilitation of the gill withdrawal reflex in APLYSIA indicate that SHORT-TERM MEMORY lasts from minutes to hours, whereas long-term memory ranges from one to many days. By contrast, studies of forgetting in human amnesic patients with deficits in long-term memory indicate that short-term memory lasts only seconds, after which information is lost, suggesting performance depends on long-term memory as of that time. On the other hand, measures of retrograde memory loss, that is the loss of memories obtained prior to brain insult, indicate that the consolidation of long-term memories is not completed for many months to years.

The proposed neurobiological mechanisms responsible for memory, both short and long term, are assumed to be similar across species, despite the differences in time course. Short-term memory, briefly, in contrast to long-term memory does not involve protein synthesis. It does, however, involve the system of SECOND MESSENGERS. Studies in *Aplysia* using SEROTONIN have led to the proposal that short-term memory is a gating action by intracellular CYCLIC AMP molecules on certain types of ION CHANNEL altering ion conductance through cell membranes. These changes act immediately to enhance or suppress the responses of postsynaptic cells in response to presynaptic neurotransmitter release thereby temporarily changing LOCAL CIRCUIT properties. Long-term memory requires greater involvement of the downstream intracellular products of ion channels coupled to G PROTEIN. These products eventually make their way into the nucleus leading to GENE EXPRESSION and, consequent on that, protein synthesis. This last step, requiring the greatest amount of time, leads to structural changes in ion channels within pre- and postsynaptic terminals which are the proposed long-lasting anatomical bases for the persistence of memories.

Long-term memory is composed of many different components, defined and supported by the distinct anatomical (and memory) systems mediating those different forms of long-term memory: declarative, or explicit, memory supported by medial temporal lobe structures; non-declarative, or implicit, memory proposed to be supported by striatal and select cortical regions. Declarative memory is described as flexible, the expression of learned items or events is not dependent upon replication of original learning event; relatively quick rate of acquisition; potential for inaccuracy (due to either ENCODING or RETRIEVAL failure). Non-declarative memory, in contrast is inflexible, expression is dependent on original learning event and the response systems used during acquisition; has slow rate of acquisition, motor skill and LEARNING of HABITS (with the exception of PRIMING) require large number of trials, despite potential for having no knowledge of learning experience; expression of implicit memories is dependable with little chance of error.

See also: engram; Hebbian synapse; long-term potentiation; long-term depression

HOWARD EICHENBAUM

long-term potentiation Long-term potentiation (LTP) is an activity-dependent form of synaptic plasticity which provides a compelling model for the synaptic basis of learning. First described in the HIPPOCAMPUS (Bliss & Lømø, 1973; see Bliss & Collingridge, 1993 for review), LTP is also found in other brain regions, including NEOCORTEX and AMYGDALA. In hippocampal slices, or in anaesthetized animals, LTP induced by brief tetanic stimulation (see TETANUS) can last for several hours; in animals with chronically implanted electrodes (see ELECTRODE) it can persist for several days. The induction of LTP requires the tetanus to be above a threshold intensity (the property of cooperativity). LTP displays two other properties which enhance its attraction as a mnemonic device: input specificity which limits potentiation to activated synapses, and associativity, which allows LTP to be induced by a weak sub-threshold tetanus to one pathway, provided it is coincident with a strong tetanus to a second, converging pathway (see HEBBIAN SYNAPSE).

In most cases, the induction of LTP is controlled by postsynaptically located NMDA RECEPTORS. (An exception is hippocampal LTP at synapses made by granule cell axons onto CA3 pyramidal cells). Specific antagonists of the NMDA receptor, such as APV (D-amino-phosphonovalerate), suppress the induction of LTP, without affecting the predominantly AMPA receptor-mediated synaptic responses evoked by single stimuli. Once LTP is induced, however, NMDA receptors appear to play no further role in its expression. At resting levels of membrane potential, the NMDA receptor channel is blocked by magnesium (Mg^{2+}) ions, and the opening of the channel requires both the binding of transmitter and strong local DEPOLARIZATION; it is this voltage dependence

of the NMDA receptor which leads directly to the properties of cooperativity, associativity and input specificity. Activation of the NMDA receptor is both necessary and sufficient for the induction of LTP. The block of LTP by APV establishes the former; the latter is shown by experiments in which LTP is induced by procedures which satisfy the requirements for activation of the NMDA receptor – for example, by repeatedly pairing single afferent stimuli with depolarizing pulses delivered to the target cell through an intracellular electrode. All this can be summarized in the following induction rule for LTP: *a synapse will be potentiated if and only if it is active at a time when the dendrite on which it is located is strongly depolarized.* Whether this rule is rigorously obeyed is not known; there are indications that input specificity, for example, is not absolute. Since the NMDA channel is permeant to calcium (Ca^{2+}) ions, and since the induction of LTP is blocked by postsynaptic injection of Ca^{2+} chelators (see CHELATING AGENT), the immediate trigger for the induction of LTP is probably the entry of Ca^{2+} through activated NMDA channels.

Two temporal components of LTP have been distinguished: early-LTP, lasting 4–6 hours, and late-LTP. Late-LTP is blocked by protein synthesis inhibitors providing these are present around the time of induction. Early-LTP is sensitive to PROTEIN KINASE inhibitors, in the presence of which only SHORT-TERM POTENTIATION (STP), lasting about an hour, survives. It is likely that early-LTP is maintained in part by postsynaptic changes, including PHOSPHORYLATION of GLUTAMATE receptors, and in part by presynaptic modifications leading to a sustained increase in transmitter release. Since induction is a postsynaptic process, any presynaptic contribution to the expression of LTP implies the existence of a mechanism which informs the presynaptic side of the synapse about the postsynaptic inductive event. A number of candidates have been proposed for the role of 'retrograde messenger', including NITRIC OXIDE and ARACHIDONIC ACID. Late-LTP may be mediated by structural changes involving both pre- and postsynaptic elements. The requirement for GENE TRANSCRIPTION in late-LTP suggests that a signal passes from the activated synapses to the soma to initiate transcription, and that a gene product then travels back from the soma to act only on the activated synapses. There is evidence that the activated synapses are tagged in some way which permits them to selectively respond to the SOMATOFUGAL message(s).

How good is the evidence that LTP is exploited by the brain to store information? Early experiments were consistent with the hypothesis: when infused into the hippocampus, the NMDA receptor antagonist APV blocked both LTP and LEARNING in the WATER MAZE. However, subsequent experiments have shown that once rats have learnt the task, APV does not prevent relearning in a different context. More recently, studies of second-generation transgenic animals, in which LTP in the hippocampus can be modulated on demand (Mayford et al., 1997), and experiments showing that in fear conditioning, the auditory CONDITIONED STIMULUS evokes a response in the AMYGDALA which is potentiated by an LTP-like process as the result of training (Rogan et al., 1997) have provided powerful new evidence in favour of the hypothesis.

See also: engram; Hebb's postulate; Hebb-like rule; Hebbian synapse; long-term depression

References

Bliss T.V.P. & Lømo T. (1973) Long-lasting potentiation of synaptic transmission in the dentate area of the anaesthetized rabbit following stimulation of the perforant path. Journal of Physiology 232: 331–356.

Bliss T.V.P. & Collingridge G.L. (1993) A synaptic model of memory: long-term potentiation in the hippocampus. Nature 361: 31–39.

Mayford M., Mansuy I.M. Muller R.U. & Kandel E.R. (1997) Memory and behavior: a second generation of genetically modified mice. Current Biology 7: R580-R618.

Rogan M.T., Staubli U.V. & LeDoux J.E. (1997) Fear conditioning induces associative long-term potentiation in the amygdala. Nature 390: 604–607

T. V. P. BLISS

longitudinal fissure Also known as the INTER-HEMISPHERIC FISSURE, this is the long FISSURE that separates the two HEMISPHERES of the BRAIN is the longitudinal fissure. Towards the posterior pole of the brain, where the right OCCIPITAL LOBE is separated from the left, it may be known as the median longitudinal fissure.

longitudinal section *see* planes of section

lordosis (from Greek, *lordos*: bent back) A distinctive curvature of the spine. The term can be applied in a variety of circumstances, but in biological psychology it generally refers to the position (frequently called the 'lordosis posture') adopted by female rats during COPULATION. It is a flexion of the spine downwards, and has the effect of presenting the vagina to the mounting male.

See also: estrus; gender

Lou Gehrig's disease Lou Gehrig's disease is AMYOTROPHIC LATERAL SCLEROSIS. Lou Gehrig (1903–1941) was an American baseball player – first base for the New York Yankees in the American League. He set a record of 2130 consecutive games played, one not bettered until 1995. He was elected to the Baseball Hall of Fame in 1939 and his life story was made into a feature film (*Pride of the Yankees*, 1942) with Gary Cooper in the lead role. Before he developed it, amyotrophic lateral sclerosis was not well-known but his popularity was such that the disease became associated with him in the public mind. The well-known mathematician, physicist and author Stephen Hawking is another well-known sufferer.

loudness Loudness is the subjective correlate of auditory stimulus intensity or AMPLITUDE. In practice, loudness also depends on the distribution of stimulus energy across the frequency domain. Thus, if the overall energy of a narrowband noise is held constant and only the bandwidth is increased, loudness remains roughly constant until the stimulus exceeds a critical bandwidth, and then begins to increase. Loudness, then, presumably depends on both the amount of activity within a frequency-specific perceptual channel, and the number of channels activated.

DENNIS P. PHILLIPS

low affinity *see* affinity

low voltage fast activity Low voltage fast activity is characteristic of ALPHA WAVES and is associated with desynchronization of the CEREBRAL CORTEX (see SYNCHRONY/DESYNCHRONY).

See also: electroencephalogram; sleep

LSD LSD (lysergic acid diethylamide) is a semi-synthetic derivative of lysergic acid, an ALKALOID found in ERGOT, a parasitic fungus (*Claviceps purpurea*) that grows on rye and wheat. In the Middle Ages, consumption of infected grains resulted in vast outbreaks of ERGOTISM, the illness that arises from ingestion of the compounds in ergot, including ERGOTAMINE and lysergic acid. One symptom of ergotism was HALLUCINATION, which may have led people to believe that such affected people were possessed by demons. In the 1940s, the chemist Albert Hofmann at Sandoz Drug Company in Basel, Switzerland, was experimenting with various derivatives of ergot compounds in hopes of finding new medicines. He synthesized a series of compounds, one of which was LSD. At the time, he had no idea he was dealing with a potent hallucinogenic drug. In 1943, after conducting several experiments, he was forced to stop work because of peculiar sensations. He recorded these impressions in his laboratory notebook and suspected they were due to accidental ingestion of LSD. Several days later he deliberately tested his theory by ingesting 0.25 mg of the substance (we know now that this is a massive dose, since LSD is an extremely potent drug). This famous description underscored the remarkable visual hallucinations and perceptual distortions induced by the drug (see Hofmann, 1968). Reports on LSD eventually found their way into the scientific literature. Although pharmacologists and psychologists were very interested in its effects, research indicated that there was little therapeutic value to the compound. In the early 1960s, the drug became illegal, although soon after, in the late 1960s and early 1970s, its use in the 'hippy' subculture reached its peak. The psychological effects of the hallucinogenic drugs such as LSD are difficult to describe because they are so subjective, varying with the individual and the person's expectations and experience with the drug. One of the most common reports is that of profound changes in sensory perception, including visual, tactile or auditory distortions. Images and sounds may be remarkably vivid or bizarre. The sense of time is also extremely altered. The neuropharmacologist Solomon Snyder, upon having ingested LSD, noted that 'two hours after having taken the drug, I felt as if I had been under its influence for thousands of years. The remainder of my life on the planet Earth seemed to stretch ahead into infinity, and at the same time I felt infinitely old' (Snyder, 1986). Sensations may be transposed from one mode to another, a phenomenon known as SYNAESTHESIA. Snyder wrote: 'I clapped my hands and saw sound waves passing before my eyes.' EMOTION and the sense of self are often affected, with a feeling of depersonalization. In many cases users report they develop special insights into themselves or the world. In some instances this feeling is experienced as positive; for others it can be quite disturbing and result in profound DYSPHORIA.

LSD is an indole compound (see INDOLEAMINE), chemically related to the neurotransmitter SEROTONIN. Although it is not known precisely how LSD causes hallucinations and sensory distortions, it is suspected that marked alterations in the serotonin system and particularly in the CEREBRAL CORTEX may underlie the phenomena. There are a number of important differences between LSD and other drugs of abuse. Unlike drugs such as COCAINE, AMPHETAMINE or HEROIN, LSD does not cause a 'rush' or strong feeling of PLEASURE, nor is it addictive. It is possible that the hallucinogens do not effect the brain REWARD system the way most other drugs of abuse do. Animals cannot be taught SELF-ADMINISTRATION of these compounds; they seem to lack true reinforcing effects in both animals and humans.

References

Hofmann A. (1968) Psychotomimetic agents. In *Drugs Affecting the Central Nervous System*, vol. 2, ed. A. Burger, pp. 169–235, Marcel Dekker: New York.
Snyder S.H. (1986) *Drugs and the Brain*, Scientific American Library: New York.

ANN E. KELLEY

lucifer yellow *see* tract tracers

lumbar puncture A technique for sampling CEREBROSPINAL FLUID in patients. A needle is inserted into the CENTRAL CANAL at the lumbar level of the SPINAL CORD and fluid drawn off. Analysis of this fluid can reveal information about the metabolic activity of the brain.

lumbar spinal cord *see* spinal cord

luminance The amount of light emitted per unit area in a given direction by a surface. It is the quantitative measure of the subjective BRIGHTNESS of an extended source, and depends on the amount of light incident on the surface (the ILLUMINENCE) and the DIFFUSE REFLECTION COEFFICIENT (ALBEDO) of the surface material. In the SI system of units (see SI UNITS) luminance is measured in candelas per metre squared, formerly referred to as a nit (nt). Surfaces that have the same apparent brightness in all directions act as perfect diffusers, and are usually referred to as Lambertian surfaces. Barium sulphate, magnesium oxide, calcium carbonate (chalk) and soot closely approximate Lambertian surfaces.

DAVID W. HEELEY

luminance mechanisms *see* opponent process theory of colour vision

luminosity *see* photometry

luminosity coefficient *see* photometry

luminosity curve *see* photometry

luminous efficiency function *see* photometry

luminous flux *see* photometry

luminous intensity *see* photometry

lurcher mutant mouse Mice with the lurcher gene in the HOMOZYGOUS condition (*Lc/Lc*) perish *in utero*: in the HETEROZYGOUS condition (*Lc/+*) mice develop but show complete loss of PURKINJE CELLS from the CEREBELLUM and consequently have an abnormal GAIT.

Luria–Nebraska neuropsychological battery (LNNB) This standardized test battery is loosely based on the examination techniques of the Russian neuropsychologist A.R. Luria (1902–1977). Form I has 269 items and Form II 279 items which are grouped first into 11 or 12 scales (such as motor functions, receptive speech and so on) and then into factor scales. Scores exceeding critical levels (based on age and education) suggest impairment on that scale. Interpretations include whether significant brain injury exists, spared and impaired abilities, and qualitative aspects of performance.

See also: neuropsychology

Reference

Golden C.J., Purisch A.D. & Hammeke T.A. (1985) *Luria–Nebraska Neuropsychological Battery: Forms I and II: Manual*, Western Psychological Services: Los Angeles.

JENNI A. OGDEN

luteinizing hormone One of the GONADOTROPHINS; see ENDOCRINE GLANDS; ESTRUS; HORMONES; HORMONES – CLASSIFICATION; MENSTRUAL CYCLE; SEX HORMONES.

luteinizing hormone releasing hormone *see* gonadotrophin-releasing hormone

luxol fast blue *see* stains

luxusconsumptie Derived from the *luxus consumption theory*, proposed in the late nineteenth century to account for excess urea production, the term luxusconsumptie refers to the hypothesis the storage of body fat is simply the consequence of excess ENERGY intake. The alternative is that body fat stores are actively monitored and regulated.

See also: adipose tissue; body weight; energy balance; leptin

LY-53857 An antagonist at the $5HT_{2B}$ receptor; see SEROTONIN RECEPTORS.

LY334370 An agonist at the $5HT_{1F}$ receptor; see SEROTONIN RECEPTORS.

lymph *see* lymphatic system

lymphatic system The lymphatic system is a network of vessels, glands and tissues that works to take fluid from the spaces between cells (the interstitial spaces or interstices) and returns both fluids and proteins to the BLOOD in veins around the shoulders (when in the lymphatic system this fluid is called LYMPH). Within the lymphatic system are several organs (Peyer's patches [around the small intestine], spleen, adenoids, tonsils, appendix) and lymph nodes. When passing through these nodes the lymph will be brought into contact with LYMPHOCYTES. These are immature forms of B CELL and T CELL, on their way to completing their development in either the THYMUS GLAND (T cells) or bone marrow (B cells) having originated from STEM CELLS in the liver and bone marrow. The actions of lymphocytes within the lymph nodes is an important part of the IMMUNE SYSTEM response to infection and disease.

lymphocytes *see* immune system

lymphotoxin A CYTOKINE; see IMMUNE SYSTEM.

Lyon–Robbins hypothesis This hypothesis is a behavioural account of the effects of PSYCHOMOTOR STIMULANTS such as AMPHETAMINE and related compounds (Lyon & Robbins, 1975). The central tenet is that these drugs, with increasing dose, cause an increased rate of responding, but in a progressively reducing number of response categories. The hypothesis accounts for the evolution of the effects of amphetamine on behaviour in experimental animals, as well as humans, from general behavioural hyperactivity to STEREOTYPY, resulting from the drug's actions to release DOPAMINE in the brain, especially within the dorsal and ventral STRIATUM.

In the rat, low doses of the drug produce typical stimulant effects such as locomotor hyperactivity, enhanced speed of behaviour such as eating, and increases in the rate of performance of learned instrumental behaviour (see INSTRUMENTAL CONDITIONING). However, at higher doses intricate behavioural sequences (for example, SOCIAL BEHAVIOUR or complex OPERANT chains) first become repetitive or perseverative in nature (see PERSEVERATION) and then disorganized and fragmented before possibly disappearing altogether from the behavioural output (see Robbins & Sahakian, 1983). The stimulation leads to repetition of individual elements of behaviour leading to aberrant phenomena such as perseverative operant responses, and then even simpler responses such as incipient head or forelimb movements, and licking, which are repeated at a high rate in a stereotyped manner. The hypothesis explains this transition to behavioural stereotypy as a consequence of progressively increasing competition between different responses within the same behavioural sequence, or from other sequences. Whereas the entire response sequence is initially facilitated, only the shorter elements (requiring the probably the least sensory feedback for performance) or the most strongly trained elements of the sequence, are evident as the dose increases. Some evidence for this viewpoint can be gleaned from observational studies of the effects of chronic amphetamine treatment on behavioural sequences in experimental animals. What ultimately may appear only as an apparently 'purposeless', stereotypy can sometimes be traced back to its origins as a component in a more complex sequence of behaviour. Evidence for behavioural competition is also provided by observations of the effects of blockade of the stereotyped head movements and oral behaviour in rats following dopamine depletion from the dorsal striatum which leads to excessive levels of locomotor activity following systemic amphetamine treatment, presumably as a consequence of reduced competition from the other stereotyped responses.

The relationship between the Lyon–Robbins hypothesis and theories emphasising the effects of amphetamine on reinforcement processes is unclear but they are probably not incompatible. The Lyon–Robbins hypothesis is quite closely related to the YERKES–DODSON LAW in experimental psychology, applied to response output, and the Broen & Storms (1977) 'response competition' hypothesis of SCHIZOPHRENIA.

References

Broen W.E. & Storms L.H. (1977) A theory of response interference in schizophrenia. In *Contributions to the Psychopathology of Schizophrenia*, ed. B. Maher, pp. 267–317, Academic Press: London.

Lyon M. & Robbins T.W. (1975) The action of central nervous system stimulant drugs: a general theory concerning amphetamine effects. In *Current Developments in Psychopharmacology*, vol. 2, ed. Essman W. & Valzelli L, pp. 80–163, Spectrum: New York.

Robbins T.W., Mittleman G., O'Brien J.P. & Winn P. (1990) The neuropsychological significance of stereotyped behaviour induced by stimulant drugs. In *The Neurobiology of Stereotyped Behaviour*, ed. S.J. Cooper and C.T. Dourish, pp. 25–63, Clarendon Press: Oxford.

TREVOR W. ROBBINS

lysergic acid diethylamide *see* LSD

lysis (from Greek, *lysis*: dissolving) The destruction or CATABOLISM (see METABOLISM) of something, particularly of cells. One speaks of an ENZYME lysing: see for an example, IMMUNE SYSTEM: EOSINOPHILS destroy by lysis parasites invading the body. (*Lysis* is a noun; the associated verb is to *lyse*.)

lysosome *see* cell

M

Mach band phenomenon Mach bands are apparent bands of light produced by a progressive increase in illumination from dark to bright. One edge of the Mach band is at the point where the illumination begins to increase and the other edge is at the point where the increase in illumination stops. It is caused by LATERAL INHIBITION across the RECEPTIVE FIELD in the RETINA.

Machiavellian intelligence *see* theory of mind

macro- (from Greek, *makros*: long or great) A prefix indicating a large size. Unlike its complementary term, micro-, macro- has no fixed meaning. It is often mistakenly equated with the prefix mega- meaning one million times; see SI UNITS.

macrocephaly (from Greek, *makros*: great, *kephale*: head) An abnormally large development of the head, and of the BRAIN. It has been associated with enlargement of the SUBARACHNOID SPACE in many cases. It is contrasted with MICROCEPHALY; MEGALENCEPHALY is a more extreme enlargement with a different pathology and prognosis.

See also: hydrocephalus

macroelectrode *see* electrode

macronutrients The main nutrients: PROTEINS, FATS and CARBOHYDRATES.

macrophage (from Greek, *makros*: great, *phagein*: to eat) Literally a 'big eater' – a description given to any large CELL engaged in phagocytosis; MONOCYTES, for example, can act as macrophages; see IMMUNE SYSTEM.

macropsia A phenomenon in which things are perceived as being larger than they actually are. It can be produced by damage in the VISUAL SYSTEM (particularly the RETINA) and is also associated with certain forms of EPILEPSY, though it is neither common nor defining in this condition.

See also: micropsia

macrosmatic A rather antique term indicating possession of well-developed olfactory organs (see OLFACTION). It was first used by Sir William Turner, in 1890, in attempting to classify MAMMALS by the development of their olfactory apparatus. Animals were classed as macrosmatic, microsmatic ('where the olfactory apparatus is relatively feeble') or anosmatic (where the sense of small appeared to be absent). There has been a tendency to describe mammals in terms of the sensory system that appears to be of primary value to them. Mice, for example, are certainly very dependent on their olfactory systems. For instance, a variety of effects of PHEROMONES (BRUCE EFFECT, LEEBOOT EFFECT, WHITTEN EFFECT, VANDENBERGH EFFECT) were first described in mice. Some have attempted to classify PRIMATES, including man, as being primarily visual, but it is clear that all of the senses are well developed, most especially in man, and that development of the CEREBRAL CORTEX has allowed assimilation of information across senses, and rapid shifting of ATTENTION from one sensory domain to another.

Reference

Turner W. (1890) The convolutions of the

brain: a study in comparative anatomy. *Journal of Anatomy and Physiology* 25: 105–153.

macula A term used to describe the surfaces of the SEMICIRCULAR CANALS (see VESTIBULAR SYSTEM) from which HAIR CELLS originate, and to which the VESTIBULAR NERVE is connected. Note that this is not the same thing as the MACULA LUTEA, which is part of the RETINA.

macula lutea *see* fovea

macular sparing This is more properly known as *macula sparing hemianopia* (or sometimes *macula splitting*). It is a restricted area of intact vision that occurs within the centre of a HEMIANOPIA: that is, the vision of the macula lutea remains intact when that of the area around it has been lost. The damage is 'crossed': damage to the visual areas of the left OCCIPITAL LOBE can produce right macular sparing. It occurs after damage not to the RETINA but to the VISUAL CORTEX. It was thought to be a function of a bilateral innervation of the cortex by the MACULA LUTEA, but it transpires that the macula lutea is not actually represented bilaterally. Instead, the explanation for macula sparing is thought to derive from the observation that, in the visual cortex, the representation of the macula is much exaggerated and so the probability of sparing following a LESION here is quite high. The most common cause of lesions that produce macula sparing is disruption of blood flow in the MIDDLE CEREBRAL ARTERY (see BLOOD) in the occipital lobe.

Reference

Hart W.M. Jr (ed.) (1992) *Adler's Physiology of the Eye*, 9th edn, Mosby Year Book: St Louis MO.

mad cow disease *see* bovine spongiform encephalopathy

magic bullet Colloquialism describing the property a DRUG might be hoped to have in treating only the target tissue – a TUMOUR for example – without having an effect on any other tissue, or developing any unwanted SIDE-EFFECTS. Such drugs are rarely available: therapeutic agents that have beneficial effects often produce unwanted side-effects. The severity of the side-effects have to be weighed against the value of the treatment being delivered. (Note also that the term side-effects is something of a misnomer: a drug only has effects: *unwanted effects* would be a more accurate term than side-effects.)

magic mushroom Some mushrooms, most notably a Mexican mushroom, *Psilocybe mexicana*, contain HALLUCINOGENS such as PSILOCYBIN.

magnesium Magnesium (Mg^{2+}) is an important MINERAL important in ADENOSINE TRIPHOSPHATE activity and in NEUROTRANS-MISSION; see NMDA RECEPTORS.

magnesium channel *see* ion channel

magnetic resonance imaging Magnetic resonance imaging (MRI) is a method for visualising brain structure and metabolism. It relies upon the technique of NUCLEAR MAGNETIC RESONANCE IMAGING, in which a large magnetic field is employed to induce atomic nuclei with 'odd' spin to align themselves in space. When subjected to brief radio-frequency pulses, such nuclei emit electromagnetic signals which can be detected and used to generate a 3-dimensional image in which the intensity is proportional to signal strength. Brain structure is imaged by tuning the scanner to detect signals from protons, which are abundant in the body bound in water and fat molecules. Depending on the scanning parameters, such images can be employed to reveal the fine-grained structure of the brain, or to highlight different kinds of pathological change, for example, those associated with STROKE or EPILEPSY. Because of its greater sensitivity, flexibility, and spatial resolution, MRI has largely supplanted COMPUTERIZED AXIAL TOMOGRAPHY (CAT) scanning for the purposes of detecting and localizing brain pathology. And because no ionizing radiation is involved, MRI can be used not just in a clinical context, but also for research in healthy volunteers. An extension of the MRI technique – FUNCTIONAL MRI – is an important FUNCTIONAL NEUROIMAGING method.

MICHAEL D. RUGG

magnetoencephalography *see* SQUID magnetometry

magnetometry *see* SQUID magnetometry

magnetoreception A sensory system that detects the earth's magnetic field. Several species appear able to do this, including electrosensitive marine fish, birds and several others. Magnetoreception has been proposed as a mechanism involved in MIGRATION and NAVIGATION, but little is known of how magnetic fields are detected by neural tissue.

Reference

Lohmann K.J. & Johnsen S. (2000) The neurobiology of magnetoreception. *Trends in Neuroscience* 23: 1531–1559

magnocellular (from Latin, *magnus*: great, large) Literally, big cells. In many paces in the CENTRAL NERVOUS SYSTEM there are NEURON groups in which the cells are described as magnocellular, being so much bigger than neighbouring cells. Magnocellular neurons are often associated with the synthesis of HORMONES (as is the case, for example, in the PARAVENTRICULAR NUCLEUS OF THE HYPOTHALAMUS) and with neurons containing MONOAMINES or ACETYLCHOLINE and which project over longs distances within the brain. For example, acetylcholine is contained within magnocellular neurons in the BASAL FOREBRAIN. There are though other examples of magnocellular neurons that are neither hormone producing not monoaminergic – in the LATERAL GENICULATE NUCLEUS for example. The opposite of magnocellular is PARVOCELLULAR.

magnocellular basal nucleus *see* nucleus basalis of Meynert

maintenance insomnia The state of INSOMNIA in which, having fallen asleep, an individual wakes frequently, disrupting normal SLEEP.

See also: onset insomnia; sleep disorders; termination insomnia

major histocompatibility complex For class I major histocompatibility complex (MHC) cells and class I major histocompatibility complex cells, see IMMUNE SYSTEM.

major tranquillizer *see* antipsychotic

malleus *see* ossicles

malnutrition Malnutrition has two type of consequences that are relevant to biopsychology. The first is the immediate effect on dietary preference, appetites and aversion, and food choice by the individual. The second is the deleterious effect malnutrition may have on brain deterioration in adults, or on brain development in a foetus or child.

Humans and animals are unable to synthesize many crucial nutrient substances, and therefore must consume them in food. If a diet lacks a particular nutrient or particular set of nutrients over a long period of time, then malnutrition may result. But when a wide array of nutrients is available, most individuals seem to eat a mostly balanced diet most of the time. The question of how an appropriate balance of nutrient intake is maintained, and whether there is a SPECIFIC APPETITE (or SPECIFIC HUNGER as it is also known) for each type of nutrient that is needed, has been the focus of much research. There are a very few nutrients for which a clear specific appetite seems to be triggered whenever a physiological deficit occurs for that nutrient. The most robust specific appetite is SALT APPETITE or SODIUM APPETITE, which is directed specifically towards salty tasting foods during states of physiological sodium depletion. Aside from salt, however, most classes of nutrients do not have distinct tastes (see GUSTATION). That poses the question of how the brain might recognize whether a food contained a particular needed mineral, vitamin or other nutrient. This problem appears to have had a major consequence: aside from salt appetite, there are very few specific appetites for nutrients that are triggered innately in states of physiological depletion. Only two other nutrients, both of which are minerals, have been indicated to have specific appetites that can stand up to rigorous experimental scrutiny: IRON and CALCIUM. All other states of specific nutrient depletion appear to act via a generalized LEARNED APPETITE mechanism rather than through innate specific appetites. Most of them produce symptoms of illness and malaise over the long term. When a particular diet is accompanied by such symptoms, two things appear to happen. First, a learned aversion (see FOOD-AVERSION LEARNING) begins to develop for the foods that are associated with the illness. This developing aversion leads individuals to try new foods, and to avoid the old one, whenever the opportunity arises. Second, if a particular new food is accompanied by dramatic recovery from the illness, which may happen if it contains the missing nutrient, a moderate preference for that particular new food may be learned. This combination of biopsychological mechanisms leads most animals and humans to consume an adequately balanced diet of nutrients over the long term.

Very dramatic cases of malnutrition, if they persist uncorrected, can in some instances lead to brain damage. The most common example of this in adults in Western society may be KORSAKOFF'S SYNDROME, which typically affects late-stage chronic alcoholics. The disease is not caused by alcohol itself, but rather results because severe alcoholics may consume almost nothing but alcoholic beverages for weeks at a time. If this dietary pattern recurs repeatedly over many months, a specific nutrient deficit for thiamine may result. THIAMINE, also known as vitamin B1, is needed by brain neurons in order to metabolize their principal fuel, glucose. Without thiamine, neurons begin to starve to death. Neurons in particular brain structures, such as the MAMMILLARY BODIES and the THALAMUS, important to MEMORY, are especially susceptible to starvation due to thiamine deficiency, and begin to die first. The result is severe memory impairment. As neural starvation continues, cognitive function is also impaired. Aside from Korsakoff's syndrome, there are relatively few types of brain damage that are known to result from specific malnutrition in human adults. The case is different for children. The brains of developing foetuses and children, in which neurons are actively multiplying, growing, becoming pruned, and establishing new connections, are much more susceptible to the effects of malnutrition than the brains of adults. For this reason, a very wide set of types of malnutrition may produce permanent changes in brain structure and function if they are allowed to occur in severe degree for any appreciable length of time (see DEVELOPMENT).

KENT C. BERRIDGE

mammals The members of the class Mammalia (see TAXONOMY) are distinguished, generally, by the presence of hair (those without hair, such as the naked mole rat, have lost their hair for specific evolutionary reasons) and, more importantly, by the presence (in females) of mammary glands for the production of milk. There are three subdivisions of the class: MONOTREMES, MARSUPIALS and the EUTHERIAN MAMMALS. The monotremes are the most primitive, distinguished by laying eggs. Platypuses and echidnas are monotremes. The marsupials – kangaroos, opossums, bandicoots and koalas – are distinguished by early birth and subsequent nursing within a maternal pouch (the marsupium). All other mammals are eutherian. The young of eutherian mammals develop for relatively long periods within the UTERUS. The eutherian mammals are divided into many orders, including PRIMATES, RODENTS and many others.

Reference

Campbell N.A., Reece J.B. & Mitchell L.G. (1999) *Biology*, 5th edn, Addison-Wesley: Menlo Park CA.

mammary gland The breast: the term MAMMA can be used to describe a milk gland or breast. The *mammilla* is the nipple of the mammary gland.

See also: lactation; maternal behaviour; suckling

mammillary bodies The mammillary bodies are located in the posterior HYPOTHALAMUS. They receive input from the SEPTAL NUCLEI and hypothalamus, and, via the postcommissural FORNIX, from the SUBICULUM, a part of the HIPPOCAMPUS. Their output, mainly from the medial mammillary nucleus, is directed to the anterior thalamic nuclei via the MAMMILLOTHALAMIC TRACT. The mammillary bodies are also interconnected with the MIDBRAIN. The medial mammillary nucleus projects, via the mammillotegmental tract, to the dorsal and ventral tegmental nuclei, which project back mainly to the lateral mammillary nucleus via the mammillary peduncle. The mammillary bodies are thus well positioned to interface the LIMBIC functions of the FOREBRAIN and MIDBRAIN.

See also: limbic system; malnutrition; Korsakoff's syndrome

KAZUE SEMBA

mammilothalamic tract *see* Korsakoff's' syndrome; mammillary bodies

mand *see* tacting

mandible *see* skull

mania Pathological elevation of MOOD, associated with overactivity, sleeplessness (see INSOMNIA), grandiosity and irritability. Mania occurs in the manic phase of BIPOLAR DISORDER, a form of AFFECTIVE DISORDER. Sufferers may develop a PSYCHOSIS, experiencing DELUSION and HALLUCINATION. The condition may result in irresponsible behaviour, such as sexual disinhibition and over-spending. A delusional sense of invulnerability may lead to injury or death. Manic illness can be treated with a mood-stabilising DRUG, such as LITHIUM salts, or an ANTICONVULSANT, such as SODIUM VALPROATE or CARBAMAZEPINE. These drugs treat both the acute symptoms of mania and act prophylactically to prevent mood swings. In addition, ANTIPSYCHOTIC drugs may be necessary to control behaviour and to treat psychotic symptoms.

IAN C. REID

manic depression Recurrent mood disorder characterised by individual episodes of pathologically elevated and pathologically depressed mood.

See also: affective disorder; bipolar disorder; depression; mania

IAN C. REID

maps Representations of the spatial configuration of objects in an organism's environment. Tolman (1886–1959) first developed and explored this construct. Animals clearly posses many spatial NAVIGATION strategies that do not require the use of a COGNITIVE MAP. For example, animals can learn to approach specific proximal cues emanating from a goal (TAXIS strategies), or to perform specific responses to reach a goal (PRAXIS strategies). However animals that possessed *only* these abilities should display limited behavioural flexibility. For instance they should be unable to move directly to an invisible goal from a novel start location, or to devise a shortcut. Demonstrations of animals solving these very problems provide the most compelling evidence for the existence of cognitive maps.

Many animals can use a direct route to reach an invisible goal when released from a novel location. This ability has been systematically examined in rats using the WATER MAZE. In these experiments rats are given experience using distal spatial cues to swim to a submerged escape platform from various start locations. On a PROBE TEST the rats are released from a novel start position. Despite being inexperienced at swimming from this position rats typically adopt the correct bearing and swim straight to the platform. In one demonstration of animals using shortcuts an experimenter carried a chimpanzee on a meandering route around a field. *En route* they saw a second experimenter periodically hide food in various locations. After a RETENTION interval this chimpanzee and several naive chimpanzees were released into the open field. The naive chimpanzees never retrieved much food. However, the experienced chimp moved directly from one food site to the next, retrieving almost all the food on every trial. Additionally, the experienced chimpanzee frequently used the shortest possible path to visit the food sites. As this chimpanzee originally visited the food sites in a random order, it appears that chimpanzees can perceive the relative positions of elements in their environment and can use this knowledge to organize their foraging behaviour.

The HIPPOCAMPAL FORMATION plays a key role in SPATIAL MAPPING. A LESION of the HIPPOCAMPUS in rodents and birds produces severe ACQUISITION impairments in a variety of map-based spatial tasks. Importantly, hippocampal lesions do not disrupt the retention of previously acquired map-based information or performance on taxis- or praxis-based tasks. This suggests the hippocampal formation is crucial for the acquisition, but not long-term storage, of spatial maps. Additionally, hippocampal size may be positively correlated with spatial ability in variety of rodents and birds. SINGLE-UNIT ELECTROPHYSIOLOGICAL RECORDING studies of PYRAMIDAL NEURONS in the hippocampal formation have found PLACE CELLS in the CA1 and CA3 subfields that increase spiking (see SPIKE) when animals enter circumscribed locations. However, PARIETAL CORTEX and FRONTAL CORTEX lesions impair performance on some spatial tasks, neurons in the NUCLEUS ACCUMBENS and SUPERIOR COLLICULUS also code location information, and HEAD DIRECTION CELLS have been found in the PRESUBICULUM. These latter findings suggest that the hippocampal formation is a component of the larger neural system that subserves spatial cognition.

See also: alternation learning; configural learning; food-storing birds; latent learning; maze learning; mazes; optimal foraging theory; receptotopic representration; spatial behaviour; spatial cognition; spatial memory; spontaneous alternation; tonotopic representation

DONALD M. WILKIE

marche à petits pas French for 'walk with little steps': a style of walking characteristic of patients with PARKINSON'S DISEASE (and some other motor disorders). Individuals take very small, shuffling steps.

marijuana The form of the hemp plant (*Cannabis sativa*) that consists of a crude mixture of dried leaves, small stems and flowering tops. The name appears to be derived from the Mexican word *maraguanquo*, 'an intoxicating plant'. Marijuana is a commonly used PSYCHOACTIVE drug in many cultures. It is usually smoked for its intoxicating properties, although it is sometimes baked in cookies or brownies and ingested orally. The active compound in marijuana is delta-9-TETRAHYDRO-CANNABINOL, or THC.

See also: addiction; cannabis; cannabinoids

ANN E. KELLEY

Marr's computational theory of vision David Marr (1945–1980) formulated an influential theory of vision in which he suggested that images progress through a series of processing steps (which he identified as representations) including the PRIMAL SKETCH which records the locations of object edges and colour and texture variations, and the TWO-AND-A-HALF-D SKETCH (or 2.5-dimensional sketch) in which

the relative distance and orientation of the elements of the visual field are identified. The final stage is the 3-dimensional model representation, although it has been pointed out the two-and-a-half D sketch contains all the information required for 3-dimensional representation. The two-and-a-half D sketch Marr believed to be useful in that it was an abstract, mental, representation of the visual world and could be used in recognition no matter what the conditions of viewing (which of course change the view of that which is being perceived). Such abstract representation is based on a projection of the external environment onto the (more or less) flat surface of the RETINA: in order to perceive in three dimensions we have to integrate information form the two retinae and create from that three dimensions. An important feature of the two-and-a-half-D visual sketch is that it lays emphasis on the creative nature of 3-dimensional perception.

See also: depth perception; stereopsis

References

Marr D. (1982) *Vision*, W.H. Freeman: San Francisco.

marsupial see mammals

masculine An adjective used to describe any physical or behavioural trait that is typically displayed by males of a given species. Physical or phenotypic traits, such as male anatomy (such as the penis) are obviously viewed as genetic in nature. However, it is less clear as to the degree to which masculine behaviours in humans are genetically programmed or learned.

See also: feminine; gender; hormones and cognition; organization effects of steroid hormones; sex differences; sexual behaviour; sexual differentiation

masking Masking refers to the occlusion of one STIMULUS by another: it is a term usually qualified by a sensory domain – *auditory masking* or *visual masking* for instance. *Backward masking* is said to occur when the mask appears after the target stimulus; *forward masking* occurs when the mask is presented before. *Brightness masking* involves presentation of a bright light which makes perception of the target difficult; *pattern masking* involves presentation of a complex pattern (in whatever sensory modality). *Metacontrast masking* involves the brief presentation of a target followed by a mask which occupies the space around where the target was (it follows the target's contours). *Paracontrast masking* is the same as metacontrast masking except that the mask is presented before the target.

mass action This term refers to the notion that the brain is not differentiated according to function; the exact area of brain damage is not the significant determinant of what cognitive deficits ensue but rather the amount of tissue damaged is critical. This view, strongly supported by Karl Lashley (1890–1958) is in direct opposition to the localizationist perspective in which specific regions of the brain perform specific functions and subsequently, the nature of the deficit is contingent on the area that is lesioned. Although localizationist views have garnered much support from recent studies (particularly in FUNCTIONAL NEUROIMAGING), many cognitive functions, such as MEMORY or word READING appear to involve a number of different brain regions diffusely organized across the brain.

See also: across-fibre pattern theory; binding problem; engram; grandmother cell; labelled-line theory

MARLENE BEHRMANN

massa intermedia Also known as the *adhesio interthalamica*, the massa intermedia is a COMMISSURE composed of fibres that run across the MIDLINE, connecting the THALAMUS in the right and left hemispheres. Curiously, it is not present in all individuals and it has been suggested that its absence might be associated with higher degrees of intelligence.

massed trials *see* trial

mast cell *see* immune system; histamine

matching law The matching law was developed by students of B.F. Skinner (1904–1990), particularly Richard Herrnstein (1930–1994) to try to bring a greater quantitative precision to the study of OPERANT behaviour. It begins with the observation that a subject (rat or human) facing one or several choices will press

a lever at a rate or allocate time in proportion to the distribution of REINFORCEMENT density across the choices. In a two-lever concurrent choice situation, if lever A is running a variable interval (VI) 20-second schedule (see SCHEDULES OF REINFORCEMENT) and lever B is running a VI 40-second schedule, lever A can be said to be twice as rich as lever B. When the experiment is properly constructed (that is, no pay-off exists for simply switching levers), lever A will receive twice as much behaviour as lever B. This observation translates into rational choice in economics and OPTIMAL FORAGING THEORY in ETHOLOGY. It has attracted numerous reward experiments in psychobiology (for example, recent choice studies using INTRACRANIAL SELF-STIMULATION).

A useful extension of the matching law has been into the single-lever situation where the choice is assumed to be between the operant (that is, lever pressing for a food reinforcement) and all other activities in which the subject can engage. If a variable interval schedule is run with trials varying from rich to lean (for example VI 5 to VI 80 seconds) a curve results relating response rate to the rate of reinforcement obtained. The curve is hyperbolic, growing out of the origin to an ASYMPTOTIC BEHAVIOURAL MAXIMUM. The mathematics for curve fitting are identical to the those for enzyme kinetics or RECEPTOR BINDING. The theory presented by Heyman (one of Herrnstein's students) is that as reinforcement on the lever grows, so does affinity for the lever in the same way a drug is more likely to be associated with a receptor if the drug concentration increases. Dissociation in the drug case occurs when the drug comes off the receptor and in the operant case is produced by the attraction of all of the other reinforcers that can not be obtained while the subject is lever pressing. As with the RATE FREQUENCY CURVE, this method has been validated by a series of tests (such as giving various doses of any drugs that is an AGONIST or ANTAGONIST at DOPAMINE receptors, or making responding more difficult through weighted levers to produce characteristic curve shifts). Like the biochemical parallels and like the rate-frequency curve-shift method, this method uses a reinforcement density required to sustain half maximal responding as its reward measure, and is able to separate reward from motor effects and measure reward effects quantitatively.

See also: behavioural economics; cost–benefit analysis

JAMES R. STELLAR

material specific amnesia In material specific amnesia there is an impairment selective for a specific type of information. It contrasts with GLOBAL AMNESIA, a complete loss or severe impairment of DECLARATIVE MEMORY.

materialism *see* monism

maternal behaviour The behavioural repertoire which mothers exhibit towards, and usually in the presence of, their offspring. These behaviours typically promote the survival, growth and DEVELOPMENT of the offspring and are generally restricted to a limited temporal period following birth. The term usually refers to behavioural features observed in mammalian species although non-mammalian species, (for example birds and reptiles) can also exhibit specific PARENTAL BEHAVIOURS during the period following the birth of their progeny. However, the lactatory (see LACTATION) function characteristic of mammals dictates that mothers are required to maintain a close physical proximity to their offspring to suckle and thus the range of maternal behaviours is most highly developed in mammals. In most (probably all) mammalian species, there are complex, dynamic, reciprocal interactions between mother and neonatal offspring which are definable with respect to specific olfactory, auditory, visual and tactile stimuli and subsequent synchronised physiological, hormonal (see HORMONES) and behavioural responses. Specific maternal behaviours vary from species to species and have probably evolved as a function of differing habitats and survival requirements. The behavioural repertoire is also determined by factors such as the degree of development and independence of the offspring at birth, the rapidity of subsequent maturation and the range of behaviours necessary for survival as an adult, particularly those required to gather food. ALTRICIAL MAMMALS are totally helpless at birth and entirely dependent upon maternal care, even for basic physiological HOMEOSTASIS, such as thermoregulation (see THERMOGENESIS). Typically the eyes are closed and they have minimal capacity to move. Specific maternal behaviours in this case include nest building and assistance with bodily waste elimination. Examples of such atricial mammals include rats, mice, cats and dogs. PRECOCIAL MAMMALS are capable of weight bearing and even walking when born. Their eyes and ears are open and they are not reliant upon their mothers for thermoregulation or waste elimination. The precocial species tend to be those which live in large social groupings, or herds, and which move over extensive areas to graze. Specific features of maternal behaviour in this instance include a very brief period of nesting and hiding of the offspring before rejoining the herd where membership of the large group confers extra protection from predators. Cows, sheep, and deer are examples of precocial mammals. The remaining group of mammals are the PRIMATES. The helpless offspring cling to the mother's body, which is typically covered by fur, and are transported around for a period of months until sufficiently independent. However, the young are able to see, to hear and to thermoregulate. These species tend to gather food by FORAGING. Humans differ by the requirement for the mother to cradle their offspring to facilitate feeding.

See also: imprinting; maternal separation/deprivation; social behaviour

Reference

Krasnegor N.A. & Bridges R.S. (1990) *Mammalian Parenting: Biochemical, Neurobiological and Behavioral Determinants*, Oxford University Press: New York.

KEITH MATTHEWS

maternal separation/deprivation Terms used to describe situations in which there is a discontinuity in an already established mother–offspring relationship, often with deleterious consequences for the offspring. Both terms are used interchangeably in clinical and scientific literature and the meaning of each term varies widely from one context, or experiment, to another. There is a consensus view that interruption of the complex reciprocal interactions between mammalian mother and offspring during development has adverse consequence for a wide range of biological functions and, ultimately, behaviour. Studies in numerous species have employed maternal separation as a manipulation of the early environment and have demonstrated that the provision of maternally specific stimuli is essential for optimal growth and DEVELOPMENT. Thus, there are enduring neuroanatomical, neurochemical and behavioural consequences of maternal separation. The most-cited work studying the effects of maternal separation in experimental animals was conducted in 1958 by Harry Harlow (1905–1981). Macaque monkeys were separated from their mothers within a few hours of birth and reared with artificial surrogate mothers built from wire mesh or from wood with a cloth covering. The monkeys greatly preferred the cloth-covered surrogates, independent of the site where milk was available, demonstrating a non-nutritionally determined 'affectional responding' (see AFFECT). This work led to a radical conceptual re-evaluation of the nature of the affective linkage between mammalian mothers and offspring. Previously this was assumed to be determined by nutritional factors. Opportunistic studies of separation in children appear to confirm that humans are also susceptible to the adverse consequences of maternal deprivation. However, provision of nurturance by non-mothers (the father for instance) or other females, may be capable of abolishing many of these effects. John Bowlby drew together theoretical constructs from ETHOLOGY and PSYCHOANALYSIS, to derive attachment theory. This theory infers an infantile motivational system in which clinging, following, searching and crying are activated by events which disturb the proximity to the attachment object, or mother. Such behaviours are observed in many species in response to maternal separation and also occur in an orderly sequence with a period of protest (vocalization and locomotion) followed by a period of despair (immobility and hyporesponsivity to external stimuli. There is enduring interest in the role for such separation experiences in the development of human PSYCHOPATHOLOGY.

See also: critical period; imprinting; maternal behaviour; neurodevelopment; social behaviour

References

Bowlby J. (1969) Attachment and Loss, vol. 1, Attachment, Basic Books: New York.
Harlow H. (1958) The nature of love. American Psychologist 13: 673–685.

KEITH MATTHEWS

mathematics and the brain On an evolutionary time scale mathematics is a very recent invention. Therefore, it is extremely unlikely that the human brain is genetically endowed with mechanisms specialized for formal mathematical knowledge and reasoning. How then are mathematical abilities implemented in the brain? Do these abilities exploit brain systems specialized for other cognitive functions, such as LANGUAGE, or do they instead draw upon very general capacities for concept formation and reasoning? Are mathematical abilities localized to particular brain systems, or are they represented diffusely? If there is at least some localization, is it consistent across individuals? These questions are far from being resolved. However, several lines of research are providing relevant information. Studies of human infants suggest that the ability to carry out rudimentary arithmetic operations is present early in life. For example, infants who see one toy and then another placed behind a screen apparently expect to see two toys when the screen is removed, and are surprised if there is only one. Research with non-human animals has similarly revealed rather sophisticated numerical abilities in many species. These lines of research offer insights into basic, and perhaps innate, capacities that may provide part of the foundation for complex mathematical knowledge and skills.

Questions concerning localization of mathematical abilities in the human brain have been addressed through studies of brain-damaged adults. These studies seek to establish relationships between damage to particular brain areas, and deficits affecting mathematical knowledge or skills (see ACALCULIA). FUNCTIONAL NEUROIMAGING methods (such as FUNCTIONAL MRI) are also being applied. Most studies have focused on basic arithmetic abilities, and have not addressed more complex mathematical skills. Some findings suggest that posterior cortical regions, especially the PARIE-TAL CORTEX, may play a role in arithmetical abilities. However, many other brain areas may also be implicated, including the FRONTAL CORTEX, THALAMUS, and BASAL GANGLIA. Several attempts have been made at a theoretical synthesis, although none has yet gained wide acceptance. The most fully developed theory assumes that arithmetic problem-solving implicates several component abilities, including a capacity for recognizing digits and other symbols, present in both hemispheres and localized to the ventral VISUAL SYSTEM; a capacity for representing numerical magnitudes, present in both hemispheres in the vicinity of the parieto-occipito-temporal junction; knowledge of arithmetic table facts (such as $6 \times 7 = 42$) represented in LEFT HEMISPHERE language areas; and procedures for carrying out multi-digit calculations, involving coordination of verbal and visuo-spatial representations.

MICHAEL McCLOSKEY

mating see copulation; sexual behaviour

maturation The developmental process involving growth and differentiation leading to adult functioning. The manner in which the term is used introduces theoretical complexities which revolve around the nature of the interaction (if any) between heredity and environment in the maturational process (see NATURE–NURTURE). Maturation can simply be viewed as that proportion of the variance in psychoneurobiological changes occurring during development attributable to genetic factors. One interpretation is that maturation represents the invariant, biologically 'unfolding' of morphological (see MORPHOLOGY) and behavioural changes related to a genetically predetermined outcome. A more contemporary view is that maturation occurs within boundary conditions. Environmental input that normally is inevitable for members of a species is necessary for 'normal' maturational change, but there are genetically regulated limits on the extent, timing, and the kind of environmental input that can influence. Environment could be seen to trigger or initiate the process of maturation or

have a more continuous and complex (albeit subtle) influence.

RICHARD C. TEES

Mauthner neuron Named after Ludwig Mauthner (1840–1894), Mauthner neurons (or Mauthner cells) are most often studied in fish and amphibia, where they are located in the BRAINSTEM. They are giant cells with sensory input arriving through EPHAPTIC TRANSMISSION: their output goes to MOTOR NEURONS that control tail activity. The speed of activation from sensory input to motor output indicates that they are important in escape responses. In higher VERTEBRATES they are found in the SPINAL CORD.

maxilla see skull

maximum concentration of available binding sites Abbreviated to B_{MAX}: this is a valuable statistic in pharmacology, used to index RECEPTOR BINDING functions: it informs one about the concentration of LIGAND required to occupy (see RECEPTOR OCCUPANCY) all available receptor sites in a particular piece of tissue.

maze learning A descriptive term for the LEARNING shown by small RODENTS in a range of different types of apparatus – MAZES – sometimes consisting of a quite complex array of alleyways and choice points leading to a goal with food or water. First studied systematically at the beginning of the twentieth century, maze learning takes advantage of the natural tendency of rodents to use well-trodden pathways during FORAGING near the burrows, or in moving around inside buildings. Several different types of learning process can be engaged and this has led to the development of a variety of specific and theoretically motivated mazes, such as the RADIAL ARM MAZE and WATER MAZE.

A key debate about the learning expressed in mazes was whether animals learned to go to specific places using some kind of internal MAP of the world that they built up by exploration (a view espoused by Edward Tolman (1886–1959)), or whether they learned simple HABITS such as approaching identifiable cues or making specific responses (such as left or right turns – a view espoused by sceptical learning theorists such as Clark Hull [1884–1952] and

Kenneth Spence [1907–1967]). The 'place vs. response' controversy reflected a division of opinion about the mental capacities of animals that was never formally resolved but has now given way to the multiple types of learning and MEMORY view of contemporary behavioural neuroscience.

RICHARD G. M. MORRIS

mazes A range of different types of apparatus that traditionally consist of a quite complex array of alleyways and choice points leading to a goal consisting of food or water and used to study learning in rodents. The key feature of all mazes is the physical movement of the animal from a starting point to the goal by a route involving choice on the part of the animal. One of the earliest was the Small maze based on a garden at the royal palace at Hampton Court near London. Others include the Hebb–Williams mazes developed in the 1940s to provide a flexible screening system for the analysis of brain dysfunction after various kinds of cerebral lesions. Mazes were widely used in the 1940s and 1950s, when early learning theorists asserted that the basic principles of learning could be worked out by studying the behaviour of rats 'at the choice point'. While this confidence is no longer shared, and many studies of learning are now carried out in automated operant chambers, mazes continue to be used. More recent examples include the RADIAL ARM MAZE and the watermaze.

Mazes have the advantage of simplicity and generally give rise to rapid learning. They have the disadvantage of needing to be run by hand and that it is not always easy to control the cues that animals use during learning. As a consequence, analysis of the reasons why a treatment such as a LESION or DRUG causes an impairment in maze learning are not always easy to unravel unambiguously. None the less, ingenious variations such as the radial arm maze have provided a way of gaining insight into the WORKING MEMORY system of the mammalian brain, while the watermaze has provided useful insights into the processes and neural mechanisms underlying spatial learning.

See also: maze learning; T maze; Y maze

RICHARD G. M. MORRIS

McGill pain questionnaire A questionnaire developed by Ronald Melzack for determining an individuals subjective experience of PAIN. It has 20 sets of verbal descriptors that probe the sensory and emotional aspects of pain as experienced by the individual. The responses are numerical rather than verbal and so can be summed to give an overall index of subjective pain. It has been a valuable tool in the management of pain, a continuing problem for modern medicine.

Reference

Melzack R. & Wall P.D. (1982) *The Challenge of Pain*, revised edn, Penguin Books: London.

McGurk effect An example of CROSS-MODAL CONFLICT: if one PHONEME is presented aurally to the ears while another is presented visually by the lips an intermediate sound will be heard.

See also: Stroop effect

MDMA MDMA (3,4 methylenedioxymethamphetamine) is one of the substances that act as HALLUCINOGENS; one of a class of drugs known as the PHENETHYLAMINES.

See also: amphetamine

mecamylamine A drug that is an ANTAGONIST at NICOTINIC ACETYLCHOLINE RECEPTORS. It is often used in studies of nicotine receptors in the CENTRAL NERVOUS SYSTEM, since it crosses the BLOOD–BRAIN BARRIER easily and has a relatively low AFFINITY for nicotinic acetylcholine receptors at the NEUROMUSCULAR JUNCTION. It does however affect nicotinic receptors in the AUTONOMIC NERVOUS SYSTEM.

mechanoreceptor A receptor for the detection of mechanical force: a MECHANOSENSORY pathway is one that is involved in the sensory detection of mechanical force. For example, see HAIR CELLS.

See also: sensory transduction; touch

mechanosensory *see* mechanoreceptor

medial Towards the middle, in contrast to LATERAL, which is away from the middle.

'Middle' in brain terms refers not to the dead centre but to the MIDLINE.

medial agranular cortex *see* shoulder cortex

medial forebrain bundle The medial forebrain bundle (MFB) proper runs through the LATERAL HYPOTHALAMUS and extends from the VENTRAL TEGMENTAL AREA posteriorly to the DIAGONAL BAND OF BROCA anteriorly. It connects systems that are neither primarily sensory or motor, but serves instead integrative functions as judged from the impact of stimulation or lesions on REWARD, MOTIVATION, and attendant physiology. If the HYPOTHALAMUS can be said to be the head ganglion of the autonomic nervous system, the MFB can be said to be the Los Angeles Freeway of the LIMBIC SYSTEM. In a parallel arrangement, a fibre system surrounding the third ventricle, called the perifornical fibre system, interconnects even more medial lying structures of the ventral forebrain. Anatomical studies of MFB constituents reveal that over 50 pathways (see Nieuwenhuys, 1982) use this bundle with origins from the entire ventral brain. These pathways make many more than 50 insertions. Consider for example, the ventral tegmental area which gives rise to the limbic forebrain dopamine inputs. While it counts as one input to the MFB, it has terminations in the NUCLEUS ACCUMBENS, AMYGDALA, PREFRONTAL CORTEX, SEPTAL NUCLEI, OLFACTORY TUBERCLE and other sites. Some pathways spread out over most of the cross-sectional area of the MFB while others may remain compact. Sub-areas of the medial forebrain bundle have also been identified on the basis of cell types. In addition to the above complexity of fibres of passage, a population of intrinsic neurons have their cell bodies in the MFB itself. They are called path neurons and have characteristic multiple branching axons and dendritic fields that extend into the axons' passage. Thus, it is no surprise that a structure as complex as this has been slow to yield the anatomical mechanisms of reward or of feeding control from lesion, stimulation and drug studies.

References

Nieuwenhuys R., Geeraedts L.M.G. & Veening J.G. (1982) The medial forebrain bundle of the rat: 1. General introduction. *Journal of Comparative Neurology* 206: 49–81.

Veening J.G., Swanson L.W., Cowan W.M., Nieuwenhuys R. & Geeraedts L.M.G. (1982) The medial forebrain bundle of the rat: 2. An autoradiographic study of the topography of the major descending and ascending components. *Journal of Comparative Neurology* 206: 82–108.

JAMES R. STELLAR

medial geniculate nucleus The medial geniculate nucleus (MGN) – also known a the medial geniculate body – is an auditory nucleus in the THALAMUS, consisting of ventral and posterior parts that connect the central nucleus of the INFERIOR COLLICULUS to the primary and anterior AUDITORY CORTEX respectively, and medial and dorsal parts that connect to secondary auditory cortical fields. The medial and dorsal parts are modifiable by LEARNING. The recurrent input from the auditory cortex exceeds the number of afferents from the midbrain by a factor of 10. Because of that and its connection with the RETICULAR ACTIVATING SYSTEM the MGN modifies its input to the cortex depending on context, AROUSAL or SLEEP.

See also: lateral geniculate nucleus

JOS J. EGGERMONT

medial lemniscus *see* dorsal column – medial lemniscal system

medial longitudinal fasciculus *see* hindbrain; vestibular complex

medial prefrontal cortex The area of FRONTAL CORTEX of the MEDIAL WALL in rats, with reciprocal connections with DORSOMEDIAL NUCLEUS OF THE THALAMUS and possibly homologous to DORSOLATERAL PREFRONTAL CORTEX in PRIMATES. The precise extent of rodent medial prefrontal cortex is disputed. Many authors (e.g. Paxinos & Watson, 1997) would include both PRELIMBIC CORTEX (PrL) and CINGULATE CORTEX (Cg1–2). Infralimbic cortex, although lacking a distinct laminar structure (see LAMINA) and having only weak connections with dorsomedial nucleus of the thalamus, nevertheless shares some characteristics of PREFRONTAL CORTEX and may be included. SHOULDER CORTEX would not be included: it also has dorsomedial nucleus connections but this area is regarded as homologous to primate secondary motor cortex and FRONTAL EYE FIELDS.

Reference

Paxinos G. & Watson C. (1997) *The Rat Brain in Stereotaxic Coordinates*, compact 3rd edn, Academic Press: San Diego.

VERITY J. BROWN

medial preoptic area *see* preoptic area

medial septum *see* septal nuclei

medial superior olive *see* auditory pathways; sound localization; superior olivary complex

medial temporal lobe *see* temporal lobe

medial terminal nucleus *see* accessory optic system

medial wall A term used in conjunction with the FRONTAL CORTEX (especially in RODENTS) when describing the MEDIAL PREFRONTAL CORTEX. The frontal cortex is developed around the anterior pole of the CORPUS CALLOSUM in an extensive arc. For example, at the top there is SHOULDER CORTEX and MOTOR CORTEX and at the bottom ORBITOFRONTAL CORTEX. Between these is the medial prefrontal cortex (including INFRALIMBIC CORTEX and PRELIMBIC CORTEX) which presents as a vertical bank of tissue immediately adjacent to the LONGITUDINAL FISSURE, which separates the two hemispheres of the brain. The term medial wall is therefore simply an architectural description of this general area of the frontal cortex.

median eminence A slightly elevated region of the tuber cinerium of the HYPOTHALAMUS at the floor of the third ventricle that surrounds the stem of the INFUNDIBULUM or pituitary stalk. It is the site of interface between the hypothalamus and the anterior PITUITARY GLAND. It is highly vascularized with fine blood vessels of the hypothalamo-pituitary system. Neurons producing hypothalamic HORMONES that regulate the production and secretion of pituitary hormones are located in certain hypothalamic nuclei, and their axons terminate on the portal vessels in the median

eminence to release their hormones into this portal circulation.

KAZUE SEMBA

median nerve A nerve innervating SKIN receptors on the ventral surface of the hand (the palm of the hand). It has been subject to some intriguing investigation. Merzenich *et al.* (1983) showed that if the nerve was cut, and regeneration prevented (for peripheral nerves will spontaneously regenerate) cortical organization changed. Following the transection, the area of the CEREBRAL CORTEX innervated by the median nerve was silent, but over a short period of time, it was found that a significant part of the cortical area previously responsive to median nerve stimulation became responsive to inputs from parts of the skin next to those that the median nerve had innervated.

Reference

Merzenich M.M., Kaas J.H., Wall J.T., Sur M., Nelson R.J. & Felleman D. (1983) Progression of change following median nerve section in the cortical representation of the hand in areas 3B and area 1 in adult owl and squirrel monkeys. *Neuroscience* 10 639–665.

median raphe nucleus *see* raphe nuclei

medical model Also known as the DISEASE MODEL; the term medical model crystallizes the belief that all illnesses must have a biological cause; that is, both physical *and* psychological illnesses must have a biological basis. Acceptance of the medical model indicates a belief that there is no psychological disorder that does not have an underlying physical cause (and typically one would suspect a brain dysfunction). Wing (1978) laid out two criteria for the medical model: (1) symptoms should group: possession of certain types of symptoms should indicate the likely presence of other types of symptoms (and indeed the absence of still others). Symptomatic classification like this is the basis of medical diagnosis. (2) A biological basis for the illness – that is, a biological basis for the SIGNS AND SYMPTOMS of the disorder – should be specifiable.

The first of these criteria tends to be true of psychological disorders: DSM-IV and ICD 10 both devote themselves to a classification of the signs and symptoms of psychological disorders, with considerable success. The second criterion is very much harder to demonstrate. In the nineteenth century, when it was discovered that the GENERAL PARESIS OF THE INSANE had a physical cause, it encouraged strongly the belief that all psychological disorders would eventually be shown to have a biological root. A great deal of research has subsequently gone in to determining the biological basis of disorders such as SCHIZOPHRENIA, DEPRESSION and ANXIETY, but there is little clear and unambiguous evidence that a specific change in either brain structure or chemistry actually *causes* any of these diseases: all of them may be associated with brain changes, but determining whether these changes are causal or not has proved exceptionally difficult. However, the belief that minds cannot have an existence separate from brains (see DUALISM) and that, at root, all psychological processes must be brain processes, has encouraged the belief that all psychological disorders must be brain disorders, treatable by physical means. The precise nature of the relationships between psychological and neural processing remains obscure though, and it may be that understanding these relationships will not prove to be in any way as simple as the medical model would have us believe.

See also: eliminative materialism; mind–body question

Reference

Wing J.K. (1978) *Reasoning about Madness*. Oxford University Press: Oxford.

medium spiny neurons These are the principal neurons in the STRIATUM, and are also the most numerous neuronal type in this region. Their DENDRITES are densely covered with DENDRITIC SPINES, as apparent in Golgi-stained sections (see DENDRITE). These spines receive synapses from the CEREBRAL CORTEX and THALAMUS. Medium spiny neurons also receive dopaminergic input from the SUBSTANTIA NIGRA (via the NIGROSTRIATAL DOPAMINE SYSTEM) and CHOLINERGIC and GABAERGIC synapses from striatal INTERNEURONS. Medium spiny neurons use GABA as a neurotransmitter. Those projecting to the GLOBUS PALLIDUS also contain the neuropeptide, ENKEPHALIN, while those projecting to the substantia nigra pars reticulata contain SUBSTANCE P and DYNORPHIN.

See also: histology

KAZUE SEMBA

medulla (from Latin, *medulla*: marrow) The term MEDULLA is a general one that refers to the inner portion of an element of tissue. Many structures have a medulla – the kidney does for example – but in neuroscience the term medulla (or the adjective medullary) invariably refers to the MEDULLA OBLONGATA.

medulla oblongata The medulla oblongata or MYELENCEPHALON is the most caudal part of the BRAINSTEM. It merges with the PONS rostrally and the SPINAL CORD caudally and contains sensory and motor nuclei that contribute to the fifth, seventh, eighth, ninth, tenth, eleventh and twelfth CRANIAL NERVES. The RETICULAR FORMATION forms the core of the medulla. Its neurons receive diverse inputs and, in turn, send ascending, descending and propriobulbar (intramedullary) connections that provide the anatomical substrates for coordinated activity of cranial nerve nuclei and AUTONOMIC integration. The sensory and motor decussations of the MEDIAL LEMNISCUS and PYRAMIDAL TRACT (see DECUSSATION) are located in the caudal medulla oblongata.

DAVID A. HOPKINS

medullary reticular formation That part of the RETICULAR FORMATION in the MEDULLA OBLONGATA. It contains four parts: (1) the PARAMEDIAN RETICULAR AREA (involved in fine MOTOR CONTROL); (2) NUCLEUS GIGANTOCELLULARIS (involved in the regulation of SLEEP and tone of MUSCLES); (3) the LATERAL RETICULAR AREA (containing the LATERAL RETICULAR NUCLEUS and PARVOCELLULAR RETICULAR NUCLEUS); and (4) INTERMEDIATE RETICULAR NUCLEUS (concerned with AUTONOMIC functions).

See also: ascending reticular activating system; midbrain reticular formation; pontine reticular formation

medullary tegmentum The upper portion (TEGMENTUM) of the MEDULLA OBLONGATA, a caudal extension of the PONTINE TEGMENTUM; see HINDBRAIN.

mega- (from Greek, *mega*: big) Prefix indicating a factor of 10^6, or one million times; see SI UNITS.

megalencephaly (from Greek, *mega*: big, *kephale*: head) Megalencephaly is an abnormally large head size (defined as being above the 98th percentile). It is a condition associated with BRAIN enlargement, not simple enlargement of the head (for example, because of thickening of the SKULL). It is more extreme than MACROCEPHALY and is associated with MENTAL RETARDATION, but not primary sensory impairment. There has been a suspicion that it is associated with AUTISM, but this is not the case: incidence of megalencephaly in autism appears to be no greater than in the non-autistic population. There is an animal model of megalencephaly: expression of a recessive (see RECESSIVE ALLELE) GENE in the HOMOZYGOUS condition (*mceph/mceph*) in a mouse is associated with megalencephaly. Examination of this has led to the suggestion that it is HYPERTROPHY of cells in the brain rather than HYPERPLASIA that causes megalencephaly. Dysfunction of GROWTH FACTORS has been suggested to be responsible for this hypertrophy.

References

Petersson S., Nordqvist A.C.S., Schalling M. & Laverbratt C. (1999) The megalencephaly mouse has disturbances in the insulin-like growth factor system. *Molecular Brain Research* 72: 80–88.

Petersson S., Pedersen N.L., Schalling M. & Laverbratt C. (1999) Primary megalencephaly at birth and low intelligence level. *Neurology* 53: 1254–1259.

Meige syndrome *see* blepharospasm

meiosis *see* cell division

Meissner's corpuscles *see* skin

melancholia Antique description of DEPRESSION.

See also: humour

melanocyte stimulating hormone One of the HORMONES released by the ADENOHYPOPHYSIS; see ENDOCRINE GLANDS; HORMONES – CLASSIFICATION.

melanocyte stimulating hormone inhibiting factor One of the HORMONES involved in the control of the release of other hormones from the PITUITARY GLAND; see ADENOHYPOPHYSIS; ENDOCRINE GLANDS; HORMONES – CLASSIFICATION.

melanocyte stimulating hormone releasing factor One of the HORMONES involved in the control of the release of other hormones from the PITUITARY GLAND; see ADENOHYPOPHYSIS; ENDOCRINE GLANDS; HORMONES – CLASSIFICATION.

melatonin A hormone produced in and released by the PINEAL GLAND (see HORMONES). Its chemical name is 5-methyoxy-N-acetyltryptamine. Melatonin is synthesized from its immediate precursor SEROTONIN. The ENZYME serotonin N-acetyltransferase (NAT) converts serotonin to N-acetylserotonin (which is the rate limiting step). This is then converted to melatonin by the enzyme 5-hydroxyindole-O-methyltransferase. Synthesis and secretion of melatonin are markedly influenced by the light–dark cycle. During the day, synthesis and secretion are reduced. At the onset of darkness, the sympathetic innervation of the pineal increases and synthesis of NAT and hence melatonin is greatly increased. The precise physiological and behavioural functions of melatonin in humans are not known. In seasonally breeding mammals, reproductive cycles are tied to the length of the PHOTOPERIOD. Melatonin may be a neuroendocrine transducer that influences secretion of reproductive hormones.

See also: biological clock; circadian rhythm

ANN E. KELLEY

membrane A skin or thin layer of tissue serving as a covering, lining or partition. A neuronal membrane is the boundary of brain cells which controls permeability and serves other functions via surface specializations. PLASMALEMMA is the term given to the membrane covering the SOMA and the dendrites (see DENDRITE) of the cell, while the membrane covering the AXON is called the AXOLEMMA. Neuronal membranes are composed of LIPIDS and PROTEINS. The characteristics of the lipids are responsible for the structure of the membrane and its permeability. The proteins are held by the structure of the lipids. Some of the proteins are intrinsic to the lipid layers and others are extrinsic, located on either the internal or external surface of the membrane. Groups of intrinsic proteins act as carriers of substances (such as sugars and amino acids or NEUROTRANSMITTERS) across the membrane. When the cell is at its RESTING POTENTIAL, some protein units are functioning as pumps, actively moving substances across the membrane against the concentration or electrical gradient to maintain the negative charge of the cell. During an ACTION POTENTIAL, the SODIUM–POTASSIUM PUMP ceases, while other groups of intrinsic proteins act as an ION CHANNEL, opening to allow the passage of sodium and potassium across the membrane. Proteins on the external surface of the membrane may be specialized for the binding of neurotransmitters. Of these, some may have an ion channel which is opened directly when a neurotransmitter chemical binds. In other cases, a receptor protein is coupled to G PROTEIN on the internal surface of the membrane, which may stimulate SECOND MESSENGERS and in turn opens an ion channel.

ERIC M. BOWMAN

membrane channel *see* ion channel

membrane potential The difference in electrical potential, measured in volts, that exists across a MEMBRANE when it is at rest (that is when it is not undergoing DEPOLARIZATION or HYPERPOLARIZATION). It is also known as the RESTING POTENTIAL and is normally about −70 mV: that is the inside of an AXON is relatively negatively charged with respect to the outside of the axon.

See also: action potential

meme (from Greek, *mimeme*: something imitated) A meme is understood to be a cultural unit, transmitted between individuals and across generations by non-genetic means. Memes are things such as practices, beliefs, icons or any other unit of CULTURE. The term was coined in 1976 by Richard Dawkins and was identified as the cultural equivalent of a GENE. It has gained an unintended usage

implying that something is ephemeral, or of passing value.

References

Blackmore S.J. (1999) *The Meme Machine*, Oxford University Press: Oxford.
Dawkins R. (1976) *The Selfish Gene*, Oxford University Press: Oxford.

memory Memory is a maintained representation of internal or external experiences constituted as modifications of neural structure and/or behaviour. Memory includes such diverse forms of plasticity as the simple processes of HABITUATION and SENSITIZATION, and the more complex abilities to recollect facts and events. However, memory recollection need not be conscious. For example, IMPLICIT MEMORY, including PRIMING and motor skills learning, can be expressed without conscious awareness of learning. Memory does not include native response tendencies, reflex adaptations, developmental processes, or temporary states of the organism such as fatigue, although it is sometimes difficult to distinguish memory from these phenomena.

Memory researchers have distinguished different forms of memory such as: DECLARATIVE MEMORY versus PROCEDURAL MEMORY, relational memory versus non-relational memory (see RELATIONAL AND NON-RELATIONAL MEMORY), SEMANTIC MEMORY versus EPISODIC MEMORY, EXPLICIT MEMORY versus IMPLICIT MEMORY, WORKING MEMORY versus reference, TAXON MEMORY versus LOCALE MEMORY, DATA BASED MEMORY versus EXPECTANCY BASED MEMORY, and FACT MEMORY versus SOURCE MEMORY. Memory is thought to be represented at the neuronal level by networks of connected cells. The modulation of cellular firing patterns and either sustained firing after a LEARNING event, or the ability to reactivate the original neuronal response to a stimulus after the stimulus is no longer present represent the cellular traces of memory. At the single-cell level, memory ENCODING can result in changes in the MEMBRANE properties that affect ION flow, SYNAPSE growth or reaction, and changes in PRESYNAPTIC and POSTSYNAPTIC NEUROTRANSMITTERS related functions. Neuronal connections between engrams and overlapping representations of memories allow the rapid association of related memories. Cortical sensory and motor areas are hypothesized to be involved in the long-term storage of memories. For example, the visual attributes of a memory may be stored in the VISUAL CORTEX, and the olfactory attributes of the same memory may be located in the OLFACTORY CORTEX. The reactivation of a complete memory is hypothesized to occur when the CELL ASSEMBLY in the sensory areas that represent the components of the memory becomes simultaneously active through synchronous firing (see ENGRAM for a more detailed discussion of the cellular components and storage of the memory trace).

Memory has been shown not to be a single process, but instead to be consist of MULTIPLE MEMORY SYSTEMS, each of which has its own neuronal network. The HIPPOCAMPUS and related medial structures in the TEMPORAL LOBE are thought to be important for the encoding of declarative memories, novelty detection, and memory CONSOLIDATION. The AMYGDALA is important for STIMULUS–REINFORCER ASSOCIATION and for encoding the emotional components of memories. STIMULUS–RESPONSE ASSOCIATION depends on the STRIATUM. The PREFRONTAL CORTEX has been shown to be involved in WORKING MEMORY and source memory (see SOURCE AMNESIA). The CEREBELLUM is involved in CLASSICAL CONDITIONING processes such as eye-blink conditioning. Finally, BRAINSTEM areas have been shown to be involved in the conditioning of motor reflexes and the adjustment of visual reflexes. The discovery of these multiple memory systems has lead some to view memory not as entity to be stored, but instead as a reflection of the plasticity within each functional system of the brain.

Memory is not immutable; it is subject to many distortions. Over time many recollections become less specific, and can even be completely forgotten (see FORGETTING). The details of a memory can be changed to fit our scripts about what would most likely happen in that type of situation. Also, studies of eyewitness testimony have demonstrated that our memory is very susceptible to suggestion, to the point that people can claim to remember things that never actually happened to them. A person's emotional status at the time of encoding can also dramatically affect the memory formation process. In some circumstances traumatic experiences such as rape can cause someone to forget the event, and sometimes they can cause a person to form vivid recollections of certain aspects of the occurrence. AGEING, diseases (see ALZHEIMER'S DEMENTIA), and brain damage also modify memory.

See also: emotion; learning

HOWARD EICHENBAUM

memory cell *see* immune system

memory deficits The global term used to describe any of a variety of memory failures, including the inability retain or store information, and the inability to recall previously stored information. Memory deficits can be transient or pervasive, and can be seen in SHORT-TERM MEMORY or LONG-TERM MEMORY. In some cases, memories can be temporarily or lastingly restored during recovery. In other situations, such as ALZHEIMER'S DEMENTIA or surgical disruption, memory is not usually restored. Damage can result from accidental injury, surgery, disease, or AGEING. The type of deficit experienced can depend on the location and extent of damaged tissue. In addition memory deficits can be induced functionally through manipulation of cognitive demands. It is notable that memory deficits can occur in the absence of other cognitive deficits, such as LANGUAGE, perceptual or motor impairments. The differential memory deficits and the sparing of other cognitive abilities has led to more complete understanding, identification, and differentiation of memory systems and the type of memories they encode.

There are two basic types of memory deficits, short term and long term. These two deficits are differentiated functionally and through task requirements. Short-term memory is time and capacity limited while long-term memory is not limited by time or capacity. These two types of memory are controlled by different areas of the brain; short-term memory is thought to be controlled by sensory NEOCORTEX, while long-term memory is distributed over various systems and regions of the brain including the medial TEMPORAL LOBE , STRIATUM and CEREBELLUM.

Short-term memory deficits are often manifested as perceptual deficits. This type of deficit occurs with damage to the sensory neocortical areas. The type of deficit is dependent on the sensory area effected. In addition to these perceptual deficits, there is evidence in the human neuropsychological literature for a short-term memory deficit in the absence of long-term memory problems. This deficit is seen after damage to the cortex between WERNICKE'S AREA and BROCA'S AREA. It is manifested by patients inability to repeat information supplied verbally. For instance, a patient would not be able to immediately repeat a test sentence. However, long-term memory of this information, the ability to recount the general content of the sentence remains intact. There is some discrepancy as to whether this is a pure language deficit or an isolated short-term memory deficit. Long-term memory deficits are diverse including not only the inability to form new memories (ANTEROGRADE AMNESIA), but also the inability to recall previously stored information (RETROGRADE AMNESIA). Both of these deficits occur as a result of damage to the medial temporal lobe and medial diencephalon. The medial temporal lobe memory system includes the HIPPOCAMPUS, the ENTORHINAL CORTEX, PERIRHINAL CORTEX, and PARAHIPPOCAMPAL CORTEX, and sometimes includes the AMYGDALA.

Studies of human AMNESIA and attempts to develop animal models of amnesia have allowed for the expansion of the understanding of long-term memory deficits. Though amnesia is a widespread and varied deficit, it is not global. Several memory domains are in fact spared. Amnesic patients are cognitively intact aside from their memory deficits. Patients have intact motor ability: they do not have problems with their basic movements. Unlike patients with short-term memory deficits amnesiac patients have normal perceptual abilities. Patients are able to perform normal perceptual tasks such as the mirror-reading task without deficit. Cognitive abilities such as speaking, seeing, hearing and writing remain intact in these patients. Thus amnesiac patients retain their skills even with very global memory problems. In addition to the retention of skills, amnesiac patients are able to acquire and retain HABITS. Habits are differentiated from other memories because of the explicit nature of the task. Habits do not require the ability to state or exhibit knowledge of the memory. Habits can be manifested as an improvement in performance of a task, such as a motor task, or even a cognitive task. For instance, both amnesic patients and normal subjects required to read a story will become increasingly faster at reading the story with increased practice. PRIMING, an increase in ability to respond or in the speed to response caused by previous exposure, is also intact in amnesic patients. Examples of this include the word stem completion task, the partial pictures task, dot completion task, and the STROOP EFFECT. Priming is dependent on cortical mechanisms and is not affected with damage to the medial temporal lobe. Despite these spared domains, there are many functions and abilities which are impaired in amnesic patients. Patients are not able to remember recent events which they are not allowed to rehearse. When demands, either memory or cognitive, exceed the load of working memory, amnesiac patients will fail the task. In addition, amnesiac patients have a graded deficit of previous memories. For instance, though they may retain information stored several years before damage is incurred, they will not remember information given to them several weeks before the damage.

In addition to these organic forms of memory deficits, memory deficits can be inorganic. These can be induced by diverting ATTENTION, increasing cognitive demands, or imposing delays. In a DIGIT SPAN TASK for instance, distracting the subject will decrease their ability to remember a list of words. In addition to the deficits in medial temporal lobe long-term memory, there are other long-term deficits caused by injury to other brain regions. For instance, CLASSICAL CONDITIONING is disrupted with a LESION of the cerebellum and emotional memory is disrupted with a lesion of the amygdala.

HOWARD EICHENBAUM

memory span Memory span refers to the number of items (typically, digits, letters or words) one can immediately repeat back in the correct serial order. It is a traditional measure of SHORT-TERM MEMORY or WORKING MEMORY capacity and depends critically on the operations of the ARTICULATORY LOOP component of working memory (see Baddeley, 1986). In the case of forward digit span – the most common form of memory span measure – the span size typically ranges from five to eight items among normal adults. Memory span has been used in various standardized tests of INTELLIGENCE, including the WECHSLER ADULT INTELLIGENCE SCALE (WAIS).

See also: recency effect; rehearsal; phonological store; primacy effect

Reference

Baddeley A.D. (1986). *Working Memory*, Oxford University Press: Oxford.

AKIRA MIYAKE

memory trace *see* engram

menarche The first menstruation: the term POSTMENARCHAL is used to indicate females who have passed this point; see MENSTRUAL CYCLE.

meninges The meninges are layers of connective tissue that surround the BRAIN and SPINAL CORD; the singular noun is *meninx*. Around the brain are three layers: the DURA MATER (Latin, hard mother) is a relatively thick, tough but flexible layer of connective tissue that surrounds the brain and other meningeal layers. The outer surface of the dura adheres to the inner surface of the SKULL. Beneath the dura is the SUBDURAL SPACE, through which blood vessels pass, and below is the ARACHNOID MEMBRANE (from Greek, *arachne*: spider – the arachnoid membrane is like a spider's web). The arachnoid is thinner and softer than the dura. It gives rise to the ARACHNOID TRABECULAE (Latin, *trabecula*: a little beam) which descend through the SUBARACHNOID SPACE to contact the PIA MATER (Latin, pious mother) a meningeal layer thinner still than the arachnoid, which contains small blood capillaries and is attached directly to the surface of the brain, following faithfully the GYRI AND SULCI. All three meningeal layers cover the brain and spinal cord but the arachnoid is not present around the SPINAL NERVES and CRANIAL NERVES, which are covered by a lining that is in effect a fusion of the dura and pia mater. The spaces between the meningeal membranes is filled with CEREBROSPINAL FLUID (CSF), which gains access to the subarachnoid space from the cerebral VENTRICLES (where it is synthesized) via three openings from the fourth ventricle: the FORAMINA OF LUSHKA (one in each hemisphere) and the FORAMEN OF MAGENDIE. The function of the meninges is effectively to suspend the brain in fluid, supporting it and absorbing shocks. The fact that it is suspended in fluid effectively decreases the weight of the brain. Moreover, the fact that it is supported in a triple layer of membranes, lubricated by fluid, means that shearing forces generated following sudden impact can be absorbed. Were it not for this, sudden blows to the head would cause tissue to shear – to tear and fragment.

The terms dura mater and pia mater are curiosities: *mater* really does derive from *mater*, Latin for mother, and should, properly, not be referred to as *matter*, as is often done. Carlson (1998) explains the origins of these terms. A Persian physician, Ali ibn Abbas, in the tenth century used the Arabic term *al umm* to describe the meninges. Literally this does mean mother, but also described covering material, there being no term for membrane. The more solid dura was called *al umm al djafiya*, the softer pia *al umm al rigiga*. A century later these were unsympathetically translated literally into Latin as hard mother and soft mother, pious being used in the sense of soft rather than having religious connotation.

See also: hydrocephalus; meningitis

Reference

Carlson N.R. (1998) *The Physiology of Behavior*, 6th edn, Allyn & Bacon:

meningioma *see* tumour

meningitis Inflammation of the membranes (MENINGES) that envelope the brain and spinal cord. The usual cause is infection by almost any of the common viruses or bacteria, the identity of which determines the course of the disease. Viral infections are usually benign and self-limiting, though suspect as a possible cause of persisting debility (see MYALGIC

ENCEPHALITIS). Bacterial infections generally respond well to prompt intervention with antibiotics, but chronic infections, by the organisms responsible for tuberculosis or syphilis, are relatively intractable. Characteristic symptoms of meningitis are due to raised intracranial pressure and include HEADACHE, neck stiffness and urinary retention.

L. JACOB HERBERG

menstrual cycle (from Latin, *menses*: months) Defined literally, a menstrual cycle is any rhythm that occurs on a monthly basis. However, the phrase has become an almost exclusive reference to the human ovulatory cycle, which is a Type 1 cycle (meaning that ovulation and PSEUDOPREGNANCY are spontaneous and not induced by copulatory stimulation). In humans, if an egg is not fertilized by sperm, or if a fertilized egg cannot impregnate itself in the blood-rich lining of the uterus, then the lining will slough off through the vagina. The act of discharging the mix of blood and dead endometrial tissue is known as MENSTRUATION, and occurs at approximately monthly intervals from puberty to menopause. Human attitudes towards menstruation, and menstrual blood in particular, have a spotty history. Ancient Middle Eastern cultures regarded the blood as dirty, and women were shunned or confined to small dark rooms for the duration of menstruation. In contrast, certain Pacific island cultures regarded the blood as a source of renewed life, and individuals would drink it as part of a ritual ceremony.

As with ovulation during estrous cycles in other mammals, the generation and release of eggs is initiated by a cascade of HORMONES moving to and from the ovaries. Like ESTROUS cycles, the human ovulatory cycle consists of phases: the menses phase, the follicular phase and the luteal phase. Menses begins the cycle on the first day of menstruation. Five days later, as menstruation subsides, the follicular phase begins. The ovaries begin to secrete ESTROGEN, which stimulates the growth of the endometrial layer of the uterus and, approximately one week later, induces the release of GONADOTROPHINS (FOLLICLE-STIMULATING HORMONE and LUTEINIZING HORMONE) from the anterior PITUITARY GLAND. Secretion of these gonadotrophins over a two- to three-day period initiates ovulation. The luteal phase begins at ovulation, when the corpus luteum ('yellow body') begins to secrete PROGESTERONE. If PREGNANCY does not occur, the corpus luteum regresses, both estrogen and progesterone levels in the blood decrease, and menstruation begins. Menstrual cycles occur spontaneously in women, as estrous cycles do in certain animals (for example, rats and guinea pigs). Like female great apes, women do not have a period of behavioural ESTRUS. However, women do experience a significant periovulatory rise in sexual desire and frequency of masturbation and sexual intercourse, usually on the weekend before or immediately following ovulation. DYSPHORIA is also experienced by some women during the late luteal phase.

See also: premenstrual tension; sex hormones; sexual motivation

JAMES G. PFAUS

menstruation *see* menstrual cycle

mental age In contrast to CHRONOLOGICAL AGE (actual age, calculated in days, months or years), mental age is an index of the level of intellectual achievement of an individual; see INTELLIGENCE TESTING.

mental chronometry The timing of the cognitive operations; see REACTION TIME.

mental handicap *see* mental retardation

Mental Health Act Legislation governing aspects of the detention, care and treatment of psychiatric patients in the UK. Legislation varies within the UK – England and Wales have the Mental Health Act 1983; Northern Ireland has the Mental Health (NI) Order 1986; in Scotland the Mental Health (Scotland) Act 1984 applies. The Republic of Ireland employs the Mental Treatment Act of 1945. Diagnostic definitions vary from Act to Act, as does the scope for detention and compulsory treatment, right of appeal, and other legal mechanisms.

IAN C. REID

mental imagery *see* image

mental representation This is not the same as either REPRESENTATION or METAREPRESEN-

TATION; but see METAREPRESENTATION for a discussion of mental representation.

mental retardation Substantial impairments in intellectual functioning which exist concurrently with related limitations in adaptive skill areas which may include communication, self care, social and interpersonal skills, community access, self direction, understanding of health and safety, functional academic skills, leisure and work skills. In order for mental retardation to be diagnosed it is widely agreed by professionals that there should be deficits in at least two of these further areas. Furthermore the combination of deficits should manifest in the main before the age of 18 years, so that people who became disabled in their functioning as a result of acquired BRAIN INJURY are not classified as mentally retarded.

This term is used throughout the United States for what is referred to in the UK as LEARNING DISABILITY, and in Australia and New Zealand as INTELLECTUAL IMPAIRMENT. Earlier terms which have been discarded as inaccurate or offensive include MENTAL HANDICAP and MENTAL SUBNORMALITY. The term LEARNING DIFFICULTY is also used in the UK although there is danger of confusion because there are identifiable specific learning difficulties, such as DYSLEXIA and DYSGRAPHIA, which are *not* associated with mental retardation. Which term to use as a description of the condition creates great controversy within professional groups and also in those advocating for people with mental retardation. For example, the term MENTAL RETARDATION is virtually never used in the UK since it is considered to be pejorative. The term LEARNING DISABILITY is thought to have more positive connotations, although the term LEARNING DIFFICULTY is often preferred by advocates and self-advocacy groups.

There are three alternative, albeit complementary, ways of defining mental retardation. The first is administrative, and is based on determining the person's level of intellectual functioning by INTELLIGENCE TESTING. IQ levels of 55 to 69 are described as moderate, and IQs below 55 as severe, mental retardation. Those with an IQ below 25 are described as having profound retardation. This method allows us to identify the prevalence of mental retardation in the population as a whole. A second way of

defining the condition is in terms of its AETIOLOGY, although in many cases the aetiology of mental retardation is unknown. There are specific organic impairments, such as DOWN SYNDROME, WILLIAMS SYNDROME, CORNELIA DE LANGE SYNDROME and PRADER–WILLI SYNDROME which may be associated to varying degrees with intellectual impairments. However the majority of people with mental retardation have no known organic impairments and in that sense are not different from other people, but are less cognitively and behaviourally developed. It is possible, therefore, that much mental retardation is a result of social or other environmental factors, such as severe cultural disadvantage or extremely poor familial circumstances. A third defining characteristic of mental retardation is that the person will need specific training in skills that most people acquire incidentally and that allow independent community living. According to this view, the level of disability is a function of the amount or intensity of instruction which would be required to establish independent community living. It is this definition which is implicit in the approach taken by most psychologists, since it leads directly to restorative or ameliorative action.

Treatment – or more accurately, intervention – involves using a wide variety of methods to increase skills and decrease behaviour problems. BEHAVIOUR ANALYSIS has had marked and dramatic effects in ameliorating the additional deficits associated with the lowered intellectual functioning, using procedures built around the concepts of SHAPING and REINFORCEMENT. The primary aim of such interventions is to give the person skills to enable them to survive in ordinary or supported communities, and to live a meaningful and valued life.

CHRIS CULLEN

mental set A predisposition or tendency, which biases STIMULUS processing or RESPONSE output.

See also: attention; attentional set; attentional set-shifting; schema

VERITY J. BROWN

mental subnormality *see* mental retardation

mentalism *see* dualism; neurophilosophy

meperidine Also known as PETHIDINE, this is a synthetic compound with properties similar to MORPHINE.

See also: opiates

mercury-in-rubber strain gauge Also known as a PLETHYSMAGRAPH; a device for estimating SEXUAL AROUSAL from measures of blood flow in the penis or vagina.

Merkel's discs *see* skin

mescaline Mescaline (chemically, 3,4,5-tri-methoxyphenethylamine – a PHENETHYLAMINE drug) is an HALLUCINOGEN, used in the Americas certainly since the time of Columbus and probably for very many centuries before that. Mescaline was derived from the mescal bean (which gives it its name) but because this preparation has unwanted toxic properties it was later extracted from the PEYOTE cactus rather more safely; mescaline is therefore also known as peyote.

mesencephalic locomotor region A region in the MESOPONTINE tegmentum which was once thought to control locomotor activity. The region was defined functionally, rather than anatomically, but was nonetheless believed to be the PEDUNCULOPONTINE TEGMENTAL NUCLEUS (PPTg). Evidence came initially from the PRECOLLICULAR–POSTMAMMILLARY TRANSECTION experiments, and subsequently from TRACT TRACERS and PPTg electrical stimulation (see ELECTRICAL BRAIN STIMULATION) or LESION studies. Although the PPTg is still thought to have a role in many aspects of motor control, it is now clear that locomotion is driven by a distributed system rather than a specific centre in the brain. Some authors have argued that the term 'mesencephalic locomotor region' no longer has any value and should be abandoned.

See also: locomotion

Reference

Allen L.F., Inglis W.L. & Winn P. (1996) Is the cuneiform nucleus a critical component of the mesencephalic locomotor region? An examination of the effects of excitotoxic lesions of the cuneiform nucleus on spontanous and nucleus accumbens induced loco-motion. *Brain Research Bulletin* 41: 201–210.

WENDY L. INGLIS

mesencephalon (from Greek, *mesos*: middle, *enkephalon*: brain) The MIDBRAIN. Many of the generally descriptive Greek and Latin terms in NEUROANATOMY, though still useful in describing the developing nervous system, have been moved aside over the years: RHOMBENCEPHALON has given way to HINDBRAIN, MESENCEPHALON to MIDBRAIN and PROSENCEPHALON to FOREBRAIN. The term *mesencephalic*, meaning 'of the mesencephalon', or 'of the midbrain', has survived rather better than the term mesencephalon itself.

mesial (from Greek, *mesos*: middle) Towards the middle. Although in certain contexts this has a specific meaning, in neuroscience it is a rarely used form of MEDIAL.

mesocortex *see* juxtallocortex

mesoderm The middle one of the three GERM LAYERS present in the developing EMBRYO (the others being ECTODERM and ENDODERM), it gives rise to tissues such as such as MUSCLES, heart (see BLOOD), KIDNEY, LIVER, BLOOD and bone (see CONNECTIVE TISSUE); see DEVELOPMENT.

mesolimbic Connecting the MESENCEPHALON and LIMBIC SYSTEM; most commonly used to refer to the MESOLIMBIC DOPAMINE SYSTEM.

mesolimbic dopamine system A chemically identified anatomical system comprising cell bodies of dopamine-containing neurons of the VENTRAL TEGMENTAL AREA (VTA), which send their axons in the medial forebrain bundle to terminate predominantly in the ventral STRIATUM. The dopaminergic neurons of this system belong to one of several populations of dopamine-containing neurons in the MESENCEPHALON (hence, 'meso-'). The cells giving rise to the mesolimbic projection have been designated the A10 group. The A10 cells project to the ventral striatum (the largest component of which is the NUCLEUS ACCUMBENS but which also includes anteromedial portions of the CAUDATE–PUTAMEN, OLFACTORY TUBERCLE, AMYGDALA and HIPPOCAMPUS, all of which are components of the LIMBIC SYSTEM hence,

'-limbic'). The mesolimbic dopamine system is activated by PSYCHOMOTOR STIMULANTS and other addictive drugs. INTRACRANIAL SELF-STI-MULATION (ICSS) in the medial forebrain bundle also releases dopamine in the ventral striatum. It is this activation of the mesolimbic dopamine system which may underlie the reinforcing properties of ICSS and drugs of abuse.

See also: mesolimbicocortical system; nigrostriatal dopamine system

VERITY J. BROWN

mesolimbicocortical system A chemically identified anatomical system comprising dopamine-containing cells of the MESENCEPHALON which project to LIMBIC and cortical areas of the FOREBRAIN. Whereas the term MESOLIMBIC DOPAMINE SYSTEM is used to refer to the projections mainly from the A10 cell group to subcortical limbic structures, the term meso-limbicocortical system is used to refer to these projections as well as to projections to cortical areas from A10 neurons and projections to limbic areas from neurons of the A9 and A8 groups. Thus, the subcortical terminal regions of the mesolimbicocortical dopamine system are the ventral striatum (comprising the NU-CLEUS ACCUMBENS and the ventral and ante-romedial CAUDATE–PUTAMEN); the OLFACTORY BULB, anterior olfactory nucleii, OLFACTORY TUBERCLE and islands of Callaja; the SEPTAL NUCLEI; the nucleus of the diagonal band; the AMYGDALA; and the HIPPOCAMPUS. The corti-cal projections are to pyriform cortex, entorh-inal, suprarhinal and perirhinal cortex and pregenual and supragenual anteromedial cor-tex. These cortical areas have in common that they are part of, or anatomically closely related, to the LIMBIC SYSTEM. The DOPAMINE theory of schizophrenia assumes there is hyper-activity of the mesolimbicocortical dopamine system.

See also: classification of Dahlström and Fuxe; nigrostriatal dopamine system

VERITY J. BROWN

mesopic *see* duplexity theory

mesopontine The term mesopontine is used to describe an area of tissue the lies around the

junction of the MESENCEPHALON (hence meso-) and PONS. The mesopontine tegmentum (see TEGMENTUM) is the dorsal area of this. The most prominent structure in this region is the PEDUNCULOPONTINE TEGMENTAL NUCLEUS.

messenger RNA *see* RNA

mesulergine An ANTAGONIST at the $5HT_{2C}$ receptor; see SEROTONIN RECEPTORS.

metabolic *see* metabolism

metabolic mapping This is a generic term which refers to techniques that measure the rate of METABOLISM within tissues. Two of the most widely used metabolic mapping techni-ques in neuroscience are radiolabelled 2-deox-yglucose autoradiography (see RADIOLABEL), and measurement of Fos (see IMMEDIATE EARLY GENES) Like GLUCOSE, deoxyglucose is phosphorylated by the enzyme GLUCOSE 6-PHOSPHATASE, whereby it becomes trapped within the cell. The amount of deoxyglucose 6-phosphate, measured by autoradiographic imaging, is proportional to the amount of glucose metabolized through the glycolytic pathway, thus indicating the energy used within a given tissue region. Fos is a protein encoded for by the immediate early gene *c-fos*; it is produced in certain neurons in response to stimulation, and can be measured by IMMUNO-HISTOCHEMISTRY. This technique indicates which specific neurons are affected by stimula-tion. Both techniques are useful in establishing how experimental manipulations may affect metabolism in neuronal tissue.

See also: cytochrome oxidase; functional ne-uroimaging; image analysis

FIONA M. INGLIS

metabolic rate The metabolic rate of an animal is the amount of ENERGY it uses in a given amount of time. It is measured in calories (cal – or in multiples of 1000 calories, kilo-calories – kcal) usually by determining the amount of heat an animal produces when placed in a CALORIMETER or by measuring OXYGEN used in RESPIRATION. Metabolic rate of course can change very much depending on what an animal is doing. BASAL METABOLIC RATE represents the amount of energy used by an ENDOTHERM at rest (across a normal range of temperatures) and with an empty stomach – that is, it represents the energy cost of simply *being*, rather than *doing* anything. For an ECTOTHERM, the metabolic rate alters as a function of the ambient temperature, so one does not calculate a basal metabolic rate but specifies a STANDARD METABOLIC RATE at specified temperatures. It is a curious and unexplained fact that metabolic rate and body size are inversely correlated. Smaller animals have much higher metabolic rates than do larger ones.

See also: metabolism

Reference

Campbell N.A., Reece J.B. & Mitchell L.G. (1999) *Biology*, 5th edn, Addison-Wesley: Menlo Park CA.

metabolic tolerance *see* drug disposition tolerance

metabolism (from Greek, *metabole*: change) Metabolism (or a METABOLIC process) is the term given to all of the chemical changes that take place inside a living organism (animal or plant). It can be broken into two opposed components: CATABOLISM (from Greek, *kata*: down, *ballein*: to throw) and ANABOLISM (from Greek, *ana*: up, and *ballein*). Catabolism (or a catabolic process) is the name given to the process of breaking down molecules (see MOLECULE) into simpler units; it releases ENERGY. Anabolism (or an anabolic process) is a process of building more complex molecules from simpler units; it consumes energy. The term METABOLITE refers to a chemical that is the product of metabolism: a CATABOLITE is the product of catabolism, an anabolite the product of anabolism. Very often the more general term metabolite is used when more strictly catabolite would be correct. Note that the study of metabolism is central to an understanding of biology, being a central property of living things.

See also: metabolic mapping; metabolic rate

Reference

Campbell N.A., Reece J.B. & Mitchell L.G. (1999) *Biology*, 5th edn, Addison-Wesley: Menlo Park CA.

metabolites *see* metabolism

metabotropic Receptors that are indirectly coupled to an ION CHANNEL through SECOND MESSENGERS are referred to as metabotropic receptors. In contrast. ionotropic receptors directly gate their ion channels, allowing the flow of selected ions (see ION) such as SODIUM (Na^+), CALCIUM (Ca^{2+}), POTASSIUM (K^+) and CHLORIDE (Cl^-).

metameric match *see* trichromatic theory of colour vision

metamorphopsias *see* face perception

metarepresentation To understand metarepresentation it is necessary to understand the concepts of REPRESENTATION and MENTAL REPRESENTATION. The term representation is used when one thing stands for another. For example, a map may stand for the layout of a place. Mental representation is used to describe the representation in the mind of external events, past events or imaginary events. Perceptions are representations of external events. For example, 'greenness' is a mental representation of light of a certain wavelength viewed under normal conditions. Recollections are mental representations of past events. Ideas and mental images are representations of how things might be, could be (or could not be), or will be. Mental representations are conscious and occur in the explicit domain; that is, they are experienced by the person and can be described or talked about. Information in the implicit domain includes skills which are acquired but which cannot be fully described. For example, musical expertise can be demonstrated but not adequately described.

Three levels of mental representation can usefully be distinguished (Leslie, 1987). Primary representations are about how the world is now, including perceptions and knowledge of constant relationships in the world. Secondary representations are decoupled from the world as it is now, in that they represent things as they could be, as they once were, or as they will be. Secondary representations are required to recollect the past as an event different from the present, to make propositions or generate ideas and to engage in pretend play. According to Perner (1993), children less than about 18 months old cannot form secondary representations and therefore live entirely in the present.

For example, a very young child may play with a toy car only as an object. Older children can form secondary representations which allow them to consider multiple alternatives: for example, they could regard a toy car as simultaneously 'being a car' and 'being a piece of plastic'. The ability to form multiple representations is a prerequisite to forming metarepresentations.

A metarepresentations depicts something as being a representation of a subject and defines the relation between the subject and its representation (Pylyshyn, 1978). This can be illustrated by considering misrepresentations. Perception requires mental representation but understanding that perceptions are mental representations, and that your perception may differ from reality, requires metarepresentation. For example, to know that you are experiencing a visual illusion requires the ability to form a metarepresentation of the relationship (and potential difference) between perception and reality. It is the understanding of the relationships between representations which constitutes the metarepresentation. Metarepresentation is necessary during cognitive processing in order to 'label' mental representations with the type of cognitive process of which they are a product. It is necessary to know, for example, which products of cognitive processing are percepts, known facts, memories, ideas, or expectations. Memories are distinguished from knowledge because the former has a 'label' or 'episodic trace information' which imbues it with the mental quality of a recollection (Tulving, 1985). Failure to attach cognitive labels may result in imagery being misinterpreted as perceptions and ideas being misinterpreted as known facts. These sorts of errors may contribute to the HALLUCINATION and DELUSION of PSYCHOSIS (Frith, 1992). For example, one form of auditory hallucination associated with SCHIZOPHRENIA is 'thought broadcast': 'It was like my ears being blocked up and my thoughts shouted out'. In this case the patient recognizes his own thoughts but experiences them as if they were perceptions of the outside world. With more extreme examples, such as 'delusions of control' and 'thought insertion', the mislabelling is complete and the patient is convinced that the products

of internal cognitive processes (thoughts and intentions) are emanating from the outside world.

Metarepresentation is particularly important for understanding that another person may hold beliefs (mental representations) that are different from your own mental representations and that neither necessarily accords with the real world. Metarepresentation is therefore necessary for the development of complex social interactions in which it is necessary to know who knows what, and, on occasions, to practice deceit. The mental ability to form metarepresentations is a prerequisite for the ability to develop a THEORY OF MIND, which includes the ability to understand that beliefs are constrained by access to information. Patients with AUTISM have a specific difficulty with theory-of-mind tasks concerning the beliefs of other people which depend upon metarepresentation. It is not yet resolved, however, whether autism is associated with a general problem of metarepresentation or whether this problem is restricted to the domain of social interactions.

See also: consciousness

References

Frith C.D. (1992) *The Cognitive Psychology of Schizophrenia*, Lawrence Erlbaum: Hove UK.

Leslie A.M. (1987) Pretense and representation: the origins of 'theory of mind'. *Psychological Reviews* 94: 412–426.

Perner J. (1993) *Understanding the Representational Mind*, MIT Press: Cambridge MA.

Pylyshyn Z.W. (1978) When is attribution of beliefs justified? *Behavioural and Brain Sciences* 1: 592–693.

Tulving E. (1985) Memory and consciousness. *Canadian Psychology* 26: 1–12.

ROSALIND RIDLEY AND CHRISTOPHER FRITH

metastases *see* tumour

metathetic continuum METATHETIC CONTINUUM and the related term PROTHETIC CONTINUUM denote phenomena of sensation. A metathetic continuum is one in which qualitative rather than quantitative changes are described. For example, as the wavelength of light changes, one describes differences in colour – red, green and so on – that fill discrete categories. A prothetic continuum has quantitative but not qualitative changes. For example, the weight of objects can be described as being 'more' or 'less' but there are no discriminable categories of weight. The difference between this is little understood: there is, for example, no description of the mechanisms that allow humans to break colour vision into discrete segments (and it is entirely unknown whether animals with COLOUR VISION have the same types of metathetic experience of colour). It is conceivable that understanding processes such as this could be valuable in explaining how brains generate conscious experience (see CONSCIOUSNESS).

See also: sensation vs. perception

metencephalon During development the RHOMBENCEPHALON differentiates into the metencephalon and MYELENCEPHALON. The metencephalon includes the CEREBELLUM and PONS, the myelencephalon becomes the MEDULLA OBLONGATA; see HINDBRAIN.

metestrus *see* estrus

methadone A synthetic opiate, used in the relief of heroin addiction by maintenance or substitution therapy; see HEROIN for a discussion of this.

See also: addiction

methoxamine An alpha-1 noradrenaline receptor AGONIST; see ADRENOCEPTORS.

3-methoxy-4-hydroxyphenylacetaldehyde *see* dopamine

3-methoxy-4-hydroxyphenylglycoaldehyde *see* noradrenaline

3-methoxy-4-hydroxyphenylglycol *see* noradrenaline

3-methoxytyramine (or methamphetamine) *see* dopamine

methylamphetamine *see* amphetamine

methylation To methylate is to replace an ATOM (typically hydrogen) on a MOLECULE with a methyl group (a -CH3 group). DNA methylation involves attachment of a methyl group to the nucleotide CYTOSINE. This serves to protect DNA and can help regulate GENE TRANSCRIPTION.

methylphenidate (Ritalin) A psychomotor stimulant DRUG that potentiates CATECHOLAMINE release from PRESYNAPTIC sites. It has similar (though not identical actions) to AMPHETAMINE and is used in the treatment of ATTENTION-DEFICIT DISORDER, in which is has a paradoxical calming effect.

methylxanthine A metabolite of CAFFEINE (one of the XANTHINES) passed in the urine.

methysergide A drug that is a non-selective SEROTONIN receptor ANTAGONIST – that is, it does not discriminate between any of the subclasses of the SEROTONIN RECEPTORS, but blocks them all.

mianserin An atypical ANTIDEPRESSANT drug, developed from the TRICYCLIC antidepressants: it has no effects on REUPTAKE processes for any MONOAMINE and has effects on a variety of RECEPTOR types. It has strong SEDATIVE properties.

See also: monoamine hypothesis of depression

micro- (from Greek, *mikros*: little) Prefix indicating a factor of 10^{-6}, or one millionth; see SI UNITS.

microcephaly (from Greek, *mikros*: little, *kephale*: head) An abnormally small development of the head, and of the BRAIN also, often (but not always) associated with MENTAL RETARDATION.

microdialysis (Often referred to as *IN VIVO* MICRODIALYSIS; colloquially [and incorrectly] referred to as DIALYSIS, which is a more general term.) A process by which neurochemical substances (see NEUROCHEMISTRY) can be extracted from brain extracellular fluid by means of a small SEMIPERMEABLE MEMBRANE. Microdialysis permits the quantitative measurement of changes in brain chemistry in behaving animals and involves the implantation into a brain structure of interest of a small metal tube attached to a short section of dialysis tubing. Artificial CEREBROSPINAL FLUID perfused through the tubing collects molecules from the extracellular fluid as they move across the dialysis membrane by DIFFU-

SION. Collected perfusate, termed DIALYSATE, is then analysed for its chemical composition using various analytical procedures (such as HIGH PERFORMANCE LIQUID CHROMATOGRAPHY).

See also: electrochemistry; no net flux; push–pull perfusion; reverse microdialysis; voltammetry

CHARLES D. BLAHA

microelectrode *see* electrode

microenvironment A term used to indicate localized areas of activity within organisms, as opposed to the environment at large in which organisms exist. One might talk for example of the microenvironment that is formed at a SYNAPSE: the SYNAPTIC CLEFT is a microenvironment in which important biological events occur.

microfilament *see* cytoskeleton

microglia *see* glial cells

micrographia A condition in which handwriting (see WRITING) is much reduced in size, though the style (that is an individual's particular style of handwriting) and content is preserved. It is associated with motor disorders, most notably PARKINSON'S DISEASE. In this condition it is thought to give evidence that existing motor programmes (see MOTOR PROGRAMMING) are intact, though their execution may be made more difficult by the disease.

microinjection A direct injection into brain of a very small amount of fluid. There are two circumstances in which microinjections are made: (1) in order to determine the effect of a DRUG or chemical acting at a particular brain site on behaviour; and (2) in order to deliver fluid into brain during STEREOTAXIC SURGERY.

Microinjection into conscious animals to study the effects of a drug on behaviour involves permanently implanting (under general anaesthesia) a guide CANNULA into the brain. This is held in place by DENTAL ACRYLIC and SKULL SCREWS. The guide cannula will be normally occluded by a STYLET (or OBDURATOR) – a pin that fits securely into the guide cannula, filling its entire length. The guide cannula does not terminate in the structure to which one is trying to gain access but above it.

To make a microinjection, the stylet is removed and a microinjection cannula inserted through the guide. The microinjection cannula extends beyond the tip of the guide to access the structure into which fluid is to be injected. The microinjection cannula will be attached by polyethylene tubing to a microlitre syringe, usually mounted in a pump. Activation of the pump drives fluid, at a suitably slow rate, into brain. After waiting for a period to allow fluid to diffuse away from the cannula tip, the microinjection cannula is withdrawn and the stylet reinserted. Animals will typically be microinjected while conscious, unless the drug has effects that make this inadvisable.

Microinjections can be made using a cannula during STEREOTAXIC SURGERY, usually to deliver NEUROTOXINS or TRACT TRACERS. In this case the animal will be anaesthetized and a guide cannula will not be used. The cannula will be inserted under stereotaxic control, fluid infused, the cannula withdrawn after a suitable interval to allow diffusion away from the cannula tip, and the wound sealed appropriately.

microiontophoresis (also spelled microionophoresis) A technique for administering ionized (see ION) chemicals near a neuron that is being electrophysiologically recorded (see SINGLE-UNIT ELECTROPHYSIOLOGICAL RECORDING). The sign of current (positive or negative) for ejection depends on the charge of the ionized chemical. The intensity of current roughly determines the amount of chemicals to be ejected. Multibarrel glass electrodes are commonly used for microiontophoresis, with each barrel containing a DRUG such as an AGONIST or ANTAGONIST of interest. One barrel can be used for recording; alternately, a separate microelectrode for recording can be glued to multibarrel electrodes. Intracellular microiontophoresis with a marker such as BIOCYTIN allows for labelling of single neurons.

KAZUE SEMBA

microneurography An technique in which minute electrodes (see ELECTRODE) are placed into a peripheral NERVE using hypodermic needles, in order to record electrical activity. This technique has been especially useful in mapping SOMATOSENSORY system activity.

micropsia A phenomenon in which things are perceived as being smaller than they actually are. It can be produced by damage in the VISUAL SYSTEM and is also associated with certain forms of EPILEPSY, though it is neither common nor defining in this condition. Pharmacological treatment of the retina with ANTICHOLINERGIC drugs produces micropsia.

See also: macropsia

microsaccade A small SACCADE; see NYSTAGMUS.

microscopy The use of a microscope for detailed examination of material. No matter what form of HISTOLOGY has been accomplished, tissue invariably must be examined under a microscope. Several important different techniques are available: these include LIGHT MICROSCOPY, CONFOCAL MICROSCOPY and ELECTRON MICROSCOPY.

See also: camera lucida; cell counting; chemical neuro-anatomy; stereology

microtome A device for cutting sections of tissue (see HISTOLOGY). There are two important parts: a block on which tissue can be held firm and a cutting blade. Microtomes work in essentially one of two ways: either the blade is moved across the tissue; or the tissue is moved across the blade. (Modern blades are disposable, in a manner analogous to scalpel blades.) In either case, each pass will move the tissue block through a predetermined distance (which will determine the thickness of the sections being cut). The tissue to be placed on the block can be processed in a variety of ways: the most common are PARAFFIN EMBEDDING (also called paraffin wax processing), PLASTIC EMBEDDING and freezing (usually achieved using dry ice or a cooled solvent). All make the tissue firm so that it can be sectioned without distortion. The thickness of the sections cut is to a large extent dependent on the method of embedding. For example, paraffin-embedded sections can be as thin as 4 μm, plastic even thinner. Frozen sections are usually in excess of 25 μm thick. Frozen sections thinner than this can be cut on a CRYOSTAT, which maintains low temperature better than a bench microtome. (When the sections are cut they warm slightly – they defrost – but in a cryostat, where the local air temperature is controlled this presents less of a problem.)

See also: fixation; vibratome

microtubule *see* cytoskeleton

micturition (from Latin, *micturire*: urination) Micturition – the passage of urine – is unusual from a neural control perspective: it involves involuntary reflexes (see REFLEX) mediated by the AUTONOMIC NERVOUS SYSTEM. PARASYMPATHETIC systems, activated by bladder distension, control contraction of the bladder wall, to force the expulsion of urine. SYMPATHETIC NERVOUS SYSTEM activation causes relaxation of the bladder, activation of this system leading to inhibition of the parasympathetic control mechanisms. The bladder is also controlled by BARRINGTON'S NUCLEUS, in the PONS: this nucleus is under the control of FOREBRAIN systems as well as input from the bladder to indicate its state of fullness. Output from Barrington's nucleus can coordinate peripheral activity, leading to voluntary bladder emptying.

midazolam A benzodiazepine drug, also available as Hypnovel.

See also: benzodiazepine-induced hyperphagia

midbrain Also called the MESENCEPHALON, the midbrain is the smallest part of the BRAINSTEM. It is sandwiched between the PONS caudally, and the DIENCEPHALON rostrally. Like the pons and MEDULLA, the midbrain is divided into the TECTUM, TEGMENTUM, and most ventrally, CEREBRAL PEDUNCLE. The tectum in the midbrain consists of the SUPERIOR COLLICULUS and INFERIOR COLLICULUS, concerned with visuomotor coordination and auditory functions, respectively. The cerebral peduncle consists of fibre tracts arising from the MOTOR CORTEX and other FOREBRAIN structures. In the tegmentum immediately dorsal to the cerebral peduncle lies the SUBSTANTIA NIGRA, which is involved in the regulation of striatal functions (see STRIATUM and NIGROSTRIATAL DOPAMINE SYSTEM). Loss of the pars compacta of substantia nigra is the principal pathological feature of PARKINSON'S DISEASE.

KAZUE SEMBA

midbrain extrapyramidal area *see* pedunculopontine tegmental nucleus

midbrain reticular formation Also known as the mesencephalic reticular formation, this is a part of the RETICULAR FORMATION. It contains three main elements: the *deep mesencephalic nucleus*, the PEDUNCULOPONTINE TEGMENTAL NUCLEUS and the CUNEIFORM NUCLEUS (including the subcuneiform nucleus).

See also: ascending reticular activating system; medullary reticular formation; mesencephalic locomotor region; pontine reticular formation

middle cerebellar peduncle A large fibre tract carrying information from the PONTINE NUCLEI to the CEREBELLUM; see HINDBRAIN.

middle cerebral artery *see* blood

middle-in/out processing *see* top-down vs. bottom-up perceptual/neural processing

middle temporal gyrus The TEMPORAL LOBE has three principal gyri (see GYRI AND SULCI) clearly visible on the outer surface: the inferior, middle and superior temporal gyri (the inferior being most ventral, the superior most dorsal).

middle temporal region The middle temporal region, or area MT (also commonly known as V5; see AREAS VI–V5) is a region in the EXTRASTRIATE CORTEX located within the SUPERIOR TEMPORAL SULCUS in the Old World monkey. It is identified by its pattern of heavy myelination (see MYELIN). It receives its major input from layers 4B and 6 of area V1 and other inputs from the thick stripes of V2 suggesting a strong dependence on the MAGNO-CELLULAR (M) pathway, and also has input from the SUPERIOR COLLICULUS. It contains a complete topographic representation of the visual field and its receptive fields are approximately 10 times larger than those of a corresponding retinal location in area V1. MT is strongly implicated in the processing of information about visual motion (see MOTION PERCEPTION) and has thus received considerable attention as an example of the notion that differing visual functions (such as motion, depth, colour and so on) are processed in separate extrastriate regions. The vast majority of cells are directionally selective and are organized into directionally selective columns (see CORTICAL COLUMNS AND HYPERCOLUMNS). In monkeys damage to this area produces a motion blindness that spares other visual functions. Recordings from individual cells show that the behaviour of the animal on tasks of motion direction judgement are well correlated to the response of appropriately tuned cells. Further the behaviour of the animal on these tasks can be altered by microstimulation of these cells suggesting a causal relationship between the firing of these cells and visual behaviour. Some cells in this area have been shown to be sensitive to the overall motion of patterns rather to the local component of motion (to which cells of area V1 are sensitive). A human homologue of area MT has been identified by myelin staining and by FUNCTIONAL NEUROIMAGING techniques that compare the response in the cortex to moving stimuli with its response to stationary stimuli. The identified area is located approximately in the junction of the TEMPORAL LOBE, PARIETAL LOBE and OCCIPITAL LOBE. Damage to this area in humans may lead to MOTION BLINDNESS (also termed CEREBRAL AKINETOPSIA) where the patient is unable to process information about motion though other visual information is spared.

See also: visual system

ROBERT J. SNOWDEN

midline The brain is divided into two hemispheres (see HEMISPHERE): the midline is an imaginary line that runs along the surface of the brain from ANTERIOR to POSTERIOR which perfectly separates the right hemisphere from the left. Though this line is imaginary in so far as there is not an actual line present dividing the hemispheres, there are physical representations of it. There is a large blood vessel that runs along the midline of the rodent brain (the MIDLINE SINUS) and the SKULL has a midline SUTURE. These give an accurate indication of the position of the midline, essential in rodent STEREOTAXIC SURGERY.

midline sinus *see* midline

migraine Classical migraine is characterized by episodes of unilateral HEADACHE ushered in by distinctive visual symptoms (scintillating FORTIFICATION SPECTRA for instance) and is usually accompanied by NAUSEA, VOMITING and PHOTOPHOBIA. In some variants one or more of these features, even the headache, may be absent. Trigger factors include hormonal (see HORMONES) disturbances (from contraceptive pills for example), certain dietary constituents (such as cheese, chocolate and chianti), drugs (such as RESERPINE or m-CPP, a serotonin 2B/2C receptor agonist – see SEROTONIN RECEPTORS) and attacks may be especially frequent at the onset or termination of a period of psychological STRESS. Heredity may sometimes contribute, but psychosocial traits and personality play little part. The pathogenesis of migraine was for long accounted for by the vascular hypothesis (Wolff, 1963). This ascribed the prodromal symptoms to cortical ISCHAEMIA produced by local or unilateral VASOCONSTRICTION, followed by a painful rebound dilatation of the blood vessels of the overlying scalp. Unfortunately this account leaves many questions unanswered. Elaborations of Wolff's theory have emphasized the possible role of the TRIGEMINAL NERVE (the fifth cranial nerve; see CRANIAL NERVES), release of NEUROTRANSMITTERS, NEUROPEPTIDES, NITRIC OXIDE (NO), and SPREADING DEPRESSION. For example, the PAIN and the successive vasomotor changes accompanying an attack have been ascribed to disordered (ANTIDROMIC) activity in the ophthalmic branch of the trigeminal, causing release of pain-inducing neuropeptides in the walls of cerebral blood vessels and in the DURA MATER. The peptides involved include SUBSTANCE P and CALCITONIN GENE-RELATED PEPTIDE (CGRP); these substances may serve also to bring about vasomotor changes by releasing an ENDOTHELIUM-relaxing factor such as nitric oxide. The prodromal cortical disturbances (which may include transient APHASIA or contralateral HEMIPARESIS) are widely believed to be caused by a process of spreading depression, but the evidence for the occurrence of spreading depression in deeply fissured human cortex remains controversial. Migraine prophylaxis is commonly sought by treatment with the serotonin receptor antagonist METHYSERGIDE, while the attacks themselves can often be aborted with serotonin receptor agonists (such as naratriptan, sumatriptan or zolmitriptan).

Unfortunately, these tend to have unwanted side-effects, they are not always effective, their mode of action is uncertain and the role of SEROTONIN in the pathogenesis of migraine remains obscure. Other drugs commonly used for treatment or prevention, with varying success, include vasoactive ergot alkaloids, CALCIUM CHANNEL blocking agents, adrenergic alpha 2 receptor agonists (such as CLONIDINE) and beta receptor antagonists, PROPRANOLOL for example (see NORADRENALINE RECEPTORS).

Reference

Wolff H.G. (1963) *Headache and Other Head Pain*, 2nd edn, Oxford University Press: New York.

L. JACOB HERBERG

migration Most if not all animals respond to two geophysical cycles: diurnal (daily) and annual periodicity, produced by the earth's rotation and tilt with respect to the sun. One response to periodicity is HIBERNATION. Poorwill birds in southwestern North America, for example, retire to caves each fall where they overwinter as their body temperature drops to 10 °C. A more common response to periodicity is migration. Many aquatic animals, such as plankton, undertake diurnal vertical migrations, moving up and down a water column in response to changes in light, temperature and food. Other animals undertake seasonal vertical migrations moving, for example, from alpine meadows in mountains to valley floors each autumn. Many animals undertake seasonal north–south movements that cover much longer distances. One prodigious migrant is the Arctic tern. Each fall this bird flies from the Arctic south along the eastern shoreline of North America, then across the Atlantic to the African coast, which is followed to the Antarctic seas. After reversing this journey in the following spring, the birds will have flown more than 20 000 miles. Many migrants exhibit increased fat deposition before migration. Some animals, especially nocturnally migrating birds, show ZUGUNRUHE (migratory restlessness) before migration. Once under way migration tends to follow fixed routes for each species. Routes often follow geological features such as coastlines and mountains, but at times also cross featureless open oceans and deserts. For many species there are traditional resting areas *en route*. Migrants maintain species-specific compass directions during their journey. This orientation sense seems to be genetically pre-programmed. Many migrants, even inexperienced animals, show spontaneous directional preferences at the onset of migration. For example, birds in a funnel-shaped cage containing an inked pad floor will mark the cage wall at a certain orientation as they hop and flit about. Directional information seems to come from several sources. Two of the most clearly established compasses are the sun and the rotation of the stars around the North Star. Orientation information may also be obtained from olfactory gradients, infrasound gradients, and the earth's magnetic field gradients – but these mechanisms remain controversial. Because the positioning of the sun and stars changes over the course of the year, animals must possess some circannual timing process successfully to use these as accurate compasses. Migration probably evolved because it permits animals to maximize resource recruitment and minimize exposure to harsh climates and barren environments.

See also: biological clock; circannual rhythm; flight; maps; navigation; neuronal migration

DONALD M. WILKIE

milli- Prefix indicating a factor of 10^{-3}, or one thousandth; see SI UNITS.

milnacipran *see* serotonin noradrenaline reuptake inhibitor

mimicry Mimicry is typically understood as a strategy in NATURAL SELECTION such that animals (mimics) take on the appearance of other animals (models). *Batesian mimicry* occurs when an animal mimics the appearance of a model that is avoided by predators. *Müllerian mimicry* occurs when several SPECIES adopt a common pattern or colouration in order to warn off predators. Note that mimicry is generally understood by ethologists (see ETHOLOGY) to relate to the mimicking of form rather than behaviour; see OBSERVATION LEARNING and EMULATION for discussion of how organisms might copy behaviour.

mind–body question The question of how mind and body, or more specifically mind and brain, are related remains one of the most difficult problems both of philosophy and of science. With fresh discoveries being reported daily of how changes in the physical substrate of the brain are correlated with changes in mental life, discussions of the mind–body and mind–brain link at times receive wide publicity. This is well exemplified by the Nobel Laureate Francis Crick's *The Astonishing Hypothesis* and by Antonio Damasio's *Descartes' Error*, both published in 1994.

The dualist (see DUALISM) view of the relation between mind and body has taken several different forms down the centuries. The classical exposition of it is usually regarded as that of René Descartes (1596–1650). For him, mind and body were both substances. Body was an extended material substance, the mind an unextended or spiritual substance. The mind was taken to be subject to quite different principles of operation from the body. There remains a variety of dualist theories of mind in the philosophical market place. Some assume that mental events and brain events run in parallel without any causal interaction (see EPIPHENOMENA). Others regard the brain as, in some undefined way, secreting mental events rather in the way that glands secrete various substances. Others hold interactionist theories recognizing that the body acts upon the mind and the mind acts upon the body. Yet another variant of dualism is the view that claims that mind is an emergent property (see EMERGENT PROPERTIES) of brain processes. By analogy, water possesses properties not evident in its constituents of oxygen and hydrogen. Equally, mind and brain are found to have very different properties. Most of those who have subscribed to one or another form of dualism have also held the view that there is some causal interaction between mental and physical events.

According to the physiologist Sir John Eccles (1903–1997; joint winner of the Nobel Prize for Medicine, 1963) the mind in a non-physical world influences what is happening at the level of the electron and the mechanics by which the happenings at a SYNAPSE take place. Although in one sense this view may fit most of the data, it raises a number of further difficult problems, such as how can an immaterial world of the mind interact with the brain and, more seriously, what evidence is there that the brain is indeed subject to influences other than those operating at the physical level. A view which finds considerable favour today assumes that there is only one set of events to be studied, denying that minds are things or collections of things to be set over against a material substance, the brain. This involves a dualism of properties since brain processes, whilst essentially being physical systems are conceived of as having further non-physical properties which are recognized as mental events. Such a view is variously labelled as a dual aspect theory or a dual attribute theory of the mind–body relationship. A variant of this view attractive to the neuroscientist has been labelled non-reductive physicalism. It denies the existence of a non-material entity, the mind, but does not deny the existence of CONSCIOUS-NESS or other mental phenomena. On this view, the human nervous system operating in concert with the rest of the body in its environment is the seat of consciousness. The neuroscientist D. M. Mackay (1922–1987) argued for duality without the extreme of dualism. He suggested that concepts such as seeing, hearing, feeling, thinking on the one hand, and concepts of neural activity belong to different categories and that there are strong logical as well as other reasons against mixing them carelessly. He called his view comprehensive realism in the sense that realism implies reckoning with what must be reckoned with, that is to say, first and foremost the data of our conscious experience but at the same time we must reckon with the physical data about our brains. He argued that the use of the word 'comprehensive' indicates an intellectual position with insists on confronting both of these things. He further argued that the interactionist and the materialist also seek to hold on to real truths about human nature; the materialist recognizing that our physical embodiment invites analysis on the same terms as the analysis of other physical events in the material world, and the interactionist recognizing that what it means to be a conscious agent is more than can be described in material terms alone. On this view we should regard conscious experience as being embodied in brain activity rather than interacting with it. Mental events and brain events are two complementary aspects of conscious human agency. Mackay differed from the neuropsychologist Roger Sperry (1913–1994; winner of the Nobel Prize for Medicine, 1981), whom he saw as accepting some sort of interference through which the mind acts on the brain, pushing and hauling the system around.

See also: neurophilosophy; reductionism

References
Crick F. (1994) *The Astonishing Hypothesis: The Scientific Search for the Soul*, Simon & Schuster: London.
Damasio A.R. (1994) *Descartes' Error*, Putnam: New York.

MALCOLM A. JEEVES

mindblindness A popular term describing the inability of people with AUTISM to represent mental states; see METAREPRESENTATION; THEORY OR MIND.

mineral Minerals are inorganic substances – for example, CALCIUM, POTASSIUM, SODIUM and ZINC. Traces of these are present in many foods and are essential components of the DIET. Many are essential for proper neural functioning; for instance, see ACTION POTENTIAL for examples of the involvement of sodium and potassium.

mineralocorticoids A class of HORMONES, including ALDOSTERONE, secreted from the ADRENAL GLAND; with the GLUCOCORTICOIDS, they represent the CORTICOSTEROIDS; see ENDOCRINE GLANDS; HORMONES – CLASSIFICATION; IMMUNE SYSTEM; OSMOREGULATION.

miniature endplate potential *see* quantal release

minimal brain dysfunction A classification applied to children with a range of behavioural and psychological disorders (but no necessary identifiable brain pathology) including HYPERACTIVITY and IMPULSIVITY. These are both features of ATTENTION-DEFICIT DISORDER, a diagnostic term that has to a large extent replaced minimal brain dysfunction.

minor tranquillizer *see* tranquillizer

miracle berry A west African tasteless berry that renders for a short period (less than an hour) sour tastes sweet. The effective agent has been named MIRACULIN, and it appears to affect sweet taste receptors on the tongue (see GUSTATION).

miraculin *see* miracle berry

mirror drawing A technique in which subjects are required to trace a drawing (often a star shape) using concurrent visual feedback of their own performance via a mirror (so that the direction of travel of the hand appears as the reverse of the actual direction of travel). It is a technique used to asses visually guided skill learning and co-ordination in humans. It is often used as part of a NEUROPSYCHOLOGICAL TEST BATTERY to assess abilities in patients who have sustained brain damage.

mirror neuron It has been suggested that a NEURON in the CEREBRAL CORTEX that is normally activated during performance of a task can also be activated, not by movement, but by the observation of an appropriate movement in another individual; such actions have been described as those of a MIRROR NEURON system. It is thought that such events reveal important information about MENTAL REPRESENTATIONS in the brain.

Reference

Nishitani N. & Hari R. (2000) Temporal dynamics of cortical representation for action. *Proceedings of the National Academy of Sciences USA* 97: 913–918.

mirror test The mirror test has been used to try to determine whether or not certain SPECIES of PRIMATES have a SELF CONCEPT. Self concept has been defined by Povinelli & Cant as involving an individuals awareness that they are (1) an object of knowledge; (2) a causal agent; (3) the subject of experience; (4) a being with a unified existence across time. Such knowledge develops in human infants by about 2 years of age: does it develop in primates? Gallup attempted to determine this by examining the interactions of chimpanzees with mirrors, especially when they had been marked on the head with a dye. He inferred that if they paid attention to the mark, having seen it in the mirror, it would mean that they recognized themselves. It has been claimed that gorillas, chimpanzees, bonobos and orang utans do this, but that species of primate below these cannot. However, criticisms of these experiments have been mounted, particularly concerning the use of ANAESTHETICS in placing the marking dye, and it has also been noted that there are considerable individual differences between animals of the same species on this test.

References

Gallup G.G. (1970) Chimpanzees self recognition. *Science* 167: 86–87.
Heyes C.M. (1994) Reflections on self-recognition in primates. *Animal Behaviour* 47: 909–919.
Povinelli D.J. & Cant J.G.H. (1995) Arboreal climbing and the evolution of self-conception. *Quarterly Review of Biology* 70: 393–421.

mitochondria (singular: mitochondrion) Small bacterium-like structures, found in most EUKARYOTE cells, which use OXYGEN and CARBOHYDRATE to fuel the production of ADENOSINE TRIPHOSPHATE (ATP). The mitochondrion is composed of two membranes, an outer and an inner (see MEMBRANE). The inner membrane is convoluted to produce more surface area and is the site of an ENZYME called ATP SYNTHASE. Within the inner membrane, electrons (see ELECTRON) released during the OXIDATION of carbohydrates are carried by a series of enzymes and cofactors called the ELECTRON TRANSPORT CHAIN and used to drive membrane-bound PROTON pumps, which extrude protons from the matrix to the intermembrane space, against a CONCENTRATION GRADIENT. At sites containing ATP synthase, the energy released when protons flow back across the inner membrane, according to their concentration gradient, is coupled to the synthesis of ATP from adenosine diphosphate and inorganic phosphate. ATP is then transported from the mitochondrion to sites within the cell which break down ATP to fuel cellular reactions.

FIONA M. INGLIS

mitochondrial Eve The DNA in MITOCHONDRIA – mitochondrial DNA – is inherited only from our mothers. Molecular biologists, knowing something of the way in which mitochondrial DNA mutates, have estimated that all modern humans (*Homo sapiens sapiens*; see HOMINID) share a single common ancestor, dubbed Eve, who lived in Africa some 200 000 years ago. More recent research has suggested that part of the Y chromosome (see X AND Y CHROMOSOMES) can be used in a similar manner to trace the male ancestor of modern man. An estimate has been made that the common ancestor – Adam – lived in Africa some 188 000 years ago, though the 95% confidence intervals for this indicate a possible range from 51 000 to 411 000 years. Hypotheses about mitochondrial Eve and Adam generated considerable excitement, suggesting a single locus of origin for modern man, but more recent research has been sceptical about these hypotheses.

mitosis *see* cell division

mitral cell Mitral cells – so called because they are shaped like a bishop's mitre – are found in the OLFACTORY BULB. Their dendrites (see DENDRITE) form the OLFACTORY GLOMERULI, receiving sensory input from the OLFACTORY EPITHELIUM, while their axons (see AXON) project through the OLFACTORY TRACT to various sites in brain; see OLFACTION.

MK801 5-methyl-10,11-dihydro-5H-dibenzo[a,d]-cyclohepten-5,10-imine; also known as DIZOCILPINE. A non-competitive ANTAGONIST at the part of NMDA RECEPTORS sensitive to PHENCYCLIDINE. MK801 was an important discovery during the 1980s, when research on AMINO ACID NEUROTRANSMITTERS was developing rapidly. Selective antagonists to a variety of amino acid receptors were being discovered or created (see for example APV) but MK801 had the apparent advantage that it could be effectively administered by SYSTEMIC INJECTION. Later research identified its more specific action at the so-called phencyclidine receptor.

mnemonic (from Greek, *mnemon*: mindful) A memory aid, or technique for improving RETENTION. Most mnemonics involve some combination of vivid VISUAL IMAGERY, organization of information into meaningful units and hierarchies, and association with well-learned information. For example, the method of loci, one of the oldest known mnemonics, involves mentally associating visual representations of the to-be-remembered items with a set of pre-established locations on an imagined landscape. At test, one mentally 'walks' through these locations, 'picking up' items along the way. Although such strategies are quite effortful at the start, they ultimately produce better memory retention than a more passive approach to LEARNING.

JENNIFER A. MANGELS

mobilization NEUROTRANSMITTERS are packaged into SYNAPTIC VESICLES in SYNAPTIC TERMINALS. In order to be released into the SYNAPTIC CLEFT, vesicles must move to DOCKING SITES on the inner surface of the presynaptic membrane. This movement through the CYTOPLASM to the docking site is called mobilization. Mobilization depends on PROTEINS associated with the CYTOSKELETON: some proteins promote mobilization, others inhibit it. CALCIUM ions (Ca^{2+}) (see ION) are also involved in this process. An ACTION POTENTIAL arriving at a terminal triggers influx of Ca^{2+} into the synaptic terminal, where it can attach to CALCIUM-BINDING PROTEINS (known as ANNEXINS). There is a great variety of presynaptic binding proteins (the so-called SNARE PROTEINS) involved in mobilization, some attached to presynaptic membranes (for example SYNTAXIN) while others are attached to synaptic vesicles (for example SYNAPTOPHYSIN and SYNAPTOTAGMIN). The differential distribution of these within and between neurons can help in identifying particular groups of neurons.

modal completion *see* pattern completion

modules and modular organization The visual system processes the incoming information in a modular fashion. The information about each object in a scene arrives in various different forms. Thus the shape of the object can be discovered from an analysis of the pattern of shading over the surface of the object, from an analysis of texture gradients across the surface of the object, from an analysis of the variation in stereoscopic disparity across the object (see DEPTH PERCEPTION), from an analysis of how the object occludes other objects or is occluded by them. These different sources of information are all relatively independent of each other and can be processed separately. Different cortical areas are specialized to deal with different sources of information. The same principle is true more generally of cortical processing, in which separate sources of information that arise from different sense organs are processed separately in different cortical areas. The difficult issue that has not been fully understood yet is how the different sources of information are brought together to form a coherent representation of a whole object, or even how far they are brought together. Occasionally, information from one module becomes mixed up with other modules. Thus there are individuals who experience apparently VISUAL IMAGERY in response to auditory stimulation. This condition is known as SYNAESTHESIA.

See also: areas V1–V5; binding problem; neural coding; pattern perception

ROGER J. WATT

molarity A measure of how concentrated a solution is. A solution is said to be one molar (1M) if it contains one MOLE of a substance in one litre of solution. Molarity is calculated as:

$$\text{molarity (M)} = \frac{\text{grams}}{(\text{molecular weight} \times \text{vol. in litres})}$$

mole (mol) The MOLECULAR WEIGHT of a substance in grams.

See also: molarity

molecular biology That branch of biology that studies the basic molecular organization of living organisms. It is very much bound up with the study of DNA and genes (see GENE). Molecular biology provides analysis of the structure of organisms and valuable tools (see GENE TRANSFER IN THE CNS for example) but whether or not it can provide insight into psychological processes remains uncertain.

molecular layer *see* cerebellum – anatomical organization

molecular taxonomy The classification of organisms based on analysis of their GENO-

TYPE) rather than their gross structure (their PHENOTYPE).

molecular weight (MW) The molecular weight of a MOLECULE is the sum of the ATOMIC WEIGHT of all the atoms of which the molecule is composed. One needs to know the molecular weight of a substance in order to be able to prepare solutions of a given MOLARITY.

See also: formula weight; waters of crystallization

molecule Composed of individual atoms (see ATOM), a molecule is the smallest quantity of a substance that retains the properties of that substance.

molindone An atypical ANTIPSYCHOTIC.

moltification *see* imprinting

monaural *see* binaural

monism The philosophical idea that reality cannot be differentiated into physical and mental substances; it is the reverse of DUALISM, which holds that minds are non-physical things, different from physical substance. For biological psychology, the difference between monism and dualism can be baldly summarized so: dualism holds that minds and brains are distinct; monism hold that they are essentially the same.

Monism has appeared in different formats. Spinoza held to a dual attribute theory in which physical and mental events were all held to be different expressions of one and the same substance, God. Berkeley formulated a related theory, known as *idealism*, in which all was held to be mental rather than physical. *Neutral monism*, a view held by Hume, suggested that all reality was of one type, but was described as neither mental nor physical. However, probably the most common general contemporary conception of monism is known as MATERIALISM, a view first proposed by Hobbes. In this theory, all is held to be physical. The central difficulty in this is the reduction of mental events to physical events; that is, how does our everyday talk of mental events (expressed using terms such as 'belief', 'justice', 'pleasure' and so on – see FOLK PSYCHOLOGY) translate into physical events? Various philosophers have wrestled with this issue: some have argue in favour of a strict form of REDUCTIONISM in which there is a close concordance between physical and mental states; others have argued for a non-reductive materialism in which any mental state can be seen as an EMERGENT PROPERTY of physical matter (that is, brains); and others, most notably Hilary Putnam, have argued for a FUNCTIONAL MENTALISM, in which mental terms are seen as having value (in so far as they predict behaviour) and in which mental states can be functionally expressed through the actions of multiple different systems, liberating them in some sense from strict physical relationships.

See also: connectionism; consciousness

monomeric acrylamide Acrylamide is used in the production of gels for GEL ELECTROPHORESIS. Monomeric acrylamide is one of the more potent NEUROTOXINS: systemic administration produces LESION of neurons in the PERIPHERAL NERVOUS SYSTEM. It is not widely used.

monoamine A class of NEUROTRANSMITTERS that possess a single amine (-NH₂) group. The term MONOAMINERGIC indicates possession of monoamines, as in MONOAMINERGIC neurons or monoaminergic systems. Monoamines consist of a central ringed structure with a side chain. There are two groups of monoamines, the CATECHOLAMINE group, in which the ringed structure is a catechol, and the INDOLEAMINE group, in which the ringed structure is an indole. The most well-known monoamines are the catecholamines DOPAMINE, NORADRENALINE (known as norepinephrine in the United States) and ADRENALINE (epinephrine) and the indoleamines SEROTONIN and MELATONIN. The monoamines dopamine, noradrenaline, and serotonin are localized in nuclei in the MIDBRAIN and HINDBRAIN, and send long projections to the forebrain where they are thought to play a critical role in modulation of neuronal activity. Functionally they have been associated with cognition, EMOTION, MOTIVATION and motor activity (see LOCOMOTION) and, pathologically, with DEPRESSION, SCHIZOPHRENIA and PARKINSON'S DISEASE.

See also: dopamine hypothesis of schizophrenia; monoamine hypothesis of depression

ANN E. KELLEY

monoamine hypothesis of depression A hypothesis about the pathophysiology of AFFECTIVE DISORDER, largely derived from the observation that many effective ANTIDEPRESSANT drugs share the property of perturbing MONOAMINE systems. The monoamine hypothesis has focused on NORADRENERGIC and SEROTONERGIC systems, though DOPAMINERGIC systems are also increasingly implicated in the biology of rewarded behaviour, and by inference, in MOOD states.

The monoamine hypothesis emerged in the 1960s when it was noted that drugs which depleted neuronal noradrenaline and serotonin, such as RESERPINE (used as an ANTIHYPERTENSIVE) appeared to cause DEPRESSION in some individuals, leading to the idea that a relative deficiency of monoamines may represent the cause of mood disorder generally. This idea was supported by the finding that serendipitously discovered antidepressant agents, such as the TRICYCLICS and MONOAMINE OXIDASE INHIBITORS cause a short-term increase in levels of monoamines at the SYNAPTIC CLEFT. Furthermore, depletion of TRYPTOPHAN, a precursor of serotonin, leads to relapse in some patients who have responded to antidepressants. There are, however, several problems for the hypothesis, at least in this simple form. (1) Though antidepressants elevate synaptic monoamine levels within hours, their antidepressant effects are delayed for two to three weeks. (2) Tryptophan depletion does not appear to cause depression in individuals who have never suffered from a depressive disorder. (3) Some very effective antidepressants, such as MIANSERIN, do not appear significantly to block monoamine reuptake. (4) Efforts to demonstrate both conclusively and exclusively that monoamine function is abnormal in depressed patients have been largely unsuccessful.

The hypothesis has been modified over the last three decades, partly to try and take account of some of these problems and partly in the light of new observations. In the 1970s and 1980s, interest centred on the possibility that persistent activation of monoaminergic receptors by antidepressants would result in adaptation responses, such that RECEPTOR sensitivity or number might be downregulated. The time course of such effects might be more in keeping with the delayed onset of antidepressant action. For example, it was observed that many antidepressants downregulate central beta- NORADRENALINE RECEPTORS following CHRONIC, rather than acute administration. The monoamine hypothesis in this form therefore postulated that depression might be caused by monoamine receptor SUPERSENSITIVITY, and that antidepressants downregulated and thus attenuated this proposed pathological state of affairs. However, not all antidepressant agents share this effect, and in any case, the time course for downregulation is still rather less than the time taken for antidepressant effects to emerge clinically. Furthermore, appropriate receptor antagonists (such as beta receptor antagonists) do not have antidepressant activity, as predicted by this new form of the hypothesis. More recent formulations have added a further dimension – the role of the inhibitory AUTORECEPTOR. It has been suggested, for example, that a serotonin specific reuptake inhibitor (SSRI; for example PROZAC) acting at the monoaminergic cell bodies in the BRAINSTEM could lead to increased activation of $5HT_{1a}$ autoreceptors. These autoreceptors shut down cell firing in the short term, acting against expected increases in synaptic serotonin in the projection field in the CEREBRAL CORTEX and LIMBIC SYSTEM caused by ongoing reuptake inhibition. Once the cell body autoreceptors desensitize in the face of chronic REUPTAKE blockade, and cell firing increases again, then the effect of reuptake inhibition at the terminals now results in an increase in synaptic serotonin availability. This version of the monoamine hypothesis now predicts once more that the depressed state is due to lack of availability of serotonin at cell terminals. None the less, the monoamine hypothesis cannot fully account for depressive disorder, and other factors must operate in the genesis and maintenance of depressive disorder. Despite this, the hypothesis has proved a useful stimulus to research into the biology of affective disorder.

See also: dopamine hypothesis of schizophrenia

IAN C. REID

monoamine oxidase Monoamine oxidase (MAO) is an ENZYME that catalyses the destruction of many types of MONOAMINE, including DOPAMINE, NORADRENALINE and SEROTONIN, the principal monoamine neurotransmitters in brain. It is present in many body tissues. In brain it is found in both neurons (see NEURON) and GLIAL CELLS. There are two forms of monoamine oxidase, A and B (MAO-A and MAO-B), separate enzymes each coded by its own independent GENE. MAO-A activity is inhibited by the drug CLORGYLINE and acts preferentially on serotonin, adrenaline and noradrenaline. MAO-B activity is inhibited by the drug DEPRENYL and acts preferentially on PHENYLETHYLAMINE. Both forms, MAO-A and MAO-B, work on dopamine, although MAO-A has primary responsibility for this.

See also: monoamine hypothesis of depression; monoamine oxidase inhibitors

Reference

Feldman R., Meyer J.S. & Quenzer L.F. (1997) *Principles of Neuropsychopharmacology*, Sinauer Associates: Sunderland MA.

monoamine oxidase inhibitors MONOAMINE OXIDASE is an ENZYME that catalyses the destruction of many types of MONOAMINE: monoamine oxidase inhibitors (MAOIs) are a class of DRUG that prevent this action, in general therefore promoting an increase in levels of monoamines. The earliest example was IPRONIAZID (one of the hydrazine group of monoamine oxidase inhibitors): later examples include PHENELZINE and NIALAMIDE (hydrazines), and PARGYLINE and TRANYLCYPROMINE (non-hydrazines), CLORGYLINE and DEPRENYL. The early monoamine oxidase inhibitors, hydrazines and non-hydrazines alike, were nonselective (that is, they acted on monoamine oxidase-A and -B equally well). Clorgyline and deprenyl are modern monoamine oxidase inhibitors, selective for MAO-A and MAO-B respectively. Monoamine oxidase inhibitors have a variety of uses: they can be given experimentally as broad spectrum enhancers of monoamine activity; and pargyline is typically given in conjunction with the catecholamine selective neurotoxin 6-HYDROXYDOPAMINE to increase its effectiveness. More importantly, monoamine oxidase inhibitors have been used in the treatment of DEPRESSION (iproniazid was one of the first ANTIDEPRESSANT drugs used – later drugs such as the TRICYCLICS however have largely replaced monoamine oxidase inhibitors) while deprenyl has been used in the management of PARKINSON'S DISEASE. Interestingly, deprenyl, like some of the other monoamine oxidase inhibitors, is metabolized to methamphetamine and AMPHETAMINE. After treatment with deprenyl for three days or more, detectable amounts of these can be found in the urine.

See also: monoamine hypothesis of depression

Reference

Feldman R., Meyer J.S. & Quenzer L.F. (1997) *Principles of Neuropsychopharmacology*, Sinauer Associates: Sunderland MA.

monoaminergic *see* monoamine

monochromatism A form of colour blindness that is characterized by the absence of functional cone photoreceptors (see CONES). The vision of monochromats is that of a system composed purely of RODS such as that experienced by normally sighted observers in dim illumination. There is a complete lack of the ability to discriminate stimuli on the basis of colour alone, and this is coupled with the rod characterization of poor ACUITY and sensitivity to bright light. It would not be strictly correct to state that monochromats perceive the world as 'black and white' or 'shades of grey'. Most cases of monochromatism are hereditary, and it is extremely rare.

DAVID W. HEELEY

monoclonal antibody An antibody produced by a cell line derived from a single B CELL (see IMMUNE SYSTEM). B cells are cells whose role in the immune system is to produce ANTIBODIES specific to a foreign ANTIGEN. Because all cells within the cell line are derived from the same cell, each molecule of antibody produced will be identical. This technique is used to produce antibodies which are highly specific to a particular antigen, and unlike POLYCLONAL ANTIBODIES, may often provide specificity

between similar antigens such as RECEPTOR subtypes.

FIONA M. INGLIS

monocular 'One eye' as distinct from BINOCULAR which means 'two eyes'.

DAVID W. HEELEY

monocular parallax *see* motion parallax

monocyte *see* immune system

monophasic vs. biphasic pulses Monophasic pulses go in only one direction, typically negative in psychobiology. Biphasic pulses have a negative phase usually followed immediately by an equal current and duration positive phase. The biphasic wave form was originally thought to be gentler on tissue, as the stimulation gave no net stimulation. However, the positive phase of the pulse may generate axonal firing on stimulation pulse onset or, if long enough, on offset (see ELECTRICAL BRAIN STIMULATION). Thus, biphasic stimulation is actually more complex and is not widely used. In addition, monophasic stimulation with a switching network can provide no net electron flow without the complexity of positive stimulation through the use of a switching network on the terminal stage of the stimulator.

JAMES R. STELLAR

monopolar electrode *see* electrode

monosaccharides *see* sugars

monosodium glutamate *see* primary tastes

monosynaptic Having one synapse: a monosynaptic pathway involves one NEURON synapsing on another: a direct connection from one structure to another is a monosynaptic pathway.

See also: disynaptic

monosynaptic reflex arc *see* reflex arc

monosynaptic stretch reflex *see* stretch reflex

monotonic In auditory perception, monotonic refers to a stimulus that is invariant, having the same frequency or PITCH. In mathematics, monotonic describes a function or sequence that neither increases nor decreases.

monotreme *see* mammals

monozygotic twins Also known as IDENTICAL TWINS; monozygotic twins share a common GENOME: they are the product of a single ZYGOTE that, for reasons that are not entirely clear, divides into two. Depending on when this occurs, monozygotic twins may or may not share the same the CHORION in the UTERUS. If the split occurs before the zygote is embedded in the PLACENTA, there will be separate development in separate chorions; if it occurs after placental embedding the twins will develop in the same chorion. About one-third of cases involve separate chorions, two-thirds a single chorion.

See also: dizygotic twins; twin studies

mood Mood is a state of EMOTION: it is not a synonym for emotion but a category of it. Ryle characterized moods as states that monopolize a person and contrasted them with feelings, states that are composed of relatively transient sensations. But the distinction between the terms 'emotion', 'mood' and 'feeling' is fraught with difficulty. In psychiatry, mood has traditionally been contrasted with AFFECT: affect has been thought of as objective while mood has been characterized as subjective, though evidently this dichotomy is forced since both mood and affect are gauged to some extent at least through behaviour, which is overt and observable. Indeed, the terms MOOD DISORDER and AFFECTIVE DISORDER are now regarded as more or less synonymous. It is perhaps best to regard mood as one of those terms, like VOLUNTARY or INVOLUNTARY, which convey meaning only imprecisely. It is a term imported into science from FOLK PSYCHOLOGY that will neither go away nor translate precisely into a scientific term.

See also: dysphoria; euthymic mood; psychotic mood disorder

Reference

Ryle G. (1949) *The Concept of Mind*, Hutchinson: London.

mood disorder Any disorder in which there is a major change in emotional state: DEPRESSION and BIPOLAR DISORDER (MANIC DEPRESSION)

are the principal types of disorder classified as mood disorders.

See also: affective disorder; emotion; mania; mood; unipolar depression

morbidity (from Latin, *morbidus*: disease) Disease, sickliness or unwholesomeness. An index of morbidity would be a frequency count of the numbers of individuals in a given sample contracting an illness or disease, or falling sick.

See also: mortality

Moro reflex A reflex movement of any body part towards the MIDLINE displayed by infants, first described by Ernst Moro (1874–1951). It can be used to detect sensory deficits in infants. The STARTLE REFLEX gradually replaces it.

See also: infant reflexes

morpheme (from Greek, *morphe*: form) A linguistic unit that has meaning but which cannot be further subdivided; see LANGUAGE; SLIPS OF THE TONGUE.

morphine The principle active ingredient found in OPIUM, the extract of the poppy plant. Morphine is named after the Greek god *Morpheus*, the god of dreams. Morphine, a NARCOTIC ANALGESIC (see ANALGESIA; NARCOTICS), is a potent opiate drug that has a number of physiological effects. It can induce sleepiness and relaxation, suppress respiration, increase PAIN threshold, and cause a profound sense of well-being and EUPHORIA. These latter reinforcing properties lead to SELF-ADMINISTRATION of morphine. Use of the opium extract for its psychological and medicinal properties may date back over 5000 years. References to opium use are found in the writings of early Egyptian, Greek, Roman, Arabic and Chinese cultures. In the nineteenth century, opium (in the form of LAUDANUM, a potion containing opium) became an important part of the pharmacopoeia in England and America. One of the most famous descriptions of the properties of morphine is provided by Thomas De Quincey (1785–1859) who wrote an essay, *Confessions of an English Opium-Eater*, in 1821. He first took opium for a toothache and wrote: 'In an hour, O heavens! What a revulsion! What a resurrection from its lowest depths, of the inner spirit!...That my pains had vanished was now a trifle in my eyes; this negative effect was swallowed up in the immensity of those positive effects which had opened before me, in the abyss of divine enjoyment thus suddenly revealed...here was the secret of happiness, about which philosophers had disputed for so many ages, at once discovered; happiness might now be bought for a penny, and carried in the waistcoat pocket; portable ecstasies might be had corked up in a pint-bottle and peace of mind might be sent down by the mail.'

However, while the pain-relieving effects of opiates were much appreciated, the dangers and addictive properties also became clear as its use spread throughout societies (see ADDICTION). Morphine has high ABUSE POTENTIAL; with repeated use, individuals can become addicted to the drug. Morphine addiction is associated with a need for the drug to function normally, intense drug craving, and a withdrawal syndrome following abstinence from the drug. Morphine is also self-administered by animals. Much of what is known about the brain's endogenous OPIOID PEPTIDES, the ENDORPHINS and ENKEPHALINS, has been derived from studies of morphine's effects in animals. Morphine is the most commonly used drug in the treatment of pain. A number of physiological symptoms result from morphine administration, which are the consequence of the drug acting in several brain regions. The main physical effects morphine has is to reduce pain perception. Morphine commonly causes NAUSEA and VOMITING, particularly with initial use. It also causes a marked constriction of the pupil, known as 'pinpoint pupil'. This sign is commonly seen in HEROIN addicts (heroin being a semi-synthetic derivative of morphine). Opiates slow the movement of food through the digestive tract and thus cause constipation. The most dangerous physiological effect is respiratory depression, respiratory arrest being the most common cause of death from overdose.

Morphine DEPENDENCE may be associated with a high degree of TOLERANCE and physical dependence. With repeated use, the dose taken by the user gradually becomes higher. However, tolerance develops to some effects of opiates and not to others. For example a remarkable degree of tolerance may be exhibited to the respiratory depressant, sedative, analgesic, nauseating and euphoric effects while little tolerance is seen to the constipating and pupil-decreasing effects. Physical dependence is also classically associated with opiate addiction, and a WITHDRAWAL SYNDROME results in dependent individuals upon cessation of the drug. It is not known what particular factors determine whether a person, once exposed to morphine or other opiates, will become dependent. As is true with all drugs with abuse potential, some people can experiment or be exposed to morphine and not develop a habit, while others become addicted. Many factors, including social environment, drug availability and psychological state may determine the pattern of drug use.

ANN E. KELLEY

morphogen *see* development

morphogenesis The physical and mechanical events governing how cells and tissues move in the embryo and mould the final shape of the various organs: see DEVELOPMENT.

morphology The internal structure or make-up of entities, such as words (in linguistics), animals, plants and their constituent cells (in biology), or the earth and its features (in geology).

ANNE CUTLER

morphometry The measurement of form; see MORPHOLOGY.

Morris water maze A frequently used description of an open-field swimming pool used to study spatial learning; see WATER MAZE.

RICHARD G. M. MORRIS

mortality (from Latin, *mortalis*: mortal) Literally, the condition of being mortal and therefore liable to death. An index of mortality would be a frequency count of the numbers of deaths in a given sample of individuals.

See also: morbidity

mossy cells These are the major cell type of the hilus of the DENTATE GYRUS; see HILAR CELLS.

mossy fibres There are two groups of mossy fibres in the brain. One is the mossy fibres in the HIPPOCAMPUS, which are axons of GRAN-ULE CELLS in the DENTATE GYRUS. They course laterally and terminate in the stratum lucidum of the CA3 region (see CA1–CA3) of the hippocampus. The second group of mossy fibres is in the CEREBELLUM. These mossy fibres represent one class of AFFERENT to the CEREBELLAR CORTEX. Their terminal endings are called rosettes. Rosettes make multiple synaptic contacts with various neuronal elements in the granular layer, in a complex nodular arrangement called a GLOMERULUS.

KAZUE SEMBA

motilin *see* endocrine glands; hormones

motion after-effect *see* opponent processes

motion blindness A rare condition where the ability to register visual movement is much more greatly impaired than other visual functions (also known as CEREBRAL AKINETOPSIA). It is believed to result from damage to the specialized motion area V5 (see AREAS VI–V5) of the EXTRASTRIATE CORTEX. Most recent knowledge of the condition comes from the patient described by Zihl *et al.* (1983).

See also: middle temporal region; motion perception

Reference

Zihl J., von Cramon D. & Mai N. (1983) Selective disturbance of motion vision after bilateral brain damage. *Brain* 106: 313–340.

OLIVER J. BRADDICK

motion parallax When the head is moved, the images of visual targets that lie at different distances from the EYE are displaced by different amounts, creating a relative motion between them that is referred to as motion parallax (or frequently, MONOCULAR PARAL-LAX). It has been demonstrated convincingly that this parallax is a sufficient cue, on its own, to DEPTH PERCEPTION. Striking impressions of 3-dimensional depth can be created in a flat 2-dimensional image that is composed of randomly placed dots if an appropriate shearing motion is introduced into the display, linked mechanically to movements of the head. The depth impression that is created in this manner

bears many similarities to that induced by STEREOPSIS.

Reference

Rogers B.J. & Graham M. (1979) Motion parallax as an independent cue for depth perception. *Perception* 8: 125–134.

DAVID W. HEELEY

motion perception Image motion is exploited for many important and diverse purposes in visual perception. We need to register and predict the trajectories of moving objects to avoid or intercept them. Common motion of visual elements provides a powerful indicator that they belong together, and so allows the VISUAL FIELD to be correctly segmented into objects and background. Characteristic motion patterns allow us to recognize the actions of other people and animals, which are socially and practically significant to us. We guide our movements (see LOCOMOTION) and POSTURE in large part through the patterns of OPTIC FLOW generated by our own movements, and these patterns can also reveal the 3-dimensional layout of the environment that we move through. Given this wealth of information it is not surprising that sensitivity to motion is a prominent feature of visual systems throughout the animal kingdom, and is served by a specialized subsystem in PRIMATES.

For a visual neuron to be involved in motion processing, it must show DIRECTIONAL SELEC-TIVITY – that is, it must respond more strongly to one direction of motion than to others. Directional selectivity can arise if a neuron is activated by combined inputs from two nearby regions A and B of the visual field; if the signal from A is delayed with respect to B, signals from a stimulus moving A–B will yield signals that coincide in time, while signals from the opposite motion B–A will be separated in time and so have a weaker effect. This configuration is called a REICHARDT DETECTOR after its discoverer in the insect visual pathway. There exist other schemes of connectivity that can yield an essentially equivalent pattern of response.

Prolonged viewing of a particular pattern of motion (for example an expanding spiral) leads to the perception of the opposite motion in a stationary pattern. This MOTION AFTER-EFFECT is taken as evidence that directionally selective neurons in the human brain are showing an adaptation effect to the motion supporting the idea of a specialized motion subsystem.

Direction selectivity has not been found among cells of the RETINA or LATERAL GENICULATE NUCLEUS in primates. However cells of the MAGNOCELLULAR pathway in these structures respond strongly to rapidly changing stimuli and provide the input to a specialized set of directional cells in cortical area V1 (see AREAS VI–V5). The 'motion pathway' of macaque VISUAL CORTEX is formed by connections of these cells directly, and indirectly through areas V2 and V3, to area V5 (also known as area MT, the MIDDLE TEMPORAL REGION). Cells in V5 are almost exclusively strongly directionally selective, and much evidence supports the idea that this is an essential brain area for the processing of motion information. Beyond V5 in the motion pathway is an adjacent area, the medial superior temporal (MST), where cells are also highly directional, but with a very large RECEPTIVE FIELD. The human brain contains an area that is apparently homologous to monkey V5, near the boundary of the OCCIPITAL LOBE and TEMPORAL LOBE. FUNCTIONAL NEUROIMAGING studies show that it is strongly activated by moving compared to static stimuli, and the condition of MOTION BLINDNESS is associated with bilateral damage in this region.

The directional cells of area V1 seem to be well adapted to measure the local motion of a limited region. The additional processing from V1 to V5, and beyond, must elaborate this information in ways that are required for it to be used effectively in perception. Studies of V5 and MST suggest several ways in which this happens. First, V1 neurons are quite limited in the range of high velocities which they can detect; this range is considerably greater in the directional response of V5 neurons. Second, V5 neurons integrate motion information over larger areas, and in some cases are organized to detect the boundaries that segment differently moving regions. Third, V1 neurons are subject to the 'aperture problem' that arises when motion is processed for short contour segments; for example upwards motion will be detected in the top edge of a square even when

the square as a whole moves diagonally. Certain V5 cells can combine information from differently oriented contours and so resolve this ambiguity. Fourthly, MST cells respond to the large scale patterns of flow that occur as a result of the animal's movement through the environment, including appropriate responses to particular image motions from objects at different distances.

The signals that encode motion in areas V5 and MST are required for the control of PURSUIT EYE MOVEMENTS. If pursuit is accurate, the image of a moving object is maintained stationary on the retina. Our perception of the object's motion in this case must depend on information about how the eyes are moving, as well as on neuronal responses to image motion. V5 is considered to be part of the DORSAL STREAM of cortical information processing, concerned with spatial relationships and the visual control of action. However, motion information is also used in the identification of objects (considered to be the function of the VENTRAL STREAM), both through 3-dimensional structural information and through the characteristic motion patterns of human beings and other biological objects. Motion information must converge with pattern and form information to provide an integrated perception of the objects, surfaces and events in our environment.

Reference

Smith A. T. & Snowden R.J. (eds.) (1994) *Visual Detection of Motion*, Academic Press: London.

OLIVER J. BRADDICK

motion sickness Motion sickness is produced by certain forms of motion under certain conditions: it is experienced typically by passengers in automobiles, trains, ships and boats, and (less typically) spacecraft. Two features stand out: first, motion sickness involves low-frequency movement generating conflicting signals to and from the VESTIBULAR SYSTEM about position in space; and second, that it is passengers that experience motion sickness, not drivers or pilots. This indicates that the foreknowledge of movement, however brief, is sufficient to allow the vestibular system to understand the nature of the movements being, and to be, experienced. The most notable account of motion sickness is the *sensory conflict theory*, which suggests that mismatches in the information about body position provided by various sensory systems, notably the vestibular system and VISUAL SYSTEM, generates NAUSEA. Various treatments are available for motion sickness, including various types of DRUG that affect HISTAMINE, ACETYLCHOLINE and SEROTONIN receptors.

Motion sickness remains somewhat enigmatic. At the heart of the enigma is the question of whether motion sickness represents an organizational principle of the nervous system – that is, that the generation of nausea by mismatched sensory signals is an adaptive response to specific conditions – or whether it is the accidental consequence of doing things to human bodies that they were not designed to do.

Reference

Yates B.J., Miller A.D. & Lucot J.B. (1998) Physiological basis and pharmacology of motion sickness: an update. *Brain Research Bulletin* 47: 395–406. (Note that this edition of *Brain Research Bulletin* – issue number 5 of volume 47 – is devoted entirely to motion sickness.)

motivation Motivation is understood as a process that moves organisms to engage in particular acts, but its exact status remains uncertain. Various explanations to account for why individuals engage in certain acts have been offered: INSTINCT, DRIVE and AROUSAL have been used to account for motivation in animals, while complex psychoanalytic (see PSYCHOANALYSIS) and psychological processes have been proposed to account for human actions. LEARNING theorists were much concerned to provide accounts of motivation. The DRIVE REDUCTION theory proposed by Clark Hull (1884–1952) suggested that the INCENTIVE behind all behaviour was elimination and avoidance of discomfort. (Early theories concerning human motivation had similarly stressed the importance of hedonism – the maximization of REWARD and minimization of PUNISHMENT.) Hull and others also distinguished between the motivation produced by an internal state of drive (referred to as PRIMARY MOTIVATION) and that produced by

the presence of an external STIMULUS (such as food or water) which was referred to as INCENTIVE MOTIVATION. Primary motivation and incentive motivation evidently interact with each other, even in very simple organisms. For example, it was shown that sugar on the chemosensory apparatus of flies always promotes neural activity, but whether or not consummatory actions follow depends on the internal state of the fly.

The neural bases of motivation were once thought to be essentially hypothalamic and were investigated in terms of basic functions: FEEDING, DRINKING, SEXUAL BEHAVIOUR and THERMOREGULATION. The DUAL CENTRES HYPOTHESIS argued that states such as hunger and satiety – the 'on' and 'off' switches of particular forms of motivation – were controlled by reciprocally acting centres in the HYPOTHALAMUS, but the notion of drive centres has been largely replaced by more distributed processing accounts. Elements of the LIMBIC SYSTEM – including the hypothalamus – are often assumed to have a fundamental role in motivation (and the related construct of reward) and some have argued that the NUCLEUS ACCUMBENS operates as a LIMBIC–MOTOR INTERFACE, translating motivation into action. In these neural accounts the idea of a CENTRAL MOTIVE STATE is typically present, either explicitly or implicitly. A central motive state is a neural representation of motivation that exists independently of the internal or external stimuli that generate it, and its strength can be used to account for the degree to which a particular activity occurs. However, this begs a fundamental question concerning the status of the term motivation itself. Is motivation an identifiable process with a designated neural system (in the way that vision is for example) and is that process common to all instances of 'motivation'? Use of the term 'motivated behaviour' is one way of circumventing this problem. By specifying a *behaviour* rather than the state or motivation, one can examine all of the processes involved in that behaviour (feeding for example) and describe sensory mechanisms, cognitive processes, and effector mechanisms that regulate it. Others have attempted to avoid the question by treating motivation as an ATTRIBUTION that individuals use to label their own actions and intentions and, by extension, those of other people and animals. In this formulation, motivation is simply a shorthand way of describing a quality of disparate conditions that need have no underlying unity.

It is realistic to assume that there is no single substrate to motivation, no single NEURON system that must be activated in order to experience it. What has to be accounted for is why certain activities are selected under particular conditions and why their strength varies. An examination of stimulus strength, cognitive processes of LEARNING and MEMORY, and mechanisms of response selection should provide a satisfactory account of behaviour without recourse to additional constructs such as motivation.

See also: behavioural economics; supervisory attentional system

motoneuron *see* motor neurons

motor adaptation Motor adaptation refers to the processes involved in regulating movements, whether whole body movements or more localized phenomena such as EYE MOVEMENTS. The ability to change or modify motor skills (see SKILL LEARNING) is believed to depend upon long term changes in the organization of synapses in the CEREBELLUM in particular and has been investigated in a variety of ways. For example, small weights can be added to body parts of experimental animals to determine how this affects movement and the organization of neural systems

motor aphasia *see* Broca's aphasia

motor apraxia An inability to perform a skilled movement despite a clear understanding of the goal and the movement sequence that is required to produce the action. For example, Kimura reports that patients with left anterior cortical lesions are impaired in producing single facial expressions while patients with left parietal lesions are impaired in producing single hand postures. Milner & Goodale report that a pathway through the dorsal cortex between the posterior cortex and anterior cortex is especially involved in making hand movements in relation to targets because if this system is damaged, objects will not be correctly grasped even though the patient is able to see the target clearly. Patients with more lateral cortical damage by report not seeing objects but may none the less GRASP them correctly.

See also: dorsal stream; ventral stream

References

Kimura D. (1999) *Sex and Cognition*, MIT Press: Cambridge MA.
Milner A.D. and Goodale M. (1995) *The Visual Brain in Action*, Oxford University Press: Oxford.

IAN Q. WHISHAW

motor aprosodia *see* aprosodia

motor control The research domain concerned with issues related to the selection, sequencing and execution of voluntary movement. One of the main issues which is central to motor control research (many of which were introduced by the Russian physiologist Bernstein) is the degrees of freedom problem. Since there is no unique solution which provides a desired movement endpoint, the central nervous system has to select a subset of all possible movement components and execute them quickly and in an appropriate order. Other areas of interest include feedback versus feedforward contributions to control, coordinate transformations, and spatial and temporal sequencing of movement subcomponents.

See also: locomotion; motor cortex; motor programming; motor system; movement deficits

DAVID P. CAREY

motor cortex The anterior regions of the CEREBRAL CORTEX which play a role in the generation of movements of the skeletal musculature. At a gross level, motor cortex is subdivided into PRIMARY MOTOR CORTEX (area 4; approximately contiguous with the precentral gyrus – see BRODMANN'S AREAS) and NON-PRIMARY MOTOR CORTEX (all of the medial and anterior cortex involved in motor preparation and planning; premotor and SUPPLEMENTARY MOTOR CORTEX). Non-primary motor cortex is five times more plentiful than primary motor cortex in *Homo sapiens*; in monkeys the ratio is 1:1. The premotor cortex (PMC) is located in the lateral part of Brodmann's area 6. The supplementary motor cortex (SMC) is located in the medial part of area 6, just anterior to the leg representation in the primary motor cortex. Recently, electrophysiological studies in non-human primates have been used to characterize a set of CINGULATE MOTOR AREAS (CMC; Brodmann's areas 23 and 24, see CINGULATE CORTEX). Subdivisions of these regions have been suggested, based on electrophysiological and anatomical grounds. For example a recent count revealed that three areas in the CMC have been proposed, two in PMC and three in SMC. Early views of primary motor cortex suggested relatively neat, independent representations of distinct muscle groups, arranged in the classical HOMUNCULUS. Single cell recordings in this area suggest that such a view is an oversimplification; there are multiple, spatially distinct representations of the muscles which control the fingers, for example. These representations are intermingled with small representations of other muscle groups of the hand, and even more distant muscle groups such as those which control rotations about the wrist, elbow and even the shoulder. In non-primary motor cortices, these motor maps are even less precise, although current theory still suggests largely separate representations of major muscle groups, such as those related to movements of the distal musculature of the hand and finger versus the more proximal musculature of the upper arm and shoulder. Other early views of the non-primary motor cortices include the notion that they influence motor activity exclusively through projects to the appropriate motor representations in primary motor cortex. This position has been refuted by numerous anatomical studies showing direct connections of SMC and PMC to motor neurons in the spinal cord. Of course, one difficulty in establishing what the different motor cortices do is that most of the data has been based on recordings of the activity of single neurons in each of the regions. Identifying that a particular neuron changes its activity before or during the movement of a particular muscle group does not provide unambiguous information about what movement-related parameters that cell may be influencing (or being influenced by). Electrophysiological studies tend to be driven by the theoretical perspective of the particular electrophysiologist: early studies have empathised the coding of relatively low-level movement parameters such as isometric force at a single joint. Later work has examined cell activity in relation to movement direction and amplitude in space. Advances of electrophysiological technology allowed for recording more complex movements in three dimensions rather than, for example, rotations about a single joint. Unfortunately complete consensus on what movement-related parameters are coded in a given region of the motor cortex has yet to be reached. Contemporary studies of premotor cortices by physiological psychologists have tended to focus on how these regions use sensory information to guide the control of actions such as reaching and grasping, and perhaps play a role in the understanding of the meaning of actions performed by others. Studies of the more medial structures of the SMC tend to focus on potential contributions in learning new movements, movement complexity (rather loosely defined) and the integration of movements made by two limbs simultaneously. Cingulate motor cortices are still being described in terms of their connectivity with other brain regions and in their exact number and location in non-human primates. Study of the organisation of the motor cortices has depended rather heavily on electrophysiology and neuroanatomy; neuropsychological contributions have been fewer, perhaps because lesions in humans seldom respect small functional boundaries. Nevertheless, the advance of recent non-invasive techniques should allow for investigations with increasing spatial and temporal resolution to be performed using human subjects. To date, imaging studies are providing evidence which contradicts some of the simple descriptions that have been attached to the different motor cortices, such as a unique role of the SMC in the preparation of movements. Many brain regions are activated in human subjects while they prepare a series of finger movements, including primary motor cortex, parietal cortex, and all three of the non-primary motor cortical zones described above. Nevertheless, since human subjects are capable of following complex instructions as well as producing many different patterns of movements to various instructional sets, these technologies will undoubtedly advance our understanding of the functions of the motor cortices in the future.

DAVID P. CAREY

motor neglect Patients with major STROKE damage affecting the cerebral arteries of the RIGHT HEMISPHERE frequently suffer from one or more symptoms within the complex known as the NEGLECT SYNDROME. One of these symptoms is variously known as MOTOR NEGLECT, DIRECTIONAL HYPOKINESIA, or PREMOTOR NEGLECT. The patient has a difficulty in voluntarily moving the affected limb or limbs within the side of space opposite their brain damage, independently of any PARESIS or motor weakness. In some severe cases this problem may be associated with a disowning of the contra-lesional limb, perhaps even a delusional belief that it belongs to someone else.

A. DAVID MILNER

motor neuron disease (Also known as MOTONEURON disease) The term motor neuron disease actually represents a constellation of disorders related principally by symptoms. The most common (at around 80% of all motor neuron disease cases) is AMYOTROPHIC LATERAL SCLEROSIS, or LOU GEHRIG'S DISEASE, which is a disorder of the CENTRAL NERVOUS SYSTEM. GUILLAIN–BARRÉ SYNDROME is the best known motor neuron disease involving damage to the peripheral nerves. There are of course also a variety of disorders of the MUSCLES, such as MUSCULAR DYSTROPHY, which impair movement.

See also: movement deficits

motor neurons (Also known as motoneurons) The type of NEURON that has the CELL BODY in the VENTRAL HORN of the SPINAL CORD that sends an AXON out via the VENTRAL HORN to make contact with a MUSCLE FIBRE at a NEUROMUSCULAR JUNCTION. These are the neurons that finally transmit neural messages from the CENTRAL NERVOUS SYSTEM to the MUSCLES. Motor neurons come in a variety of sizes: large ones have wide diameter axons that transmit fast action potentials and innervate

fast muscles. Smaller motor neurons have thinner axons, transmit more slowly and innervate slower muscles.

See also: final common path; motor unit

motor pool The term motor pool refers to the collection of MOTOR NEURONS that innervate a particular MUSCLE. Co-ordination across motor pools is thought to be necessary for the production of normal movement of any type, from VOLUNTARY movements to REFLEX actions.

motor programming The preparation of a set of instructions for movement. Borrowed from computing, the term encapsulates the idea that the high-level decision to move must be translated into low-level commands for synchronized contractions and relaxations of muscles. It is unlikely that the program itself contains specification of muscle activity: rather, like a computer program which must be compiled into machine code, the motor program has a representation of current (start) state and goal state and it contains the specification of the translation of one to the other via muscular activity. Thus, when 'compiled' it specifies which muscles contract or relax in order, the relative timings of these contractions (specifically, the onset and duration of specific muscular activity) and finally, the degree of force.

Although it appears to make intuitive sense that these aspects of the program would be hierarchically organized (for example, with the first specification being which muscles to move, the second being the sequence to move them in and the third being the duration or force of their activity), this does not appear to be the case. Rather, any of these aspects of the program can be composed in advance. For example, when subjects are given knowledge, prior to the signal to move, of one or more of the parameters (limb to be moved, direction of movement or extent of movement), the movement is initiated with a shorter latency following the signal to move (that is to say, there is a REACTION TIME advantage). This indicates that it is possible to program, say, the extent of a movement in advance of specifying which muscles will move. By measuring the reaction time advantage and manipulating the availability of information about the forthcoming movement prior to the signal to move, it is possible to infer the nature and timing of motor programming processes. For example, it is possible to measure how long it takes to program sequences of movements of different complexity or length. From such experiments, it has been demonstrated that although it is not possible to state exactly how long motor programming takes, it takes longer to make a more complex or a longer motor program.

It is a widely held view that once initiated, the program runs through to the goal state without modification. Indeed, some definitions of a motor program refer to the control of movements executed in the absence of peripheral feedback. Although it is possible to use feedback to change movement during the execution of a motor program, these kinds of modifications are most likely to be themselves defined within the program as a potential contingency. Thus, the program still runs to completion and could be said to be unmodified. For example, when lifting an object, if the anticipated weight is greater than the actual weight, the object will initially be moved with the force required to lift the anticipated weight and, therefore, will fly up. Within about 50 msec (too short a period to halt execution and initiate a revised program) there will be a correction of the force and compensation for the unanticipated outcome of the movement. Other kinds of corrections require the termination of the running motor program and the initiation of an entirely new program. Therefore, these corrections take longer (perhaps as long as 200 msec) to make. Indeed, even before the series of muscular contractions begins, there is a point, estimated to be about 100 msec prior to movement onset, after which initiation cannot be terminated and execution of the program is inevitable. Slips of action (such as pouring orange juice on one's breakfast cereal, or heading for the telephone when the door bell is ringing) are often compounded because the unfortunate subject cannot swiftly terminate the inappropriately initiated motor program.

VERITY J. BROWN

motor readiness A cognitive state of preparation for action, in which the motor system is primed in expectation of the requirement for specific responses; see ALERTNESS.

VERITY J. BROWN

motor strip That part of the FRONTAL LOBE controlling action; see MOTOR CORTEX.

motor system The motor system is a very large tranche of tissue extending from the CEREBRAL CORTEX to the NEUROMUSCULAR JUNCTION. The cerebral cortex contains three main motor areas: the PRIMARY MOTOR CORTEX (number 4 of BRODMANN'S AREAS), the PREMOTOR CORTEX (Brodmann area 6) and the SUPPLEMENTARY MOTOR CORTEX, all in the posterior part of the FRONTAL LOBE. Several motor pathways run from the cerebral cortex: the CORTICOSTRIATAL runs to the BASAL GANGLIA (see CORTICOSTRIATAL LOOPS) the CORTICOTECTAL to the SUPERIOR COLLICULUS, CORTICOPONTINE to the PONS (including the CORTICORUBRAL pathway to the RED NUCLEUS) and the CORTICOBULBAR to the MEDULLA OBLONGATA. Note that none of these pathways leaves the BRAIN. Information travels from the brain to the SPINAL CORD by a number of routes: the CORTICOSPINAL TRACT (the PYRAMIDAL TRACT) travels from the cerebral cortex direct to the spinal cord, but most of the innervation of the spinal cord travels from the BRAINSTEM. There is a medial and a lateral pathway from the brainstem to the spinal cord: the lateral pathway is made up of the RUBROSPINAL TRACT (from the red nucleus) while the medial pathways include the TECTOSPINAL TRACT (from the superior colliculus), the RETICULOSPINAL TRACT (from the RETICULAR FORMATION) and the VESTIBULOSPINAL TRACT (from the VESTIBULAR SYSTEM). There are also descending pathways from the CEREBELLUM and from a variety of AMINERGIC neurons: for example, the cell groups in the ASCENDING RETICULAR ACTIVATING SYSTEM often send axons down into the spinal cord. These pathways from the brain terminate on INTERNEURONS in the spinal cord, which funnel information to the 31 pairs of SPINAL NERVES: nerves exit via the VENTRAL ROOT, issuing motor instructions that will arrive at the neuromuscular junctions.

It is important to realize that all actions are not generated by the cerebral cortex. Instead it has been argued that the higher levels of the system issue rather general commands which do not lay out in precise detail the exact muscular operations that must take place. While very precise, controlled movements appear to demand the use of higher centres, it is clear that coordinated actions can be organized from positions very low in the motor system (see Tresch *et al.*, 1999) while actions that demand very rapid responses following processing of sensory information can be generated from the brainstem (see STARTLE REFLEX for example). It seems to be the case that actions are organized by the lowest level of the motor system that can do so.

See also: motor control; motor cortex; motor neurons; motor programming; reflex; voluntary

Reference

Tresch M.C., Saltiel P. & Bizzi E. (1999) The construction of movement by the spinal cord. *Nature Neuroscience* 2: 162–167.

motor theory of speech perception The theory that holds that speech is perceived via recognition of the speaker's intended phonetic gestures; early statements of the theory proposed invariant motor commands underlying the articulatory gestures corresponding to the PHONEME being uttered, but later the invariant feature was proposed to be the (more abstract) intentional structures controlling articulatory movements. Heterogeneity and interdependence of gestural cues to a single phoneme however pose serious problems for the model (see Klatt, 1989).

See also: speech perception

Reference

Klatt D.H. (1989) Review of selected models of speech perception. In *Lexical Representation and Process*, ed. W.D. Marslen-Wilson, pp. 169–226, MIT Press: Cambridge MA.

ANNE CUTLER

motor unit A composite comprising a single motor neuron (see MOTOR NEURONS and all the muscle FIBRES which it makes contact with via the NEUROMUSCULAR JUNCTION.

See also: innervation ratio

motor–limbic handshaking *see* limbic–motor interface

mounting behaviour The species-specific manner in which males mount females prior to INTROMISSION and EJACULATION.

mouth The term MOUTH (or oral cavity) barely requires definition, but it is important to recognize the several different parts in and around the mouth. The PALATE is the roof of the mouth and is divided into the soft palate (at the rear) and the hard palate (at the front). The OROPHARYNX is that part of the mouth between the soft palate and the EPIGLOTTIS. Receptors in the oropharynx are important in signalling information about the foods and fluids present in the mouth to the brain. Behind the oropharynx is the PHARYNX – which is what, in everyday language, one would call the throat. It is obviously involved in the mechanics of swallowing food and water but, unlike the oropharynx, is not involved in detecting the composition of foods and fluids. The pharynx leads to both the TRACHEA (the windpipe) and the OESOPHAGOUS (esophagus in American spelling) The epiglottis is the flap of cartilage that covers the GLOTTIS – which is the opening to the LARYNX and the TRACHEA. The larynx is the upper part of the windpipe and is important in SPEECH PRODUCTION; the trachea connects to the bronchi in the lungs. The epiglottis functions to guard the trachea during swallowing of food, which is of course destined to travel down the oesophagous to the STOMACH.

See also: digestive system; gustation; tongue

moveable electrode *see* electrode

movement deficits Impairments in the initiation or execution of movement as a result of neurological injury or disease. There are many levels in the NEURAXIS at which dysfunction can result in movement deficits and the type of movement deficit often reveals the nature of the injury. The table overleaf indicates the nature of the dysfunctions that follow damage at various levels of the neuraxis.

In addition, there are many progressive degenerative disorders of the central nervous system – for example, PARKINSON'S DISEASE and HUNTINGTON'S CHOREA – that also involve deficits in the ability to initiate and execute voluntary movements. Such degenerative disorders often involve damage to anatomically or neurochemically identifiable systems but the impact of this loss may be felt in multiple CNS systems. There are also many diseases – such as MYASTHENIA GRAVIS and MULTIPLE SCLEROSIS – that impact on movement by affecting the peripheral nervous system and neuromuscular junction.

VERITY J. BROWN

MPP⁺ (1-methyl-4-phenyl-pyridinium ion) The neurotoxic metabolite of MPTP. MPTP penetrates from the blood to the brain without difficulty and is then is oxidized to MPP⁺ which is thought to enter DOPAMINERGIC neurons via REUPTAKE processes. Exactly how MPP⁺ kills neurons is not clear: it is presumed to interfere with MITOCHONDRIA.

See also: neurotoxins

MPTP MPTP (1-methyl-4-phenyl-1,2,3,6-tetrahydropyridine) is an extremely selective and species-specific neurotoxin (see NEUROTOXINS).

Its toxic effects are almost exclusively limited to the dopaminergic neurons of the SUBSTANTIA NIGRA of PRIMATES. MPTP-induced loss of nigral dopamine neurons results in an irreversible Parkinsonian condition which is virtually identical to the IDIOPATHIC condition. The discovery of the toxic effects of MPTP has had a pronounced effect on research into PARKINSON'S DISEASE. It has both enabled the development of an excellent animal model of the condition and given insights into the mechanisms which may cause the degeneration of nigral dopaminergic neurons.

The cardinal symptoms of Parkinson's disease are BRADYKINESIA, RIGIDITY and TREMOR. The disease is progressive and typically affects the aged. The condition results from degeneration of DOPAMINE cells in the substantia nigra which consequently results in loss of dopamine within the STRIATUM. As the disease progresses dopaminergic neurons in the VENTRAL TEGMENTAL AREA may also degenerate along with NORADRENERGIC neurons in the LOCUS COERULEUS. In general, the symptoms can be alleviated in a dose-dependent manner by the

Human Movement Disorders

Location	Dysfunction	Description
Spinal cord	Paraplegia	Loss of sensation and movement in lower torso and legs
	Paralysis	Loss of movement
	Paresis	Some loss of movement (either general low grade loss or total loss but in a restricted area of the body)
Cerebellum	Ataxia	Loss of control of posture, balance and gait (fine movements preserved)
Primary motor cortex	Hemiplegia	Loss of movement on one side only (movement control is lateralized, therefore will only get paraplegia with a bilateral lesion)
Secondary and/or tertiary motor cortex	Apraxia	Loss of purposeful movements (such as movements on command or copying)
	Neglect	Loss of directed to movements to parts of space
Basal ganglia	Athetosis	Writhing movement
	Chorea	Involuntary jerky movement
	Dyskinesia	Disordered movement
	Akinesia	Absence of movement initiation
	Bradykinesia	Slow execution of movement

systemic administration of dopaminergic agents such as L-DOPA. Parkinson's disease typically occurs in the absence of obvious precipitating factors hence the term idiopathic Parkinson's disease. A single, relatively small dose of MPTP is sufficient to induce a profound, irreversible Parkinsonian condition in humans which is virtually identical to the idiopathic condition in terms of its symptomology, pathology and response to treatment. The toxic effects of the compound were discovered by chance when drug abusers self-administered MPTP as a contaminant in a batch of a synthetically produced 'designer drug'. There are however subtle differences between MPTP-induced Parkinsonism and Parkinson's disease. MPTP patients can be much younger and their response to dopamine agonist therapy more problematic. There is a tendency for these patients to experience severe side-effects to dopamine agonists much sooner than idiopathic patients. These side-effects include 'end of dose deterioration', DYSKINESIA at peak effect and psychiatric complications. It is also debatable whether LEWY BODIES, that is inclusion bodies which are characteristic of the degenerating substantia nigra in the brains of idiopathic Parkinsonian patients, are seen following MPTP-induced neurotoxicity.

MPTP shows remarkable species specific toxicity. It is extremely toxic to humans and certain species of monkey. The macaque monkeys, *Macaca fascicularis*, are particularly susceptible to the toxic effects of MPTP, doses in the range of 1 mg/kg being sufficient to induce a marked Parkinsonian syndrome. This syndrome is virtually identical to the idiopathic human condition with the exception of resting tremor which is not always observed. The drug is far less toxic to marmosets where it tends to induce a milder syndrome which is reversible to some extent. In contrast, MPTP has virtually no toxic effects in rats and guinea pigs though certain strains of mice, for example C57 black mice, are susceptible to large doses of the drug. There is anecdotal evidence to suggest that older monkeys are more vulnerable to the toxic effects of MPTP than young ones. Degeneration of dopaminergic neurons in the ventral tegmental area and noradrenergic neurons in the locus coeruleus have been reported following the administration of large doses of MPTP to aged macaques. However, it appears that the full behavioural syndrome can be elicited following MPTP doses which result in selective degeneration of nigral dopaminergic neurons and where striatal dopamine depletions are limited to the CAUDATE NUCLEUS and the PUTAMEN.

MPTP itself is a relatively harmless compound. Its toxic properties arise from its conversion into the highly toxic compound MPP$^+$. MPTP is a small lipid soluble molecule which can penetrate the BLOOD–BRAIN BARRIER with ease. Once in the brain it is thought to be oxidized to MPP$^+$, the reaction being catalysed by the enzyme MONOAMINE OXIDASE-B (MAO-B), which is found in the MITOCHONDRIA of GLIAL CELLS. This proposed mechanism is supported by the observation that DEPRENYL, a selective inhibitor of MAO-B, can protect experimental animals from the toxic effects of MPTP. This observation has led to clinical trials where MAO-B inhibitors have been administered in attempts to slow the progression of the idiopathic human condition on the assumption that the degeneration that occurs in Parkinson's disease is mediated by an MPTP-like compound. Results to date remain contentious. MPP$^+$, once formed, is thought to enter dopaminergic neurons via the dopamine REUPTAKE system. This hypothesis is supported by the observation that blockers of the dopamine transporter reduce the toxic effects of MPP$^+$ on cultured dopaminergic neurons. The species specific nature of MPTP-induced toxicity may reflect an action of neuromelanin. This pigment tends to be present in nigral neurons of species which are susceptible to MPTP. It is thought that neuromelanin may actively bind MPP$^+$ and thus act as a depot for it. The precise manner in which MPP+ kills nigral neurons is unclear but it is assumed that the compound interferes with mitochondrial functioning.

See also: free radicals; 6-hydroxydopamine

IAN J. MITCHELL

Muller cell A specialized form of GLIAL CELL (see EPENDYMOGLIAL CELLS) in the RETINA.

Müllerian internal genitalia Male and female foetuses have the capacity to develop both female and male internal genitalia; these being, for females, the oviducts, UTERUS, cervix and (possibly) the upper VAGINA, and for males, the epididymis, vas deferens and seminal vesicles. The female internal genitalia arise from the Müllerian ducts, the male from the Wolffian ducts. (It is from these ducts that the terms Müllerian internal genitalia and WOLFFIAN INTERNAL GENITALIA arise.) In females, the Wolffian ducts naturally become functionless but in males, the presence of ANDROGENS from the TESTES prevent this, and allow for the development of male internal genitalia. If a foetus is castrated (see CASTRATION) female internal genitalia will develop, in even a male foetus. Male HORMONES are critical for the maintenance and proper development of the male internal genitalia: what one might call the natural state is for the development of female internal genitalia.

See also: sexual differentiation

Reference

Johnson M. & Everitt B.J. (1980) *Essential Reproduction*, Blackwell Scientific Publications: Oxford.

multi-infarct dementia *see* vascular dementia

multi-layer perception *see* neural networks

multimodal Used synonymously with POLYMODAL, but in fact multimodal refers to a distribution with more than one peak.

multiparous (from Latin, *multus*: much, *parere*: to bring out) Multiparous refers to the production of more than one offspring at birth: RATS for example are multiparous, litters of fifteen pups at a single birth not being uncommon. Humans are not normally multiparous.

multiple memory systems A concept suggesting distinguishable cognitive operations and processes underlying MEMORY. Memory systems are divided broadly into those involving conscious and explicit expression of memories and those involving non-conscious learning of biases and skills that demonstrated by implicit expression. Three initial criteria have been proposed by which a memory system is deemed a separate and experimentally supportable memory system. The first criterion is CLASS INCLUSION OPERATIONS. This system enables one to perform a number of tasks independent of the material content – for instance, PRIMING using either picture fragments, word stems or categories. The second is properties and relations. This requires a coherent list of features within that system, in addition to any relations with already existing systems those features have. The third criterion is CONVERGENT DISSOCIATIONS. This is the ability to show that distinct systems are responsible for the performance of separate tasks, such as in double dissociations.

There are five memory systems defined and outlined by Schacter & Tulving (1994) which are derived from work on humans. PROCEDURAL MEMORY consists of the non-conscious processes of motor skill and habit learning (see HABITS), CONDITIONING and ASSOCIATIVE LEARNING. Retrieval of this type of information is implicit. The neuroanatomical structures mediating these types of memory are proposed to be the STRIATUM and select parts of the CEREBRAL CORTEX involved in the acquisition of these specific responses. The second, a PERCEPTUAL REPRESENTATION SYSTEM, includes the various priming abilities of visual and auditory word forms, and structural descriptions. Method of retrieval for this type of information is implicit and depends on the unimodal neocortical structures (see NEOCORTEX) involved in the original learning event. SEMANTIC MEMORY is the third system. Within this system exists generic, FACT MEMORY and KNOWLEDGE BASED MEMORY. Modes of processing include spatial and relational memory for which retrieval is an explicit, cognitive event. Structures within the medial TEMPORAL LOBE, which include the HIPPOCAMPAL FORMATION and surrounding cortical structures, are responsible for this memory system. Fourth is the PRIMARY MEMORY SYSTEM, also known as WORKING MEMORY. It includes information retrieved explicitly through the visual and auditory modalities. The fifth system is EPISODIC MEMORY. This encompasses personal, autobiographical and event memory all retrieved explicitly. Medial temporal lobe structures are responsible for this memory system.

The following classification has been offered to account for the animal learning literature, consisting predominantly of rodents and non-human primates. The major distinction is between DECLARATIVE MEMORY versus NON-DECLARATIVE MEMORY. Subsystems within this classification scheme involve the dichotomy of hippocampal dependent (which includes FORNIX, hippocampal formation and surrounding cortical areas, diencephalic structures such as thalamic nuclei [see THALAMUS; DORSOMEDIAL NUCLEUS OF THE THALAMUS] and MAMMILLARY BODIES) versus hippocampal independent memory. Declarative memory includes all that is expressed explicitly, such as semantic, episodic and working memory. Non-declarative, or procedural, memory consists of conditioning, skill and habit learning. There also exists an anatomically driven classification scheme for animals which suggests the existence of AMYGDALA, hippocampal, and dorsal STRIATUM memory systems. These break down into an emotional or conditioning system; a relational or mnemonic memory system; a habit memory system.

In addition to these relatively well defined memory systems, some suggest that distinct POLYMODAL association cortices represent an even further distinction among memory systems. However, if one chooses to define a memory system based on the three criterion mentioned above, then the following may be no more than a descriptive of the functions of those cortical areas. The PERIRHINAL CORTEX and ENTORHINAL CORTEX have been implicated in OBJECT RECOGNITION MEMORY and the ability to make STIMULUS–STIMULUS ASSOCIATIONS. Select regions of the PREFRONTAL CORTEX are thought to be primarily involved in working memory, which in and of itself is a polymodal function.

References

Schacter D.L. & Tulving E. (eds.) (1994) *Memory Systems*, MIT Press: Cambridge MA.
Sherry D.F. & Schacter D.L. (1987) The evolution of multiple memory systems. *Psychological Review* 94: 439–454.

HOWARD EICHENBAUM

multiple sclerosis A neurodegenerative disorder involving loss of MYELIN from axons (see AXON). The loss is often patchy, with DEMYELINATION occurring at small points in different parts of the nervous system. A GLIAL SCAR marks the site of each demyelinating LESION. It is the most common form of neurological disorder in individuals under 50 years of age (the age of onset is typically around 30 years) having a prevalence of approximately 1 in 2000 (and being rather more common in women than men). The precise form of the disease obviously reflects the sites of greatest pathology. Multiple sclerosis typically presents as a muscular disorder, with weakness in the limbs, though visual disturbances are also very common. Cognitive deficits have also been reported, intellectual function being impaired in anything from 30–70% of patients.

multiple system atrophy This is a generalized term used to indicate a form of brain damage that has affected a number of different systems. Under this heading neurologists have included SHY–DRAGER SYNDROME (which involves AUTONOMIC NERVOUS SYSTEM damage), OLIVOPONTOCEREBELLAR ATROPHY (which features ATAXIA) and STRIATONIGRAL DEGENERATION (which has some of the features of PARKINSON'S DISEASE). Parkinson's disease itself, typically thought of as involving specific loss of the neurotransmitter DOPAMINE from within the BASAL GANGLIA, actually involves loss of a variety of neurons from many sites in the MIDBRAIN and BRAINSTEM. It is not generally considered as a form of multiple system atrophy though there are clear relationships between Parkinsonism, multiple system atrophy and other conditions such as PROGRESSIVE SUPRANUCLEAR PALSY and AMYOTROPHIC LATERAL SCLEROSIS (LOU GEHRIG'S DISEASE).

multiple trace model A model of the organization of MEMORY in the HIPPOCAMPUS involving multiple but related memory traces distributed throughout this structure. One effect of this is to make memory resistant to hippocampal damage, unless the damage is very extensive.

References

Moscovitch M. & Nadel L. (1998) Consolidation and the hippocampal complex revisited:

in defense of the multiple trace model. *Current Opinion in Neurobiology* 8: 297–300.

Nadel L. & Moscovitch M. (1997) Memory consolidation, retrograde amnesia and the hippocampal complex. *Current Opinion in Neurobiology* 7: 217–222.

multipolar neuron *see* bipolar neurons

multitrode electrode

multiunit recording *see* single-unit electrophysiological recording

Munchausen's syndrome Named after a fictional character, Baron von Munchausen, whose adventures were chronicled by R.E. Raspe (1737–1794): this syndrome describes individuals who feign injury in order to obtain medical attention. It has no known cause.

See also: neurosis

muricide (from Latin, *mus*: mouse) Mouse killing; in the past – but not now – muricidal behaviour has been used as a measure of AGGRESSION in rats.

muscarine The definitive AGONIST at MUSCARINIC ACETYLCHOLINE RECEPTORS. (Muscarinic refers to a property: a muscarinic receptor is one that binds muscarine.) Muscarine is a toxin found in the fly agaric mushroom (*Amanita muscaris*) – these are easily recognized mushrooms with white stalks, topped by bright red caps with white spots. The inocybe and clitocybe mushrooms also contain muscarine. Symptoms of muscarine poising include sweating, salivation, constricted pupils, abdominal PAIN, cramping of muscles in the VISCERA, diarrhhoea, VOMITING, CONVULSIONS, COMA and death. The effects of muscarine can be reversed by ATROPINE an ANTAGONIST at acetylcholine receptors, but it is better not to consume muscarine at all, thereby avoiding the need for an antidote.

See also: muscimol; nicotine; psychomotor stimulants

muscarinic acetylcholine receptors *see* acetylcholine receptors

muscimol The best known and most often used AGONIST for the GABA-A RECEPTOR (see GABA RECEPTORS). Muscimol is a breakdown product of IBOTENIC ACID, which is found (like MUSCARINE) in the fly agaric mushroom, *Amanita muscaris*. Muscimol does not have fatal effects in humans, but high doses do produce unpleasant effects similar to muscarine, as well as HALLUCINATION. It reinforces the belief that eating fly agaric mushrooms is to be avoided in all circumstances.

muscle fibre *see* muscles

muscle spindle Information from MUSCLES (proprioceptive information, or PROPRIOCEPTION) is provided principally by two structures: the GOLGI TENDON ORGAN and muscle spindles. Rather obviously, muscle spindles are concerned with information coming from muscles, the Golgi tendon organs with information from tendons. Less obviously, the muscle spindles provide information about muscle *stretching*, while the Golgi tendon organs provide information about muscle *contraction*. The sensory information provided by these structures is of great importance. If the connections to the CENTRAL NERVOUS SYSTEM from them are cut – deafferented (see DEAFFERENT) – it will lead to a relative disuse of the affected muscles. For example, if the muscles of one arm are deafferented it will lead not to paralysis but to relative incapacitation. LEARNING new motor tasks with the deafferented muscles will be more difficult than it would have been.

Muscle spindles are shaped like the spindles used to twist thread: relatively long, and wider in the middle than at the ends. They are made up of INTRAFUSAL FIBRES and EXTRAFUSAL FIBRES. (These terms are derived from Latin *fusus*, meaning spindle: the extrafusal fibres lie on the outside of the muscle spindle, the intrafusal fibres on the inside.) Within the muscle spindle are two sensory receptors: one is called the PRIMARY SENSORY ENDING (or CENTRAL SENSORY ENDING; or ANNULOSPIRAL ENDING) and is found within the core of intrafusal fibres. The second type is the SECONDARY SENSORY ENDING (or DISTAL SENSORY ENDING; or FLOWER SPRAY ENDING) which are found towards the ends of the spindle. These two types of sensory ending are reactive to different things. Both respond when muscles change their shape – it is the deformation of spindle shape that triggers the neural activity that will be relayed to the central nervous system – but the primary endings show an initial large change in activity which adapts quickly, while the secondary endings react more consistently and slowly. As such the primary endings provide information about the moment-by-moment changes in muscle activity while the secondary endings provide information about the force being exerted.

Muscle spindles have as their main function the transmission of sensory information to the central nervous system but their activity is modified by two types of MOTOR NEURONS. GAMMA MOTOR NEURONS have their cell bodies in the VENTRAL HORN of the SPINAL CORD, their axons exiting via the VENTRAL ROOTS (see AXON; CELL BODY). These contact a region adjacent to the extrafusal muscle fibres called the MYOTUBE region. ALPHA MOTOR NEURONS (which also come from the ventral horns) contact the extrafusal fibres themselves. Alpha motor neurons conduct impulses more quickly and are more numerous than gamma motor neurons. By controlling the activity of the myotube region and the extrafusal fibres, alpha and gamma motor neurons can affect the ability of extrafusal fibres to contract, effectively setting their sensitivity to changes in muscle stretching.

See also: locomotion

Reference

Rosenzweig M.R., Leiman A.L. & Breedlove S.M. (1996) *Biological Psychology*, Sinauer Associates: Sunderland MA.

muscles The study of muscles might at first seem to have little to do with biological psychology. But it is very important not to forget that an animal has a BRAIN to assess sensory input, comparing current input with what has been learnt and memorized, and to organize reactions to that input. Those reactions involve control of the musculature (a term that describes systems of muscles in groups or in total) and it is therefore important that biological psychologists should have at least a rudimentary acquaintance with what muscles are and how they work. Muscles come in three types: SKELETAL MUSCLE (or striated muscle) is attached to bone (by tendons) and is

responsible for the overt movement of the body; CARDIAC MUSCLE is found (obviously enough) only in the heart; SMOOTH MUSCLE makes up blood vessels and the organs of the digestive tract.

A skeletal muscle is a bundle of long fibres, each the length of the muscle. Each MUSCLE FIBRE grows from MYOBLASTS (cells that produce muscle fibres) which develop into MYO-TUBES (muscle cells with a cylindrical shape) and finally into MYOFIBRILS. Each muscle fibre is actually a multinucleated CELL, created by combining smaller cells – the MYOFIBRILS – early in DEVELOPMENT. Myofibrils are made of two kinds of MYOFILAMENT: thin or THICK FILAMENTS. The filaments contain PROTEINS: the thin filaments possess ACTIN, while thick filaments possess MYOSIN. Skeletal muscle appears striped or striated because of the way in which the myofilaments are organized into units that repeat (each unit being called a SARCOMERE). When muscles contact the thin and thick filaments slide past each other, changing the sizes of the sarcomeres. This sliding is based on an interaction between myosin and actin, the two binding together to form transient CROSS BRIDGES, a process critically dependent on ADENOSINE TRIPHOSPHATE. Muscle contraction is initiated by the arrival of ACTION POTENTIAL at the NEUROMUSCULAR JUNCTION. It is important to note that, actively, muscles only contract: muscle extension is passive. Note also that skeletal muscles can be described using various different terms. (1) Muscles that act in coordination together – both contracting to produce a specific effect for example – are said to be SYNERGISTIC MUSCLES. (2) Muscles that act in reciprocal pairs (when one contracts the other must extend) are said to be ANTAGONISTIC MUSCLES. One of these will be an EXTENSOR MUSCLE, the other a FLEXOR MUSCLE. The best known example of this is biceps–triceps relationship. (Bend your arm in the classic body-building pose: the biceps on top of the arm swells: it has contracted and flexed the arm: it is a flexor muscle. On the underside of the same arm, the triceps muscle has passively elongated – it is the extensor muscle here. To extend your arm again, the triceps must contract, your biceps muscle passively extending.) (3) There are FAST

MUSCLE FIBRES and SLOW MUSCLE FIBRES. The difference between the two depends essentially on the duration for which a high concentration of CALCIUM ions (Ca^{2+}) is maintained following activation of the neuromuscular junction. Fast muscle fibres mediate rapid and powerful muscle contractions: the movement of muscles in locomotion (see LOCOMOTION) – walking or running, or the wing beats of birds – depend on these. Anything that requires repeated muscle contraction to occur without fatigue developing needs fast muscle fibre activation. Slow muscle fibres can manage long contractions: they are important for POSTURE. Control of skeletal muscles depends on being able to send signals from the brain that activate muscles via the neuromuscular junction, and by sensory information being relayed from the musculature back to the brain. The major sensory receptors that monitor muscle activity are the MUSCLE SPINDLE and the GOLGI TENDON ORGAN.

Cardiac muscle is essentially skeletal muscle but with certain specific differences to do with the electrical and MEMBRANE properties of individual cells. Cardiac muscles cells have INTERCALATED DISCS (which normal skeletal muscle cells do not have) that provide the opportunity for direct electrical coupling of cells. Action potentials arriving at one site in the heart can be communicated across all cells very quickly, ensuring uniformity of action in generating heartbeats. In addition, cardiac cells can generate their own action potentials without input, being in possession of PACEMAKER CELLS with oscillatory properties (see OSCILLATION). The entire mass of cardiac muscle can be referred to as the MYOCARDIUM, which gives rise to terms such as myocardial and myocardiac: terms such as this simply refer to the musculature of the heart. Smooth muscle is not striated, the myosin and actin containing myofibrils not being organized in the same way as in skeletal muscle. It lacks the contractile power of skeletal muscle but can maintain contraction over great lengths, allowing it to develop peristaltic movements (see PERISTALSIS) to move blood through vessels or gut contents through the digestive tract.

References

Campbell N.A., Reece J.B. & Mitchell L.G. (1999) *Biology*, 5th edn, Addison-Wesley: Menlo Park CA.

Rosenzweig M.R., Leiman A.L. & Breedlove S.M. (1996) *Biological Psychology*, Sinauer Associates: Sunderland MA.

muscular dystrophy A disorder of the MUSCLES impairing movement; contrast with MOTOR NEURON DISEASE. There are various types: Duchenne MUSCULAR DYSTROPHY is a sex-linked heritable condition affecting only males; other types (facioscapulohumoral, inherited, and myotonic) are also heritable, affect both males and females, and differ in their precise pattern of symptoms. Duchenne and facioscapulohumoral are characterized by muscle weakness; inherited and myopathic also feature altered muscle tone (MYOTONIA).

muscular rigidity *see* rigidity

music and the brain Just as the human brain has regions specialized for LANGUAGE, so there are regions specialized for different aspects of music. Understanding this process is, however, complicated by the fact that the different attributes of music (such as melodies, rhythms and timbres) are not processed in the same way. Furthermore, the processing of these attributes may differ between expert and non-expert musicians. One thing is clear however: the neural systems underlying music are different from those for language.

Striking evidence has come from cases of musicians who suffered brain damage severely affecting language but sparing musical abilities. The Russian composer Shebalin suffered severe APHASIA following a STROKE in the LEFT HEMISPHERE yet was successfully able to continue his work as a composer. Similarly, the French composer and organist Langlais suffered a left hemisphere vascular accident resulting in aphasia, ALEXIA and AGRAPHIA yet could read musical notation and continued to compose. Similar distinctions between musical and verbal abilities are also seen among people with no special musical training. It is, for example, often observed that people with BROCA'S APHASIA can sing with good melody in spite of severe speech handicaps. While these examples of aphasia without AMUSIA (loss of musical functions), as well as those of amusia without aphasia are rarely, if ever, pure, the relative differences do support a DOUBLE DISSOCIATION between language and music. This indicates a division of the neural substrates responsible for critical aspects of the verbal and musical communication systems.

This division has often been taken to mean that the left hemisphere is vital for language processes while the RIGHT HEMISPHERE is vital for music. Such a distinction is an oversimplification. A review of patients with localized brain damage or with unilateral sodium amylobarbitone injections (Wada technique) does indicate that the right hemisphere contributes more than the left for singing. Consistent with this, DICHOTIC LISTENING TASKS also show left ear superiority for musical stimuli (the reverse is found for verbal stimuli). These findings depend, however, on the elements of music being tested. In general, when musical excerpts are processed as entities then there is a right hemisphere advantage (for example, for melody). In contrast, step-by-step or elemental analyses of music show either no hemispheric difference or a left hemisphere advantage. Thus the left hemisphere may be more important for those musical abilities that share properties with speech, namely temporal order, duration, simultaneity and rhythm. There is also evidence that the right hemisphere advantage for melody is lost in people with extensive musical training, in whom a left hemisphere advantage may be found.

The SUPERIOR TEMPORAL GYRUS is a principal recipient of auditory information and right, but not left, TEMPORAL LOBE excision can impair pitch judgements. The involvement of this region is also implicated by PET (positron emission tomography) studies of people hearing melodies or making pitch judgements. The results suggest that specialized systems exist in the right superior temporal cortex for the perception of melodies and that pitch comparisons involve interactions between the right frontal and right temporal cortices. Finally, there has been much interest in the possible relationship between HANDEDNESS and musical abilities. It is easy to cite famous musicians who were left-handed (from C.P.E. Bach to Cole Porter and Paul McCartney) and surveys among professional musicians do indicate a slight increase in left-handedness. This is supported by evidence that left-handers can show superior pitch recognition judgements, and tentative links have been made with the relative importance of the right hemisphere for melody.

JOHN P. AGGLETON

mutant A mutant is the product of a MUTATION: whole animals can be referred to as mutants, as can component parts (a CELL, or a GENE for example). Mutant animals can be created by deliberate experimental procedure or can arise spontaneously. Examination of mutants with known genetic changes can reveal information about the relationships between genes and performance (of either behaviour or of some biological process).

mutation An alteration in a genetic sequence, caused by a change in the order of NUCLEOTIDES in a piece of DNA. Because DNA sequences are inherited between generations, mutations will also be inherited.

FIONA M. INGLIS

mutism The absence of speech; it can occur as a psychological condition with no physical cause and also occurs in an ORGANIC condition known as *akinetic mutism*. In this patients are conscious and aware, but emit no speech (see SPEECH PRODUCTION) and show a generally restricted range of responses in any dimension. It has been associated with brain damage around the third ventricle (see VENTRICLES).

mutual parasitism *see* symbiosis

myalgic encephalitis (ME) Chronic muscular PAIN and FATIGUE supposedly associated with an inflammatory process in BRAIN and/or SPINAL CORD. Evidence for organic pathology has been widely accepted by legislative bodies, the law courts and patient support groups but scientific support is unconvincing. Neurological studies (see Thomas, 1993) have instead indicated central subjective fatigue after minimal exertion without verifiable evidence of inflammatory immunological (see IMMUNE SYSTEM) or degenerative change. The condition is more accurately subsumed as CHRONIC FATIGUE SYNDROME but is associated with many other distressing symptoms especially – in over 75% of cases – DEPRESSION and ANXIETY and it presents a serious clinical challenge.

Reference

Thomas P.K. (1993) The chronic fatigue syndrome: what do we know? *British Medical Journal* 306: 1557–1558.

L. JACOB HERBERG

myasthenia gravis Relapsing muscular weakness due to autoimmune inflammatory damage to CHOLINERGIC receptors at the NEUROMUSCULAR JUNCTION. The onset is marked by muscular fatigue ('myasthenia') and drooping eyelids, especially following exertion. The condition may be progressive and after some years lead to terminal respiratory paralysis. Central cholinergic neurotransmission and cognitive function are spared. Effective palliation can be achieved with ANTICHOLINESTERASE drugs such as PHYSOSTIGMINE which prolong the excitatory action of ACETYLCHOLINE at surviving receptors, while the autoimmune process itself may be slowed by treatment with GLUCOCORTICOIDS and other IMMUNOSUPPRESSANT drugs, or by surgical removal of the THYMUS GLAND.

L. JACOB HERBERG

myelencephalon Duriung development the RHOMBENCEPHALON differentiates into the METENCEPHALON and myelencephalon. The metencephalon includes the CEREBELLUM and PONS, the myelencephalon becomes the MEDULLA OBLONGATA; see HINDBRAIN.

myelin Myelin is the fatty substance that provides AXON insulation in the nervous system. In the CENTRAL NERVOUS SYSTEM myelin is provided by OLIGODENDROGLIA; in the PERIPHERAL NERVOUS SYSTEM it is supplied by SCHWANN CELLS. In both cases, cell processes wrap around axons forming a multilayer insulating sheath (see PROCESS). Gaps in the myelin sheath (NODE OF RANVIER) permit ionic

flow across the axon MEMBRANE. Since such activity is only present at limited points on myelinated axons, ACTION POTENTIAL speed is greatly accelerated compared to the speed along UNMYELINATED axons. Myelin has a complex structure. It is composed of LIPIDS (70–85%), PROTEINS (15–30%) with a small GANGLIOSIDE component. Most of the protein – some 80% – is made either PROTEOLIPID or MYELIN BASIC PROTEIN (though note that myelin basic protein is a term that actually covers a complex group of proteins, all derived from a single GENE). Many fibres in the nervous system are normally unmyelinated (also called non-myelinated). Obviously, this presents no problem for normal neural activity. However, loss of myelin (DEMYELINATION) or the failure to form myelin properly (DYSMYELINATION) has important functional consequences. MULTIPLE SCLEROSIS is the best known of the demyelinating disorders.

See also: glial cells

Reference

Newman S., Saito M. & Yu R.K. (1995) Biochemistry of myelin proteins and enzymes. In *Neuroglia*, ed. H. Kettenmann & B.R. Ransom, pp. 535–554, Oxford University Press: Oxford.

myelin basic protein In fact, not a single protein but a group of PROTEINS, derived from a single GENE, that form an important part of the protein component of MYELIN. ANTIBODIES to myelin basic protein are available, making immunohistochemical examination (see IMMUNOHISTOCHEMISTRY) of myelin possible.

myenteric plexus The myenteric plexus is a composite of neurons (see NEURON), ganglia (see GANGLION) and FIBRES that line the walls of the GASTROINTESTINAL SYSTEM (especially the small intestine). It functions with relative independence from the CENTRAL NERVOUS SYSTEM and AUTONOMIC NERVOUS SYSTEM to regulate intestinal ENDOCRINE functions and MUSCLES.

myoblast *see* muscles

myocardium *see* muscles

myoclonus (from Greek, *mys, myso*: muscle, *klonos*: tumult) Myoclonus is a term that describes and involuntary spasm of the skeletal muscle (see MUSCLES); myoclonic is the adjectival form of myoclonus.

See also: convulsions; dyskinesia; epilepsy; tonic–clonic

myofibril *see* muscles

myofilament *see* muscles

myopia *see* refractive error

myosin *see* muscles

myotonia Altered muscle tone: there is delayed relaxation after contraction. Myotonia features in several conditions, notably certain forms of MUSCULAR DYSTROPHY.

myotube *see* muscles

N

NADPH diaphorase Nicotinamide adenine dinucleotide phosphate (NADPH) diaphorase is an ENZYME that can operate as a NITRIC OXIDE SYNTHASE inhibitor. It is commonly used in HISTOCHEMISTRY to stain any type of NEURON that synthesizes the novel neurotransmitter NITRIC OXIDE.

naja naja The term naja naja relates to the venoms of various cobras: *Naja naja* is the Indian cobra, *Naja naja siamensis* the Thailand cobra and *Naja naja atra* the Formosan cobra. These venoms are of interest because they bind to NICOTINIC ACETYLCHOLINE RECEPTORS. Radiolabelled (see RADIOLABEL) venom of *Naja naja siamensis* has been used to map nicotinic receptors in the CENTRAL NERVOUS SYSTEM (though other more selective – and slightly safer – agents are used now). The bite of cobras is deadly because of the action of the venom at nicotinic acetylcholine receptors in the NEUROMUSCULAR JUNCTION and in the central nervous system

See also: cone snails; bungarotoxin: neurotoxins

naloxone A drug that is a selective blocker of OPIATE RECEPTORS. Naloxone is a well-known opiate ANTAGONIST as is the structurally similar compound NALTREXONE. Naloxone binds to opiate receptors and blocks them until the drug is metabolized, preventing opiate drugs or ENDOGENOUS OPIATES from stimulating the receptors. It binds non-selectively (that is, it binds to all opiate receptor subtypes). It is used extensively in research on opioid systems, opiate drugs, and ADDICTION. Administration of naloxone to an opiate-dependent individual will result in immediate precipitation of WITHDRAWAL symptoms, since in PHYSICAL DEPENDENCE, the opiate receptors need the presence of the drug to function normally.

ANN E. KELLEY

naltrexone A morphine derivative related to NALOXONE and, like naloxone, used to treat individuals recovering from ADDICTION to OPIATES. It is therapeutically more useful than naloxone because it is easily administered (it can be given orally), has few side effects and has a long-lasting (approximately 24 h) effect on OPIATE RECEPTORS.

nano- Prefix indicating a factor of 10^{-9}, or one thousand millionth; see SI UNITS.

narceine *see* opium

narcolepsy Narcolepsy is a disorder of SLEEP characterized by excessive daytime sleepiness, and by sudden, irresistible SLEEP ATTACK. The sleep attacks are particularly problematic when they are accompanied by CATAPLEXY, a loss of muscle tone leading to partial or complete postural collapse. While these two daytime symptoms tend to occur together, they can be dissociated from one another. The daytime, narcoleptic sleep attacks may be spontaneous and unexpected or be triggered by a strong EMOTION such as surprise, humour, or erotic pleasure. When studied in the laboratory, narcoleptic patients typically show onset REM SLEEP periods and the sleep recorded during attacks has the electrographic (see ELECTROENCEPHALOGRAM) signs of REM.

Narcolepsy is also characterized by two related anomalies of nocturnal REM sleep: (1) HYPNAGOGIC HALLUCINATION and terrifying dreams at sleep onset; and (2) HYPNOPOMPIC HALLUCINATION and sleep paralysis on awakening later in the night. Like the daytime symptoms, these nocturnal signs are the expression of the intensification of REM sleep generator which produces REM sleep signs at sleep onset and which continues to produce REM sleep signs after arousal. This physiological hypersensitivity of the REM sleep generator has been shown to be familial with genetic transmission linked to HLA ANTIGEN complex. It is mediated via the DOPAMINE system which resulting CHOLINERGIC hypersensitivity. This explains the success of treatment with drugs which enhance aminergic synaptic efficacy and/or which antagonize the cholinergic system. Patients with narcolepsy may also develop SLEEP APNOEA and should be treated by a sleep disorders specialist.

The four cardinal symptoms of classical narcolepsy are sleep attacks, cataplexy, hypnagogic and hypnopompic hallucinations and sleep paralysis. Together they constitute the tetrad first described by Gellineau in 1887. But only recently has narcolepsy been understood as physiological hypersensitivity of the REM sleep generator. Relaxation of these diagnostic criteria has often resulted in the over-treatment of excessive daytime sleepiness with stimulants. This should be guarded against because of the addictive potential of these drugs. Moreover, because the attacks may be precipitated by emotional stimuli, it has been equally erroneously assumed that this syndrome was psychogenic and could be reversed by psychodynamic psychotherapy. Now that our psychopharmacological armamentarium contains less addictive and more versatile agents such as the biogenic amine reuptake blockers, the treatment of narcolepsy can be rational, safe and efficacious.

J. ALLAN HOBSON

narcosis (from Greek, *narke*: sleep, numbness) A state of unconsciousness; high doses of NARCOTIC drugs such as OPIATES can cause narcosis.

ANN E. KELLEY

narcotic analgesics *see* narcotics

narcotics (from Greek, *narke*: sleep, numbness) A group of compounds, derived from OPIUM or synthesized, with similar structure and pharmacological actions. Narcotics are also known as NARCOTIC ANALGESICS or OPIATES. This term was originally meant to distinguish narcotic analgesics, drugs which relieve PAIN and cause sleepiness, from nonnarcotic analgesics such as aspirin. However, the term is somewhat misleading since many lay people and law-enforcement officials refer to all illegal drugs as narcotics. In medical and scientific literature, the term narcotic refers only to opiates. Narcotics have many physiological and subjective effects; they cause a feeling of well-being, relaxation and drowsiness, cause respiratory depression and constriction of the pupils, and are potent analgesics. Narcotics have a high ABUSE POTENTIAL. Examples of narcotics are MORPHINE, HEROIN, CODEINE, METHADONE and FENTANYL.

ANN E. KELLEY

narcotine *see* opium

nasal bone *see* skull

nasal hemianopia *see* hemianopia

nasal visual hemifield *see* hemifield

nasal–anal length The nasal–anal length is used as an index of body size in rats and is an important statistic in the determination of normal development. For example, genetically obese ZUCKER RATS, while having hugely elevated body weight, have a shorter nasal–anal length than normal, indicating abnormal body development.

natriuresis The excretion of SODIUM; see NATRIURETIC PEPTIDES.

natriuretic peptides The term natriuresis refers to the excretion of sodium: the first natriuretic peptide to be discovered (in the heart) was ATRIAL NATRIURETIC PEPTIDE (ANP), which is a hormone whose production is triggered by increased BLOOD pressure (see HORMONES; PEPTIDES). It is released into the blood stream from the heart, travels to the kidneys and promotes water and sodium loss (by excretion). Two other types of natriuretic peptide have subsequently been discovered: BRAIN NATRIURETIC PEPTIDE (BNP) which is also found in the heart as well as the brain, and a C-TYPE NATRIURETIC PEPTIDE (CNP) found in the CENTRAL NERVOUS SYSTEM, where it is thought to have neurotransmitter properties. Two types of RECEPTOR for natriuretic peptides have been characterized, referred to as ANP_A and ANP_B. At the former, ANP has greater affinity than BNP which in turn has greater affinity than CNP; at the ANP_B receptors, CNP has the highest affinity, followed by ANP and, with equal affinity, BNP.

natural killer cells *see* immune system

natural reinforcer *see* reinforcer

natural selection Alfred Russel Wallace (1823–1913) and Charles Darwin (1809–1882) independently devised the same theory of how species could automatically change, without human or divine intervention, providing a plausible mechanism for EVOLUTION to take place. This theory, natural selection, depends upon differential survival to provide the selective agent, which is provided by human choice in the artificial selection long practised by stock breeders and agriculturalists. Inherited traits which increase the survival chances of their possessors increase FITNESS, causing more descendants to be left in subsequent generations. Automatically, therefore, species tend to evolve whose individuals are well fitted to the challenges of the environment: this process is called ADAPTATION. Adaptation depends upon the existence of heritable variation between individuals, yet its mechanism – differential death – inexorably uses up this variation. At the time the theory was proposed, inheritance was thought to be a process of blending characters of parents, thus diminishing variation in every generation. Darwin later realized this difficulty and concluded he had been wrong; however, the discovery by Gregor Mendel (1822–1884) that inheritance was particulate largely solved the problem. The 'particles' (the modern term is ALLELE) do not blend and reduce variation, but maintain their status and change only in their frequency in the population: the code is digital. In addition, we now know that errors in passing genetic material (DNA) from generation to generation

cause new alleles very occasionally to be added to the pool of variation. There are several sorts of error, or MUTATION, that can occur; for instance, a single NUCLEOTIDE base may be wrongly substituted in a replicated DNA molecule, a simple copying error. Many mutations are thought to be neutral, with no effect on the PHENOTYPE, and most others interfere with normal processes and are lethal. However, occasionally one may have an effect that confers advantage. Species change was originally believed to be continuous, since no general agent of environmental change was known (and indeed the objection of many churchmen to Darwin's presentation was the suggestion that God's creatures were imperfect, rather than to the idea of species change *per se*). Modern theory has instead found it useful to treat species as optimized to a particular environment by natural selection, as a way of understanding how specific adaptations work to enable success. (Note: the optimization is local, rather than attaining any abstract perfection, since natural selection is constrained to work on existing genetic material, which encodes a necessarily limited range of variation.) In stable environments, this is probably a good approximation; species change then occurs largely as a result of global environmental change, such as pollution (for example by OXYGEN produced by blue-green algae in early phases of geological history), plate tectonic movements and associated volcanic activity (the creation of islands for example), climate change (global desiccation leaving isolated islands of forests for instance) and in response to mass extinctions caused by extraterrestrial impacts (such as comet collisions).

RICHARD W. BYRNE

nature–nurture A phrase encapsulating the ancient debate between those who favour genetic explanations (nature) for individual differences and those who favour environmental explanations (nurture). In psychology, this debate has been most marked when considering INTELLIGENCE. Although MOLECULAR BIOLOGY is providing better explanations of the mechanisms by which any GENE might act and affect the organism's DEVELOPMENT, it is a problem never likely fully to be resolved.

nausea *see* vomiting

Nauta–Gygax stain A silver STAIN used to demonstrate the presence of degenerating axons after damage in the nervous system. The staining of normal fibres is actively suppressed, allowing a picture of only degenerating axons to be developed. This technique was improved by Fink & Heimer in the 1960s, developing the FINK–HEIMER STAIN.

navigation LOCOMOTION to a goal in space. Animals have several navigation strategies. The strategy used depends on factors such as goal properties, landmark availability and goal distance. BEACON HOMING entails travelling up a stimulus gradient emanating from the goal. The use of landmarks to coordinate goal-directed locomotion is called PILOTING. During DEAD RECKONING a homeward trajectory is computed from a record of the bearing, speed and length of each leg of the outbound journey. In map and compass navigation a MAP is used to estimate current position, and a compass is used to estimate orientation and to hold a course.

See also: foraging; migration; path integration; spatial behaviour

DONALD M. WILKIE

NBQX *see* CNQX

necrosis (from Greek, *nekros*: dead body) The death of a CELL, or a group of cells, or elements of tissue or organs. Necrotic cells show PYKNOSIS and disintegration of their NUCLEUS. Many different things can bring about necrotic cell death: application of an agent such as an EXCITOTOXIN to make a LESION produces necrosis. Necrosis is unwanted: it is contrasted with APOPTOSIS (programmed cell death).

negative contingency A contingency that associated with NEGATIVE REINFORCEMENT.

See also: conditioned inhibition

negative patterning A discrimination problem in which two conditioned stimuli (CSs) (see CONDITIONED STIMULUS) are reinforced when presented separately but are not reinforced when presented together in compound. Intuitively, the combined CSs should produce more, not less, responding. However, Rescorla (1973) has provided evidence that the combination of the two CSs might generate a third CONFIGURAL CONDITIONED STIMULUS which acts to inhibit the responding which would otherwise occur to each separately-presented CS.

See also: configural learning

Reference

Rescorla R.A. (1973) Evidence for 'unique stimulus' account of configural conditioning. *Journal of Comparative and Physiological Psychology* 85: 331–338.

JASPER WARD-ROBINSON

negative priming Negative priming occurs when a stimulus which immediately precedes a target results in a delayed response time. For example, if the colour *red* preceded the word *blue* it could have a negative priming effect when one wished to record REACTION TIME to respond to the word blue.

See also: interference; Stroop effect

negative reinforcement The four basic procedures in OPERANT CONDITIONING are POSITIVE REINFORCEMENT, NEGATIVE REINFORCEMENT, PUNISHMENT and OMISSION. Reinforcement processes, whether positive or negative, change response probability. If a response occurs, and it is followed by the removal of a stimulus, and this results in an increase in response probability, then it is said that negative reinforcement has occurred. According to the behaviourist tradition, negative reinforcement has typically been defined simply in empirical terms. However, it has become more common to view operant conditioning procedures in terms of their motivational or regulatory consequences. Thus, with negative reinforcement, it is evident that the type of stimulus being removed, which results in an increase in response probability, is an AVERSIVE STIMULUS. According to the motivational view, negative reinforcement involves the organism behaving so as to decrease the probability of aversive events.

See also: motivation

JOHN D. SALAMONE

negative reinforcer *see* reinforcer

negative symptoms *see* schizophrenia; type II schizophrenia

negative transfer The term given to the disruption of performance on a task that can be produced by practice on a different task. It is a phenomenon demonstrable in animals and in humans. An (almost) everyday example given for humans is that of negative transfer between playing treble and descant recorder – the same fingering on each instrument produces different notes.

See also: interference

neglect alexia Many patients with hemispatial NEGLECT SYNDROME show an impairment in reading such that information on the CONTRALATERAL side of a page, of a paragraph or even of a single word may be misread. For example, following a right-sided lesion, a patient may read the word *this* as *his* or the word *discount* as *mount*. As with neglect, this is not attributable to a primary sensory or motor deficit nor to an APHASIA. Patients with neglect typically read words better than they read pronounceable non-words, suggesting that information on the contralateral side of the stimulus is not entirely abolished in neglect and can be used to differentiate lexical status. Longer words are misread more often than shorter words and the further to the ipsilesional side the word is presented, the greater the probability of correct reading.

MARLENE BEHRMANN

neglect dyslexia An acquired reading disorder affecting the READING of letters at one end of the word, usually the left. Associated with SPATIAL NEGLECT.

ELAINE FUNNELL

neglect syndrome A condition in which there is unawareness of, and failure to respond to, stimuli on one side of the body, despite sensory and motor systems being undamaged. The term UNILATERAL NEGLECT also describes this. The neglect syndrome as described in patients is typically a form of CONTRALATERAL NEGLECT – that is, patients fail to respond to stimuli presented in space on the side of their bodies

contralateral to a lesion (see SPATIAL NEGLECT for a full discussion of this). Dysfunction of ATTENTION has been thought to be a critical process involved in the production of neglect. In animals, both cortical and subcortical mechanisms of neglect have been investigated. Unilateral damage to the NIGROSTRIATAL DOPAMINE SYSTEM produces what some have described as a form of neglect.

See also: motor neglect

nematode (from Greek, *nema, thread, eidos*: form) A class (see TAXONOMY) of worms, including threadworms and roundworms. In neuroscience, undoubtedly the most famous type of nematode is CAENORHABDITIS ELEGANS.

neocerebellum *see* cerebellum

neocortex In evolutionary terms, the youngest part of the CEREBRAL CORTEX. Neocortex is discriminated from ALLOCORTEX and JUXTALLOCORTEX by virtue of having six distinct cell layers (see CORTICAL LAYERS). It is the largest part of the human brain, though of course it is functionally divided into distinct territories concerned with sensory, motor or associate functions. In essence, all of the cortical tissue visible on a human brain is neocortex: the allo and juxtallocortex is buried below it. Neocortex is also known as the ISOCORTEX or (in older literature) ECTOPALLIUM or neopallium.

neocortex ratio *see* nervous system

neologism (from Greek, *neo*: new, *logos*: word) Literally, a new word (or phrase).

neonate (from Greek, *neo*: new, and Latin, *natus*: born) Literally, a neonate is a new-born infant; neonatal describes the time immediately after the birth and the events taking place therein.

neonate neurological syndrome *see* drug effects *in utero*

neophobia (from Greek, *neo*: new, *phobos*: fear) Fear of novelty. Placed in a novel situation, most animals show a degree of neophobia. For example, a rat placed in an OPEN FIELD with an attractive food in the centre will not immediately go to the food. Typically, it will explore the circumference of the open field, REARING to gain additional information, before venturing in to the centre of the arena to investigate the food. Neophobia serves a purpose in minimizing the risks that animals run in their environments, though too great a degree, or insufficient, are not helpful strategies. Certain brain systems have been associated with neophobia, including the DORSAL NORADRENERGIC BUNDLE and the AMYGDALA.

neoplasia; neoplastic Neoplasia is the production of a neoplasm (see TUMOUR). The term neoplastic is one that refers to neoplasms – they produce neoplastic disorders.

neoplasm see tumour

neostigmine An acetylcholinesterase inhibitor; a synthetic form of PHYSOSTIGMINE (ESERINE). It differs from physostigmine in being unable to cross the BLOOD–BRAIN BARRIER and in having weak actions at ACETYLCHOLINE RECEPTORS.

neostriatum Archaic term that refers to the CAUDATE NUCLEUS and the PUTAMEN.

See also: archistriatum; palaeostriatum

nephron see osmoregulation

Nernst equation After Walther Nernst (1864–1941): the Nernst equation is a formula for calculating the MEMBRANE POTENTIAL at which ions present on both sides of a MEMBRANE are in equilibrium (the EQUILIBRIUM POTENTIAL of a given ION). In regard to POTASSIUM ion concentration for example it is given as:

$$E_K = \frac{RT}{ZF} \log_e \frac{[K^+]_o}{[K^+]_i}$$

where E_K is the membrane potential at which potassium ions (K^+) are in equilibrium (which is known as the potassium ion *Nernst potential*); R is the gas constant; T the temperature in degrees Kelvin; Z the valence of K^+; F the Faraday constant and $[K^+]_o$ and $[K^+]_i$ the concentrations of potassium ions inside and outside the membrane.

Reference

Keynes R.D. & Aidley D.J. (1981) *Nerve and Muscle*, Cambridge University Press: Cambridge.

nerve A nerve is a collection of NEURONS (nerve cells): the terms NEURON and NERVE CELL are interchangeable, but the term NERVE is different to these. Nerves in the PERIPHERAL NERVOUS SYSTEM are composed of several elements. The essential components are bundles of axons. Each individual AXON within bundles is insulated from the others by the NEURILEMMA, a sheath of cells: MYELIN-producing SCHWANN CELLS lie around the axon itself. Outside these is a layer of fibrous connective tissue called the ENDONEURIUM. Individual fibres, wrapped in these layers, are then collected together in bundles, bound in another layer of connective tissue, the PERINEURIUM. Many bundles, and blood vessels are collected into nerves, bound by a final layer of connective tissue, the EPINEURIUM. Within the brain itself one does not talk about nerves: axons are gathered into what are variably called bundles, tracts or pathways which are not bound by neurilemma (myelin is provided by oligodendroglia in the CENTRAL NERVOUS SYSTEM, not by Schwann cells), perineurium or epineurium.

See also: cranial nerves; spinal nerves

nerve cell see neuron

nerve cord see nervous system

nerve crush Following a crush or cut, axons degenerate distal to the LESION site, and macrophages remove the axonal debris by phagocytosis (see DEGENERATION; MACROPHAGE). Proximal to the lesion site axons regenerate new branches (SPROUTING). Regeneration is often successful in the PERIPHERAL NERVOUS SYSTEM; axon GROWTH CONES re-enter the degenerating tubes of the distal nerve stump, now consisting of SCHWANN CELLS lined by BASAL LAMINA, and may re-innervate their targets. In the mammalian CENTRAL NERVOUS SYSTEM, however, most axons do not regenerate long distances. This may be the result of inadequate supplies of TROPHIC molecules and the presence of growth-inhibitory molecules.

ROGER J. KEYNES

nerve deafness Nerve deafness is an essentially incorrect expression that indicates hearing loss not originating in the external or middle ear. DEAFNESS resulting from damage to the AUDITORY NERVE is rare, the most common cause being tumours of the VESTIBULOCOCHLEAR NERVE (the eighth cranial nerve). Most nerve deafness cases result from damage to the HAIR CELLS, induced by factors such as noise trauma, OTOTOXIC DRUGS such as certain AMINOGLYCOSIDES, and viral or bacterial infections. The outer hair cells are most susceptible to damage, rarely are the inner hair cells selectively damaged in the presence of normal outer hair cells. Nerve deafness is often accompanied by LOUDNESS recruitment.

JOS J. EGGERMONT

nerve growth factor One of the GROWTH FACTORS involved in the DEVELOPMENT and survival of NEURONS. The discovery of nerve growth factors has been one of the landmarks of modern neuroscience, a discovery pioneered by the work of Samuel Detwiler and Viktor Hamburger in the 1920s, and developed further by Rita Levi-Montalcini from the 1940s on to the present day. Nerve growth factor is involved in development and maintenance of neurons in the SYMPATHETIC NERVOUS SYSTEM, sensory neurons in the GANGLIA of the DORSAL ROOT and CHOLINERGIC neurons in the NUCLEUS BASALIS OF MEYNERT. Other types of growth factor such as BRAIN-DERIVED NEUROTROPHIC FACTOR, NEUROTROPHIN-3 and CILIARY NEUROTROPHIC FACTOR are involved in other parts of the nervous system. Nerve growth factor binds to RECEPTORS, and while it initiates a variety of SECOND MESSENGERS, works slightly differently to standard NEUROTRANSMITTERS, in that the nerve growth factor, bound to the receptor, is internalized by the receiving neurons. Once within the neuron nerve growth factor is transported to the CELL BODY from the TERMINALS where it was first bound.

See also: endocrine glands; neurodevelopment; saporin; transplantation; tyrosine kinase receptors

Reference

Kandel E.R., Schwartz J.H. & Jessell T.M. (2000) *Principles of Neural Science*, 4th edn, McGraw-Hill: New York.

nerve net *see* nervous system

nerve nets *see* neural networks

nerve ring *see* nervous system

nervous breakdown Lay term applied to an episode of psychiatric disorder; commonly associated in the public eye with precipitation by STRESS. Despite widespread use, the term is of little value as it has no specific meaning, and it is not used professionally.

IAN C. REID

nervous system In thinking of the nervous system one typically describes that found in VERTEBRATES, which includes the CENTRAL NERVOUS SYSTEM (BRAIN and SPINAL CORD, and associated cranial and SPINAL NERVES); and the PERIPHERAL NERVOUS SYSTEM, which includes the SOMATIC NERVOUS SYSTEM and the AUTONOMIC NERVOUS SYSTEM (which is divisible into the SYMPATHETIC NERVOUS SYSTEM, PARASYMPATHETIC NERVOUS SYSTEM and the ENTERIC NERVOUS SYSTEM). Vertebrate nervous systems may differ in detail (see for example RODENT VS. PRIMATE PREFRONTAL CORTEX) but all work to this common plan. But of course, the INVERTEBRATES also have nervous systems. The simplest form of nervous system is the NERVE NET, a system of neurons (see NEURON) that branch throughout an organisms' body: *cnidarians* (hydras) have these. Slightly more complex are NERVE RINGS, which are centralized within a body, with RADIAL NERVES extending away from this: *echinoderms* – such as the starfishes – have these. Many invertebrates have bodies that are bilaterally symmetrical and have nervous systems that reflect this. NERVE CORDS – thick bundles of neurons – are frequently present, either singly, running along the middle of the animal (as is the case with, for example, leeches) or with two nerve cords, one on either side of the body (as is the case with flatworms such as *Planaria*). More complex invertebrate nervous systems show the development of GANGLIA (singular, GANGLION), which are clusters of neurons. In some species there may be multiple ganglia, often systematically reflecting different body segments. From ganglia, rudimentary brains develop. Just as in mammalian NEURODEVELOPMENT, the brain develops as an extension of the NEURAL TUBE and is enclosed with the CRANIUM, ganglia that are gathered in the head end of an invertebrate body are sometimes referred to as brains, or head ganglia. The degree to which this occurs is referred to by the term CEPHALIZATION: the flatworms are the most primitive group of invertebrates to show any degree of cephalization, while the most encephalized invertebrates are the *cephalopods* (cuttlefish, squid and octopus – the term cephalopod is from Greek, *kephale*: head, and *podos*: foot – cephalopods have a highly cephalized head, and the feet have been specialized into tentacles radiating from that).

Note well that there are some difficulties with terminology: CEPHALIZATION is used to indicate the degree to which an animal has developed a head, with specialized sensory receptors, feeding organs and, perhaps most importantly, a concentration of neural tissue (either a head ganglion or a brain). The term ENCEPHALIZATION has been used in three ways. (i) It is a simple index of the degree to which the CEREBRAL CORTEX has developed. (ii) Encephalization has been used to describe the degree to which more recently evolved tissue – the cerebral cortex and particularly the NEOCORTEX – has taken over functions that were previously regulated by structures further down the NEURAXIS. It remains uncertain to what degree functions are 'taken over' as opposed to 'made more sophisticated' (that is, do older and newer structures combine with each other or do newer structures comprehensively take over the functions of older ones?). (iii) The word encephalization features in the ENCEPHALIZATION QUOTIENT (EQ) which is the ratio of log brain mass to log body mass. The encephalization quotient assumes that animals that are in some sense more intelligent (see INTELLIGENCE) have brains that are relatively larger in proportion to their body size compared to rather less intelligent animals. It is a measure that was introduced in the 1970s by H.J. Jerison, and was initially used in assessment of the likely intelligence of extinct animals, principally, of course, of dinosaurs (see PALAEONEUROLOGY; DINOSAUR BEHAVIOR). It is a relatively crude measure: later authors interested in determining the relative intelligence of different species have taken measures such as a NEOCORTEX RATIO, the ratio of neocortical mass to the total brain mass.

Similar measures could be taken for any identifiable brain structure.

See also: peripheral nerves and spinal nerves

References

Macphail E.M. (1982) *Brain and Intelligence in Vertebrates*, Clarendon Press: Oxford.

network nodes Network nodes are components of artificial NEURAL NETWORKS. A node is typically represented by a section of a computer program written to behave like a simplified NEURON. Inputs to the node are delivered via synaptic 'weights' (see SYNAPSE) and the activation of the node is usually taken as the sum of the weighted inputs. This activation then determines the node's output, according to the node's input–output function. The point of this arrangement is that the weights can be altered, so that the same inputs can produce entirely different outputs depending upon the rule used to change the weights.

PAUL DEAN

network oscillation *see* oscillations

neural adhesion molecules These are molecules that guide GROWTH CONE development. They are present on the growth cone and interact with the local environment to guide cellular DEVELOPMENT and extension. Neural adhesion molecules, like ADHESION MOLECULES in general, are GLYCOPROTEINS. There are three major classes: (1) the IMMUNOGLOBULINS (of which NEURAL CELL ADHESION MOLECULE is the most abundant); (2) the CADHERINS; (3) the INTEGRINS (of which FIBRONECTIN and LAMININ are the best known).

See also: extracellular matrix; neurodevelopment

Reference

Kandel E.R., Schwartz J.H. & Jessell T.M. (2000) *Principles of Neural Science*, 4th edn, McGraw-Hill: New York.

neural assembly A neural assembly – or more generally, CELL ASSEMBLY – is a term used to describe a collection of neurons in the CENTRAL NERVOUS SYSTEM that operate in concert (see NEURON). An assembly is not the same as a NEURAL NETWORK: assemblies operate on a smaller scale with 'local' rather than 'global' functions. In artificial NEURAL NETWORKS as-semblies can be specifically characterized with both structure and function within the net-work, but in the central nervous system exact specification is harder to achieve. ASSEMBLY CODING is the theory that features of a stimulus or state group together according to rules specified by the architecture of the assembly processing those stimuli or states.

See also: binding problem; ensemble coding and population coding

neural cell adhesion molecule *see* neural adhesion molecules

neural coding The way in which a NEURON codes information is not clear: ENSEMBLE COD-ING and POPULATION CODING are processes that have been identified. Population codes operate though numbers of neurons while ensemble codes operate by patterns of activity. In the context of NEURAL NETWORKS, three different types of coding are identified: (1) LOCAL REPRESENTATIONS, in which individual neurons code functions; (2) DENSE DISTRIBU-TED REPRESENTATIONS, in which more than half the units in a network must be activated to represent a particular construct; and (3) SPARSE CODING, in which only a few neurons in a network are required to represent a particular construct.

See also: binding problem; grandmother cell

Reference

Földiák P. & Young M. (1995) Sparse coding in primate cortex. In *The Handbook of Brain Theory and Neural Networks*, ed. M.A. Arbib, pp. 895–898, MIT Press: Cam-bridge MA.

neural crest A group of cells that arises from the dorsal part of the newly formed NEURAL TUBE in the EMBRYO of all VERTEBRATES. Neural crest cells migrate away from the developing CENTRAL NERVOUS SYSTEM to popu-late many regions of the developing body. Below the level of the head they differentiate into the SENSORY NEURONS comprising each DORSAL ROOT GANGLION, the neurons of the AUTONOMIC NERVOUS SYSTEM, pigmented cells, cells of the ADRENAL GLAND and supporting cells of the PERIPHERAL NERVOUS SYSTEM (SCHWANN CELLS). In the head they also give

rise to a major portion of the bones of the SKULL and face.

See also: neurodevelopment

ROGER J. KEYNES

neural Darwinism A proposition made by Gerald Edelman (winner, with Rodney Porter, of the Nobel Prize for Physiology or Medicine in 1972) which suggests that synapses (see SYNAPSE) form during DEVELOPMENT but that only those that are functionally important are retained – that is, the synapses that are left have exhibited 'survival of the fittest'. It is an hypothesis consistent with much of what is known about NEURODEVELOPMENT, in which there is an initial overexpression of synapses followed by SYNAPTIC PRUNING. Since many synaptic connections are formed and strength-ened (see LONG-TERM POTENTIATION; PERFO-RATED SYNAPSES) as a result of experience in the world, it enables a dynamic and interactive view of neural functions.

Reference

Edelman G.M. (1999) *Neural Darwinism: Theory of Neuronal Group Selection*, Basic Books: New York.

neural induction *see* neurodevelopment

neural networks Neural networks are com-puting machines, with an internal organization partially resembling that used in the brain. Often termed ARTIFICIAL NEURAL NETWORKS (ANNs) to distinguish them from real thing, they may be constructed from special purpose silicon chips, but at present usually exist as computer programs. They can be visualized as a number of NETWORK NODES, analogous to NEURONS, connected together in a particular way. The connections form the architecture of the net. The purpose of this organization is that connections between nodes have 'weights', similar to SYNAPSES, that can be altered in value. The calculation performed by a neural network therefore depends both on its present inputs, and on the way its weights have been altered by past inputs. In this regard its behaviour resembles human LEARNING, and procedures for altering weights are often re-ferred to as learning rules.

There are two main classes of learning rule. In UNSUPERVISED LEARNING, the weights in a net are altered according to the pattern of its inputs. The net, which may consist of a single layer of interconnected nodes, learns a method for classifying its inputs that depends on the precise nature of the learning rule, but does not require continuous external prompting. Such nets are described as self-organizing, and an example would be a KOHONEN NETWORK which learns input mappings resembling those observed in SENSORY CORTEX. In SUPERVISED LEARNING, by contrast, the net is trained to produce correct answers by using the difference between its output and an externally specified target output. The DELTA RULE is a procedure for computing the desired change in weights from this difference, called the error, for nets that have two layers. The nodes in the input layer receive input from an external source, and are connected only to nodes in the output layer, which communicate the results of the network's calculations. However, a more powerful and popular architecture, the MULTI-LAYER PERCEPTION, has at least one additional layer of 'hidden' nodes. These receive input from the input nodes, and in turn are connected only to nodes in the output layer. For a multilayer perception the delta rule must be generalized, because the error signal needs to be propagated back to the hidden layer so the weights from the input layer can be altered correctly (see BACKPROPAGATION).

Supervised learning would be of limited use if it only reproduced already known correct answers. However, appropriately trained neural networks can generalize their behaviour to give correct answers to inputs never previously encountered. The power to generalize is a critical feature of ANNs and underlies both their applied and theoretical importance. It has been proved mathematically that multi-layer perceptrons are able to approximate a very wide range of input–output functions. Yet further capabilities are added, in recurrent nets, by allowing connections from between nodes in the same layer, and from one layer to a preceding one. It is not only the computational power of ANNs that is relevant to psychology though: the distinctive way in which the computations are done is also of interest. In contrast to traditional computing procedures, whereby a single stream of instructions is executed one step at a time, processing in ANNs is distributed over the nodes and (in theory) carried out in parallel. PARALLEL DISTRIBUTED PROCESSING has intriguing resemblances to human learning and performance. ANNs can carry out tasks requiring complex statistical calculation with no explicit mathematical knowledge. They may continue to produce approximate answers when damaged, or when their inputs are corrupted. They are particularly suited to 'real-world' problems, such as PATTERN PERCEPTION and ASSOCIATIVE LEARNING, which have many constraints no single one of which is decisive (see ARTIFICIAL INTELLIGENCE).

As models of human processing, ANNs are used at different levels of fidelity. In COMPUTATIONAL NEUROSCIENCE, network nodes can be made similar to real neurons in intrinsic structure, the connections between them made to conform to known neuroanatomy, and the weight modification rules made to resemble those governing the efficacy of real synapses (the equivalent of, for instance, LONG-TERM POTENTIATION). Such networks may be useful for understanding the detailed organization of particular regions of the brain, such as CEREBRAL CORTEX, HIPPOCAMPUS and CEREBELLUM. In CONNECTIONISM, more abstract neural networks are used as existence proofs that a biologically plausible organization can be used to perform certain classes of computation. Areas studied include VISUAL PERCEPTION, MOTOR CONTROL, MEMORY and LANGUAGE. The networks used for these studies typically consist of highly simplified nodes in architectures whose relation to those used by the brain is unknown. Debates about their processing capacities are wide ranging, including topics such as the nature of human DECISION-MAKING and CONSCIOUSNESS. One prominent area of dispute is whether neural networks can generate precise symbolic representations whose behaviour is governed by formal logical, grammatical or mathematical rules (see ARTIFICIAL INTELLIGENCE again).

See also: neural coding

References

Churchland P.S. & Sejnowski T.J. (1992) *The Computational Brain*, Cambridge MA: MIT Press.

Gurney, K. (1997) *An Introduction to Neural Networks*, London: UCL Press.

PAUL DEAN

neural plasticity The degree to which the CENTRAL NERVOUS SYSTEM is plastic is uncertain. It was thought that, once in adult form, the mammalian central nervous system could not regenerate or develop further – all it could do was degenerate and die. This may not be the case. Some degree of reconnection may be possible following damage, and neurons (see NEURON) in the HIPPOCAMPUS for example appear to be produced in adult life. Certain species of animal with distinct seasonal patterns in their behaviour also show a seasonal plasticity. For example, the circuitry controlling BIRDSONG in many species changes, with changes in the numbers and size of neurons reflecting seasonal changes in behaviour and LEARNING.

See also: recovery of function; sensitization (receptor); supersensitivity

Reference

Tramontin A.D. & Brenowitz E.A. (2000) Seasonal plasticity in the adult brain. *Trends in Neuroscience* 23: 251–258.

neural plate In the EMBRYO of VERTEBRATES the entire CENTRAL NERVOUS SYSTEM and most of the PERIPHERAL NERVOUS SYSTEM originates from a thickened sheet of ECTODERM cells occupying the MIDLINE of the embryo, the neural plate, while the remainder of the ectoderm differentiates (see DIFFERENTIATION) into skin cells. The neural plate consists of presumptive NEURONS and glia, and its cells are directed to neural fates and away from the skin differentiation pathway as a result of molecular signals that arise from midline cells (MESODERM) lying deeper in the embryo. The neural plate subsequently folds into the NEURAL TUBE.

See also: neurodevelopment

ROGER J. KEYNES

neural tube The primordium of the brain and spinal cord in the EMBRYO of VERTEBRATES. The neural tube results from the folding of the MIDLINE sheet of proliferating neural cells, the NEURAL PLATE, into a hollow tube, a process known as NEURULATION. During subsequent development, its cells proliferate, migrate and differentiate to generate mature NEURONS and glia. The overall shape of the tube alters dramatically as it expands and folds at the head end of the embryo, where it subdivides into FOREBRAIN, MIDBRAIN and HINDBRAIN, while the SPINAL CORD retains a cylindrical appearance. The VENTRICLES of the brain originate from the central canal of the neural tube, and the CHOROID PLEXUS is also derived from its wall.

See also: neurodevelopment

ROGER J. KEYNES

neuralgia Pain caused by malfunctioning sensory pathways. Notable examples are trigeminal and postherpetic or posttraumatic neuralgia. In trigeminal neuralgia ('TIC DOULOUREUX') paroxysms of intense PAIN occur in the distribution of the ophthalmic branch of the TRIGEMINAL NERVE (the fifth cranial nerve). Attacks may be triggered by pressure on the nerve at its exit from the skull, and may cease after surgery. Postherpetic neuralgia follows destruction of fast-conducting sensory neurons by herpes virus, releasing abnormal activity in surviving pain fibres (see GATE THEORY OF PAIN). The term NEURALGIA is also commonly used in a non-technical sense to refer to pain of unknown origin.

L. JACOB HERBERG

neuraxis An imaginary line that runs through the dead centre of the CENTRAL NERVOUS SYSTEM, from the FOREBRAIN to the CAUDA EQUINA. Structures are often said to be high or low in the neuraxis: CEREBRAL CORTEX is higher, SPINAL CORD lower.

neurilemma *see* nerve

neurin NEURIN and STENIN are PROTEINS: neurin (and other related proteins) is found on MICROTUBULES and stenin on SYNAPTIC VESICLES. The interaction of these proteins enables movement of vesicles through PRESYNAPTIC TERMINALS; see SYNAPSE; SYNAPTIC TRANSMISSION.

neurinoma A form of TUMOUR, most often associated with the BRAINSTEM.

neurite An axon or DENDRITE: the adjective neuritic is often encountered describing something associated with these.

neuroactive A term used to identify any DRUG, chemical or other agents or proces that has effects on nervous tissue. For example, a neuroactive compound is one that effects the NERVOUS SYSTEM.

neuroadaptation The complex biological changes that occur in the brain with repeated or chronic exposure to a DRUG. Drugs by their very definition induce some change in the NEUROCHEMICAL environment of the brain; one exposure to a particular drug will cause a specific effect (for example, increased levels of a particular neurotransmitter). However, with repeated exposure, the body and brain often adapt to the presence of the drug. Through homeostatic or 'self-corrective' mechanisms, the nervous system attempts to compensate for the effects of the drug. Observable signs of neuroadaptation include the presence of TOLERANCE, PHYSICAL DEPENDENCE or SENSITIZATION. In tolerance, progressively more drug is needed in order to obtain the same effect. In physical dependence, there is a need for the presence of the drug in order to function normally, and a WITHDRAWAL SYNDROME may result upon cessation of the drug. Sensitization ('REVERSE TOLERANCE') is another neuroadaptive phenomenon, in which an increase in the response to the drug occurs with repeated use. What has become more apparent in recent years, however, is that these behavioural or physiological changes are often accompanied by profound and long-lasting alterations in neuronal circuits within the brain. With the advent of modern molecular biological techniques, many studies have shown that addictive drugs (such as ALCOHOL, COCAINE, NICOTINE, and MORPHINE) induces changes at the level of RECEPTORS, content of NEUROTRANSMITTERS, G PROTEIN, SECOND MESSENGERS, GENE EXPRESSION, and even MORPHOLOGY of NEURONS. Many of these changes occur in the brain's reinforcement system. Thus it is believed that these underlying, long-term neuroadaptive changes are associated with the ADDICTION process.

Reference

Hyman S.E. & Nestler E.J. (1996) Initiation and adaptation: a paradigm for understanding psychotropic drug action. *American Journal of Psychiatry* 153: 151–162.

neuroanatomy Neuroanatomy is the study of the structure of the nervous system, and is a sub-discipline of anatomy as well as of neuroscience. Neuroanatomy provides an understanding of the morphological detail of neural structures such as NEURONS and nuclei (see NUCLEUS), as well as their organization including synapses, projections, and systems (see PROJECTION NEURONS; SYNAPSE). As such, neuroanatomy is the basis for physiological and behavioural studies of the nervous system. Modern neuroanatomy started late in the nineteenth century with the establishment of the notion, known as the NEURON DOCTRINE, that the nervous system is made of individual cells as units. Another prevalent view, known as the RETICULAR THEORY, held that the nervous system consists of a mesh of fused tissues. Golgi (1843–1926) was among the strong supporters of this view. Ironically, however, it was the silver impregnation method developed by Golgi that Ramon y Cajal (1852–1934) used to study nervous tissues and proved the neuron doctrine. This doctrine was further supported by von Waldeyer (1836–1921) who coined the term neuron in 1891, and by Sherrington (1857–1952) who recognized the gaps between neurons and called them synapses in 1897. Ramon y Cajal, Golgi and Sherrington received Nobel Prizes for their work.

The understanding of neural structures has progressed in parallel with the advances in neuroanatomical techniques. Early investigators used various dyes to delineate structural organization of the brain. By far the most commonly used was CRESYL VIOLET, which stains NISSL BODIES and clearly demarcates cell bodies of neurons and glia. By using the Nissl stain, variations in the size and density of cells were examined and these cytological measures were used to identify cellular groupings in the brain, thus delineating nuclei. This approach is called cytoarchitectonics. In the CEREBRAL CORTEX, five types of CYTOARCHITECTURE were identified by von Economo (1876–1931). The cerebral cortex was also cytoarchitectonically divided into 52 regions by Brodmann (1868–1918) and the map of BRODMANN'S AREAS is now widely used as a reference.

A major advance in neuroanatomy took place with the advent of sensitive TRACT TRACERS in the early 1970s. Although degeneration methods were used earlier to study connections between different parts of the brain, the extraordinary sensitivity of HORSERADISH PEROXIDASE as a tract tracer was unprecedented, and virtually all known pathways were re-examined and new projections identified using this new tracer. Re-examination usually confirmed previous findings, but revealed much greater detail. Horseradish peroxidase was followed by other equally or more sensitive tracers in ensuing years. Many of them are PLANT LECTINS or their conjugates with horseradish peroxidase. In addition to these tracers that are visible with bright- or dark-field MICROSCOPY, FLUORESCENT TRACERS have also become available. Fluorescent tracers provide the opportunity to investigate axonal branching with two or even three labels that fluoresce at mutually distinguishable wavelengths. Another major advance in neuroanatomy occurred with the emergence and growth of CHEMICAL NEUROANATOMY since the early 1970s. Chemical neuroanatomy is the study of the brain from a neurochemical point of view. Initially histochemical techniques, then immunohistochemistry as well as receptor binding AUTORADIOGRAPHY and, most recently, IN SITU HYBRIDIZATION have been used to map the distributions of various substances, particularly NEUROTRANSMITTERS and related enzymes in the nervous system. Various subtypes and subunits of neurotransmitter receptors have also been mapped. A few interesting issues have emerged from these studies. One is that the distribution of neurotransmitters does not necessarily follow nuclear boundaries defined by cytoarchitectonics or Nissl staining. More often than not, neurons containing a given neurotransmitter are distributed across such classically defined nuclei. On the other hand, neurochemical markers often reveal borders that are not obvious with Nissl staining. These observations have raised the issue of the definition of a nucleus. A second issue is that the distributions of a given neurotransmitter and its receptors are not always matched even at macroscopic levels. There can be both technical and theoretical explanations for this discrepancy, but the paradox is not completely solved.

One of the most significant advances in neuroanatomy is the functional mapping of the brain. Various activity markers have been developed for animal studies. In particular, C-FOS and other products of IMMEDIATE EARLY GENES, which are transcription factors that can cause alteration in GENE EXPRESSION, are commonly used as neuronal activation markers. However, these markers cannot be used for human brains for obvious reasons, and until recently, much of our understanding of the human brain was based on inferences from animal studies. However, the development of FUNCTIONAL NEUROIMAGING techniques has made it possible for the first time to investigate the structural basis of various psychological functions directly in the human brain. Existing brain imaging techniques still do not provide information about the connectivity or the nature of increased activity, but there appears to be rapid progress in improving time resolution. This represents one exciting avenue of research in human neuroanatomy.

See also: double labelling; histology; stereotaxic surgery

KAZUE SEMBA

neuroaugmentation *see* deep brain stimulation

neuroblast An embryonic neuron; see EMBRYO; BLAST; NEURODEVELOPMENT.

neuroblastoma A neoplasm (see TUMOUR) containing immature, partially differentiated NEUROBLASTS. The cells are typically rather small and may aggregate in a variety of ways (sheets or clumps for example). They occur particularly in children and most commonly are associated with the ADRENAL GLANDS.

neurochemistry Neurochemistry is the study of the chemistry of the nervous system. Used as a noun, neurochemical refers to a chemical having a neural function. All NEUROTRANSMITTERS are neurochemicals, for instance. As an adjective neurochemical is used to described processes, events, or mechanisms that pertain to chemical transmission in the nervous system. Neurochemical processes therefore pertain to the events that are associated with this process, including modulation of release of the transmitter, control of extracellular levels, action of the neurochemical on receptors, such as POSTSYNAPTIC RECEPTORS, PRESYNAPTIC autoreceptors, and REUPTAKE sites, and intracellular events. Such things are the subject matter of neurochemistry. Researchers in the fields of NEUROPHARMACOLOGY and PSYCHOPHARMACOLOGY also investigate neurochemical processes.

ANN E. KELLEY

neurocranium *see* skull

neurocrine Neurocrine transmission is the opposite of PARACRINE transmission; neurocrine transmission is synonymous with WIRING TRANSMISSION. Paracrine transmission is synonymous with VOLUME TRANSMISSION.

See also: neurotransmission

neurodegeneration The degeneration of neural tissue, whether occurring spontaneously in a neurodegenerative disease (such as PARKINSON'S DISEASE), induced experimentally (by making a LESION), or as part of naturally occurring PROGRAMMED CELL DEATH (see APOPTOSIS).

See also: necrosis

neurodevelopment The anatomical complexity of the nervous system of VERTEBRATES presents a special challenge for the mechanisms of embryonic DEVELOPMENT. Diverse types of NEURON are assembled into characteristic positions, arranged as nuclei, columns or layers (laminae) (see LAMINA; NUCLEUS), from which they project axons to their appropriate targets and where they receive a particular AFFERENT input. Several stages are distinguished: presumptive neural cells in the early embryo are first committed to a neural fate (neurons and glia); they then show PROLIFERATION until their last MITOSIS (see CELL DIVISION), during

which they may acquire regionally appropriate instructions for subsequent DIFFERENTIATION; after this they may migrate variable distances to their final positions (see NEURONAL MIGRATION), where they differentiate further, SPROUTING axons that are guided to their targets, elaborating dendrites and receiving synaptic inputs (see DENDRITE; SYNAPSE). Neurons are over-produced, and many may die at this stage (see APOPTOSIS). The later stages of development include synapse formation (SYNAPTOGENESIS), further apoptosis as PRESYNAPTIC and POSTSYNAPTIC cell populations are matched in size, and SYNAPTIC PRUNING, when the final adjustments to connectivity are made.

The beginnings of the nervous system are recognizable with the NEURAL PLATE, a thickened sheet of ECTODERM cells occupying the MIDLINE of the EMBRYO. These cells are directed to neural fates by molecular signals that arise from midline (MESODERM) cells lying deeper in the embryo, a process known as NEURAL INDUCTION. A number of neural-inducing proteins have been identified in amphibian embryos, and these appear to work by antagonizing the action of molecules that would otherwise direct ectoderm cells towards an epidermal (skin) fate. Further NEUROGENIC GENES have been identified that cells need to express in order to achieve their neural fates. The neural plate subsequently folds into the NEURAL TUBE, which subdivides in turn into a series of vesicles arranged in a head-to-tail (rostral to caudal) direction, the FOREBRAIN, MIDBRAIN and HINDBRAIN, and continues caudally as the SPINAL CORD. The early hindbrain then subdivides further into a series of repeat-units, or segments (RHOMBOMERES). These early vesicular and segmental patterns in the neural tube represent the ground plan for the later development and regional specialization of the CNS. The peripheral nervous system is largely derived from the neural crest, a migratory cell population that arises from the dorsal part of the neural tube.

Regional diversity along the rostro-caudal axis of the nervous system is dependent on local variations in the expression of genes that specify cell position in the embryo. Crucially, a cluster of HOMEOTIC SELECTOR GENES in the fruit fly (*DROSOPHILA*), which plays a key role in imparting different fates to the body segments by regulating other genes, has been shown to be conserved in vertebrates. These genes have duplicated during animal evolution so that mammals deploy four copies of each equivalent Drosophila gene, probably allowing for greater diversity of pattern. These mammalian Hox genes are expressed in overlapping domains along the rostro-caudal embryonic axis, a pattern that is especially clear in the neural tube. In the hindbrain, moreover, the boundaries of individual Hox gene expression correspond precisely with the boundaries between adjacent segments (rhombomeres); as in the fly, each rhombomere expresses a unique combination of Hox genes, and it is likely that its particular pattern of differentiation is determined by this combination. Consistent with this, rhombomere differentiation may be severely perturbed in Hox GENE KNOCKOUT mice. The Hox genes are not expressed rostral to the developing hindbrain, but the midbrain and forebrain show regional expression patterns of other genes that are homologous to homeotic selector genes specifying head segments in the fly. For all these genes, it remains to be determined how their protein products direct subsequent cell differentiation.

Patterning in the dorso-ventral axis of the CNS is dictated by interactions between the neural tube and the NOTOCHORD, a midline rod of cells that lies immediately underneath the neural tube at all levels caudal to the forebrain. Notochord removal prevents MOTOR NEURONS from differentiating in the ventral region of the developing spinal cord, and ventral cells express genes characteristic of dorsal fates instead. A protein (SONIC HEDGEHOG) secreted by the notochord appears to be critical in establishing dorso-ventral cell fates in the spinal cord, ventral fates being induced by high concentrations of sonic hedgehog, and dorsal fates by low concentrations. In some regions of the developing CNS, cell lineage has been analysed in detail by labelling individual precursor cells IN VIVO. In general this has shown that a cell's fate is sealed late in its lineage, usually around the time of the final mitosis, and that interactions with the environment are important in determining it. In the developing CEREBRAL CORTEX, for example,

presumptive neurons retain their original laminar fates when transplanted just before their last mitosis to a new position in the cortex, but change their fates in accordance with this new position if transferred at an earlier stage in their history. Region-specific fates (for example VISUAL CORTEX versus SOMATOSENSORY CORTEX) are determined later in development, possibly via the pattern of connections received by the different cortical areas.

Growing axons are guided to their targets by a variety of cues. Their tips (growth cones) respond to attractive and repulsive molecules which are attached to the surfaces of neighbouring cells or diffuse in the EXTRACELLULAR space from more distant regions. Guidance is not always accurate, however, and many examples exist where inappropriate or 'exuberant' connections are made. These may be removed later by apoptosis or branch retraction (synaptic pruning). The CRITICAL PERIOD of each cortical development represents an example of synaptic pruning where final connectivity is shaped by patterns of electrical activity. The capacity of the mature mammalian CNS to modify its synaptic connectivity – its plasticity – is a reflection of the retention of developmental mechanisms into adulthood. Such retention does not, however, extend to damaged CNS axons, which are unable to regenerate following injury and disease. The resulting disability may be ameliorated by repair strategies such as TRANSPLANTATION of developing CNS tissue, and a deeper understanding of neurodevelopment will be critical for their success.

ROGER J. KEYNES

neuroendocrinology The study of the relationships between the NERVOUS SYSTEM and the ENDOCRINE system.

neuroenergetics A term used to describe the study of ENERGY consumption by neurons (see NEURON). It is of interest to basic neuroscientists interested in how neurons develop and maintain themselves, and to those scientists and clinicians using FUNCTIONAL NEUROIMAGING techniques based on analysis of REGIONAL CEREBRAL BLOOD FLOW. This is the most common usage of the term in biological psychology, but note (1) that Freud (see PSYCHO-

ANALYSIS) had a neural energy model of DREAMING that has been described as 'neuroenergetic'; and (2) Neuroenergetic Release ® is a technique used in complementary medicine.

See also: neurofibrillary tangles

neurofibrillary tangles Pathological markers present in the brains of patients with ALZHEIMER'S DEMENTIA and DOWN SYNDROME. They are derived from NEUROFIBRILS and are composed of PROTEINS (in particular a protein known as *paired helical filament*). They are believed to be markers of CELL BODY damage, in contrast to PLAQUES (another pathological marker for these, and other disorders) which are thought to indicate AXON TERMINAL degeneration. They are not evenly distributed in the brains of Alzheimer patients but are found predominantly in the CEREBRAL CORTEX and HIPPOCAMPUS.

neurofibrils Neurofibrils are intracellular structures forming part of the CYTOSKELETON: they are aggregations of NEUROFILAMENTS and MICROTUBULES.

neurofilament *see* cytoskeleton

neurogenic genes These are the type of GENE that a NEURON needs to express in order to achieve its neural fate; see NEURODEVELOPMENT.

neurohormone A term used synonymously with *either* neuromodulator; *or* to indicate a conventional NEUROTRANSMITTER acting via VOLUME TRANSMISSION; *or* indicating a conventional HORMONE acting in the CENTRAL NERVOUS SYSTEM as a neurotransmitter. It is not a particularly helpful term.

neurohypophysis *see* adenohypophysis

neuroimmunology The study of the relationships between the NERVOUS SYSTEM and the IMMUNE SYSTEM.

neuroinformatics A term used to describe the union of information technology and NEUROSCIENCE. The emerging discipline of neuroinformatics has been drive n buy a growing realization that solutions to information handling problems made by the mammalian BRAIN are exceptionally clever, and that it is more profitable for computer scientists to model artificial computers on natural ones – brains – rather than using computers as inadequate models of brains.

neurokinins Neurokinin A and neurokinin B are NEUROPEPTIDES related to SUBSTANCE P; they act at the same receptors as does substance P; see TACHYKININ.

neuroleptanalgesia The combined administration of a NEUROLEPTIC and analgesic agent (see ANALGESIA) to sedate prior to minor surgery.

neuroleptic The term neuroleptic is to all intents and purposes synonymous with the term ANTIPSYCHOTIC. The derivation of 'neuroleptic' is a little obscure. It appears to be come from the Greek *neuron*: nerve, and *lambanein* (*lepsis*): to seize. Strictly speaking therefore, neuroleptic could be used to refer to any DRUG that affects the nervous system and induces an effect. Some authors suggest that the term neuroleptic actually refers to the fact that neuroleptics 'in addition to their beneficial effects have side-effects similar to the behavioural manifestations of neurological diseases' (Davison & Neale, 1996 p. 414). It is hardly ideal to refer to a class of drugs in terms of their side-effects. The term antipsychotic, relating simply to the ability of a drug to combat PSYCHOSIS, is more accurate and should be used in preference to neuroleptic.

Reference

Davison G.C. & Neale J.M. (1996) *Abnormal Psychology*, 6th edn, Wiley: New York.

neurology Neurology literally refers to the study of nervous tissue (*neuron* being Greek for nerve) but it has come to mean the branch of medicine that concerns itself with the diagnosis and treatment of disorders of the nervous system. It is expressly medical: NEUROSCIENCE is the scientific study of the NERVOUS SYSTEM and does not have special medical focus, although it evidently has medical value.

neuromodulation When a neuropeptide is co-localized with a classical or small-molecule neurotransmitter in the same PRESYNAPTIC TERMINAL, the neuropeptide is often found to have no effect of its own on the postsynaptic neuron (see NEUROTRANSMITTERS). However, when co-applied or co-released with the small-molecule transmitter, it alters the effect of the latter by enhancing, reducing or prolonging its action. This process is NEUROMODULATION and substances with such actions, usually (but not always) neuropeptides, are called neuromodulators. A classical example is VASOACTIVE INTESTINAL POLYPEPTIDE (VIP) co-localized with ACETYLCHOLINE in the presynaptic terminals of the submandibular salivary gland. VIP alone has little effects but it augments the secretory action of acetylcholine.

KAZUE SEMBA

neuromuscular junction The neuromuscular junction is the point at which a motor neuron (also known as a MOTONEURON; see MOTOR NEURONS) meets a MUSCLE FIBRE: it is a specialized form of SYNAPTIC TERMINAL. It is the point at which neuronal activity is translated into muscular action. Motor neurons have their cell bodies in the ventral horns of the SPINAL CORD, where they receive thousands of different synaptic inputs which may be transformed into ACTION POTENTIAL activity travelling along the AXON (which leaves at the VENTRAL ROOT). Shortly before arrival at a muscle, the axon branches extensively, each branch making contact with a different muscle fibre within the target muscle. The various points of contact are of course the neuromuscular junctions. Arrival of the action potential at these produces (in VERTEBRATES) liberation of the neurotransmitter ACETYLCHOLINE. The DEPOLARIZATION produced by acetylcholine is large and effective enough to generate an action potential in each of the muscle fibres innervated: the depolarization is called the ENDPLATE POTENTIAL. The critical effect of the endplate potential is to permit influx of CALCIUM ions (Ca^{2+}) into a MYOFILAMENT.

Muscle contractions are caused by the interaction of MYOSIN (on the THICK FILAMENTS) and ACTIN (on the THIN FILAMENTS) (see MUSCLES). ACTIN molecules have myosin binding sites that are normally covered by a protein called TROPOMYOSIN. The thin filaments also have a protein called TROPONIN COMPLEX which controls the positioning of tropomyosin. Calcium ions bind to the troponin complex, effectively relocating the troponin and expos-

ing the myosin binding sites on the actin molecules. Under these conditions, thin and thick filaments can move relative to each other, producing muscle contractions. If calcium ion concentration falls, the myosin binding sites on the actin molecules are once again obscured by tropomyosin. Calcium concentration is closely controlled by two things: the arrival of action potentials, and the SARCOPLASMIC RETICULUM (a specialized form of ENDOPLASMIC RETICULUM), which acts as a reservoir for calcium, releasing it in response to action potential stimulation.

The neuromuscular junction can be affected by specific illnesses: MYASTHENIA GRAVIS is the best-known example of such a disorder.

See also: motor unit

References

Campbell N.A., Reece J.B. & Mitchell L.G. (1999) *Biology*, 5th edn, Addison-Wesley: Menlo Park CA.

Rosenzweig M.R., Leiman A.L. & Breedlove S.M. (1996) *Biological Psychology*, Sinauer Associates: Sunderland MA.

neuron (also: neurone) Neurons are elementary units of the nervous system that are specialized for communication. For this purpose, neurons have excitable membranes and, in response to various signals such as NEURO-TRANSMITTERS, generate action potentials and conduct them to their targets (see ACTION POTENTIAL). In contrast, GLIAL CELLS, which are the other main cell type in the nervous system, do not generate action potentials. Another unique feature of a neuron is that their final MITOSIS (see CELL DIVISION) occurs mostly before birth. The brain has only limited abilities to generate new neurons after birth. The notion that the nervous system is not a mesh of tissues but consists of individual nerve cells is called the NEURON DOCTRINE and established in the late nineteenth century. This discovery involved many scientists, and Ramon y Cajal (1852–1934), Golgi (1843–1926) and Sherrington (1857–1952) played a major role. The term neuron was coined by von Waldeyer (1836–1921) in 1891.

A neuron consists of the SOMA or cell body, dendrites (see DENDRITE) and the AXON. The soma is the site of the synthesis of PROTEINS, and contains the NUCLEUS and various subcellular organelles including MITOCHONDRIA, RIBOSOMES, ENDOPLASMIC RETICULUM, GOLGI APPARATUS and LYSOSOMES. The term PERIKARYA is often used interchangeably with the soma, but strictly speaking, it refers to the CYTOPLASM around the nucleus. From the soma emerge a number of dendrites, usually two to five, which branch into secondary and higher-order dendrites. The function of dendrites is to receive synaptic inputs. The axon emerges from either the soma or a main dendrite. Although a neuron usually has a single axon, axons may branch to innervate multiple targets. The function of the axon is to conduct action potentials, and release neurotransmitters at axon terminals. Axons can be myelinated (see MYELIN) or unmyelinated. Myelinated axons have the NODES OF RANVIER, which are gaps in myelin that allow faster conduction of action potentials. The action potential is generated at the AXON HILLOCK, the cone-shaped site where the axon originates.

Individual neurons display characteristic morphologies which have fascinated neuroanatomists for a century, and these morphological features have been used to classify neurons. Neurons with a single process ('processes' being axons and dendrites) are found in the peripheral ganglia (see GANGLION), and are called PSEUDOUNIPOLAR NEURONS because the process eventually divides into two. Neurons with two processes 180° apart are called BIPOLAR NEURONS, and in the CEREBRAL CORTEX they are INTERNEURONS. Neurons that have multiple, branching dendrites are called MULTIPOLAR NEURONS and usually have long axons that project to other regions of the CENTRAL NERVOUS SYSTEM. Certain neurons are known for their characteristic dendritic morphologies. PURKINJE CELLS in the CEREBELLUM have unmistakable patterns of dendritic trees which look like flattened orange trees. Large PYRAMIDAL NEURONS in the cerebral cortex have a triangle-shaped cell body, a long APICAL DENDRITE which ascends toward the surface of the cortex, and shorter, BASAL DENDRITES. MEDIUM SPINY NEURONS in the STRIATUM are known for their extremely dense DENDRITIC SPINES.

Neurons have two principal functions: the generation and conduction of action potentials, and neurotransmission. Action potentials are generated in response to various inputs received by the soma and dendrites, mostly at synapses. The probability of generating action potentials is determined by the temporal and spatial summation of excitatory, inhibitory and modulatory inputs as well as the intrinsic membrane properties that are unique to individual neurons. The pattern of dendritic branching has a crucial role in determining the electrophysiological properties of neurons. For neurotransmission, neurons have elaborate systems to synthesize NEUROTRANSMITTERS and release them from their terminals. Neurons are also themselves a target of neurotransmitters, and transmitter receptors are present on dendrites, soma and axon terminals. It should noted that although neurotransmission is a unique property of neurons, the uniqueness lies in the direct apposition of target cells against the signalling cell – that is, the SYNAPSE. Secretion of chemical messengers *per se* is not unique to neurons but occurs in ENDOCRINE cells as well. The difference is that HORMONES secreted by endocrine cells are released into circulation (the blood or CEREBROSPINAL FLUID) which delivers them to distant target cells. Therefore, neurotransmission can be viewed as one end of a spectrum of chemical communication used by cells, with the endocrine action at the other end, and the PARACRINE action or VOLUME TRANSMISSION in the middle of the spectrum.

There are aspects of neuronal functions that add complexity to the concept of the neuron as a functional unit. First, there is evidence that components of dendrites in a single neuron can represent separate functional units in certain mammalian neurons including cerebellar Purkinje cells. Second, although DALE'S PRINCIPLE stipulates that all terminals of the same neuron release the same set of neurotransmitters, differential release of transmitters has been demonstrated in invertebrate neurons. Third, a variety of GAP JUNCTIONS is now known to exist between neurons, allowing passage of small molecules and electrical coupling of two and more neurons. Although these new findings do not refute the NEURON DOCTRINE, they provide further complexity to the function of neurons.

See also: neuroanatomy; neurophysiology

KAZUE SEMBA

neuron doctrine *see* neuroanatomy; neuron

neuronal filling *see* tract tracers

neuronal migration An important stage in the development of the CENTRAL NERVOUS SYSTEM, when presumptive neurons (see NEUROBLAST) have undergone their last CELL DIVISION and migrate to their final positions in the NEURO-PIL. Most neuroblasts arise at the region of the NEURAL TUBE lining the VENTRICLES, and migrate both radially, towards the PIA MATER (see MENINGES) on the external surface of the brain and spinal cord ('inside-out'), and tangentially, along the long axis of the CNS. Radial migrations take place on specialized glial cells (RADIAL GLIAL CELLS) that span the full thickness of the neural tube. Some radial migrations in the developing CEREBELLUM take an ('outside-in') direction.

See also: neurodevelopment

ROGER J. KEYNES

neuropathology Neuropathology is the branch of medicine and research concerned with the study of NEUROPATHY.

neuropathy Neuropathy is a generalized term for all physical disorders of the nervous system (both CENTRAL NERVOUS SYSTEM and PERIPHERAL NERVOUS SYSTEM).

neuropeptide hormones Peptides (for example SOMATOSTATIN) are known as HORMONES when secreted from ENDOCRINE GLANDS, and NEUROPEPTIDES when produced by neurons (see NEURON) in the CENTRAL NERVOUS SYSTEM. The NEUROPEPTIDE HORMONES can be considered as synonymous with the protein hormones: see HORMONES – CLASSIFICATION.

neuropeptide gamma *see* tachykinins

neuropeptide K *see* tachykinins

neuropeptide Y (NPY) One of the peptide NEUROTRANSMITTERS. It is found in the CENTRAL NERVOUS SYSTEM, but particularly large

concentrations in the ARCUATE NUCLEUS OF THE HYPOTHALAMUS and has potent actions in the PARAVENTRICULAR NUCLEUS OF THE HYPOTHALAMUS – microinjection of neuropeptide Y here promotes FEEDING strongly. It is coexistent with in brainstem NORADRENALINE neurons (especially those of the VENTRAL NORADRENERGIC BUNDLE) that are known to be associated with the control of feeding. Moreover, arcuate neurons that synthesize it posses LEPTIN receptors, and it has been suggested that circulating leptin can trigger neuropeptide Y activation to influence feeding. Five RECEPTOR subtypes for neuropeptide Y have been described (designated $Y_1–Y_5$), all G PROTEIN coupled, and all activated by both neuropeptide Y and a related molecule, NEUROPEPTIDE YY.

neuropeptide YY (NPYY) One of the GUT–BRAIN PEPTIDES, closely related to NEUROPEPTIDE Y. Peptide YY is synthesized in the PANCREAS in neurons that control INSULIN and GLUCAGON synthesis and release. When present in brain it is known as neuropeptide YY. It acts at the same types of RECEPTOR as neuropeptide Y but its functions remain obscure.

neuropeptides These are peptides found in the nervous system that act as NEUROTRANSMITTERS or neuromodulators (see NEUROMODULATION). Until the mid-1970s or so, it was generally believed that there were six or seven neurotransmitters in the nervous system, with relative small, simple structures, such as acetylcholine, noradrenaline, GABA and glutamate. Ground-breaking work during this decade on hypothalamic peptide control of pituitary function, largely through development of RADIOIMMUNOASSAY and techniques in IMMUNOHISTOCHEMISTRY, led to the eventual discovery and characterization of scores of neuropeptides. In 1977, the Nobel Prize was awarded to Roger Guillemin, Andrew Schally and Rosalyn Yalow for their work on neuropeptides. It is now known that neuropeptides play an important functional role in many areas of the central and peripheral nervous system. Neuropeptides differ from classical transmitters in many aspects of their synthesis, action, and degradation. For example, neuropeptides are synthesized from large precursor molecules in the cell body and transported to the terminal; classical transmitters can be synthesized in the terminal. Examples of well-known neuropeptides include SUBSTANCE P, ENKEPHALIN, ENDORPHIN, NEUROPEPTIDE Y, NEUROTENSIN, CHOLECYSTOKININ and CORTI-COTROPIN-RELEASING FACTOR.

See also: gut–brain peptides

ANN E. KELLEY

neuropharmacology The study of the effects of any DRUG on the nervous system. In the discipline of neuropharmacology, drugs are used as tools to elucidate mechanisms and functions at the level of neurotransmitters, receptors, molecular and intracellular processes. This is also an important field of study for investigating mechanisms underlying therapeutic drugs and drugs used to treat neurological and psychiatric disorders.

ANN E. KELLEY

neurophilosophy The interface between neuroscience and the philosophy of mind. Assuming that minds are activities of brains, then, according to neurophilosophers, understanding how the brain works is needed to understand how the mind works (see MATERIALISM and REDUCTIONISM). Opposed by traditional philosophers, neurophilosophy is a development of the later half of the twentieth century. It is engendered by advances in the study of the brain together with disappointment with the tradition that favoured non-empirical methods for understanding the mind. As part of a more general trend in philosophy of science toward naturalism, neurophilosophers generally emphasize the co-evolution of psychology and neuroscience. Questions addressed in both neurophilosophy and by non-empirical philosophy include: what is the nature of knowledge, and how do we learn and remember? What is the nature of perception? of CONSCIOUSNESS? What is it to be in control of one's behavior, to act in a voluntary fashion? What is the self?

To illustrate, consider the possibility that your visual experiences might be systematically inverted relative to mine – where you see red, I see green, and so on. Traditional philosophers have often assumed that the inverted spectrum

problem, as this is called, demonstrates that consciousness is intractable scientifically. Neurophilosophers opt to study behaviour along with the visual system to discover what the wiring for colour discrimination is like, how colour information is processed, and whether differences in neuronal structure map on to differences in colour perception. Science so far suggests that the causal mechanisms subserving colour perception can be successfully explored, and hence the possibility for comparison between individuals is not foreclosed. As long as awareness of colour *has* a causal structure in the brain – as long as it is not a property of soul-stuff detached from all causal interaction with the brain – data from psychology (that is, the colour-hue relationships) and neuroscience (tuning curves for the three types of CONES in the RETINA, wiring from the retina to CEREBRAL CORTEX and intracortically) predicts that genuine differences in colour perception will correlate with genuine differences in wiring and in neuronal activity. In context of a more detailed of the brain in general, the question of comparisons between individuals will be settled, one way or another, by the data.

Objections to the relevance of neuroscience to understanding the nature of psychological functions take essentially three forms. (1) It is conceivable that cognition could be instantiated in very different kinds of brains, and even in structures other than brains – something made of copper and silicon perhaps. What matters is only the *organization* of components, not the components themselves. (2) cognition is analogous to the software, the brain to the hardware. It is no more necessary to look at the brain to understand the nature of, for example, LEARNING, than it is necessary to understand my computer's microchips in order to understand how Microsoft Word constitutes a word processor. (3) Cognition that involves awareness is essentially subjective. Neuroscience is necessarily objective; it cannot break the subjectivity barrier. Replies are as follows. (1) The premises are fine, but the conclusion does not follow. First, even if other kinds of devices could have our psychology, we still want to know what exactly our psychology is, and how brains work such as to produce psychological states. Additionally, there are many conceivable solutions to how a cognitive operation might be accomplished, and neuroscience helps narrow the search space. This is now clear from the combined 'top-down' and' bottom-up' studies on the VISUAL SYSTEM and on LANGUAGE (see TOP-DOWN VS. BOTTOM-UP PERCEPTUAL/NEURAL PROCESSING). Second, important characteristics of psychological functions are in fact constrained by the nature of neural components. That many processes run in parallel, that WORKING MEMORY has a limit of about seven chunks of data, and GESTALT phenomena such as perceptual grouping, appear to be directly related to brain structure and organization. Third, some characteristics, such as how visual perception avoids smear with saccadic EYE MOVEMENTS (about three per second), or that there is a multiplicity of systems for spatial cognition, cannot be revealed by behavioural tests, and are discernible only neurally. (2) The structure and organization of psychological capacities cannot be assumed to be well understood at this stage. Doing COGNITIVE NEUROSCIENCE is like doing REVERSE ENGINEERING when you do not know exactly *what* the device really does. Traditional psychological assumptions specifying the taxonomy of capacities and how they interconnect can prove inadequate given data from cognitive neurobiology. For example, that there is a multiplicity of systems for memory and for attention. (3) This objection is correct but without significance. Suppose a neuroscientist observes activity in a subject's brain which is experienced by the subject as the smell of peppermint. The neuroscientist will not herself thereby smell peppermint. In that limited respect, neuroscientific knowledge does not capture subjectivity. This concession, however, is neither metaphysically nor scientifically interesting. It merely notes that being aware of a smell is different from knowing the neurobiological basis of smell-awareness, which is rather obvious when stated explicitly.

References

Akins K. (1996) Of sensory systems and the 'aboutness' of mental states. *Journal of Philosophy*: 337–372.

Clark A. (1993) *Sensory Qualities*, Oxford.

Churchland P.M. (1994) *The Engine of Reason; The Seat of the Soul*, MIT Press: Cambridge MA.

Crick F. (1994) *The Astonishing Hypothesis: The Scientific Search for the Soul*, Simon & Schuster: London.

Churchland P.S. (1986) *Neurophilosophy*, MIT Press: Cambridge MA.

Passingham, R. (1993) *The Frontal Lobes and Voluntary Action*, Oxford.

PATRICIA S. CHURCHLAND

neurophysin A peptide, the product of the synthesis of both VASOPRESSIN and OXYTOCIN, and released with these in the NEUROHYPOPHYSIS. The precise form of neurophysin depends on whether it is formed in vasopressin or oxytocin neurons.

neurophysiology The branch of neuroscience involved in studying the function of the nervous system studied primarily using electrophysiological techniques. This is in contrast with NEUROANATOMY which is primarily involved in the study of structure. The subject matter of neurophysiology has gradually changed with the advance of knowledge. The earliest successes occurred soon after the development of improved electrophysiological recording techniques in the 1920s and 1930s. Some of these advances include the discovery of the ACTION POTENTIAL and its ionic basis; the mechanisms underlying transmission of information across a chemical SYNAPSE; the mechanisms of SENSORY TRANSDUCTION and the encoding of information in sensory AFFERENT neurons; the components of SPINAL REFLEXES; the changes on the ELECTROENCEPHALOGRAM (EEG) changes associated with SLEEP and waking; and the topographic representation (see TOPOGRAPHY) of sensory cortical areas. Other advances came from the application of mathematical modelling, most notably the HODGKIN–HUXLEY EQUATIONS describing the flow of ions during an action potential.

During the last 50 years, much of neurophysiology has concentrated on understanding the CNS mechanisms underlying areas identified by traditional psychology, such as perception, movement, motivation, and learning. One approach has been to study function in terms of systems, for example the visual system or motor system, which extend across multiple levels of the nervous system. Each system can be studied in terms of the information processing that occurs at each relay in the system. The response properties of NEURONS within a nuclear region can be analysed in order to study the input–output relationships for each relay. The organization of such response properties within a brain region can reveal the organizational principles underlying this processing. Changes which occur in response properties over time have been used to study the mechanisms underlying NEUROPLASTICITY. Other changes during pathological states such as PARKINSON'S DISEASE and ALZHEIMER'S DEMENTIA have been used to understand and test therapeutic approaches to these diseases. The study of neurophysiology has been greatly enhanced by recent techniques which allow the FUNCTIONAL NEUROIMAGING of brain activity in conscious humans during motor behaviours or various cognitive tasks. The advances in computer technology have also led to an expansion in mathematical modelling on many of these topics (see NEURAL NETWORKS). Many discoveries of importance to neurophysiology have been made in INVERTEBRATES because of specialized features (such as the giant axon of the squid) or the advantages offered by a simplified nervous system (such as motor programming in the leech or learning in the APLYSIA).

Neurophysiology has also expanded greatly in the reductionistic (see REDUCTIONISM) analysis of the CNS, following the discovery that many functions are carried out by single PROTEINS. For example, the development of the PATCH CLAMP technique has made it possible to study the properties of single channels, such as the VOLTAGE-SENSITIVE ION CHANNELS responsible for the action potential or transmitter-specific channels at synapses. The interaction between neurophysiology and NEUROPHARMACOLOGY has permitted a detailed description of different types of neurotransmitters and their receptors as well as the intracellular consequences of receptor activation (see SECOND MESSENGERS). Advances in MOLECULAR BIOLOGY have made it possible to study the precise structure of these receptor proteins and the relationship between structure and function. There has also been significant interaction between these various fields in the

understanding of the growth and development of the nervous system, for example with respect to GROWTH FACTORS, cell–cell signalling during axonal growth and synapse formation (SYNAPTOGENESIS), and selective cell death (APOPTOSIS).

DOUGLAS D. RASMUSSON

neuropil (from Greek, *neuron*: nerve, *pilos*: hair) This is simply a description given to any neuronal network made up of the following items: AXON, DENDRITE, CELL BODY and SYNAPSE, and associated GLIAL CELLS.

neuropsychological test battery To assess function after brain injury a battery of tests is often used. An effective neuropsychological battery will include tests of a range of cognitive functions – including ATTENTION, MEMORY, visual-perceptual functions (see SENSATION VS. PERCEPTION; VISUAL SYSTEM), PLANNING and PROBLEM SOLVING and REACTION TIME – without unnecessary duplication. A neurological battery would include these tests, as well as additional tests for a wider range of brain function. The reason for using a battery of tests is to identify a profile of preserved and impaired performance, which is more informative than knowledge of performance on any individual test. To enable comparison of subtests, typically all the tests within a single battery will employ a similar subject interface (such as the use of a touch-screen computer). Additionally, performance norms for a variety of patient groups and control subjects are often available. There are many commercially available test batteries. Some of these are pencil and paper tests, for example, the LURIA–NEBRASKA NEUROPSYCHOLOGICAL BATTERY, but there is increasing interest in automated test batteries, such as the CAMBRIDGE AUTOMATED NEUROLOGICAL TEST BATTERY (CANTAB).

See also: fixed battery; sensorimotor test battery

VERITY J. BROWN

neuropsychology Neuropsychology is an area of scientific research common to neurologists, psychologists, neurophysiologists and psychiatrists. It originally focused mainly, though not exclusively, on the CEREBRAL CORTEX. Topics of concern in the early days of the discipline were disorders of language, perception and action. Although certain of these disorders only occur in humans, neuropsychologists believe that findings relevant to human pathology are available through animal experimentation. Today research in human and animal neuropsychology complement one another.

Attempts to localize mental processes to particular bodily structures can be traced back at least to the fifth century BC, when Hippocrates identified the brain as the organ of intellect and the heart as the organ of the senses. Around the same time, Empedocles, concerned with the relationship of mind to body (see MIND–BODY QUESTION; NEUROPHILOSOPHY) located mental processes in the heart. For the next 2000 years, the relative merits of 'the brain hypothesis' and 'the cardiac hypothesis' were debated. Although by 1900 a field similar to modern neuropsychology had developed which in many ways anticipated modern concepts, it virtually disappeared from view for more than 50 years. This may have been because much of the early work was published in German when English-speaking scientists were dominating NEUROLOGY and experimental psychology. Some believe that experimental psychology, so long a strength of North American psychology, was so heavily biased towards behaviourist ways of thinking that any reference to mental processes was shunned and this inhibited the development of neuropsychology there. Others argue that over concern with localization of function leading to the so-called 'diagram makers' led to loss of interest in the neural mechanisms of cognitive functions. It seems generally accepted that the word was first used by Sir William Osler (1849–1919) in 1913, from when it was used occasionally by neuroscientists such as D.B. Lindsley, Heinrich Klüver, Karl Lashley and Donald Hebb. Lashley seemed to use the term synonymously with PHYSIOLOGICAL PSYCHOLOGY. Hebb, however, used it to refer to an interdisciplinary approach to behaviour which involved neurology and physiological psychology. He gave the term wide publicity as a subtitle to his hugely influential book *The Organization of Behaviour: A Neuropsychological Theory* published in 1949.

Different disciplines have their own methods to study how brain function relates to changes in behaviour and mental life. The contribution of experimental psychology, and particularly cognitive psychology, has been crucial in all these endeavours. Whilst most neuropsychological techniques involve the study of overt behaviour and responding, they need to be supplemented by the contributions that can be made by those who study EVENT-RELATED POTENTIALS, which open a time and space window into covert steps in brain information processing which may not necessarily be accompanied by any overt behaviour or reported as private experiences.

The question of whether and to what extent particular mental functions can be localized in particular parts of the brain remains an enduring issue in neuropsychology. Today research in neuropsychology centres around the functions of circumscribed areas of or systems within the brain. Whilst the contribution from NEUROPHYSIOLOGY to neuropsychology remains important, a clear distinction can be made between the primary question for the physiologist of 'How does the nervous system work?' and that of the neuropsychologist 'How does the working of the nervous system produce behaviour, including inferred cognitive processes?'. Both anatomical and physiological work related to neuropsychology have thus contributed to one of the most intensively studied issues, namely differences in the structure and function of the cerebral lobes. This took a great step forward with the work of Roger Sperry on his split-brain animals and human commissurotomy patients (see SPLIT BRAIN). Today neuropsychologists recognize that to talk about LATERALIZATION of function in a simplistic way begs a number of important questions, such as, what is it that is lateralized? Is it that they are differently organized? Is it that they have two distinct ways of processing information? Answers to these questions are well illustrated by the intensive work on how speech (see SPEECH PERCEPTION; SPEECH PRODUCTION) and LANGUAGE are organized in the brains of respectively right- and left-handed individuals.

As the young science of neuropsychology grew up in different parts of the world, it developed its own distinctive emphases and techniques. In the USA, the emphasis was largely, though not entirely, on quantitative and psychometric techniques. In some instances batteries of tests were applied to large groups of patients. In the UK, the approach tended to be more qualitative and less psychometric, paying more attention to the in-depth study of crucial single cases, an approach more evident recently in North America. In Russia (or the USSR as it then was) the leadership of A. Luria using qualitative and non-psychometric techniques was dominant. Currently some of the most rewarding developments are taking place as a direct result of developments in FUNCTIONAL NEUROIMAGING of the active and alert human brain. The use of magnetic resonance imagery techniques, of positron emission tomography and of human cerebral blood flow are producing major new results. Molecular biological approaches are also used in, for example, the study of CHOLINERGIC systems and their changes in relation to the onset of DEMENTIA.

References

Jeeves M.A. & Baumgartner G. (1986) *Methods of Investigation in Neuropsychology*, Pergamon: Oxford.

MALCOLM A. JEEVES

neuroscience The scientific study of NERVOUS SYSTEM and all the tissues that compose it. Because it is such a large field of study, qualifying terms are often added such as BEHAVIOURAL NEUROSCIENCE, COGNITIVE NEUROSCIENCE or invertebrate neuroscience (the study of the nervous systems of INVERTEBRATES, obviously). NEUROLOGY refers to the branch of medicine that concerns itself with the diagnosis and treatment of disorders of the nervous system. It is expressly medical: neuroscience is the scientific study of nervous systems and does not have special medical focus, although it evidently has medical value. The neurosciences have expanded enormously over the past few decades, perhaps best indexed by the growth of organizations dedicated to neuroscience: see for example the websites maintained by the Society for Neuroscience (www.sfn.org) or the Federation of European Neuroscience Societies (www.fen-

s.org). Intellectually, it is of considerable interest to see the effect that neuroscience has had on psychology, in which biological explanations for many psychological phenomena are routinely sought, where in the past mental explanations (MENTALISM) would have been identified. The impact of neuroscience has also been felt in philosophy with the advent of NEUROPHILOSOPHY (and see also DUALISM). While there is great enthusiasm at the moment for neuroscientific explanations of psychological phenomena (see for example CONSCIOUSNESS) doubts have been expressed about the cogency of the explanations offered and indeed the ability of neuroscience to provide explanations for all forms of psychological process.

See also: behaviourism; cognitive psychology

neurosecretion Although there is a sense in which one can consider every NEURON as a neurosecretory cell (since they all secrete neurochemicals of one sort or another; see NEUROCHEMISTRY) this term is generally reserved for neurons that secrete HORMONES, NEUROTRANSMITTERS or other factors within the PITUITARY GLAND (principally within the NEUROHYPOPHYSIS). For example, neurons in the PARAVENTRICULAR NUCLEUS OF THE HYPOTHALAMUS project into the pituitary and release VASOPRESSIN into the BLOOD stream there: this action can be described as neurosecretion.

neurosis An obsolete term. The disease classification system DSM-IV has abandoned the term, though ICD 10 still uses the 'neurotic' as an adjective in subclassification. It was used to refer to conditions in which patients did not lose touch with reality, did not have any organic state, and did not have PERSONALITY DISORDER, and which were considered to be less serious than PSYCHOSIS. Inappropriate use of so-called 'mental defence mechanisms' was believed to play a role in the development of neurotic disorders. As the classification was made by exclusion, and the disorders were not necessarily mild, and the status of mental defence mechanisms uncertain, it became preferable instead to group relevant disorders by common descriptive characteristics. Such disorders include: ANXIETY disorders; OBSESSIVE

COMPULSIVE DISORDER; DISSOCIATIVE DISOR-
DERS; and SOMATIZATION DISORDERS.

IAN C. REID

neurosurgery Clinical or experimental surgery
directed at the nervous system.

See also: stereotaxic surgery; neurology

neurosyphilis Organic state following infection of the central nervous system (CNS) by
the organism responsible for syphilis (the
spirochaete *Treponema*). The commonest CNS
complication is the disorder once known as
GENERAL PARESIS OF THE INSANE. Onset is
usually 10–15 years after primary infection.
Principal features include personality change,
disinhibition, mood swings and dementia.
Neurosyphilis may mimic other disorders. The
disorder is treated with penicillin.

IAN C. REID

neurotensin One of the NEUROPEPTIDES: there
are two RECEPTOR types – NTS1 is a high
AFFINITY receptor, NTS2 low affinity; both are
G PROTEIN coupled. Neurotensin is found in
the CENTRAL NERVOUS SYSTEM and has been
most extensively studied as a neurotransmitter
in COEXISTENCE with DOPAMINE in VENTRAL
TEGMENTAL AREA neurons. Neurotensin is
stored in large, dense core SYNAPTIC VESICLES
(as is another coexistent neuropeptide, CHOLE-
CYSTOKININ) whereas dopamine is stored in
smaller vesicles. It is thought likely that the
neuropeptide transmitters and dopamine can
be differentially released from terminals. Low
rates of stimulation are associated with dopamine release, higher rates with release of the
neuropeptide. The postsynaptic effects of these
are complex, while the presynaptic effects
involve reciprocal modulation of further neurotransmitter release.

neurothelium *see* blood–brain barrier

neurotoxins Poisons that have an action
against neurons (see NEURON) are known as
neurotoxins. Some are tools used in neuroscience to make a LESION in neural tissue
while others (such as CONOTOXINS) occur
naturally and are used by predators to capture
prey. Many substances can destroy neurons
non-selectively – copper sulphate for example

– while other chemicals have more specific
effects on tissue. EXCITOTOXINS act at GLUTA-
MATE RECEPTORS and destroy cell bodies but
not other local tissue elements; GLIOTOXINS
destroy GLIAL CELLS. Still other neurotoxins
have effects against chemically identified neurons: 6-HYDROXYDOPAMINE destroys CATECHO-
LAMINE containing neurons while 5,7-
DIHYDROXYTRYPTAMINE destroys those containing SEROTONIN. MPTP (1-methyl-4-phenyl-
1,2,3,6-tetrahydropyridine) is an extremely selective and species specific neurotoxin with
actions on the DOPAMINE containing neurons
of the SUBSTANTIA NIGRA of PRIMATES. In using
neurotoxins, the goal of neuroscientists is to
make lesions as selective for a particular type
of neuron as possible: IMMUNOTOXINS offer the
possibility of being able to generate highly
selective lesions.

See also: AF 64A; monomeric acrylamide;
saporin

neurotransmission A broad term, neurotransmission indicates communication between cells
in the NERVOUS SYSTEM (and between cells of
the nervous system and other tissues; see
NEUROMUSCULAR JUNCTION). Neurotransmission can be chemical or electrical: chemical
communication between neurons can involve
the release of NEUROTRANSMITTERS at specialized synapses (SYNAPTIC TRANSMISSION) or
may involve the release of neurotransmitters
in a diffuse manner, without specialized synapses (which is known as VOLUME TRANSMIS-
SION). Direct electrical communication
between neurons is known as EPHAPTIC TRANS-
MISSION.

See also: chemical transmission; neuron

neurotransmitters Chemical substances used
for signalling between neurons in the nervous
system. Transmitters are released at the SY-
NAPSE by the PRESYNAPTIC neuron into the
SYNAPTIC CLEFT. They then bind to RECEPTORS
on the POSTSYNAPTIC neuron or an effector
organ such as muscle, to evoke a variety of
postsynaptic effects. The nature of this response depends on the properties of the receptor activated, rather than the transmitter itself.
Thus, the same neurotransmitter can have
different effects depending on the receptor

present on the postsynaptic neuron, and by the same token, different transmitters can have similar effects if the properties of the activated receptors are similar. Transmitters also bind to presynaptic receptors to modulate further release from the axon terminal. A substance is accepted as a transmitter when the following four criteria are met: synthesis and presence in the presynaptic terminal, release from the presynaptic terminal, mimicking of the postsynaptic action by exogenous administration, and inactivation mechanisms to terminate its action.

Neurotransmitters are classified into two categories: small-molecule transmitters, and peptide transmitters. Small-molecule transmitters are relatively few in number, and include, among others, ACETYLCHOLINE, BIOGENIC AMINES (the CATECHOLAMINES, DOPAMINE, NORADRENALINE and ADRENALINE; and the INDOLEAMINES, SEROTONIN and HISTAMINE), and AMINO ACIDS (GLUTAMATE (or glutamic acid), GABA (gamma aminobutyric acid) and GLYCINE). More than 50 peptide transmitters are known to date, although only several of them have so far satisfied all four criteria as a neurotransmitter. Peptide transmitters usually contain 3 to 36 amino acids. They include hypothalamic releasing HORMONES such as SOMATOSTATIN, pituitary hormones such as VASOPRESSIN, OXYTOCIN and BETA ENDORPHIN, and gastrointestinal peptides such as CHOLE-CYSTOKININ, SUBSTANCE P and ENKEPHALINS (see GUT–BRAIN PEPTIDES). Small-molecule transmitters and peptide transmitters differ in several ways. Small-molecule transmitters are usually synthesized at the TERMINAL. Their precursors are supplied locally, while their synthesizing enzymes are transported from the CELL BODY. At the terminal, small-molecule transmitters are packaged into SYNAPTIC VESI-CLES by VESICULAR TRANSPORTERS. In contrast, peptide transmitters are not synthesized at the terminal, but rather derive from precursor proteins that are synthesized in the cell body. The precursors are packaged into vesicles along with the cleaving enzymes and transported along the axon to terminals. The final processing of neuropeptides occurs during the transport. Therefore, once a neuropeptide is depleted at the terminal, further release re-

quires a new supply of the peptide from the cell body.

The mechanism of release is the same for all transmitters. The arrival of action potentials at the axon terminal causes an increase in the intracellular CALCIUM (Ca^{2+}) concentration. This causes synaptic vesicles to fuse with the cell membrane, and transmitters are released into the synaptic cleft. This process is called EXOCYTOSIS. Once transmitters are released, timely removal or inactivation is crucial for terminating their action. Amino acids and biogenic amines are removed from the synaptic cleft by high-affinity REUPTAKE transporters located at the presynaptic terminal or in GLIAL CELLS, whereas acetylcholine is degraded enzymatically by ACETYLCHOLINESTERASE. Neuroactive peptides are removed more slowly, by diffusion and degradation by peptidases in the extracellular space. Transmitters internalized by the high-affinity reuptake mechanisms are recycled for subsequent release.

Small-molecule transmitters and peptide transmitters can coexist in the same neuron, and be co-released. Numerous examples of such co-localization have been reported in the nervous system. For example, vasoactive intestinal polypeptide is present in the cholinergic presynaptic terminals in the parasympathetic ganglia (see GANGLION). The release of co-localized neuropeptides appears to be activity-dependent in that they are released only when the neuron is highly active, as during bursts, whereas the release of small-molecule transmitters is usually proportional to the activity of the neuron. Certain small-molecule transmitters and neuropeptides also interact at the presynaptic terminal to regulate transmitter release. These presynaptic and postsynaptic actions of co-localized transmitters permit an extraordinary diversity of information transfer at one synapse. In addition to these classical neurotransmitters, non-classical transmitters have been identified. These include ATP and NITRIC OXIDE (NO). Although ATP has an important role in energy metabolism, it is also packaged into synaptic vesicles and released synaptically in a Ca^{2+}-dependent manner. Nitric oxide is a gaseous neurotransmitter that diffuses across the cell membrane. Because of this diffusibility, nitric oxide has been suggested to play a role as a retrograde messenger (a messenger that is released by the postsynaptic neuron to act on the presynaptic terminal) during LONG-TERM POTENTIATION. Carbon monoxide (CO) may act in a similar manner to NO.

Many drugs work by influencing the synthesis, release, reuptake and receptor binding of neurotransmitters. For example, stimulants such as AMPHETAMINE and COCAINE are known to enhance dopamine release in the MESOLIMBIC DOPAMINE SYSTEM. MORPHINE works by acting at endogenous OPIOID RECEPTORS. Biogenic amines and acetylcholine are also implicated in neurological disorders such as PARKINSON'S DISEASE and ALZHEIMER'S DEMENTIA, as well as SCHIZOPHRENIA and AFFECTIVE DISORDERS. Drugs that affect the action of these transmitters at various strategic sites have been developed for therapeutic purposes. The L-DOPA therapy for Parkinson's disease is well known in which L-DOPA acts as a precursor for dopamine.

See also: neuromodulation; neuron; neuropharmacology; neurophysiology

KAZUE SEMBA

neurotrophic (from Greek, *neuron*: nerve, *trophos*: a feeder) Something that enables a NEURON to grow and survive, either by nourishing a neuron directly; by guiding development properly; or by suppressing harmful processes and factors; see GROWTH FACTORS. Neurotrophic is not the same thing as NEUROTROPIC.

neurotrophin-3 *see* nerve growth factor

neurotropic (from Greek, *neuron*: nerve, *tropos*: turning) Having a partiality for neural tissue. For example, a neurotropic VIRUS is a virus that targets the CENTRAL NERVOUS SYSTEM (see for example RABIES). It is not the same thing as NEUROTROPHIC.

neurulation *see* neural tube

neutrophil *see* immune system

niacin Also known as nicotinic acid: one of the essential VITAMINS.

nialamide *see* monoamine oxidase inhibitors

niche competition A term that describes the competition between SPECIES for resources: organisms may fit an ECOLOGICAL NICHE uniquely (for example when on a small island) or they may have to compete with other species within an ecological niche for the resources it contains.

nicotine The active ingredient in TOBACCO. Tobacco has been used by humans for several thousand years. Native peoples in North and South America were the first to grow the tobacco plant and smoked its leaves for its PSYCHOACTIVE effects. New World explorers first observed tobacco smoking in the time of Columbus and it was introduced into Western cultures and other parts of the world in the sixteenth century. In most present human societies, delivery of nicotine through smoking tobacco is a common, legal and (relatively) socially acceptable form of psychoactive drug consumption. Although there are over 3000 chemical components in cigarette smoke, it is now believed that nicotine is the active and addictive compound. Thus, nicotine is one of the most widely consumed psychoactive drugs in the world. A one-pack-per-day smoker will administer hundreds of nicotine doses to himself daily (about 200 puffs), which amounts to over 70 000 doses of nicotine per year. Nicotine can be administered in a variety of ways, but smoking is by far the most common route of administration. As smoke is drawn into the lungs via particles of 'tar' (condensate), nicotine is absorbed rapidly into the circulatory system. Blood concentrations rise rapidly, and it is estimated that nicotine enters the brain in approximately 7 seconds. Ingestion of nicotine via oral routes (chewing tobacco, nicotine gum, snuff) results in a much slower rise in blood nicotine concentrations, and levels persist for longer periods. Nicotine has a variety of complex effects on the PERIPHERAL NERVOUS SYSTEM and CENTRAL NERVOUS SYSTEM. It can act as both a stimulant and a depressant. In studies of subjective effects of smoking, people say that they smoke for both its arousing and relaxation effects.

The principal actions of nicotine on neurotransmitters involve effects at CHOLINERGIC, DOPAMINERGIC, and GLUTAMATERGIC synapses. In the central nervous system NICOTINIC ACET-

YLCHOLINE RECEPTORS are activated, and there is also increased release of DOPAMINE. There is recent evidence that nicotine facilitates glutamatergic transmission as well. It is thought that effects on dopamine may underlie the rewarding and addictive properties of nicotine, while effects on acetylcholine in the cerebral cortex may be related to the cognitive-enhancing effects in smokers. Moreover, since glutamate receptors are critically involved in plasticity, interaction of nicotine with glutamate receptors may mediate the long-term addictive process. Nicotine stimulates cholinergic receptors in the autonomic nervous system, and at the NEUROMUSCULAR JUNCTION. Nicotine also induces the release of catecholamines in the periphery, which results in cardiovascular activation (accelerated heart rate, increased blood pressure and cardiac output, and vasoconstriction).

DEPENDENCE on nicotine is by far the greatest cause of disease and death in Western societies, not because of the dangers of nicotine itself, but because of the fact that nicotine is addictive and is inhaled along with many other toxic compounds in cigarette smoke. For example, it has been estimated that there are 400 000 smoking-related deaths per year in the United States alone. There are a number of diseases causally linked to smoking, including lung cancer, coronary heart disease, hypertension, and chronic lung disease such as emphysema. People continue to smoke despite current widespread knowledge of the adverse health consequences of smoking, and experts state that nicotine is as addictive as heroin. In fact, most people who smoke would like to quit. However, of those smokers trying to quit, approximately 70–80% relapse within three months, as is true for HEROIN and ALCOHOL. Smoking cessation often results in a distinct WITHDRAWAL SYNDROME. The most common SIGNS AND SYMPTOMS are irritability, ANXIETY, restlessness, impaired concentration, and a strong CRAVING for tobacco. HEADACHE, drowsiness, INSOMNIA, and gastrointestinal complaints are also common. Neuropsychological tests in smokers undergoing withdrawal show decreases in VIGILANCE, ATTENTION and psychomotor performance, and increases in hostility. The syndrome gradually subsides within days or weeks, but the craving and desire for a cigarette often far outlast the physical complaints.

Why do people smoke? Social factors are probably very important in the teenage years, when smoking dependence most often develops. Eighty percent of all smokers start before the age of 18. Peer pressure, parental modelling, and experimentation may contribute to initiation of the behaviour. When the habit is well established, it is likely that other factors related to the biological effects of nicotine contribute to the maintenance of the behaviour. Perhaps most important of these are nicotine's positive reinforcing effects. Like all drugs of abuse, nicotine affects mood, emotion and cognitive functions. Self-administration tests in animals have shown that rats and monkeys will press a lever to deliver intravenous nicotine. However, it does not appear that nicotine produces the powerful EUPHORIA or 'rush' that is experienced with other drugs that are smoked or delivered intravenously, such as heroin or cocaine.

See also: addiction; dependence; reward

ANN E. KELLEY

nicotine patch *see* transdermal drug delivery

nicotinic acetylcholine receptors *see* acetylcholine receptors

nictitating membrane (from Latin, *nictitare*: to wink) A layer of SKIN that covers the CORNEA and forms a second eyelid in certain species – amphibia and birds have this, as do a few MAMMALS, most notably cats and rabbits. Nictitating membrane closure has been used as an UNCONDITIONED RESPONSE in studies of CLASSICAL CONDITIONING, typically in rabbits.

night blindness Night blindness refers to poor vision in dim light. Everyone experiences temporary night blindness when moving suddenly from high to low illumination conditions (see SCOTOPIC VS. PHOTOPIC) – strong sunlight to a dark room for example. More permanent night blindness arises from vitamin A deficiency (vitamin A being an enzyme necessary for the regeneration of isomerized (see ISOMER) RHODOPSIN in RODS in the RETINA) or by any condition that weakens rod vision, since scotopic vision is mediated by rods. Poor photopic vision, or 'DAY BLINDNESS,' also occurs, either when moving from scotopic to photopic conditions or because of deficiencies in the CONES.

LAWRENCE M. WARD

night terrors (*pavor nocturnis*) DREAMING of a vivid and unpleasant nature that cause individuals – usually children – to wake in a fright. They are a form of SLEEP DISORDER associated with SLOW-WAVE SLEEP. Their cause is not known, but fortunately, in general, night terrors disappear as children grow older.

nigrostriatal dopamine system The nigrostriatal dopamine system is composed of relatively few neurons (about 2000 per HEMISPHERE in the rat brain) having their SOMA are in the SUBSTANTIA NIGRA pars compacta and axons (see AXON) travelling in the medial forebrain bundle. The terminals are principally in the CAUDATE NUCLEUS and PUTAMEN, where they release DOPAMINE (see Smith & Bolam for review of nigrostriatal system anatomy and connections). Degeneration of the nigrostriatal pathway is the principal pathological feature of PARKINSON'S DISEASE. It has also been associated with MOTOR PROGRAMMING, the control of REACTION TIMES, MOTIVATION, and the formation of HABITS and stereotyped behaviour.

See also: mesolimbic dopamine system; mesolimbicocortical system; tubero-infundibular dopamine system

Reference

Smith A.D. & Bolam J.P. (1990) The neural network of the basal ganglia as revealed by the study of synaptic connections of identified neurons. *Trends in Neurosciences* 13: 259–265.

nigrotectal pathway *see* superior colliculus

nine-hole box This operant box consists of a square chamber which has a curved rear wall with an horizontal array (1.5 cm above the grid floor) of nine poke-holes. When used for testing rats, each hole will have an approximately 1.5 cm square opening and be about 3 cm deep. There is a recessed light at the back of each hole and a photocell beam is directed vertically across the opening to detect nose

poke responses into the hole. On the opposite wall of the chamber is a reward hopper, occluded by a hinged flap, into which liquid reward or food pellets are dispensed once they have been earned. This apparatus provides an alternative to the more commonly used OPERANT CHAMBER, the SKINNER BOX. It has been very successfully used in studies of REACTION TIME performance and to detect lateralized deficits in response organization.

See also: nose poke vs. lever press

VERITY J. BROWN

Nissl bodies The nineteenth-century German neurologist Franz Nissl (1860–1919) discovered that the histological stain methylene blue stained the CELL BODY of all cells in nervous tissue: the elements stained became known as Nissl bodies or Nissl substance (or, colloquially, just Nissl). Nissl substance in fact is made of PROTEINS, DNA and RNA in the cell NUCLEUS. Staining for Nissl substance is a very simple and common histological procedure because it stains effectively all cells in the nervous system. The most common stain used to do this is CRESYL VIOLET.

See also: histology

nitric oxide (NO) One of the highly reactive and readily diffusable FREE RADICALS, found in many tissues in the body. Nitric oxide may act either locally at its site of synthesis, or at adjacent cells, where it binds to a wide variety of cellular components such as ENZYMES, ION CHANNELS and RECEPTORS, thereby altering their function.

In the brain, nitric oxide is synthesized upon demand by NITRIC OXIDE SYNTHASE (NOS), the activity of which is highly regulated by a requirement for CALMODULIN. Increases in intracellular calcium concentrations allow calmodulin to bind to NOS, causing conversion of ARGININE TO CITRULLINE, with a concomitant release of nitric oxide. NOS also requires the presence of cofactors including nicotinamide adenine dinucleotide phosphate (NADPH), flavine mononucleotide, flavine adenine dinucleotide, and tetrahydrobiopterin, and an iron-containing HEME element, which act as an electron transport chain in the synthesis of nitric oxide. Several isoforms of NOS have been isolated, of which neuronal NOS and endothelial NOS (named after the tissues from which they were first isolated) are found throughout the brain, co-localized with several transmitter systems. NOS is found in high concentrations in HIPPOCAMPUS, CEREBRAL CORTEX, OLFACTORY BULB, STRIATUM, CERE-BELLUM, and several structures in the BRAIN-STEM. It is co-localized with CHOLINE ACETYLTRANSFERASE in the PEDUNCULOPON-TINE TEGMENTAL NUCLEUS and LATERODORSAL TEGMENTAL NUCLEUS, and with SOMATOSTATIN and NEUROPEPTIDE Y in cortical neurons. NOS is also found in cells of many blood vessels throughout the body, including the CEREBRAL VASCULATURE, and mediates SMOOTH MUSCLE relaxation, leading to increased blood flow.

In many cells, nitric oxide mediates its effect through binding with the heme element of guanylyl cyclase, resulting in increased production of CYCLIC GMP, one of the SECOND MESSENGERS which activates cyclic GMP-dependent PROTEIN KINASE. Protein kinases catalyse the phosphorylation of many cellular enzymes, altering their rate of activity, and may induce such effects as increased transmitter release and altered ion channel permeability. In the hippocampus, nitric oxide release is associated with the stimulation of NMDA RE-CEPTORS, and has been shown to augment LONG-TERM POTENTIATION (LTP), possibly by acting trans-synaptically to increase transmitter release, suggesting a role in LEARNING and MEMORY. Similarly, nitric oxide has also been implicated in activity-dependent modification of synapses in some areas of the central nervous system during development, by augmenting and preserving synchronously firing neuronal inputs on target neurons or tissues.

Some tissues in the body use the toxic free-radical properties of nitric oxide to alter irreversibly the function of cellular components in order to destroy them. MACROPHAGE cells in the IMMUNE SYSTEM contain an isoform of nitric oxide synthase known as INDUCIBLE NOS. This is used to produce large amounts of nitric oxide which destroys foreign matter phagocytosed by the macrophage cells. Similarly, nitric oxide may be toxic to neurons, if it is produced in large quantities. In ISCHAEMIA and some disease processes, alterations in intracellular calcium concentrations may lead to synthesis of excess nitric oxide which would result in dysfunction, and possibly death of the neuron.

See also: sodium nitroprusside

FIONA M. INGLIS

nitric oxide synthase The novel neurotransmitter NITRIC OXIDE (NO) is not stored in a prepared form, as conventional NEUROTRANS-MITTERS are: it is synthesized on demand by nitric oxide synthase (NOS): see NITRIC OXIDE for details. Determining which neurons contain nitric oxide synthase is therefore the principal means for defining which of them can synthesize nitric oxide.

nitrous oxide There are four important things to know about nitrous oxide (N_2O). (1) It is *not* NITRIC OXIDE (NO). Nitric oxide is found in many neurons and has some of the properties of NEUROTRANSMITTERS or neuromodulators (see NEUROMODULATION). Nitrous oxide (N_2O) and nitric oxide (NO) should *never* be confused. (2) Nitrous oxide is an anaesthetic agent, given by inhalation, and typically used as an ADJUVANT to other forms of ANAESTHE-SIA. Alone, it does not appear to produce true anaesthesia. (3) It has analgesic properties (see ANALGESIA): a mixture of 20% N_2O in air can produce analgesia equivalent to that of MOR-PHINE. (It is often given during labour, and is colloquially known as 'gas and air'.) (4) It has been popularly known as 'laughing gas'. It does not stimulate HUMOUR; it does have a relaxing effect similar to morphine.

NMDA (N-methyl-D-aspartate) A synthetic organic compound exhibiting a highly selective BINDING AFFINITY for a subtype of IONOTRO-PIC GLUTAMATE RECEPTORS found in the CNS.

See also: NMDA receptors

CHARLES D. BLAHA

NMDA receptors One of three IONOTROPIC GLUTAMATE receptor subtypes found in the central nervous system (CNS) that is activated by NMDA (N-methyl-D-aspartate) (though note that NMDA does not occur naturally in the brain). Other ionotropic glutamate receptors are activated by AMPA and KAINIC ACID.

NMDA acts only at NMDA receptors, AMPA at AMPA and so on. NMDA- and AMPA-gated channels mediate the bulk of fast excitatory CNS synaptic transmission and are permeable to SODIUM (Na$^+$), POTASSIUM (K$^+$), and CHLORIDE (Cl$^-$) ions. Inward ionic current through NMDA receptors is voltage-dependent due to MAGNESIUM (Mg^{2+}) block at a negative resting MEMBRANE POTENTIAL. NMDA receptors have been extensively studied in recent decades and it has been found that they play a critical role in many processes, including LONG-TERM POTENTIATION (LTP) for which calcium (Ca^{2+}) entry into neurons via NMDA-gated ion channels is critical. Areas rich in NMDA receptors include limbic regions such as the HIPPOCAMPUS and AMYGDALA, NEOCORTEX, and the BASAL GANGLIA.

See also: excitotoxins

CHARLES D. BLAHA AND ANN E. KELLEY

no net flux In vivo determination of the quantity of NEUROTRANSMITTERS in a localized brain region of an experimental animal is often achieved using MICRODIALYSIS. Determination of the absolute level of transmitter normally present in an area is difficult though: fluid is continually perfused through the dialysis probe, so that the interface between the fluid being perfused and brain INTERSTITIAL FLUIDS always presents a CONCENTRATION GRADIENT across which molecules will flow. Microdialysis will tend therefore to remove any molecules that will cross the SEMIPERMEABLE MEMBRANE of the dialysis probe, reducing dramatically their concentration in the part of brain being dialysed. (To put it more colloquially, dialysis sucks.) This can be avoided using the no net flux procedure: one can determine the normal resting concentration of a molecule in a given area by adding known amounts of that molecule to the perfusion fluid going through the dialysis probe. If the concentration added is less than that in brain, more of that molecule will be found in the extracted DIALYSATE than was initially present (ENDOGENOUS molecules having diffused in, following the concentration gradient); but if the concentration added to the perfusate is more than that in brain, less of that molecule will be found in the extracted dialysate than was initially present (EXOGEN-

OUS molecules having diffused into brain, following the concentration gradient). The concentration of the molecule added to the dialysate that produces no net flux across the dialysis membrane can be taken to be a reasonable estimate of the concentration of that molecule normally present in the area being dialysed.

See also: high-performance liquid chromatography

nociception (from Latin, nocere: to hurt, and perception) Nociception is the detection of pain; nociceptive is sensitivity to pain; a nociceptor is a sensory receptor sensitive to painful stimuli. See PAIN for further discussion.

nocturnal (from Latin, nocturnes: happening at night) A nocturnal animal is one that is active at night and rests during the day. Many small animals – rats and mice for example – are nocturnal. Predators – such as cats and owls – have developed sensory systems (vision and hearing in these examples) to help catch nocturnal prey.

See also: crepuscular; diurnal

nocturnal enuresis Nocturnal enuresis (or, more prosaically, BEDWETTING) is a loss of bladder control during the night. It occurs in children more often than adults and is a problem associated with SLOW-WAVE SLEEP (see SLEEP DISORDERS). It has been associated with ANXIETY and with hormonal disturbances (see HORMONES). It is often treated by BEHAVIOUR THERAPY: an ENURETIC BLANKET is used. The presence of only a few drops of urine on this completes an electrical circuit and causes a bell to ring. Quite quickly, children can learn to associate the initiation of bladder emptying with waking, after which of course, the bladder can be emptied. Nocturnal enuresis resistant to such therapy and not associated with anxiety can persist into adulthood.

nocturnal myoclonus Also known as REST-LESS LEG SYNDROME or PERIODIC LIMB MOVEMENT IN SLEEP, this is a disorder of SLEEP in which there is MYOCLONUS. It can be a debilitating condition because of the disruptive effect on sleep. Treatments designed to achieve relaxation of MUSCLES and alleviation of STRESS are often recommended.

See also: REM without atonia; sleep disorders

nocturnal penile tumescence *see* impotence

node of Ranvier A gap in the MYELIN sheath of a NEURON; the presence of the nodes of Ranvier allows for the development of SALTATORY conduction, which is much faster than CABLE TRANSMISSION; see ACTION POTENTIAL and GLIAL CELLS for further information.

nodose ganglion The VAGUS NERVE has two sensory GANGLIA, the JUGULAR GANGLION (superior) is one and the NODOSE GANGLION (inferior) the other. Neurons of the nodose ganglion provide general visceral afferent input from the upper alimentary tract (oesophagus, stomach, small intestine), respiratory system (larynx, trachea, lungs) and heart.

noise Noise has two types of meaning. (i) It refers to any random , uninformative component in communication that contrast with a defined signal (see INFORMATION THEORY; signal detection theory; SIGNAL TO NOISE RATIO). (ii) Noise is also used as a term in acoustics and refers to an auditory stimulus without a definite PITCH. COLOURED NOISE is any noise other than WHITE NOISE (and is achieved by passing white or pink noise through a frequency filter). PINK NOISE is a noise with both random FREQUENCY and AMPLITUDE, with the power for each octave being equal. WHITE NOISE is a noise with both random frequency and amplitude with equal power per bandwidth. White noise is typically encountered as a masking noise, either in psychological experiments where the effects of masking are examined, or in experiments where a constant meaningless acoustic background is required.

nomifensine A drug that inhibits the REUPTAKE of CATECHOLAMINES: both DOPAMINE and NORADRENALINE reuptake are inhibited, though nomifensine has greater potency for noradrenaline .

nominal aphasia An alternative name for ANOMIA.

non-contingent *see* contingency

non-declarative memory *see* multiple memory systems

non-fluent aphasia Part of a clinical dichotomy (vs. FLUENT APHASIA) (Goodglass, 1993). A widely-used clinical description of APHASIA that provides a general characterization of the patient's LANGUAGE disorder based on spontaneous SPEECH PRODUCTION. Speech is slow and effortful. Associated with lesions anterior to the ROLANDIC FISSURE.

See also: Broca's aphasia; transcortical motor aphasia; global aphasia

Reference

Goodglass H. (1993) *Understanding Aphasia*, Academic Press: San Diego.

CHARLOTTE C. MITCHUM

non-NMDA receptors *see* glutamate receptors

non-primary motor cortex *see* motor cortex

non-propositional memory Also known as IMPLICIT MEMORY.

See also: hippocampus

non-pyramidal neuron *see* pyramidal neurons

non-relational memory *see* relational and non-relational memory

non-REM sleep Non-REM sleep is one of the two basic states of SLEEP. The other is REM SLEEP. Non-REM sleep represents the larger portion of total sleep, except in NEONATES. It is characterized by large slow waves in the cortical EEG, absence of movements, elevated sensory thresholds, and decreased autonomic activity. Non-REM sleep is classified into four stages according to the pattern of the EEG, in particular, the amount of slow waves and SLEEP SPINDLES. (Some authors use the term non-REM sleep to refer to all of these stages, reserving the term SLOW WAVE SLEEP for stages 3 and 4, the deepest stages of sleep. Others use the terms non-REM sleep and slow wave sleep as synonyms, each referring to all four stages.) Non-REM sleep is controlled by both FOREBRAIN and MEDULLA, as well as humoural factors. The function of non-REM sleep is thought to be the restoration of bodily functions.

KAZUE SEMBA

non-shivering thermogenesis *see* brown adipose tissue; thermoregulation

non-specific projections Non-specific projections refer to those projections that are neither sensory nor motor in nature. The concept was originally introduced by Moruzzi (1910–1986) and Magoun (1907–1991) in 1949 in their proposal of the ASCENDING RETICULAR ACTIVATING SYSTEM, and further expanded by Jasper (1906–1999), who proposed that the association nuclei of the THALAMUS represent the thalamic reticular system. The general picture that emerged was that AROUSAL is maintained not by specific sensory or motor systems, but by the non-specific system consisting of the reticular structures in the brainstem and the thalamus which provide tonic (sustained) and phasic (short-lasting) arousing influences, respectively, on the CEREBRAL CORTEX.

See also: reticular formation

KAZUE SEMBA

non-synaptic transmission *see* volume transmission

noogenesis (from Greek, *noos*: the mind, *genesis*: creation) Noogenesis is the study of the EVOLUTION of the mind and intellect.

noology (from Greek, *noos*: the mind, *logos*: discourse) Noology is the study of the mind and intellect.

nootropic (from Greek, *noos*: the mind, *tropos*: turning) A nootropic is a DRUG thought to enhance cognition; see COGNITIVE ENHANCERS. Note that it is considered that a nootropic drug should exert its maximal effect in conditions of neural impairment. They are intended to restore function in patients who have some form of neural disability. They are not intended to produce an increase in cleverness and there is little substantive evidence that they have any benefit for healthy individuals

noradrenaline (NA) An alternative name, which originated in the United States, is NOREPINEPHRINE: the names noradrenaline and norepinephrine refer to exactly the same chemical. It is also known as ARTERENOL. Noradrenaline and ADRENALINE were named this way in the United Kingdom, because they

were first synthesized there from tissue taken from the ADRENAL GLAND; the terms epinephrine and norepinephrine were used in the United States because they was first synthesized from tissue taken from the KIDNEY (from Greek, *nephros*: kidney).

Noradrenaline is one of the NEUROTRANSMITTERS; neurons that contain noradrenaline are said to be NORADRENERGIC. It is a CATECHOLAMINE neurotransmitter and therefore a member of the even larger family of MONOAMINE neurotransmitters. The full chemical name for noradrenaline is 3,4-DIHYDROXYPHENYLETHANOLAMINE. Noradrenaline, like DOPAMINE, is synthesized from the amino acid L-TYROSINE. The enzyme TYROSINE HYDROXYLASE catalyses the conversion of tyrosine to L-DOPA (L-3,4-dihydroxyphenylalanine). L-DOPA is then converted by AROMATIC L-AMINO ACID DECARBOXYLASE to dopamine. In dopaminergic neurons, this is as far as the conversion goes, dopamine being transported and packaged for use as a neurotransmitter. However, further conversion of dopamine produces noradrenaline. The presence of the enzyme DOPAMINE BETA-HYDROXYLASE, involved in the conversion of dopamine to noradrenaline, is the principal way to discriminate noradrenaline- from dopamine-containing neurons. In other neurons a further conversion can occur: the enzyme PHENYLETHANOLAMINE-N-METHYLTRANSFERASE is involved in the production of adrenaline from noradrenaline. There are multiple receptors for noradrenaline (see ADRENOCEPTORS). The synaptic action of noradrenaline is terminated in two ways: destruction by enzymes or by REUPTAKE, for which there are specific noradrenaline transporters. As with dopamine catabolism, enzymatic destruction can be achieved by either of two enzymes: MONOAMINE OXIDASE (MAO) or CATECHOL-O-METHYLTRANSFERASE (COMT). (Both MONOAMINE OXIDASE-A and MONOAMINE OXIDASE-B effectively degrade noradrenaline.) Monoamine oxidase destruction of noradrenaline leads to formation of the metabolite 3,4-DIHYDROXYPHENYLGLYCOACETALDEHYDE (DHPGA): ALDEHYDE DEHYDROGENASE further con-verts this to 3,4-DIHYDRODXYMANDELIC ACID (DHMA), which COMT then degrades to VAN-ILLYMANDELIC ACID (VMA).

DHPGA can also be converted by ALDEHYDE REDUCTASE to 3,4-DIHYDROXYPHENYLGLYCOL (DHPG) which COMT converts to 3-METHOXY-4-HYDROXYPHENYLGLYCOL (MHPG). COMT destruction of noradrenaline itself leads to production of the metabolite NORMETANEPHRINE (NMN) which monoamine oxidase can convert to 3-METHOXY-4-HYDROXYPHENYLGLYCOALDEHYDE (MHPGA). MHPG-A can be further converted by aldehyde dehydrogenase to produce a VMA and MHPG. Measurement of the metabolites of noradrenaline (or indeed any other neurochemical) can give important information regarding its synthesis in brain.

In the CENTRAL NERVOUS SYSTEM, noradrenaline neurons have their cell bodies in the PONS and MEDULLA, but axons ascend to innervate an exceptionally large proportion of the central nervous system. There are three principal groups of noradrenaline neurons: the LOCUS COERULEUS complex; the lateral tegmental noradrenaline neurons; and the dorsal medullary noradrenaline neurons. (An older terminology discussed these in terms of the DORSAL NORADRENERGIC BUNDLE [from the locus coeruleus] and the VENTRAL NORADRENERGIC BUNDLE [including the lateral tegmental and dorsal medullary neurons]). These neurons were first characterized using HISTOFLUORESCENCE techniques and were catalogued using the CLASSIFICATION OF DAHLSTRÖM & FUXE. The functions of noradrenaline neurons are many and varied, as one would expect for neurons that project so widely through the central nervous system. In biological psychology, the neurons of the locus coeruleus have been associated with ATTENTION, MEMORY and with the regulation of SLEEP, while the pontine and medullary neurons have been associated with a variety of AUTONOMIC processes, including the control of FEEDING. Noradrenaline neurons *en masse* are though to be an essential component of the ASCENDING RETICULAR ACTIVATING SYSTEM. In the PERIPHERAL NERVOUS SYSTEM, noradrenaline is the neurotransmitter for the postganglionic sympathetic neurons (see AUTONOMIC NERVOUS SYSTEM). In addition, the CHROMAFFIN CELLS of the ADRENAL GLAND secreted both noradrenaline and adrenaline. The action of noradrenaline released from here is more like that of a hormone rather than a neurotransmitter, in that it diffuses around the body in the blood, binding to any appropriate receptors contacted (see FIGHT-OR-FLIGHT; STRESS).

Reference

Feldman R., Meyer J.S. & Quenzer L.F. (1997) *Principles of Neuropsychopharmacology*, Sinauer Associates: Sunderland MA.

noradrenaline receptors *see* adrenoceptors

noradrenergic Relating to the neurotransmitter NORADRENALINE. For instance, a neuron that synthesizes and releases noradrenaline is said to be noradrenergic.

norepinephrine *see* noradrenaline

norepinephrine receptors *see* adrenoceptors

normetanephrine *see* noradrenaline

Northern blotting *see* blotting

nose poke vs. lever press Rats are trained in OPERANT paradigms to explore a wide variety of psychological functions. The classic operant response is a lever press, popularized by the SKINNER BOX, but any trained behaviour can be the operant response. In a NINE-HOLE BOX, rats are trained to make nose pokes, which can be advantageous: even requiring that the rat hold a lever down does not greatly restrict its movement, but in making a nose poke, the rat must maintain a relatively still posture and is in a known orientation. This is particularly useful for measuring REACTION TIME or for observing reactions to lateralized stimuli.

VERITY J. BROWN

nosology (from Greek, *nosos*: disease, *logos*: discourse) The systematic study and classification of diseases.

6/6 notation This notation expresses the ability to resolve visually fine details (see VISUAL ACUITY). It is commonly used to indicate how well an observer performs in a standardized eyesight test (see SNELLEN LETTERS). The numerator is the distance in metres at which the test was conducted (here standardized at 6 metres) and the denominator the distance at which the smallest resolvable letters would subtend 5 minutes of arc. The pre-metrication notation was referenced on a standardized viewing distance of 20 feet and led to the common expression '20/20 vision'.

DAVID W. HEELEY

notochord *see* neurodevelopment

nuclear magnetic resonance imaging *see* magnetic resonance imaging

nuclei of the lateral lemniscus *see* auditory pathways; lateral lemniscus

nucleic acid A nucleic acid is composed of a string of NUCLEOTIDES connected by chemical bonds (specifically, phosphodiester bonds). RI-BONUCLEIC ACID (RNA) and DEOXYRIBONU-CLEIC ACID (DNA) are nucleic acids.

nucleolus A component of the NUCLEUS of a CELL; it is composed of CHROMOSOMES and important for the generation of RIBOSOMES.

See also: subcellular organs

nucleosides Five-carbon SUGARS with a phosphate base; do not confuse these molecules with NUCLEOTIDES.

nucleotides Nucleotides are the building blocks of a NUCLEIC ACID, of which the most notable are RIBONUCLEIC ACID (RNA) and DEOXYRIBONUCLEIC ACID (DNA). The latter contains the nucleotides adenine, thymine, guanine, and cytosine: in RNA, thymidine is substituted by uracil. They are five-carbon sugars bonded to nitrogen bases with phosphate groups attached; not to be confused with NUCLEOSIDES.

nucleus of the optic tract *see* accessory optic system

nucleus (i) *Cellular*: A large dense structure within a EUKARYOTE cell, in which the DEOX-YRIBONUCLEIC ACID (DNA) is separated from the CYTOPLASM. The nucleus is enveloped by two semipermeable membranes (see MEM-BRANE). The nucleus is the site at which DNA is translated into RIBONUCLEIC ACID (RNA). The RNA then enters the cytoplasm, where PROTEINS are made. See also, GENE.
(ii) *Anatomical*: A cluster of neuronal cell bodies within the brain. Cells within a nucleus may be defined on the basis of a common feature, such as histochemical staining, or biochemical marker, or by a common function. (iii) *Atomic*: The nucleus of an ATOM contains a proton and a neutron; see ATOM.

FIONA M. INGLIS

nucleus abducens The nucleus abducens is a motor nucleus in the caudal PONS that contains cell bodies of MOTOR NEURONS whose axons form the abducens or sixth cranial nerve (see CRANIAL NERVES). The abducens nerve innervates the lateral rectus muscle of the eye, which is involved in deviating the eyeball laterally (abduction). The nucleus abducens receives input from the vestibular nuclei and the paramedian pontine RETICULAR FORMATION which are involved in balance and control of head and eye movement. Injury to the abducens nerve causes paralysis of the lateral rectus muscle on the side of injury, causing DIPLOPIA or double vision due to strong deviation of the eye.

KAZUE SEMBA

nucleus accumbens The nucleus accumbens is the prominent component of the ventral striatum (the others being the olfactory tubercle and ventral parts of the caudate and putamen) (see STRIATUM). It is now accepted that the nucleus accumbens is a heterogeneous structure containing at least three distinct sub-territories. These are: (1) a central 'core' which envelops the ANTERIOR COMMISSURE and has a CYTOARCHITECTURE identical with that of the overlying dorsal striatum with which it merges imperceptibly. (2) A medial 'shell' which surrounds the core on its medial, ventral and lateral sides. The core and shell are found predominantly in the caudal three-quarters of the nucleus accumbens in the rat brain. (3) A 'rostral pole' which is characterized by a blend of histochemical features, afferent and efferent connections that suggest it is comprised of both core and shell components. Within the core, populations of GABAERGIC MEDIUM SPINY NEU-RONS having the phenotype of similar neurons in the caudate and putamen are found, namely those expressing SUBSTANCE P and the D1 dopamine receptors (see D1–D5 DOPAMINE RECEPTORS) and others expressing ENKEPHALIN and the D2 receptor. There is some evidence of a patch and matrix organization within the nucleus accumbens, but this is not as readily visible as it is in the dorsal striatum.

Cortical afferents to the nucleus accumbens arise in the allocortical (see ALLOCORTEX) or 'limbic cortical' sites, particularly the basolateral AMYGDALA, ventral and dorsal subiculum components of the HIPPOCAMPAL FORMATION and specific parts of the anterior cortex, such as the PRELIMBIC CORTEX, and also the anterior CINGULATE CORTEX. These afferents terminate in distinct subterritories of the nucleus accumbens. For example, the basolateral amygdala projects mainly, but not exclusively, to the core region of the nucleus accumbens; the ventral subiculum projects especially to the dorsal parts of the medial shell region. The nucleus accumbens receives a dense dopaminergic innervation arising in the dopamine neurons of the VENTRAL TEGMENTAL AREA (via the MESOLIMBIC DOPAMINE SYSTEM) and also afferents from the intralaminar and midline nuclei of the THALAMUS. There is a significant serotoninergic input to the nucleus accumbens arising from the midbrain RAPHE NUCLEI and also a noradrenergic innervation arising in the LOCUS COERULEUS. The core and shell compartments of the nucleus accumbens have distinctive efferent connections. Fibres from the core project to the dorsolateral ventral pallidum, the ENTOPEDUNCULAR NUCLEUS (in the rat and which is homologous to the internal pallidal segment in the primate) and SUBSTANTIA NIGRA pars compacta. The shell of the nucleus accumbens, and also the rostral pole, project to ventromedial parts of the ventral pallidum, entopeduncular nucleus, ventral tegmental area and substantia nigra pars compacta. The shell also gives rise to 'atypical' (so far as the striatum is concerned) projections that reach the EXTENDED AMYGDALA and lateral PREOPTIC AREA – lateral hypothalamic continuum. The rostral pole and shell also project to the MESOPONTINE portions of the RETICULAR FORMATION and midbrain PERIAQUEDUCTAL GREY.

BARRY J. EVERITT

nucleus ambiguus The nucleus ambiguus is a motor nucleus of the CRANIAL NERVES located in the ventrolateral MEDULLA OBLONGATA. It is so named because it lacks clear boundaries that distinguish it from the surrounding medullary RETICULAR FORMATION. The nucleus consists of four main sub-nuclei or formations: the compact (oesophageal motor neurons), the semi-compact (pharyngeal motor neurons), the loose (laryngeal motor neurons) and external (cardiopulmonary) formations. The nucleus innervates the striated musculature of the upper respiratory and alimentary tracts via the ninth and tenth cranial nerves and the cranial rootlets of the eleventh cranial nerve and is involved in swallowing, respiration and cardiopulmonary functions.

DAVID A. HOPKINS

nucleus basalis of Meynert Named after the German neuroanatomist Meynert (1833–1892) the nucleus of Meynert is a nucleus in the caudal part of the BASAL FOREBRAIN. It is also referred to as the MAGNOCELLULAR BASAL NUCLEUS because it contains a cluster of magnocellular or large neurons with multiple dendrites. These are CHOLINERGIC neurons, and are part of the cholinergic cell column in the basal forebrain. The cholinergic neurons in the nucleus basalis of Meynert innervate the NEOCORTEX through medial and lateral pathways, and provide the major source of ACETYLCHOLINE to the cortex. The degeneration of these cholinergic neurons is a neuropathological hallmark of ALZHEIMER'S DEMENTIA.

KAZUE SEMBA

nucleus cuneatus The nucleus cuneatus, in the lower MEDULLA, is a SOMATOSENSORY nucleus that relays information about discriminative TOUCH and PROPRIOCEPTION. Together with the NUCLEUS GRACILIS, it forms the posterior column nuclei, with the nucleus gracilis being the smaller and more medially located of the two. Both nuclei receive axons from the first-order sensory neurons in the DORSAL ROOT GANGLIA. The nucleus cuneatus receives information from the information from the upper part of the body; information from the lower part (the trunk and lower limbs) is directed to the nucleus gracilis. The axons of the second-order neurons in these nuclei give rise to the MEDIAL LEMNISCUS which ascends to the THALAMUS.

nucleus gigantocellularis *see* medullary reticular formation

nucleus gracilis The nucleus gracilis is a SOMATOSENSORY nucleus in the lower MEDULLA that relays information about discriminative TOUCH and PROPRIOCEPTION. Together with the NUCLEUS CUNEATUS, it forms the posterior column nuclei, with the nucleus gracilis being the smaller and more medially located of the two. Both nuclei receive axons from the first-order sensory neurons in the DORSAL ROOT GANGLIA. The nucleus gracilis receives information from the lower part of the body (the trunk and lower limbs), while information from the upper part is directed to the nucleus cuneatus. The axons of the second-order neurons in these nuclei give rise to the MEDIAL LEMNISCUS which ascends to the THALAMUS.

KAZUE SEMBA

nucleus of the solitary tract (nucleus tractus solitarius) A nucleus (actually a pair of nuclei) in the MEDULLA that receives and integrates taste sensation (see GUSTATION) as well as visceral sensory signals. The nucleus of the solitary tract belongs to a class of integrative BRAINSTEM nuclei which combine together diverse sources of information from several nuclei of the CRANIAL NERVES. The information is integrated to a degree within the nucleus, and then passed on either to other structures within the brainstem that control reflexive responses, or upwards to the forebrain for further processing.

The solitary tract, in which the nucleus of the solitary tract sits, is a band of fibres near the midline at the top of medulla oblongata. The nuclei themselves are positioned like a pair of cigars laid at the top of the medulla, within the solitary tract, running from front to back. The two nuclei almost converge together at the midline at their most caudal points, but angle outwards slightly as they run forward, forming a V shape together. The front section of the nucleus of the solitary tract is sometimes referred to as the gustatory or taste nucleus. Taste sensory neurons project from the tongue and palate to this section of the nucleus of the solitary tract through two cranial nerves. The FACIAL NERVE (seventh cranial nerve) carries fibres from taste receptors located in the front and middle regions of the tongue. The GLOSSOPHARYNGEAL NERVE (ninth cranial nerve) carries fibres from receptors located at the back of the tongue and the palate. Both nerves project to gustatory neurons within the anterior one-third of the nucleus of the solitary tract. Within this nucleus, an array of neurotransmitters are found: glutamate, GABA, ENKEPHALIN, CHOLECYSTOKININ, and NEUROPEPTIDE Y, among others.

Electrophysiological recording studies have shown that neurons in the anterior nucleus code sweet, salty, sour, and bitter taste qualities in a FUZZY SET fashion. A given neuron is likely to respond to more than one taste quality, and often responds to several. Such a degree of broad tuning for gustatory neurons has been interpreted to mean that taste quality, unlike other sensory features such as auditory pitch or visual space, is not precisely coded within the brain according to a labelled-line coding scheme (see LABELLED-LINE THEORY) in which a particular taste would only activate a narrow set of neurons or 'labelled lines' corresponding to its taste quality. However, although each gustatory neuron within the nucleus can be activated by many different tastes, each neuron is activated to a higher degree by certain tastes than by others. There exist sucrose-best, salt-best, sour-best and bitter-best classes of neurons within the nucleus of the solitary tract, in the sense that these classes of neurons are activated to the greatest degree by that particular taste quality. This has given rise to the fuzzy set or ACROSS-FIBRE PATTERN THEORY of taste coding, which suggests that it is the particular pattern of firing across all gustatory neurons which determines the taste that is perceived. Although almost all tastes will activate almost all neurons, the pattern of firing across neurons will be slightly different and specific to each taste. This is a considerably more complex type of sensory code than simple labelled lines, and it is not yet clear how forebrain gustatory structures translate the fuzzy set code, although they must do so.

The nucleus of the solitary tract not only codes taste sensory quality, but may also begin to process taste palatability or pleasantness.

There are two types of evidence that indicate palatability is recognized to some degree by neurons in or around the nucleus of the solitary tract. One type of evidence is electrophysiological: neurons in the nucleus of the solitary tract that code a sweet taste may alter their firing patterns to that taste if it has been made less palatable, either by making the animal less hungry by prior feeding, or by producing a conditioned aversion to that taste by pairing it associatively with nausea. The second type of evidence is behavioural: DE-CEREBRATE animals, which lack all FOREBRAIN structures and can only respond reflexively using their brainstem, including the nucleus of the solitary tract, are still able to discriminate in their behavioural responses to basic palatability. Such decerebrates still swallow a sweet taste and lick their lips if the taste is placed on their tongue, but they violently reject a bitter taste. This behavioural discrimination indicates that neurons within the brainstem, including those within the nucleus of the solitary tract, are still able to decode acceptable from unacceptable taste qualities, and to make a rudimentary decision to respond appropriately.

The caudal parts of the nucleus of the solitary tract receive sensory inputs via the VAGUS NERVE from the visceral organs: intestines, liver, kidneys, heart and so on. For example, illness that produces gastrointestinal distress can activate neurons in the middle portion of the nucleus of the solitary tract. Perhaps most important among the physiological functions of the nucleus, however, are the control of basic functions such as heartbeat and breathing. The respiratory rhythm of ordinary breathing is controlled to a large degree by neural circuits originating in the nucleus of the solitary tract. Lesions of the caudal portion of the nucleus are typically fatal in consequence because they disrupt the rhythm and produce suffocation.

KENT C. BERRIDGE

nucleus raphe magnus The nucleus raphe magnus is a raphe nucleus located in the ventral tegmentum of the caudal PONS and rostral MEDULLA. Like other RAPHE NUCLEI, the nucleus raphe magnus contains SEROTONIN neurons, and these are part of the B3 serotonin cell group (see CLASSIFICATION OF DAHLSTRÖM AND FUXE). A small percentage of these neurons also contain GABA. Serotonin neurons in the nucleus raphe magnus project, via the dorsolateral fasciculus, to the superficial layers (laminae one and two) of the DORSAL HORN of the SPINAL CORD. This pathway is involved in antinociception or suppression of PAIN, and mediates the supraspinal antinociceptive actions of MORPHINE and certain ENDOGENOUS OPIATES or opioids.

KAZUE SEMBA

nucleus raphe pontis *see* raphe nuclei

nucleus ruber Latin name for the RED NUCLEUS.

nutrients (from Latin, *nutrire*: to nourish) A nutrient is any substance that feeds or nourishes an organism, including PROTEINS, FAT, CARBOHYDRATE and others. An animal's DIET must include material necessary for the continued production of a wide variety of MOLECULE types that are internally synthesized. There are in addition *essential nutrients* that cannot be synthesized by a body and which must therefore be ingested in 'ready made' form. What constitutes an essential nutrient varies across species: for humans vitamin C (ASCORBIC ACID) is an essential nutrient, but many other animals it is not. There are a variety of ESSENTIAL AMINO ACIDS, ESSENTIAL FATTY ACIDS, VITAMINS and MINERALS that fall into the category of essential nutrients.

nychthemeron (from Greek, *nyktos*: night, *hemera*: day) A nychthemeron is one complete day–night cycle; nychthemeral is the adjective describing this.

See also: biological clock

nystagmus (from Greek, *nystazein*: to nap) A regular involuntary repetitive movement of the EYES. There are various forms. *Caloric nystagmus* is produced by placing hot or cold water in the ear, generating a vestibulo-ocular reflex (see VESTIBULAR-OCULAR INTERACTIONS). *Central nystagmus* is caused by damage to the CENTRAL NERVOUS SYSTEM components of the VESTIBULAR SYSTEM. *Jerk nystagmus* features alternating fast and slow movements.

Labyrinthine nystagmus is caused specifically by damage to the vestibular labyrinth (see VESTIBULAR SYSTEM). *Optokinetic nystagmus* describes the switching between a SMOOTH FOLLOWING MOVEMENT and a SACCADE in the opposite direction that operate when the VISUAL FIELD is in constant motion (for example, when observing from a moving vehicle): smooth movements allow FIXATION to be retained as long as possible, saccades permit fixation on another object as the original visual target disappears from view. *Pendular nystagmus* features movements of the same speed in each direction (like a pendulum). *Physiological nystagmus* involves involuntary movements that occur during fixation, composed of short drifts and TREMOR-like movements that occur randomly, plus MICROSACCADE returns to the FIXATION POINT. *vestibular nystagmus* describes any form of nystagmus associated with the vestibular system.

O

ob/ob mouse A mutant, genetically obese mouse: *ob* is a RECESSIVE ALLELE, *Ob* a DOMINANT ALLELE. Only the *ob/ob* homozygous recessive displays OBESITY. This mutant has been important in showing that BROWN ADIPOSE TISSUE dysfunction contributes to obesity, and that LEPTIN is an important signal from fat cells to brain.

See also: Zucker rats

obdurator *see* microinjection

obesity State characterized by an excess of body fat. Clinical measures of obesity are achieved using methods including skinfold thickness, underwater weighing, total body potassium, bioelectrical impedance, computer imaging (for example COMPUTERIZED AXIAL TOMOGRAPHY or MAGNETIC RESONANCE IMAGING scans) and the Quetelet or BODY MASS INDEX (BMI). Measures of adiposity may provide either whole-body composition or specific organ values (see Heymsfield *et al.*, 1995). However, for convenience, body mass index [wt (kg) / ht (m)^2] and standard height and weight tables are typically consulted to assess level of obesity relative to the general population. Normal weight is defined as BMI between 20 and 24.9, overweight from 25 to 29.9, obese from 30 to 40 and morbid obesity greater than a BMI of 40. Standard weight tables identify normal or ideal weight according to the population average for gender, height, and age with overweight as a percentage of ideal between 110 and 120% and obese as greater than 120% of ideal. Problems with these definitions arise when applied to indivi-

duals since some tables do no accurately reflect population norms (many are from North America and apply less well elsewhere, and some are from insurance companies) and they fail to take account of changes in body weight as a function of AGEING. Also, a BMI greater than 30 can occur in athletes who have a significant proportion of body composition as fat-free mass. Nevertheless, in the general population morbidity and mortality rates increase as a function of degree of overweight.

The prevalence of obesity is increasing in Western countries. In Great Britain from 1980 to 1987, the proportion of overweight or obese adults (aged 16–64) increased from 39% to 45% of men and from 32% to 36% of women. In the USA the prevalence of frank obesity increased between 1980 and 1995 from 25% to 34%. The medical consequences associated with obesity include DIABETES, HYPERTENSION, hypercholesterolemia, hypertriglyceridemia, cardiovascular disease, gallbladder disease, arthritis, and respiratory disease. However, regional adiposity is a better predictor of risk to health than BMI. ENERGY stores are determined by the balance between the amount of energy expended (in physical activity, THERMOGENESIS and resting METABOLISM) and the amount of energy consumed. Thus, during a static state of weight maintenance, energy intake is equal to energy expenditure, whereas during weight loss or weight gain, negative or positive energy balance is achieved by changes in the rates of energy intake to energy expenditure. For example, long-term energy restriction coupled with increased physical activity should result in negative energy balance and therefore weight loss. However, this relationship is influenced by genetic endowment and differential rates of oxidation and storage of different nutrients.

Studies of the aetiology of obesity have focused on both metabolic abnormalities and on evidence of overeating which might underlie pathogenesis. Psychological approaches to the treatment of obesity focus on changing eating behaviour and increasing physical activity. Clear evidence that the obese overeat relative to the non-obese has not been forthcoming. However, in part this may be due to methods of measuring food intake both in the laboratory where the demand characteristics of the study might produce artificially lower intakes and in free living conditions, where diet records, dietary recall and weighed intakes might result in under-reporting.

Classic studies by Stanley Schachter in the 1960s proposed that obese consumers differ from normal weight consumers in their responsiveness to external factors in determining when and how much to eat rather than responding to internal cues such as changes in blood glucose levels (see INTERNALITY). However, studies by Judith Rodin later concluded that EXTERNALITY is not determined by BODY WEIGHT, rather external responsiveness occurs across body weight categories. In addition, work by C. Peter Herman and his colleagues further refined assumptions about obese/normal weight differences by focusing on RESTRAINED EATING. Thus, differences in eating behaviour may be accounted for by the degree to which consumers restrict their eating below a desired level. Restrained eating can be associated with successful dieting and long-term normal weight maintenance, but it is also associated with episodes of overeating and lack of restraint. It has been suggested that chronic dieting, overeating and long-term weight fluctuations may characterize a sub-population of the obese and that there is no evidence of an obese eating style. Obesity involves excess body fat and is linked to increased risk of ill health. Behavioural therapies for obesity focus on reducing energy intake and increasing exercise, however, the success of such treatments may be influenced by genetic predisposition,

metabolic inputs as well as the psychological effects of chronic dieting.

See also: feeding; hunger

Reference

Heymsfield S.B., Allison D.B., Heshka S. & Pierson R.N. (1995) Assessment of Human Body Composition. In *Handbook of Assessment Methods for Eating Behaviors and Weight-Related Problems*, ed. D.B. Allison, pp. 575–560, Sage: Thousand Oaks CA.

MARION M. HETHERINGTON

object agnosia The ability to derive meaning from what we see is a fundamental part of the world we experience. Object identification requires an exceedingly complex series of operations beginning with the image on the RETINA: our VISUAL SYSTEM must take the very restricted sensory input falling on a tiny patch of neural tissue at the back of the eye, extract edges and visible surfaces, and from this representation produce a geometric description of what is seen that is not limited to any particular vantage point of the observer. The extraction of invariant object form that remains independent of viewpoint is only one half of the problem; to identify what is seen, visual form must be imbued with meaning. In order to better construe the nature of the difficulty, we can think of the task facing the brain as one that entails a mapping from one kind of abstract mathematical space – in which the physical structure of the object is specified, regardless of orientation and shading precisely enough to distinguish it from all other solid objects that also have a possible representation in this space – to another kind of abstract space in which the significance of the object as a concept is determined, again in such a way as to distinguish it from the representation of every other object concept that also exists in this space. Furthermore, this mapping can operate bi-directionally: we can take a word referring to an object, and from the meaning access some kind of description of the object's physical structure which we can then visualize, either by drawing it or by an internal process commonly referred to as mental imagery.

Object agnosia refers to a disorder of the higher-level mechanisms that extract a coherent percept of the object and map this representation to meaning. Our preliminary remarks suggest two broad subtypes: (1) impairments of the mechanism responsible for perceptual synthesis of the form of an object across different viewpoints, resulting in an agnosia that is traditionally designated as apperceptive visual agnosia, and (2) ASSOCIATIVE AGNOSIA, in which the fully integrated percept of the object is not assigned the correct meaning. In addition, agnosia can occur in other modalities besides vision; cases have been described with TACTILE AGNOSIA, in which objects cannot be recognized by TOUCH despite normal sensory capabilities, with no corresponding impairment observed in the visual modality, or AUDITORY AGNOSIA, where the disturbance in confined to the identification of sounds.

See also: object recognition

DANIEL N. BUB

object constancy Object constancy refers to a perceptual phenomenon: particular objects are always seen as being those particular objects despite changes in the conditions in and under which they are perceived. (For example, the location or lighting conditions under which they are seen.) SHAPE CONSTANCY refers to the fact that the shape of the object is always perceived correctly, despite changes in the angle from which it is viewed; SIZE CONSTANCY relates to the fact that knowledge about the size of an object is always correctly detected, despite the fact that the size of the image on the RETINA will vary with distance.

See also: colour constancy; sensation vs. perception

object primitives *see* haptic

object recognition The environment that we live in has a wide spread of things that we can readily identify. This act of identification is called object recognition. It does not necessarily mean that we can name the thing in question, but does mean that we are able to make an appropriate response to it. We use the term 'object' to refer to a wide assortment of different types of visual event, but they all share some common attributes. All visual objects are spatially defined and circumscribed so that they occupy volume in the scene; they tend to be solid and bounded by a distinct surface.

The process of recognition of an object essentially involves the action of matching an incoming perceptual representation of an object with an internally held specification. For example, in recognizing some object as a chair the perceptual process will generate a description of the image of the object in terms of the surfaces that it has and their spatial arrangement. This description will then be compared against a set of features that all (or at least the majority of) chairs have, such as a flat horizontal surface of appropriate size held at an appropriate height by a number of upright legs. If the description compares well then, a judgement that the object is a chair can be made with reasonable confidence. There is a specific problem in the process of object recognition. The image of an object, and its visual appearance, depend to a very considerable extent on the circumstances of the object: how it is illuminated, what direction it is being viewed from; what its surroundings are. Thus the information that is to be used to recognize the object is highly variable.

There are various possible versions of the process of object recognition which differ in the types of information that is being compared. At one extreme it is possible that the comparison process could involve matching 2-dimensional templates of objects against the image to find the template that matches best. In this case the template is effectively a single complex feature. The drawback with this approach is that the natural variability of objects would far exceed the capacity of any template. Thus a specific chair might well be recognizable from its match to a template of itself, but not any other. At the other extreme, it is possible that a description of the object made up of a large number of small features could be computed from the incoming information and then this compared with an equivalent full internal structural description. The drawback to this approach is that the process of creating a full structural description of the image of the object is itself highly complex.

See also: object agnosia; object constancy

ROGER J. WATT

object recognition memory *see* multiple memory systems

observation learning The acquisition of some novel behaviour solely by observing the behaviour of another animal, usually a CONSPECIFIC. There are many potential causes. The presence of a conspecific may produce social facilitation – for example, a satiated chick will eat if it sees others doing so; it may also direct the observer's ATTENTION to some aspect of the environment, thus aiding LEARNING. An animal may also form a PAVLOVIAN ASSOCIATION between a CONDITIONED STIMULUS (CS) and an UNCONDITIONED STIMULUS (US) by observation. There is little evidence that an instrumental association between a response and a US can form this way, possibly because this would require the observer to identify the observed response with its own actions. Nevertheless, the occurrence of vocal imitation in animals suggests that observational learning of an instrumental association between a vocal response and reward might be possible, perhaps as here this identification process is easier. Some investigators treat observation learning synonymously with PERCEPTUAL LEARNING.

See also: instrumental conditioning; Pavlovian conditioning

CHARLOTTE BONARDI

obsession A recurrent, intrusive thought that, though recognized as senseless, foolish or unpleasant, cannot be banished from consciousness, despite the sufferer's wish and efforts to do so. Thoughts may take any form, but often have a sexual or violent content that the sufferer finds repugnant. As a rule, such thoughts are not acted upon.

See also: obsessive compulsive disorder

IAN C. REID

obsessive compulsive disorder (OCD) A neurotic disorder (see NEUROSIS) characterized by OBSESSION, often associated with compulsive ritual acts. Sufferers experience repeated thoughts which intrude on their consciousness unbidden. The thoughts are often unpleasant, and though recognized as foolish or pointless, the subject feels compelled to act them out. The content of obsessional thoughts varies widely, ranging across sexual or violent impulses, fears of contamination and pathological doubting to more vague, meaningless preoccupations. Compulsions are repeated actions based on the obsessional thoughts, which suffers again try, but are unable, to resist. Compulsions may take the form of counting rituals, checking rituals, cleaning rituals (such as repeated handwashing) and obsessional slowness. The carrying out of compulsive acts is not in itself pleasurable. Rather, such acts are frustrating and may prove highly time-consuming and disabling. Sufferers prevented from pursuing rituals may become extremely anxious, though any relief from ANXIETY by engaging in a compulsive act is short-lived.

The condition usually begins in early adulthood, and most surveys indicate that women are slightly more likely to be affected than men. OCD tends to be a chronic, continuous, condition. It is likely that many sufferers do not come to medical attention, and estimates of prevalence vary widely. Contemporary surveys suggest that the disorder may be more common than previously thought, with a lifetime prevalence of between 2 and 3%. The aetiology of the condition is unknown. FUNCTIONAL NEUROIMAGING studies implicate fronto-striatal abnormalities, and successful treatment with ANTIDEPRESSANT drugs – particularly serotonin selective reuptake inhibitors (SSRI) – suggests SEROTONERGIC dysfunction may play a role. Treatment is usually a combination of pharmacological and psychological therapies. SSRI antidepressants, and the TRICYCLIC clomipramine are frequently used. Exposure therapy (response prevention) with relaxation training, and COGNITIVE THERAPY have been employed with success. Though estimates of outcome vary, approximately 50% of sufferers appear to respond well to treatment. Severely disabling, chronic and intractable OCD is one of the few indications for PSYCHOSURGERY. There are recognized associations with DEPRESSION and TOURETTE'S SYNDROME.

IAN C. REID

obstructive apnoea Brief episodes of APNOEA produced by relaxation of MUSCLES in the throat obstructing passage of air. It is typically associated with snoring or other breathing difficulty (see BREATHING, NEURAL CONTROL OF) and, while not usually life-threatening, causes SLEEP disruption which can badly affect daily routines.

occipital bone *see* skull

occipital lobe The cerebral CORTEX is divided into four LOBES. The occipital lobe is located at the posterior end of the cortex and is separated from the PARIETAL LOBE by the parietal-occipital sulcus. The very posterior pole of the lobe contains the PRIMARY VISUAL CORTEX and damage to this region leaves primates (including humans) phenomenally blind though residual visual function can be demonstrated (termed BLINDSIGHT). The rest of the lobe also contains areas that process visual information (though visual areas are not confined to this lobe).

See also: areas V1–V5; visual system

ROBERT J. SNOWDEN

occluding contour *see* edge detection

occlusion (from Latin, *occludere*: to shut) To occlude something is to block it; an occlusion is that which forms the blockage, regardless of whether that something is in (for example) a BLOOD vessel or a CANNULA.

occupancy Occupancy describes the proportion of RECEPTORS to which a DRUG is bound: maximal occupancy implies binding to all available receptors.

See also: efficacy

octopamine Octopamine is a MONOAMINE neurotransmitter but, very unusually, it is present only in INVERTEBRATES. It appears to act in a way homologous with NORADRENALINE in the nervous system of VERTEBRATES; noradrenaline is not functionally active in invertebrate nervous systems. This point of difference between vertebrate and invertebrate nervous systems is most unusual. There are no other differences in either monoamine or amino acid NEUROTRANSMITTERS between vertebrates and invertebrates, and many NEURO-

PEPTIDES are commonly used by both. Why there should be a difference in this instance is not entirely clear.

Reference

Roeder T. (1999) Octopamine in vertebrates. *Progress in Neurobiology* 59: 533–561.

ocular Literally 'of the eye'.

DAVID W. HEELEY

ocular apraxia An inability to maintain visual FIXATION on an object: poor visual scanning in which the eyes wander off-target.

See also: ataxia; Balint's syndrome

ocular dominance Nerves from CORRESPONDING RETINAL POINTS in each eye converge onto BINOCULAR cells in the VISUAL CORTEX. Cells with strong ocular dominance receive excitatory inputs from only one eye and inhibitory inputs from the other. Other cells have weak ocular dominance while others have equal inputs from the eyes. Cells with right-eye and left-eye dominance form alternating ocular-dominance columns (see CORTICAL COLUMNS AND HYPERCOLUMNS) across the visual cortex. Columns develop from competition between left and right eye inputs in the infant. SQUINT disrupts their development and the development of STEREODEPTH PERCEPTION.

Reference

Howard I.P. & Rogers B.J. (1995) *Binocular Vision and Stereopsis*, Oxford University Press: New York.

IAN P. HOWARD

oculomotor The oculomotor system is the neuromuscular complex involved in the control of the position and tension of the eye muscles and hence the degree of convergence and direction of the optic axes and the accommodative state of the eye.

DAVID W. HEELEY

oculomotor apraxia An inability to shift gaze to an object when it appears in the visual field; sometimes referred to as part of PSYCHIC PARALYSIS OF GAZE which also involves OPTIC ATAXIA.

oculomotor nerve The third cranial nerve (see CRANIAL NERVES) controls EYE MOVEMENTS, including muscular movement of the eyelid and pupillary movements.

oddball task (Also known as the *oddball test* or *oddball paradigm*, or the *oddity problem*.) This is a discrimination test in which subjects are required to detect a low-probability target stimulus randomly presented amongst other more frequent stimuli. The stimuli can be presented in any modality, though auditory and visual stimuli are the most commonly used. Studies of EVENT-RELATED POTENTIALS using the ELECTROENCEPHALOGRAM have shown that the P300 occurs in response to significant low-probability events. It is a widely used task, suitable for testing both adults and children and has been used to examine both normal subjects and patients with a variety of different conditions.

odorant (typically spelled using the American version: *odor* rather than *odour*) An ODORANT is any substance which stimulates the OLFACTORY SYSTEM (see STEREOCHEMICAL THEORY OF ODOUR DISCRIMINATION).

See also: odorimetry

odorimetry The measurement of the strength and quality of odours. It is an important field of activity, both experimentally and practically. The following terms are encountered: an ODORANT is the substance which stimulates the OLFACTORY SYSTEM (see STEREOCHEMICAL THEORY OF ODOUR DISCRIMINATION); the *odour character* (or *odour quality*) is the property of one odorant that permits it to be discriminated from other odorants; the *odour descriptor* is a term used in human olfactory discrimination that describes the odour (perfume manufacturers have many terms which describe the scents they produce); *odour pervasiveness* describes the rate of decline in odour concentration that accompanies reduction in the concentration of the odorant. This is a quality that can be objectively discriminated in animals as well as in humans using a discrimination task in which responses are required when odours are detected; *odour threshold* is defined as the concentration of an odorant required for

half of a sample of testers (human or animal) to detect the odor.

odour aversion learning Odour aversion learning is the same thing as FOOD-AVERSION LEARNING, but relates to the presentation of an odour rather than the ingestion of food.

See also: olfaction

oedema (American spelling: EDEMA) (from Greek, *oidema*: swelling) A pathological accumulation of fluid in tissue; the adjective used to describe such accumulation is oedematous (or American, edematous).

oesophagous *see* mouth; digestive system

oestradiol *see* estradiol

oestrogens *see* estrogens

oestrus *see* estrus

off the baseline *see* baseline

7-OH-DPAT 7-hydroxydipropylaminotetralin; in speech this is usually referred to as '7 hydroxy d pat'. It is an AGONIST at the D3 dopamine receptor; see D1–D5 DOPAMINE RECEPTORS.

See also: 8-OH-DPAT

8-OH-DPAT 8-hydroxydipropylaminotetralin; in speech this is usually referred to as '8 hydroxy d pat'. It is an agonist at the 5HT1A receptor.

See also: serotonin receptors; 7-OH-DPAT

oleic acid One of the FATTY ACIDS.

See also: triglycerides

olfaction Commonly known as the sense of smell, olfaction is the sensory process that detects and responds to airborne chemical stimuli. The human sense of smell is very sensitive to certain odourants with detection levels as low as a few parts per trillion parts of air (green pepper odour for example). Thresholds for odour detection span approximately 10^{12} orders of magnitude. The physicochemical events that determine human olfactory sensitivity apply equally well to animal sensitivities. However the absolute sensitivity of most mammals is orders of magnitude greater than in humans. This is primarily related to the number of receptors in the olfactory mucosa, being in the order of 100 million in rabbit contrasting with 10 million in human.

The structure of the nose varies from a simple sac in salamanders, frogs and tortoises to a more complex structure in mammals, almost completely occupied by the TURBINATE BONES, which bear the OLFACTORY EPITHELIUM. Within this epithelium the receptor neurons are arranged in a mosaic between supporting cells, and overlie a single layer of basal cells. The receptor neurons have apical cilia entering the mucous layer which is secreted from the Bowman's glands, and their unmyelinated axons synapse in complex GLOMERULI in the OLFACTORY BULB. Cilia have long been established as a feature of the olfactory neuron and emphasis has been placed on their role in the perception of odours. They increase the surface area of the receptor-cell surface, and are believed to contain the seven-transmembrane receptors for odorant ligands (see LIGAND).

Most mammals, the exceptions being higher primates, possess a functionally well-developed dual olfactory system. The main olfactory system has its neural receptors located in the nasal cavity. These give rise to axons which ascend into the cranial cavity through the CRIBRIFORM PLATE to synapse on MITRAL CELLS in the olfactory bulbs. Behaviour that is initiated by olfactory cues but can be modified by complex variables, such as past experience, requires integrative NEURAL NETWORKS, and is probably represented neuroanatomically by this main olfactory pathway which relays in PYRIFORM CORTEX, THALAMUS and ORBITO-FRONTAL CORTEX. This allows for a degree of plasticity in the behavioural response and, in contrast to insects, mammals rarely show fixed actions patterns of behaviour in response to odour cues. A second set of chemoreceptor neurons located in the VOMERONASAL ORGAN send axons via the VOMERONASAL NERVE to the ACCESSORY OLFACTORY BULB. In contrast to that of the main bulb, the projection of the accessory bulb is directly into the limbic brain with connections to the AMYGDALA and HY-POTHALAMUS. The accessory olfactory pathway has, therefore, a fairly direct connection with those neural structures involved in pri-

mary motivated behaviours such as FEEDING and SEXUAL BEHAVIOUR and neuroendocrine function, but unlike the main olfactory bulb appears not to have access to the thalamus and in turn neocortical regions that integrate sensory information.

Although it is generally accepted that most mammals use all sensory systems to assess their environment, some clearly rely on olfactory information more than others, especially in the context of REPRODUCTION. Thus, not only do mice identify the sex of an individual by its odour, but their physiological reproductive state is determined largely by chemical cues. Mice, like most nocturnal mammals, are categorized as MACROSMATIC. PRIMATES, on the other hand, including man, have all of their senses well developed and with the evolutionary enlargement of the NEOCORTEX have the capacity to assimilate and integrate information rapidly from a number of sensory channels simultaneously. More pertinently, primates possess the ability to attend to whichever sensory channel is most relevant at the time and behaviour is not dominated by any one sense.

The olfactory neurons of VERTEBRATES, including mammals, are continuously replaced, the turnover occurring even in adult life. The BASAL CELLS, located close to the BASAL LAMINA, serve as STEM CELLS for mature neurons. Active division of these cells is stimulated following damage to the olfactory mucosa. Complete experimental section of the olfactory sensory axons induces degeneration of the olfactory neurons which is followed by an outburst of mitotic activity in the basal cells which subsequently differentiate into mature neurons. Their axons establish anatomical and functional synaptic connections with the apical dendrites of the mitral cells, their first relay in the olfactory bulb. The continual regeneration of olfactory receptor neurons poses some special problems for olfactory LEARNING and MEMORY. To complicate matters further, cells from the SUBVENTRICULAR ZONE of the cortex migrate rostrally to reach the olfactory bulb, where they differentiate into intrinsic neurons called GRANULE CELLS. These granule cells form dendro-dendritic synapses with mitral cells which are crucial to the role of the olfactory bulb in olfactory learning. This migration occurs not only in the postnatal period, but is also observed in the adult. These regenerative events raise the question as to how this instability in the organization of the neural network can sustain olfactory memories for any length of time. Perhaps this accounts for why olfactory memories are difficult to recall in the absence of the cue, and even the process of recognition may require continual updating.

See also: limbic system; pheromones

BARRY KEVERNE

olfactory bulb A large structure on the ventral surface of the anterior pole of the brain, whose relative size compared to the rest of the brain varies greatly across species. It is for example relatively small in humans, relatively large in RODENTS and other animals for whom OLFACTION is a major source of sensory input. It receives information from the OLFACTORY EPITHELIUM via the OLFACTORY NERVE. It sits on a bone at the base of the brain called the CRIBRIFORM PLATE. From the olfactory bulbs, neurons project via the OLFACTORY TRACT to various structures important for integrating olfactory information with other sources of information, including the PYRIFORM CORTEX, THALAMUS and ORBITOFRONTAL CORTEX.

See also: accessory olfactory bulb; olfactory glomeruli

olfactory cortex *see* olfactory system; pyriform cortex

olfactory epithelium Found at the top of the nasal cavity, the olfactory epithelium contains the olfactory receptor cells; see OLFACTION.

olfactory glomeruli The olfactory glomeruli are found in the OLFACTORY BULB; they are clusters of the AXONS and DENDRITES of MITRAL CELLS. The olfactory glomeruli receive information from the OLFACTORY EPITHELIUM and project to various sites in the brain; see OLFACTION.

olfactory mucosa A layer of mucous covering the OLFACTORY EPITHELIUM into which the OLFACTORY RECEPTORS extend; see OLFACTION;

STEREOCHEMICAL THEORY OF ODOUR DISCRIMINATION.

olfactory nerve The first cranial nerve (see CRANIAL NERVES), concerned with relaying information from olfactory CHEMORECEPTORS in the nasal cavity to the OLFACTORY BULB.

See also: olfaction; gustation

olfactory prism There have been several attempts to classify olfactory stimuli (ODORANT) into primary odours analogous to the primary colours (see COLOUR VISION). Carolus Linnaeus (1707–1778) attempted to do this (as well as introducing a fundamentally important system of biological classification – see TAXONOMY). He classified odours into seven types: *camphor*, *musk*, *floral*, *peppermint*, *ethereal*, *pungent* and *putrid*. This system was expanded by Hendrik Zwaardemaker (1857–1940) to include nine categories: *ethereal*, *aromatic*, *fragrant*, *ambrosaic*, *alliaceous*, *empyreumatic*, *hircine*, *foul* and *nauseous*. In the twentieth century this rather unrealistic list was replaced by an OLFACTORY PRISM (or SMELL PRISM) devised by Hans Henning. The prism can be conceived of as a triangular block, having six corners. Each corner was classified by an odour: *flowery*, *foul*, *fruity*, *spicy*, *burnt* and *resinous*. Henning proposed that all odorants could be classified using these six primaries. A complex odour would be represented within the prism, its position dependent on how much of each of the six primaries was present in it. The most recent attempt to classify odours is the CROCKER–HENDERSON SCALE (available commercially as the Crocker–Henderson Odor Classification Set including samples with which to make comparison judgements). This scale used only four primaries: *fragrant*, *acid*, *burnt* and *caprylic* (smelling like a goat, caprine being the adjective that describes goats [from Latin, *caprinus*: a goat – which is where the term Capricorn comes from]). None of these classification systems has been universally accepted: it is doubtful whether primary odours exist in the way in which primary colours do.

See also: olfaction; stereochemical theories of odour discrimination

olfactory receptors *see* stereochemical theory of odour discrimination

olfactory system The olfactory system is different to other sensory systems such as the AUDITORY SYSTEM and VISUAL SYSTEM, in that it does not project through the THALAMUS. Instead, information is relayed directly to parts of the oldest cortical tissue (the PALAEOCORTEX – see CEREBRAL CORTEX) in the MEDIAL TEMPORAL LOBE. The OLFACTORY EPITHELIUM transmits information via the OLFACTORY NERVE to theOLFACTORY BULBS. Neurons project from here via the OLFACTORY TRACT to structures referred to collectively as the OLFACTORY CORTEX. These areas are (1) the ANTERIOR OLFACTORY NUCLEUS, which projects (via the ANTERIOR COMMISSURE) to the contralateral OLFACTORY BULB; (2) the OLFACTORY TUBERCLE; (3) the PYRIFORM CORTEX (thought of as the main region for olfactory discriminations and the single area most often referred to as olfactory cortex); (4) the AMYGDALA (the cortical nucleus); and (5) the ENTORHINAL CORTEX.

This evolutionarily old system is complemented by another which does involve the neocortex. The olfactory tubercle, sitting at the base of the brain below the striatum (initial studies included the olfactory tubercle with the NUCLEUS ACCUMBENS and the BED NUCLEUS OF THE STRIA TERMINALIS in the designation VENTRAL STRIATUM – see STRIATUM) projects to the DORSOMEDIAL NUCLEUS OF THE THALAMUS, which also has input from the olfactory regions of the amygdala, and which sends olfactory information on to the ORBITOFRONTAL CORTEX for higher analysis. The orbitofrontal cortex (the lateral posterior portions) also receives olfactory information from the HYPOTHALAMUS (which uses olfactory information with respect to the control of MOTIVATION), which receives information from the pyriform cortex and amygdala. The amygdala is also able to present olfactory information to sites lower in the NEURAXIS concerned with FEAR.

See also: olfaction; stereochemical theory of odour discrimination

olfactory tract Olfactory bulb neurons project via the OLFACTORY TRACT to various structures important for integrating olfactory information with other sources of information, including the PYRIFORM CORTEX, THALAMUS and ORBI-TOFRONTAL CORTEX; see OLFACTION; OLFACTORY GLOMERULI.

olfactory tubercle *see* olfactory system

oligodendroglia *see* glial cells

oligonucleotide (from Greek, *oligos*: few or little) A compound composed of a small number of NUCLEOTIDES.

olivocochlear bundle *see* auditory pathways; top-down vs. bottom-up perceptual/neural processing

olivopontocerebellar atrophy A form of MULTIPLE SYSTEM ATROPHY involving loss of tissue in the olivary complex, PONS and CEREBELLUM. There is difficulty with the initiation and the completion of movements.

See also: ataxia

omission Omission is a word in everyday use that indicates the act of omitting – leaving something out. In biological psychology it has a rather more specific meaning: it is most commonly encountered in the context of REINFORCEMENT delivery, where omission refers to the failure to deliver reinforcement following and appropriate RESPONSE.

See also: autoshaping; conditioning; extinction

omnivore (from Latin, *omnis*: all, *vorare*: to devour) An animal that eats both other animals and plants.

See also: carnivore; herbivore

on the baseline *see* baseline

on-line, off-line memory *On-line* and *off-line* are terms derived from computer use: on-line refers to the state in which a device is directly connected to a processing unit; off-line indicates the disconnected state. The term on-line memory has been used to indicate that information is being manipulated by active processes. Off-line memories are those held in some form of storage and not currently activated.

See also: working memory

on—off effects *see* antiparkinsonian

on—off paradigm Tests that employ a design in which a test condition is interleaved with either a no-test or different test condition (an A–B–A–B–A–B design) are sometimes labelled as using an 'on–off paradigm'. This is an example of the inappropriate use of the word PARADIGM: what is meant is an on–off experimental design or method.

oncogene A GENE found in a VIRUS that can affect the METABOLISM of a CELL and cause cancer.

ondansetron An antagonist at the 5HT$_3$ receptor; see SEROTONIN RECEPTORS.

one-trial learning One-trial learning is, as it says, learning that occurs with only one trial. The term *one-trial learning theory* has been applied to the belief that, in ASSOCIATIVE LEARNING, associations are not strengthened gradually over repeated trials but are learned immediately. As a general principle this is incorrect: associations do strengthen with repetition.

oneirism The experiencing of a visual HALLUCINATION, rich in content and highly organized. Such hallucinations may be caused by a variety of states, including DELIRIUM TREMENS and NARCOLEPSY.

See also: dreaming

onset insomnia The state of INSOMNIA in which an individual fails to fall asleep.

See also: maintenance insomnia; sleep; sleep disorders; termination insomnia

ontogeny (from Greek, *ontos*: to be, *genesis*: creation) Ontogeny means the DEVELOPMENT of an individual (though note that in customary use, ontogeny makes reference to the development of a whole individual while *ontogenesis* is taken typically to refer to the development of a particular aspect of an individual). In contrast, PHYLOGENY (from Greek, *phylon*: race, *genesis*: creation) refers to the development of a SPECIES.

oocyte An immature OVUM: a primary oocyte undergoes MEIOSIS (see CELL DIVISION) to become a secondary oocyte. This undergoes a second meiotic division which is completed if fertilization occurs.

open field A large arena, usually square and with walls, into which animals can be placed. In an open field, a rat will typically move around the perimeter (possible showing THIGMOTAXIS) before venturing into the centre. Initially activity includes LOCOMOTION and REARING but HABITUATION is followed by the appearance of other activities, such as GROOMING. Open field tests are occasionally used just to measure locomotion but are more commonly employed to discriminate states of ANXIETY ('anxious' rats will remain at the periphery), NEOPHOBIA (neophobic rats will not venture into the centre, even if enticements such as novel foods are placed there) and EXPLORATION.

open loop *see* closed loop, open loop

open study *see* double blind study

operant Responses, typically voluntary skeletal responses, acquired by REWARD or REINFORCEMENT processes; or similar responses suppressed by PUNISHMENT processes. Operants, also called instrumental responses, were first studied by Edward L. Thorndike (1874–1949), an early stimulus–response (S–R) learning psychologist. Thorndike placed a hungry cat in a puzzle box with a latch device which opened a door, allowing the cat to ESCAPE and eat. Over successive trials latency to operate the latch and consequently escape decreased, which became to be known as a LEARNING CURVE. Decreased latency to escape was interpreted as demonstrating the growth in strength of a S–R bond between the stimuli emanating from the puzzle box and the act of operating the escape device. S–R bond strengthening was thought to be produced by the rewarding effects of escape and eating. Thorndike formalized his observations into the LAW OF EFFECT, which states that S–R connections which are followed by rewards are strengthened whereas S–R connections which are followed by punishment are weakened. One criticism of Thorndike's law of effect was that it violated the temporal rules of causality – that cause precede effect. How, asked critics at the time, can escape and eating affect the S–R bond when they follow rather than precede it?

B.F. Skinner (1904–1990), who coined the term operant, reformulated Thorndike's basic notion in a way that circumvented the causality issue. Rewards, or reinforcers (see REINFORCEMENT VS. REWARD) as Skinner preferred to call them, did not retroactively strengthen S–R bonds but rather simply increased the future probability of the response that produced the reinforcer. In Skinner's view operant responses such as latch operation did not have eliciting stimuli such as the constellation of cues in the puzzle box. Rather operant responses were controlled by their consequences, by rewards and punishments that increased or decreased the future probability that the response would be emitted. Skinner identified two basic ways in which operant responses could be strengthened. Some responses spontaneously occur at some low but detectable level, the so-called OPERANT LEVEL. Reinforcing these responses will lead to an increased frequency. Other responses never spontaneously occur. For these to be conditioned, successive approximations to the target response are first reinforced, a process referred to as SHAPING.

Skinner contrasted operant learning with the type of learning studied by I.P. Pavlov (1849–1936). Pavlov studied how S–R reflexes could be modified by learning. In his classic experiment Pavlov followed the presentation of a neutral stimulus such as a buzzer with a stimulus that elicited a reflexive response (in this famous case, dry food in the mouth elicits salivation). After several pairings of buzzer and food the previously neutral buzzer also elicited salivation. Dry food was called the UNCONDITIONED STIMULUS (US) and salivation to the dry food was called the unconditioned reflex (UCR). The buzzer was called the CONDITIONED STIMULUS (CS) and salivation to the buzzer was called the CONDITIONED REFLEX (CR).

Modern views of learning do not treat operant and Pavlovian conditioning as separate entities but rather as two processes that are intertwined in most instances of LEARNING. Two developments have lead to the position that learning is a blend of processes. The first was the recognition that there is an implicit operant reinforcement relationship in Pavlovian conditioning. Salivation as a CR is followed by food, the same stimulus that could be used to reinforce lever pressing for example.

Thus a component of the salivation response could be an operant. The other development was the discovery of a phenomenon called AUTOSHAPING. A typical operant conditioning procedure is to reward hungry pigeons with grain for pecking a lit circular key mounted on the wall of an OPERANT CHAMBER. In a typical experiment the key peck response would by shaped by rewarding successful approximations to the final response of striking the key. In 1968 Brown and Jenkins discovered that key pecking could be conditioned by pairing key light presentation with a presentation of food, a Pavlovian conditioning procedure. Thus one factor responsible for key pecking is Pavlovian conditioning. But it is not the only factor: If key pecks are made to cancel food – the so-called omission procedure – key pecking decreases, showing that the food reward that follows the key peck is important as well.

Modern research has also discovered that it is not the CONTIGUITY or pairing of CS and US per se, or the pairing of operant response with reward per se, that is important in learning. Rather it is the statistical correlation or CONTINGENCY between CS and US, and between response and rewards that is important. Learning seems to occur when animals detect that food is more probably after a CS than it is at other times when the CS is absent. Learning seems to occur when animals detect that food is more probably at times when they emit a response that at times in which they do not.

See also: associative learning; aversive conditioning; conditioning; discrimination learning; discriminative cue; extinction; go/no-go learning; matching law; negative reinforcement; passive avoidance; positive reinforcement; schedules of reinforcement; stimulus generalization

DONALD M. WILKIE

operant chamber An apparatus for use in OPERANT CONDITIONING (see INSTRUMENTAL CONDITIONING; OPERANT). The most common, and best known, is the apparatus developed by B.F. Skinner (1904–1990) commonly called the SKINNER BOX. The NINE-HOLE BOX is a different type of operant chamber.

See also: nose poke vs. lever press

DONALD M. WILKIE

operant conditioning Operant conditioning is the term B.F. Skinner (1904–1990) used to describe INSTRUMENTAL CONDITIONING.

See also: operant

operant level *see* operant

opercula of the insula *see* insula cortex

opercular cortex (from Latin, *operire*: to cover) An operculum is a cover or lid and is a term encountered in several biological contexts. The opercular cortex is composed of those parts of the FRONTAL CORTEX, PARIETAL CORTEX and TEMPORAL LOBE that are adjacent to the LATERAL SULCUS (see LATERAL FISSURE) and which cover the INSULA CORTEX. (It is also known as the opercula of the insula.) Damage to this part of the brain can produce a variety of effects including the OPERCULAR SYNDROME (which involves difficulty in moving the MUSCLES of the face and mouth), NON-FLUENT APHASIA and EPILEPSY.

opercular syndrome *see* opercular cortex

opiates The opiate drugs consist of a class of compounds that are extracted from the poppy plant (*Papaver somniferum*), including OPIUM, MORPHINE, and CODEINE, as well as synthetic derivatives such as HEROIN and MEPERIDINE (Demerol). Traditionally, this group of drugs has also been called NARCOTICS, after the Greek word for 'stupor' or 'benumbing'. Use of the extracts of the poppy plant for its psychological and medicinal properties may date back over 5000 years. Opiates are extensively used in medicine for pain relief, and they are effective cough suppressants and anti-diarrhoeal agents. Opiates are also a major class of drugs that lead to ADDICTION.

ANN E. KELLEY

opioid peptides These are peptide NEUROTRANSMITTERS (see NEUROPEPTIDES) related to the OPIATES. For example ENKEPHALIN, ENDORPHIN, and DYNORPHIN are all opioid peptides. They are derived from three PROHORMONES: PRODYNORPHIN (which produces dynorphin), PROOPIOMELANOCORTIN (which produces endorphin and the hormone ADRENOCORTICOTROPIC HORMONE [ACTH]) PREPROENKEPHALIN and PROENKEPHALIN

(which produces enkephalin). These three hormones are each coded by a separate GENE and are differentially located through the CENTRAL NERVOUS SYSTEM. Enkephalin is the most abundant of them.

See also: morphine

opioid receptors There are three main classes of RECEPTOR for the OPIOID PEPTIDES: delta, kappa and mu. All are G PROTEIN coupled but each has a distinct pharmacology and the various opioid peptides show different affinity for each type. For example, ENDORPHINS have the highest AFFINITY for delta receptors, DYNORPHIN for kappa receptors. It should be noted though that all the opioid peptides can act at all of the receptors: it is only the degree of affinity that discriminates them.

opioids *see* opioid peptides

opium Opium is archetypal among the OPIATES. It is made from the seed pods of the poppy *Papaver somniferum* and has a variety of active constituents: MORPHINE, CODEINE, THEBAINE, PAPAVERINE, NARCOTINE and NARCEINE are all active ALKALOIDS found in opium.

Reference

Feldman R., Meyer J.S. & Quenzer L.F. (1997) *Principles of Neuropsychopharmacology*, Sinauer Associates: Sunderland MA.

opponent process theory of colour vision The theory holds that colour appearance is determined by two opponent mechanisms: red–green and blue–yellow. It also includes a black–white mechanism. Within each of these opponent pairs, responses to one colour are inhibited (opposed) by those to the other colour. For example, responses to a red light are inhibited by those to a green one, and vice versa. The concept of opponent colours was first described in 1878 by Hering (1834–1918) and later verified quantitatively by Hurvich & Jameson in the 1950s using hue-cancellation methods, on the basis of observations that while some pairs of colours can coexist in one sensation, others cannot. For example, a colour can be seen as blue-green, green-yellow, yellow-red or red-blue, but a blue-yellow or a red-green is never perceived. Thus these latter two colour pairs are termed opponent. Since red, green, blue and yellow cannot be described in terms of any other colour, they are also called UNIQUE HUES. It was argued that each opponent pair must originate neurally from a single mechanism responding in a bipolar fashion to the two colours. The colour-opponent basis of colour appearance is thought to begin in the RETINA with the combination of the three types of CONES (L, M and S) into different subtractive mechanisms (termed CONE OPPONENT) and additive mechanisms (termed achromatic or LUMINANCE MECHANISMS). Both neurophysiological and psychophysical data demonstrate the existence of a so-called 'red–green' cone opponent mechanism which differences the L and M cone outputs (L − M or M − L), a so-called 'blue–yellow' cone opponent mechanism which differences the S cones from the L and M in combination (S − [L + M] or vice versa), and an achromatic mechanism which sums cone outputs (L + M + S) and does not encode colour. Individual neurons which respond to these cone opponent combinations are found in the retina, the LATERAL GENICULATE NUCLEUS, and in areas V1 and V2 (see AREAS V1–V5) of the primate VISUAL CORTEX (see CORTICAL BLOBS).

Although these cone opponent mechanisms form the early neural stages of primate colour vision, they cannot directly correspond to the colour opponent mechanisms described by Hering. This is because colour appearance based on the activity of a single cone opponent mechanism does not correspond to the colour opponent unique hues described by Hering. For example, colour stimuli which are seen only using the 'blue–yellow' cone opponent mechanism are purplish and greenish in appearance rather than blue and yellow, moreover stimuli which isolates the so-called 'red–green' cone opponent mechanism are pinkish or bluish in appearance. Thus it is likely that colour opponency and the unique hues, which form the basis of our cognitive experience of colour, arise from interactions between the cone opponent mechanism occurring at a higher visual stage. These interactions are likely to be complex as the colour-opponent mechanisms are non-linear in their behaviour. At present, the linking hypotheses required to describe colour appearance quantitatively in terms of the activity of the early cone opponent mechanisms remain to be elucidated.

See also: colour vision; trichromatic theory of colour vision

KATHY T. MULLEN

opponent processes Certain perceptual phenomena can be characterized by a mutually exclusive pairing of sensations. Some of the best known examples occur in vision, and in particular in the case of COLOUR VISION where such pairing lead to the development of the influential OPPONENT PROCESS THEORY OF COLOUR VISION. Similar pairings of sensations also occur in visual MOTION PERCEPTION. Adaptation to motion in one direction will induce a perception of motion in the opposite direction in subsequently viewed static objects, indicating the existence of at least two, mutually opponent motion mechanisms. This MOTION AFTER-EFFECT is frequently referred to as the WATERFALL ILLUSION in recognition of a nineteenth century report of the phenomenon at the Falls of Foyers in Scotland.

DAVID W. HEELEY

opsin Opsin is the protein that forms the majority part of the light-sensitive PHOTOPIGMENT (see PROTEINS; VISUAL PIGMENT).

DAVID W. HEELEY

optic (from Greek, optos: seen) Relating to vision (see VISUAL SYSTEM) or to the EYE.

optic agnosia An inability to name objects when they are presented visually but with an intact ability to name them when they are touched.

See also: agnosia; optic aphasia

optic aphasia A condition in which it is possible to name an object from a verbal description or from TOUCH, but with an inability to name the object when presented visually.

See also: aphasia; optic agnosia

Reference

Chanoine V. & Nespoulous J.L. (1999) Visual object recognition in optic aphasia: A review of the syndrome. *Revue de Neuropsychologie* 9: 3–42.

optic ataxia An inability to reach for an object when it is in sight: sometimes referred to as part of PSYCHIC PARALYSIS OF GAZE which also involves OCULOMOTOR APRAXIA.

See also: ataxia; Balint's syndrome

optic chiasm The point at which the axons of each OPTIC NERVE cross the midline of the brain, named for its resemblance to the Greek letter chi (χ). It is located just anterior to the PITUITARY GLAND on the underside of the brain. Each hemisphere of the brain receives information from the opposite visual hemifield. Axons of retinal ganglion cells in the right (nasal) half of the left eye (which images the left half of the VISUAL FIELD) must therefore cross the midline to the right hemisphere, while axons from the left half of the right eye cross in the opposite direction. Axons from the right (temporal) half of the right eye and left half of the left eye do not cross the midline.

DAVID L. FERSTER

optic disc *see* blind spot

optic flow J. J. Gibson (1904–1979) defined optic flow as the motion of the visual surroundings relative to the head as we move or the scene moves. With self-rotation, optic flow occurs about the axis of rotation. With self-translation, the scene straight ahead expands from the direction of heading, while the scene to the sides, above or below flows along great arcs. Optic flow is analysed by cells in the MIDDLE TEMPORAL REGION and indicates our speed and direction of motion. In interpreting optic flow from motion of the retinal image, we must allow for effects of EYE MOVEMENTS.

IAN P. HOWARD

optic nerve The second cranial nerve (see CRANIAL NERVES), relaying visual information from the GANGLION cells of the RETINA to a variety of subcortical sites (SUPRACHIASMATIC NUCLEUS, LATERAL GENICULATE NUCLEUS, PRETECTAL NUCLEUS, SUPERIOR COLLICULUS). Axons of the optic nerve are partially crossed at the OPTIC CHIASM.

See also: visual system

optic tectum *see* superior colliculus; tectum

optical densitometry In biological psychology, optical densitometry can be used to obtain objective measures from histological material (see HISTOLOGY). Optical densitometry involves shining a light on the material and measuring the amount of light that passes through (that is, compare source intensity with the amount of light that passes through the material). It is a difficult procedure: staining intensity (see STAINS) in histological material can vary for a number of procedural reasons: appropriate standardization of each section has to be made in order to calibrate densitometric measures properly. Objective measurement in histology is more often achieved using cell counting measures (see STEREOLOGY) but there are occasions when this is not the most appropriate technique.

optical fractionator A technique used in STEREOLOGY, based on the DISECTOR, used to estimate the numbers of cells (neurons or glial cells, for example) in a given piece of tissue. It involves sampling from a known section thickness in a known fraction of the section area and then combining the outcome of these sampling procedures to estimate cell numbers.

Reference

West M.J., Slomianka L. & Gundersen H.J.G. (1991) Unbiased stereological estimation of the total number of neurons in the subdivisions of the rat hippocampus using the optical fractionator. *Anatomical Record* 231: 482–497.

optimal foraging theory Adaptationist model that specifies which FORAGING behaviours would be optimal. Optimal foraging models assume that the reproductive fitness (see NATURAL SELECTION) of the forager increases linearly with foraging efficiency. The optimal forager maximizes its rate of food energy intake. Foraging models have primarily studied two basic foraging problems: which prey items to consume and when to leave a patch. Field and labaoratory studies with birds, mammals and insects are generally in accordance with qualitative rather than quantitative predictions of optimality models. The need to minimize predation risk, to fulfil specific nutritional needs and CONSPECIFIC competition may constrain the forager from optimality.

See also: food-storing birds; hoarding behaviour

DONALD M. WILKIE

optokinetic Relating to EYE MOVEMENTS.

Optotrack Optotrack ® is a device for measuring movement without making contact with that which is being monitored. It uses infrared markers on the surface of an object or organism as position sensors to track motion.

oral administration of drugs *see* drug administration

oral pons *see* pontine reticular formation

orality A tendency to examine objects with the MOUTH (see for example, KLÜVER–BUCY SYNDROME). The *oral stage* is a critical part of the development of a child according to Freud (see PSYCHOANALYSIS). The passive oral phase involves a child simply suckling and lasts for about eight months. After this comes the aggressive oral phase in which the mouth is used more interactively to explore the world. Freud's *oral triad* describes the desire first to suck at the breast, then to be devoured by it, then finally to sleep with it.

orbitofrontal cortex An area of PREFRONTAL CORTEX, occupying the ventral aspect of the FRONTAL LOBE, named for its proximity to the orbit of the EYE in the brain of PRIMATES. Although orbitofrontal cortex in the primate brain is granular, the GRANULAR LAYER is less well developed than that of DORSOLATERAL PREFRONTAL CORTEX. Thus, cytoarchitectonic considerations (see CYTOARCHITECTURE) as well as patterns of connectivity have led to orbitofrontal cortex being considered LIMBIC ASSOCIATION CORTEX. As limbic association cortex extends to other lobes, this area of the frontal lobe is also part of a functionally defined LIMBIC LOBE.

VERITY J. BROWN

orbits of the eye The eye sockets, in the SKULL; the term orbit occurs in anatomical terms (such as ORBITOFRONTAL CORTEX) and always indicates proximity to the orbits of the eye.

orexigenic (from Greek, *orexis*: appetite, and *genesis*: creation) An orexigenic agent is one that stimulates APPETITE.

orexin *see* hypocretin/orexin

organ of Corti A receptive organ, part of the auditory apparatus. It includes the BASILAR MEMBRANE, HAIR CELLS and TECTORIAL MEMBRANE. The hair cells are fixed to the basilar membrane by DEITER'S CELLS. The tips of the hair cells contact the tectorial membrane which, unlike the basilar membrane, is quite rigid. Movement of the basilar membrane causes the hair cells to bend against the inflexible tectorial membrane, the movements of the hair cells being converted into neural impulses.

See also: auditory perception; cochlea; hearing theories

organelle *see* subcellular organs

organic (from Greek, *organon*: instrument) In biological sciences *organic* refers to the body; to any of the organs of the body. It is an important discriminator in psychology: one can talk of organic states as being those disorders that have a physical cause within the body. These are contrasted with psychological dysfunctions that appear to have no organic cause. This distinction is coming under pressure, since it is now often held that all psychological events are manifestations of brain states, implying that any disease or dysfunction must have an organic cause (see MIND–BODY QUESTION; NEUROPHILOSOPHY). However, one can still at least discriminate between disorders with very obvious organic causes, and those that have no discoverable organic cause at present.

organization effects of steroid hormones STEROID HORMONES organize the gender-specific development of GONADS and BRAIN during foetal and perinatal periods, literally setting the stage for their gender-specific activation by steroid hormones at PUBERTY. In males, the secretion of testicular ANDROGENS both defeminizes and masculinizes the development of the gonads and brain during critical pre- and postnatal periods. Male rats castrated after birth will not show masculine SEXUAL

BEHAVIOUR unless androgens are replaced exogenously, whereas female rats administered androgens after birth will display masculine sexual behaviours. The masculinizing and defeminizing effects of androgens occurs by aromatization into ESTROGEN in different regions of the brain.

See also: sex differences; sexual differentiation; sexual dimorphism

JAMES G. PFAUS

organophosphates Several organophosphorous compounds are irreversible ACETYLCHOLINESTERASE inhibitors: they bind to acetylcholinesterase for what are essentially indefinite periods, rendering it functionally useless. Agents such as NEOSTIGMINE and PHYSOSTIGMINE, in contrast, are not irreversible, having actions measurable in terms of a few hours. The insecticide *parathion* was the first such compound to be developed. This was widely used but found to have very harmful, even fatal, effects on VERTEBRATES, including humans. A derivative, *malathion*, was found to have no effect on mammals or birds and has continued in use. Several related compounds have been developed as agents of chemical warfare: sarin, soman and tabun are all organophosphates related to, and much stronger than, parathion. These were developed in Germany; DIISOPROPYLFLUOROPHOSPHATE (DFP) was developed in the United Kingdom and United States. All of these compounds can be absorbed into the BLOOD through the SKIN or by inhalation since they are highly lipid soluble (see LIPIDS). Likewise, they cross the BLOOD–BRAIN BARRIER without difficulty: symptoms include breathing difficulties, sweating, VOMITING and defaecation, CONVULSIONS and paralysis. Agents to combat the actions of organophosphates have been developed also: pralidoxime (pyridine-2-aldoxime methiodide) and trimedoxime can cause separation of the organophosphate from endogenous acetylcholinesterase, restoring normal function.

Reference

Feldman R., Meyer J.S. & Quenzer L.F. (1997) *Principles of Neuropsychopharmacology*, Sinauer Associates: Sunderland MA.

organum vasculosum of the lamina terminalis This is one of the CIRCUMVENTRICULAR ORGANS; it is thought to have sensory functions related to OSMOREGULATION.

orgasm Orgasm is a profoundly rewarding release of accumulated sexual excitement and tension and is generated after a requisite amount of somatosensory sexual stimulation has been achieved. It is referred to colloquially as 'climax' or 'coming', and is the shortest phase of the human sexual response cycle, usually lasting a few seconds. Orgasms vary in physiological and psychological intensity, not only between individuals but also at different times for the same individual. Although defining 'an orgasm' is difficult, there are several common physiological and psychological events that occur regularly during orgasm: The intense release of sexual excitement and arousal is accompanied by rhythmic contractions of pelvic floor muscles and is typically followed by an extended period of relaxation, during which SEXUAL AROUSAL is inhibited and further sexual stimulation can be aversive.

In women, orgasms are accompanied by simultaneous rhythmic contractions of the uterus, outer third of the vagina, and the anal sphincter that are felt as a warm tingling or throbbing sensation. The first contractions occur quickly and are intense, whereas subsequent contractions are spaced out in time and less intense. A subjectively mild orgasm may consist of fewer, less intense, and more temporally spaced contractions compared to a subjectively intense orgasm. Feelings of subjective pleasure usually start in the clitoris and spread throughout the entire pelvic region, muscles in the body contract and flex, and breath comes in deep gasps, often along with moans or other vocalizations. Unlike women, orgasms in men occur in two phases. The first consists of a series of contractions of the vas deferens, prostate and seminal vesicles that force semen into the urethra. This leads to a feeling of ejaculatory inevitability, a loss of inhibitory control over EJACULATION. In the second phase, contractions of the urethra, penis and prostate combine to expel the seminal fluid from the urethra during ejaculation. There is always a slight delay between the first and second phases of orgasm in men, due to the distance that semen must travel in the urethra. Men experience orgasm as a deep pressure or throbbing followed by intensely pleasurable and sharp pumping sensations which correspond to contractions of the anal sphincter, rectum, perineum and genitals, as ejaculation occurs. Unlike men, women do not typically experience a feeling of orgasmic inevitability, and can 'lose' their orgasms due to external distractors or abrupt changes in the pattern of genital stimulation. Although orgasm and ejaculation usually occur together in men, they are not identical. Ejaculation can occur in men with spinal cord injury without any perception of sexual stimulation or orgasm, and orgasm can occur without ejaculation in prepubertal boys or in men with prostate disease, following the use of certain drugs, or if several prior ejaculations have been experienced in fairly rapid succession.

Orgasms are typically generated by somatosensory stimulation of the genitals during masturbation or sexual intercourse, and the pattern of preferred stimulation differs for different individuals. Some women prefer gentle and indirect massaging of the CLITORIS, whereas others prefer quick and direct clitoral contact. Still other women may prefer vaginal stimulation to achieve orgasm. Some women prefer a single, intense orgasm whereas others prefer many quick orgasms of small intensity. Likewise, in some men, repeated stimulation of the glans penis may lead to orgasm, whereas for others the entire penile shaft must be stimulated. Some men prefer quick and intense genital stimulation, whereas others prefer less intense genital stimulation and more whole-body touching. Delayed or inhibited orgasm can occur in both men and women following use of any DRUG that inhibits SYMPATHETIC AROUSAL, or if STRESS or control issues pervade the relationship or the sexual act.

Although it is not yet known definitively what makes orgasms feel pleasurable, the brain plays a critical role. Orgasms induce profound changes in cortical EEG (see ELECTROENCEPHALOGRAM) activity, and are usually followed by THETA WAVES. Interestingly, HEROIN users refer to the rush of EUPHORIA induced by heroin as 'orgasm-like', and often use sexual terms to refer to the insertion of the needle into a vein and the spurting out of solution that produces the euphoria. Heroin euphoria is also followed by a period of relaxation. In male rats, ejaculation induces the release of endogenous OPIOIDS into different brain regions. Opioid antagonists, like NALOXONE or NALTREXONE have also been reported to diminish the experience of orgasm in men and women. It is possible, therefore, that the euphoria experienced during orgasm involves the release of endogenous opioids, which, like heroin, activates many neural systems, including those that underlie REWARD, SLEEP, and PAIN modulation. Orgasm also induces the release of OXYTOCIN and VASOPRESSIN from the POSTERIOR PITUITARY. These NEUROPEPTIDE HORMONES are involved in many physiological and psychological processes, among them pair bonding or feelings of closeness. A desire for close facial contact after orgasm may involve the release of these substances.

See also: pregnancy; reproduction; sexual motivation

JAMES G. PFAUS

orientation To orient strictly means to turn to the east. In practice, to orient, or ORIENTATION, refers to the process of moving into a particular position with respect to something – orienting to a STIMULUS means simply turning towards it.

See also: classical conditioning; orientation selective neurons

orientation selective neurons A type of NEURON whose activity is determined by the orientation of a STIMULUS: the RECEPTIVE FIELDS are maximally sensitive to edges and to lines in a particular orientation; see CORTICAL COLUMNS AND HYPERCOLUMNS and FEATURE DETECTOR.

orienting reflex Automatic turning REFLEX to orient to the source of an external sensory stimulus.

orofacial dyskinesia Disorders of movement involving the musculature of the musculature in the OROPHARYNX and face. In TARDIVE DYSKINESIA, the dyskinetic movements typically occur in the form of repetitive involuntary movements of the orofacial region (that is, the mouth, lips, tongue and eyes). Similar movements have been shown to occur in animals maintained on NEUROLEPTIC drugs over long periods. In such animals, administration of CHOLINOMIMETIC drugs can produce exaggerated orofacial dyskinesias. DOPAMINERGIC drugs are also known to have effects on the orofacial musculature: APOMORPHINE (a dopamine receptor AGONIST) given systemically can induce biting and licking. AMPHETAMINE, which promotes the release of dopamine rather than stimulating receptors directly, does not produce orofacial activity when given systemically, but direct microinjection into the rat ventrolateral CAUDATE–PUTAMEN (a homologue of the primate PUTAMEN) does produce compulsive biting and licking. Other disorders of the BASAL GANGLIA, such as PARKINSON'S DISEASE, can also involve orofacial dyskinesias, indicating that these systems, and the neurotransmitters acting in them, are important for the production of orofacial movements.

JOHN D. SALAMONE

oropharynx *see* mouth

orthodromic *see* antidromic

orthodromic activation *see* antidromic activation

orthography (from Greek, *ortho*: straight, correct, right, *graphia*: writing) Orthography is spelling, in particular, spelling correctly; see ACQUIRED DYSLEXIA; WRITING.

orthopsychiatry (from Greek, *ortho*: straight, correct, right) Preventative psychiatry; orthopsychiatry is that branch of psychiatry concerned with the prevention of mental illness before it has taken hold.

oscillations Oscillatory activity is a pattern of rhythmic activity that can be generated within NEURAL NETWORKS either by intrinsic mechanisms within neurons, the direct interaction of adjacent neurons (see NEURON) or by the intervention of intermediate systems which lock together the firing of neurons, often at a distance from each other. (The influence of BRAINSTEM systems on the THALAMUS is an example of this – see BURST FIRING.) Oscillations are related to burst firing: BURST FIRING describes the rhythmic activity of a single

neuron, OSCILLATION describes the rhythmic activity of a population of neurons. Oscillations are important in a number of ways. For examples, (1) many elements of movement depend on simple rhythmic muscular activity: the oscillatory activity of CENTRAL PATTERN GENERATORS, located in the SPINAL CORD provides that rhythm. Similarly, PACEMAKER CELLS in the heart, controlling rhythmic beating, can be described as oscillatory (see MUSCLES). (2) Oscillatory activity is important in the SUPRACHIASMATIC NUCLEUS of the HYPOTHALAMUS, involved in the regulation of CIRCADIAN RHYTHM. (3) Oscillations in at the NEURAL ASSEMBLY level have been associated with the generation of synchronization (see SYNCHRONY/DESYNCHRONY). While there is an association between oscillation and synchrony, it appears not to be absolute: the oscillatory activity of a single neuron does not guarantee that adjacent neurons will be synchronized to that pattern of activity. (4) Oscillations have also been associated with information processing. It has been suggested that the coding of information by the CENTRAL NERVOUS SYSTEM is dependent on the synchronization of neurons, and that oscillatory activity is one means for binding these neurons functionally together (see Singer, 1996).

References

Singer W. (1996) Neuronal synchronization: a solution to the binding problem? In *The Mind–Brain Continuum*, ed. R. Llinás & P.S. Churchland, pp. 101–130, MIT Press: Cambridge MA.

oscillator *see* central pattern generator

oscillopsia A failure of VISUAL SUPPRESSION that is caused by disease of the VESTIBULAR SYSTEM. Vestibular disease can cause small oscillations in the position of the eye (known as NYSTAGMUS). These movements are not anticipated by the visual system as they are not centrally initiated, and therefore there is no central visual suppression. Consequently a spinning or oscillating of the visual world is perceived which is said to be similar to postrotatory VERTIGO. It is sometimes referred to as DANDY'S SYMPTOM.

DAVID W. HEELEY

osmometric thirst *see* osmoregulation

osmoreceptor *see* osmoregulation

osmoregulation Osmoregulation is the term given to the control of WATER BALANCE in the body. It is a complex process involving the integrated actions of a variety of tissues, chemical processes, and of course behaviour. Animal bodies contain four fluid compartments: about two thirds of body water is contained within cells (INTRACELLULAR FLUID), the remaining one-third being outside cells (EXTRACELLULAR FLUID). There are three types of extracellular fluid: CEREBROSPINAL FLUID (which has relatively little to do with osmoregulation, forming only about 1% of the total body fluid volume); INTRAVASCULAR FLUIDS (that is, blood plasma; see BLOOD) which forms about 7.5% of the body fluid volume); and, making up the bulk of the extracellular fluids, INTERSTITIAL FLUID (the fluid found in the spaces between cells – about 25% of total body fluid volume). Intracellular, interstitial and intravascular fluids are separated by a SEMIPERMEABLE MEMBRANE: cell walls divide intracellular from interstitial fluids, and the walls of blood vessels separate intravascular fluids from all others. Interstitial fluids normally are ISOTONIC with the others so water remains in whatever compartment it is already in: if the interstitial fluids lose water (that is, become HYPERTONIC), fluid will be drawn out of cells (by a process of OSMOSIS). If the interstitial fluids become too diluted (that is, become HYPOTONIC), cells will gain water (again, by osmosis). The maintenance of an appropriate amount of water in the various body compartments uses two systems: osmometric thirst (the production of physiological changes and DRINKING following cellular dehydration) and VOLUMETRIC THIRST (which involves the production of physiological change and drinking following intravascular fluid maintenance).

Osmometric thirst. The KIDNEYS control the amount of water and SODIUM present in body fluids. NEPHRONS – a million or so individual functional units present in the kidney – take fluid from the blood and pass it to the ureter, which in turn connects to the bladder, from where excess fluid is released as urine. The

volume of water retained or released by the kidney is under the control of the hormone VASOPRESSIN (which is also known as ANTIDIURETIC HORMONE). Vasopressin is synthesized in the PARAVENTRICULAR NUCLEUS OF THE HYPOTHALAMUS and the SUPRAOPTIC NUCLEUS. Neurons here are under complex neural control from a variety of different sites (see below under *Neural mechanisms*). Paraventricular and supraoptic neurons transport vasopressin along their axons to terminals in the posterior PITUITARY GLAND, where it is liberated into the blood stream. Vasopressin circulates in the blood and has an action on the kidney, causing water retention. Drinking too much water reduces vasopressin release; dehydration produces increased vasopressin release. Just as vasopressin acts on the kidney to preserve water; ALDOSTERONE (released from the ADRENAL GLAND) causes kidneys to retain sodium: if there is too much salt present in body fluids, aldosterone levels fall; if there is too little salt, aldosterone levels increase, to aid sodium retention.

Volumetric thirst. This is concerned with the control of blood volume. If blood volume is too high, increased blood pressure follows; if blood volume is too low (a state known as HYPOVOLAEMIA) cellular dysfunction and heart failure follow. Loss of blood is the commonest cause of hypovolaemia, but conditions such as vomiting and diarrhoea can also produce it. The kidneys are able to detect loss of blood flow: if this happens, kidney cells secrete a substance called RENIN into the blood. Renin is an ENZYME that converts ANGIOTENSINOGEN (which is present in the blood) to ANGIOTENSIN I (see ANGIOTENSIN). This is further converted by the enzyme ANGIOTENSIN CONVERTING ENZYME (ACE) to a highly active molecule, ANGIOTENSIN II which has an action on the brain, leading quickly to release of vasopressin, which in turn acts on the kidneys to prevent further water loss. Angiotensin II also has an action on the adrenal gland to stimulate aldosterone secretion, and stimulates contraction of blood vessels to increase blood pressure. In addition, angiotensin II is one of the most potent DIPSOGENS – chemicals that stimulate drinking – known to exist. Volumetric thirst is also stimulated by BARORECEPTORS in the heart: stretch receptors in the atria detect loss of blood volume when blood is returning to the heart after circulation. The atria also secrete atrial natriuretic peptide (ANP), which has a reverse action: baroreceptors work to detect hypovolaemia; ANP is released when there is too much water, working to inhibit secretion of renin, aldosterone and vasopressin, and to suppress drinking.

Neural mechanisms. There are three essential signals to brain that stimulate drinking. Volumetric thirst is signalled (1) via atrial baroreceptors (which transmit via the VAGUS NERVE to the NUCLEUS OF THE SOLITARY TRACT in the MEDULLA) and (2) by angiotensin II (which has an action on the AREA POSTREMA [which is intimately connected to the nucleus of the solitary tract] and SUBFORNICAL ORGAN, TWO CIRCUMVENTRICULAR ORGANS); osmometric thirst is be signaled by (3) OSMORECEPTORS. Osmoreceptors are neurons in the brain whose firing rate is affected by their level of hydration. Their precise location is still uncertain: osmoreceptors were not identified and named, but were predicted by theories of osmoregulation. It seems likely that the circumventricular organs (in this case the ORGANUM VASCULOSUM OF THE LAMINA TERMINALIS) are critically involved.

The subfornical organ, organum vasculosum of the lamina terminalis and nucleus of the solitary tract are all connected to the median preoptic nucleus. This in turn is connected to the paraventricular and supraoptic nuclei of the hypothalamus, which control vasopressin secretion. The nucleus of the solitary tract and preoptic areas are also connected to the lateral hypothalamus, which appears not to be involved in vasopressin regulation, but is involved in the initiation of drinking (see Clark *et al.*, 1991). Clearly, this neural machinery is capable of responding independently to either osmometric or volumetric thirst, as it often must. It is quite conceivable to have for example, blood loss (due to wounding) without there being loss of fluid from the intracellular compartments. It is however also the case that both osmometric and volumetric thirst occur together (as happens when water is lost from the skin by evaporation). Brain processes involved in drinking – which are still not completely understood – are able to deal effectively with these various contingencies.

See also: sodium appetite; thirst; drinking

References

Carlson N.R. (1998) *Physiology of Behavior*, 6th edn, Allyn & Bacon: Needham Heights MA.

Clark J.M., Clark A.J.M., Warne D., Rugg E.L., Lightman S.L. & Winn P. (1991) Neuroendocrine and behavioural responses to hyperosmolality in rats with lesions of the lateral hypothalamus made by N-methyl-D-aspartate. *Neuroscience* 45: 625–629.

osmosis (from Greek, *othismos*: impulse) Osmosis is a term describing the movement of molecules in SOLUTION; osmotic is the adjectival form. Osmosis is particularly important in regard to the movement of molecules across a SEMIPERMEABLE MEMBRANE (that is, any membrane that is permeable to certain molecules but not others). A small amount of a solute (plain salt, sodium chloride [NaCl] for example) added to a solvent (water in a beaker for example) will, even without stirring, DIFFUSE and come to a more-or less even concentration throughout the solution. This represents osmotic movement. Of more interest is the situation that develops – OSMOTIC PRESSURE – when a semipermeable membrane is present. If there was a semipermeable membrane dividing the beaker into two equal halves and NaCl was added to only one half, then for a brief period there would be NaCl solution on one side of the semipermeable membrane and only water on the other. Because molecules will always try to move *down* a CONCENTRATION GRADIENT (that is from a high concentration to a low one) water molecules are drawn across the membrane from the pure water side to the salty water side – that is from a high concentration (only water present) to a lower concentration (water and NaCl molecules present). The molecules of NaCl would make the reverse journey, though again, one that took molecules *down* a concentration gradient. The movement of solutes across membranes – or more properly, the force that solutes bring to bear on membranes – is known as osmotic pressure. (Note this is not the same thing as HYDROSTATIC PRESSURE: if one had a beaker with a semipermeable partition and poured 100 ml of water into one half and 50 ml into the other, very quickly the volume of water on either side would equalize at 75 ml each side. This is because of hydrostatic pressure: the pressure exerted by water, in this case, by the pull of gravity.)

See also: electrostatic pressure; membrane potential; microdialysis

osmotic minipump This is a small device surgically fitted to experimental animals (usually rats) that will deliver small amounts of DRUG over an extended period (a process referred to colloquially as SLOW RELEASE). The pump – a small cylinder – is placed, under general ANAESTHESIA, beneath the SKIN. A CATHETER leads from this and can be placed either into a BLOOD vessel (as one would do for intravenous SELF-ADMINISTRATION) or it can be connected , using the standard procedures in STEREOTAXIC SURGERY, to a CANNULA aimed at a particular site in BRAIN (either tissue or VENTRICLES). The minipump is filled with a known concentration of drug. Over about 14 days this will diffuse out of the system into the animal. It provides a method for the continuous infusion of a drug at a constant rate and has two advantages over repeated injections: first, it is much less stressful to an animal to undergo one operative procedure under general anaesthesia rather than have serial injections; and second, it produces a much more constant level of drug in PLASMA or at the site of infusion than can be achieved with a series of injections. In humans, TRANSDERMAL DRUG DELIVERY achieves the same ends.

See also: drug administration

osmotic pressure *see* osmosis

ossicles The ossicles are the bones of the middle ear: the MALLEUS (hammer), INCUS (anvil) and STAPES (stirrups). Sound waves are funnelled by the PINNA to the TYMPANIC MEMBRANE (the eardrum). Vibration of this membrane is transmitted via the malleus onto the incus and onto the stapes, which then contact the OVAL WINDOW in the COCHLEA. The ossicles represent a phenomenally efficient means for the transduction of sound. If airwaves contacted the oval window directly most

would be reflected away. Working through the ossicles prevents this.

See also: auditory perception; hearing theories

otoacoustic emissions Otoacoustic emissions are low level sounds emitted by the healthy ear, either spontaneously or in response to a sound, and can be recorded by a microphone inserted in the ear canal. Spontaneous otoacoustic emissions are only present in normal ears and result from abnormally strong positive mechanical feedback from the outer HAIR CELLS to the BASILAR MEMBRANE. They only occur for a few frequencies, typical for the ear in question, and rarely exceed 20 dB SPL. Stimulated otoacoustic emissions in response to clicks comprise of a combination of frequencies with relative levels depending on the patency of the outer hair cells along the basilar membrane. The absence of stimulated otoacoustic emissions in a certain frequency range is a strong indication for outer hair cell loss in that range and therefore of hearing loss. Distortion product otoacoustic emissions are produced in response to a pair of low level tones with frequencies F1 and F2 (F2 about 1.2 times F1), the strongest distortion product otoacoustic emission has a frequency equal to $2F1-F2$. If F2 corresponds to a region on the basilar membrane with outer hair cell-loss distortion product otoacoustic emissions are absent. Otoacoustic emissions are extensively used to screen for hearing loss and to study the physiology of the human inner ear.

JOS J. EGGERMONT

otoconia Synonymous with otoliths; see VESTIBULAR SYSTEM.

otolith Otoliths are small bone-like crystals found in the SEMICIRCULAR CANAL of the ear. Their function is to alter RECEPTOR sensitivity on HAIR CELLS. Examination of otoliths has also been used to examine diet composition. Otoliths are not usually wholly digested by animals. Seabirds, for instance, regurgitate them in pellets and, because the otoliths present in the auditory apparatus of different species of fish are different, examination of relative numbers of different otoliths present in the birds' pellets can be used as an index of the amounts of various types of fish in their diets.

Reference

Johnstone I.G., Harris M.P., Wanless S. & Graves J.A. (1990) The usefulness of pellets for assessing the diet of adult shags. *Bird Study* 37: 5–11.

otolithic membrane *see* vestibular system

ototoxic drugs A class of drugs that damage the ears. Kanamycin is used experimentally to make a LESION in the COCHLEA, specifically the OUTER HAIR CELLS. It is possible to destroy completely the outer hair cells over large areas of the cochlear without damaging INNER HAIR CELLS. Tuning of the nerve fibres arising from the inner hair cells is greatly broadened if outer hair cells are removed.

See also: nerve deafness

ouabain Pronounced wah-bain: the name ouabain is a French spelling of the Somali, *wabayo*, the tree whose seeds yield ouabain. Ouabain is a potent toxin that blocks the SODIUM–POTASSIUM PUMP. Because SODIUM is cotransported across membranes with a various types of CATECHOLAMINE, INDOLEAMINE, CHOLINE and other substances, ouabain has a profound effect on neurochemical activity.

outer hair cells *see* hair cells

oval window *see* cochlea

ovariectomy Removal, by surgery, of an OVARY. In experiments concerned with SEXUAL BEHAVIOUR in animals (typically rats or mice) ovaries may be removed and injections of PROGESTERONE and ESTROGEN given, in order the better to control the hormonal state of the female animal involved.

ovary The structure in female animals that produces female GAMETES – eggs. These are passed to the UTERUS (in VERTEBRATES) via the oviduct (or, in invertebrates, via the oviduct to the VAGINA).

overdose A term used to denote the presence or administration of an abnormally high amount of drug, which results in unwanted toxic or lethal effects. In relation to DRUG ABUSE, people sometimes administer to themselves too much of the drug in question, resulting in dangerous or fatal consequences, such as heart arrhythmias or respiratory de-

pression. Therapeutic drugs can also result in overdose, if a wrong dose is mistakenly administered, or purposely, as in the case of a suicide attempt. It has been suggested that various CONDITIONING factors affect an individual's TOLERANCE of drugs. Included in these factors are the place in which drugs are administered: PLACE CONDITIONING for example appears to play a part in determining tolerance to drugs. It is thought that overdose is more likely to occur if these various conditioning factors are not present, or if drugs are administered in places different to those normally used.

See also: dependence; LD50; therapeutic index

Reference

Siegel S. (1999) Drug anticipation and drug addiction. The 1998 David Archibald Lecture, *Addiction* 94: 1113–1124.

ANN E. KELLEY

overselectivity This is a term most often associated with the literature relating to MENTAL RETARDATION and AUTISM. It refers to limitations on LEARNING imposed by overselecting from available stimuli or stimulus features. It is concentration on a restricted range of attributes (rather than, as the term could imply, an *over*-inclusion of attributes to concentrate on) impairs learning. It is a difficulty that can be ameliorated by appropriate behavioural programmes.

Reference

Dube W.V. & McIlvane W.J. (1999) Reduction of stimulus overselectivity with nonverbal differential observing response. *Journal of Applied Behaviour Analysis* 32: 25–33.

overshadowing The attenuation of PAVLOVIAN CONDITIONING found when the CONDITIONED STIMULUS (CS) is presented in compound with a second stimulus during its pairings with the UNCONDITIONED STIMULUS (US). For example, a tone will govern fear responding (see CONDITIONED FEAR) if it has been paired with a shock; but that same tone will produce only weak responding if it has been conditioned in compound with a strong light (note: the light is absent during the test). Overshadowing experiments have proved to be informative about the ways that animals process stimuli during LEARNING.

See also: attention

JASPER WARD-ROBINSON

overt rhythm Overt rhythms are measurable periodic outputs shown by an organism. Output can be in the form of behaviour (a rhythmic pattern of activity for example) or physiology (for instance a rhythmic pattern of hormone release). ENTRAINMENT is the process by which the BIOLOGICAL CLOCK (which is ENDOGENOUS) is synchronized with a ZEITGEBER (an external 'time giver') to produce an overt rhythm. The period of an overt rhythm may be about a day (a CIRCADIAN RHYTHM), shorter than a day (an ULTRADIAN RHYTHM) or longer than a day (an INFRADIAN RHYTHM).

See also: circannual rhythm

overtraining This is also know as overlearning; it is the continued use of training or practice TRIALS on a task that has already been learned to a satisfactory standard. No additional benefit to performance of the task is achieved through overtraining, though two beneficial effects are present. First, animals that have been overtrained show more rapid EXTINCTION of responding when REINFORCEMENT is no longer available (the overtraining extinction effect). Second, if challenged with a reversal (see REVERSAL LEARNING) animals that have been overtrained switch their responding more rapidly (the overtraining reversal effect).

ovulate To OVULATE is to generate and release eggs (ova; see OVUM); ovulation describes this process: see MENSTRUAL CYCLE; PREGNANCY; PSEUDOPREGNANCY; REPRODUCTION.

ovum (from Latin, *ovum*: egg) An ovum (plural: ova) is a female sex cell, which when fertilized by SPERMATOZOA has the capacity to develop into a new individual.

See also: oocyte; reproduction

OX-42 *see* chemical neuroanatomy; glial cells

oxidation A process by which molecules in their reduced form may lose valence electrons to more electronegative compounds. Also as an anodic reaction measured using VOLTAMMETRY.

See also: reduction

CHARLES D. BLAHA

oxidative enzymes A type of ENZYME that engages in OXIDATION; see CELL.

oxidative stress Molecular oxygen can be converted to hydrogen peroxide and a free radical such as SUPEROXIDE. FREE RADICALS are agents that can oxidize (see OXIDATION) other substances, destroying them. The term OXIDATIVE STRESS refers to the damage imposed on a CELL by this process. It is a process under investigation as a cause of neurodegenerative disorders such as PARKINSON'S DISEASE.

oxotremorine Oxotremorine is an AGONIST at MUSCARINIC ACETYLCHOLINE RECEPTORS; it is a PARASYMPATHOMIMETIC DRUG that has the capacity to induce strong TREMOR attacks in animals.

oxygen The eighth element of the periodic table, designated O. Oxygen is a gas which combines with most other elements to form oxides. It shares electrons with other atoms in covalent bonds of molecules, attracting these shared electrons close to its nucleus, thereby producing a polar bond (for instance in water). In organic molecules, polar bonds with oxygen are unstable and highly reactive. Given these properties, it is not surprising that oxygen plays a role in so many biological reactions, from the dissolving of ions in aqueous solutions to providing energy for metabolism. In neuroscience, oxygen plays several roles. Perhaps the most important is its function in GLYCOLYSIS in the nervous system. Without oxygen (for example, if the blood supply to the brain is interrupted by STROKE or HAEMORRHAGE), the brain suffers from the effects of ANOXIA resulting in cell death. Brain areas of high cellular activity have increased blood flow to supply the necessary oxygen as well as glucose. Therefore, a measure of oxygen levels can be used as an indirect indicator of neural activity. Radioactive oxygen (^{15}O), produced by a cyclotron, emits positrons and has a half-life of two minutes. Therefore, it is used in FUNCTIONAL NEUROIMAGING as a marker for neural activity.

ERIC M. BOWMAN

oxygenase An ENZYME that catalyses reactions in which OXYGEN is incorporated into a substrate.

oxymetazoline An alpha-2 noradrenaline receptor AGONIST; see ADRENOCEPTORS.

oxytocin One of the HORMONES released into the BLOOD stream from the NEUROHYPOPHYSIS (posterior PITUITARY GLAND). It is synthesized in MAGNOCELLULAR neurons of PARAVENTRICULAR NUCLEUS OF THE HYPOTHALAMUS and the SUPRAOPTIC NUCLEI OF THE HYPOTHALAMUS: axons of these extend down into the pituitary gland and liberate hormones there. As a hormone, it is involved in LACTATION and the production of SMOOTH MUSCLE contraction in the UTERUS (see PREGNANCY). It also facilitates the ascent of sperm following INTROMISSION and EJACULATION. It is also contained in some neurons (for example, paraventricular nucleus neurons that project to the AMYGDALA, SEPTAL NUCLEI, LATERAL HYPOTHALAMUS and many parts of the BRAINSTEM and SPINAL CORD) that use it as one of their NEUROTRANSMITTERS; it acts at the same receptors as VASOPRESSIN.

P

P300 The P300 (also known as the P3) is a class of EVENT-RELATED POTENTIALS (ERP) of positive polarity, with a peak latency which can vary anywhere from 300 to 600 or more msec, and which is elicited by relatively rare or salient stimulus events in any sensory modality. Among the most common of the experimental procedures employed to elicit the P300 is the ODDBALL TASK in which relatively rare stimuli must be discriminated from more frequently occurring background stimuli. In such tasks, the amplitude of the P300 is inversely proportional to the probability of the eliciting stimulus and its peak latency co-varies with the time required to classify the stimulus. These properties, along with the fact that it can as well be elicited by the OMISSION of an expected stimulus as by the presentation of an unexpected one, have led to the P300 being regarded as a truly ENDOGENOUS component, reflecting the engagement of high-level cognitive processes. The P300 does not represent the activity of only one brain region. Experimental and neuropsychological studies indicate that the component reflects the activity of multiple regions, including inferior PARIETAL CORTEX and DORSOLATERAL PREFRONTAL CORTEX, and that the relative contributions of these regions varies according to stimulus and task factors. The cognitive functions indexed by the P300 have been much debated, but remain uncertain. Because of its relatively large size and reliability, and the simplicity of the procedures required to elicit it, the P300 has received much interest as a possible measure of cognitive impairment in studies of neurological and psychiatric illness. This interest was fuelled by the finding that the peak latency of the component lengthens with age, and is even more prolonged in individuals with dementing illnesses such as ALZHEIMER'S DEMENTIA. The variation in the P300 measures within the population is however too great to permit them to be used reliably as an aid to diagnosis. While the P300 is undoubtedly a valuable marker of cognitive function in the context of group studies, uncertainty about its neural origins, and the cognitive functions it reflects, limit its usefulness.

See also: electroencephalogram; neuropsychology

MICHAEL D. RUGG

pacemaker cells Cells in any part of the body (though the term is typically associated with cells in the heart) that have a rhythmic activity: see BURST FIRING; MUSCLES; OSCILLATIONS

Pacinian corpuscles *see* skin

pain An unpleasant sensory and emotional experience associated with actual or potential tissue damage, or described in terms of such damage (see Merskey, 1991). This definition includes three elements common to most definitions: (1) pain is a sensory experience distinguishable from other sensory modalities – such as temperature or touch; (2) this sensory experience is normally accompanied by an aversive emotional state; and (3) the distinctive sensory–emotional experience of pain sometimes occurs in the absence of tissue damage or physical stimulation that would lead to tissue damage. It is sometimes assumed that pain is subjective and can only be unequivocally identified by self-report. This view has been strongly opposed on the grounds that human adults, human infants and many species of mammals respond to tissue injury in a similar manner. Psychophysical studies (see PSYCHOPHYSICS) of pain show that the sensory experience, and the aversive state, are to some extent dissociable in that a DRUG and brain LESION can modify the emotional state without altering the magnitude of the pain sensation proportionately. This implies that the sensory and emotional aspects of pain depend on pathways in the brain that are, at some level, different.

Neurological theories of pain fall into two classes. SPECIFICITY theories hold that pain is associated with activation of a specific class of sensory afferent neurons (nociceptors; see NOCICEPTION). Pattern theories hold that pain arises when a particular pattern or level of sensory input is detected by the brain, and that the sensory input may be provided by a variety of sensory receptors, not specific nociceptors. In normal tissue, pain is evoked by stimuli which activate a subclass of small myelinated (A-delta fibres; see A FIBRES) and unmyelinated (C FIBRES) neurons with very high thresholds for activation. These neurons, like other sensory neurons, have their cell bodies in the DORSAL ROOT GANGLIA. The nociceptive cells have two processes, one projects distally and terminates as a FREE NERVE ENDING. The other terminates in lamina 1 or lamina 5 of the DORSAL HORN of the SPINAL CORD on relay cells which project to the THALAMUS and BRAINSTEM by two routes. The nociceptive afferents also synapse on INTERNEURONS in layer 1 and 2 that inhibit or excite the relay cells. Relay cell axons cross over to the ascending tracts on the contralateral side of the cord. One group of pathways ascends in the ventrolateral white matter of the cord, and runs through the medial brainstem to the posterior and intralaminar groups of thalamic nuclei, then to the FRONTAL CORTEX and posterior PARIETAL CORTEX. Many fibres in this pathway terminate in the RETICULAR FORMATION and PERIAQUEDUCTAL GREY which have heavy connections with the LIMBIC SYSTEM.

This pathway is thought to be important for the emotional aversive aspect of pain, and for stimulating descending inhibitory pathways. The other group of pathways ascend in the ventrolateral tract and the dorsal columns of the cord, and run through the MIDBRAIN in the MEDIAL LEMNISCUS to the ventrobasal group of thalamic nuclei. The ventrobasal thalamus in turn projects to the SOMATOSENSORY CORTEX. This pathway is thought to be important for the localization and identification of painful events. The role of the cortex in pain remains uncertain as no cortical region essential for pain perception has been discovered.

When a brief, noxious stimulus is applied to a limb, pain is felt in two waves. The first pain has a sharp stinging quality, while the second pain has a burning quality, and the sensation is longer lasting. This represents the waves of excitation from the faster conducting A-delta fibres and the slow conducting C fibres. They are thought to release the neurotransmitters GLUTAMATE and SUBSTANCE P, respectively. Stimulation that would normally be innocuous, may elicit pain from injured tissue because substance P, and other mediators of inflammation, sensitize the injured tissue and the cells in the dorsal horn. The cells of the dorsal horn do not simply relay information from nociceptors to the brain. They integrate information from nociceptors with information from other classes of sensory AFFERENT in the spinal cord, and from the brain, particularly the brainstem. STRESS and drugs such as MORPHINE activate a neural system, which includes the periaqueductal grey and RAPHE NUCLEI, that sends descending fibres down the cord to the dorsal horn. This system acts to inhibit the transmission of information from nociceptors to the dorsal horn relay cells. The descending inhibitory controls are though to explain the fact that humans or animals may appear insensitive to normally painful conditions, such as broken bones, when they are in a state of FEAR or extreme excitement. The neural circuits of descending inhibitory controls contain ENDOGENOUS OPIATES, and it is thought that analgesics (see ANALGESIA) like morphine act by mimicking the actions of the endogenous opiate neurotransmitters in these systems.

See also: emotion; gate control theory of pain

Reference

Merskey H. (1991) The definition of pain. *European Journal of Psychiatry* 6: 153–159.

KEITH B. J. FRANKLIN

pain asymbolia Inappropriate responding to PAIN. Ramachandran has described a recent case in which STROKE damage in the INSULA CORTEX resulted in a condition in which painful stimuli evoked laughter.

See also: phantom limb pain

paired associate learning Procedure for MEMORY testing in humans. It requires the acquisition of associations between pairs of items (for example word pairs like 'horse – pen'). The goal of LEARNING is to recall the associate (pen in this case) in response to the first member of the pair. This procedure is used to examine PROACTIVE INTERFERENCE and RETROACTIVE INTERFERENCE.

STEFAN KÖHLER

palaeocortex *see* allocortex; cerebral cortex

palaeoneurology The study of fossil brains. Obviously, soft tissue such as brain does not fossilize. However, it is often possible to construct an ENDOCAST within a SKULL (fossilized or not) which can reveal information about the gross appearance of the tissue beneath the skull. Comparison with endocasts from the skulls of living CONGENERS can then help in determining the relationships between brain and skull to give an indication of the morphology of the brains of animals long extinct. Such studies in the first half of the twentieth century established that increasing brain size does not offer a particular evolutionary advantage. Nineteenth-century dogma had it that evolution produced a gradual increase in brain size, but the relationship between brain size and body size had not been properly accounted for. The studies of Tilly Edinger established that the brains of extinct animals were similar in size and gross morphology to living congeners.

See also: comparative anatomy

Reference

Buchholtz E.A. & Seyfarth E.-A. (1999) The gospel of the fossil brain: Tilly Edinger and the science of palaeoneurology. *Brain Research Bulletin* 48: 351–3621.

palaeocerebellum *see* cerebellum

palaeopallium *see* juxtallocortex

palaeostriatum Archaic term that refers to the GLOBUS PALLIDUS.

See also: archistriatum; neostriatum

palate *see* mouth

palatine bone *see* skull

palilalia *see* echolalia

palipraxia *see* echopraxia

pallidum *see* globus pallidus

pallidotomy Surgical removal of the GLOBUS PALLIDUS, or part of it. The internal segment of the globus pallidus may be surgically lesioned to provide relief from intractable PARKINSON'S DISEASE.

See also: psychosurgery; thalamotomy

pallium (from Latin, *pallium*: a large square cloak) In NEUROANATOMY, the term pallium refers to a covering and has been used as a synonym for the CEREBRAL CORTEX, with other terms deriving from this – NEOPALLIUM for example is synonymous with NEOCORTEX. Dorsal pallium is term used in the neuroanatomy of birds, reptiles, amphibia and fishes to refer to the cerebral cortex, which is not as well developed in these as it is in MAMMALS.

palmitic acid One of the FATTY ACIDS.

See also: triglycerides

palpation (from Latin, *palpare*: to stroke) Palpation is a light TOUCH. It is a term used in studies of touch (see TACTILE AGNOSIA for example) and in medical and veterinary practice to describe touching a subject in order, for instance, to test for reactivity to SOMATOSENSORY stimulation or encourage recovery from ANAESTHESIA.

palsy Palsy is a rather dated term that indicates the presence of PARALYSIS. It is a term that is still used to described some conditions – CEREBRAL PALSY and PROGRESSIVE SUPRANUCLEAR PALSY for example – but in other cases it has ceased to be used. For instance, PARKIN-

son's disease was once known as the SHAK-
ING PALSY.

pancreas An endocrine organ important to the
metabolism of food and to the regulation of
HUNGER and SATIETY. At the beginning of a
meal GLUCOSE is absorbed into the blood
stream from food in the intestine. When
glucose reaches the pancreas, it causes the
pancreas to secrete the hormone INSULIN into
the blood. Insulin is required into order to
allow muscle cells and other body tissue to
take up glucose and use or store it. Without
insulin, glucose cannot be used as a source of
energy by the body, and levels of glucose build
up in the blood. This condition occurs in some
forms of DIABETES. Low levels of insulin in the
blood stream, which would normally be produced by eating a meal, act on the brain to
induce satiety. Very high levels of insulin cause
body cells to take up all available blood
glucose, depleting the level of glucose available
to the brain, and creating a cue for hunger.
Conversely, the pancreas may secrete a second
hormone, GLUCAGON, under fasting conditions.
This hormone causes body stores of ENERGY,
GLYCOGEN and fat cells (ADIPOCYTES) to release glucose and other fuel components into
the blood.

See also: digestive system; feeding

KENT C. BERRIDGE

pancreatic beta cells *see* insulin

pancuronium A synthetic form of CURARE,
marketed as Pavulon.

pandysmaturation A term used to indicate the
presence of various developmental problems in
childhood that are thought might be an indicator of possible development of SCHIZOPHRE-
NIA in adult life. Pandysmaturation covers
developmental changes in motor, sensory and
cognitive processes. The changes are always
delays with respect to normal controls and are
associated with dysfunction rather than advanced functioning. The delay need not be
permanent: functions may be normalized as
development progresses, but there will have
been at least a delay in maturation.

Reference
Fish B., Marcus J., Hans S.L., Auerbach J.G. &

Perdue S. (1992) Infants at risk for schizophrenia: sequelae of a genetic neurointegra-
tive defect. *Archives of General Psychiatry*
49: 221–235.

panic State of extreme fearfulness, usually of
acute onset, characterized by psychological and
physical effects. Panic may, of course, be an
appropriate response to a threatening stimulus:
in clinical terms, pathological panic occurs
either in the absence of a threat or as a
reaction out of proportion to its cause. Psychological manifestations include severe ANXIETY
and FEAR of loss of CONSCIOUSNESS or death;
physical symptoms reflect activation of the
SYMPATHETIC NERVOUS SYSTEM and include
dry mouth, palpitations, hyperventilation,
sweating, trembling and nausea amongst many
others. The physical effects of panic may
mimic many clinical disorders, including the
symptoms of heart attack. Hyperventilation
may lead to rapid reduction of blood CARBON
DIOXIDE resulting in neurological symptoms
such as tingling. Re-breathing expired air from
a bag may therefore sometimes help. Panic
disorder is a form of anxiety disorder in which
spontaneous episodic attacks of panic occur
several times in a week. Attacks last from a
few minutes to hours. The attacks may have no
specific trigger, though may be initiated by
crowded or social situations. Avoidance of
situations which may trigger a panic attack
may lead to social phobia or agoraphobia (see
PHOBIA). The condition is thus potentially very
disabling. ANXIOLYTIC drugs, such as the BEN-
ZODIAZEPINES, may abort attacks, but do not
cure the condition. ANTIDEPRESSANT drugs are
more effective in treating the disorder, as is
COGNITIVE–BEHAVIOURAL THERAPY.

IAN C. REID

panprotopsychic identism Panprotopsychic is
derived from Greek *pan*: all, *protos*: first and
psyche soul (though *psyche* has come to stand
for psychology without reference to soul).
Identism is a philosophical proposition, developed by Frederich von Schelling (1775–1854)
which suggests that matter and mind are at a
fundamental level identical. Panprotopsychic
identism holds that there is only one reality;
that mind and matter are not dividable; and

that CONSCIOUSNESS is universally present (see PANPSYCHISM).

See also: mind–body question; neurophilosophy

panpsychism The proposition that all elements of the material world possess, in however small a degree, CONSCIOUSNESS. The combination of elements can lead to the development of higher forms of this.

See also: emergent properties; mind–body question; neurophilosophy; panprotopsychic identism

Panum's fusional area The region that straddles the HOROPTER and within which retinal images are perceived as single and fused. Disparate retinal images caused by objects that lie within this region are normally perceived as possessing depth.

DAVID W. HEELEY

papaverine *see* opium

Papez circuit The American neuroanatomist James Papez (1883–1958) proposed that a closed neuronal circuit through inner structures of the CEREBRAL CORTEX is a neuroanatomical substrate for the expression of EMOTION. This circuit is known as Papez circuit. Starting with the HIPPOCAMPUS, the circuit is relayed through the MAMMILLARY BODY, anterior thalamic (see THALAMUS) nuclei, CINGULATE CORTEX, and back to the hippocampus. Although the details of these pathways have been revised, the concept that these structures are intimately involved in emotion greatly influenced neurobiological studies of emotion, leading to the proposal by Paul MacLean in the 1950s of the concept of the LIMBIC SYSTEM.

papillae *see* taste buds

para- *see* peri

para-chlorophenylalanine A drug that blocks the synthesis of the neurotransmitter SEROTONIN: administration of 100 mg/kg to rats can reduce brain serotonin concentration to 5% of normal.

parabigeminal nucleus A small nucleus at the border of the PONS and MIDBRAIN containing the Ch1–8 cholinergic neurons. These project to the SUPERIOR COLLICULUS and LATERAL GENICULATE NUCLEUS.

parabiosis (from Greek, *para*: beside, *biosis*: a type of life) Parabiosis is the joining of two organisms (at any stage in development) occurring naturally or achieved through surgical intervention. It is not a common state. The best known natural condition is that of *parabiotic twins*, colloquially known as SIAMESE TWINS. This is a developmental condition in which there has been incomplete separation of MONOZYGOTIC TWINS during development, leaving them joined and possibly sharing organ functions. In experimental studies, *parabiotic animals* have been surgically created. For example, rats have been joined symmetrically so that parts of their intestines are crossed: food eaten by one rat will pass through its GASTROINTESTINAL SYSTEM but will then cross into the other rat for a short passage before returning to the original animal. In this way it was thought that one could determine the functions of discrete sections of the digestive tract on FEEDING and SATIETY. It is not a common procedure.

parabiotic *see* parabiosis

parabrachial nuclei The parabrachial nuclei (medial and lateral; visceral and gustatory) form some of the most important links between the BRAINSTEM and SPINAL CORD and the FOREBRAIN. The rich diversity of inputs and widespread efferent projections implicate the parabrachial nuclei in neural systems subserving and integrating GUSTATION, visceral and AUTONOMIC function and NOCICEPTION. The parabrachial nuclei consist of groups of cells located in the dorsolateral PONTINE TEGMENTUM, positioned medially and laterally adjacent to the SUPERIOR CEREBELLAR PEDUNCLE (BRACHIUM CONJUNCTIVUM) with which they are not, however, functionally related. Up to 12 distinct parabrachial sub-nuclei have been identified according to cell morphology, relationships to the superior cerebellar peduncle and neuroanatomical connectivity. The subnuclei receive specific afferent connections from many levels of the NEURAXIS and, in turn, send widespread ascending projections to the DIENCEPHALON and forebrain, and descending projections to the brainstem and spinal cord.

Anatomical and physiological studies point to specific functions for individual sub-nuclei but substantial overlap and reciprocal connections also indicate that the parabrachial nuclei play integrative roles.

Gustatory regions of the rostral NUCLEUS OF THE SOLITARY TRACT project to the external medial, medial and ventral lateral sub-nuclei. Respiratory and cardiovascular regions of the nucleus of the solitary tract project most strongly to the central lateral and external lateral sub-nuclei while cardiorespiratory regions of the ventrolateral medullary reticular formation are reciprocally connected with the KÖLLIKER–FUSE sub-nucleus. General visceral sensory (gastric) regions of the caudal nucleus of the solitary tract project to the dorsal lateral and central lateral sub-nuclei. The AREA POSTREMA, a circumventricular organ involved in body fluid HOMEOSTASIS and blood pressure regulation, projects rather discretely to the external lateral sub-nucleus. Nociceptive neurons in superficial and deeper laminae of the SPINAL CORD and DORSAL HORN of the MEDULLA send topographically organized projections to the superior lateral and external lateral sub-nuclei. The ascending projections of the various parabrachial sub-nuclei have functionally significant connections to gustatory regions of the THALAMUS, the ventromedial nucleus of the HYPOTHALAMUS, the central nucleus of the AMYGDALA, and the INSULA CORTEX and lateral FRONTAL CORTEX. These connections and physiological studies indicate that the parabrachial nucleus is involved in gustatory, cardiorespiratory and visceral functions as well as nociception. Thus, the parabrachial nuclei represent an important anatomical and functional link between gastric, visceral and nociceptive afferent signals that modulate or are important for autonomic components of emotion.

See also: paraventricular system

DAVID A. HOPKINS

paracrine Paracrine transmission is the opposite of NEUROCRINE transmission; neurocrine transmission is synonymous with WIRING TRANSMISSION. Paracrine transmission is synonymous with VOLUME TRANSMISSION.

See also: autocrine; neurotransmission

paradigm (from Greek, *para*: beside, *deiknynai*: to show) The term paradigm was introduced into science by Thomas Kuhn (1922–1996). Kuhn used the term to refer to an overarching conceptual framework within which scientific theories could be developed and tested. The theory, outlined in his book *The Structure of Scientific Revolutions* published in 1962, was based on his study of the history of science, and in particular his analysis of the shift from an astronomy that placed the earth at the centre of the universe (a geocentric universe) to one that placed the sun at the centre of the universe (a heliocentric universe). The revolution brought about by Copernicus in establishing the sun as the centre of our universe took on the status of a paradigm: astronomy is understood wholly in Copernican terms. Within neuroscience and psychology paradigms can be identified too: for example the NEURON DOCTRINE is paradigmatic within neuroscience, universally accepted. In psychology it is a little harder to establish paradigms that are recognized by everyone. BEHAVIOURISM can make a good claim to have established a paradigm in which theories and hypotheses can be formulated and tested, as can PSYCHOANALYSIS, but neither of these has achieved universal regard. However, Kuhn did not specify precisely what conditions had to be met in order for a theory to mutate into a paradigm. While neither of these examples, behaviourism or psychoanalysis, is universally recognized, both do provide large-scale conceptual frameworks in which research can proceed, which is sufficient for them to be described as paradigmatic.

Note that the term paradigm is also used in a smaller way to describe a method or procedure (see ON–OFF PARADIGM for example). It should not be. The term paradigm should be reserved for describing the overarching conceptions – Kuhn's 'conceptual boxes' – into which we fit our observations of the world.

Reference

Kuhn T.S. (1970) *The Structure of Scientific Revolutions*, 2nd edn, University of Chicago Press: Chicago.

paradoxical sleep *see* REM sleep

paraesthesia (American spelling is *paresthesia*) (from Greek, *para*: beyond, *aisthesis*: sensation) The term paraesthesia is used to describe an abnormal sensation of the SKIN arising from any part of the body but which is not caused by an external agency such as the application of heat or pressure. A DRUG, a LESION within the nervous system, and EPILEPSY can induce paraesthesia.

parafascicular nucleus of the thalamus One of the intralaminar nuclei of the THALAMUS, this has complex functions: it has been associated with LEARNING, MEMORY and REWARD. It receives innervation from (and returns projections to) the ASCENDING RETICULAR ACTIVATING SYSTEM and has connections, often reciprocal, with the BASAL GANGLIA, AMYGDALA, HIPPOCAMPUS and CEREBRAL CORTEX.

paraffin embedding *see* microtome

paraformaldehyde *see* fixation

paraganglion (plural *paraganglia*) Paraganglia are small GANGLIA (see GANGLION) composed of CHROMAFFIN CELLS; see VAGUS NERVE.

parahippocampal cortex *see* parahippocampal gyrus

parahippocampal gyrus A large area of the ventromedial cortex of the primate brain that consists of areas TH and TF of von Bonin and Bailey. It receives direct projections from visuospatial processing areas of the posterior PARIETAL CORTEX and substantial input from other polymodal areas and has reciprocal connections with the DORSOLATERAL PREFRONTAL CORTEX. It projects to the ENTORHINAL CORTEX and, together with entorhinal cortex and PERIRHINAL CORTEX, it interacts with the AMYGDALA, HIPPOCAMPUS and STRIATUM in mediating distinct forms of MEMORY.

See also: temporal lobe

References

Suzuki W.A. & Amaral D.G. (1994) Topographic organization of the reciprocal connection between the monkey entorhinal cortex and the perirhinal and parahippocampal cortices. *Journal of Neuroscience* 14: 1856–1877.
Von Bonin G. & Bailey P. (1947) *The Neocortex of Macaca Mulatta*, University of Illinois Press: Urbana IL.

RICHARD G. M. MORRIS

parahormones These are chemicals such as HISTAMINE, ANGIOTENSIN and the PROSTAGLANDINS that are similar to HORMONES but which are not produced in ENDOCRINE GLANDS, though they have all of the other characteristics of a 'true' hormone. The distinction between endocrine gland produced hormones and non-endocrine gland produced parahormones is not one made by all neuroscientists: many use the term hormone to refer to all of these.

paralimbic cortex The term paralimbic means literally 'beside (*para-*) the limbic system (*limbic*)'. It is used to describe various areas of the CEREBRAL CORTEX associated with the LIMBIC SYSTEM. The terms limbic system and LIMBIC CORTEX are both rather imprecise: the term paralimbic even more so. In the absence of clear and unambiguous meaning it would be better not to use this term.

parallel distributed processing *see* parallel vs. serial processing

parallel processing *see* parallel vs. serial processing

parallel fibres *see* cerebellum – anatomical organization

parallel vs. serial processing This dichotomy refers to the number of operations that a processor can perform at the same time. When processing is strictly serial, only one operation can be performed at a time on a single input. When processing is parallel, multiple operations can be performed simultaneously on either a single input or on multiple inputs. The serial/parallel dichotomy is fundamental to characterizing how a system processes information. A major research emphasis in psychology therefore has been to identify the serial and parallel operations in human perception and cognition.

This dichotomy was initially explored by experiments investigating how humans recognize objects or patterns (see OBJECT RECOGNITION; PATTERN PERCEPTION). Subsequently, in his seminal investigation, Saul Sternberg

(1966) developed a set of diagnostic analysis techniques which revealed that people engage in a serial process of MEMORY scanning. Sternberg measured the time it took someone to recognize whether an item was one of a list of items held in memory for a few seconds. He found that as the length of the memorized list increased, the time taken to decide whether or not an item was on that list increased linearly. This systematic result involving REACTION TIME is the type of performance expected from a process that compares the to-be-recognized item with members of the list in a serial or sequential manner. In contrast, if the comparison process were carried out in parallel, then reaction time should be the same for lists of varying lengths, assuming that each of the individual comparisons has the same duration. Represented graphically, reaction time plotted for each of a range of list lengths would produce a flat function (that is, a slope approximating zero) which is one of the diagnostic indicators of parallel processing. If the function relating list length to reaction time increases linearly, then serial processing can be inferred. It is important to point out, however, that considerable debate has surrounded the use of these and other diagnostic techniques to make inferences about whether the underlying system is serial or parallel (see Townsend, 1990).

The serial/parallel dichotomy has also been important for characterizing the operations used when humans search their visual environments. Laboratory experiments using VISUAL SEARCH tasks have measured the time required for an observer to detect the presence of a target item in a display of distracters (Treisman & Gelade, 1980). The target and distracters can vary along a number of dimensions such as colour, form or size. When the target differs from the distracter items in terms of a simple feature such as colour, as in the case of a red target in a display of green distracters and blue distracters, then typically target detection time is unaffected by how many distracters are present in the field. The processing of items in the display takes place in parallel. In contrast, when the target must be distinguished from the distracter items by the conjunction of two features, such as a red circle in a field of blue

circles and red squares, then search time increases linearly as the number of distracter items increases. In this case the search process is serial, with items in the display inspected sequentially until the target is detected. Once again the shape of the function relating reaction time to the number of display items is key for making inferences about the nature of the underlying processing operations.

The serial/parallel distinction is closely related to the distinction between discrete and continuous processing. In a processing system that consists of a number of successive stages, the time course associated with information transmission between stages can be discrete in the sense that output is transmitted from one stage to the next only when processing is complete. In this case, the processing stages operate in a strictly serial manner. Alternatively, one stage could provide continuous output to the next thereby transmitting partial products and permitting temporal overlap between the processing of two stages. This is a case of parallel processing because multiple operations are performed simultaneously. In the ARTIFICIAL INTELLIGENCE field, the serial/parallel distinction pertains to the processing architecture used in computerized knowledge systems. Standard computer simulations which dominated the field initially were strictly serial and performed sequential operations on information represented symbolically. The 1980s brought with it the PARALLEL DISTRIBUTED PROCESSING (PDP) architecture in which DISTRIBUTED REPRESENTATIONS are used rather than symbols, and computations are carried out across numerous parts of a network simultaneously.

See also: neural coding

References

Sternberg S. (1966) High-speed scanning in human memory. *Science* 153: 652–654.

Townsend J.T. (1990) Serial vs. parallel processing: sometimes they look like Tweedledum and Tweedledee but they can and should be distinguished. *Psychological Science* 1: 46–54.

Treisman A.M. & Gelade G. (1980) A feature-integration theory of attention. *Cognitive Psychology* 12: 97–136.

PATRICIA A. REUTER-LORENZ

parallelism Relating to parallel distributed processing; see PARALLEL VS. SERIAL PROCESSING

paralysis Paralysis is a loss of control over the movement of MUSCLES, though it has come to have a more general use describing the loss of any function. It has replaced the antique term PALSY. Medical science identifies a variety of types of palsy and paralysis, usually naming either the structures responsible for the paralysis or the form it takes.

paralysis agitans An antique term for PARKINSON'S DISEASE.

paramedian reticular area see medullary reticular formation

paranoia A clinical construct referring to a psychological state characterized by excessive self-reference. In day-to-day use the term is increasingly restricted in meaning to the harbouring of persecutory ideas or DELUSION, but technically may include any abnormality of belief such as grandiose delusions, delusions of guilt or religious delusions. Abnormal persecutory content of thought is encountered in a variety of clinical conditions, including paranoid SCHIZOPHRENIA, PSYCHOTIC MOOD DISORDERS, certain PERSONALITY DISORDERS and any organic state such as DELIRIUM TREMENS.

IAN C. REID

paraphasia The erroneous addition or substitution of a sound (phonemic or literal paraphasia; for instance, *pepter* for *pepper*) or word (global or VERBAL PARAPHASIA; for example, *salt* for *pepper*) in speech. It is a common symptom of APHASIA. A full word substitution that is related in meaning or by SEMANTIC category to the intended target is a SEMANTIC paraphasia. An unrelated word substitution is a random paraphasia. Excessive production of VERBAL paraphasias may result in jargon. Paraphasic errors that render a novel or nonsense word may be described as neologistic paraphasia. A mixture of verbal and literal paraphasias may yield speech described as neologistic jargon.

See also: anomia

CHARLOTTE C. MITCHUM

paraplegia Paralysis of the lower parts of the body, typically including the legs and possibly including also the lower part of the trunk of the body.

See also: hemiplegia

parasagittal The prefix para- indicates something being beside something else; the term SAGITTAL indicates a PLANE OF SECTION through the brain longwise, parallel with the MIDLINE. The term parasagittal is used synonymously with the term sagittal: it simply indicates planes of section parallel with the sagittal axis.

parasite see symbiosis

parasympathetic As an adjective, indicative of the activity or involvement of the SYMPATHETIC NERVOUS SYSTEM in an effect or process.

parasympathetic ganglia Ganglia (singular GANGLION) are clusters of neurons (see NEURON): the parasympathetic and sympathetic ganglia are ganglia that form an integral part of the AUTONOMIC NERVOUS SYSTEM. The basic organization of the autonomic nervous system is a short chain of two neurons: one is a PREGANGLIONIC neuron in the CENTRAL NERVOUS SYSTEM that projects to the second, a postganglionic neuron in one of the peripheral autonomic ganglia. The sympathetic ganglia are found near the spinal column while parasympathetic ganglia are located in or near the target organs. see AUTONOMIC NERVOUS SYSTEM for comprehensive details.

parasympathetic nervous system One of the major divisions of the autonomic nervous system, the others being the SYMPATHETIC NERVOUS SYSTEM and the ENTERIC NERVOUS SYSTEM; see AUTONOMIC NERVOUS SYSTEM for a comprehensive description.

parasympathomimetic drugs These are drugs such as OXOTREMORINE, PILOCARPINE, ARECOLINE and MUSCARINE (all having AGONIST action at MUSCARINIC ACETYLCHOLINE RECEPTORS) which have potent effects on structures innervated by PARASYMPATHETIC neurons that are postganglionic.

parasynaptic transmission *see* volume transmission

parathyroid gland *see* endocrine glands; hormones

parathyroid hormone *see* endocrine glands; hormones

paraventricular nucleus of the hypothalamus A prominent nucleus in the HYPOTHALAMUS. It sits adjacent to the third ventricle (see VENTRICLES), with neurons bordering almost the whole dorsoventral extent of this, reaching as far down as the ARCUATE NUCLEUS. At the more dorsal part of the third ventricle, the paraventricular nucleus extends out into a butterfly wing shape. It contains MAGNOCELLULAR and PARVOCELLULAR components, arranged in a variety of subnuclei. The magnocellular neurons, like those of the SUPRAOPTIC NUCLEUS OF THE HYPOTHALAMUS, synthesize OXYTOCIN and VASOPRESSIN, which are released from axon terminals that extending the PITUITARY GLAND. The outputs of the parvocellular portion extend into many parts of the CENTRAL NERVOUS SYSTEM, including other hypothalamic nuclei, SEPTAL NUCLEI, AMYGDALA, MAMMILLARY BODIES, HIPPOCAMPUS and many nuclei in the BRAINSTEM (including the DORSAL MOTOR NUCLEUS OF THE VAGUS) and SPINAL CORD. These neurons also use vasopressin and oxytocin, but as NEUROTRANSMITTERS rather than HORMONES. Inputs to the paraventricular nucleus come from a variety of sites, including hypothalamic nuclei, CEREBRAL CORTEX, NUCLEUS ACCUMBENS, and the PERIAQUEDUCTAL GREY. There are substantial NORADRENALINE-containing inputs from the VENTRAL NORADRENERGIC BUNDLE. However, the most closely studied input comes from the NUCLEUS OF THE SOLITARY TRACT, the sensory nucleus of the VAGUS NERVE. The position of the hypothalamic paraventricular nucleus, with input from the vagus and output directed to the dorsal motor nucleus of the vagus and pituitary gland, puts it in a key position for the integration of AUTONOMIC and ENDOCRINE events. Functionally, the paraventricular nucleus ahas been associated with the OSMOREGULATION, FEEDING, SEXUAL BEHAVIOUR and responses to STRESS. In biological psychology the most closely investigated pro-

cess has been feeding. Leibowitz and her colleagues have shown that noradrenergic stimulation (or stimulation with NEUROPEPTIDE Y) produces a strong feeding response, especially of CARBOHYDRATES. Similar injections of GALANIN promote intake of FAT, while injections of OPIOIDS promotes protein intake. It has been argued that this nucleus has a critical function in the regulation of MACRONUTRIENTS, though the precise mechanism of these effects remains to be elucidated.

References

Leibowitz S.F. (1992) Neurochemical neuroendocrine systems in the brain controlling macronutrient intake and metabolism. *Trends in Neurosciences* 15: 491–497.

Swanson L.W. & Sawchenko P.E. (1983) Hypothalamic integration: organization of the paraventricular and supraoptic nuclei. *Annual Review of Neuroscience* 6: 269–324.

paraventricular nucleus of the thalamus A nucleus in the THALAMUS, adjacent to the DORSOMEDIAL NUCLEUS OF THE THALAMUS. It has output to the INFRALIMBIC CORTEX and input from the HYPOTHALAMUS and PREOPTIC AREAS, and from sites in the BRAINSTEM associated with AUTONOMIC functions. It is of interest to note that the VENTRAL NORADRENERGIC BUNDLE sends autonomic related information to the PARAVENTRICULAR NUCLEUS OF THE HYPOTHALAMUS and the paraventricular nucleus of the thalamus. In the RAT, the balance of these is in favour of the hypothalamus, but in the brain of PRIMATES, much more of the projection travels to the thalamus. It is thought to be a part of the thalamus with autonomic and integrative functions.

See also: paraventricular system

paraventricular system A system defined by Lawes (1988), identified by connections with the AREA POSTREMA: all component parts of the system are govern by the rules that they must be within two extrinsic SYNAPSES of the area postrema, and be connected to at least two other component parts. What is revealed is an organized tranche of tissue that extends along the VENTRICULAR SYSTEM, with a high density of neurons containing ATRIAL NATRIURETIC PEPTIDE and NORADRENALINE. The area postrema, NUCLEUS OF THE SOLITARY

TRACT PARABRACHIAL NUCLEI, PARAVENTRICU-
LAR NUCLEUS OF THE HYPOTHALAMUS, PARA-
VENTRICULAR NUCLEUS OF THE THALAMUS and
central nucleus of the AMYGDALA are all
included. Lawes argues that this system has
evolved to detect changes in the internal milieu
and effect responses to those changes.

Reference

Lawes I.N.C. (1988) The central connections
   of area postrema define the paraventricular
   system involved in antinoxious behaviors. In
   *Nausea and Vomiting: Recent Research and
   Clinical Advances*, ed. J. Kucharczyk, D.J.
   Stewart & A.D. Miller, pp. 77–101, CRC
   Press: Boca Raton FL.

parenchyma A rarely used term: the parenchyma are those cells (see CELL) specific to a
structure, held in place by a supportive framework. In the CENTRAL NERVOUS SYSTEM, neurons (see NEURON) can be identified as
parenchymal, held in place by GLIAL CELLS.

parental behaviour *see* maternal behaviour

parenteral (from Greek, *para*: beside, *enteral*:
relating to the intestine) The term parenteral is
typically used with reference to the delivery of
a DRUG or chemical to a body, usually by
injection. It indicates that the delivery has been
made by a route other than one involving the
GASTROINTESTINAL SYSTEM – that is, not by
oral means, and not by cannulation of the
digestive system.

See also: drug administration

paresis Reduced muscular activation without
loss of sensation; see HEMIPARESIS; GENERAL
PARESIS OF THE INSANE.

pargyline *see* monoamine oxidase inhibitor

parietal bone *see* skull

parietal cortex The parietal cortex only becomes clearly defined within the brains of
PRIMATES, since only in primates is there a
clearly defined LATERAL (or Sylvian) SULCUS
and a clearly defined central (or Rolandic)
SULCUS. These major sulci form the inferior
and anterior borders, respectively, of the PAR-
IETAL LOBE. The parietal lobe is conventionally
divided into two parts: the POSTCENTRAL
GYRUS lying immediately behind the central

sulcus, and the remainder of the lobe, collectively designated POSTERIOR PARIETAL CORTEX
(PPC). Within the postcentral strip is the
primary SOMATOSENSORY CORTEX (S1), in
which the different modalities of tactile sensation are represented in a largely homuncular
layout (see HOMUNCULUS). This postcentral
region contains BRODMANN'S AREAS 1, 2 and
3. Other purely somatosensory areas are now
known to exist elsewhere in the parietal lobe,
notably area S2, which is found in the upper
lip of the lateral sulcus adjacent to the TEM-
PORAL LOBE.
   Most of the parietal cortex contains areas
whose sensory inputs are either purely visual or
multimodal (usually visual and somatosensory). In the Brodmann system, there were
only two main areas in the monkey parietal
cortex beyond the postcentral gyrus, numbered
5 and 7, and these two were supplemented in
the human by areas 39 and 40. We now know
that there are many areas in the monkey PPC,
with area 7 splitting into at least five: 7a, 7b,
LIP, AIP, and VIP; and area 5 into at least four:
MIP, PO(=V6), V6A, and 5. Also there are
several adjacent areas within occipital cortex
and temporal cortex that are closely related to
PPC areas and may reasonably be included
with them, notably the MIDDLE TEMPORAL
REGION, INCLUDING AREA MT (OR V5) and
areas MSTd, MSTl, V3A, and Tpt. In monkeys, the PPC is mainly concerned with sensorimotor integration, particularly the on-line use
of visual and tactile information in guiding
action. Thus many PPC neurons respond during visually-guided movements of the arm,
hand or eyes. Accordingly many need information about the spatial relationship between the
observer and the target object. But other
neurons need only to know the size and shape
of objects, in order to guide manipulative
movements (notably in area AIP). Lesions of
PPC impair REACHING and grasping skills (see
GRASP), as well as EYE MOVEMENTS and accurate jumping. In fact reversible lesions of AIP
alone will cause impaired visually guided
grasping. PPC lesions also impair the monkey's
ability to use information displaced from the
focus of attention. Thus the monkey fails to
make use of a discriminative cue to help it
decide which of two foodwells to choose. This

difficulty in attending to peripheral cues probably explains the failure of monkeys with PPC lesions to solve the LANDMARK TASK. In this task, the location of a cue (rather than its nature) determines the rewarded foodwell.

In the human brain, the visuomotor functions that largely characterize the monkey PPC seem to be concentrated in the upper parts of the lobe, in and around the INTRAPARIETAL SULCUS. Thus damage here causes visuomotor difficulties in the directing the arm in space, in controlling the orientation and grip of the hand with respect to visual targets, and in making saccadic (see SACCADE) eye movements to visual targets. Complementary studies using FUNCTIONAL NEUROIMAGING show that these areas are activated during a range of visually guided motor acts. More anterior damage, in the postcentral gyrus, unsurprisingly causes loss of somatic sensation confined to the opposite side of the body.

More surprisingly, the lower half of the human parietal lobe (the INFERIOR PARIETAL LOBULE, IPL; areas 39 and 40) seems to have differentiated not only to do new things, but to do them asymmetrically. Thus damage to the right IPL can produce a variety of cognitive disorders, the most common of which is SPATIAL NEGLECT. It may also cause perceptual difficulties such that the patient will have difficulty perceiving an array as a whole, and will be unable to reproduce its structure by drawing. These high-level visuospatial problems are still poorly understood. Brain imaging studies show that the right IPL is active during complex visuospatial tasks, e.g. involving mental rotation, but its precise function remains mysterious. The IPL in the left hemisphere is equally unknown territory. Damage here causes problems with calculation, and with the comprehension of written and spoken language. Although these striking disorders are the most obvious signs of UNILATERAL parietal damage in humans, there is a well-documented syndrome that follows BILATERAL parietal damage, known as the BALINT'S SYNDROME (or occasionally Balint–Holmes) syndrome. This syndrome is characterized by three features. Two of these constitute global versions of the VISUOMOTOR CONTROL disorders (of hand and eye respectively) discussed earlier. The third

disorder is of ATTENTION, incorporating aspects of spatial neglect, and in addition a narrowed focus of attention, making it very difficult for the patient to shift attention to other objects in their visual environment.

A. DAVID MILNER

parietal lobe Each cerebral HEMISPHERE is divided into four LOBES, of which the parietal lobe is one. It only becomes clearly defined within the brains of PRIMATES, since only in primates is there a clearly defined LATERAL (or Sylvian) SULCUS and a clearly defined central (or Rolandic) SULCUS. These major sulci form the inferior and anterior borders, respectively, of the parietal lobe. The parietal lobe is conventionally divided into two parts: the POSTCENTRAL GYRUS lying immediately behind the central sulcus, and the remainder of the lobe, collectively designated POSTERIOR PARIETAL CORTEX (PPC). Within the postcentral strip is the primary SOMATOSENSORY CORTEX (S1), in which the different modalities of tactile sensation are represented in a largely homuncular layout (see HOMUNCULUS). This postcentral region contains BRODMANN'S AREAS 1, 2 and 3. Other purely somatosensory areas are now known to exist elsewhere in the parietal lobe, notably area S2, which is found in the upper lip of the lateral sulcus adjacent to the TEMPORAL LOBE. For information concerning parietal function, see PARIETAL CORTEX.

A. DAVID MILNER

Parkinsonism The same as PARKINSON'S DISEASE

See also: Parkinsonian-like conditions

Parkinson's disease A disorder resulting from the loss of function of neurons in the MIDBRAIN. The classic symptoms of the disease are TREMOR, muscular RIGIDITY, BRADYKINESIA and AKINESIA (respectively, slowness of and failure to initiate movement) and postural instability, including loss of coordination and a stooped posture. The affected cells are the DOPAMINE-containing cells of the SUBSTANTIA NIGRA, which form the NIGROSTRIATAL DOPAMINE SYSTEM. This projects to the dorsal STRIATUM, a major component of the BASAL GANGLIA, a group of nuclei in the basal forebrain involved in the control of movement. The disease is progressive and the cellular degeneration may begin many years before there are any symptoms. Consequently, the age of patients at the onset of the symptoms of Parkinson's disease is typically 55 to 60 years. There is no gender bias, with equal numbers of men and women suffering from the disease, and neither are there known to be any socioeconomic or cultural effects. There is no known cause of Parkinson's disease, hence the disease is termed IDIOPATHIC. Recent research has suggested that accumulation of FREE RADICALS within the substantia nigra might be neurotoxic (see NEUROTOXINS), though it is not clear yet whether this hypothesis will be verified (see SUPEROXIDE DISMUTASE). However, there are other forms of Parkinsonism, also resulting in loss of midbrain dopamine cells and sharing many of the symptoms, but of which the cause is known. The most well-known of these include POST-ENCEPHALITIC PARKINSONISM, in which the symptoms follow viral ENCEPHALITIS; GUAM DISEASE; and Parkinsonism resulting from MPTP toxicity.

One of the earliest symptoms of the disease is a loss of facial expression, which has been termed masked face. However, it is the tremor which usually causes the patient to seek medical attention. The characteristic features of the tremor are that it occurs at rest, when the limbs are relaxed, and there is often a rhythmic rolling of the hand, at a rate of approximately three per second, known as PILL-ROLLING. The muscular rigidity is due to non-synergistic contraction of muscles. If an attempt is made to move the patient's limb passively, the movement will be jerky, resembling a ratchet movement and giving this feature the term COGWHEEL RIGIDITY. The bradykinesia and akinesia render the patient unable to move freely, particularly when there is no salient stimulus to prompt the movement, and this can result in FREEZING. In more advanced and severe cases, patients may have problems walking: for example, they may be unable to initiate the next step and hence they freeze or they may fall; it has been noticed that their arms do not swing normally with their step, again leading to loss of balance and an uncoordinated gait; they may walk with a series of small, shuffling steps, which is known as FESTINATION. There are cognitive deficits also. For example, patients are impaired on tests measuring ATTENTION and the ability to plan a sequence of action. In some cases, there are also psychiatric consequences of the disease, most typically DEPRESSION but sometimes SUBCORTICAL DEMENTIA.

There is no known cure for the disease and treatments are aimed at slowing the progression of the disease and alleviating the symptoms. The most common treatment for Parkinson's disease is the drug L-DOPA (levo-DOPA), a precursor of dopamine which can increase the availability of dopamine in the brain to compensate for the reduction in dopamine due to neuronal loss. Selegiline® (DEPRENYL), chemically related to AMPHETAMINE (see PSYCHOMOTOR STIMULANTS), is a MONOAMINE OXIDASE B (MAO-B) inhibitor and is often given in conjunction with L-DOPA as it not only relieves present symptoms, but there is some indication that it also slows the progression of the disease. There are treatments, many of which are still considered experimental, which involve surgical intervention. For example, it is possible to implant dopamine-producing nerve cells, either derived from foetal brain tissue or from the patient's own chromaffin cells of the adrenal medulla, which will secrete dopamine when in the brain (see AUTOGRAFTS; TRANSPLANTATION). There has also been a resurgence of interest in the benefits of surgical LESION of the structures on the output circuits of the basal ganglia, which are known to be overactive in the disease. By silencing these overactive cells, many of the more disabling symptoms of the disease can be ameliorated. It is also possible to silence these overactive cells by application of high-frequency stimulation: deep brain stimulation can be applied with good effect for Parkinsonism in several areas of the brain, including the GLOBUS PALLIDUS internal segment, the THALAMUS and the SUBTHALAMIC NUCLEUS. This technique also has the advantage that it is reversible (the stimulator can be turned on and off) and carries less risk of unintended damage than making a lesion. It was believed that the dopamine-containing cells were destroyed and that once lost, the only chance for replacement of the cells was by surgical grafting of tissue. However research suggests that, if appropriately stimulated with NERVE GROWTH FACTORS, the cells might be able to regain function.

See also: movement deficits

Reference

Sacks O. (1973) *Awakenings*, revised edition, Pelican Books: Harmondsworth.

VERITY J. BROWN

Parkinsonian-like conditions Most cases of PARKINSON'S DISEASE are known as idiopathic Parkinson's disease (IDIOPATHIC being a term indicating that the disease has arisen spontaneously with no known cause). There are other forms of PARKINSONISM, collectively known as Parkinsonian-like conditions, which also involve loss of DOPAMINERGIC neurons from the MIDBRAIN and which share many of the SIGNS AND SYMPTOMS of idiopathic Parkinsonism, but for which the cause is known. The best known are POST-ENCEPHALITIC PARKINSONISM, GUAM DISEASE; and Parkinsonism resulting from MPTP toxicity.

paroxysm (from Greek, *para*: beyond, *oxys*: sharp) The term PAROXYSM can refer to any sudden sharp PAIN, but the term *paroxysmal disorder* is used in NEUROPSYCHOLOGY to describe any short but severe disturbance. It is a term that has been used to describe EPILEPSY (which features SEIZURES) and NARCOLEPSY (which does not feature seizures). What both have in common is sudden onset and relatively short duration. CATALEPSY may also be described as a paroxysmal disorder.

pars tuberalis of the pituitary *see* adenohypophysis

parthenogenesis (from Greek, *parthenos*: a virgin, *genesis*: production) The process of reproduction in unisexual species; see REPRODUCTION.

partial agonist *see* agonist

partial pictures task A task in which subject is asked to identify the item represented in a series of partial line drawings. Pictures are initially presented in a highly degraded form (such as fragments of the lines). The object is then presented in more and more complete forms until the subject is capable of identifying the represented object. Many such pictures comprise a series, and the series is presented repeatedly. If subjects have intact PRIMING, they will be able to identify the picture at earlier stages as the test progresses. This ability will remain even with significant delays between the series presentations.

HOWARD EICHENBAUM

partial reinforcement When a REWARD is not given after every OPERANT response, the REINFORCEMENT is said to be partial. A typical partial reinforcement schedule would be a variable interval schedule (see SCHEDULES OF REINFORCEMENT) where after a certain time interval (which varies from trial to trial) the next operant behaviour is followed by a reinforcement. Animals and humans working under partial reinforcement schedules are well known to be more persistent in responding after being switched to EXTINCTION (all reinforcement withheld). One theory for why this occurs is that the partial reinforcement schedule makes it harder to judge when extinction has begun as there are normally periods were responding is not reinforced interspersed between ones where reinforcement is forthcoming.

See also: partial reinforcement extinction effect

JAMES R. STELLAR

partial reinforcement acquisition effect An effect related to the PARTIAL REINFORCEMENT EXTINCTION EFFECT: animals trained to complete a particular task using PARTIAL REINFORCEMENT (as opposed to CONTINUOUS REINFORCEMENT) show faster rates of performance once the task has been acquired. This effect has been less well-studied than the partial reinforcement extinction effect. Presumably whatever hypotheses account for he one will account for the other.

partial reinforcement extinction effect Animals trained to complete a particular task using PARTIAL REINFORCEMENT (as opposed to CONTINUOUS REINFORCEMENT) show resistance to extinction (see EXTINCTION): that is they persist in responding when the REINFORCEMENT is no longer being delivered for greater lengths of time than animals that were trained with continuous reinforcement. It is a phenomenon shown by all animals, and by humans. Various theories have been proposed to account for it: the *discrimination hypothesis* suggests that it exists because it is harder for partially reinforced animals to tell when the period of reinforcement has ended. (This is perhaps the most intuitively plausible hypothesis.) The *frustration hypothesis* suggests that the conflict between expecting a REWARD on some trials and not on others is critical in developing the effect, while the *sequential hypothesis* suggests that animals learn that a non-rewarded trial is a cue for a subsequent rewarded trial, keeping responding going for longer (see Domjan for further discussion of these). Neurologically, the partial reinforcement extinction effect is known to be dependent in part at least on the HIPPOCAMPUS (Jarrard *et al.*, 1986).

See also: partial reinforcement acquisition effect

References

Domjan M. (1993) *The Principles of Learning and Behavior*, 3rd edn, Brooks Cole: Pacific Grove CA.

Jarrard L.E., Feldon J., Rawlins J.N.P., Sinden J.D. & Grey J.A. (1986) The effects of intra-hippocampal ibotenate on resistance to extinction after continuous or partial reinforcement. *Experimental Brain Research* 61: 519–530.

partial seizure Generalized SEIZURES involve both hemispheres (see HEMISPHERE) of the brain and the skeletal MUSCLES on both sides of the body: it is to a large extent a whole body event. A partial seizure in contrast will have a single specific focus (hence the term FOCAL SEIZURE) in the brain and involve spasm of particular muscles. Partial seizures with a focus in the TEMPORAL LOBE may also involve sensory phenomena – olfactory sensations are often present (see OLFACTION).

parturition (from Latin, *parere*: to bring out) The act of childbirth.

parvalbumin *see* calcium-binding proteins

parvocellular (from Latin, *parvus*: little) Literally, small cells. In many paces in the CENTRAL NERVOUS SYSTEM there are groups of neurons (see NEURON) described as MAGNOCELLULAR – big cells. The neighbouring, smaller, neurons are often referred to as parvocellular. Both the PARAVENTRICULAR NUCLEUS OF THE HYPOTHALAMUS and LATERAL GENICULATE NUCLEUS for example have parvocellular and magnocellular components.

parvocellular reticular nucleus *see* medullary reticular formation

passive avoidance Avoidance behaviour occurs when organisms behave in such a way as to decrease the probability of aversive stimuli being presented or encountered. Avoidance is distinguished from ESCAPE by the occurrence of the aversive event; escape occurs when the animal escapes from or terminates an aversive stimulus, whereas avoidance occurs when the animal avoids the aversive stimulus altogether. Passive avoidance is characterized by the animal's not engaging in a response (hence passive) that leads to the presentation the aversive stimulus. For example, in 'step-through' passive avoidance, the animal can avoid shock that is delivered in a particular chamber by simply not stepping through the doorway into the chamber. Passive avoidance is sometimes used as a simple ONE-TRIAL LEARNING test for MEMORY experiments.

JOHN D. SALAMONE

passive transport Unlike ACTIVE TRANSPORT, passive transport is movement across a MEMBRANE that does not require the expenditure of energy.

See also: osmosis

patch and matrix organization of the striatum The NEOSTRIATUM can be divided into two components: patches (known as STRIOSOMES in primates) and matrices, the patches occupying some 15% of the total volume, the matric-es 85%. The patches are in effect a 3-dimensional complex embedded within the matrix, the two components being distinguishable using a number of neurochemical indices. Patches are comparatively low in ACETYLCHO-

LINESTERASE activity, CALCIUM-BINDING PRO-TEIN content and SOMATOSTATIN levels but have higher densities of MUSCARINIC ACETYL-CHOLINE RECEPTORS and OPIOID RECEPTORS. Patch and matrix components are also discriminable by virtue of their anatomical connections, different CORTICAL LAYERS projecting to each.

Reference

Hanley J.J. & Bolam J.P. (1997) Synaptology of the nigrostriatal projection in relation to the compartmental organization of the neostriatum in the rat. *Neuroscience* 81: 353–370.

patch clamp A technique used in NEUROPHY-SIOLOGY which involves the use of micropip-ettes to seal a small patch of MEMBRANE. Events at a single ION CHANNEL can then be examined in this patch. It is a significant advance on the VOLTAGE CLAMP technique, enabling experiments to be conducted on a variety of CELL types in a variety of tissues. Erwin Neher and Bert Sakmann developed the technique in the 1970s and were rewarded with the Nobel Prize for Physiology or Medicine in 1991.

path integration A term that refers to the integrative computations made in order to navigate by DEAD RECKONING. Colloquially, the intuitive process of path integration is called 'sense of direction'.

See also: allothetic navigation

pathogen *see* pathology

pathogenesis *see* pathology

pathognomy *see* pathology

pathology PATHOLOGY is the study of the changes brought about in the tissues and organs of the body by disease or accident; a PATHOGEN is an agent that causes disease; PATHOGENESIS is the process by which changes are brought about; something is said to be pathognomic if it causes disease; and PATHOG-NOMY is the description of such changes. The prefix path- is indicative of a word having something to do with disease; as a suffix it can indicate either someone suffering from a disease (as in PSYCHOPATH).

pattern completion In visual perception, the contours of an object or pattern are rarely fully visible. One object may occlude another or it may self-occlude its own contours. In these cases, the viewer generally understands that contours continue even when they are hidden. For instance, if you place a pencil on top of this page, you will infer the continuity of text under the pencil. Two types of completion are distinguished: in AMODAL COMPLETION, completed contours are assumed but not seen (pencil example). In modal completion, the mind perceives a contour that is not physically present (SUBJECTIVE CONTOUR).

JEREMY M. WOLFE

pattern perception An essential task of the VISUAL SYSTEM is to represent the geometrical relationships between elements in the field of view. This process of pattern perception leads to the neural description of shape, a key requirement for OBJECT RECOGNITION. It is also closely related to TEXTURE PERCEPTION. Retinal GANGLION cells respond to contrast between the centre and surround of their RECEPTIVE FIELD. Thus they are well activated by geometrical features such as spots and edges, but convey little explicit information about what feature has activated them. Rather, they provide an essential preliminary to the more specific analysis conducted in the VISUAL CORTEX. SINGLE-UNIT ELECTROPHYSIOLOGICAL RECORDING in cats and monkeys shows that cells in area V1 (see AREAS V1–V5) have oriented receptive fields; that is, they integrate contrast signals from the retina so as to respond selectively to line or edge segments of specific orientations (see ORIENTATION SELECTIVE NEURONS). Many of these receptive fields are end-stopped, responding best to a contour segment which terminates at one or both ends of the receptive field. The visual input contains significant patterns at many different scales, from fine details to the broadest distribution of light and dark. These provide visual information in different bands of spatial frequency. Individual neurons in area V1 appear to act as SPATIAL FREQUENCY CHANNELS each responding optimally to a particular band, and so allowing the representation of pattern features at a range of scales.

Psychophysical experiments testing selective ADAPTATION, and interactions at THRESHOLD, demonstrate that human vision has the same orientation-selective and spatial-frequency selective mechanisms found in cat and monkey cortex. Experiments on texture perception, and computational analysis, concur that oriented contour segments at various scales and their terminations form the primitive elements in the visual representation of pattern. However, any such element cannot be signalled purely by activity in cells with a single receptive field orientation, but must depend on the distribution of activity across a wide range of cortical cells.

The PATTERN PRIMITIVES signalled by cortical cells cannot be processed as unrelated elements. At some level, the neural representation must make explicit the relationships between elements that belong to an extended contour, region, or object. This process is apparent in the phenomena of perceptual grouping first described by the GESTALT psychologists: elements tend to appear grouped according to their proximity, similarity, colinearity ('good continuation'), and common movement ('common fate'). These laws may reflect interactions between cells with separated receptive fields that respond to similar or geometrically related pattern elements.

The processing of pattern is believed to be a function principally of the VENTRAL STREAM in EXTRASTRIATE CORTEX. This transmits information from areas V1 and V2 through area V4 to the INFEROTEMPORAL CORTEX and areas lying in the SUPERIOR TEMPORAL SULCUS in the monkey. In these areas, individual neurons are best activated by more complex pattern structures than the elementary contour segments which activate area V1. Research is still at an early stage in exploring how patterns are represented at these higher levels. However, a general feature is that receptive fields become progressively larger at higher levels of the ventral stream. Related to this, the cells show an increasing degree of position invariance – that is, they respond to their preferred pattern configuration regardless of where it appears within the large receptive field. The highest levels in the TEMPORAL LOBE are believed to integrate pattern information to provide the neural basis of object perception and FACE PERCEPTION.

The description of any visual object includes many different features or pattern properties, as well as other properties such as colour and motion. Different cortical cells, often in different areas, are involved in representing these different properties. This raises the BINDING PROBLEM: what determines that these properties are perceived as belonging to a common object? VISUAL SEARCH experiments show that a target object defined by a conjunction of features (for example, a red circle) can only be identified among others sharing the individual features (for example, green circles, red triangles) if visual ATTENTION is focused on each object in turn. This led Anne Triesman to propose the 'feature integration theory' – that solving the binding problem depends on visual attention, activating together the representations of the various features of an object. Some recent neurophysiological experiments have led to the hypothesis that perceptual binding is based on synchronization of nerve impulses among a set of neurons signalling the features that are linked together.

Major unresolved questions are concerned with how pattern processing is integrated with other aspects of visual perception. First, we have considered only 2-dimensional pattern relationships; it is uncertain how far in the brain these can be processed independently of the representation of the third dimension of space (DEPTH PERCEPTION). Second, the early stages of pattern processing are organized retinotopically; each cell signals the pattern properties of a particular region of the VISUAL FIELD. At higher levels, it is unlikely that patterns are represented in a fixed spatial matrix; rather each pattern element must be specified in terms of the object to which it belongs. Despite this, information about the object identity ('what?') and its location ('where?') must be bound together in some way. How the transition is made in the brain from retinotopic to object-based representations, and how the latter are coupled to spatial information, are quite unknown.

See also: feature detector; feature search

References

Spillman L. & Werner J. (1990) *Visual Perception: The Neurological Foundations*, Academic Press: San Diego.

Treisman A. (1998) Feature binding, attention and object perception, *Philosophical Transactions of the Royal Society of London Series B* 353: 1295–1306.

OLIVER J. BRADDICK

pattern primitives *see* pattern perception

pattern self-similarity A form of VISUAL SYMMETRY that has generated much interest recently is that of self-similarity (repetition) over size-scaling. A new branch of mathematics was defined by Benoit Mandelbrot to describe the relative roughness or smoothness of functions over scale, even when the functions were not classically differentiable (requiring that they become smoother at smaller scales). The self-similarity of these 'fractal' functions provides a better match to many natural textures and event sequences than the patterns of traditional random generators, and has inspired a new view of the constraints determining visual processing mechanisms.

Reference

Mandelbrot B. (1982) *The Fractal Geometry of Nature*, W.H. Freeman: San Francisco.

CHRISTOPHER TYLER

pattern theories As relating to SOMATOSENSORY experience; see SKIN.

Pavarine One of the brand names for PAPAVERINE, a DRUG used to increase BLOOD flow. It is typically given in cases where there is poor circulation of the blood, and as a treatment for IMPOTENCE.

Pavlovian association A Pavlovian association is one formed between a CONDITIONED STIMULUS (CS) and an UNCONDITIONED STIMULUS (US); see PAVLOVIAN CONDITIONING; OBSERVATION LEARNING.

Pavlovian conditioning A form of ASSOCIATIVE LEARNING, originally demonstrated by the Russian physiologist I. P. Pavlov (1849–1936) in studies of the salivary response of dogs. From his earlier work on the physiology of digestion, Pavlov knew that the secretion of

digestive juices could be elicited by psychological factors. A dog (Pavlov's usual experimental subject) would salivate not just when it took food into its mouth, but in response to a range of other events – for instance, at the approach of the laboratory attendant who supplied the food. Food in the mouth evokes salivation automatically and is referred to as an UNCONDITIONED STIMULUS (or unconditional stimulus, US) and the response it evokes is thus an unconditioned reflex (UR). The ability of other events to evoke this reflex depended, Pavlov suspected, on the animal's having experienced them in association with food, that is, on learning through experience. To demonstrate this in the laboratory he set up a special training procedure in which he could control exactly what events a lightly restrained dog experienced. From time to time a small portion of food was dispensed automatically and each presentation was preceded by a neutral event, such as the flashing of a light. Salivation occurred to the food itself from the outset but also, after a few pairings of light and food, the animal came to salivate when the light flashed. The light was described as a CONDITIONED STIMULUS (or conditional stimulus, CS), as its ability to evoke salivation was conditional on its having been paired with food. Salivation to the light was referred to as a CONDITIONED REFLEX (CR). This terminology led to the whole procedure being described as CONDITIONING. Since other forms of training, introduced subsequently, were also regarded as being instances of conditioning, the version devised by Pavlov is often distinguished by the label classical conditioning.

The defining feature of the Pavlovian conditioning procedure is that the animal is exposed to paired presentations of two stimuli (although in Pavlov's, as in most other experiments on classical conditioning, the onset of the conditioned stimulus usually preceded that of the unconditioned stimulus by a short interval (see DELAY CONDITIONING). This feature is found in many other procedures used for the study of learning in laboratory animals. In the conditioned-emotional-response procedure, the subject, usually a rat, receives pairings of an initially neutral stimulus, such as the sounding of a tone, and an aversive event, such as a brief shock. After a few such pairings the rat begins to show a conditioned response – to show signs of fear when the tone is sounded and before any shock occurs. In the AUTOSHAP-ING procedure a freely moving hungry animal – a pigeon say – experiences presentations of a light followed by food. In this case the response conditioned is that of approaching and pecking at the light. Although these procedures differ in many ways from those used by Pavlov for dogs, the same essential feature is present: all involve the paired presentation of two environmental events.

Pavlov interpreted his conditioning in terms of the formation of an association between (to pursue our original example) the part of the brain that was activated by the flashing light and the part of the brain that responded to food. The formation of this new link between these two brain 'centres' was supposed to allow activation of the first (produced by presentation of the light) to evoke activity in the second (the food centre) even when food itself had not been presented. It will be noted that the fact that the unconditioned stimulus elicits a response is incidental to the process of conditioning. Indeed, subsequent research has shown that conditioning can occur perfectly well when the unconditioned response is prevented from occurring (for instance by pharmacological manipulations that prevent salivation) or when the stimuli used are both neutral so that neither evokes any obvious unconditioned response. From this perspective, Pavlovian conditioning is the process by which animals learn about the co-occurrence of certain events. The fact that a change in behaviour often follows is useful both to the animal (salivation prior to feeding makes food more digestible) and to the experimenter (who can use the magnitude of the conditioned response to monitor the formation of the association); responding is not, however, an essential component of the procedure.

It is none the less true that Pavlovian conditioning frequently does result in a change in behaviour and it remains to explain why this should be. According to the STIMULUS SUBSTI-TUTION HYPOTHESIS the existence of a link between the centre for the CS and that for the US allows the former event to take on some of the properties of the latter. The animal then treats the CS as if it were the US (to the extent that the physical properties of the former allow this). This hypothesis supplies a satisfactory account of some examples of conditioned responding (for example the autoshaped pigeon that approaches and pecks at a light CS appears to have transferred to the light the behaviour that it normally shows to food). Whether it can apply to all cases of classical conditioning remains a matter for debate.

GEOFFREY HALL

Pavlovian fear Fear evoked by a CONDITIONED STIMULUS as a consequence of PAVLOVIAN CONDITIONING in which an initially motivationally neutral stimulus is paired with an unconditioned aversive event.

See also: aversive conditioning; conditioned fear

A. SIMON KILLCROSS

Pavlovian to instrumental transfer Pavlovian to instrumental transfer is of theoretical interest because it addresses the question of whether these two forms of LEARNING (PAVLO-VIAN CONDITIONING and INSTRUMENTAL CONDITIONING) are mediated by common processes. It has also been of practical interest in studying the abilities of animals, both normal and those with an experimental treatment of some sort, to learn and to use information about their environments appropriately. A typical experimental procedure would involve three stages: (1) presentation of a CONDITIONED STIMULUS with REINFORCE-MENT (such as the delivery of food pellets) but no instrumental requirement (for example, no lever pressing). In this stage therefore animals are simply being trained to make a Pavlovian association between a STIMULUS and REINFOR-CER. (2) In the second stage, the same animals would be trained in a standard instrumental procedure – for example, to lever press for the reinforcement. (3) In the third stage, the instrumental response (lever pressing) would continue but without the PRIMARY REINFORCER (no pellets would be delivered – the animals would be responding in EXTINCTION) but the conditioned stimulus from stage (1) can be presented again. The degree to which this conditioned stimulus now invigorates performance of the instrumental act of lever pressing reflects the degree of Pavlovian to instrumental transfer.

pavor nocturnis Latin term for NIGHT TERROR.

paw preference Animals often show a consistent preference for using one or other paw in tasks involving reaching for food or to LEVER PRESS. This is assumed to indicate the existence of LATERALIZATION of function in species other than humans, where lateralization is typically very marked, with strong side biases (right handedness for example) and lateralized functions within the central nervous system (see LEFT HEMISPHERE for examples). Animals also will often show side biases if given the choice of two locations (in a T MAZE for example) that are apparently identical. Such ASYMMETRY in animals is thought to reflect changes in subcortical and well as (or even instead of) cortical asymmetry.

pecking order *see* dominance

pedal reflex A reflex often used to determine the depth of ANAESTHESIA in rodents. Pressure on a rat's hindlimb ankle joint causes the foot to be withdrawn, a reflex absent in deeply anaesthetized animals.

peduncle (from Latin, *pedis*: the foot) In plant biology, a peduncle is the stalk of a solitary flower; in marine biology it is the stalk by which animals such as barnacles cling to rocks and other objects; in neuroanatomy, a peduncle is a tract of myelinated (see MYELIN) FIBRES; for examples see CEREBRAL PEDUNCLES, CEREBELLAR PEDUNCLES.

pedunculopontine tegmental nucleus (PPTg) Also called the pedunculopontine nucleus (PPN) or tegmental pedunculopontine nucleus (TPP). A nucleus situated in the MESOPONTINE TEGMENTUM, caudal to the SUBSTANTIA NIGRA and rostral to the PARABRACHIAL NUCLEUS. It is best known as the site of the Ch5 CHOLINERGIC neurons (see CH1–CH8), which constitute the largest cholinergic input to the THALAMUS. The nucleus is also the target of the major GABA output from the substantia nigra zona reticulata, and receives innervation from every other site in the BASAL GANGLIA, as well as the NUCLEUS ACCUMBENS and VENTRAL PALLIDUM. Neurons in the PPTg atrophy during the course of PARKINSON'S DISEASE and PROGRESSIVE SUPRANUCLEAR PALSY. What role this loss has in generating the symptoms of these disorders is not clear, though the anatomical reciprocity between the PPTg and STRIATUM provides evidence for a fundamental role in the behavioural deficits in basal ganglia diseases.

The boundaries of the PPTg have been drawn with respect to the location of the cholinergic neurons. These are most densely packed in the posterior part of the nucleus – the pars compacta – but are more scattered further anteriorly – the pars dissipata. The cholinergic neurons are also contain other transmitters, including SUBSTANCE P and GLUTAMATE, and NITRIC OXIDE, a novel neuromodulator. Together with the Ch6 neurons of the LATERODORSAL TEGMENTAL NUCLEUS, they form the cholinergic component of the ASCENDING RETICULAR ACTIVATING SYSTEM. They have long projection neurons and influence activity in many structures in the FOREBRAIN, most notably the thalamus, through which they can also influence the CEREBRAL CORTEX. Functionally, mesopontine cholinergic neurons interact with those in the dorsal RAPHE NUCLEI and LOCUS COERULEUS, locally and at the level of the thalamus, for the regulation of BEHAVIOURAL STATE. Within the PPTg, the terminal fields of basal ganglia and ventral striatal-ventral pallidal output neurons are found in the MIDBRAIN EXTRAPYRAMIDAL AREA. This area is located in the medial aspect of the PPTg, adjacent to the decussation of the SUPERIOR CEREBELLAR PEDUNCLE. In human and primate brains, the cholinergic neurons form a crescent around the striatal output neurons at this level, characteristic of the relationship between the substantia nigra pars compacta and zona reticulata. In the rat, the location of the cell bodies and terminal fields partially overlap (although output neurons do not project to the cholinergic cell bodies). Behavioural data suggest the importance of interactions between ascending (cholinergic/glutamatergic) and descending (striatal outflow) neurons. It is possible that the small GABA neurons in the PPTg are the link between these systems.

Reference

Inglis W.L. & Winn P. (1995) The pedunculopontine tegmental nucleus: where the striatum meets the reticualr formation. *Progress in Neurobiology* 47: 1–29.

WENDY L. INGLIS

pellet A rather general word that has different meanings dependent on the context. In biological psychology the two most likely meanings of the term pellet are: (i) the solid formed during centrifugation; see SUBCELLULAR FRACTIONATION. (ii) More commonly, it refers to a food pellet. Many OPERANT tests require delivery of a food REWARD, and the most common used is a 45 mg food pellet containing a balance of nutrients that an animal can maintain itself on satisfactorily. (Different pellet compositions to suit different species are commercially available; see LAB CHOW.) Pellets can also be obtained in flavoured forms, which further encourages operant responding.

penetrance In genetics, penetrance is the degree to which a DOMINANT ALLELE (or RECESSIVE ALLELE in the HOMOZYGOUS condition) is expressed as a PHENOTYPE in a given population: that is, what proportion of individuals in a given population actually show a particular feature that is coded genetically?

penis Male external genitalia, used for COPULATION and for the passage of urine; see also VAGINA.

pentobarbital (Nembutal) Short-acting barbiturate used frequently for rapid induction of HYPNOTIC SLEEP in humans and for general ANAESTHESIA in experimental animals.

See also: phenobarbital; sodium amobarbital; thiopental

CHARLES D. BLAHA

pentobarbitone This is exactly the same as PENTOBARBITAL: in the United States the barbiturate drugs have '-tal' endings, but in Europe, pharmacologists have classified them using '-one' endings.

pepsin *see* digestive system

peptidase A type of ENZYME that breaks down PEPTIDES (by breaking the peptide links in the molecule).

peptide neurotoxins Rather obviously, PEPTIDES that are NEUROTOXINS; CONOTOXINS are the best-known example.

peptides Chains of two or more AMINO ACIDS. Adjacent amino acids are linked together by a chemical bond called a peptide bond (a single bond between a nitrogen and carbon molecule). Peptides are different from PROTEINS only in that they are smaller; a peptide is considered to be less than 10 kilodaltons in molecular weight. In terms of structure, one end of the peptide has an amino group at one end (referred to as the N-terminus) and a carboxyl group at the other. Since all peptides have these structural features in common, the individual chemical identity of different peptides is rendered by the existence of differing side-chains. Like proteins, peptides are synthesized in the RIBOSOMES of cells, where MESSENGER RNA codes for their structure. Peptides are broken down by a type of ENZYME called PEPTIDASE. Peptides in the nervous system, called NEUROPEPTIDES, act as NEUROTRANSMITTERS and neuromodulators (see NEUROMODULATION) and have an important role in neural signalling.

ANN E. KELLEY

percent solution A term used to describe concentration. A 20% solution is one in which there is 20 g of a solute per 100 ml solvent. So for example, rats given 20% sucrose to drink are being presented with a solution that contains 20 g of sucrose in 100 ml water. Percent preparations may also carry the notations w/v or w/w: 'w' stands for weight and 'v' for volume. This defines on what basis the percentage calculation has been carried out: in g per ml (w/v) or g per g (w/w) for example. Most solutions are made on a w/v basis – that is a weight of solute added to a volume of solvent, but pastes and gels, for example, are more likely to be w/w preparations.

See also: SI units

perception *see* sensation vs. perception

perception of second languages The DEVELOPMENT OF LANGUAGE-SPECIFIC PHONOLOGY in childhood is highly efficient, and effectively tailors SPEECH PERCEPTION to the native language. In consequence, perception of second languages acquired beyond childhood becomes inefficient: PHONETIC contrasts absent from the native language are not easily perceived (for example, English [r] and [l] for Japanese-speakers) and segmentation of continuous speech into individual words is difficult (subjectively, the second-language speech seems too fast to keep up with). Listeners use segmentation procedures which exploit aspects of language-specific PHONOLOGY such as rhythm, and where native and second languages differ in rhythm, these procedures are inefficient, even counter-productive.

See also: word recognition

ANNE CUTLER

perceptual fluency A characteristic of perceptual processing related to the ease of the identification of perceptual objects. The perceptual fluency of a given stimulus can be enhanced by recent, previous exposure to that stimulus, regardless of whether the individual is consciously aware of this repetition or not. This facilitation is hypothesized to result from temporary, residual activation of the processes involved in perceptual identification (see PERCEPTUAL PRIMING). Dual-process theories of MEMORY propose that processes associated with perceptual fluency exert non-conscious, or automatic influences on tests of EXPLICIT MEMORY. These automatic influences generate feelings of familiarity (for instance, items that are easier to perceive are thought to have been seen before), but do not provide information about the spatio-temporal context in which the information was previously encountered.

See also: implicit memory

JENNIFER A. MANGELS

perceptual learning Perceptual learning occurs when subjects come to perceive or recognize particular environmental stimuli differently after repeated exposure to them. INCENTIVE MOTIVATION is not necessary and, while it is likely to occur during DISCRIMINATION LEARNING training, it arises only indirectly. Perceptual learning is a process whereby long lasting alterations occur to the percepts (that is, conscious experiences) and their neural

substrates, such that stimuli are subsequently perceive differently. D. O. Hebb (1904–1985) (see CELL ASSEMBLY THEORY) did propose a putative neural mechanism for this type of learning. Some investigators treat OBSERVATION LEARNING synonymously with perceptual learning. It also shares important features with LATENT LEARNING. For example, in both cases the learning of a new discrimination is modified by the organism's stimulation history.

RICHARD C. TEES

perceptual priming In priming phenomena, the presentation of prime stimulus alters the detection or identification of a subsequent PROBE STIMULUS. A distinction is made between perceptual and SEMANTIC PRIMING. In perceptual priming, detection of a probe is facilitated by the visual or auditory properties of the prime, not by its meaning. Perceptual priming can be seen as a form of IMPLICIT MEMORY since the subject need not be consciously aware of the prime. It is preserved in amnesiac patients (see AMNESIA). There are multiple loci of priming reflecting multiple perceptual sub-systems.

See also: explicit memory; episodic memory; semantic memory

Reference

Schacter D.L. (1994) Priming and multiple memory systems: perceptual mechanisms of implicit memory. In *Memory Systems*, ed. D.L. Schacter & E. Tulving, pp. 233–268, MIT Press: Cambridge MA.

JEREMY M. WOLFE

perceptual representation system *see* multiple memory systems

perforant path One of three major pathways of excitatory FIBRES in the HIPPOCAMPUS (the others being the mossy fibre pathway [see MOSSY FIBRES]) and the SCHAFFER COLLATERALS). The perforant path travels from the SUBICULUM to GRANULE CELLS in the HILUS of the DENTATE GYRUS. Fibres from the ENTORHINAL CORTEX (layer II) travel to CA3 (see CA1–CA3) via the perforant path also.

perforated synapses A conventional SYNAPSE is non-perforated. Perforated synapses are synapses that appear to have divided into two portions, forming two daughter synapses from one parent synapse. There is some suggestion that this is a process involved with synaptic plasticity and that the numbers of perforated synapses changes following tetanic stimulation (see TETANUS), giving rise to the possibility of an association with LONG-TERM POTENTIATION or LONG-TERM DEPRESSION.

Reference

Itarat W. & Jones D.G. (1993) Morphological characteristics of perforated synapses in the latter stages of synaptogenesis in rat neocortex – stereological and 3-dimensional approaches. *Journal of Neurocytology* 22: 753–764.

perfusion *see* infusion

pergolide An ergot-derived drug which acts as an AGONIST at DOPAMINE receptors with greater effect at D2 rather than D1 receptors. It is used as an adjunct to L-DOPA in the treatment of PARKINSON'S DISEASE. BROMO-CRIPTINE and LISURIDE are similar ergot-derived drugs.

peri-; para- Peri- and para- are two commonly encountered prefixes: peri- (from Greek, *peri*: around) indicates that something is around something else, while para (from Greek, *para*: beside) denotes that something is beside something else. So for example, the periventricular white matter (see BROCA'S APHASIA) is the WHITE MATTER around the cerebral VENTRI-CLES; the PARAVENTRICULAR NUCLEUS OF THE HYPOTHALAMUS is a nucleus in the HYPOTHA-LAMUS beside the third ventricle.

periaqueductal grey (PAG) Also known as the CENTRAL GREY or midbrain central grey, this structure is wrapped around the CEREBRAL AQUEDUCT as it travels through the MIDBRAIN and BRAINSTEM. It is composed of small neurons, with some larger cell groups embedded with in it (such as the LATERODORSAL TEGMENTAL NUCLEUS, which contains the Ch6 cell group [see CH1–CH8]).The largest inputs come from structures higher along the NEUR-AXIS. Principal inputs are from the HYPO-THALAMUS, PREOPTIC AREA, ZONA INCERTA, AMYGDALA, SUPERIOR COLLICULUS and INFER-IOR COLLICULUS, with BRAINSTEM sites (for example RAPHE NUCLEI, PARABRACHIAL NUCLEI

and LOCUS COERULEUS) making a smaller contribution. There are also some inputs from both the CEREBRAL CORTEX (mainly FRONTAL CORTEX) and the SPINAL CORD. There are also a great many intrinsic connections between different parts of the PAG. The outputs are for the most part reciprocal with the inputs: the largest outputs go to the hypothalamus and related structures such as the preoptic areas and zona incerta. Numbers of sites in the PONTINE RETICULAR FORMATION and MEDUL-LARY RETICULAR FORMATION also receive input from the PAG, as does the PEDUNCULOPON-TINE TEGMENTAL NUCLEUS. The PAG has been associated with a variety of integrative and AUTONOMIC functions, many to do with the control of AGGRESSION, DEFENCE and FEAR. VOCALIZATION and RAGE reactions can both be stimulated from here. Hormonal release is also to some extent regulated by the PAG, and it has been associated strongly with ANALGESIA and the perception of PAIN.

See also: fight-or-flight

periarcuate Literally, around (PERI-) the ARC-UATE SULCUS.

peribrachial area The area around the BRA-CHIUM CONJUNCTIVUM (also called the SUPER-IOR CEREBELLAR PEDUNCLE) that is important in the generation of PGO WAVES during REM SLEEP. The organization of this area appears to be relatively complex, with different areas have differing functions: neurons in the caudo-lateral part of the peribrachial area appear to be the most important for PGO wave production.

perifornical hypothalamus A part of the LATERAL HYPOTHALAMUS adjacent to the FOR-NIX. It has been argued that stimulation in this area by DOPAMINE is involved with FEEDING and REWARD and that the ANOREXIA produced by AMPHETAMINE is mediated here: evidence for and against this has been presented. It has also been associated with the control of BLOOD pressure.

periglomerular dopamine neurons *see* classification of Dahlström and Fuxe; dopamine

perikaryon (perikarya) Perikaryon and SOMA are both used as alternative terms for a CELL BODY. However, the term perikarya strictly refers to the CYTOPLASM surrounding the NUCLEUS of a CELL.

See also: neuron

perimetry The measurement of retinal sensitivity (see RETINA) achieved using a perimeter. The perimeter is a hemisphere onto any part of which a stimulus can be presented. The task given to the subject is to fixate (see FIXATION) on the centre of the hemisphere and attempt to detect the presented stimuli. Failure to detect in particular places is indicative of problems with localized retinal sensitivity.

perinatal (from Latin, *natus*: to be born) The period around birth.

perineum That part of the body between anus and genital organs; see SPINAL CORD.

perineurium *see* nerve

periodic limb movement in sleep *see* nocturnal myoclonus

periodic table of the elements The periodic table of the elements was formulated by Dmitri Ivanovich Mendeleev (1834–1907) a Siberian and one of Russia's most famous and influential scientists. The periodic table arranges each ELEMENT by its ATOMIC NUMBER: by doing this it effectively categorizes the elements into groups that have similar properties. The organization works remarkably well: when Mendeleev devised the table he was able to accommodate all of the known elements and leave spaces for those that had not been discovered. Subsequent research has filled gaps and confirmed the organizational principle of the table. There are a number of websites, and commercial software, that present the periodic table. Many do so in an informative and interactive way. The website www.chemicool.com (maintained by David Hsu) is helpful, and there are others than fulfill the same function just as well.

peripheral dyslexia Various types of ACQUIRED READING DISORDER – ATTENTIONAL DYSLEXIA, NEGLECT DYSLEXIA, PURE ALEXIA – that arise when the written word form is not processed effectively.

ELAINE FUNNELL

peripheral nerves and spinal nerves Peripheral nerves and spinal nerves both are, and are not, the same thing. Peripheral nerves are composed of individual neurons (see NEURON) which interact directly with body tissues. These neurons aggregate together to form peripheral nerves. As these FIBRES are traced back towards the SPINAL CORD, they group to form peripheral nerves. As these are traced back still further towards the spinal cord, they combine to an even greater degree to form spinal nerves. Of course, in both the peripheral and the spinal nerves there are in fact neurons projecting in each direction: some from the spinal cord to the body tissues and some from the body to the spinal cord. Close to the spinal cord these are separated: the AFFERENT fibres (bringing information in to the spinal cord form the body) enter the spinal cord through the DORSAL ROOT GANGLIA and the DORSAL ROOTS. The EFFERENT fibres (those fibres that travel from the spinal cord to the body) exit the spinal cord via the VENTRAL ROOTS.

See also: dermatome

peripheral nervous system The organized NERVOUS SYSTEM beyond the CENTRAL NERVOUS SYSTEM (the BRAIN and SPINAL CORD). The peripheral nervous system contains the CRANIAL NERVES and SPINAL NERVES; peripheral nerves (see PERIPHERAL NERVES AND SPINAL NERVES) and two major divisions: the AUTONOMIC NERVOUS SYSTEM (also known as the INVOLUNTARY NERVOUS SYSTEM), which further divides into the SYMPATHETIC NERVOUS SYSTEM and PARASYMPATHETIC NERVOUS SYSTEMS; and the SOMATIC NERVOUS SYSTEM (alternatively known as the VOLUNTARY NERVOUS SYSTEM).

peripheral reading disorder The term peripheral reading disorder can be taken to be synonymous with PERIPHERAL DYSLEXIA; it is therefore a term that can also be applied to the categories of dyslexia that come under this general heading: see DYSLEXIA for a description of these.

See also: pure alexia

peripheral vision Vision with the non-foveal regions of the eye (see FOVEA).

DAVID W. HEELEY

perirhinal cortex The perirhinal cortex (BRODMANN'S AREAS 35 and 36) is found in the ventromedial part of the TEMPORAL LOBE, located around the RHINAL SULCUS: it is part of the INFERIOR TEMPORAL CORTEX. It has substantial cortical connectivity, receiving input from auditory, visual and somatosensory systems and is a every early point at which polymodal information coalesces together. It has output to various suite, including HIPPO-CAMPUS, AMYGDALA, STRIATUM and to many of the cortical areas that project to it. It has been implicated in OBJECT RECOGNITION, ASSOCIA-TIVE LEARNING and MEMORY.

Reference

Murray E.A. & Bussey T.J. (1999) Perceptual-mnemonic functions of the perirhinal cortex. *Trends in Cognitive Sciences* 3: 142–151.

peristalsis Peristalsis is a form of movement of material in tubes produced by rhythmic contraction. It is used most commonly to describe the movement of material through the GASTRO-INTESTINAL SYSTEM, where rhythmic contractions of SMOOTH MUSCLE forming the walls of the gut force material along. The term can be more generally applied: a *peristaltic pump* for example is one that operates by rhythmically squeezing tubing to force fluid through.

peristriate cortex An area of CORTEX around (peri-) the STRIATE CORTEX. There has been some debate about the nature of visual processing in these areas. It appears likely that areas of cortex adjacent the striate cortex proper possesses visual functions and are to some extent at least functionally divisible.

Reference

Spatz W.B., Vogt D.M. & Illing R.-B. (1991) Delineation of the striate cortex, and the striate-peristriate projections in the guinea pig. *Experimental Brain Research* 84: 495–504.

periventricular dopamine system *see* classification of Dahlström and Fuxe; dopamine

periventricular nucleus of the hypothalamus A small nucleus at the base of the HYPOTHALAMUS, adjacent to the ARCUATE NU-CLEUS. It is most notable as a source of the TUBEROINFUNDIBULAR DOPAMINE SYSTEM. It is not the same as the PARAVENTRICULAR NU-CLEUS OF THE HYPOTHALAMUS.

peroxisomes Subcellular organs that are important in the metabolic (see METABOLISM) activity of the CELL. They contain OXIDATIVE ENZYMES which produce hydrogen peroxide for some cellular functions and are involved in breaking down FATTY ACIDS into smaller molecules that MITOCHONDRIA can use. In the LIVER, peroxisomes are important in the CATA-BOLISM of ALCOHOL.

perseveration Perseveration describes behaviour (including mental behaviour such as thinking) which, though not excessive in quantity, is restricted to a few behavioural options, and which appears to be functionless. STEREO-TYPY, in contrast, describes apparently functionless behaviour which is highly repetitive, because it is both restricted in quality and excessive in quantity. For example, only ever eating one item of diet from a wide choice would be a form of perseveration whereas excessive, continuous chewing, particularly of inedible objects would be a form of stereotypy. Perseveration can be regarded as resulting from the failure of a neural system which inhibits a pre-potent behaviour and permits a change from that behaviour to another. Such changes in behaviour usually occur in ADAPTATION to a changing environment or as the result of self-generated variations in behaviour. Perseveration may occur as a result of damage to a theoretical mechanism, the SUPERVISORY AT-TENTIONAL SYSTEM, postulated to exist in the FRONTAL LOBE of higher mammals (Shallice, 1988) although perseveration may also occur as the result of failure of other neural mechanisms. Perseveration can occur at any level of cognitive organization (Goldberg, 1986). Motor perseveration occurs when a person fails to inhibit a behaviour (and start another) when an action has been completed. For example, a person may continue to draw round and round in a circular motion having been asked to draw a circle. Task perseveration is said to occur when one task is repeated when another is requested. For example, a person may draw two, separate circles when asked to draw a circle and a square. Set perseveration is said to occur when one aspect of a task is carried over to the next task even though other aspects of the two tasks are completed differently. For example, a person may draw a circle and then draw a square having been asked to draw a circle and then write the word square. Perseveration can be demonstrated using the WIS-CONSIN CARD-SORT TEST. Perseveration frequently involves stimulus bound behaviour. This is behaviour which is determined by the most salient (perceptually striking), but not necessarily the most important, or meaningful, environmental event within the context of ongoing circumstances. For example, perseverative ATTENTION to novel acoustic events may result in distraction from conversation. Distractibility is therefore a superficially paradoxical accompaniment to perseveration. Perseveration is seen in many patients with frontal lobe damage, SCHIZOPHRENIA, AUTISM, ASPERGER'S SYNDROME and some patients with MENTAL RETARDATION.

References

Goldberg E. (1986) Varieties of perseveration: a comparison of two taxonomies. *Journal of Clinical and Experimental Psychology* 8: 710–726.

Shallice T. (1988) *From Neuropsychology to Mental Structure*, Cambridge University Press: Cambridge.

CHRISTOPHER FRITH AND ROSALIND RIDLEY

persistent vegetative state Patients in the persistent vegetative state go through a cycle of sleeping and waking but they show no meaningful response to changes in their environment except at a reflex level. They differ from patients in COMA who do not open their eyes and who fail to show REFLEX responses to stimulation. The condition is a common result of trauma: as many as 1000 beds may be occupied by patients in a vegetative state in the United Kingdom alone, and they place an exceptionally heavy burden on nursing services. The management of this condition is fraught with unanswered social, ethical, forensic and medical problems. It was formerly believed that patients who had remained in a vegetative state for more than a few months would never recover, and the ethical and clinical issues may then have seemed less daunting. More recently, however, instances have been documented where patients have started to respond and communicate in a primitive but appropriate manner after four months or more. Before this point they had failed to initiate even the simplest eye-tracking movements (Andrews, 1993). A few patients, after several years, have become able to feed themselves and to laugh at humorous situations. It remains debatable, however, whether the quality of life after 'recovery', in even the most favourable cases, would have been deemed acceptable if the patient had been able to choose beforehand (see Gillon, 1993). Critics have questioned whether heroic treatment of the persistent vegetative state can result in substantial benefit other than a sense of achievement for the medical staff. The likelihood or otherwise of future recovery is bound to be of decisive importance. Unfortunately, neurological investigation can offer scant guidance. The pathological basis of the condition is destruction of the CEREBRAL CORTEX or underlying WHITE MATTER, with sparing of the vital centres in the BRAINSTEM. The possible role of intact structures in the THALAMUS and brainstem in cognition, or in the ability to suffer PAIN, in decorticate patients, is quite unknown. This uncertainty has important implications – for example in implementing judicial decisions in North America and the UK that have authorized withdrawal of assisted nutrition and other forms of life-support when clinical circumstances seemed to warrant it.

References

Andrews K. (1993) Recovery of patients after four months or more in the persistent vegetative state. *British Medical Journal* 306: 1597–1600.

Gillon R. (1993) Patients in the persistent vegetative state: a response to Dr Andrews. *British Medical Journal* 306: 1602–1603.

L. J. HERBERG

personality Personality is a complex construct that can be construed in the most general way as the traits (both of behaviour and psychological process) that characterize an individual. Various measures of personality have been developed (such as the well known intraversion and extraversion scales, though many others exist also). A comprehensive analysis of personality is beyond the scope of this edition; interested readers are referred to a standard textbook of psychology such as Eysenck (1998). The concept of personality has impact on biological psychology only in so far as it is used in clinical settings, where the notion of PERSONALITY DISORDER is used.

Reference

Eysenck M. (1998) *Psychology: An Integrated Approach*, Longman: Harlow UK.

personality disorder DSM-IV identifies a number of personality disorders, on an axis (axis II) defined for these and MENTAL RETARDATION. They group into three clusters: cluster A can be characterized as eccentric or odd, cluster B as dramatic or erratic and C as anxious or fearful. The component conditions are indicated in the table on page 598.

Treatment for these conditions focuses on PSYCHOTHERAPY, typically the various forms of BEHAVIOUR THERAPY, COGNITIVE THERAPY and COGNITIVE–BEHAVIOURAL THERAPY.

perspective Perspective is one of a class of cues to DEPTH PERCEPTION that are generally referred to as pictorial or MONOCULAR cues in that they do not require BINOCULAR vision or observer motion, and are thus often employed by artists. With ATMOSPHERIC PERSPECTIVE, objects that are distant appear to be less sharply defined than those that are near due to light scattering in the intervening atmosphere (this also causes changes in the colour of distant objects). LINEAR PERSPECTIVE is the apparent convergence of parallel lines with increasing distance and the associated reduction in the size of a visual image as an object recedes. This is an extremely powerful cue to relative distance which is frequently exploited in painting.

DAVID W. HEELEY

pertussis toxin A bacterial toxin isolated from the bacterium *Bordetella pertussis*, the causative agent in whooping cough. The use of pertussis toxin as an experimental tool has been key to the discovery and understanding of the G PROTEIN group, membrane-bound proteins that are responsible for transducing external signals to cellular events within neurons. Pertussis toxin inactivates inhibitory G proteins (G_i), thus blocking the ability of the G protein to inhibit ADENYLATE CYCLASE, or to influence ION CHANNEL activity. To be activated, a subunit in the G_i protein must exchange a guanine diphosphate molecule (GDP) for a guanine triphosphate (GTP). Pertussis toxin catalyses the ADP-ribosylation (the addition of an adenosine diphosphate-ribose group) of an amino acid (see AMINO ACIDS) residue within the subunit, and prevents GTP from binding. This reaction is covalent, and thus the G protein is permanently inactivated until new protein can be synthesized.

ANN E. KELLEY

pervasive developmental disorder A broad category of developmental disorders that includes CHILDHOOD DISINTEGRATIVE DISORDER, AUTISM, RETT SYNDROME, ASPERGER'S SYNDROME and other disorders of DEVELOPMENT.

PET PET (positron emission tomography) is a method for generating images showing the uptake into the brain of RADIOACTIVE TRACERS from the bloodstream. The spatial precision of the method is high, allowing tracer uptake to be localized with an accuracy of less than 1 cm. This degree of precision is achieved by employing as tracers positron-emitting isotopes (for example $^{15}O_2$, ^{11}C). When such isotopes decay, each emitted positron travels only a short distance before meeting an electron. The ensuing annihilation event gives rise to the emission of two high-energy photons, which travel on paths that are exactly 180° apart. A PET scanner consists of several rings of coincidence detectors, which surround the head and register the simultaneous arrival of pairs of photons on opposite sides, thus fixing the plane along which each annihilation event occurred. This information can be used, much like X-ray data in COMPUTERIZED AXIAL TOMOGRAPHY (CAT) to construct a 3-dimensional image of the relative concentration of the tracer within the brain. By using different tracers, it is possible to image, and obtain

Principal forms of personality disorder

CLUSTER A

paranoid personality disorder	suspicious, angry, hostile; higher rates in relatives of individuals with SCHIZOPHRENIA
schizoid personality disorder	asocial, unemotional, indifferent to the comments of others, a degree of ANHEDONIA
schizotypal personality disorder	odd beliefs and magical thinking; flattened AFFECT; eccentric behaviour

CLUSTER B

antisocial personality disorder	
borderline personality disorder	unstable MOODS, relationships and self-image (was once thought of as on the border of schizophrenia and NEUROSIS - this is no longer held to be the case, though the name survives)
histrionic personality disorder	ATTENTION seeking; HYSTERIA
narcissistic personality disorder	inflated perception of self-worth; egocentric

CLUSTER C

avoidant personality disorder	oversensitive to criticism or the possibility of rejection or disapproval, with consequent poor social functioning
dependent personality disorder	low self-confidence and self-reliance; dependent behaviour and attachment difficulties
obsessive compulsive personality disorder	obsession with rules and schedules; not the same as OBSESSIVE
personality disorder	COMPULSIVE disorder

In addition:

antisocial personality disorder	see PSYCHOPATH

quantitative estimates of, several different aspects of brain function, including metabolic rate, RECEPTOR density, and blood flow. The short HALF-LIFE (approximately 2 minutes) of $^{15}O_2$ means that several scans can be obtained during a single scanning session. With modern scanners, up to 12 scans, each requiring approximately 1 minute to obtain, can be collected from a volunteer without exceeding radiation dosimetry guidelines. PET has found wide application in the study of both abnormal and normal brain function, and is an important method for FUNCTIONAL NEUROIMAGING studies of brain function.

MICHAEL D. RUGG

petal *see* fugal

pethidine Also known as MEPERIDINE, this is a synthetic compound with properties similar to MORPHINE.

See also: opiates

petit mal seizure *see* absence seizure

peyote *see* hallucinogens; mescaline

PGO waves PGO (pontine-geniculate-occipital) waves or SPIKES are hallmarks of REM SLEEP in certain mammals such as cats. They are monophasic spikes of about 200–300 microvolts recorded from the dorsolateral PONS, which contains the generator, the LATERAL GENICULATE NUCLEUS of the THALAMUS and the OCCIPITAL LOBE, hence their name. At the onset of REM sleep, the appearance of

PGO waves slightly precedes muscle atonia, ELECTROENCEPHALOGRAM changes, and rapid eye movements. PGO waves continue throughout a REM sleep period. The function of PGO waves is not clear, but is thought to be related to internal generation of visual stimuli and startle behaviour.

See also: sleep

KAZUE SEMBA

pH In solution, an acid has a greater concentration of hydrogen ions (H$^+$) (see ION) rather than hydroxide ions (OH-); a BASE has the reverse. The pH scale is used to measure the degree to which a solution is an acid or a base: the pH of any solution is defined as:

$$pH = -\log[H^+]$$

That is, pH is the negative log of the concentration of hydrogen ions in a solution. In a neutral solution the concentration of hydrogen ions is 10^{-7} M (M stands for molar) yielding a pH of 7. Values less than 7 indicate increasing acidity, more than 7 decreasing acidity (and hence increasing alkalinity – the term ALKALI is a synonym for base). The largest value is 14 (the most basic), the lowest 0. Each point on the scale represent a change of a factor of 10: a change in pH of one points represents a 10× change in acidity, a change of two points a 100× change, three points a 1000× change and so on. The degree of acidity was once measured using a litmus test, though this is rarely used now. Most laboratories will possess a pH meter that will have a special pH electrode which, when placed in a solution, will determine the pH, registering this on a meter. Most physiological fluids have a pH between about 6 and 8, though there are exceptions. Some examples of solutions and their pH are: pure water has a pH of 7; human BLOOD and CEREBROSPINAL FLUID have a pH of a little over 7. Ammonia and bleach are strong bases with pH values over 11. Urine has a slightly acid pH of about 6; black coffee has a pH of around 5. GASTRIC ACID has a pH of about 2.

The technicalities of pH are of less concern to biological psychologists than are the practicalities. Strong acids and bases burn and damage tissue (unless there are specialized protective arrangements, as is the case for highly acidic gastric acid). It is therefore of critical importance when preparing solutions for delivery to subjects – human or animal – to know what the pH is. Extremes of acidity or alkalinity can be avoided by preparing solutions in a BUFFER.

Reference

Campbell N.A., Reece J.B. & Mitchell L.G. (1999) *Biology*, 5th edn, Addison-Wesley: Menlo Park CA.

phagocyte (from Greek, *phagein*: to eat, *kytos*: a vessel) A phagocyte is a CELL that engages in a process called phagocytosis: it is a cell that eats other cells.

See also: glial cells; immune system

phantom limb pain Pain that appears to originate in an area of the body, usually a limb, that has been amputated or is congenitally absent. Phantom limb sensations occur in most patients who suffer an amputation. Approximately two-thirds of patients experience pain in the phantom at some time after the loss of the limb. Of these, 5–10% experience severe and continuing pain, the cause of which remains uncertain. The phantom limb appears to be a normal response to a loss of sensory input to the CENTRAL NERVOUS SYSTEM, since removing all the sensory input from limb by LOCAL ANAESTHETIC block of a nerve can induce the phenomenon in intact individuals, and stimulation of other body areas may be felt in the phantom limb. The location of body areas in which touch evokes touch sensations in the phantom limb may be understood in terms of their positions in the CORTICAL MAP on the SOMATOSENSORY CORTEX. The cortical map of the body surface represents the 3-dimensional surface of the body on a 2-dimensional surface. This transformation requires some distortion, and one consequence is that there are portions of the map where there are adjacent representations of body regions are not adjacent in 3-dimensional space. It is thought that the fine structure of the map is maintained by competition between the incoming sensory neurons so that, when amputation removes input from some region of the map, the innervation of the adjacent regions may take over. The result is that neural input from body areas supplying cortical regions adjacent to the representation of the amputated limb will be misinterpreted as coming from the missing limb. One of the adjacent regions is necessarily the stump remaining after the amputation, and it is suggested that pain in the stump region is referred to the phantom limb. Other potential causes of pain referred to the phantom are nociceptive (see NOCICEPTION) input from the CONTRALATERAL intact limb, and memories of previous pain stored in the brain. These suggestions derive from evidence that pain in the phantom limb is correlated with sensory and physiological changes in the contralateral intact limb, that the risk of developing phantom limb pain is increased when prolonged intense pain in the limb precedes the amputation, and that episodes of pain can be triggered by contemplation of distressing memories.

KEITH B. J. FRANKLIN

pharmacodynamic tolerance *see* cellular tolerance

pharmacodynamics The study of the actions of drugs within an organism; see DRUG.

pharmacokinetics The study of the disposition and movement of DRUGS within an organism; see DRUG; PHARMADYNAMICS.

pharmacological dose *see* physiological dose

pharynx *see* mouth

phase dependent reflexes *see* locomotion

phase timing *see* timing

phaseolus vulgaris leucoagglutinin *see* tract tracers

phasic *see* tonic–phasic

phencyclidine (PCP; Sernyl) An arylcycloalkylamine compound with anaesthetic (see ANAESTHESIA) and anti-nociceptive (see NOCICEPTION) properties. Abuse of PCP in humans may evoke toxic PSYCHOSIS.

See also: angel dust; dissociative anaesthetics; ketamine

CHARLES D. BLAHA

phenelzine *see* monoamine oxidase inhibitors

phenethylamine A class of HALLUCINOGENS including MESCALINE and the methoxylated amphetamines, the best-known of which is MDMA (3,4 methylenedioxymethamphetamine).

See also: amphetamine

phenobarbital (Luminal) Long-acting barbiturate most frequently used as an oral or intravenous hypnotic with excellent ANTI-CONVULSANT properties in humans and animals.

See also: pentobarbital; sodium amobarbital; thiopental

CHARLES D. BLAHA

phenobarbitone This is exactly the same as PHENOBARBITAL: in the United States the barbiturate drugs have '-tal' endings, but in Europe, pharmacologists have classified them using '-one' endings.

phenothiazines A class of DRUG, including CHLORPROMAZINE, used to treat SCHIZOPHRENIA; see ANTIPSYCHOTIC.

phenotype The genetic constitution of an individual is called the GENOTYPE. The PHENOTYPE in contrast is the actual observable characteristics, produced by an interaction between genetic composition and its modification by experience and the environment. A genotype is a blueprint; a phenotype is what one actually gets.

phenoxybenzamine An alpha 1 NORADRENALINE receptor ANTAGONIST; see ADRENOCEPTORS.

phentolamine A non-specific alpha NORADRENALINE receptor ANTAGONIST. It also has potassium ION CHANNEL blocking abilities.

phenylephrine An alpha-1 noradrenaline receptor AGONIST; see ADRENOCEPTORS.

phenylethanolamine-N-methyltransferase The enzyme responsible for the conversion of NORADRENALINE to ADRENALINE (in American English, norepinephrine to epinephrine). Possession of this enzyme therefore identifies those neurons capable of synthesizing adrenaline.

phenylethylamine A false neurotransmitter (see NEUROTRANSMITTERS): phenylethylamine can be taken up by noradrenaline TERMINALS and will replace NORADRENALINE in the SYNAPTIC VESICLES, before being liberated in a normal manner. It is not however particularly potent at noradrenaline receptors.

phenylketonuria A relatively rare inherited disorder, involving a recessive GENE (see RECESSIVE ALLELE): an ENZYME in the LIVER, phenylalanine hydroxylase, fails early in life. Phenylalanine is consequently not converted and accumulates, as does phenylpyruvic acid, a derivative. If undetected it can lead to brain damage (by interfering with MYELIN formation in the FRONTAL LOBE). However it is detectable: there are blood tests for parents and, in the affected infants, urine has a characteristic musty smell. Blood tests in the affected infants will also reveal excess quantities of phenylalanine. It is treated by means of low phenylalanine diet.

phenytoin One of the most commonly used ANTICONVULSANT drugs, commercially available as Dilantin. It is thought to act by inhibition of VOLTAGE-SENSITIVE ION CHANNELS for sodium (Na^+) and possibly calcium (Ca^{2+}) in neuronal membranes.

pheromones Pheromones are chemical messengers which are secreted to the outside environment where they act on other individuals, usually of the same species, to stimulate behavioural or physiological changes, by stimulating their olfactory (smell) or gustatory (taste) receptors. The term PHEROMONE was proposed by Karlson & Lüscher in 1959 to refer to substances previously called 'external hormones' (ECTOHORMONES). Other terms, such as TELERGONES, ALLOMONES and KAIROMONES have been proposed for special subsets of pheromones, but have not become popular. Pheromones have two general effects on the receiving individual: releaser effects which result in rapid behavioural changes (they 'release' behaviour) and primer effects, which alter the neuroendocrine system, resulting in a later behavioural change (they 'prime' the behavioural change). Invertebrate pheromones are detected by special CHEMORECEPTOR cells which, in many insects, are located on special hair-like antennae. Invertebrate pheromones serve as sexual attractants, stimulate aggrega-

tion or dispersal, inhibit reproduction and excite alarm reactions. There are trail pheromones, alarm pheromones and pheromones which regulate maturation. The queen bee, for example, produces a mandibular gland pheromone which inhibits ovarian development in other bees. Many invertebrate pheromones, such as bombykol, the sex attractant pheromone of the female silkworm, have been identified chemically and are used to control reproduction artificially. In vertebrates, pheromones are detected by the main olfactory receptors and the VOMERONASAL ORGAN, which stimulate the OLFACTORY NERVES causing neurotransmitter release in the OLFACTORY BULB and other brain areas. This can release an immediate change in behaviour or prime a later behavioural change by activating the neuroendocrine system and influencing the release of hypothalamic, pituitary and gonadal HORMONES. Vertebrate pheromones serve as sex attractants, maternal odours and alarm odours, and can regulate reproduction by facilitating or inhibiting puberty and adult reproductive behaviour. The pheromone concept has been criticized as most pheromones consist of a complex mixture of chemicals rather than a single chemical; the responses to the odour may be learned through experience rather than innate and there are may chemical signals which serve no specific function. For example, individual-specific odours and odours that distinguish males from females do not 'trigger' any specific response. Thus, pheromones should be characterized by the information they contain as well as by the responses that they elicit. Terms such as CHEMOSIGNALS and SOCIAL ODOURS have been used to circumvent the problems with the use of the term pheromone, but the concept of 'pheromones' has been resistant to change.

See also: gustation; olfaction; reproduction; sexual behaviour

Reference

Karlson P. & Lüscher M. (1959) 'Pheromones': a new term for a class of biologically active substances. *Nature* 183: 55–56.

RICHARD E. BROWN

Phineas Gage On 13 September 1848, Phineas Gage suffered a bizarre accident in which a tamping iron was propelled through the front part of his head. The iron entered his left cheek just under the eye, pierced the frontal lobes (see FRONTAL LOBE) of his brain and exited through the top front part of his head. Gage's medical recovery was nothing short of astonishing, as he survived this massive onslaught with normal INTELLIGENCE, MEMORY, speech, sensation and movement. However, Gage displayed a profound change in personality and social conduct that established him as a landmark case in the history of neuroscience. Formerly responsible, socially well adapted, and well liked by peers and supervisors, after the accident Gage became irresponsible and untrustworthy, irreverent and capricious, with markedly unreliable behaviour and little regard for social convention.

John Harlow, Gage's physician, astutely surmised that there was a causative relationship between the damage to the front part of Gage's brain and the profound change in his personality and social conduct. Harlow's observations, which were never fully appreciated by his contemporaries, hinted at a conclusion that was both radical and prescient: there are structures in the front part of the human brain that are dedicated to the planning and execution of personally and socially adaptive behaviour, and to the aspect of reasoning known as rationality. A number of subsequent case reports supported Harlow's contention, and modern neuropsychological investigations have documented that the PREFRONTAL CORTEX is crucial for social conduct, planning, and decision-making. Relatedly, this region plays a key role in emotional behaviour, and in particular, the link between EMOTION and reasoning. Studies have shown, for example, that reasoning with too little emotion can be as detrimental for good decision-making as reasoning with too much emotion. The role of emotions in DECISION-MAKING, at both conscious and non-conscious levels, is more important than previously believed.

The tools of modern neuroscience enabled scientists to perform a careful reconstruction of the injury to Gage's brain. Specifically, using measurements of Gage's skull and the tamping iron (which are part of the Warren Anatomical Medical Museum at Harvard University), scientists were able to deduce the precise path of the tamping iron through Gage's brain, and to confirm that the damage included the left and right prefrontal regions, anterior to structures required for motor behaviour and speech, and in precisely the location that has been confirmed in modern studies as the key neural underpinning of rational decision-making and the processing of emotion.

See also: executive functions; social behaviour; somatic marker hypothesis

DANIEL TRANEL

phobia Irrational and persistent FEAR of certain objects, animals or situations. Descriptions of phobic behaviour have been known throughout history – for example Hippocrates described a man who had an irrational fear of bridges. Usually a fear is described as a phobia only when it has a significant impact on a person's life. For example many people have a fear of poisonous snakes, but this does not usually impact on everyday functioning unless the person is in an environment where poisonous snakes are commonly found. If a person living in Ireland (where there are no snakes at all) spent a significant amount of time worrying about coming into contact with snakes, then this would be described as phobic.

A question which has exercised clinicians and researchers for decades is how phobias come into existence. Why is one person terrified of spiders when another person has no fear of them at all? One of the earliest theories was an explanation in terms of CLASSICAL CONDITIONING. The stimulus or situation which is to become phobic is one which, initially, the person has no fear of. It is accidentally or adventitiously paired with an aversive stimulus in a typical classical conditioning paradigm (see AVERSIVE CONDITIONING), and thus acquires many of the same fear inducing properties as the aversive stimulus. A report published in 1920 by the American behaviourist John B. Watson (1878–1958) in which he described establishing a conditioned emotional reaction (see CONDITIONED REFLEX) in Albert B., an 11-month-old child, is the basis for this theory. Albert was invited to stroke a white rat, whereupon an iron bar was struck behind his head. Eventually he came to fear the rat, and this generalized (see STIMULUS GENERALIZATION) to a rabbit, a dog, a fur (seal) coat, Watson's hair and a Santa Claus mask. However most investigators do not now consider this to be an adequate general explanation of the AETIOLOGY of phobias for two main reasons. First, it is rarely the case that a clear conditioning process can be identified for individuals who have phobias. Second, it is known that some stimuli and situations are much more likely to enter into phobias than others. For example, very rarely would anyone become afraid of electric plug sockets (even though they are potentially dangerous) whereas it is very common for people to be afraid of snakes, even when it is highly unlikely that a person has ever directly come into contact with a snake. One explanation of this incorporates the notion that humans might be biologically prepared to be phobic of some situations, especially those likely to threaten our survival. These would obviously include many situations such as heights and potentially dangerous animals, and this also allows us to see why it is difficult or even impossible to condition fears to other, non-threatening situations or stimuli. In order to preserve the classical conditioning theory of phobias, theorists have also invoked the involvement of more complex aspects of the conditioning paradigm such as EXPECTANCY BASED MEMORY, HIGHER-ORDER CONDITIONING, SENSORY PRECONDITIONING, BLOCKING, and LATENT INHIBITION. Thus modern understandings of the aetiology of phobias bring in cognitive factors.

Competing psychological approaches, such as those based on PSYCHOANALYSIS, view phobias as the SIGNS AND SYMPTOMS of underlying psychic conflict and treatment under these paradigms involves dealing with the conflicts rather than with the symptoms alone. This debate between BEHAVIOUR THERAPY and psychoanalysis was humorously portrayed in the paper describing the 'Little Albert' experiment: 'The Freudians twenty years from now, unless their hypotheses change, when they come to analyse Albert's fear of a seal skin coat … will probably tease from him the recital of a dream which upon their analysis will show that

Albert at three years of age attempted to play with the pubic hair of the mother and was scolded violently for it' (Watson & Rayner, 1920). Behavioural and COGNITIVE THERAPY approaches are generally the treatments of choice with direct exposure to the fearful stimuli being the method most likely to reduce the phobia.

Reference

Watson J.B. & Rayner R. (1920) Conditioned emotional reactions. *Journal of Experimental Psychology* 3: 1 – 14.

CHRIS CULLEN

phobic anxiety *see* anxiety

phonagnosia A form of AGNOSIA relating to the SPEECH PERCEPTION.

phoneme A speech sound such as a vowel or a consonant; the smallest independent unit capable of distinguishing two WORDS – for example, *grammar* from *glamour*.

See also: phonetics; phonology

ANNE CUTLER

phonemic cueing *see* anomia

phonemic paraphasia *see* anomia

phonetics (from Greek, *phone*: voice) Phonetics is a branch of linguistics concerned with the sound of spoken LANGUAGE.

See also: phonic; phonology; speech production; speech percep-tion; word recognition

phonetic memory *see* short-term memory

phonic (from Greek, *phone*: voice) The term phonic is always used in relation to sound, especially speech. For example, the phonic method (or more colloquially, PHONICS) is a method of teaching READING by appreciation of the sounds words (or their component parts) have.

See also: phonology; speech perception; speech production

phonological dysgraphia *see* agraphia

phonological dyslexia An ACQUIRED READING DISORDER in which the oral READING of unfamiliar words and novel letter strings is most affected and often completely removed.

Familiar words are read more successfully and, in general, words with irregular spelling–sound correspondences (for example, *pint*, *yacht*) are read as successfully as regular words (for example, *mint*, *throng*). Frequently occurring written words are read better than less frequent and, sometimes, concrete words are read better than abstract words. Visual errors (for instance, *campaign* – *camping*) but not semantic errors, occur. The brain LESION associated with phonological dyslexia affects the LANGUAGE areas of the dominant HEMISPHERE. Theoretical models of normal reading can account for phonological dyslexia as an impairment to the sublexical phonological processes involved in decoding novel letter strings into sound.

See also: central dyslexia; deep dyslexia; developmental dyslexia; surface dyslexia

Reference

Coltheart M. (ed) (1996) Phonological Dyslexia. Special issue. *Cognitive Neuropsychology* 13: 749–887.

ELAINE FUNNELL

phonological loop *see* articulatory loop

phonological store A limited-capacity SHORT-TERM MEMORY system that briefly retains spoken information. The memory traces of information held in this store fade and disappear within one to two seconds, but a process of REHEARSAL can ensure continued retention. The phonological store is assumed to play an important role in LANGUAGE acquisition, spoken-language comprehension, and learning to read.

See also: articulatory loop; central executive; working memory

Reference

Baddeley A.D. (1990). *Human Memory: Theory and Practice*, Laurence Erlbaum: Hove UK.

ANNE CUTLER

phonology (i) The system and patterns of sounds occurring in a given language. Phonology includes both segmental (see PHONEME) and supra-segmental patterning (see PROSODY). (ii) A branch of linguistic science: the study of

(i). Phonology is distinguished from PHONETICS. Phonology tells us that *leaping* and *reaping* are different words in English (but such a contrast does not exist in the phonology of Japanese); and that the first phoneme of *leaping* is the same as the last phoneme of *ball*. Phonetics tells us that in most English dialects these two realizations of the same phoneme are pronounced quite differently.

See also: speech production; speech perception

ANNE CUTLER

phosphate buffer A buffer solution; it is typically made in a form known as Sörensen's buffer, with sodium phosphate (dibasic) and potassium acid phosphate. It is used as a VEHICLE for many substances (EXCITOTOXINS for example) administered to the CENTRAL NERVOUS SYSTEM.

phosphoinositide *see* inositol

phospholipase An ENZYME involved in the regulation of PHOSPHOLIPIDS. There are two varieties, phospholipase C and phospholipase A_2, that are important in the generation of SECOND MESSENGERS.

Reference

Kandel E.R., Schwartz J.H. & Jessell T.M. (2000) *Principles of Neural Science*, 4th edn, McGraw-Hill: New York.

phospholipids *see* lipids

phosphorylation The donation of a phosphate group from ADENOSINE TRIPHOSPHATE (ATP) to another MOLECULE is called PHOSPHORYLATION; the receiving molecule is said to have been phosphorylated. It is an important part of energy metabolism.

Reference

Campbell N.A., Reece J.B. & Mitchell L.G. (1999) *Biology*, 5th edn, Addison-Wesley: Menlo Park CA.

phosphotidylinositol *see* inositol

photic (from Greek, *photos*: light) An adjective indicating a relation to light. For example, photic driving describes the rhythmic firing of the ELECTROENCEPHALOGRAM caused by flickering light (which can cause EPILEPSY in susceptible people).

photometry The radiant flux of a source is the total amount of energy emitted as electromagnetic radiation, integrated across all wavelengths. RADIOMETRY is the assessment of this quantity. In practical terms, radiometric measurements pose many challenges due to the fact that no single detector device has a uniform response to all wavelengths. PHOTOMETRY (from Greek, *photos*: light) is a special case of radiometry and is concerned with measuring the radiant energy that stimulates the human eye, and is conducted with a photo-detector that has the same SPECTRAL SENSITIVITY as a hypothetical 'standard observer'. This spectral sensitivity is defined by the LUMINOUS EFFICIENCY FUNCTION, a curve of LUMINOSITY COEFFICIENTS (the proportion of incident light energy absorbed at the retina) for the range of visible wavelengths. These coefficients are derived from measurements of the intensity of the sensation of BRIGHTNESS or LUMINOSITY at different wavelengths, induced by a source of constant energy (the LUMINOSITY CURVE). Luminous efficiency functions have been defined for the light adapted eye (the photopic curve) and the dark adapted EYE (the scotopic curve) (see SCOTOPIC VS. PHOTOPIC) corresponding to the visual response mediated by the photoreceptor systems of CONES and RODS respectively.

There are four photometric quantities. The LUMINOUS FLUX is the total radiant flux adjusted for the luminous efficiency function and is expressed in lumens. The LUMINOUS INTENSITY is the luminous flux per unit of solid angle. It is expressed in lumens per steradian or candelas. This is much more convenient measure than luminous flux as few if any sources radiate equally in all directions (isotropically). LUMINANCE is a measure of the brightness of an extended source of surface, expressed in candelas per metre squared and is typically the measure used to define the brightness of surfaces such as VDU screens, and finally ILLUMINENCE is a measure of the luminous flux density that is incident on a surface, expressed in lumens per square metre.

DAVID W. HEELEY

photon For many purposes, light can be considered as a form of wave. However, quantum theory shows that, particularly with respect to the interaction of light with matter (as in the photoelectric effect), light energy is not continuously distributed throughout the wave but is carried in discrete bundles of energy known as photons. The energy carried by a photon is not divisible but is of a specific amount or quantum and remains concentrated in the photon throughout its journey across space.

DAVID W. HEELEY

photon noise A photon is a unit of light (or of other electromagnetic radiation). Light is quantal in nature: photon production obeys the laws of quantum physics, and photons arriving at any photoreceptive surface can be described only in terms of an average number arriving in a given period of time. The uncertainty is therefore referred to as photon noise.

photoperiod The period in every 24-hour cycle when an organism is exposed to light. Photoperiodism describes the physiological response to light shown by organisms; see BIOLOGICAL CLOCK; MELATONIN.

photophobia (from Greek, *photos*: light, *phobos*: fear) A desire to avoid light – literally a fear of light. Photophobia is a phenomenon particularly associated with MIGRAINE, in which exposure to light is painful. Photophobia is not a fear of having one's photograph taken.

photopic *see* scotopic vs. photopic

photopigment *see* spectral sensitivity; visual pigment

photoreceptor (from Greek, *photos*: light, and RECEPTOR) A receptor for a specific form of sensory transduction – the conversion of photic energy (light) into neural activity; see CONES; RETINA; RODS; SENSORY TRANSDUCTION; SPECTRAL SENSITIVITY.

phrenic nerve (from Greek, *phrenos*: midriff) The phrenic nerve is involved in the control of activity in the diaphragm; it has a role in the control of breathing (see BREATHING, NEURAL CONTROL OF).

phrenology Phrenology is a system of brain–behaviour relationships articulated by Franz Josef Gall (1758–1828) and Johann Spurzheim

(1776–1832) in the late eighteenth and early nineteenth centuries. Gall and Spurzheim outlined in detail how 27 different cognitive functions and personality traits were subserved by specific brain regions. Phrenology was based on skull saliencies: that is, bumps on the skull were used as clues about underlying brain specialization. For example, Gall noted that his schoolmates with superior MEMORY had prominent eyes, and reasoned that this was the result of overdevelopment of underlying brain regions important for memory. The notion of phrenology has always been controversial. Not only did the phrenological maps contain a degree of detail about cerebral localization that far outstripped empirical evidence, but the evidence itself – correlations between skull bumps and mental capacities – bordered on the absurd. Another problem with phrenology was the inclusion of traits such as 'God and religion' and 'love for one's offspring' which not only had poor consensus about their meaning, but also religious connotations that attracted rancorous criticism, especially from those disturbed by the anti-dualistic nature of Gall's position. Marie-Jean-Pierre Flourens (1794–1867) for example, conducted ABLATION experiments in which he demonstrated that the crucial factor in how an organism was affected by brain damage was the extent of tissue removed (the size of the lesion) and not the location of damage. There ensued a long-running debate between 'localizationists' and 'anti-localizationists', the latter of whom insisted that the CEREBRAL HEMISPHERES operated as a unity, without specific specialization of function. This debate has been regularly revisited throughout the last century of neuroscience, often in ways that resembled the polemics of the early nineteenth century. For example, discoveries such as those of Paul Broca (1824–1904) and Carl Wernicke (1824–1880)which showed that we speak with the LEFT HEMISPHERE, were countered by the experiments of Shepherd Ivory Franz (1874–1983) and Karl Lashley (1848–1904) which demonstrated that all areas of the cerebral cortex were equally important for complex learning and memory. As a system of cerebral localization, phrenology earned a rather robust negative connotation but in retrospect, the phrenologists deserve credit for initiating a highly productive debate which has fuelled the advance of neuroscience, stimulating empirical studies of brain–behaviour relationships and important discoveries about neural plasticity and recovery of function.

See also: equipotentiality; localization of function; plasticity; dualism

DANIEL TRANEL

phylogenetic scale A term used in the late nineteenth century to indicate a linear hierarchy of SPECIES. It was assumed that there was orderly evolutionary progression from the simplest animals to humans. Modern approaches to EVOLUTION do not emphasize linearity but attempt instead to engage in cladistic (see CLADE) analysis of species.

phylogeny *see* ontogeny

physical dependence A state in which an organism needs the presence of a DRUG in order to maintain physiological HOMEOSTASIS. In physical dependence, as blood levels of the drug subside and eventually disappear, characteristic physical WITHDRAWAL signs appear that can vary from relatively mild to life-threatening. A number of drugs have the potential to cause physical dependence, the most well-known ones being ALCOHOL, OPIATES (such as MORPHINE and HEROIN) and BARBITURATES. Individuals physically dependent on these drugs must take the drug in order to feel well and function normally. An example of the type of physical signs observed when the drug is removed might include sweating, diarrhoea, tremor, changes in body temperature and weight loss, which are accompanied by intense DRUG CRAVING in order to restore equilibrium. The precise mechanisms underlying the development of physical dependence are not yet known, but it is the subject of intense study. It is believed that with chronic exposure to the drug, major neuroadaptive changes take place at the level of intracellular signalling proteins and GENE EXPRESSION.

See also: addiction; neuroadaptation

ANN E. KELLEY

physiological challenge The term physiological challenge was originally applied to a series of injections given to rats to promote EATING or DRINKING following LESION of the LATERAL HYPOTHALAMUS (see LATERAL HYPOTHALAMIC SYNDROME). Systemic injections of 2-DEOXY-GLUCOSE (which generate an apparent state of cellular GLUCOSE depletion) were given to stimulate feeding; injections of HYPERTONIC SALINE (5.0% saline) were given to generate INTRACELLULAR DEHYDRATION and injections of POLYETHYLENE GLYCOL were given to stimulate EXTRACELLULAR DEHYDRATION; both these last two stimulated drinking. Later studies have used other stimulants: ANGIOTENSIN II for example also stimulates drinking. In each case the stimulus was given to produce a change in body physiology which would in turn promote a specific behavioural act. Rats with lesions of the lateral hypothalamus were found to be defective in responding to these challenges, even though they were capable of independent feeding and drinking under normal circumstances.

physiological dose A term used to indicate the scale of a dose of drug or chemical: a physiological dose is one that is within the range of concentrations found naturally in an organism; a PHARMACOLOGICAL DOSE is one that goes beyond this.

physiological psychology *see* biological psychology

physiological saline *see* isotonic saline

physiological tremor tremor

physostigmine A reversible anti-ACETYLCHO-LINESTERASE drug, found in the Calabar bean, the seed of *Physostigma venenosum*. During the nineteenth century and before, it was used in Africa (where the Calabar bean comes from) as an 'ordeal poison' in identifying witches; in contemporary science it is used in experimental animals to block the actions of acetylcholinesterase, thereby potentiating the effects of ACETYLCHOLINE, which will not be broken down if acetylcholinesterase function is impaired; and it is used clinically to treat MYASTHENIA GRAVIS. It is closely related to NEOSTIGMINE, a synthetic form of physostigmine first used in 1931: the principal difference is that neostigmine does not cross the BLOOD–BRAIN BARRIER, while physostigmine does.

phytohormones Plant hormones; see HORMONES.

pia mater *see* meninges

pica (from Latin, *pica*: a magpie) A craving for unsuitable food.

Pick's disease A dementing illness, distinct from ALZHEIMER'S DEMENTIA, often presenting with signs of FRONTAL LOBEdysfunction. The condition is extremely rare, affects women twice as often as men, and peak onset is in the fifth and sixth decades of life. Hereditary transmission as a dominant trait may occur, though many cases appear to be sporadic. Pathologically, severe and selective atrophy of frontal and anterior temporal lobes is observed. Pick's disease is a cause of PRESENILE DEMENTIA. There is no effective treatment.

IAN C. REID

pico- Prefix indicating a factor of 10^{-12}, or one million millionth; see SI UNITS.

picrotoxin A drug that acts at GABA-A RECEPTORS (see GABA RECEPTORS), where it is a noncompetitive ANTAGONIST (see COMPETITIVE–NONCOMPETITIVE BINDING). Picrotoxin is made of two components, picrotin and pictoxinin, the latter being the active component.

pill rolling *see* Parkinson's disease; tremor

pilocarpine *see* parasympathomimetic drugs

piloerection The raising of body hair, a process controlled by smooth MUSCLES (under the control of the SYMPATHETIC NERVOUS SYSTEM) operating on HAIR FOLLICLES (see SKIN). Raising and lowering of body hair has a role in THERMOREGULATION, since compacted hair traps air, which can be kept reasonably warm: straightening the hairs liberates this air and has a cooling effect. Piloerection is also important as an index of EMOTION, though it is difficult to quantify and is therefore rarely measured formally. The hair along dogs' backs, for example, rises during threat and prior to ATTACK. (In dogs it is known as raising the hackles, these being the hairs on a dog's neck. The term is part of colloquial English: 'making hackles rise' is an expression describing making someone angry.) The haplorhine PRIMATES (including chimpanzees and baboons for example) raise the hairs along their neck when threatened and about to engage in AGGRESSION (as indeed do other MAMMALS – dogs for example). Indeed, the ALPHA MALE in a group of chimpanzees will maintain a more-or-less permanent state of piloerection, possibly to give an appearance of greater size. Piloerection *per se* is controlled by smooth MUSCLES under SYMPATHETIC NERVOUS SYSTEM control. What processes produce this effect in emotional states though is not at all clear – but then the physiological basis of emotion itself in general is far from understood. The vestiges of piloerection in man might account for the common (but little investigated) phenomenon of shivers down the spine (see SHIVERING).

piloting *see* navigation

pimozide An atypical ANTIPSYCHOTIC drug.

pindolol A non-selective beta NORADRENALINE receptor ANTAGONIST; see ADRENOCEPTORS.

pineal gland Also known as the pineal body, this is a small gland located above the THALAMUS, along the MIDLINE, adjacent to the third ventricle (see VENTRICULAR SYSTEM). It has no apparent connection with the CENTRAL NERVOUS SYSTEM but is part of the AUTONOMIC NERVOUS SYSTEM. It contains relatively high concentrations of MELATONIN and SEROTONIN and is thought to have a role in the control of CIRCADIAN RHYTHM, especially in lower animals such as amphibia; in MAMMALS this function has been assumed by the SUPRACHIASMATIC NUCLEUS. Once at the centre of attention – Descartes thought it the seat of the soul – it is now merely a puzzle, having no apparent significant function.

pink noise *see* noise

pinna (from Latin, *pinna*: a feather) Strictly, pinna (plural pinnae) refers to any wing, fin, feather or similar projection from the body. In practice, it commonly (unless specified otherwise) refers to the external part of the auditory system: the ear.

See also: hearing theories; sound localization

pinocytosis A form of ENDOCYTOSIS in which MEMBRANE fragments are used in SYNAPTIC TERMINALS to create SYNAPTIC VESICLES.

piperazine The piperazines are a type of DRUG (for example, FLUPHENAZINE and TRIFLUOPERAZINE) related to the PHENOTHIAZINES, with ANTIPSYCHOTIC activity. They have quite significant EXTRAPYRAMIDAL SIDE-EFFECTS and are not commonly used.

pipradrol Pipradrol is one of the PSYCHOMOTOR STIMULANTS, an analogue of AMPHETAMINE with considerable potency. It is a drug rarely used any longer, but a number of classic studies examining the way in which environmental stimuli can modify the effects of drugs were conducted with pipradrol.

References

Robbins T.W. (1976) Relationship between reward-enhancing and stereotypical effects of psychomotor stimulant drugs. *Nature* 264: 57–59.
Robbins T.W. (1978) The acquisition of responding with conditioned reinforcement: effects of pipradrol, methylphenidate, *d*-amphetamine and nomifensine. *Psychopharmacology* 58: 79–87.

piracetam Piracetam is a NOOTROPIC drug – indeed it is the prototypical nootropic, from which several others have been derived. It is a PYROLIDONE derivative; its mechanism of action remains unclear.

See also: cognitive enhancers

piriform cortex *see* pyriform cortex

pitch Pitch is the subjective perceptual correlate of stimulus frequency. For simple sinusoidal sounds, pitch is determined entirely by signal frequency. For complex, periodic waveforms, pitch is determined largely by the FUNDAMENTAL FREQUENCY, while the distribution of the harmonic frequencies contributes to the TIMBRE of the sound. Indeed, the pitch of a complex harmonic tone remains close to that of the fundamental, even if the fundamental frequency itself is missing. This suggests that for complex sounds, a pattern recognition process may contribute to pitch perception. A percept of pitch can also arise from the temporal spacing within inherently noisy sounds (for example, clicks).

DENNIS P. PHILLIPS

pituitary gland The pituitary has been called the 'master endocrine gland'. It lies immediately below the brain, tucked into the bony portion of the skull that serves as the floor that supports the brain, and in one sense is almost an extension of the brain itself. Direct connections exist between it and the bottom structure of the DIENCEPHALON, the HYPOTHALAMUS. These connections are of two types. The first is direct neural projections, in which neurons that lie in the hypothalamus(in particular within the PARAVENTRICULAR NUCLEUS OF THE HYPOTHALAMUS and the SUPRAOPTIC NUCLEUS OF THE HYPTHALAMUS) send their axons (projection fibres) directly through the stalk (INFUNDIBULUM) that connects the brain to the pituitary and into the anterior portion of the pituitary gland, where they may stimulate endocrine cells to secrete HORMONES into the general BLOOD circulation. The second type of connection involves a special set of blood vessels that travel from the hypothalamus to the pituitary (HYPOTHALAMO-PITUITARY PORTAL SYSTEM) which acts as a porter to allow chemical neurosecretory signals secreted by neurons in the hypothalamus (see NEUROSECRETION) to be passed directly to cells in the anterior portion of the pituitary gland. These chemicals stimulate cells in this portion of the pituitary to secrete their own hormones into the general blood supply. In this way, groups of neurons in the hypothalamus can activate the pituitary as fingers playing upon a keyboard: causing a particular combination of pituitary hormones to be released, and any combination can be produced depending only upon the combination of hypothalamic command neurons that are activated. Thus the pituitary acts as an interface between the brain and the rest of the body, broadcasting signals via chemical hormones to receptors that may lie anywhere else. Pituitary hormones are particularly important for controlling physiological events relevant to set of basic motivational states such as SEXUAL BEHAVIOUR, MATERNAL BEHAVIOUR, STRESS, THIRST, and SALT APPETITE. For example, the secretion of SEX HORMONES by the OVARIES of females or the TESTES of males is regulated by groups of cells in the anterior pituitary, which secrete LUTEINIZING HORMONE when the hypothalamus commands. In females, luteinizing hormone secretion occurs in cyclic pulses, and leads to the conditions required for conception. In males, the hormone has a different name but is released continuously to stimulate the testes. The difference between luteinizing hormone secretion in males and females is not caused by differences in their pituitary glands themselves, but instead by differences in their hypothalamic signals that control the pituitary. Other endocrine cells in the anterior pituitary secrete the stress hormone, adrenocorticotropin (ACTH) when stimulated by the hypothalamic-pituitary portal system. Conversely, in the posterior pituitary some cells secrete VASOPRESSIN (also known as antidiuretic hormone) which can stimulate thirst and cause the body to retain fluid, when neurally stimulated by the hypothalamus. Others secrete OXYTOCIN, which promotes lactation, maternal behaviour, and may also be activated in sexual behaviour.

KENT C. BERRIDGE

pituitary stalk Also known as the INFUNDIBULUM; see ADENOHYPOPHYSIS; PITUITARY GLAND.

pK$_a$ A measurement taken in chemistry: pK$_a$ is the PH at which 50% of an ACID dissociates into hydrogen ions (H+) (see ION) and BASE. Strong acids have a low pK$_a$ and weak acids high pK$_a$.

place aversion In general place conditioning studies have had animals (or humans) conditioned (see CONDITIONING) to develop a positive preference for a place in which POSITIVE REINFORCEMENT was available. Place aversion involves the reverse of this: the learned avoidance (see AVOIDANCE LEARNING) of a place in which NEGATIVE REINFORCEMENT was presented; see PLACE CONDITIONING for further information.

place cells A type of NEURON in the HIPPOCAMPUS. Place cells increase their activity when an animal is oriented to a particular region in SPACE. The discovery of place cells was important in the development of O'Keefe &

Nadel's theories concerning the hippocampus as a COGNITIVE MAP.

See also: head direction cells; spatial behaviour

Reference

O'Keefe J. & Nadel L. (1978) *The Hippocampus as a Cognitive Map*, Clarendon Press: Oxford.

place code *see* hearing theories; tonotopic representation

place conditioning (conditioned place preference) A form of ASSOCIATIVE LEARNING that requires an animal to approach a location that has been previously associated with a REWARD or avoid a location hat has been associated with PUNISHMENT. The general conditioned place preference paradigm consists of an apparatus with two compartments, each compartment exhibiting distinct visuo-spatial and tactile cues (for instance, black vs. white compartment; smooth vs. rough floor). During the initial phase of positive place preference conditioning, the animal is confined to one of the compartments either where a reward is administered (which will be the paired compartment) or the compartment where no reward is administered (the unpaired compartment) on separate days. This procedure is normally repeated over four to ten days (though in some cases, for even longer). The compartments that are paired and unpaired with reward remain consistent over the course of training. On the test day, no reward is presented. The animal is placed in a neutral compartment that is connected to both the paired and unpaired sides of the apparatus, and is allowed to move freely through both compartments. The presence of a conditioned place preference is observed when the animals spend a greater amount of time in the compartment that was previously paired with the reward, relative to the compartment where no reward was administered. Thus, the compartment where reward was received previously becomes a conditioned reinforcer (see CONDITIONED REINFORCEMENT) to the animal. Place conditioning can be established using a variety of natural and artificial rewarding stimuli, such as food, water, sexually receptive mates, PSY-

CHOMOTOR STIMULANTS and OPIATES. This paradigm is useful in assessing the rewarding effects of drugs of abuse. LESIONS or pharmacological manipulations are said to effect the ACQUISITION of place conditioning if administration of such treatments during the conditioning phase has an effect on the magnitude of place preference exhibited on the test day. Alternatively, treatments effect the expression of place conditioning if they effect the magnitude of place preference exhibited on the test day when administered after the conditioning phase.

Studies on the neurobiology of place conditioning have determined that the lateral nucleus of the AMYGDALA plays a crucial role in mediating this behaviour. Lesions to the lateral nuclei of the amygdala prevent both the acquisition and the expression of place conditioning for food, water or psychostimulant reward. In addition, expression of place conditioning for a natural reward is mediated by a neural circuit linking the basolateral amygdala to the NUCLEUS ACCUMBENS. For example, DISCONNECTION between the amygdala and the nucleus accumbens disrupted the expression of place conditioning for a sucrose solution. In addition, psychopharmacological studies suggest that the MESOLIMBIC DOPAMINE SYSTEM is also involved in place conditioning. Depletions of DOPAMINE in the nucleus accumbens using 6-HYDROXYDOPAMINE disrupts the acquisition of place conditioning for psychomotor stimulant reward. Likewise, microinfusions of dopamine AGONISTS directly into the nucleus accumbens can elicit a conditioned place preference.

One debate regarding place conditioning is whether or not animals actually condition to the place where they received reward (that is, is recognition of which compartment to approach based on spatial cues?) or whether they approach other types of stimuli that were present in the paired compartment (for example, tactile or visual cues). For this reason, some authors have proposed that this behaviour should be referred to as 'CUE CONDITIONING'. Also, there remains a considerate debate as to whether this form of learning should be classified as PAVLOVIAN CONDITIONING or as INSTRUMENTAL CONDITIONING. Another controversy is whether place conditioning for psychomotor stimulant reward results in a place preference or PLACE AVERSION. In one study, chronic administration of AMPHETAMINE ($\geqslant 10$ administrations) resulted in a preference for the unpaired compartment (a conditioned place avoidance). The studies have suggested that administration of amphetamine can have both rewarding and aversive properties, depending on the administration schedule, and on how often the drug is administered. Studies on place conditioning are especially valuable in understanding how conditioned stimuli associated with drug taking can trigger relapses in drug SELF ADMINISTRATION behaviour. Drug addicts frequently report that presentation of stimuli that have been associated with drug taking (for example, their crack house, bent spoon, hypodermic syringe) can elicit WITHDRAWAL symptoms and lead to the re-initiation of drug use. It is thought that by understanding the psychological and neural dynamics of phenomena like place conditioning, we may be able to better understand the role that external stimuli play in drug taking behaviour.

See also: drug abuse; place learning; state dependence

STANLEY B. FLORESCO

place learning Place learning is contrasted with RESPONSE LEARNING: response learning requires use of a specific RESPONSE to solve a problem or execute a task; place learning involves learning to proceed to a particular place (or in a particular direction). The term place learning is also used more orless synonymously with PLACE CONDITIONING.

place preference Also known as CONDITIONED PLACE PREFERENCE, but better described as PLACE CONDITIONING.

place theory *see* hearing theories

placebo A pharmacological inert compound administered to a subject instead of the active DRUG. The original meaning of the term, from the Latin placebo: *I shall please*, referred to an inactive substance given to satisfy a patient's demand for medicine. The relationship between the patient or subject, the experimental or physician, and the experimental setting can influence expectations, motivations, and most importantly, the actual response to a drug. The response that a subject may have to a placebo (when he or she actually believes the drug is being administered) is called a placebo effect. The placebo effect is a very real phenomenon. For example, a person may believe that a drug is being administered to relieve PAIN. If the pain threshold is then measured, there may a statistically significant reduction in pain threshold, although it would likely be much less than the effect of the real drug. The phenomenon in large part reflects the power of suggestibility, and it has been estimated that approximately 30% of the population is susceptible to placebo effects. In research, the placebo is an essential part of experimental design, in order to account for any placebo effects. A double blind placebo controlled study is one in which neither the subject nor the experimenter are aware of what treatment the subject receives.

Reference

Brown W.A. (1998) The placebo effect. *Scientific American* 278: 68–73.

ANN E. KELLEY

placenta The placenta is formed from tissue lining the UTERUS and MEMBRANE tissue from the embryo(s). The function of the placenta is to deliver NUTRIENTS from the mother to offspring gestating (see GESTATION) in the WOMB. Most MAMMALS gestate within the mother's womb: the term EUTHERIAN MAMMALS is applied to those mammals that do this.

In humans, the placenta is present from the fourth week of gestation until birth. Maternal BLOOD, coming from arteries in the maternal portion of the placenta, runs intro pools in an area of the placenta known as the *endometrium*; it exist from here via veins. The FOETUS or EMBRYO is able to extract OXYGEN and nutrients from the endometrium via extensions called the chorionic villi (the CHORION being the foetus's portion of the placenta). The foetus connects to the placenta via the umbilical cord, though which umbilical arteries and veins flow. At birth the placenta is delivered with the baby still attached to it via the umbilical cord: cutting this cord gives rise to the belly button.

It is possible for a DRUG or toxin present in the maternal blood circulation to penetrate to the foetus via the placenta (see CRACK BABIES; FOETAL ALCOHOL SYNDROME). This is an important consideration during PREGNANCY.

placode (from Greek, *plakos*: flat) A thickened sheet of cells found in epithelia (see EPITHELIAL CELLS) during DEVELOPMENT that can serve as a PRIMORDIUM for a structure: the olfactory placode for example is a placode from which elements of the OLFACTORY SYSTEM will develop.

See also: neurodevelopment

planes of section When cutting through brain tissue, most commonly to generate sections (in layman's terms, very thin slices) of tissue for HISTOLOGY, there are different planes that can be used, each at right angles to the other. (1) coronal (or transverse): a cut across the brain, at 90° to the MIDLINE working from ANTERIOR to POSTERIOR (or vice versa). In terms of the human head, this would involve taking sections from the face through to the back of the head. (2) Horizontal: a cut through the brain taking sections from the top through to the bottom (DORSAL to VENTRAL) (or vice versa). In human terms this would involve taking sections from the scalp through to the neck. (3) SAGITTAL (longitudinal): a cut through the brain longwise, parallel with the midline. In human terms this would involve taking sections from ear to ear.

planning Planning can be defined for the purposes of biological psychology as a scheme for accomplishing a purpose. The idea of planning actions – giving behaviour a structure and organization, slaving actions to a purpose – is a relatively straightforward one. Psychological mechanisms involved in planning in one form or another have been described in detail. MOTOR PROGRAMMING is an example of a process by which simple actions can be built into a new coherent system of complex action, allowing complex actions to proceed automatically; that is, the CENTRAL NERVOUS SYSTEM has a programming mechanism that allows complex actions to be executed efficiently. Similarly, the term SCHEMA has been applied to mental models that are in a sense plans (or at least things that allow plans to be formulated). The SUPERVISORY ATTENTIONAL SYSTEM

is an example of a mechanism involved in the selection of actions, and the notion of EXECUTIVE FUNCTIONS has selection and planning as a central feature.

There are two broad questions that are of interest in considering planning. First, is it necessary to show CONSCIOUSNESS and INTENTION in order to exhibit planning or is planning a natural feature of central nervous system function that does not require self-awareness: can planning be explained solely in terms of the appropriate selection of learnt actions? If it can, then we can clearly say that all animals plan their actions, but if it cannot, and consciousness and intention are essential, then whether animals plan becomes more doubtful. Second, are there brain mechanisms specifically dedicated to the planning of actions? The answer appears to be yes, in so far as damage to structures such as those in the FRONTAL LOBE does affect the planning of actions. Other structures are almost certainly involved in this however. Note that the DYSEXECUTIVE SYNDROME features planning deficits and has been associated with many structures other than those in the frontal lobes.

See also: decision-making; voluntary

plant lectins *see* tract tracers

planum temporale The planum temporale is a part of the TEMPORAL LOBE, and is thought to have functions related to LANGUAGE comprehension. It is typically asymmetric in the human brain. It has been claimed that this ASYMMETRY is not present in the brains of schizophrenic patients (see SCHIZOPHRENIA), and that this absence of asymmetry was specific to the planum temporale, other normally asymmetric structures being no different in schizophrenics compared to non-schizophrenics. However, further studies have failed to replicate this effect.

plaques Plaques (also called neuritic plaques [see NEURITE] or senile plaques) are pathological markers present in the brains of patients with ALZHEIMER'S DEMENTIA and DOWN SYNDROME (and other disorders). They contain large amounts of AMYLOID and are believed to be markers of AXON TERMINAL damage, in contrast to NEUROFIBRILLARY TANGLES (another pathological marker for these disorders) which are thought to indicate the presence of CELL BODY degeneration.

plasma *see* blood; serum

plasma cell *see* immune system

plasmalemma *see* membrane

plasmid A circular, double-stranded molecule of DNA, commonly found in bacteria. Plasmids are able to self-replicate in bacteria and often confer a useful property on them, such as resistance to antibiotics. Because of their high frequency of replication, and the ease with which genes may be artificially inserted, plasmids are used extensively in molecular biology as a method of quickly producing large amounts of DNA containing a GENE of interest.

See also: clone

FIONA M. INGLIS

plastic embedding *see* microtome

plasticity *see* neural plasticity

platelet *see* blood

play Play in animals is very easily recognized but very difficult to define precisely. It consists of exaggerated fragments of chases, hunting or fighting behaviour commonly with rapid switches between one pattern and the next. It has no obvious short-term function. Play is effectively confined to mammals and some few birds and is particularly characteristic of young primates, carnivores and ungulates. Some adults play, especially when rearing young. Play may be costly in terms of energy, injury and inattentiveness – all are documented from the wild. Thus biologists assume that there must be real benefits to offset them. Many have been suggested, acquisition of physical fitness, motor skills, hunting techniques and social skills amongst them, but it has not been possible to demonstrate any large scale effects.

See also: social behaviour

AUBREY W. G. MANNING

pleasure Pleasure is generally defined as a feeling of contentment, happiness or EU-PHORIA. Pleasure is a term that is widely used by both the general public and the scientific community. However, the utility of this term for scientific investigation remains uncertain. It is sometimes said that organisms seek to obtain pleasure and avoid PAIN. Yet, it also has been suggested that pleasure is simply an internal stimulus generated when we obtain a goal or restore an equilibrium; thus, it is not clear if the organism is striving for pleasure *per se*, or if pleasure is merely one of several internal signals generated when a particular goal is reached. Although pleasure and REINFORCE-MENT are sometimes used interchangeably, this is an egregious error. Pleasure is an internal subjective state (that is, a feeling or EMOTION) while reinforcement is defined in terms of effects of stimuli upon behavior, and the relation between the feeling and the behavioral effect is unclear. In addition, although it is common in human research to study subjective reports of pleasure, it is very difficult in animals to determine whether 'pleasure' is being experienced.

JOHN D. SALAMONE

plethysmagraph Also known as a MERCURY-IN-RUBBER STRAIN GAUGE; a device for estimating SEXUAL AROUSAL from measures of blood flow in the penis or vagina.

plexiform (from Latin, *plexus*: weaving) A descriptive term indicating the existence of a complex network; hence the plexiform layer in the RETINA.

plexiform primordium *see* cortical development

plexus (from Latin, *plexus*: weaving) A network of tissues, usually of NERVE cells or BLOOD vessels.

pluripotent The term pluripotent is used in biological psychology to refer to CELLS, tissues or organisms that are capable of developing in any one of several different ways. It is a term most commonly used in describing STEM CELLS: pluripotent stem cells are those that can develop into various types of cell; once development along a particular line has been initiated, they are described as committed stem cells.

plus maze Also known as a cross maze, this is literally, a maze shaped like a plus sign. To start, animals can either be placed at the centre (giving them a choice of four arms to enter) or at the end of one of the arms, allowing them to proceed to the centre of the maze, at which point they will have a choice of the remaining three arms to enter. Plus mazes have been used in a wide variety of experiments looking at LEARNING and MEMORY and many other processes. Elevated plus mazes have been used to test ANXIETY in rodents (see ELEVATED MAZES).

See also: radial arm maze; spontaneous alternation; T maze; water maze; Y maze; mazes

Pöetzl effect An effect named after Otto Pöetzl who, in 1917, first described the phenomenon: a complex picture is shown to subjects who are then required to reproduce in a drawing as much of the picture as they can recall. Subjects then go home, having been asked to have a dream that night (Pöetzl was a Viennese psychiatrist working with the new Freudian theories) and report back the following day. On return subjects are asked to report their dream and instructed to draw a picture related to the dream. The Pöetzl effect is the reproduction in the 'dream drawing' of elements of the previously shown complex picture that were not reproduced in the first drawing. It is suggested that this shows how MEMORY can be subject to unconscious forces. It is an effect that has been used to examine HYPERMNESIA.

See also: psychoanalysis

poikilotherm *see* ectotherm

point mutation The substitution of one of the NUCLEOTIDES within a DNA sequence. Point mutations in the region of DNA encoding specific PROTEINS may cause an altered protein structure, and a consequent change in its function. Point mutations may occur during damage of DNA by environmental factors such as ultraviolet light, or during the process of DNA replication, where bases may be incorrectly inserted into a growing strand of DNA. It is believed that point mutations may be responsible for many evolutionary changes in species.

FIONA M. INGLIS

poliomyelitis (from Greek, *polios*: grey, *myelos*: marrow) A disorder affecting the GREY MATTER contained within the SPINAL CORD. Two forms mediated by viral infection (see VIRUS) are *acute anterior poliomyelitis*, an INFLAMMATION within the spinal cord, causing a variety of generalized effects (fever, pains and so on) followed by ATROPHY of nervous tissue and PARALYSIS, and *acute bulbar poliomyelitis*, affecting neurons in the MEDULLA OBLONGATA. In chronic anterior polio-myelitis there is muscular atrophy in the neck, which may undergo periods of respite; this is not virally mediated.

polyclonal antibody An antibody produced by more than one B CELL (see IMMUNE SYSTEM). Polyclonal antibodies are often produced by injecting a foreign ANTIGEN into an animal, often a rabbit, and harvesting the antibodies produced. These antibodies, derived from several B-cells within the animal's immune system, will differ in the precise part of the antigen that they recognize, and therefore often lack specificity between similar antigens, such as receptor subtypes.

See also: monoclonal antibody

FIONA M. INGLIS

polyethylene glycol Injections of this stimulate EXTRACELLULAR DEHYDRATION and, consequently, DRINKING; see PHYSIOLOGICAL CHALLENGE. It should be noted that large volumes of this need to be given by subcutaneous injection to stimulate drinking in rats: it is not a pleasant procedure and is best avoided if at all possible.

polygene A term used to describe any one GENE from a set of genes which all contribute to the control of a given function or trait

polygraph An instrument for simultaneous recording of multiple physiological variables such as ELECTROENCEPHALOGRAM (EEG), ELECTROMYOGRAM (EMG), ELECTRO-OCULOGRAM (EOG), blood pressure, heart rate, local blood flow, respiratory motion, and galvanic skin resistance (see SKIN CONDUCTANCE). These physiological measures are commonly used to monitor SLEEP states and to study emotional reactions, as in 'LIE DETECTION'. Technically, a polygraph consists of a series of amplifiers suitable for recording physiological measures under investigation, and a device for display such as a pen recorder or a screen monitor.

KAZUE SEMBA

polymer A POLYMER is any larger MOLECULE, natural or synthetic, that is composed of repeating smaller units; polymerase is an ENZYME present in the cell NUCLEUS engaged in polymerization of DNA; polymerization is the combining of molecules to form larger molecules with the same formula as the smaller ones combined (that is, polymer formation).

polymerase chain reaction labelling (PCR) A biochemical method to amplify DNA probes. In simple terms, it involves taking a sample of DNA and adding it to a solution containing the elements necessary to replicate it. The DNA undergoes polymerization (see POLYMER) and the fragments can be duplicated from the OLIGONUCLEOTIDE primers present in the solution. This process can be repeated serially to produce an increased volume of the DNA sample, without ever having had to use biological vectors to do so. It is a valuable technique in the experimental science and has practical applications. For example, if one wishes to use DNA FINGERPRINTING in the course of a forensic investigation, one might have only a small sample to use: PCR allows the sample size to be increased.

polymodal A term used to describe tissue (or a single NEURON) that is responsive to stimulation in more than one sensory dimension. Neurons in PRIMARY SENSORY CORTEX will respond to one type of STIMULUS – vision in PRIMARY VISUAL CORTEX for example – but neurons in ASSOCIATION CORTEX are often responsive to stimuli in more than one dimension.

polymorph (from Greek, *polymorphos*: many-formed) A polymorph is an organism or substance able to exist in many different forms; *polymorphism* describes the property of being polymorphic.

See also: isomer; enantiomer

polypeptide A peptide can be formed by the union of two AMINO ACIDS; a polypeptide is formed by the union of a large number of amino acids.

polysaccharide A complex sugar composed of over one thousand monosaccharides (see SUGARS); GLYCOGEN is a notable polysaccharide.

polysomnograph A device that will allow simultaneous recordings of such things as ELECTROENCEPHALOGRAM (EEG), ELECTRO-OCULOGRAM (EOG) and other electrical measures taken during SLEEP.

See also: polygraph

polysubstance abuse A term used to indicate the observation that many users of any particular DRUG will also be users of other drugs. The use (and abuse – see ABUSE POTENTIAL) of NICOTINE and ALCOHOL for example is very often paired. Relatively little experimental work has examined responses to more than one drug (with the exception of work aimed at DRUG DISCRIMINATION processes, in which the abilities of animals to discriminate one drug from another can be tested: but this is not work aimed at understanding mechanisms of polysubstance abuse). Individuals who abuse one drug are likely to be willing to use and abuse other drugs also: this is an issue of theoretical interest (do the drugs of abuse have to have a common mechanism of action in order for an individual to abuse them?) and also an important matter of public policy. Does the use of one drug encourage the use of another, and if so, does this present an argument for restricting the range of legally available drugs?

See also: self administration; substance abuse

polysynaptic A monosynaptic pathway is one with a single SYNAPSE; DISYNAPTIC indicates the involvement of two synapses; polysynaptic indicates involvement of multiple neurons and synapses.

ponophopbia (from Greek, *ponos*: toil, *phobos*: fear) Ponophobia is an irrational fear of working. It is rarely diagnosed formally.

pons The pons (bridge in Latin) or METENCE-PHALON is a BRAINSTEM structure that is located rostral to the MEDULLA and caudal to the MIDBRAIN. The dorsal portion is known as the PONTINE TEGMENTUM, which is the rostral extension of the MEDULLARY TEGMENTUM. The ventral portion consists of the PONTINE NUCLEI and the motor pathways, including the CORTICOSPINAL TRACT, and is highly developed in the human brain. Four CRANIAL NERVES (fifth, sixth, seventh and eighth) enter or exit the pons, and their sensory and motor nuclei are located in the pontine, as well as medullary, tegmentum. The pontine tegmentum also contains sensory and motor pathways.

The VESTIBULOCOCHLEAR NERVE (the eighth cranial nerve) enters the caudal pons. The nerve has a cochlear (see COCHLEA) branch, concerned with hearing, and a VESTIBULAR branch, concerned with equilibrium or balance. These primary afferent fibres have their cell bodies in the spiral and vestibular ganglia (see GANGLION), respectively, in the inner ear. The cochlear afferents terminate in the cochlear nuclei in the upper medulla, which give rise to central auditory pathways. Most of the vestibular afferents terminate in the vestibular nuclear complex in the caudal pons, while some enter the CEREBELLUM. These structures, in conjunction with the cranial nerves and their nuclei involved in EYE MOVEMENT control and the vestibulospinal pathways, play a key role in maintaining both static and dynamic balance. The FACIAL NERVE or the seventh cranial nerve also enters the caudal pons. The largest, motor branch enters the facial nucleus, which contains the cell bodies of facial MOTOR NEURONS. The facial motor nerve is involved in the control of superficial facial muscles that are important in facial expression. The taste fibres in the facial nerve descend to the medulla and terminate in the NUCLEUS OF THE SOLITARY TRACT, the origin of central gustatory (see GUSTATION) pathways. The cell bodies of taste fibres in the facial nerve are located in the geniculate ganglion in the temporal bone. The autonomic fibres of the facial nerve are involved in the secretion of saliva and tears, and originate from the superior salivatory nucleus in the pontine tegmentum. The ABDUCENS NERVE (the sixth cranial nerve) is a motor nerve innervating the lateral rectus muscle of the eye involved in rolling the eyeball laterally (abduction). The abducens nucleus is located dorsally in the pontine tegmentum, and the nerve exits the caudal pons from its ventral aspect.

The TRIGEMINAL NERVE (the fifth cranial nerve) is among the largest cranial nerves. It consists of both motor and sensory branches, and enters the rostral pons from its ventrolateral aspect. The motor trigeminal nerve originates from the motor trigeminal nucleus. It innervates jaw muscles and is involved in the opening and closing of the jaws and mastication. The sensory trigeminal nerve carries information on TOUCH, PAIN and TEMPERATURE sensations on the skin of the face, oral cavity and the teeth, as well as PROPRIOCEPTION of jaw muscles. Proprioceptive afferents have their cell bodies in the mesencephalic trigeminal nucleus. All of the other afferents have their cell bodies in the trigeminal ganglion, and terminate in the sensory trigeminal complex, which is distributed in a longitudinal column through the lower brainstem.

In addition to the cranial nerves, the pons contains various descending and ascending tracts carrying motor and sensory fibres originating or terminating in nuclei in the pons, or coursing through the pons en route to the upper brainstem, FOREBRAIN, medulla, or SPINAL CORD. The pons is also connected with the cerebellum via three large fibre bundles: the superior, middle and inferior cerebellar peduncles. These fibre bundles interconnect the cerebellum with various brainstem and thalamic nuclei (see THALAMUS) involved in balance and motor co-ordination. The PONTINE RETICULAR FORMATION refers to the areas of the pontine tegmentum that are neither sensory nor motor. These so-called non-specific nuclei (see NON-SPECIFIC PROJECTIONS) include the oral and caudal reticular nuclei, as well as several neurochemically coded nuclei. All these nuclei have widespread projections to the forebrain as well as to other brainstem regions, in particular the reticular formation at other levels. The PEDUNCULOPONTINE TEGMENTAL NUCLEUS and the LATERODORSAL TEGMENTAL NUCLEUS contain CHOLINERGIC neurons that project to the thalamus and other forebrain structures, as well as more caudal regions of the BRAINSTEM RETICULAR FORMATION. The LOCUS COERULEUS in the dorsolateral pontine tegmentum is the major source of NORADRENALINE in the brain and spinal cord. The pons also contains the RAPHE NUCLEI along the midline in the tegmentum, including the caudal part of the DORSAL RAPHE NUCLEUS and the NUCLEUS RAPHE PONTIS. The raphe nuclei contain SEROTONIN neurons. Collectively, these reticular neurons appear to be involved in integrated functions such as maintenance of CONSCIOUSNESS and awakening from SLEEP, VIGILANCE and ATTENTION, and the modulation of sensory and motor functions according to the BEHAVIOURAL STATE.

KAZUE SEMBA

pontine nuclei *see* hindbrain

pontine reticular formation That part of the RETICULAR FORMATION that lies in the PONS. It has two divisions: the *pontis caudalis* (caudal pons – an extension of the gigantocellular nucleus of the MEDULLARY RETICULAR FORMATION) and the *pontis oralis* (ORAL PONS – it is associated with the TRIGEMINAL NUCLEUS which has much to do with control of the MUSCLES of the face and mouth). The LOCUS COERULEUS is also in the pontine reticular formation.

See also: ascending reticular activating system; midbrain reticular formation

pontine tegmentum The upper portion (TEGMENTUM) of the PONS; see HINDBRAIN.

population attributable risk *see* risk

population coding *see* ensemble coding and population coding

pontomesencephalic tegmentum *see* mesopontine tegmentum

porphyria A disease of the METABOLISM of *porphyrins*, natural pigments found in many plant and animal cells (see CELL), characterized typically by excessive amounts of porphyrins in the urine. There are various types of porphyria: HYPERTENSION and damage to NERVE tissue may be present in more extreme cases. The reaction of the SKIN to light may be a feature in certain cases.

Porsolt test This is a test for the ANTIDEPRESSANT activity of a DRUG. One measures the time rats spend trying to escape from a beaker of water. This may have little to do with the state of depression, but (perhaps surprisingly) it does predict the likely antidepressant properties of novel compounds.

portal vein The vein that carries BLOOD from the intestines, spleen and STOMACH (see DIGESTIVE SYSTEM) to the LIVER; the term portal system, or hepatic portal system, describes this system of blood vessels.

positive cooperativity A phenomenon of RECEPTOR binding in which binding of a LIGAND to one site facilitates binding at another site on the same receptor.

See also: acetylcholine receptors

positive patterning The opposite of NEGATIVE PATTERNING: positive patterning involves REINFORCEMENT of a compound STIMULUS but not of the individual elements that compose it.

positive reinforcement The four basic procedures in operant conditioning are positive reinforcement, NEGATIVE REINFORCEMENT, PUNISHMENT and OMISSION. Reinforcement processes, whether positive or negative, increase response probability. If a response occurs, and it is followed by the presentation of a stimulus, and this results in an increase in response probability, then it is said that positive reinforcement has occurred. According to the behaviorist tradition, positive reinforcement has typically been defined simply in empirical terms. However, it has become more common to view OPERANT CONDITIONING procedures in terms of their motivational or regulatory consequences. Thus, with positive reinforcement, it is evident that the type of stimulus being removed, which results in an increase in response probability, is an appetitive stimulus. According to the motivational view, positive reinforcement involves the organism behaving so as to increase the probability of appetitive events.

JOHN D. SALAMONE

positive reinforcer *see* reinforcer

positive symptoms *see* schizophrenia; type I schizophrenia

positron emission tomography *see* PET

Posner effect Michael Posner designed a task in which COVERT ORIENTING of SPATIAL ATTENTION can be measured. Stimulus detection or discrimination is more rapid when a cue (for example a brief flash of light or an arrow indicating the stimulus location) directs attention to the location of the subsequent stimulus (a so-called VALID CUE) than when attention is misdirected to another location by an INVALID CUE. The reaction time difference between these two conditions is called the validity effect.

See also: attention

VERITY J. BROWN

post mortem (from Latin, *post*: after, *mors*: death) After death. The term describes the condition of being 'after death' and the process of conducting a *post mortem* examination, which is more properly called an AUTOPSY.

post- Prefix meaning after or behind: the POST-CENTRAL GYRUS is the GYRUS (see GYRI AND SULCI) immediately behind the CENTRAL SULCUS; POST NATAL is the period immediately after birth. The opposite term is PRE.

post-central gyrus *see* central sulcus

post-concussion syndrome *see* concussion

post-ejaculatory refractory period This describes the time immediately following EJACULATION in which male rats exhibit very little active behaviour, detectable neuronally by very low levels of activity in DOPAMINE-containing neurons (see NEURON) in the MIDBRAIN.

post-encephalitic Parkinsonism A form of PARKINSON'S DISEASE attributable to an infection by a VIRUS, *Encephalitis lethargica* (see ENCEPHALITIS). The patients described in Oliver Sacks's book *Awakenings* were the victims of this.

Reference

Sacks O.W. (1976) *Awakenings*, Pelican Books: Harmondsworth UK.

post-ictal From the term ictus (itself as Latin term, a blow) which refers to a sudden attack. Post-ictal is a term that is normally used to describe the period after a epileptic attack; see EPILEPSY.

post-reinforcement interval *see* post-reinforcement pause

post-reinforcement pause (also POST-REINFORCEMENT INTERVAL) In OPERANT tests, this is the interval that occurs between the delivery of REINFORCEMENT and the resumption of responding (typically lever pressing – though see NOSE POKE VS. LEVER PRESS). The length of the post-reinforcement pause is dependent on the value of the REINFORCER and the effort required to obtain it. In PROGRESSIVE RATIO tests for example, the post-reinforcement pause grows longer as the ratio schedule increases. This relationship holds good if such things as food or water are used as the reinforcer. In studies using a DRUG as the REWARD (typically involving SELF-ADMINISTRATION) the stimulant properties of the drug *per se* can have an effect on the post-reinforcement pause.

post-tetanic potentiation A tetanus is a sustained burst of ACTION POTENTIAL activity. Following this, for a short period, single action potentials release more NEUROTRANSMITTERS than normal. Post-tetanic potentiation can be seen at SYNAPTIC TERMINALS in the CENTRAL NERVOUS SYSTEM and at the NEUROMUSCULAR JUNCTION.

See also: long-term depression; long term potentiation

post-traumatic amnesia *see* concussion

post-traumatic stress disorder Trauma may cause psychological as well as physical disability. A variety of trauma-related syndromes with similar features have been described over the last 300 years, culminating most recently in the concept of post-traumatic stress disorder (PTSD). The disorder was first included in the third revision of DSM (see DSM-IV) in 1980, and appeared in ICD 10 in 1992. Though early studies focused on war veterans and survivors of major civilian disasters, contemporary practice extends the concept to include 'everyday', personal traumatic events, such as road traffic accidents and assault.

The core symptoms of PTSD include recurrent and intrusive recollections (nightmares and flashbacks); avoidance of stimuli related to the original trauma; and abnormal AROUSAL phenomena (an exaggerated STARTLE REFLEX response and SLEEP disturbance). The condition is often associated with other psychological disorders, such as generalized ANXIETY, PHOBIA, DEPRESSION and DRUG ABUSE, in addition to increased rates of physical illness. The disorder represents a significant healthcare issue – community surveys suggest a lifetime prevalence rate between 1% and 10% in Western communities. Untreated, PTSD may lead to illness and disability lasting many years – perhaps lifelong – with an as yet unquantified extended psychosocial impact. While trauma is, by definition, an essential aetiological factor in PTSD, well-conducted hormonal, physiological, neuropsychological and FUNCTIONAL NEUROIMAGING studies suggest a firm biological grounding for many aspects of the illness. Sufferers exhibit abnormal HYPOTHALAMIC-PITUITARY-ADRENAL AXIS function; altered CATECHOLAMINERGIC metabolism; disturbed MEMORY function and unusual CONDITIONING responses. Hippocampal abnormalities have proved of special interest, with structural and functional neuroimaging investigations revealing both anatomical and physiological changes. Recent research has identified a range of stress-related molecular, cellular and physiological responses in the HIPPOCAMPUS that may account for some of the cognitive and affective changes seen in trauma sufferers.

Although many different psychological and chemical treatments have been proposed for PTSD, systematic evaluation has been limited and the evidence base is meagre. A wide range of psychotherapeutic procedures has been advocated, including exposure therapy, COGNITIVE THERAPY, group and family therapies and HYPNOSIS. An entirely novel procedure, EYE MOVEMENT desensitization and reprocessing therapy, has captured considerable interest in recent years. With regard to chemical treatments, BENZODIAZEPINES, ANTICONVULSANT and NEUROLEPTIC drugs, CLONIDINE and BETA BLOCKERS have all been explored, but ANTI-DEPRESSANT therapy appears especially promising, with preliminary evidence that SELECTIVE SEROTONIN REUPTAKE INHIBITORS may be of particular value. Further trials are needed to directly compare competing therapeutic strategies, and to evaluate the combination of chemical and psychological therapy.

IAN C. REID

posterior Backward; at the back. Posterior is contrasted to ANTERIOR, at the front. The terms ROSTRAL (front) and CAUDAL (back) are synonymous with anterior and posterior.

posterior lobe *see* cerebellum – anatomical organization

posterior parietal cortex The PARIETAL LOBE is divided in two: the POST-CENTRAL GYRUS behind the CENTRAL SULCUS, the rest of the lobe being called POSTERIOR PARIETAL CORTEX; see PARIETAL CORTEX.

posterior pituitary *see* adenohypophysis; pituitary gland

posterolateral fissure *see* cerebellum – anatomical organization

postganglionic neuron The basic organization of the AUTONOMIC NERVOUS SYSTEM is a two-neuron chain consisting of a PREGANGLIONIC NEURON in the CENTRAL NERVOUS SYSTEM that projects to postganglionic neurons in a peripheral autonomic GANGLION.

postmenarchal *see* menarche

postmitotic *see* cell division

postnatal (from Latin, *natus*: born) The period after birth.

See also: postpartum

postnatal depression Depression that occurs in following the birth of a child: estimates vary, but up to 12% of mothers and 6% of fathers may experience this. Onset may be immediate following the birth of a child or may occur at some time later (up to and even beyond a year). Postnatal depression is indistinguishable from major depression *per se*: it is the timing of the episode rather than its nature that distinguishes it. There is no reliable evidence indicating that changes in levels of HORMONES or obstetric variables have an impact on the incidence of the disorder – indeed, there is no discriminable difference between parents who do, and parents who do not, develop postnatal depression. Factors that have some predictive power for postnatal depression include previous depressive illness, concurrent difficult life events and poor support from relationships and social systems. The additional burden of coping with an infant, the change in social circumstance and relationships brought about by parenthood, and such straightforward things as lack of SLEEP, appear to be factors placing individuals at risk.

postpartum (from Latin, *parere*: to bring out) Parturition is the process of childbirth; postpartum refers to the period immediately after this. This is more or less synonymous with POSTNATAL. If a discrimination between the two terms were to be made it would be in terms of duration: postpartum typically refers to period immediately following childbirth whereas the term postnatal is the counterpoint to prenatal. Pre- and postnatal can refer to points in time months before and after birth.

postsynaptic Communication at a synapse involves three elements: a SYNAPTIC TERMINAL; SYNAPTIC CLEFT and postsynaptic MEMBRANE: postsynaptic is therefore a general term referring to the postsynaptic side of this communication; postsynaptic membrane, postsynaptic neuron are typical uses.

postsynaptic density Examination of the structure of a SYNAPSE often shows either a continuous or discontinuous area of thickening along the POSTSYNAPTIC membrane. The function of this is unclear.

See also: synaptic cleft

postsynaptic receptors Receptors found at any point on a POSTSYNAPTIC site on a neuronal MEMBRANE, in contrast to PRESYNAPTIC RECEPTORS, found at PRESYNAPTIC sites.

See also: synapse

posture The position of a multi-segmented body part or the torso. In MOTOR CONTROL, posture refers to the maintenance of upright stance despite inertial and gravitational forces, fluctuations in muscle tone and so forth.

Research questions focus on how descending neural pathways modulate the SPINAL CORD circuitry which control the muscles of the trunk and legs. In general these circuits function by providing excitatory inputs to neurons in the spinal cord which activate leg/torso extensor muscles. In addition these descending circuits are able to modify spinal cord reflexes as, for example, when visual information is used to mimic the effects of body sway.

DAVID P. CAREY

potassium (K) Potassium is an ALKALI metal; potassium ions (K+) (see ION) are critical for the proper functioning of brain tissue (see for example ACTION POTENTIAL; ION CHANNEL).

See also: periodic table of the elements

potassium channel *see* ion channel

potency Drugs (often from the same class of compounds – BENZODIAZEPINES for example) that have the same types of effects can be compared in terms of their ability to produce a particular, measurable effect (either physiological or behavioural). They can then be ranked in terms of POTENCY: which drug requires the smallest dose to achieve a given degree of effect? Potency is a function of the ability of a drug to get to a target site and once there, the AFFINITY it has for receptors and the EFFICACY with which it engages in RECEPTOR BINDING.

See also: relative potency

power stroke *see* locomotion

Prader–Willi syndrome A rare AUTOSOMAL DOMINANT disorder caused by disruption of one GENE (or more) on the long arm of chromosome 15 (see CHROMOSOMES). The PHENOTYPE is characterized by diminished activity *in utero*, hypotonia of the newborn infant, non-INSULIN-dependent DIABETES, severe OBESITY, cognitive impairment (IQ range usually 50–80; see INTELLIGENCE), short stature, hypogonadotrophic hypogonadism (small GONADS produced by lack of gonadotropic hormone), and small hands and feet. The HYPERPHAGIA and accompanying diabetes with impaired fat METABOLISM have been likened to that of the mutant *OB/OB* mouse, defective in the fat-signalling protein LEPTIN. The syndrome occurs sporadically, and affected individuals seldom survive for more than 35 years.

L. JACOB HERBERG

prandial drinking Drinking immediately before, during or after the ingestion of food. Although calorie regulation, pursued through eating food, and fluid regulation, pursued through drinking liquids, are logically and physiologically independent, they appear to be psychologically linked. Just as humans often both eat and drink during a meal, animals to tend to blend eating and drinking when this is possible. One partial reason may be because the physiological consequences of eating food that is either dryer or saltier than body tissues may themselves give rise to cues for thirst. ELECTROLYTIC LESIONS (see LESION) of the LATERAL HYPOTHALAMUS were found to disrupt prandial drinking: lesioned rats would drink quite well if food and water were presented simultaneously but not if they were presented separately. This was regarded as a key feature of LATERAL HYPOTHALAMIC SYNDROME. EXCITOTOXIC LESIONS (see EXCITOTOXINS) of the lateral hypothalamus do not however produce this effect

KENT C. BERRIDGE

praxis (from Greek, *prassein*: to do) The doing of something; the practical as opposed to theoretical side of science.

See also: apraxia

prazosin An alpha-1 noradrenaline receptor ANTAGONIST; see ADRENOCEPTORS.

pre- Prefix meaning before or in front of: the PRECENTRAL GYRUS is the GYRUS (see GYRI AND SULCI) immediately in front of the CENTRAL SULCUS; PRENATAL is the period immediately before birth. The opposite term is POST-.

preattentive vision A level of visual processing analyzing features only at a low level. It is a mechanism that allows rapid searching of an array of stimuli for a single stimulus discriminated in some fundamental way; see TEXTURE PERCEPTION.

precategorical acoustic store *see* iconic memory

precentral gyrus *see* central sulcus

precocial mammals *see* maternal behaviour

precollicular–postmammillary transection
A cut completely through either one HEMISPHERE or both, along the anterior edge of the SUPERIOR COLLICULUS, at an angle such that the MAMMILLARY BODIES are caudal to the section. The technique was used in cats around the mid twentieth century, to test the hypothesis that stepping activity was coordinated wholly by the lower BRAINSTEM. Following transection, the so-called 'mesencephalic' cats could not initiate motor activity voluntarily, or upon exteroceptive stimulation. However, upon electrical stimulation (see ELECTRICAL BRAIN STIMULATION) of a particular region of the midbrain (the so-called MESENCEPHALIC LOCOMOTOR REGION) normal locomotor activity appeared, which could be made faster by increasing the strength of stimulation.

WENDY L. INGLIS

preconscious processing A term derived from PSYCHOANALYSIS: the expression PRECONSCIOUS describes mental content that is not at this moment conscious, but can be made so; it is not the same as the unconscious mind. Given the vast amount of information being processed all the time, most processing can probably be described as preconscious.

See also: attention

precuneus An area on the MEDIAL surface of the CEREBRAL CORTEX, adjacent to the CUNEATE REGION OF THE OCCIPITAL LOBE and between the subparietal and cingulate sulci (see GYRI AND SULCI). It is thought to be activated by EPISODIC MEMORY and shifting ATTENTION (see DISENGAGE AND SHIFTING ATTENTION).

precursor cells A type of CELL from which other cells will develop; see STEM CELLS.

predator confusion *see* aggression

preferred goal object A target of MOTIVATION. Since motivation cannot be directly observed, it is necessary to infer it from patterns of behaviour. Identification of a preferred goal object is one means of establishing motivation that can be applied even to animals. A preferred goal object may be a type of food, a sexual partner, a particular place, or anything else. Given a choice between it and another object, the individual will choose it. If the object is not present, the individual will seek it. If it is used as the reward in an INSTRU-MENTAL CONDITIONING procedure, the individual will work to work to obtain it.

KENT C. BERRIDGE

prefrontal cortex The broadest inclusion criteria used in the literature for prefrontal cortex is the receipt of projections from the DOR-SOMEDIAL NUCLEUS OF THE THALAMUS. In the brain of PRIMATES, the dorsomedial nucleus of the thalamus (MD) sends projections to two areas that have been called classic prefrontal cortex, namely, DORSOLATERAL PREFRONTAL CORTEX and ORBITOFRONTAL CORTEX. ANTE-RIOR CINGULATE CORTEX also receives dorsomedial nucleus projections. In the primate brain, frontal cortex can be divided into areas with a granular layer 4 and agranular areas (see AGRANULAR CORTEX; CORTICAL LAYERS). Prefrontal cortex has also been defined as the granular areas of the primate FRONTAL LOBE, which would include dorsolateral prefrontal cortex and orbitofrontal cortex but may exclude anterior cingulate, which has a less well developed granular layer.

In the RAT brain, there is no area of FRONTAL CORTEX with a granular layer, such that the definition of prefrontal cortex is more problematic. Areas with dorsomedial nucleus projections are on the MEDIAL WALL (from SHOULDER CORTEX [M2] to INFRALIMBIC COR-TEX and, on the ventral surface, VENTRAL ORBITAL CORTEX [VO], an area related to the orbitofrontal cortex of the primate brain). The projections to infralimbic cortex are sparse and from the only the most medial portion of the dorsomedial nucleus, leading to some querying the inclusion of this area. Dorsally, M2 is thought to be homologous to secondary motor cortex of the primate and therefore not prefrontal. Ventral to M2, areas Cg1 and 2 (see CG1/2/3), and possibly PRELIMBIC CORTEX, may be homologous to primate anterior cingulate cortex and not, therefore, classical prefrontal cortex.

There is some confusion about the function of prefrontal cortex, due to several factors. There is the most obvious problem of defining the extent of prefrontal cortex in the primate brain. There is reasonably good agreement about the inclusion of some areas (for example, dorsolateral prefrontal cortex). This problem mainly concerns anterior cingulate cortex, which some authors include as prefrontal cortex and others group as LIMBIC CORTEX, acknowledging the projection from dorsomedial nucleus but citing the less well-developed granular layer in primate anterior cingulate. Given that there is no consensus about the boundaries of prefrontal cortex in the primate brain, let alone the location of homologous areas in the brains of other species, it is difficult to make cross-species comparisons. This problem is compounded because the functions of prefrontal cortex are complex, so that there is difficulty in designing tasks suitable for making comparisons between species and demonstrably measuring equivalent function. In addition, the complexities of species-specific cognitive abilities means that at least some of the functions of prefrontal cortex may have to be defined in species-specific terms (LANGUAGE and verbal reasoning being the most obvious examples). Finally, as different regions of prefrontal cortex appear to process different kinds of information, proposing a single function of prefrontal cortex might be too general to be empirically useful.

The term EXECUTIVE FUNCTIONS is often applied to the functions of the prefrontal cortex, but this term is usually defined so broadly as to have limited practical use in predicting deficits following lesion damage of specific regions of prefrontal cortex. Furthermore, in its broadest use, the term executive function is applicable to other brain areas and therefore is not useful as a definition of prefrontal cortex. The alternative to using such an embracing term is to list the individual tasks on which impairments are found. This approach is inherently unsatisfying: it might be that task complexity *per se* is the reason for impairments in performance. Alternatively, if the task depends upon several fundamental cognitive abilities, performance impairments might indicate a problem with any one of a variety of different functions. Furthermore, an impairment of some fundamental cognitive operation might result in impairments on seemingly disparate tasks.

Nevertheless, with this caveat, it is possible to specify tasks on which performance impairments associated with damage to prefrontal cortex are commonly reported. For example, performance of tasks that involve making a spatial discrimination based on information presented at some prior time (for example, SPATIAL MEMORY) is impaired when the area around the PRINCIPAL SULCUS is functionally compromised. Damage to the cortex between the principal sulcus and the ARCUATE SULCUS impairs any delayed response task (that is, tasks involving WORKING MEMORY), even without a spatial component. Holding different kinds of information 'on-line' in working memory would seem to be an important requirement for anticipating outcomes, response planning and initiating goal-directed behaviour. Thus it is reasonable to suggest that a working-memory deficit following damage to prefrontal cortex is fundamental, with implications for a variety of complex behaviours. Nevertheless, impairments in ATTENTIONAL SET-SHIFTING following lesions of dorsolateral prefrontal cortex cannot be explained by a working-memory deficit, so either there is another, yet more fundamental, deficit or there must be multiple deficits.

See also: rodent vs. primate prefrontal cortex

Reference

Fuster J.M. (1997) *The Prefrontal Cortex*, 3rd edn, Lippincott-Raven: Philadelphia.

VERITY J. BROWN

preganglionic neuron The basic organization of the AUTONOMIC NERVOUS SYSTEM is a two-neuron chain consisting of a preganglionic NEURON in the CENTRAL NERVOUS SYSTEM that projects to a POSTGANGLIONIC NEURON in a peripheral autonomic GANGLION.

pregnancy Pregnancy is the period during which one or more foetuses develop inside the UTERUS prior to parturition. Pregnancy begins with the implantation of a fertilized egg into the blood-rich endometrial lining of the uterus. There are extensive changes that occur in the uterus to support and protect the growing foetus, provide it with GROWTH FACTORS, HORMONES and NUTRIENTS, and to induce parturition. Pregnancy can be divided into three phases (in humans, these are referred to as TRIMESTERS) which correspond to epochs of foetal development and different amounts of STEROID HORMONES and NEUROPEPTIDE HORMONES in circulation.

In humans, the fertilized egg implants in the endometrial lining of the uterus within a week of ovulation. Layers of endometrial cells begin to differentiate as a result of chemical signals received from the growing embryo into trophoblast cells, some of which eventually form the PLACENTA. Continued secretion of progesterone by the corpora lutea serves to maintain the uterine lining, grow the decidua (mucous membrane) and allow the invading embryo to be enclosed by endometrial cells by the eleventh day. The amnion, or foetal sac, forms out of the placenta, fills with amnionic fluid, and surrounds the embryo. Although the corpus luteum is the major source of PROGESTERONE during the first six to eight weeks of pregnancy, the placenta is the major source of progesterone and other hormones thereafter, such as HUMAN CHORIONIC GONADOTROPHIN (hCG), ESTRADIOL (from conversion of the ANDROGEN dehydroepiandrosterone sulphate, DHEA-S), HUMAN PLACENTAL LACTOGEN (hPL), and several chorionic polypeptides nearly identical in structure to CORTICOTROPIN RELEASING HORMONE (CRH), GROWTH HORMONE RELEASING HORMONE (GHRH) and THYROTROPIN. In fact, during pregnancy, the placenta is the major source of steroid and peptide hormones, nutrients and metabolism for the foetus. The hormone hCG regulates several important processes early on during pregnancy, including the maintenance of the corpora lutea to ensure continued progesterone release, and the stimulation of steroidogenesis (in particular, progesterone) from the trophoblast. This function may be critical for the development of foetal testes and the secretion of testosterone. Indeed, SEXUAL DIFFERENTIATION of the male gonadal system occurs when foetal serum hCG levels are highest and LH levels are lowest. The foetal adrenal gland is also a major source of steroid hormones, especially DHEA-S. The hormone hPL exerts several metabolic actions, including the stimulation of lipolysis which results in increased free fatty acids in the foetal circulation, inhibition of GLUCOSE uptake and increased INSULIN levels in the mother, and a shunting of placental proteins and glucose to the foetus.

A SEMIPERMEABLE MEMBRANE, the placental barrier, exists between the circulatory systems of the mother and foetus. Although this barrier keeps the mother's IMMUNE SYSTEM from attacking the foetus, it allows many substances to cross both ways, including nutrients, hormones and drugs. Steroids produced by the placenta or the foetal adrenal find their way into the mother's circulation, and STRESS HORMONES (such as CORTICOSTEROIDS) induced in the mother can find their way into the foetal circulation. The permeability of the placental barrier to drugs of abuse (see DRUG ABUSE) is of particular concern because of the potential for teratological effects during foetal development (such as birth complications, FOETAL ALCOHOL SYNDROME, delayed skills and language development).

Hormone levels in the mother's circulation show particular patterns during pregnancy that are critical for maternal behaviour. In pregnant women, levels of progesterone increase during the first trimester and stay elevated through parturition, but fall thereafter. In contrast, levels of estradiol show a less steep rise throughout pregnancy, but fall just prior to parturition. This pattern is reversed in the rat, where levels of progesterone rise in two phases, one during the first trimester (days 2–8) and one during the third trimester (days 13–20), but fall just before parturition. In contrast, estradiol levels begin to rise in the third trimester, peak during parturition, and remain elevated throughout the next week of lactational diestrus. However, in both humans and rats, PROLACTIN levels rise dramatically just before parturition. The particular levels of these steroids in blood are necessary not only to support proper foetal development, but also to generate a variety of maternal responses. Transfusing the blood of a new mother rat directly to a nulliparous rat (one that has never given birth) results in her showing MATERNAL BEHAVIOUR (for example, nest building, pup retrieval, nursing) within 24 hours in response to pups. In contrast, nulliparous rats require at least four to six days needed to sensitize maternal behaviour in response to pups only. Moreover, injecting estradiol, progesterone and prolactin to nulliparous female rats in a manner that mimics the pattern observed in blood during pregnancy is sufficient to induce a full range of maternal behaviours. Finally, OXYTOCIN is released from the PITUITARY GLAND in response to vaginocervical stimulation received during parturition. Release of oxytocin during parturition is necessary in a variety of species for maternal bonding.

See also: drug effects *in utero*; menstrual cycle; reproduction; sex hormones; estrus

JAMES G. PFAUS

pregnenolone *see* sex hormones

prehension (from Latin, *praehendere*: to seize) Prehension is the act of grasping (see GRASP).

prelimbic cortex An area of FRONTAL CORTEX of the RAT, located on the medial wall. In the atlas of Paxinos & Watson (3rd edn, 1997), prelimbic cortex is found on coronal sections between 4.2 mm to 2.2 mm anterior to BREGMA, located dorsal to INFRALIMBIC CORTEX and ventral to CINGULATE CORTEX (designated Cg1). Prelimbic cortex is given the designation PrL. PrL roughly corresponds to Cg3 in the atlas of Paxinos & Watson (2nd edn, 1986), which follows the nomenclature of Zilles (1985). This area is has certain characteristics suggesting that it might be homologous to primate DORSOLATERAL PREFRONTAL CORTEX. In particular, it receives input from DORSOMEDIAL NUCLEUS OF THE THALAMUS and a DOPAMINERGIC projection from the MIDBRAIN. Moreover, like the dorsolateral prefrontal cortex in PRIMATES, prelimbic cortex is implicated in WORKING MEMORY. However, there are also dissimilarities, leading to suggestions that it should be considered the functional equivalent of the ANTERIOR CINGULATE CORTEX of primate brain.

References

Paxinos G. & Watson C. (1986) *The Rat Brain in Stereotaxic Coordinates*, 2nd edn, Academic Press: San Diego.
—— (1997) *The Rat Brain in Stereotaxic*

Coordinates, compact 3rd edn, Academic Press: San Diego.

Zilles K. (1985) *The Cortex of the Rat: A Stereotaxic Atlas*, Springer-Verlag: Berlin.

VERITY J. BROWN

premenstrual tension Also known as perimenstrual syndrome (PMS) or late luteal dysphoric disorder (in the DSM-IV), premenstrual tension refers to an increase in emotionality, sensitivity and dysphoria experienced by some women in the week before menstruation (between 20 and 90%, depending on the study and the definition of symptoms). The symptoms include increased breast pain, weight gain, swelling (due to water retention or oedema), backaches, dysmenorrhea, fatigue, DEPRESSION, HEADACHE, INSOMNIA, ANXIETY, skin irritation and blemishes, increased appetite (with cravings for salty or sweet foods), dizziness, AGGRESSION, moodiness, medical complications (such as herpes outbreaks, EPILEPSY, conjunctivitis, FEVER) and decreased sexual desire. Obviously, not all women experience the same symptoms, nor is any one symptom experienced to the same degree. Most of the women who experience some form of premenstrual tension rate their symptoms as mild; however, approximately 3 to 5% rate them as severe enough to interfere with normal functioning. As one might expect, everyday stressors can augment the severity of symptoms.

The notion of premenstrual tension remains controversial. On one hand, it is perhaps the most obvious set of symptoms with a 'hormonal basis' besides menstruation itself. During the late luteal phase, blood ESTROGEN levels decrease whereas PROGESTERONE levels increase. However, there is little evidence that the syndrome is actually caused by the differential activity of these steroids (although individual symptoms, such as weight gain, can be linked to the actions of progesterone). Psychological reactions to individual symptoms (for example increased food intake and water retention leading to weight gain, constant breast pain) could just as easily lead to moodiness or depression. On the other hand, PMS has become political, with some groups rejecting the idea that minor irritability prior to and during menstruation must be pathologized and given a biological basis (thereby reinforcing the idea that women are not emotionally stable enough to hold positions of political or economic power). Indeed, PMS can be treated successfully in some women by vastly different regimens, for example, one that inhibits hormonal cycles altogether, or another that replaces estrogen and diminishes progesterone action. Moreover, administration of a PLACEBO can 'treat' PMS in over 50% of cases. Nevertheless, some women do experience debilitating symptoms for which placebos do not work. Many of the individual symptoms can be treated with certain drugs (for example BENZODIAZEPINES to treat depression, drugs that block REUPTAKE of SEROTONIN to treat depression [see PROZAC], aspirin to treat headaches, breast pain, and swelling, and so on.).

See also: hormones and cognition; menstrual cycle; sex differences; sexual motivation

JAMES G. PFAUS

premorbid Something that occurs in the period before the onset of a disease or sickness can be said to be PREMORBID. Data from the premorbid period can give baseline measures against which to compare performance or abilities during a period of illness; see MORBIDITY.

premotor cortex *see* motor cortex

premotor neglect *see* motor neglect

prenatal (from Latin, *natus*: born) The period before birth.

preoptic area A nucleated structure (divisible into MEDIAL and lateral preoptic nucleus and the SEXUALLY DIMORPHIC NUCLEUS OF THE PREOPTIC AREA) with input from the NUCLEUS ACCUMBENS, AMYGDALA and SEPTAL NUCLEI and output to the HYPOTHALAMUS, amygdala, SUBSTANTIA NIGRA, VENTRAL TEGMENTAL AREA and several parts of the BRAINSTEM, including LOCUS COERULEUS, CUNEIFORM NUCLEUS, RAPHE NUCLEI, PARABRACHIAL NUCLEI and CENTRAL GREY. The preoptic area is difficult to position. Some authors consider it to be an anterior part of the HYPOTHALAMUS and include the SUPRACHIASMATIC NUCLEUS within it, while others consider that the preoptic area is anterior to the hypothalamus, not in it.

Although the preoptic area blends into adjacent structures (such as the anterior hypothalamus and BED NUCLEUS OF THE STRIA TERMINALIS), developmental evidence suggests that it is an independent entity, the PRIMORDIUM being in the FOREBRAIN, cells migrating to their final position at the border of the TELENCEPHALON and DIENCEPHALON. Functionally, the preoptic area is associated with motivated behaviours such as DRINKING (lesions in the lateral preoptic area affect responding to PHYSIOLOGICAL CHALLENGE or dehydration), SEXUAL BEHAVIOUR (the sexually dimorphic nucleus of the preoptic area [in the medial part of the preoptic area] is larger in males than females – see SEX DIFFERENCES; SEXUAL DIMORPHISM) and THERMOREGULATION (there are neurons whose activity reflects body temperature here).

preplate *see* cortical development

preproenkephalin *see* opioid peptides

preprotachykinin *see* tachykinins

prepulse inhibition If a loud sound (pulse), which normally elicits a large STARTLE REFLEX, is preceded by a weak sound (prepulse), which does not elicit startle, the amplitude of startle will be reduced. This prepulse inhibition effect is maximal about 60–120 msec after the onset of the prepulse (lead interval) and decays in about 1 sec. Cross-modal prepulse inhibition also occurs (that is, a visual prepulse will inhibit startle to a auditory pulse and vice versa). Prepulse inhibition is believed to be a measure of SENSORY GATING, may be abnormal in SCHIZOPHRENIA and can be disrupted by many drugs. Prepulse inhibition of the startle reflex ha been associated with both LIMBIC SYSTEM structures such as the NUCLEUS ACCUMBENS and BRAINSTEM structures such as the PEDUNCULOPONTINE TEGMENTAL NUCLEUS.

MICHAEL DAVIS

prepyriform cortex An area at the anterior edge of the PYRIFORM CORTEX; it has been associate with a variety of functions, as diverse as DIET selection and the generation of SEIZURES.

presbyacusis *see* deafness

presbyopia *see* lens

presenile dementia *see* senile dementia

presenilins Presenilins are proteins whose regulation is thought to be disturbed in inherited forms of ALZHEIMER'S DEMENTIA. Mutations of a GENE on chromosome 1 (which codes presenilin-2, a 28 000 MOLECULAR WEIGHT protein) or on chromosome 14 (which codes presenilin-1, a 43 000–48 000 molecular weight protein) produce changes in presenilin formation. It has been suggested that increased presenilin produces excess AMYLOID, which is implicated in the formation of PLAQUES.

preserved learning Learning capacities that are spared in humans and non-human animals with impairments of MEMORY. Which learning abilities are impaired and which ones are spared depends on the neurological condition or the type of brain damage that produces the behavioural deficits. For example, patients with an AMNESIA following damage to the medial TEMPORAL LOBE show impaired declarative learning (see DECLARATIVE MEMORY) but preserved PROCEDURAL LEARNING and preserved PRIMING effects. By contrast, in patients with damage to the BASAL GANGLIA (for example PARKINSON'S DISEASE), procedural learning can be impaired whereas declarative learning capacities may be relatively preserved. That different types of brain damage produce distinct patterns of preserved and impaired learning capacities is taken as strong support for the notion of MULTIPLE MEMORY SYSTEMS.

See also: explicit memory; implicit memory; skill learning

STEFAN KÖHLER

pressor (from Latin, *premere*: to press) The term pressor describes anything that causes an increase in blood pressure (see BLOOD). A VASOPRESSOR is a substance that increases blood pressure. VASOPRESSIN is one of the HORMONES that does this (amongst other things).

prestriate cortex *see* extrastriate cortex

presubiculum An area immediately adjacent to the SUBICULUM with a layered organization. It has connections with the HIPPOCAMPUS and a dense internal connectivity, including connections across the midline to the contralateral presubiculum. Functionally it is closely related to the subiculum.

presymptomatic test A test of any sort given before the appearance of the SIGNS AND SYMPTOMS of an illness or other condition. Presymptomatic tests can often give valuable information relating to the severity (how much worse is the something now compared to before?) and progression (how much worse or better is something getting?) of a condition. Generic information about such things as body size and occasionally function, and some psychological indices (such as IQ performance; see INTELLIGENCE TESTING) are often available, but information relevant to specific conditions is often unavailable.

presynaptic Communication at a SYNAPSE involves three elements: a SYNAPTIC TERMINAL, SYNAPTIC CLEFT and POSTSYNAPTIC membrane: presynaptic is therefore a general term referring to the presynaptic side of this communication; PRESYNAPTIC membrane, PRESYNAPTIC neuron are typical uses.

presynaptic receptors Receptors found at any point on a PRESYNAPTIC site on a neuronal MEMBRANE, in contrast to POSTSYNAPTIC RECEPTORS, found at POSTSYNAPTIC sites.

See also: synapse

presynaptic terminal The PRESYNAPTIC element of a SYNAPSE; also referred to as synaptic bouton, bulb or knob.

pretectum A midbrain structure immediately anterior to the SUPERIOR COLLICULUS. It controls reflex constriction of the PUPIL: GANGLION CELLS in the RETINA project to the pretectum, which in turn projects to PREGANGLIONIC NEURONS in the EDINGER–WESTPHAL NUCLEUS. These neurons send axons to the OCULOMOTOR NERVE (the third cranial nerve; see CRANIAL NERVES) via the CILIARY GANGLION.

priapism (from Greek, *Priapos*: a male god of sexual potency) *Priapic* refers to an unhealthy preoccupation by men with their sexual potency. *Priapism* is a pathological condition in which the penis is persistently erect.

See also: impotence

primacy *see* short-term memory; serial position effect

primacy effect Superior recall performance for items presented at the beginning of a list, relative to items in middle positions. The primacy effect is thought to index the privileged transfer of earlier list items into LONG-TERM MEMORY, given that it is robust even when a 15–30 sec delay is interposed between study and test. Active memorization strategies (for example elaborative REHEARSAL) may underlie this privileged transfer, given that primacy effects are reduced under conditions where such strategies are less likely to occur, such as when the presentation rate is relatively fast (< 2 sec), or when another task must be performed concurrently. The primacy effect is also reduced in patients with ANTEROGRADE AMNESIA.

See also: recency effect; serial position effect

JENNIFER A. MANGELS

primal sketch The earliest stages of vision process variations in raw intensity value in the retinal image. The product of these early stages was described as a primal sketch by David Marr (1945–1980). The primal sketch extracts significant variations in image intensity, mainly those that are likely to be due to significant aspects of the scene rather than insignificant aspects of the illumination of the scene, or coincidental arrangements within the scene. Thus the primal sketch records the locations of object edges and colour and texture variations. This information is then used by later stages to build up a representation of the surfaces and objects in the scene.

See also: object recognition; texture perception; visual system

References

Marr D. (1982) *Vision*, W.H. Freeman: San Francisco.

ROGER J. WATT

primary fissure *see* cerebellum – anatomical organization

primary memory system This is also known as WORKING MEMORY; see MULTIPLE MEMORY SYSTEMS.

primary motivation *see* incentive motivation

primary motor cortex That part of the CEREBRAL CORTEX having most direct control over motor activity; see MOTOR CORTEX.

primary reinforcer *see* reinforcer

primary sensory cortex The areas of CERE-BRAL CORTEX that receive the most direct and principal input from the sense organs – though many of these regions are rather ill-defined. In most cases this input is via thalamocortical projections (see THALAMUS), the exception being the olfactory area (see OLFACTION). Such areas have been established for vision, audition, somaesthesia, gustation and olfaction. The size of these areas varies between species and may reflect the relative importance of each of these senses. Indeed in experimental animals overtrained on a particular task the size of these areas may change to reflect their new-found status. Near each primary area there are other less extensive zones that receive input from the primary cortex, as well as the thalamus, and are termed secondary sensory areas.

See also: auditory cortex; gustatory cortex; olfactory cortex; somatosensory cortex; visual cortex

ROBERT J. SNOWDEN

primary sensory ending *see* muscle spindle

primary somatosensory cortex The primary somatosensory cortex (SI) is the portion of the CEREBRAL CORTEX that receives the most direct input from SOMATOSENSORY systems. It is located around the POSTCENTRAL GYRUS and can be divided into three (mostly) parallel strips designated SI1, SI2 and SI3. SI1 is closest to the CENTRAL SULCUS, SI3 to the postcentral sulcus, with SI2 in between them. The body is represented somatotopically through this tissue: the various parts of the body trunk, the various parts of the face, genitalia, limbs, hands and feet are all represented in the primary somatosensory cortex. The SECOND-ARY SOMATOSENSORY CORTEX (SII) is much smaller, receives a smaller volume of direct

somatosensory input (it is principally concerned with information from the throat, tongue teeth and jaws – see MOUTH) and is located in the LATERAL FISSURE.

See also: parietal cortex; somatosensory cortex; somatosensory pathways

primary tastes The primary tastes (also called PROTOTYPICAL TASTES) are sweet, sour, salty and bitter. In experimental studies, reactivity to sweet is measured by responses to GLUCOSE; sour by weak hydrochloric acid (HCl); salty by common salt (sodium chloride – NaCl); and bitter by QUININE (quinine hydrochloride). Whether there are only four primary tastes or not is a matter of increasing conjecture. UMAMI (a Japanese word) describes a taste common to several foodstuffs and which is thought to be represented by GLUTAMATE (typically MONOSO-DIUM GLUTAMATE). It has been shown that glutamate applied to the tongue of a primate produces selective neuronal responding in the GUSTATORY CORTEX strikingly similar to that produced by application to the tongue of the other primary tastes. This suggests that there may well be a recognition system specific to umami. It is thought that umami might represent a detection system for PROTEINS.

See also: gustation

Reference

Rolls E.T., Critchley H.D., Browning A. & Hernardi I. (1998) The neurophysiology of taste and olfaction in primates, and Umami favour. In *Olfaction and Taste*, vol. 12, ed. C. Murphy. *Annals of the New York Academy of Sciences* 855: 426–437.

primary visual cortex Also known as area V1 (see AREAS V1–V5), STRIATE CORTEX or area 17 (see BRODMANN'S AREAS). This is a large region of cortical tissue in the OCCIPITAL LOBE that receives direct input from the LATERAL GENI-CULATE NUCLEUS. The RECEPTIVE FIELD of the neurons are topographically organized (see TOPOGRAPHY) with a large weighting factor favouring the central field. The properties of many neurons in this area differ from the lateral geniculate nucleus in showing input from both eyes – they are BINOCULAR – orientation selectivity and DIRECTIONAL SELEC-TIVITY. Neurons are arranged in columns so that the response preferences of the cells are invariant perpendicular to the cortical surface and systematically vary parallel to the cortical surface (see CORTICAL COLUMNS AND HYPERCOLUMNS). Neurons have response properties that can be classified as simple, complex and hypercomplex (see SIMPLE, COMPLEX AND HYPERCOMPLEX CELLS). Many of these discoveries are associated with the work of David Hubel and Torsten Wiesel who shared the 1981 Nobel Prize for Medicine.

ROBERT J. SNOWDEN

primates Biologists classify species into a nested series of groups or taxa (see TAXONOMY); the term primate labels one such taxon, at the classification level called an Order, a group within the more inclusive Class Mammalia. The primate order presents great variation within it, which some have treated as an evolutionary trend towards greater reliance on the VISUAL SYSTEM rather than OLFACTION, increased postnatal dependence (see MATERNAL BEHAVIOUR), and increased size and complexity of the CEREBRAL CORTEX. While retaining a kernel of truth, this gives an unfortunate impression of evolution directed at progressively closer approaches to human capability, which is of course nonsense. The simplest, and unique, defining feature of all primates is the possession of a fingernail on at least one digit. This ADAPTATION allows greater support for the pad of the digit, and so enables the extreme dexterity with which some primates can manipulate delicate objects, while retaining great power in the GRIP. (The five-fingered hand, another crucial element in primate dexterity, is a retained primitive feature, anatomically rather similar to that of many reptiles.)

Generalization about characteristics becomes a little easier for the main subgroups of the primates. The main division is between strepsirhines (lemurs and lorises) and haplorhines (monkeys and apes). Strepsirhines retain the wet RHINARIUM (nose-tip) and long snouts of many other mammals, relying extensively on olfaction, and the reflective TAPETUM of the eye indicates their generally nocturnal adaptation. The haplorhines possess many derived characteristics, with (in general) enhanced COLOUR VISION and DEPTH PERCEPTION, far less reli-

ance on smell, and larger brains. Those species found in the New World form a separate CLADE (see EVOLUTION), and many of them have been far less studied than Old World forms. The latter are called catarrhines (the term refers to their close-set nostrils, with nasal septum), and include monkeys and apes. Most species are relatively large-brained and highly social, living typically in semi-permanent groups; unlike any New World monkeys, some are quite terrestrial and large-bodied. The apes differ strikingly from any other mammal in their LOCOMOTION, since their motile shoulder-blades permit suspension below a branch and clambering or swinging (BRACHIATION) through trees. This taxon also includes humans, separated from their nearest ape relatives by surprisingly short spans of independent evolution (very approximately: chimpanzee 6 million years, gorilla 8 million, orangutan 16 million, gibbon 18 million).

RICHARD W. BYRNE

priming (i) *Memory*: Priming of hypothetical connections is made between memories or other cognitive operations along some dimension of similarity. For example, the word 'red' primes the word 'fire truck' for people who are familiar with red fire trucks. *See also*: SEMANTIC PRIMING

(ii) *Brain stimulation*: When the delivery of a stimulus causes a reinstatement of behaviour, or the appearance of more vigorous behaviour, priming has said to have occurred. For example, in the 1970s the term pre-trial priming was used to express the ability of ELECTRICAL BRAIN STIMULATION applied non-continently just before an INTRACRANIAL SELF-STIMULATION task to enhance the vigour of responding. Currently, priming has a use in drug ADDICTION research where a small NON-CONTINGENT drug infusion can set off extinguished (see EXTINCTION) SELF-ADMINISTRATION behaviour.

JAMES R. STELLAR

primipara (from Latin, *primus*: first, *parere*: to bring out) The term primipara is used to describe a female who has just given birth for the first time. *Primiparous* is the adjectival form.

primitive streak An important element in the DEVELOPMENT of reptiles, birds and MAMMALS. The organizer node of the primitive streak influences neural development (see NEURODEVELOPMENT) by inducing the overlying ectoderm to form neural tissue (neural induction), and it directs the establishment of the definitive head–tail and dorsal–ventral axes.

primordium The rudimentary tissue or cells from which a structure develops.

See also: anlage; neural tube

principal sulcus A major sulcus (see GYRI AND SULCI) in the FRONTAL LOBE. The tissue around it has, in the brains of PRIMATES, been described as the DORSOLATERAL PREFRONTAL CORTEX.

prion disease A fatal neurodegenerative disease in which there is SPONGIFORM ENCEPHALOPATHY and an accumulation in brain of the abnormal, non-degradable form of PRION PROTEIN (PrPsc). The primary pathogenic event is the autocatalytic, post-translational modification of PrPc to PrPsc. (note that PrP is the standard abbreviation for prion protein of any type. PrPc is the normal product of the PrP gene and is sensitive to enzymatic destruction by PROTEASE. Prp27-30 [the numbers indicate MOLECULAR WEIGHT in kiloDaltons] is the core of a larger prion protein, Prpsc, which is the disease-specific protein.) Any rare MUTATION in the PrP gene leads inevitably to disease in middle age. Conversion of PrPc to PrPsc may be spontaneous (see CREUTZFELDT–JAKOB DISEASE) or triggered by contamination with PrPsc either by ingestion (see BOVINE SPONGIFORM ENCEPHALOPATHY [BSE]) or by medical accident or experimental injection.

See also: scrapie

Reference

Prusiner S.B. (1991) Molecular biology of prion disease. *Science* 252: 1515–1522.

ROSALIND RIDLEY

prion protein Prions are though responsible for several diseases (see PRION DISEASE) but exactly how prions come to have the properties of pathogens is still rather conjectural.: prions are PROTEINS and so, unlike a VIRUS, cannot reproduce themselves. It has been suggested that a prion is a mis-folded form of a normal neuronal protein. If such a mis-folded form could gain access to a NEURON, it might then be able to convert normal protein to the prion form, which of course would disrupt normal cellular function and lead possibly to neuronal death. Stanley Prusiner was awarded the Nobel Prize for Physiology or Medicine for the discovery of prions.

proactive interference A process by which previously learned information disrupts MEMORY for new information. The degree of INTERFERENCE is related to the degree of semantic similarity between the new and old information. Proactive interference can build up across learning trials. As one attempts to learn successive lists of items that are from the same semantic category (for example: list 1: *cat, pigeon, horse*; list 2: *dog, rhino, rabbit*; list 3: *pig, giraffe, mouse*), there is a progressive decline in FREE RECALL performance as proactive interference increases. However, if a subsequent list is semantically dissimilar to the previous lists (list 4: *chair, desk, table*), performance on this list will dramatically improve. This improvement is referred to as the release from proactive interference.

See also: retroactive interference

JENNIFER A. MANGELS

proband In studies of genetic relatedness, PROBAND is the term used to describe the individual who acts as the starting-point for the investigation. One might define a characteristic – for example, diagnosed SCHIZOPHRENIA or some other illness, a behavioural capacity or physical trait – in a proband and then look for the degree to which that characteristic is shared by siblings, other living relatives or the proband's ancestors or descendents.

probe stimulus A stimulus used to explore a particular function following prior exposure to a range of stimuli; see PERCEPTUAL PRIMING.

probe test A technique used in NEUROPSYCHOLOGY and more generally in experimental psychology to investigate MEMORY: subjects are given multiple items to remember and are later presented with a single item and asked to indicate whether or not this probe item was part of the list or not. Subjects could be either humans or experimental animals – the required response need not be verbal.

problem solving Psychologists use the term problem solving to refer to tasks that require a sequence of operations to be performed to arrive at a solution: the TOWER OF HANOI is an example of such a problem solving task. The term reasoning is also used but can be considered to all intents and purposes synonymous with problem solving. Tests of animal problem solving, such as the PUZZLE BOX, can also involve such sequences but might require the operation of insight (see EMULATION) or the observation of other organisms solving the task (see OBSERVATION LEARNING).

See also: decision-making; learning

procaine Procaine is a LOCAL ANAESTHETIC, related to LIDOCAINE and indeed to COCAINE (which has local anaesthetic properties).

procaterol An beta-2 noradrenaline receptor AGONIST; see ADRENOCEPTORS.

procedural learning Procedural learning refers to LEARNING in which what is learned is a sequence of production rules rather than a set of propositions. Procedural learning refers most often to SKILL LEARNING and the learning of HABITS where learning is gradual and where the learner incrementally discovers invariance in the stimulus environment across many trials. MEMORY is embedded in the procedure and one demonstrates the memory, as in the case of a newly acquired skill, by expressing it in performance. In contrast to DECLARATIVE MEMORY, which stores propositions about facts and events, procedural memory is a form of IMPLICIT MEMORY that stores procedures inaccessible to conscious awareness. Procedural learning is expressed through performance.

LARRY R. SQUIRE

procedural memory Procedural memory is a form of MEMORY that includes the non-conscious processes of motor skill and the learning of HABITS, CONDITIONING and ASSOCIATIVE LEARNING. It is contrasted with DECLARATIVE MEMORY.

See also: long-term memory; multiple memory systems

proceptivity see appetitive vs. consummatory phases

process The term PROCESS obviously has many uses in standard English. In neuroscience, the term refers to the AXONS and DENDRITES that develop from the CELL BODY of a NEURON and to the extensions of various GLIAL CELLS.

See also: bipolar neuron

prodromal symptoms Prodromal symptoms are symptoms that occur before the main phase of an illness. For example, the DSM-IV diagnosis of SCHIZOPHRENIA requires a period in which there are various typical SIGNS AND SYMPTOMS present. But there are in addition other lesser symptoms that can occur in the period before the onset of these principal ones: these are prodromal. Similarly, there may be lesser symptoms that occur after the main active phase of the illness – these are called RESIDUAL SYMPTOMS.

prodynorphin see opioid peptides

proenkephalin opioid peptides

proestrus see estrus

progestogens A set of SEX STEROIDS including PROGESTERONE (see PROGESTINS) secreted from the ADRENAL GLAND and the OVARIES.

See also: corticosteroids; endocrine glands; hormones; estrus; hormones – classification; menstrual cycle; organization effects of steroid hormones; pregnancy; sex hormones

progesterone see progestogens; sex steroids

progestins A set of SEX HORMONES including PROGESTERONE secreted from the ADRENAL GLAND and the OVARIES.

See also: corticosteroids; endocrine glands; hormones; estrus; hormones – classification; menstrual cycle; organization effects of steroid hormones; pregnancy; sex hormones

programmed cell death see apoptosis

progressive diseases As their name implies, these are diseases (also known as progressive disorders) that become progressively worse as time goes by. Examples of progressive diseases in the central nervous system are PARKINSON'S DISEASE and ALZHEIMER'S DEMENTIA. (Regrettably there are very many more examples.) In these two disorders there is progressive NEURON loss from sites in the BRAIN that produces an ever-worsening state. Such disorders can be contrasted with other disorders which, having appeared, do not get worse: a STROKE for example can be a unique event in which sudden damage causes neurological impairment. With a stroke the impairment may actually ameliorate over time, as the immediate impact of the damage is corrected by various brain processes, and of course by the effects of medical care.

progressive fluent aphasia An alternative name for SEMANTIC DEMENTIA.

progressive non-fluent aphasia *see* semantic dementia

progressive ratio A schedule of REINFORCEMENT that is characterized by requiring the subject to make progressively more responses in order to obtain reinforcement. The subject is required to work for a reinforcement on a fixed-ratio (FR) schedule that consistently gets longer. The pattern of increment is determined in advance by the experimenter. For example, the schedule may start at FR 2 (two responses must be made), then FR 4, FR 8, FR 16, and so on. At some point, the demand of the schedule will be too high, and the subject will quit responding. This point is called the BREAKING POINT, which is defined as the last completed ratio. So, if the subject made 64 responses, got the reinforcement, but then stopped responding, the breaking point would be 64. The progressive ratio schedule is a very useful measure of how motivated the subject is to obtain the reinforcement, particularly because the actual measure of MOTIVATION, the breaking point, is independent of rate of response. This schedule is commonly used in ADDICTION research in animals, to ascertain how hard animals will work for drugs obtained by SELF-ADMINISTRATION (see DRUG ABUSE). In this case, the reinforcement is an intravenous injection of the drug.

ANN E. KELLEY

progressive supranuclear palsy A rare akinetic–rigid syndrome (see AKINESIA; RIGIDITY) also known as STEELE, RICHARDSON & OLSZEWSKI DISEASE. It differs from PARKINSON'S DISEASE in being unresponsive to L-DOPA and in primarily affecting EYE MOVEMENTS, with a characteristic loss of voluntary (non-reflexive) downward gaze. The underlying BRAINSTEM pathology does not directly affect the cranial eye-movement nuclei nor the CEREBRAL CORTEX (hence the condition's name). The onset, in middle age, is followed by relentless progression with spreading DYSTONIA and TREMOR, and death follows in 5–7 years. MEMORY, INTELLIGENCE and cognition may be affected in the later stages but this has been difficult to establish.

L. JACOB HERBERG

prohormones Prohormones are large PEPTIDES that, when processed by a proteolytic ENZYME (see PROTEOLYSIS), produce smaller peptides that can act as NEUROTRANSMITTERS or HORMONES. For an example of this, see OPIOID PEPTIDES.

projection neuron Neurons sending their AXONS to distant locations are called PROJECTION NEURONS; a collection of these is referred to as a PROJECTION (that is, a projection from one structure to another).

See also: interneurons

prokaryote *see* eukaryote

prolactin A hormone released by the ADENOHYPOPHYSIS.

See also: endocrine glands; hormones; hormones – classification; pregnancy; sex hormones

prolactin inhibiting factor One of the HORMONES involved in the control of the release of other hormones from the PITUITARY GLAND.

See also: adenohypophysis; endocrine glands; hormones – classification

proliferation (from Latin, *proles*: offspring, *ferre*: to bear) To proliferate is to grow by increasing the numbers of cells (see CELL) (or other parts); proliferation is the process of generating these cells (or other parts). *Neuronal proliferation* refers to an increase in NEURON numbers; *glial proliferation* refers to an increase in the numbers of GLIAL CELLS.

See also: hyperplasia; neurodevelopment; reactive gliosis

proopiomelanocortin *see* opioid peptides

propagation Propagation is a term in biological psychology generally applied to ACTION POTENTIAL induction.

See also: backpropagation

prophylactic A prophylactic is an object, chemical or procedure that has protective properties of one sort or another. It originally was used to describe protection against disease. In the United States, the term prophylactic is used more or less synonymously with condom, but this usage is less common in the United Kingdom. Prophylaxis describes the process of being prophylactic.

propositional memory Also known as EXPLICIT MEMORY.

See also: hippocampus

propranolol A non-selective beta NORADRENALINE receptor ANTAGONIST; see ADRENOCEPTORS.

propriobulbar A term indicating a relationship almost exclusively with the MEDULLA OBLONGATA: propriospinal systems are those that interconnect within it.

proprioception (from Latin, *proprio*: own, *recipere*: to receive) Proprioception is an animal's sense of the position of its own body; proprioceptive is the adjective describing this sense. Proprioception is a sense that relies on information coming to the CENTRAL NERVOUS SYSTEM from the MUSCLES of the body. The GOLGI TENDON ORGAN and MUSCLE SPINDLE are the principal sources of sensory information (PROPRIOCEPTORS) from the SKELETAL MUSCLES.

See also: dorsal column – medial lemniscal system; haptic; locomotion; motor control; nucleus gracilis; nucleus cuneatus; pons; spinal cord; touch

proprioceptors Proprioceptors are the sensory organs involved in PROPRIOCEPTION. Principally these are the GOLGI TENDON ORGAN and MUSCLE SPINDLE.

propriospinal A term indicating a relationship almost exclusively with the SPINAL CORD: propriospinal systems are those that interconnect within it.

prosencephalon (from Greek, *pro*: before, *enkephalon*: brain) Synonymous with the term FOREBRAIN. It includes both the TELENCEPHALON and the DIENCEPHALON.

prosody This term is used to refer to the norms of verse metrics (by students of poetry); to the abstract organizational structure which determines the grouping and relative salience of phonological units (mainly by phonologists); to the linguistic structure expressed in the supra-segmental properties of utterances (mainly by phoneticians and psycholinguists); and to the supra-segmental properties themselves – the PITCH, tempo, LOUDNESS and TIMING patterns of speech (mainly by speech researchers in applied PHONETICS and engineering). All definitions relate to the original Greek meaning of a sung accompaniment, and all would include accent, stress and rhythm as aspects of prosody.

See also: phonology

ANNE CUTLER

prosopagnosia (from Greek, *prosopos*: face) An inability to recognize faces caused by brain injury. Prosopagnosic patients must rely on voice, context, name, or sometimes clothing or gait to achieve recognition of people they know. The problem in FACE PERCEPTION is not due to blindness (VISUAL ACUITY and CONTRAST SENSITIVITY are sometimes well preserved) or general intellectual impairment (people are still recognized from non-facial cues, and SEMANTIC MEMORY can be normal). Yet even the most familiar faces may go unrecognized; famous people, friends, family, and the patient's own face when seen in a mirror. Common correlates of prosopagnosia are a visual field defect (upper left QUADRANTANOPSIA), loss of colour perception (ACHROMATOPSIA), and problems in finding one's way around (TOPOGRAPHICAL MEMORY). However, cases have been reported without any or all of these co-occurring symptoms. The usual cause of prosopagnosia is damage to ventro-medial regions of the OCCIPITAL LOBE and TEMPORAL LOBE. It is likely that there is more than one form of the disorder; one type involves impaired perception of the face, preserved IMAGERY for the appearances of familiar people, and no evidence of non-conscious (covert) recognition. The second type of prosopagnosia involves unimpaired face perception, loss of imagery for familiar faces, and evidence of COVERT RECOGNITION in the form of AUTONOMIC and non-conscious behavioural reactions.

ANDREW W. YOUNG

prostaglandin *see* immune system

protanomaly *see* colour blindness

protanopia *see* dichromatic colour blindness

protease An enzyme that degrades PROTEINS.

protein hormones *see* hormones – classification

protein kinase Any ENZYME that transfers phosphate groups from ADENOSINE TRIPHOSPHATE (ATP) to PROTEINS is called a PROTEIN KINASE. These are widely involved in mechanisms of communication between cells (see SECOND MESSENGERS).

Reference

Campbell N.A., Reece J.B. & Mitchell L.G. (1999) *Biology*, 5th edn, Addison-Wesley: Menlo Park CA.

protein kinase A A specific form of PROTEIN KINASE; one of the SECOND MESSENGERS. It features as part of a cascade of intraneuronal events that follow RECEPTOR BINDING: PROTEINS activate ADENYLATE CYCLASE which converts ADENOSINE TRIPHOSPHATE (ATP) to CYCLIC AMP which activates protein kinase A to phosphorylate (see PHOSPHORYLATION) proteins associated with ION CHANNEL activity.

protein kinase C A form of PROTEIN KINASE; one of the SECOND MESSENGERS: it is activated by CALCIUM.

See also: inositol

protein phosphorylation The donation of a phosphate group from ADENOSINE TRIPHOSPHATE (ATP) to a protein (see PROTEINS) is called PROTEIN PHOSPHORYLATION; the receiving protein is said to have been phosphory-

lated. It is an important feature of the process of communication between cells (see SECOND MESSENGERS).

Reference

Campbell N.A., Reece J.B. & Mitchell L.G. (1999) *Biology*, 5th edn, Addison-Wesley: Menlo Park CA.

proteins (from Greek, *proteios*: primary) A protein is a complex MOLECULE, composed of various combinations of any of the twenty AMINO ACIDS (each made of carbon, hydrogen, oxygen and nitrogen) with a side chain, usually containing sulphur and often phosphorous. Approximately half the dry weight of any animal CELL is made of proteins, which are critical for a range of functions including structure, transport and signalling – a neurotransmitter RECEPTOR for example consists of protein molecules embedded in a neuronal MEMBRANE. Proteins are the product of GENE activity (see DNA).

Proteins are a class of nutrients, separate from CARBOHYDRATES and FATS or LIPIDS, which consist mainly of amino acids. Many of the twenty amino acids in humans can be produced by the body itself out of other compounds. However, nine amino acids cannot be manufactured by the human body. These types must be obtained in food, and are called ESSENTIAL AMINO ACIDS for that reason: they are essential in any diet.

See also: peptides; polypeptides

KENT C. BERRIDGE

proteoglycan A glycoprotein that forms an integral part of the EXTRACELLULAR MATRIX.

proteolipid *see* lipids

proteolysis The destruction of PROTEINS by ENZYME activity.

proteome Just as the GENOME is the total amount of genetic material an individual organism has, the proteome is the complete amount of PROTEIN. Recent advances in the analysis of proteins have made it possible to conduct large scale, detailed analysis of protein content of tissues; this is known as proteomics (or proteinomics).

prothetic continuum *see* metathetic continuum

proton *see* atom

prototypical tastes *see* primary tastes

proximal Close to, in contrast to DISTAL, at a distance. In anatomical terms, proximal means nearer to the midline of the body; thus the hip is proximal to the thigh.

proximal dendrite A DENDRITE found near the CELL BODY in contrast to a DISTAL DENDRITE, found at a greater distance from the cell body.

Prozac Trade name for the SELECTIVE SERO-TONIN REUPTAKE INHIBITOR (SSRI) ANTIDE-PRESSANT FLUOXETINE. Used world-wide in the treatment of DEPRESSION, and at time of writing, the most commonly prescribed SSRI. Clinical trials indicate that Prozac is no more and no less effective than other chemical antidepressants. Though safe in clinical use, it has gathered media notoriety as a drug of abuse (see ABUSE POTENTIAL) or recreation, particularly in the USA. There is no evidence, however, that physical DEPENDENCE can occur. Distinguished from other SSRIs by the long half-life of active metabolites, which means that its action is prolonged for some weeks after the drug is stopped.

IAN C. REID

pseudagnosia *see* apperceptive agnosia

pseudinsomnia Many individuals who complain of poor SLEEP show physiologically normal sleep patterns when they are studied in the sleep laboratory. Thus it is not atypical to record 6–7 hours of polygraphically (see POLY-GRAPH) robust sleep in subjects who claim not to have slept at all! This syndrome is an extreme example of the normal tendency to exaggerate the duration of time spent in bed awake. Even for good sleepers who usually require only 5–10 minutes to fall asleep, 30–45 minutes may seem like an eternity. In studies of awakening from early morning normal sleep subjects may claim to have been awake indicating a possible dissociation of subjective and objective sleep signs at certain times of the day.

J. ALLAN HOBSON

pseudobulbar (from Greek, *pseudes*: false, *bolbos*: an onion) The term bulbar is used as an adjective to describe the MEDULLA OBLON-GATA: pseudobulbar refers to PARALYSIS of the nerves (see NERVE) connecting to this.

pseudocholinesterase *see* acetylcholinesterase

pseudoconditioning It is often observed that following presentation of a strong, or motivationally significant, stimulus responding to another stimulus may change in the sense that it resembles some aspect of the response elicited by the strong stimulus. This qualitative change in responding to other stimuli is termed PSEUDOCONDITIONING, since the behavioural change is similar to that observed during conditioning (see ALPHA AND BETA CONDITION-ING). However, unlike CONDITIONING the change in responding does not require contiguous pairing of the two stimuli. This example of LEARNING has been largely neglected by students of learning, although it may well be a ubiquitous phenomenon.

MARK A. UNGLESS

pseudohermaphrodite *see* hermaphrodite

pseudopregnancy An unusual phenomenon observed in rats and mice: if a female rat or mouse engages in SEXUAL BEHAVIOUR with an infertile male at the time of ovulation, the luteal phase of the MENSTRUAL CYCLE will be extended to 11–12 days, instead of 2–3 days if no mating occurs. The effect is generated by mechanical stimulation of the cervix by the male's penis during copulation, activating PRO-LACTIN release from the PITUITARY GLAND. Pseudopregnancy significantly extends the period during which a female rat or mouse is fertile, increasing reproductive efficiency considerably.

See also: reproduction

Reference

Johnson M. & Everitt B.J. (1980) *Essential Reproduction*, Blackwell Scientific Publications: Oxford.

pseudounipolar neuron *see* bipolar neuron

psilocybin N,N-Dimethyl-4-phosphoryltrypta-mine: an hallucinogen derived from the mushroom *Psilocybe mexicana*.

psychedelic drugs (from Greek, *psyche*: soul (or, in more contemporary terms, psychology), *delos*: visible) The term *psychedelic* (rarely, *psychodelic*) was introduced in 1957 as a general term to describe any DRUG that induces altered states of perception (see SENSATION VS. PERCEPTION) such as HALLUCINATION and SYNAESTHESIA. The term HALLUCINOGEN (see HALLUCINOGENS) can be taken to be synonymous.

psychiatry Psychology defies simple definition, but is clearly much concerned with understanding how people and animals function normally. In contrast, PSYCHIATRY is the branch of medicine concerned with the diagnosis and treatment of mental disorders, encompassing mental illness, LEARNING DISABILITY, and PERSONALITY DISORDER. Psychiatrists are medically qualified doctors who have undergone additional postgraduate training in psychiatry. Sub-specialties include general adult psychiatry, child and adolescent psychiatry, forensic psychiatry, learning disability, psychiatry of old age and psychotherapy. Although all psychiatrists receive some training in PSYCHOTHERAPY, not all psychiatrists are psychotherapists, nor are all psychotherapists psychiatrists. Psychiatrists are distinguished from psychologists by their ability to prescribe drugs and other physical treatments, their general medical training, and generally, their salaries.

IAN C. REID

psychic blindness This is the same as VISUAL AGNOSIA; see AGNOSIA.

psychic paralysis of gaze *see* oculomotor apraxia; optic ataxia

psychoactive A term, usually applied to a DRUG, indicating an ability change psychological processing or behaviour; HALLUCINOGENS, COCAINE, MARIJUANA and NICOTINE are examples of drugs that can be called psychoactive. Drugs that induce sedation, such as the OPIATES and other NARCOTICS, can also be described as psychoactive, because, although rather stupefying, they do change psychological processes.

See also: psychomotor stimulants; psychopharmacology; psychotropic

psychoanalysis Psychoanalysis is a form of PSYCHOTHERAPY. It is a term describing any of a number of systems for analysing psychological problems, but the root of all of these is the system of psychoanalysis developed by Sigmund Freud (1856–1939). The essence of Freud's theories lies in a number of critical points. (1) The belief that the mind is structured into various components: the *id* is a basic unconscious, biological force, present at birth; the *ego* is a conscious part of the mind, developing in the first year of life and concerned with operations such as DECISION-MAKING; and the *superego*, the third and last part to develop, is concerned with moral processes. These three elements can all be divided still further, and can interact, the relationships between them being a potential source of psychological conflict. (2) Freud believed that psychological problems in adulthood stem from childhood experiences. (3) Trained analysts can access psychological processes taking place using a variety of techniques, including, famously, the interpretation of dreams (see DREAMING). Later theorists built on the foundations laid by Freud, sometimes in agreement with him, sometimes not. Biological psychology is often thought of as being antithetical to psychoanalysis, but it is not the intention here to engage in a discussion of the merits and demerits of psychoanalysis. Readers who are interested in learning more about it should consult, as a starting point, a standard reference (e.g. Davison & Neale, 1996). A recent review (Horgan, 1996) also highlights a number of interesting points, comparing the so-called 'talk therapies' such as psychoanalysis, with pharmacological and brain systems approaches to psychological disturbance.

What is worth considering briefly is Sigmund Freud himself. Freud's early career, up to and including the 1880s, was in neurology, at which he excelled. His special skill was in NEUROPATHOLOGY and he contributed to the development of histological techniques (see HISTOLOGY) for analysing brain tissue. In this work he collaborated and corresponded with many of the great nineteenth-century neurologists such as Meynert who were to have a profound effect on the description and analysis of brain function and on the development of the neurosciences. He also made a specialization in paediatric neurology, writing for example about paralysis in children, on which he was considered to be a leading authority. While disappointed with the pace of his career (advancement for Jewish doctors and scientists was not as rapid as might have been hoped) it is unambiguous that Freud was one of the leading neurologists in Europe and looked set to enjoy a long and productive career. The interesting question to ask, therefore, is why did he make such a dramatic leap away from conventional neurology?

Freud's biographer and colleague, Ernest Jones, offers some interesting insights into this. In the 1860s and 1870s, new understanding of APHASIA had been developed with the findings by Broca and Wernicke of different types of aphasia produced by the occurrence of LESION in different parts of the brain. Detailed maps of the connections between these areas – BROCA'S AREA and WERNICKE'S AREA – were drawn, with differences in the aphasia that would result from damage to them hypothesized. However: 'in a subtle case of aphasia Bastian [the leading English authority on aphasia] postulated a minute lesion between the supposed associative fibres below the cortex, but when the autopsy revealed a huge cyst that had destroyed a good part of the left hemispheres of the brain, he was so stunned that he resigned from the hospital' (Jones, 1961, p. 196). Freud argued that the detailed and minute localization of brain function being proposed to account for the aphasia was wrong, not just in dramatic cases such as this, but wrong in principle. Freud, like all other nineteenth-century neuroscientists, was a product of a tradition that originated with PHRENOLOGY: all psychological functions must be localized to specific areas of brain tissue. Meynert, for example, proposed that memories were in some way attached to an individual NEURON, a single cell coding an individual unit of MEMORY. Freud rejected such ideas and argued that psychological and neurological data were being confounded when they should not be. He pointed out that Broca's and Wernicke's areas had a 'significance' [that]

was purely anatomical, not physiological, and simply due to their neighbourhood, in the former case to the motor areas of the brain, and in the latter to the entry of the fibres from the acoustic nuclei. The centres are therefore nothing more than nodal points in the general network' (Jones, 1961, p. 197). This is a remarkable statement by Jones. His huge biography of Freud was complied in the 1950s, being condensed for the 1961 edition. His use of the terms 'nodal points' (see NETWORK NODES) and 'network' (see NEURAL NETWORKS) to describe Freud's opinions are prescient. What Freud had grasped was that the relationships between psychological and neural processes are very much more complex and ambiguous than had been anticipated. Accounts of psychological life couched purely in terms of neural processes, particularly in the highly localized actions of individual cells or nuclei, appeared to him to be limited, a fact now acknowledged in the development of network theories that account for processes such as LEARNING and PATTERN PERCEPTION by the use of various types of neural networks (see also PARALLEL VS. SERIAL PROCESSING). Lacking a fundamental understanding of how neurons communicate (an appreciation of NEUROTRANSMISSION at the SYNAPSE would have to wait until the 1950s and beyond) and without a modern awareness of how neurons, real or artificial (see ARTIFICIAL INTELLIGENCE) can operate together, Freud opted instead for explanations of psychological events expressed in terms of conscious and unconscious forces. What, one wonders, would Freud have been able to do with the knowledge and techniques of modern neuroscience available to him?

References

Davison G.C. & Neale J.M. (1996) *Abnormal psychology*, 6th edn, Wiley: New York.

Horgan J. (1996) Why Freud isn't dead. *Scientific American* 275: 74–79.

Jones E. (1961) *The Life and Work of Sigmund Freud*, condensed edn, Penguin Books, London.

psychobiology Synonymous with BIOLOGICAL PSYCHOLOGY.

psychodynamic (from Greek, *psyche*: soul [though it has come to stand for psychology without reference to soul], *dynamis*: power) The term psychodynamic is used to describe theories and approaches to psychology and behaviour that provide accounts couched in psychological terms: psychodynamic means that psychological forces have dynamic power and can be used to account for psychological events without any necessary reliance on other forces (such as biological events). Psychodynamic theories operate at a purely psychological level, without regard to (for example) neuroscience. The best-known psychodynamic theory is of course the system – PSYCHOANALYSIS – developed by Sigmund Freud.

See also: consciousness; medical model; mind–body question; psychotherapy

psychogenic (from Greek, *psyche*: soul [or, in more contemporary usage, mind], *genesis*: formation) Literally, something that is formed by the mind. Of course, this rather begs the question as to whether or not one has a mind from which to form anything; see MIND–BODY QUESTION; NEUROPHILOSOPHY.

psychohydraulic *see* ethology

psychomotor epilepsy A form of EPILEPSY involving the automatic execution of complex movements; sufferers may be confused but do not lose CONSCIOUSNESS during these SEIZURES. AMNESIA about the events is usually found. GRAND MAL SEIZURE may also be shown by psychomotor epileptics.

psychomotor seizure *see* psychomotor epilepsy

psychomotor stimulants Drugs which increase motor output and mental functions. The stimulation of the AUTONOMIC NERVOUS SYSTEM caused by the psychomotor stimulants results in increases in heart rate, respiratory rate and blood pressure. The pupils are dilated and there is decreased APPETITE. There may be sweating, blurring of vision, dizziness, agitation and ANXIETY. Stimulants also increase alertness and improve mental and physical performance, particularly on tasks which can benefit from high arousal, such as REACTION TIME tasks, involving high-speed responses.

As a class, psychomotor stimulants can be further subdivided according to their chemical action in the brain. The SYMPATHOMIMETIC type, such as AMPHETAMINE and COCAINE, interferes with DOPAMINE function by stimulating dopamine release and/or blocking reuptake; the CHOLINOMIMETIC type, such as NICOTINE and MUSCARINE, has AGONIST action at CHOLINERGIC receptors; the XANTHINES, such as CAFFEINE (found in coffee) and THEOPHYLLINE (found in tea) act at the ADENOSINE receptor or are GABA antagonists; while the convulsants, such as strychnine, block the GLYCINE receptor.

Some stimulants, such as nicotine and caffeine, are freely available and their use to combat fatigue is well known and legally condoned. Others are regulated because they have potential for abuse: they produce EUPHORIA and a sense of well-being. Medicinal use of psychomotor stimulants include the treatment of NARCOLEPSY and as APPETITE SUPPRESSANTS in the treatment of OBESITY. The psychomotor stimulant RITALIN ® is used to treat ATTENTION-DEFICIT DISORDER. Stimulants may be taken orally, administered via the mucus membranes (sniffing, or 'snorting', and chewing), inhaled (smoking) or injected intravenously. Route of administration effects the nature of the 'high', with smoking, snorting or injecting producing the fastest 'rush'. Possible dangers associated with high doses include rapid or irregular heartbeat, tremors, loss of coordination, a rapid increase in blood pressure which may lead to stroke or heart attack. Prolonged use of amphetamines can lead to amphetamine-induced psychosis, which is a syndrome resembling SCHIZOPHRENIA, with hallucinations, delusions and paranoia. Symptoms usually abate when the drug is withdrawn. TOLERANCE to stimulants develops rapidly and psychological DEPENDENCE is common. WITHDRAWAL following sustained use or even a single binge can result in fatigue and psychomotor depression (known as a 'crash'), increased anxiety and DRUG CRAVING.

See also: drug abuse

VERITY J. BROWN

psychoneuroimmunology A field of study that investigates the relationships between psychological processes, the nervous system and the immune system; see IMMUNE SYSTEM.

psychopath This term is often used rather loosely in everyday speech and writing. Central to the clinical conception of psychopathy are two fundamental traits: the first is a lack of EMOTION. Psychopaths exhibit no concern for others and do not give evidence of experiencing any personal feelings. Thus their behaviour towards others will show indifference to them and the psychopath will experience no sense of shame, guilt or responsibility for the effects their own actions have on others. Second, the behaviour of psychopaths can be exceptionally antisocial. Psychopathy is at present best regarded as an essentially emotional personality disorder rather than a brain disorder. Although there has been some evidence of changes in ELECTROENCEPHALOGRAM activity, evidence for a dysfunction unique to psychopaths is not present.

Reference

Davison G.C. & Neale J.M. (1996) *Abnormal Psychology*, 6th edn, Wiley: New York.

psychopathology The study of the nature and development of abnormal behaviour, thoughts and feelings. Psychopathology and the virtually identical area of abnormal psychology is the basic science underlying CLINICAL PSYCHOLOGY and PSYCHIATRY. It has two basic components: description and explanation. There are various carefully developed schedules for making a reliable and possibly valid psychiatric diagnosis. The most widely used for clinical and many research purposes is the *Diagnostic and Statistical Manual of the Mental Disorders* (currently DSM-IV) developed by the American Psychiatric Association. This manual provides detailed and generally agreed criteria for diagnosing virtually all the conditions seen by psychiatrists and psychologists. These range from the widely recognized MOOD and ANXIETY disorders, SCHIZOPHRENIA and psychotic disorders to organic conditions and conditions related to substance abuse and various personality disorders.

There are two general classes of explanation of abnormal behaviour, the psychological and the biological. Psychological explanations are concerned with learning and cognition. Psychoanalysts from Sigmund Freud (1856–1939) and behaviourists from J.B. Watson (1878–1958) and B.F. Skinner (1904–1990) are united in maintaining that abnormal behaviour is rooted in faulty LEARNING. Of course they disagree markedly on what is wrongly learned and how it affects behaviour. More recently cognitive theorists, such as Beck, have extended this by claiming that this faulty learning leads to faulty thinking and that this is the cause of abnormal behaviour. Cognitive theories now dominate psychological thinking on abnormal behaviour. These range from Beck's view that a negative triad of negative views of the self, the world and the future underlie depression to detailed experimental studies suggesting a tendency for depressed mood to be associated with memory abnormalities while anxiety is associated with abnormal deployment of attention to negative events or bodily symptoms. Biological theories concentrate on the underlying pathophysiology. For the non-degenerative conditions abnormalities in neurotransmitters are often posited, such as the DOPAMINE HYPOTHESIS OF SCHIZOPHRENIA or MONOAMINE HYPOTHESIS OF DEPRESSION. The main support for such theories is often indirect and based on the effects of pharmacological treatment or studies of animal models of the mental illness.

While psychological and biological theories are offered for many abnormal conditions, psychological theories dominate the study of anxiety and biological theories that of schizophrenia. Both views are strongly held in depression. There is an increasing interest in both camps in the genetic basis of abnormal behaviour and in the interaction of GENE and environment.

See also: behaviour therapy; cognitive–behavioural therapy; cognitive therapy

DEREK W. JOHNSTON

psychopharmacology The study of the pharmacological, neurochemical, and behavioural effects of PSYCHOACTIVE drugs. A psychoactive DRUG is one that has direct effects on the brain, and somehow alters psychological and/or behavioural processes. The field of psychopharmacology had its beginnings in approximately the late 1950s and early 1960s, when the science of NEUROPHARMACOLOGY was developing. While neuropharmacology focused on effects of drugs on the nervous system, psychopharmacology tended to emphasize the effects of drugs on behaviour and the mind. Indeed, the term is derived from the Greek words for mind, drug, and study. (The term behavioural pharmacology describes the field in which examination of the effects of drugs on behaviour – not mental processes – is made. Behavioural pharmacology and psychopharmacology are however used almost synonymously.) Researchers within the field of psychopharmacology study these drugs for a number of reasons. First, investigators in psychopharmacology study the effects and actions of drugs. For example, people have taken certain mind-altering drugs for thousands of years, such as CANNABIS, TOBACCO, COCAINE and HALLUCINOGENS. In recent years, a quite detailed understanding of the underlying neural mechanisms associated with these drugs has emerged. Second, drugs are used as tools in order to probe the brain and to understand the physiological or functional role of a particular neurochemical system. Some drugs have very specific effects of neural systems or receptors, and thus can be used as a tool in studying that system. The OPIATES, for example MORPHINE and HEROIN, directly act as agonists on endogenous opiate receptors, while NALOXONE specifically blocks such receptors. A great deal has been learned about the normal biological function of endogenous opioid systems (for example in PAIN transmission, STRESS, REWARD, FEEDING) through use of these drugs in research. Another example would be using the psychostimulant drugs AMPHETAMINE or cocaine, both of which potently activate DOPAMINE systems, to understand the role of this system in biological reinforcement. A third goal of psychopharmacology research is to understand mental illness and mental disorders and to develop better treatments for these conditions. Researchers attempt to understand what neural substrates and what brain regions may be involved in such disorders. For example, considerable progress in the understanding and treatment of depression has been made in the past two decades, much of which as emerged in the field of psychopharmacology.

References

Dews P.B. (1978) Origins and future of behavioural pharmacology. *Life Sciences* 22: 1115–1122.

Feldman R.S., Meyer J.S. & Quenzer L.F. (1997) *Principles of Neuropharmacology*, Sinauer Associates Inc.: Sunderland MA.

ANN E. KELLEY

psychophysics (from Greek, *psyche*: mind, *physike*: natural world) The study of the relationship between the physical world, including the brain, and the mind; founded by Gustav Teodor Fechner (1801–1887) in 1860. Also a collection of methods (many invented by Fechner) for precisely measuring sensory, perceptual and cognitive functioning in whole animals, especially humans. These include both measures of performance in various experimental paradigms as well as measures of subjective responses to stimuli. Characterized by four major problems: detection, discrimination, identification, and scaling. Absolute (detection) and differential (discrimination) thresholds (minimal stimulus levels or differences, respectively, that can be responded to) are measured by methods of constant stimuli, limits, or adaptive testing. Modern methods nearly always use forced-choice paradigms, based on SIGNAL DETECTION THEORY, in which decision bias is controlled. The signal detection theory measure of performance, d' (d prime) is often used in lieu of absolute or differential threshold measurements. Identification performance is measured in bits of information (base 2 logarithm of number of alternatives) successfully transmitted from stimulus to response. Subjective psychological magnitudes are measured by several scaling methods, the most popular of which is magnitude estimation in which numbers are assigned directly to perceived psychological magnitudes. Laws established using psychophysical methods include: *Weber's law*, $\Delta I = kI$ where ΔI is differential threshold, I is the stimulus intensity at which it is measured and k is a constant). A different value of k characterizes each sensory continuum, being relatively large for light and sound intensity and relatively small for painful stimuli. *Fechner's law*, $S = (1/k) \ln (I/I_0)$ where

S is the magnitude of sensation given rise to by a stimulus of intensity I (relative to the absolute threshold intensity, I_0), and k is the constant from Weber's law, incorporates an indirect scaling of sensation. *Stevens's law*, $S = kI^b$ (where b is different for different sensory continua and k is a scaling constant), is confirmed by direct scaling methods, such as magnitude estimation. Examples of laws describing the dependence of thresholds on stimulus conditions include the *Bloch–Charpentier law*, $I_0\ t = b$ where t is stimulus duration less than about 100 msec and b is a constant that represents the minimal amount of light energy needed for detection, and *Ricco's Law*, $I_0\ A = c$ where A ($< 10'$ of visual angle) is an area stimulated on the retina and c is a constant.

LAWRENCE M. WARD

psychophysiological disorders A number of physical disorders and conditions – HEADACHE and MIGRAINE, HYPERTENSION, cardiovascular illness (see CARDIOVASCULAR PSYCHOPHYSIOLOGY) – are made worse by psychological factors. The general term used to describe this interaction is psychophysiological disorders. This term replaces an older one, PSYCHOSOMATIC DISORDERS, which had come to have a rather pejorative meaning, having the implication that such disorders were illusory or 'all in the mind'. Contemporary approaches to psychophysiological disorders de-emphasize mental explanations and simply seek to relate psychological and physiological processes, regardless of whether, at some more fundamental level, all psychological functions could possibly have a physical explanation themselves (see MIND–BODY QUESTION). Two primary factors that are central to psychophysical disorders are STRESS and personality variables (see TYPE A AND TYPE B BEHAVIOUR). Managing the impact of psychological processes in physical disorders generally requires use of an appropriate PSYCHOTHERAPY.

See also: health psychology

Reference

Davison G.C. & Neale J.M. (1996) *Abnormal Psychology*, 6th edn, Wiley: New York.

psychophysiology The study of the relationship between behaviour and/or mental states and physiological responses in humans using non-invasive methods. Behaviour, cognition and, most strikingly, emotion are accompanied by physiological changes across the bodily systems. Psychophysiology describes these processes, analyses their functional significance and uses the knowledge to increase understanding of the psychological processes involved. Much of psychophysiology is concerned with responses under the immediate control of the AUTONOMIC NERVOUS SYSTEM (ANS), although measures of the CENTRAL NERVOUS SYSTEM (CNS) and, less frequently the PERIPHERAL NERVOUS SYSTEM (PNS) are also examined. The independent variables in psychophysiological studies most commonly relate to STRESS, EMOTION, LEARNING, information processing, ATTENTION and MEMORY. Occasionally behaviour is the dependent variable and the physiological responses are manipulated, as in BIOFEEDBACK. Traditionally psychophysiological investigations were carried out under controlled laboratory conditions but advances in technology have enabled most physiological responses to be measured in real life using multi-purpose ambulatory recorders and there is increasing use of such measurement.

The ANS mediated responses studied included cardiovascular responses such as heart rate, blood pressure and peripheral blood flow (see CARDIOVASCULAR PSYCHOPHYSIOLOGY), skin conductance and gut motility. Respiratory activity is often studied both in its own right and because of its powerful effects on autonomic systems. Many aspects of immune functioning are currently under study. Numerous studies have shown that diverse stressors, such as challenging or fearful tasks, lead to profound changes such as increases in heart rate, blood pressure, peripheral resistance and skin conductance. It is often difficult to determine the branch of the ANS involved since many systems, such as the heart are under dual SYMPATHETIC and PARASYMPATHETIC control. Pharmacological blockade studies can be helpful in clarifying mechanisms. Rather helpfully sweating, and hence skin conductance, is under purely sympathetic control. While many attempts have been made to determine the differential physiological effects of different tasks (such as those involving active and passive coping; see CARDIOVASCULAR PSYCHO-PHYSIOLOGY) it is clear that individuals respond idiosyncratically irrespective of the task. This has lead to the twin concepts of stimulus stereotyping (similarity of psychophysiological response across tasks *between* individuals) and response stereotyping (similarity of response *within* individuals across tasks). It is held by some that response stereotyping may determine which organ system is vulnerable to psychosomatic or stress-related physical illness. This is consistent with the highly influential stress-diathesis model. It is also clear that different individuals respond in widely varying degrees to the same stimulus. Such hyper-reactors may be more vulnerable to disease in the organ systems involved. Other important areas of study of ANS mediated responses are emotion and learning. The three factor theory of emotion which hold that emotions can be usefully separated into behavioural, subjective and physiological components is based on psychophysiological studies. I.P. Pavlov (1849–1936) and his successors have demonstrated that autonomic responses can be classically conditioned (see CLASSICAL CONDITIONING) and the claim of B.F. Skinner (1904–1990) that such responses cannot be instrumentally conditioned has been vindicated (see INSTRUMENTAL CONDITIONING and BIOFEEDBACK). The study of classical conditioning of autonomic responses to fear inducing stimuli has provided the main support to the important preparedness theory of fear acquisition. Immune activity can be classically conditioned and is affected by stress in complex ways, with both immune suppression and enhancement being demonstrated (see IMMUNE SYSTEM). The activity of the CNS is typically studied with the ELECTROENCEPHALO-GRAM (EEG). While studies of the basic frequencies of the EEG, using filtering and spectral analytic techniques, are conducted, most investigators concentrate on EVENT-RELATED POTENTIALS (ERP) which provide information with high temporal resolution on brain activity associated with attention, memory and information processing. Information on the localization of such processes in the brain is

also acquired, although this is may be done more effectively using imaging processes such as MAGNETIC RESONANCE IMAGING (MRI). Physiological systems controlled by the PNS are less commonly studied. Muscle activity, measured with the ELECTROMYOGRAM (EMG) is used to examine the covert behavioural correlates of cognitive activities such as silent reading or imagery and considerable insights into fear related attentional processes have been acquire through studies of the STARTLE REFLEX, determined from eye blinks. EMG activity is also used to determine the likely metabolic determinants of autonomically mediated responses, such as the decrease in heart rate that follows the warning signal in the signalled REACTION TIME paradigm. EMG activity can be used to provide statistical control for movement during ambulatory studies of ANS mediated responses, such as heart rate, that are metabolically linked.

Reference

Cacioppo J.T. & Tassiary L.G. (eds.) (1990) *Principles of Psychophysiology: Physical, Social and Inferential Elements*, Cambridge University Press: Cambridge.

DEREK W. JOHNSTON

psychosis General term referring to a cluster of symptoms (usually the presence of DELUSION and HALLUCINATION), rather than a specific disease state. Subjects who are psychotic often lack insight into their situation, and are considered to be 'out of touch with reality': amongst psychiatric syndromes, psychosis accords most closely with the lay concept of 'madness'. Psychotic symptoms occur in a wide range of conditions. Most commonly encountered in SCHIZOPHRENIA, they may also be seen in severe DEPRESSION, MANIA, PARANOIA, DEMENTIA and DRUG ABUSE.

See also: neurosis

IAN C. REID

psychosomatic disorders *see* psychophysiological disorders

psychostimulant *see* stimulants

psychosurgery A term to describe a range of neurosurgical procedures conducted with the intention of minimizing or alleviating disabling psychological and emotional symptoms. Although crude behaviour modifying brain operations have been performed throughout human history (see TREPANNING) the introduction of modern neurosurgical procedures into the management of intractable mental disorders is generally attributed to the Portuguese neurologist Antonio Egas Moniz. His collaboration with the neurosurgeon Almeida Lima led to the therapeutic use of a widespread destructive LESION of WHITE MATTER tracts connecting the FRONTAL LOBE with posterior brain regions. Such was the reported success of these LEUCOTOMY (cutting the connections between frontal lobe and THALAMUS) or LOBOTOMY (disconnecting the frontal lobes from the remainder of the brain – also called FRONTAL LOBOTOMY) procedures in a previously untreatable population of psychiatric patients, particularly those with SCHIZOPHRENIA, Moniz was awarded the Nobel Prize for Physiology or Medicine in 1949. Unfortunately, adaptations of the Moniz and Lima procedure were enthusiastically and uncritically adopted across the world and many thousands of operations were conducted for a broad range of problems that strayed far beyond the original therapeutic remit, including criminal behaviour, AGGRESSION, childhood defiance and political opposition. As a consequence of such widespread and injudicious use of a poorly evaluated and irreversible treatment, a forceful and sustained opposition evolved that resulted in the abolition, or near-abolition, of such treatments in most developed countries. Around the same time, the first effective chemical ANTIPSYCHOTIC and ANTIDEPRESSANT treatments were discovered, substantially alleviating the pressure to consider surgery.

Despite the disreputable history of psychosurgery, the combination of advances in modern FUNCTIONAL NEUROIMAGING and STEREOTAXIC SURGERY with an enhanced understanding of the anatomy and functional relationships between the FRONTAL CORTEX and other brain structures has resulted in the re-emergence of neurosurgery as a viable and ethical treatment option in intractable mental disorder. Stereotaxic neurosurgery is performed in a number of treatment centres around the world; reserved as an option for patients with severe DEPRESSION, ANXIETY or OBSESSIVE COMPULSIVE DISORDER that is considered unresponsive to all conventional treatments. Despite its original use, it is not considered as a treatment option for schizophrenia. As a refinement of earlier, indiscriminate procedures, two specific target sites appear to offer maximal benefit with relatively minimal adverse effects: the white matter fibres in the anterior limb of the INTERNAL CAPSULE (anterior CAPSULOTOMY) and the anterior cingulate cortex (anterior CINGULOTOMY). As evidence accumulates from structural and functional brain imaging studies that both the MEDIAL PREFRONTAL CORTEX and the ANTERIOR CINGULATED CORTEX are involved in the pathophysiology of depression, a potential rationale is emerging for neurosurgical treatments. Although definitive data on treatment efficacy are lacking, a proportion of patients within this otherwise untreatable population derives significant benefit from neurosurgical treatment. Despite well-founded concerns about the likely adverse effects, evidence for impairments in cognitive and intellectual performance and for personality change post-surgery is absent.

See also: deep brain stimulation; pallidotomy; split brain; thalamotomy

KEITH MATTHEWS

psychotherapy Psychotherapy is an umbrella term that refers to any treatment regime – a therapy – that relies upon a psychological technique or theory. It does not refer only to PSYCHOANALYSIS (though it includes this: the terms psychotherapy and psychoanalysis are not synonyms: psychoanalysis is a form of psychotherapy). Psychotherapy can include COGNITIVE–BEHAVIOURAL THERAPY, a structured, flexible and time-limited approach to the treatment of a broad range of clinical problems, and COGNITIVE THERAPY, a short-term, focused form of treatment placing emphasis is on examination and modification of the patient's thoughts and beliefs. It can also include BEHAVIOUR THERAPY, an approach to maladaptive or unwanted behaviour based on CLASSICAL CONDITIONING procedures. From the perspective of biological psychology the critical point to consider here is that any form of psychotherapy can be conducted without reference to neuroscience: it is based on an understanding and use of psychological processes.

See also: medical model

psychotic mood disorders *see* schizoaffective disorder

psychotomimetic (from psychosis and Greek, *mimesis*: imitation) A DRUG that can produce the effects of, or like those of, psychosis is said to be psychotomimetic.

psychotropic A rather old term, synonymous with PSYCHOACTIVE.

puberty The phase of sexual maturation during which the stimulation of adult activity of the GONADS (ANDROGEN and ESTROGEN secretion) leads to spermatogenesis and oogenesis, development of secondary sex characteristics, and crystallization of adult behavioural patterns. Although the precise genetic or experiential events that initiate puberty remain unknown, puberty begins when gonadotrophin releasing hormone is first secreted from the HYPOTHALAMUS into the anterior PITUITARY GLAND, causing it to release follicle stimulating hormone and luteinizing hormone into the blood (see HORMONES). The onset of puberty in humans is approximately 11 years for girls and 13 years for boys. Precocious puberty in children can occur with some genetic abnormalities or following extreme trauma.

See also: estrus; feminine; masculine; menstrual cycle; organization effects of steroid hormones; sex differences; sexual dimorphism

JAMES G. PFAUS

pulmonary circuit *see* blood

pulvinar nucleus A nucleus of the THALAMUS important in visual processing; see GENICULOSTRIATE AND TECTOPULVINAR VISUAL PATHWAYS.

punch drunk syndrome *see* concussion

punding *see* stereotypy

punished locomotion The reduction in normal spontaneous locomotor activity around a test environment due to PUNISHMENT of move-

ment across that environment by presentation of an aversive event.

See also: animal models of anxiety; aversive conditioning; conditioned fear; conditioned punishment; locomotion

A. SIMON KILLCROSS

punishment The four basic procedures in OPERANT CONDITIONING are POSITIVE REINFORCEMENT, NEGATIVE REINFORCEMENT, punishment and OMISSION. Punishment and omission are said to decrease response probability. If a response occurs, and it is followed by the presentation of a stimulus, and this results in a decrease in response probability, then it is said that punishment has occurred. According to the behaviourist tradition, punishment has typically been defined simply in empirical terms. However, it has become more common to view operant conditioning procedures in terms of their motivational or regulatory consequences. Thus, with punishment, it is evident that the type of stimulus being presented, which results in a decrease in response probability, is an aversive stimulus. According to the motivational view, negative reinforcement involves the organism behaving so as to decrease the probability of aversive events. Thus, the punished response not being repeated removes an occasion for the possible presentation of an aversive stimulus. Essentially, punishment is another term for PASSIVE AVOIDANCE.

JOHN D. SALAMONE

pupil An adjustable opening in the IRIS of the EYE through which light passes to the RETINA. Changes in the size of the aperture are the product of REFLEX muscular actions (the pupillary reflex).

pure alexia An ACQUIRED READING DISORDER in which the processing of complete word forms is impaired. Instead, individual letters are processed in series across the word, and the alphabetic name of each letter may be pronounced aloud. The disorder is commonly referred to as LETTER-BY-LETTER READING. Print is easier to read than handwriting. The written word is often read correctly following the identification of the letters, but mistakes occur if letters have been misidentified. Short words are read faster than long words and reading time increases regularly with the number of letters in the word. WRITING is spared, but the subject has great difficulty READING back what has been written.

The disorder is believed to affect the ability to process letters in parallel. Naming the individual letters allows the word form to be assembled using verbal processes. Some cases of pure alexia appear to have rapid access to knowledge of the complete word form and to the word's meaning. This can be observed in a LEXICAL DECISION TASK and SEMANTIC CATE-GORIZATION TASK (for instance, does the written word name an animal or not?) when the written word is displayed for periods too short for letter-by-letter reading, although subjects deny that they can 'see' the entire letter string. This rapid processing of the whole word form and access to meaning is thought to take place through the automatic activation of subconscious reading processes in the RIGHT HEMISPHERE. The type of brain LESION associated with pure alexia affects posterior areas of the dominant HEMISPHERE which isolate the visual processing areas (see VISUAL SYSTEM) from the LANGUAGE areas involved in normal reading. The prognosis for the disorder varies; some cases resolve quickly; others develop into a mild form of SURFACE DYSLEXIA; yet others endure.

See also: attentional dyslexia; deep dyslexia; neglect dyslexia; peripheral reading disorder; phonological dyslexia

pure anomia *see* anomia

pure word deafness Pure word deafness is the label given to the auditory imperception following focal bilateral lesion of the primary AUDITORY CORTEX. It is most likely a defect in the perceptual elaboration of brief, closely spaced sounds, and not a formal AGNOSIA restricted to spoken LANGUAGE. The discrimination deficit, which is most obvious and debilitating for SPEECH PERCEPTION, is most profound for any PHONEME whose identity depends on the temporal resolution of sound elements less than a few tens of milliseconds apart (for example, consonants), and it extends

to the perception of non-speech sounds with comparable temporal grains.

DENNIS P. PHILLIPS

purine ADENOSINE TRIPHOSPHATE (ATP) and some derivatives (ADENOSINE and ADENOSINE DIPHOSPHATE [ADP] for example) appear to have the properties of NEUROTRANSMITTERS. These are known as purines because purine is the substance from which adenine is derived; this form of transmission is therefore called purinergic. Purinergic transmission is important in several peripheral structures and in certain parts of the CENTRAL NERVOUS SYSTEM. The receptors for purines are divided into the P2X group (P2X$_1$, P2X$_2$, P2X$_3$, P2X$_4$) which are ligand gated, and P2Y group (P2Y$_1$, P2Y$_2$, P2Y$_3$, P2Y$_4$, P2Y$_5$) that are G PROTEIN coupled. CAFFEINE and THEOPHYLLINE are thought to act at adenosine receptors.

purinergic A form of neurotransmission mediated by substances of the PURINE group.

Purkinje cells *see* cerebellum – anatomical organization

Purkinje shift The change in SPECTRAL SENSITIVITY from CONES to RODS that occurs during dark adaptation, named after Johann Purkinje (1787–1869) who first described the effect in 1825. In daylight, human vision is mediated by the cone receptors of the RETINA, but at night is mediated by the rods. Cones and rods absorb light from slightly different regions of the VISIBLE SPECTRUM: cones absorb more effectively in the yellow to orange spectral regions, compared to rods which absorb blue-green wavelengths maximally. Thus as day-vision shifts to night, reds and yellows become relatively darker and blues and greens relatively brighter in appearance.

See also: spectral sensitivity curves

KATHY T. MULLEN

purposeless chewing *see* jaw movements

pursuit eye movements *see* motion perception

push–pull perfusion A process in which neurochemical substances (see NEUROCHEMISTRY) can be extracted from brain EXTRACELLULAR fluid by means of a push–pull CANNULA. This is composed of two concentric cannulae, one inside the other. Fluid is pushed down the centre cannula and recovered by negative pressure applied to the outer cannula, the cannula tip presenting a moving fluid surface directly to brain at which molecules from the extracellular space can be collected. Collected perfusate is then analysed for its chemical composition using various analytical procedures (such as HIGH-PERFORMANCE LIQUID CHROMATOGRAPHY). Push–pull perfusion is less commonly used now than MICRODIALYSIS, which places a SEMIPERMEABLE MEMBRANE between the perfusate and brain, reducing significantly the potential for mechanical damage to tissue. Push–pull perfusions is preferred to dialysis only when trying to recover from brain very high MOLECULAR WEIGHT substances which would not pass through a semipermeable membrane with ease.

See also: electrochemistry; voltammetry

putamen The putamen is a major part of the dorsal STRIATUM) receiving cortical afferents mainly from the sensorimotor cortex. It is distinguished from the CAUDATE NUCLEUS only by this pattern of cortical connectivity and only becomes separated from it by the internal capsule in those species where this fibre pathway is well-developed.

See also: basal ganglia

BARRY J. EVERITT

puzzle box A box with one or more locking mechanisms (for primates typically bolts or clasps) which an animal must learn to manipulate in order to obtain a reward. Puzzle boxes have been used to asses LEARNING in a very wide variety of species, including primates and rats, and even invertebrates.

pyknosis (from Greek, *pyknos*: thick) A process of thickening or condensing. When used to describe a CELL it is generally applied to the cell NUCLEUS and is an indication that a cell is dying.

pyramidal motor system *see* extrapyramidal motor system

pyramidal neurons One of two principal types of NEURON in the CEREBRAL CORTEX (the other being NON-PYRAMIDAL NEURONS). A pyramidal neuron has a CELL BODY shaped (unsurprisingly) like pyramids, with the apex of the pyramid aimed at the outer surface of the brain. Arising from the apex of the pyramid is a DENDRITE – the APICAL DENDRITE – that ascends more or less at right angles through the CORTICAL LAYERS to layer 1. Branches of the apical dendrite penetrate into the layers it passes through. The base of the pyramidal cell body (typically around 30 μm across) gives rise to multiple dendrites – the BASAL DENDRITES – that move off laterally through the cortical layer in which the neuron sits. The cell body also gives rise to an AXON that might make local connections but will also leave the area of the cell body, projecting to other parts of the cerebral cortex or to sites elsewhere in the brain, as far away as the SPINAL CORD. The density of pyramidal neurons, and the proportion of pyramidal to non-pyramidal neurons, varies from layer to layer and from region to region within the cortex. Output layers (layers 5 and 6) usually have the most pyramidal neurons. In contrast to pyramidal neurons, non-pyramidal neurons are not shaped like pyramids but have cell bodies that are much rounder, or possibly star-shaped (stellate). Non-pyramidal neurons are smaller than pyramidal, having a diameter of about 10 m. They do not have identified apical and basal dendrites, but have dendritic fields that spread locally. Their axons do not leave the cerebral cortex, but project locally, within the same cortical layer as the cell body and into adjacent layers. They are in effect cortical INTERNEURONS that receive cortical input and process it locally, influencing the actions of other cortical neurons.

pyramidal tract Synonymous with CORTICOSPINAL TRACT.

See also: extrapyramidal motor system

pyrexia (from Greek, *pyr*: fire) A medical term for FEVER, which involves the production of heat (see THERMOGENESIS).

pyriform cortex (from Latin, *pirum*: a pear, *forma*: form) The common spelling is *pyri-*

form, though *piriform* is also used, and is more closely related to the Latin root: piriform means pear-shaped. The pyriform cortex is the area most commonly identified as the OLFACTORY CORTEX (see OLFACTORY SYSTEM). It has direct input from the OLFACTORY TRACT and projects to the ENTORHINAL CORTEX and AMYGDALA. It is found on the ventral surface of the brain, immediately behind the OLFACTORY BULB and below the OLFACTORY TUBERCLE.

pyrogen *see* immune system

pyrolidone A group of chemicals one of which, PIRACETAM, is a noted NOOTROPIC.

See also: cognitive enhancers

pyruvate A product of GLUCOSE metabolism; see RESPIRATION.

Q

quadrant One quarter of the RETINA (or of the VISUAL FIELD). Retinal quadrants are defined by horizontal and vertical axes passing through the FOVEA; see QUADRANTANOPSIA; QUADRANTACHROMATOPSIA.

quadrantachromatopsia *see* achromatopsia

quadrantanopsia A visual defect in a specific QUADRANT.

See also: quadrantachromatopsia

quadriplegia Complete paralysis of both arms and legs; HEMIPLEGIA is a paralysis restricted to one side of the body only.

quadruped A four-legged animal – that is, one that has its spinal column more or less parallel to the ground and engages in LOCOMOTION with all four feet (hooves, paws or whatever they might be) on the ground. Humans and many primates are BIPEDS: only two feet are used for locomotion.

quaking mutant mouse *see* jimpy mutant mouse

qualia (*Qualia* is plural; singular is *quale*) Qualia are the qualities or properties of mental states that allow individuals to define the nature of the sensory input. It is a relatively complex philosophical term around which there is some debate: qualia do not have INTENTIONALITY and are not REPRESENTATIONS, but are features of that which possesses them. Qualities such as 'redness' or 'squareness' have been proposed as qualia. However some philosophers have argued that there is no possibility of sharing qualia – can one properly describe to another 'what it is like' to experience a quale? – and that they are therefore of no value.

quanta *see* quantal release

quantal flux *see* quantal release

quantal release The release of NEUROTRANSMITTERS from SYNAPTIC TERMINALS is not a matter of inducing continuous flow: it is not analogous to turning on a tap and having water flow out. Instead, neurotransmitters are released in discrete packets called QUANTA (singular, quantum). This was observed first by Fatt & Katz in 1952. They observed that at the NEUROMUSCULAR JUNCTION, without PRESYNAPTIC stimulation, a series of small potentials could be recorded at POSTSYNAPTIC sites: these were not as large as the ENDPLATE POTENTIAL and so were called MINIATURE ENDPLATE POTENTIALS. Fatt & Katz realized that these potentials were directly related to discrete amounts of neurotransmitter being released, ACETYLCHOLINE in this case. The term QUANTAL FLUX also describes the flow of quanta.

References

Fatt P. & Katz B. (1952) Spontaneous subthreshold activity of motor nerve endings. *Journal of Physiology (London)* 117: 109–128.

Feldman R., Meyer J.S. & Quenzer L.F. (1997) *Principles of Neuropsychopharmacology*, Sinauer Associates: Sunderland MA.

quantitative trait loci *see* candidate gene analysis

questionnaire studies Questionnaires form an important part of psychological testing, being essentially a form of structured self-report. The design and construction of questionnaires is a complex process: inappropriate design will lead to misleading responses and poor data analysis. Biological psychology has maybe less interest in questionnaires than other forms of psychological study, but they are nevertheless valuable. Such tests as the MCGILL PAIN QUESTIONNAIRE, the EATING ATTITUDES TEST, the general health questionnaire and the HERMAN & POLIVY RESTRAINT SCALE are invaluable in providing information about the behaviour and experiences of individuals. A NEUROPSYCHOLOGICAL TEST BATTERY can provide valuable objective data about the *performance* of individuals, but questionnaire studies can provide valuable information about their *experiences*.

There are many different types of structure that can be employed in constructing a questionnaire. These include simple open-ended questions (tell me about your relationship with your mother), or questions requiring a simple response (who is the Prime Minister of Great Britain?) or multiple-choice questions. Rating scales are also used: these include bipolar ratings (also known as the SEMANTIC DIFFERENTIAL) in which subjects are required to mark on a scale running between polar extremes where they judge themselves to be. (The poles might be, for example, *very happy* and *very sad*: a subject would have to indicate where on a line between these poles their current state was.) The LIKERT SCALE is similar, but more structured, subjects being able to choose between several categories stretching between polar opposites (such as *very sad, sad, neither happy nor sad, happy* and *very happy*). Other forms of question include instructions to the subject to rank order items that describe themselves, and simple check box questionnaires (which are very familiar from market research: which brand of soap do you buy – tick all the boxes that apply).

Reference

Eysenck M (1998) *Psychology: An Integrated Approach*, Addison-Wesley-Longman: New York.

Quetelet index A measure of body mass; see OBESITY.

quiet biting attack *see* aggression

quiet sleep *see* slow-wave sleep

quinine Quinine, extracted from the bark of cinchona trees, is one of the ALKALOIDS. In the past it has been used medically in the treatment of malaria. In biological psychology, quinine hydrochloride is used to adulterate food and water in experiments interested in taste perception (see GUSTATION) and related processes such as FINICKINESS: it has no significant nutritive content, is colourless and odourless, but does have a characteristic bitter taste which, at appropriate concentrations (around 0.5%) causes rejection of quinine adulterated food and water. The effects of quinine on taste are typically contrasted with those of SACCHARIN, which is also non-nutritive, but has a sweet taste that (in low concentrations) animals typically find pleasant. Quinine is also the ingredient that gives tonic water its characteristic bitter taste.

quinolinic acid (quinolinate) An EXCITATORY AMINO ACID that is a rigid structural analogue of GLUTAMATE, which has been used extensively as an excitotoxin. Like other EXCITOTOXINS, quinolinic acid causes prolonged DEPOLARIZATION of neurons, which at a high enough dose results in cell death. Fibres of passage are spared. Quinolinic acid has been used as a pharmacological tool to destroy selectively specific neuronal populations, in a manner similar to KAINIC ACID, IBOTENIC ACID, and NMDA. It appears to act in part at least, at NMDA RECEPTORS. Studies using quinolinic acid injections into the STRIATUM have been proposed as an animal model for HUNTINGTON'S CHOREA. Since quinolinic acid is also produced endogenously from tryptophan, one theory proposes that quinolinate might be an endogenous excitotoxin responsible for the massive striatal cell death observed in this disease.

See also: drug ionization; kynurenic acid

ANN E. KELLEY

quisqualic acid (quisqualate) Alpha-amino-3,5-dioxo-1,2,4-oxadiazolidine-2-propanoic acid: one of the EXCITOTOXINS, which binds to GLUTAMATE RECEPTORS and is used to produce lesions (see LESION) in experimental animals. It is not commonly used, though some evidence exists to suggest that it has, in certain parts of brain, selectivity for specific neurons.

See also: drug ionization

R

rabies An infectious disease caused by a NEUROTROPIC RNA VIRUS endemic in rodents and canines world-wide. Infection ordinarily follows the bite of a rabid animal, and multiplication of the virus in the CHOLINERGIC NEUROMUSCULAR JUNCTION is followed by centripetal AXONAL TRANSPORT to the brain and from there to virtually every organ of the body. Brain symptoms develop after an incubation period of days or years. *Furious rabies* is typically associated with severe affective disturbances and painful spasms of the larynx and pharynx, traditionally interpreted as 'hydrophobia' (fear of water); *paralytic rabies* is less common. Both variants are invariably fatal without early post-exposure vaccination.

L. JACOB HERBERG

racemate A racemate, or racemic mixture, is a substance in which the D ISOMER and L isomer of a MOLECULE are present in equal amounts. BENZEDRINE, for example, is a racemic mixture of D,L-AMPHETAMINE.

racemic mixture *see* racemate

Racine's five stages of kindled seizures In the RAT, kindled seizures usually evolve through Racine's five stages: (1) facial twitching, (2) head movement, (3) forelimb clonus (see TONIC–CLONIC), (4) clonus plus REARING on hind legs, (5) rearing plus falling; see KINDLING.

radial arm maze An apparatus used for studying MEMORY primarily in the RAT. The apparatus generally consists of a circular centre platform, with anywhere from four to seventeen arms radiating out of the centre at equidistant angles from each other. In the original version, the ends of each arm on the maze are baited with a food REWARD. The rat is required to use spatial cues around the room to visit each of the arms in a non-repetitive manner. Different variants of this task can assess WORKING MEMORY, REFERENCE MEMORY and SPATIAL MEMORY. The 'delayed spatial win-shift' and 'optimal foraging' tasks have been used to investigate the functions of the HIPPOCAMPUS, PREFRONTAL CORTEX and NUCLEUS ACCUMBENS.

See also: foraging; maze learning; spatial behaviour; win–stay, lose–shift

Reference

Floresco S.B., Seamus, J.K. & Phillips A.G. (1997) Selective roles for hippocampal, prefrontal cortical, and ventral striatal circuits in radial arm maze tasks with or without a delay. *Journal of Neuroscience* 17: 1880–1890.

STANLEY B. FLORESCO

radial glial cells An alternative name for radial astrocytes; see GLIAL CELLS.

radial nerve *see* nervous system

radiant flux *see* photometry

radioactive tracer *see* tract tracers

radiofrequency lesion *see* lesion

radioimmunoassay (RIA) An *in vitro* technique for detecting the presence of a specific MOLECULE in samples of homogenized tissue, based on the binding of an ANTIBODY to an

ANTIGEN, but unlike immunoassay, the antigen is tagged with a RADIOLABEL.

See also: autoradiography

Reference

Feldman R., Meyer J.S. & Quenzer L.F. (1997) *Principles of Neuropsychopharmacology*, Sinauer Associates: Sunderland MA.

radioisotope *see* isotope

radiolabel A radiolabel is an ISOTOPE (alternatively known as a RADIOISOTOPE) attached to a chemical allowing that chemical subsequently to be detected using an appropriate technique (such as AUTORADIOGRAPHY or RADIOIMMUNOASSAY). When the radiolabel is attached to a LIGAND for identification of RECEPTOR binding, it is known as a RADIOLIGAND. Radiolabelling techniques are less used than they used to be, having largely been overtaken by techniques such as IMMUNOHISTOCHEMISTRY and IN SITU HYBRIDIZATION.

radioligand A ligand that has been radiolabelled; see RADIOLABEL.

radiometry *see* photometry

rage *see* aggression

random dot stereogram A technique for presenting depth information through BINOCULAR DISPARITY without correlated monocular information. A field of random dots (or other small pattern elements) is presented to one eye, together with a similar field in the other eye whose elements have been shifted to conform to the binocular disparities of the desired depth profile. Any gaps left by the disparity shifts are filled with new random elements, so that the pattern in the second eye remains completely random; no information about the depth profile is logically present in either eye. The process by which the depth profile is gradually perceived to emerge from the random array has held continued fascination in visual science.

See also: stereodepth perception

Reference

Julesz B. (1971) *Foundations of Cyclopean Perception*, University of Chicago Press: Chicago.

CHRISTOPHER TYLER

raphe nuclei (from Latin, *raphe*: seam) The raphe nuclei form a column of neurons (see NEURON) along the MIDLINE of the BRAINSTEM. The raphe is divisible into component nuclei with projections to virtually all parts of the CENTRAL NERVOUS SYSTEM: the more posterior nuclei have descending projections while the more anterior nuclei have ascending projections. SPINAL CORD, BRAINSTEM, CEREBELLUM and virtually all parts of the MIDBRAIN, DIENCEPHALON and FOREBRAIN have serotonin inputs. The various raphe nuclei are all associated with populations of SEROTONIN-containing neurons, labeled as cell groups B1–B9 in the CLASSIFICATION OF DAHLSTRÖM AND FUXE. The various raphe nuclei and serotonin cell groups are as follows: *nucleus raphe pallidus* (B1); *nucleus raphe obscurus* (B2); NUCLEUS RAPHE MAGNUS (B3); MEDIAN RAPHE NUCLEUS (pontine portion) (B5); DORSAL RAPHE NUCLEUS, pontine portion (B6); dorsal raphe nucleus, midbrain portion (B7); median raphe nucleus, midbrain portion (B8). Cell group B4 is in the CENTRAL GREY (the portion in the MEDULLA OBLONGATA) and B9 in the MEDIAL LEMNISCUS; the NUCLEUS RAPHE PONTIS incorporates elements of both B5 and B6. Functionally, the raphe nuclei have been associated with many processes: the dorsal and medial nuclei, and the nucleus raphe magnus (important in pain suppression) have been the most closely investigated. The dorsal and medial raphe nuclei have both been associated with SLEEP (especially SLOW-WAVE SLEEP): lesions in these structures, or local inhibition of serotonin synthesis, produce INSOMNIA. The dorsal raphe also has a role in the regulation of HIPPOCAMPAL THETA, which is prominent during the waking state. In addition, the dorsal raphe has connections with the BASAL GANGLIA: it sends serotonin containing afferents to the SUBSTANTIA NIGRA pars compacta, GLOBUS PALLIDUS and STRIATUM.

rapid eye movement sleep *see* REM sleep

rapid scan voltammetry Electrochemistry technique in which rapid voltage scans (10–15 msec duration) are applied to an ELECTRODE to measure OXIDATION and/or REDUCTION of electroactive compounds.

CHARLES D. BLAHA

rate dependent The term rate dependent describes an important point made by the LYON–ROBBINS HYPOTHESIS: that the baseline rate of responding affects the response to a DRUG (though the hypothesis was formulated with specific regard to the actions of AMPHETAMINE). Thus an action having a high baseline rate of responding can be reduced by amphetamine, but an action with a low baseline rate might be increased by the same dose of the drug. It is an important point, for it emphasizes that behaviour (and psychological processes) affect the response to drugs – that is, drugs do not have fixed and given effects but have effects dependent on the state of the subject receiving them.

rate frequency curve Rewarding ELECTRICAL BRAIN STIMULATION, particularly of the LATERAL HYPOTHALAMUS, produces strong INTRACRANIAL SELF-STIMULATION behaviour. However much the strength of this behaviour attracted early researchers to the field, it is not of great interest today. What is of current interest is the strong rewarding effects that the brain stimulation generates. Unfortunately, measuring these reward effects is not a simple matter. They cannot be directly inferred from behavioural vigour as non-reward factors such as immediacy of stimulation delivery, stimulation-induced motivational or PRIMING effects, and lack of satiation also contribute to behavioural vigour. These effects are generally not seen with natural stimuli. But, even with natural stimuli, reward effects cannot be inferred directly from the behavioural vigour as non-reward factors also contribute (for example consider the effort needed for the OPERANT response, the SCHEDULES OF REINFORCEMENT, the presence of alternative REINFORCEMENT and so on). Many techniques have been invented to allow an inference about stimulus reward strength and many of these techniques involve finding a stimulus threshold of some type. The rate frequency curve is generated by varying over a number of trials the stimulation pulse frequency used to comprise the burst

given as a reinforcement. This leads to corresponding changes in behaviour so that when stimulation pulse frequency (x axis) is plotted against rate of operant behaviour (y axis) a sigmoidal (or lazy S) curve results. In most common usage, the rate frequency curve method takes as its threshold the stimulation pulse frequency required to produce half of the asymptotic maximal behaviour seen at high pulse frequencies. This point is called LOCUS OF RISE (LOR) after the notion that the half-maximal point depicts the location where the curve rises from zero to maximum behavioural levels and it is comparable to the ED50 from a pharmacological DOSE RESPONSE CURVE. Locus of rise has been shown by studies to change when factors effecting reward change (for example stimulation current) but not to change, at least to a first approximation, when lever-throw weight or other motor performance variables are altered. Thus, the locus of rise is said to have been validated as a measure of brain stimulation reward. Motor performance variables typically do change the asymptotic maximal behaviour observed and this statistic is sometimes reported along with locus of rise to indicate the effect of the manipulation (a DRUG OR LESION for example) on operant response capacity independently of any effect on brain stimulation reward.

The number of trials in a rate frequency curve is typically about six or more. Pulse frequencies typically are chosen on a log scale starting at high level (for example, 251 Hz or log 2.4) and dropping systematically (in 0.2 log Hz steps for instance) to a low level (10 Hz or log 1.0). The trials are often short (around 90 sec), and may contain a brief warm-up period (of 30 sec for instance) to allow for the subject to adjust its responding to the new pulse frequency. With seven trials of 90 sec duration and a few seconds between trials, it is possible to get an entire rate frequency curve in 10–15 minutes, depending on the schedule of reinforcement used and whether the schedule is temporarily suspended during stimulation delivery to prevent contamination of the responding by false positive (stimulation-elicited level biting) or false negative (interfering motor effects). With such a fast reward measure and the ability to repeat it without satiation effects altering the estimate, the rate frequency curve is very useful in studying potentially addictive drugs where the time course of action is often 30 minutes to 1 hour. On a technical level, modern researchers often keep the burst duration constant (for example 0.5 sec) so that the number of pulses varies with the pulse frequency. Also, many researchers feel that a short pulse width (such as 0.1 msec) prevents multiple axonal firing and simplifies the interpretation. Higher currents are required with shorter pulse duration, so that at 0.1 msec pulse duration, current ranges of 100–1,000 A are used. No damage is done to tissue and no changes in threshold are observed over many months of testing if the stimulator is designed with a switching network on the output stage to allow current delivered during a pulse to be pushed back by the tissue's natural capacitance between pulses by employing a switching network on the output stage to connect the stimulation electrode to ground.

Finally, a key feature of brain stimulation reward as measured by the rate frequency method is that it is quantitative or psychophysical (see PSYCHOPHYSICS). That is, large effects (of a drug for instance) can be separated from small ones and assigned a number (such as percent stimulation frequency change in locus of rise calculation). This also helps avoid ceiling or cellar effects where a drug or other manipulation might appear to be without effect, but actually would have one if the test were properly conducted. These properties combined with the separation of reward and motor performance factors make the rate frequency method one of the premier methods for assessing reward enhancing or degrading effects of drugs.

JAMES R. STELLAR

rate limiting step The rate limiting step is that step in a series of chemical reactions that is effectively the slowest. If, in order to produce a substance, C, one has to start with a substance A, convert that to another substance, B, and then convert that to C (each conversion being catalysed by a particular ENZYME) the conversion (A to B, B to C) that is effectively the slowest is known as the RATE LIMITING STEP (because the rate of production

of the substance, C, is limited by this step). In chemistry there are *rate laws* which allow for the formal, mathematical, calculation of the comparative rates of production of the various components parts in a series of chemical reactions: the rate limiting step is not simply a conventional term meaning 'slow' but a component in a process that can be empirically determined.

ratio run *see* schedules of reinforcement

ratio schedule *see* schedules of reinforcement

rats Rats are rodents – that is, members of the order *Rodentia* (see TAXONOMY). Rodents are further classified into the suborder *Simplicidentata* (with one pair of incisor teeth), these then being divided into three infraorders: the *Sciuromorpha* (beavers, chipmunks, woodchucks and others); *Myomorpha* (including the genera *Mus*, mice, and *Rattus*, rats); and *hystricomorpha* (guinea pigs, porcupines, capybaras and other large South American rodents). Rabbits and hares are classified separately into the order *Lagomorpha duplicidentata* (having an extra pair of upper incisors). Rodents are by far the largest order of the class Mammalia, accounting for an estimated 40% or so of all mammals, with rats accounting for over 60% of these. Rodents are classified together by various features, by far the most prominent of which is their dentition. (The name rodent derives from Latin, *rodere*: to gnaw.) Rodents possess large incisors at the front of the jaw which are edged like chisels: the enamel of the incisors is not present to a significant degree at the back of the tooth, which therefore wears away much faster than the front, allowing the enamelled front edge to become sharpened. The incisors also have no roots and grow continually: all rodents must gnaw on hard objects in order to prevent excessive growth of their incisors. Behind the incisor teeth is a gap (rodents have no canine teeth) filled by a hairy pad (that projects in from the cheek). Behind this are the molar teeth; premolars are also absent.

There are various species of rat: *Rattus rattus* (the black rat) and *Rattus norvegicus* (the Norway rat, or common brown rat) are the most common. The name Norwegian rat is something of a misnomer. The brown rat is thought to come originally from Asia, arriving in Great Britain in about 1730, before it reached Norway. Since its arrival in Great Britain, the brown rat has steadily displaced the indigenous black rat, which is now found only in a few parts of the western British Isles, most notably on some of the Western Isles off the coast of Scotland. Sadly, unlike the disappearance of the red squirrel, under pressure from the non-indigenous grey, no one seems to care about the loss of the British native black rat. In the scientific literature, rats are typically identified by their English names: Lister hooded rats have a white body and black hood around their heads. SPRAGUE-DAWLEY and WISTAR RATS are albinos (white fur, red eyes) much used because their genetic constitution is relatively invariant. There are also a variety of rats with specific genetic mutations: for example, there are spontaneously hypertensive rats and rats with movement disorders; ZUCKER RATS are obese.

Rats have become the animal of choice in most behavioural experiments for a variety of reasons: at a mundane level they are inexpensive to purchase and to maintain; they are of a suitable size for housing in large colonies; and they are an appropriate size for behavioural testing. (Mice, in contrast, are so small that behavioural testing equipment requires too great a degree of miniaturization.) More importantly, rats are behaviourally agile and can accomplish a wide variety of tests (in contrast to pigeons, for example, which do little other than flap their wings and peck); and rats have what might be considered a prototypical mammalian brain. They possess all of the major structures of the brain of PRIMATES, including an extensive development of the CEREBRAL CORTEX, unlike birds, reptiles or amphibia. Similarly, their general physiology replicates closely that of the higher orders of the class Mammalia. These features do not make them identical to primates and humans, but they make rats acceptable experimental substitutes. While one would not leap directly to clinical trials in humans after studying only rats, what one learns from studying a rat's brain provides a good approximation of what one can expect to find in a primate or human brain.

See also: animal models; animal welfare

Rattus norvegicus *see* rats

Rattus rattus *see* rats

rauwolscine An alpha-2 noradrenaline receptor ANTAGONIST; see ADRENOCEPTORS.

Raven's progressive matrices These are tests of analytic INTELLIGENCE. They involve presentation of a series complex patterns followed by a blank: subjects are required to select which of several alternatives completes the sequence. Versions are available for children (the coloured progressive matrices), adults (the standard progressive matrices) and more able adults (advanced progressive matrices).

See also: intelligence testing

Raynaud's syndrome A condition (also known as *Raynaud's disease*) in which the small BLOOD vessels at the extremities of the fingers and toes are overly sensitive to low temperatures: the constrict, obstructing blood flow and leading to an absence of sensation (numbness) and TINGLING.

reaching The act of moving the hand (or one digit of the hand) towards a position in space. In PRIMATES, reaching is often referred to as the transport component of the 'reach-to-grasp' movement. Reaching is thought to be relatively independent of the systems which control the precise positioning and movements of the hand which grasps the target (see GRASP). Recent neuropsychological evidence suggests that patients with a different LESION in the PARIETAL CORTEX can have deficits with either the control of the grasping portion of the movement or with the control of the reaching part of the movement.

See also: grip; motor control

DAVID P. CAREY

reacquisition Reacquisition self-evidently refers to a second ACQUISITION of a task or information following an initial LEARNING experience. There is interest in the rate of reacquisition following EXTINCTION of responding – the rate of reacquisition varies as a function of previous learning experiences – and there is interest in the reacquisition of information in patients who have suffered brain damage.

Reference

Parkin A.J., Hunkin N.M. & Squires E.J. (1998) Unlearning John Major: the use of errorless learning in the reacquisition of proper names following herpes simplex encephalitis. *Cognitive Neuropsychology* 15: 361–375.

reaction time The time from the onset of a signal (the imperative signal) to the subject's response, in a detection or identification task. The imperative signal can be presented in any sensory modality and, generally, it is temporally unpredictable to minimize the possibility of the subject anticipating the signal. The response is usually the measured onset of movement, but may be verbal or the onset of muscular activity on an ELECTROMYOGRAM.

In a SIMPLE REACTION TIME task, the response can be selected and prepared in advance of the signal. In the most straightforward case of simple reaction time, there is only one signal and one response and the task is one of signal detection. In a variant of simple reaction time, there are two or more possible signals, corresponding to two or more responses, but prior to each signal a cue is given, positively indicating which signal will be presented. Although this is more accurately referred to as a CUED CHOICE REACTION TIME, it is often regarded as being functionally equivalent to simple reaction time. In the CHOICE REACTION TIME task, there are different signals corresponding to different responses. The signal may or may not be temporally unpredictable but it does change, unpredictably, from trial to trial. The subject must decode the signal and select the appropriate response. It is less important to include temporal unpredictability in the choice reaction time task, as the possibility of anticipatory reactions is reduced: even if the subject knows the exact time of the stimulus, they must still wait for the signal in order to select and initiate the appropriate response. Fastest reaction times are generally obtained with finger lift responses to a compatible (that is, the same finger is used) VIBROTACTILE STIMULUS. Slowest reaction times are obtained when the signal is degraded, the response is incompatible with the stimulus, there are many stimulus and response possibilities or the response is particularly difficult.

Reaction times are used to infer the timing of mental operations. Reaction time is the product of the time for the signal from the stimulated receptor to reach the brain, plus the time taken by each mental operation or manipulation of the information, plus the time for the signal to leave the brain and reach the muscles to effect the response. Hence, reaction time is proportional to the number of mental operations performed in a task and therefore reaction times can been used to infer something of the neural and psychological architecture which underlies cognitive operations. In the mid-nineteenth century, shortly after the demonstration by Hermann von Helmholtz that nerve conduction was not instantaneous but took a finite and measurable length of time, F.C. Donders (1818–1889) applied a SUBTRACTIVE LOGIC to the study of mental operations. He reasoned that by comparing reaction times in tasks which differed in their composition by exclusion of one or more processing stages, one could infer the timing of those processing stages. He developed three tasks, the A, B and C reactions. In the A reaction, a single stimulus is detected and the response is the same on every trial. Thus, the A task is a classic simple reaction time and requires only stimulus detection and not stimulus decoding or response selection. In the B reaction, there are two stimuli each of which is associated with a different response. Thus, the B task is a classic choice reaction time and requires stimulus detection, stimulus decoding and response selection. The C reaction is a GO/NO-GO LEARNING task: there are two stimuli but the subject is required to respond to only one of them so, although stimulus detection and stimulus decoding are required, the response can be selected in advance. According to the subtractive logic, the difference in time between A and C represents the time to decode the stimulus, while the difference in time between B and C represents the time to select the response. This approach has been very influential, although the fundamental assumptions have been challenged, with the most damning criticism being that inserting or deleting stages is likely to influence the timing of the remaining stages or fundamentally to alter the nature of the task. Nevertheless, the principle of comparing reaction times under different circumstances in order to infer the timing of cognitive operations is firmly established and modification of the original approach has strengthened its impact. For example, processing time within a stage can be manipulated by varying the complexity or volume of computation of that stage. In this manner, the timing of the cognitive operations can be estimated without resorting to attempts to delete the entire stage. MENTAL CHRONOMETRY, as the field is called, continues to have a significant impact in cognitive science.

See also: signal detection theory

References

Brown V.J. & Robbins T.W. (1990) The role of the striatum in the mental chronometry of actio: a theoretical review. *Reviews in the Neurosciences* 2:181–213.

VERITY J. BROWN

reactive depression *see* endogenous depression; exogenous depression

reactive disorders Psychological disorders caused by external events (that is, they are disorders that are a reaction to events) rather than disorders caused by a bodily dysfunction. For example, DEPRESSION is often a reactive disorder, triggered by (for instance) bereavement or some other form of personal loss. PARKINSON'S DISEASE, on the other hand, is caused by NEURON loss in the SUBSTANTIA NIGRA (and elsewhere in the BRAIN).

reactive gliosis A process (also known as GLIAL SCARRING) that occurs following injury to the nervous system. Reactive gliosis involves a complex variety of events, occurring over a period of several days, that involves activation of all the major forms of GLIAL CELLS: MICROGLIA take on the PHAGOCYTE function, OLIGODENDROGLIA precursor cells can be activated to repair MYELIN, and ASTROCYTES proliferate to restore normal neural functioning. The glial scar, in its final form, is composed principally of astrocytes that have multiplied in the damaged area. The process of reactive gliosis occurs naturally in response to brain injury, whether that injury is of an accidental nature or a deliberately placed experimental lesion.

The presence of reactive gliosis is an effective indicator of brain injury and so, for example, the location and size of experimental lesions can be effectively mapped by examining, immunohistochemically, GLIAL FIBRILLARY ACIDIC PROTEIN (GFAP) reactivity (which identifies selectively, astrocytes).

References

Fawcett J.W. & Asher R.A. (1999) The glial scar and central nervous system repair. *Brain Research Bulletin* 49: 377–391.

reading Reading is most often of interest within biological psychology when presenting as a problem (see DYSLEXIA). The normal mechanisms by which reading is acquired and maintained are generally of more interest to COGNITIVE PSYCHOLOGY. Models of reading, such as that proposed by Ellis & Young, involve (1) a visual analysis system for the recognition of material (a mechanism for GRAPHEME–PHONEME conversion is also required: auditory analysis has to feature for integration of spoken words); (2) a LEXICON for WORD RECOGNITION; (3) a SEMANTIC analysis system (for recognition of word meaning); (4) a system of SPEECH PRODUCTION.

See also: acquired reading disorder; central reading disorders; developmental reading disorder; language; peripheral reading disorder; reading age; speech perception

Reference

Ellis A.W. & Young A.W. (1996) *Human Cognitive Neuropsychology*, Psychology Press: Hove UK.

reading age Reading age refers to the age at which children normally begin to read. It is not an especially helpful term, except in the negative: children who are failing to read can be contrasted with other, younger, children who have learned to read. A 10-year-old child for example who can only read as well as a 5-year-old can be said to have a reading age of 5. The term READING READINESS is more commonly used to describe the acquisition of skills necessary to begin reading in early childhood.

See also: dyslexia; reading

reading readiness *see* reading age

reafference An alternative term for proprioceptive feedback; see LOCOMOTION; PROPRIOCEPTION.

rearing (i) The raising of offspring; see MATERNAL BEHAVIOUR.

(ii) A motor act frequently engaged in by rats. Rats rear up on their hind legs, with their backs straight, in order to increase their sensory input; a simple form of EXPLORATION. It is often measured (by a simple count) in experiments examining unconditioned behaviour. Rats that are neophobic or showing ANXIETY-like symptoms may show changes in the amount of rearing and other activities (see NEOPHOBIA).

reboxetine *see* selective noradrenaline reuptake inhibitor

recall Two similar MEMORY processes are RECALL, the bringing to mind of information, and RECOGNITION, the identification of items presented to a subject.

See also: free recall; forgetting; long-term memory; short-term memory; on-line, off-line memory; recovered memory; retrieval-induced forgetting; word recognition; working memory

recency *see* short-term memory; serial position effect

recency effect *see* serial position effect

receptive field The area of a receptor surface feeding into a defined nerve cell. For example, the GANGLION CELLS of the RETINA receive inputs from receptors arranged in concentric excitatory and inhibitory regions. Colour-opponent types code colour, non-opponent types are achromatic. Ganglion-cell receptive fields are small and closely packed in the FOVEA and large in the periphery of the retina. Cells in the VISUAL CORTEX have elongated receptive fields and respond to stimuli with a particular orientation, motion or size (spatial frequency). Cells in higher cortical visual areas (see AREAS VI–V5) are even more selective and serve as FEATURE DETECTORS for PATTERN PERCEPTION, MOTION PERCEPTION and COLOUR VISION.

IAN P. HOWARD

receptivity *see* appetitive vs. consummatory phases

receptor An ambiguous term used most often to describe PROTEINS that possess a BINDING SITE for a small molecule or LIGAND. Receptor is also used to describe cells specialized for sensory transduction, such as a PHOTORECEPTOR or ELECTRORECEPTOR. Receptor proteins are usually found in the cell MEMBRANE. The binding site is typically localized on the extracellular side – the outside – of the membrane. Receptor proteins are folded so that they may traverse neuronal membranes a number of times: for example 7-transmembrane domain receptor proteins contain seven separate domains that span the entire width of the membrane. When a ligand binds to the protein, the receptor is activated resulting in a conformational change in the protein which may open a membrane channel (see ION CHANNEL) or initiate ENZYME activity in the same or an adjoining protein. An AGONIST activates receptors, an ANTAGONIST blocks them.

See also: receptor subunits; second messengers

JOHN E. DOWLING

receptor binding A term describing the interaction of a LIGAND and RECEPTOR; in biological psychology, when one discusses receptor binding one is referring to NEUROTRANSMITTERS or a DRUG acting at a receptor BINDING SITE on the MEMBRANE of a NEURON, though there are many other forms of chemical–receptor interaction that can be described (see, for example, STEREOCHEMICAL THEORY OF ODOUR DISCRIMINATION). Receptor binding occurs in a 'lock and key' manner: there are specific receptors to which specific molecules can bind. The stereochemical structure of a MOLECULE (see STEREOCHEMISTRY) will determine whether or not it can bind to a receptor. Note that normally one finds REVERSIBLE BINDING: that is, the receptor and ligand do not form permanent chemical bonds, but only weak ones that can easily be broken. IRREVERSIBLE BINDING, when a ligand forms a more or less permanent bond with a receptor can occur. Binding obeys the LAW OF MASS ACTION and should show a dose–effect relationship (see DOSE EFFECT CURVE).

See also: affinity; allosteric binding; autoradiography; competitive – non-competitive binding; dose response curve

References

Feldman R., Meyer J.S. & Quenzer L.F. (1997) *Principles of Neuropsychopharmacology*, Sinauer Associates: Sunderland MA.

receptor occupancy The proportion of the RECEPTOR population to which a DRUG (or LIGAND) has bound is known by the term RECEPTOR OCCUPANCY. Pharmacologists calculate receptor occupancy using the DISSOCIATION CONSTANT and drug concentration.

receptor potential *see* electrotonic conduction

receptor reserve A drug with a high AFFINITY for its RECEPTOR might need only to a bind to a relatively small proportion of receptors available in a particular piece of tissue in order to achieve a maximal effect. The remaining unoccupied receptors are known as a receptor reserve.

receptor subunits Many receptors for NEUROTRANSMITTERS are composed of individual subunits. For example, NICOTINIC ACETYLCHOLINE RECEPTORS, NMDA RECEPTORS and GABA-A receptors (see GABA RECEPTORS) are all composed of identifiable subunits, often with distinctive BINDING SITES.

receptotopic representation The general principle that neurons within a sensory nucleus (or cortical field) are spatially arrayed according to their RECEPTIVE FIELD locations – that is, according to the portion of the peripheral receptor sheet from which they ultimately derive their input. This results in the generation of MAPS of the CONTRALATERAL body surface in the SOMATOSENSORY CORTEX, and of the contralateral VISUAL FIELD in the VISUAL CORTEX. The afferent pathways to different points within such a representation are relatively independent, which is why focal lesions of a representation may result in equally focal functional deficits.

See also: tonotopic representation

DENNIS P. PHILLIPS

recessive allele An allele of a particular GENE on one CHROMOSOME of an autosomal pair, which will only contribute to the PHENOTYPE of its encoded protein (see PROTEINS) if the allele present on the second chromosome is the same recessive allele.

See also: autosomal chromosome; dominant allele

FIONA M. INGLIS

recessive gene *see* recessive allele

reciprocal altruism *see* altruism; sociobiology

reciprocal inhibition Sherrington (1857–1952) identified RECIPROCAL INNERVATION as a key process in muscle activation: that is, activation of one group of muscles produces inhibition of antagonist muscles (see MUSCLES). The concept of reciprocal inhibition is a neurophysiological extension of this, involving mutual inhibition of two neurons (see NEURON). In psychology, *reciprocal inhibition therapy* is a BEHAVIOUR THERAPY procedure in which an attempt is made to strengthen a response antagonistic to a response that one wants eliminated.

reciprocal innervation *see* reciprocal inhibition

reciprocal interaction model of brain state control *see* dreaming

recognition *see* recall

recombinant DNA A molecule of DNA that is formed by joining separate pieces of DNA. For example, recombinant DNA is used in the engineering of PLASMID vectors in order to deliver a specific GENE to host cells.

FIONA M. INGLIS

recording electrode *see* electrode

recovered memory Recall by an individual of a traumatic event from their past for which they have shown little or no previous awareness. Such memories are typically of childhood sexual or physical abuse and emerge during therapy which the patient has sought for personal problems. Such allegations are a source of anguish for both parties: the accused carers feel tainted by the allegations of their children and the accusers believe their freshly discovered past is being devalued by those who have wronged them. The origin and reliability of such memories are a matter of continuing debate and controversy among experimental psychologists and mental health professionals.

Those who believe all recovered memories to be false see them as IATROGENIC in origin: fabrications, stemming from inappropriate suggestions made by over-zealous or incompetent therapists. They point to the popularity of such books as *The Courage to Heal* which urges its readers to seek reasons for their personal difficulties in a childhood history of sexual abuse : 'If you think you were abused and your life shows the symptoms then you were' (Bass & Davies, 1988, p. 22) The USA-based False Memory Syndrome Foundation claims to represent over 7000 parents who have been wrongly accused of abuse by their children and similar organizations now exist in Britain, Australia and elsewhere. Supporters can point to research which demonstrates the malleability of memory and its vulnerability to repeated suggestion. In one study, students who wrote a contemporaneous note of how they heard of the 'Challenger' space shuttle disaster were asked three years later to recall the circumstances. Only 7% of the sample recalled their original experiences correctly and 25% gave entirely fictitious accounts, in some instances maintaining their belief in these accounts even when confronted with their original notes. In another study, 25% of an adult sample were prepared to believe that they had experienced a fictitious incident as a child, when this was put to them repeatedly in the context of genuine events from their past; in some instances acceptance was accompanied by the recall of spurious detail (Lindsay & Read, 1994). FALSE MEMORY SYNDROME supporters point to the fundamental implausibility of claims of recovered memories from the first two years of life or of alien abduction which they see as proof of the fictitious nature of all such 'memories'.

Those who argue for the fundamental plausibility of the recovered memory concept argue that it is not incompatible with the known mechanisms of MEMORY. Most memory theories recognize the distinction between information which is available and that which is accessible at any time. Memory is context-dependant and requires specific cues to trigger RETRIEVAL of particular memories. It is not necessary to accept the Freudian view of repression to believe that memories of past events might only emerge into consciousness when triggered by the appropriate cue. Such memories would be just as subject to distortion and fabrication as conventional memories but like the latter normally contain a kernel of truth. Supporters of the recovered memory concept point to the ubiquity of the phenomenon in therapy. A working party of the British Psychological Society conducted a survey of its members who were therapists and found that over 20% of the respondents had seen clients who claimed to have recovered memories of child sexual abuse during the last year. One-third had recovered memories of abuse before entering therapy, a finding incompatible with a simple iatrogenic interpretation; nor had they read *The Courage to Heal*. Nearly one-third of the therapists had seen clients who recovered memories of a physical trauma (a car accident; waking up during an operation) underlining the fact that memory recovery was not confined to sexual memories, though in general all memories were of a traumatic nature. Two-thirds believed that false memories were possible but over 90% maintained that the memories recovered by their clients were 'essentially accurate' (British Psychological Society, 1994).

Such findings led the British Psychological Society Working Party to conclude that partial or complete loss of memory was a common consequence of trauma during childhood and that such memories could be recovered after a period of years. The Report went on to acknowledge that the production of false memories by inappropriate therapy was also possible and there was a need for rigorous guidelines to obviate this risk. These conclusions were attacked by false memory syndrome supporters who argued that the figures for recovered memories in therapy merely underlined the inability of even trained therapists to appreciate the vulnerability of their clients to memory distortion (Pendergast, 1996). However, the parallel report of the American Psychological Society's Working Party (1996) reached similar conclusions. Key issues still to be addressed include: establishing a data base of apparently false and genuine recovered memories and examining whether there are neuropsychological correlates linked to the retrieval of true and false memories. The debate continues.

References

American Psychological Association (1996) *Working Group on Investigation of Memories of Childhood Abuse: Final Report*, American Psychological Association: Washington DC.

Bass E. & Davies L. (1988) *The Courage to Heal: A Guide to Woman Survivors of Sexual Abuse*, Harper & Row: New York.

British Psychological Society (1994) *Recovered Memories: The Report of the Working Party of the British Psychological Society*, British Psychological Society: Leicester UK.

Lindsay D.S. & Read J.D. (1994) Psychotherapy and memories of childhood sexual abuse: a cognitive perspective. *Applied Cognitive Psychology* 8: 1–42.

Pendergast M. (1996) *Victims of Memory*, HarperCollins: London.

GRAHAM DAVIES

recovery of function This refers to the observation that following accidental brain damage in humans, or an experimental LESION in animals, cognitive, sensory or motor functions that were initially lost can be recovered, either spontaneously or with specific forms of training. What remains unclear in this is whether recovery of function involves the restoration of function to a damaged area, the transfer of function to a different system (that is, NEURAL PLASTICITY) or the re-learning of a process using entirely different neural systems. It appears to be the case that recovery of function is better if the damage is early rather than late (the KENNARD PRINCIPLE) though this doctrine is less regarded now than it formerly was. It is also clear that recovery from a series of small lesions is more readily achieved than is recovery from one large lesion – the SERIAL LESION EFFECT.

recruitment In neurophysiology this refers to the addition of neurons (see NEURON) FIRING in response to a excitatory stimulus as the duration of stimulation lengthens. In psychology, recruitment refers to the sudden increase in LOUDNESS of an auditory stimulus following an increase in intensity just above the threshold for detection.

rectum *see* digestive system

recurrent inhibition A condition in which the FIRING of a NEURON produces a feedback effect that inhibits its firing.

recurrent neural nets A term for NEURAL NETWORKS having both feed forward and feedback connections.

See also: artificial intelligence; reductionism

red nucleus A prominent nucleus in the RETICULAR FORMATION of the MIDBRAIN. The name derives from its rich blood supply which gives the structure a reddish colour in the human brain; its original Latin name, NUCLEUS RUBER, reflects this. The input to the red nucleus originates from the CEREBELLUM, via the SUPERIOR CEREBELLAR PEDUNCLE, and from the MOTOR CORTEX, via the corticorubral pathway. The red nucleus projects to the SPINAL CORD via the rubrospinal tract, as well as to the cerebellum and BRAINSTEM. These connections place the red nucleus as a relay station interposed in a variety of extrapyramidal pathways involved in motor coordination.

KAZUE SEMBA

reduction A process by which molecules in their oxidized (see OXIDATION) form may gain valence electrons from less electronegative compounds; also as an cathodic (see CATHODE) reaction measured using VOLTAMMETRY.

CHARLES D. BLAHA

reductionism The main claim of reductionism is that the goal of science in the long run is to discover reductive explanations of macro phenomena. Reduction is a relation between scientific theories about some natural phenomenon. The macro-level theory describes the phenomenon in high-level terms, and the micro theory aims to characterize the lower-level constituents and their interactions. A reduction is achieved when the macro phenomenon can be explained in terms of the microstructure and its dynamics. According to logical empiricists, this required that the macro theory be logically deducible from the micro, together with suitable 'bridge laws'. This is generally recognized as inappropriately strong. First, because reductions, like explanations, are usually partial and incomplete; second, because getting the theories to fit explanatorily typically involves conceptual modification to one or the other, or sometimes both. Achieving reductive integration between macro and micro theories does not imply that there is anything wrong or unscientific about the macro level theory, only that it is to be explained in micro terms.

The classical examples of reductive integration with minimal modifications to the theories are two-fold: thermodynamics to statistical mechanics (temperature in a gas is reductively explained as mean kinetic energy of the constituent molecules) and theory of optics to theory of electromagnetic radiation (visible light is explained as an electromagnetic phenomenon). The reduction of macro genetics to molecular biology is incomplete and is a good example of the diachronic aspect of theory integration. That is, the macro and micro level theories co-evolve, each providing constraints and corrections for the other. It is also complicated for many reasons, including the fact that a GENE can be distributed over separate chunks of DNA and a given segment of DNA can be involved in the production of distinct traits. Additionally, traits are the product of many interactions, including epigenetic (see EPIGENESIS) conditions.

In the course of co-evolution of theories, sometimes the conceptual modifications (high and low level) are made. This is easiest to see after a long passage of time and scientific evolution. Thus central concepts in Aristotelian physics, such as natural place and impetus, end up having no role whatever in Newtonian physics. In biology, the notion of 'vital spirit' dropped out of the science as cell biology and molecular biology flourished. These sorts of revisions are often accompanied by revisions in the formulation questions in science. For example, at the onset of Harvey's seventeenth-century investigation of the heart, his question was 'Where are the animal spirits concocted?' After his discovery that the heart was actually a mechanical pump, the original question faded from view, replaced by new questions, such as 'What causes the heart to change beating rates?'

Explanation of psychological phenomena in terms of the underlying neuronal mechanisms is a goal of reductionism in COGNITIVE NEUROSCIENCE. The favoured is the strategy that research should proceed at many levels of brain organization simultaneously. A purely 'bottom-up' or purely 'top-down' research (see TOP DOWN VS. BOTTOM UP PERCEPTUAL/NEURAL PROCESSING) strategy is generally considered unnecessarily restrictive. The interaction between experimental psychology and neuroscience has been enabled good progress on a number of questions, including the nature of MEMORY, ATTENTION, perceptual systems, DRIVE and EMOTION, for example FEAR. Typical aspects of macro–micro co-evolution are already evident. For example, conceptual revision has been required to accommodate the data. Memory turns out not to be a single undifferentiated function, but a complex set of partially dissociable functions. One area of impressive progress has been the phenomenon of WORKING MEMORY for spatial location. Particular neurons that hold spatial information in the absence of a the stimulus have been identified, and computer models suggest how networks of neurons might function to receive, hold and deliver spatial information. Another problem that has begun to yield concerns the REWARD system and how new information can be used to make predictions about future events. In this instance, bumblebee neurobiology has been successfully modelled to explain FORAGING behaviour and the bee's ability to predict which type of flower will be a good source of nectar, as well as remember which individual flowers of that type have been already visited. Models of NEURAL NETWORKS have provided insights into various mechanisms, and are important in suggesting experiments for PSYCHOPHYSICS or NEUROPHYSIOLOGY. RECURRENT NEURAL NETS (having both feed-forward and feedback connections) explore the dynamical properties of nervous systems, and suggest mechanisms for such functions as generating representational sequences, decomposing sequences, storing information in the short term, and using stored information to interpret a degraded stimulus.

Much remains to be discovered, and the co-evolution of neuroscience and psychology is still in the very early stages. Whether a reduction can be achieved, and how much conceptual revision will be needed, will depend on the facts of the case.

See also: dualism; eliminative materialism; folk psychology

References

Bechtel W. & Richardson R. (1993) *Discovering Complexity*, Princeton University Press: Princeton NJ.

Churchland P.S. (1986) *Neurophilosophy*, MIT Press: Cambridge MA.

Wimsatt W. (1976) Reductionism, levels of organization, and the mind–body problem. In *Brain and Consciousness: Scientific and Philosophic Strategies*, ed. G. Globus, G. Maxwell & I. Savodnik, pp. 199–267, Plenum Press: New York.

PATRICIA S. CHURCHLAND

reductive materialism *see* eliminative materialism

redundancy A term used in INFORMATION THEORY to describe the degree to which a message can be reduced without loss of content. It is a term used in analysis of NEURAL CODING and, in a related way, in neuroanatomy. During NEURODEVELOPMENT, many more synapses (see SYNAPSE) are established than will be maintained – SYNAPTIC PRUNING reduces their number. Thus a number of the contacts made initially prove to be redundant.

reduplication The DELUSION that things – people or objects, typically of significance to the person suffering the delusion – have been replaced by exact doubles. A specific form involving close family members is CAPGRAS SYNDROME. Typically, reduplication involves changes in RIGHT HEMISPHERE function. It may occur after a LESION of the right hemisphere and appears also in ALZHEIMER'S DEMENTIA.

reentrant A reentrant pathway or system is one in which a particular structure or region provides input to a second, this one in turn sending a projection to the first. CORTICOSTRIATAL LOOPS incorporate cortical reentrant systems, the CEREBRAL CORTEX supplying input to the STRIATUM, the output of which then is funnelled back to the cortex.

See also: reverberating circuit; topography

reference electrode *see* electrode

reference memory An operationally defined MEMORY process for which responses to specific stimuli are consistent across trials and used to guide choices. This is in contrast to information relevant only during single trials as in a WORKING MEMORY task. The task used most to test reference memory is the RADIAL ARM MAZE, in which some arms are never rewarded, while some are rewarded only the first time they are visited. The reference memory component in the radial arm maze task is the knowledge about those never-rewarded arms. Responses that include only those arms that are known to sometimes contain REWARD are a strategy useful across trials.

HOWARD EICHENBAUM

referred pain Pain that is perceived as being located at a site that is distant from the actual site of injury or disease. It most commonly arises from disorders in the internal organs. It occurs because the brain contains no representation of the internal organs. Sensory fibres from internal organs mingle with those from regions of the body surface to which they are adjacent during embryological development, and terminate on the same relay cells. Thus AFFERENT fibres from the VISCERA can excite cells in the brain's representation of the body surface or SOMATOSENSORY HOMUNCULUS.

See also: gate control theory of pain

KEITH B. J. FRANKLIN

reflectance Where there is boundary between two substances with different optical densities (refractive indices), such as the junction between air and water, a beam of incident light will not be completely transmitted across the interface. A certain proportion of the light will be reflected, the reflectance, and some will be transmitted, the TRANSMITTANCE. There will also be other losses due to scattering and absorption.

DAVID W. HEELEY

reflex A specific movement resulting from a specific sensory input. The exact nature of the response is determined by the sensory AFFERENT fibres that are activated by the sensory stimulus and the connections within the brain or SPINAL CORD that the sensory afferents make with MOTOR NEURONS or INTERNEURONS. In the case of the MONOSYNAPTIC STRETCH REFLEX (also known as the knee jerk or tendon tap reflex) these are direct connections, but in the case of all other reflexes there is at least one central interneuron between input and output.

DOUGLAS D. RASMUSSON

reflex arc In neural terms, the simplest form of behavioural organization. A NEURON carries information from a MUSCLE SPINDLE via the DORSAL HORN to the spinal grey matter (see SPINAL CORD) where it synapses on a spinal efferent neuron which leaves the spinal cord via the VENTRAL ROOT, activating muscle tissue. This forms a MONOSYNAPTIC REFLEX ARC (two neurons with one synapsing on to the other); a DISYNAPTIC REFLEX ARC would involve an interneuron between the sensory neuron and the motor neuron.

See also: reflex; stretch reflex

refractive error Condition where the far point of the eye (that is, the distance that is in focus when ACCOMMODATION is completely relaxed) is not at infinite distance. Refractive error results from a mismatch between the length of the eye, the curvature of the CORNEA and the power of the LENS. In MYOPIA (short sightedness) focusing is limited to close distances, while in HYPEROPIA (long sightedness) the far point is beyond optical infinity and an effort of accommodation is required to focus even on distant objects. In ASTIGMATISM, the cornea of the eye is not a spherical curve but is more sharply curved in one direction, so that vertical and horizontal contours are in focus at a different distances. In each case sharp vision can be restored by corrective spectacles.

OLIVER J. BRADDICK

refractory (from Latin, *refractarius*, stubborn) Refractory refers to resistance. For example, the *refractory period* (or *refractory phase*) is the very short interval following an ACTION POTENTIAL when a NEURON cannot fire again. In the very short term, no firing is possible (the ABSOLUTE REFRACTORY PERIOD) though this

ameliorates with time. The *psychological refractory period* is the interval following stimulation during which reactions to a second stimulus are longer than normal. The term refractory can also be used adjectivally to describe a variety of conditions: during intervals such as the POST-REINFORCEMENT PAUSE an animal could be described as refractory.

See also: post-ejaculatory refractory period

regional cerebral blood flow (rCBF) BLOOD flow varies in different regions of the CENTRAL NERVOUS SYSTEM: the density of blood vessels is not uniform (areas where there are high SYNAPSE concentrations have the greatest vascular innervation) and the amount of blood present depends on the metabolic demands of the local tissue. The fact that blood flow is 'demand driven' and therefore proportionally highest in areas of highest metabolic activity is the basis for many functional neuroimaging techniques: see FUNCTIONAL NEUROIMAGING for further discussion of this.

rehearsal A term common in MEMORY research: it describes the repetition of material during LEARNING and the maintenance of material in SHORT-TERM MEMORY.

See also: articulatory loop; phonological store

Reichardt detector *see* motion perception

reinforcement Reinforcement is a term coined by B.F. Skinner (1904–1990) to refer to the property of a STIMULUS in strengthening an operant response made by an organism. An example of a reinforcer would be a food pellet and an example of an OPERANT behaviour would be lever-pressing by a hungry rat. Reinforcement leads to very predictable behaviour such as the pause after reinforcement on a schedule where a rat is given a reinforcement after a fixed interval (see SCHEDULES OF REINFORCEMENT). If the reinforcement is made available on a variable interval schedule, the response rate is steady. Another example, comes from the resistance to EXTINCTION observed in partial schedules of reinforcement versus continuous reinforcement, where every response triggers a reinforcement. Such observations apply equally well to animals and humans, making reinforcement one of the central concepts of PSYCHOBIOLOGY. Skinner originally intend this bond between behaviour and the reinforcing stimulus to be seen as a reflected in operant behaviour in the same way that the bond between a CONDITIONED STIMULUS and UNCONDITIONED STIMULUS in CLASSICAL CONDITIONING is reflected in the strength of the conditioned stimulus. However, this hope was dashed by the ability of the subjects to learn to display low rates of behaviour to a reinforcer, as in the DIFFERENTIAL REINFORCEMENT OF LOW RATES schedule of reinforcement. In current research, some direct studies of the biological basis of reinforcement processes are made, such as in ELECTRICAL BRAIN STIMULATION or in studies involving the SELF-ADMINISTRATION of a DRUG. Often reinforcement is used as a device to get subjects to behave in desired ways for other studies of motor or sensory or cognitive function. Given that reinforcement can elicit instinctive behaviour directly or relation to conditioned stimuli set up in association (even accidentally) with reinforcement, interpretation of when reinforcement is operating can be difficult. For example, is the rate of food response decrease seen after administration of a drug that blocks DOPAMINE receptors due to a loss of reinforcement strength or a motor impairment? In drug reinforcement, an increase in the dose provided in a self-administration situation typically results in a decrease in response rate as the subject attempts to maintain an optimal blood level. This optimal blood level indicates that two forces are acting to constrain behaviour: one which pushes up responding and is probably the reinforcing effects of the drug, and the second which pushes down responding and is probably the aversive or toxic effects of the drug. While methods exist to measure the reinforcing strength of a drug reward, they must be validated against experimental tests. The mistake in generalizing from food 'self-administration' reinforcement (the larger the reinforcement the more the response until satiety) to drug self-administration is an illustration of face-valid intuition-based conclusions.

JAMES R. STELLAR

reinforcement vs. reward These terms have the same basic meaning in many situations. A STIMULUS (such as food to a hungry animal) that will support operant behaviour (for instance, lever-pressing) when given as an outcome of that behaviour is a reinforcer and thus can be said to provide reinforcement. Food given to a hungry animal would be thought of as a pleasurable or positive hedonic experience and would likely be described as such if the animal were a human. Thus, the concept of PLEASURE and the ANTHROPOMORPHISM it brings becomes part of the connotation of the term 'reward' but not part of the term 'reinforcement'. On the other hand, the agent (for instance aspirin) that terminates a painful event (a HEADACHE for instance) is considered a NEGATIVE REINFORCER and can also be said to provide reinforcement which increases the display of behaviour (in this example, the taking of the aspirin). Typically, one does not apply the term 'reward' here as the subject is in a negative hedonic state (headache) and is returned to normal without crossing over into the positive range.

One place where the term reward has found fairly frequent use is in the field of ELECTRICAL BRAIN STIMULATION (ESB) where rats engage in self-stimulation or what is often referred to as INTRACRANIAL SELF-STIMULATION (ICSS). Here the positive hedonic state connotation applies. Another reason for using the term 'reward' is a political one. The most well-developed study of rewarding stimuli especially in North America was the Skinnerian tradition which was attached to the notion that any anthropomorphism was scientifically incorrect. Because the researchers studying ICSS also were probing the brain and some Skinnerians also independently opposed research on neural mechanisms before a more complete understanding of behaviour was produced, the term 'reward' provided an opportunity to distinguish themselves from the Skinnerian tradition, even though they used many of its operational principles. Finally, the ICSS researchers were biologically inclined and some of them had trained as biologists. Thus they did not feel the sting of the criticism of anthropomorphism which struck hard at the then emerging field of psychology. And at the most practical level, the term 'reward' is shorter and easier to say than 'reinforcement'. In such case, and where broad equivalence is perceived, the shorter term is referred. Even the short CAT scan (COMPUTERIZED AXIAL TOMOGRAPHY) became CT scan.

JAMES R. STELLAR

reinforcer Something that provides REINFORCEMENT is a reinforcer. Thorndike, in 1911, proposed the LAW OF EFFECT, in which a reinforcer was defined as something that an animal would do nothing to avoid, but would often do something to get, or to maintain. This effectively, though rather circularly, defined a POSITIVE REINFORCER. A NEGATIVE REINFORCER can be defined in reverse as something which an animal will act to avoid, or will do things in order not to get or maintain. Clearly, both positive and negative reinforcers can increase behavioural output. Reinforcement is often described in terms of being primary or secondary: a PRIMARY REINFORCER is one that has an intrinsic reinforcing quality. Food and water are typically used in experiments as primary reinforcers (and indeed are often referred to as examples of NATURAL REINFORCERS). Reinforcers are also spoken of as being conditioned or unconditioned: a conditioned reinforcer is something that has acquired reinforcing property through conditioning (see CONDITIONED REINFORCEMENT). An UNCONDITIONED REINFORCER is one that has reinforcing properties of its own: it is a primary or natural reinforcer such as food or water. A secondary reinforcer is something not reinforcing in and of itself, but predictive or symbolic of it. An animal might learn that a switching on a light a given number of times by pressing a lever produces a primary reinforcer. The light would be a secondary reinforcer; tertiary reinforcers (and so on) are also possible. Money can be considered as a secondary reinforcer: it has value only in terms of what it can buy, not in itself. It is worth considering that reinforcement is rarely if ever a standard property of an object or state: for example, a positive reinforcer may very well lose its value following repeated exposure. While one fudge doughnut may be a very potent reinforcer, the fourth or fifth in succession will have lost a considerable amount of its capacity for reinforcement.

See also: appetitive conditioning; conditioning; instrumental conditioning; negative reinforcement; positive reinforcement; stimulus–reinforcer association

reinnervation *see* innervate

Reitan trail-making test *see* Halstead–Reitan test battery

relational and non-relational memory Relational memory is synonymous with CONFIGURAL LEARNING.

See also: memory

relational representation A representation of the relations between stimuli or categories: tests of TRANSITIVE INFERENCE determine whether subjects are capable of relational representations.

relative efficacy *see* efficacy

relative potency A pharmacological concept: relative potency is a ratio describing the effectiveness (comparing EC50 for example) of one DRUG measured against a standard.

relative risk *see* risk

relaxin A hormone secreted from the OVARIES.

See also: endocrine glands; hormones; hormones – classification

release *see* efflux

REM-on, REM-off neurons *see* REM sleep

REM sleep Also known as paradoxical or active sleep, REM (rapid eye movement) sleep is the stage of SLEEP characterized by the activated cortical ELECTROENCEPHALOGRAM (EEG), bursts of saccadic (see SACCADE) EYE MOVEMENTS known as rapid eye movements, and ATONIA or the absence of muscle tone. Minor intermittent twitches also occur in the face and extremities. Autonomic activities are elevated but tend to be irregular. Thus, the blood pressure and heart rate are raised, while respiration is shallower and more irregular, compared to during NON-REM SLEEP. Temperature regulation is lost (poikilothermia), and penile erections occur in males. In cats, spiky waves called PGO WAVES are recorded in the

PONS, LATERAL GENICULATE NUCLEUS of the THALAMUS, and OCCIPITAL LOBE (VISUAL CORTEX). AROUSAL thresholds to external stimuli are raised. DREAMING is also associated with REM sleep, although some dreaming occurs during non-REM sleep. During nocturnal sleep in humans, REM sleep occurs periodically every 90 minutes. Each episode of REM sleep lasts about 20 minutes initially, but its proportion within each cycle increases towards dawn. REM sleep comprises about 20–25% of the total sleeping time in adult humans.

The earliest reports of periodic REM sleep episodes in both humans and cats were made in the 1950s by Aserinski, Kleitman & Dement. These studies put forward the notion that sleep is not a single uniform state but consists of two qualitatively different states. The active EEG pattern suggests an active state of the brain, leading early investigators to coin the terms PARADOXICAL SLEEP and ACTIVE SLEEP. The question that followed was which of the two represented the deeper state, but the answer seemed to be ambiguous as the two types of sleep indeed represent two qualitatively different states. In 1962, Jouvet localized the timing and triggering mechanisms of REM sleep to the lower BRAINSTEM by demonstrating that periodic episodes of atonia, rapid eye movements and PGO waves appear in cats in which all forebrain structures rostral to the pons were removed. A great deal of work followed to delineate the mechanisms for different components of REM sleep. The site important for muscle atonia has been localized to an area of the PONTINE TEGMENTUM ventral to the LOCUS COERULEUS, and it was found that neurons in this area project to the MEDULLARY RETICULAR FORMATION whose descending projection in turn actively inhibits motor neurons during REM sleep. PGO wave generator neurons have been localized to the dorsolateral tegmentum, and their projections to the thalamus were confirmed by ANTIDROMIC ACTIVATION.

These neurophysiological data led scientists to propose various models of REM sleep generation. A reciprocal interaction model was proposed by Hobson & McCarley in the 1970s. According to this model, the cyclic occurrence of REM sleep is regulated by the interaction of so-called REM-OFF AND REM-ON NEURONS. MONOAMINERGIC neurons are thought to represent REM-off neurons, and to have a permissive role for REM sleep induction by disinhibiting REM-on neurons as they become silent towards the onset of REM sleep. The identity of REM-on neurons was thought to be GIGANTOCELLULAR tegmental neurons initially, but they have since been replaced by CHOLINERGIC neurons in the MESOPONTINE TEGMENTUM. These neurons are thought to be responsible for REM sleep induction by releasing ACETYLCHOLINE in the area of PONTINE RETICULAR FORMATION near the site for atonia. Injections of the drug CARBACHOL, which mimics the action of acetylcholine, into this pontine site induce a REM-sleep-like state in animals. Thus, REM sleep induction appears to involve the interaction of cholinergic and monoaminergic neurons. However, mechanisms for the cyclic occurrence as well as the abrupt cessation of REM sleep remain unknown.

The function of REM sleep is a matter of speculation. Selective deprivation of REM sleep induces irritability, ANXIETY and the lack of concentration in humans, and the cessation of REM sleep deprivations is followed by a 'rebound' of REM sleep, suggesting that there is a biological need for REM sleep. Phylogenetically, REM sleep is a relatively recent phenomenon and appears to be restricted to mammals. Of all the mammalian species studied so far, placental and marsupial species show REM sleep, as well as two monotremes, echidna and platypus, whereas no convincing evidence for REM sleep exists in sub-mammalian species. Developmentally, the total amount of REM sleep is much greater in newborn babies than in adults. It reaches adult levels by adolescence, and remains about the same throughout life although the total sleep time gradually decreases with age. The high proportion of REM sleep time in immature organisms is taken to suggest that REM sleep is important in stimulating the developing brain when environmental stimuli are minimal. The occurrence of dreaming during REM sleep in humans has suggested to some authors that the brain needs to be activated periodically to maintain its HOMEOSTASIS even during sleep.

See also: narcolepsy

References

Steriade M. & McCarley R.W. (1990) *Brainstem Control of Wakefulness and Sleep*, Plenum Press: New York.

KAZUE SEMBA

REM sleep behaviour disorder *see* REM without atonia

REM without atonia One of the principal features of REM SLEEP is ATONIA – loss of muscle tone. As such, DREAMING during REM sleep is not accompanied by movement despite much activity within brain MOTOR SYSTEMS. The complex actions that occur while dreaming may therefore be acted out which, given that the individual is asleep, can be rather dangerous. REM without atonia is in effect the opposite of CATAPLEXY: cataplexy is the inappropriate presence of atonia during the waking state. REM without atonia is the absence of atonia during REM sleep.

remyelination The restoration of MYELIN following loss; see DEMYELINATION.

renal Relating to the kidneys or kidney function.

renin *see* angiotensin; osmoregulation

Renshaw cells Renshaw cells are inhibitory INTERNEURONS found in the VENTRAL HORN of the SPINAL CORD. They have excitatory input from the MOTOR NEURONS and form synapses (see SYNAPSE) with these (suppressing the actions of neurons that have just signalled to them) and with adjacent motor neurons, suppressing their activity also.

See also: ventral root

repetition blindness A reduced sensitivity to the second occurrence of a visual stimulus (for example a letter or word) compared to the sensitivity to a non-repeated stimulus occurring at a comparable place and time. Repetition blindness is most readily demonstrated in *rapid serial visual presentation* tasks where successive stimuli are presented in a single location at a relatively high rate (8 Hz for example). Repetition blindness may result from the inability of the VISUAL SYSTEM to individuate two identical items occurring so close to each other in space and time.

Reference

Kanwisher N. (1987) Repetition blindness: Type recognition without token individuation. *Cognition* 27: 117–143.

JEREMY M. WOLFE

replacement therapy General term for any treatment that attempts to replace something that is missing: L-DOPA is given to patients with PARKINSON'S DISEASE in an attempt to restore levels of the neurotransmitter DOPAMINE. Attempts have been made to give drugs to patients with ALZHEIMER'S DEMENTIA in order to restore levels of the neurotransmitter ACETYLCHOLINE. The latter attempts have been less successful than those using L-DOPA in Parkinsonism.

reporter gene A foreign GENE, which is used to signal the insertion, for experimental purposes, of a piece of DNA into a cell. The presence of reporter genes may be detected by purification of cellular DNA and separation by GEL ELECTROPHORESIS, or in some cases, by assay for function of its encoded protein.

See also: gene knockout; gene transfer in the CNS; viral vector

FIONA M. INGLIS

representation *see* metarepresentation

reproduction The process by which an individual is created from the GAMETES of one or more parents. Reproductive behaviours are those which aid in this process, from SEXUAL BEHAVIOUR to parental behaviour (see MATERNAL BEHAVIOUR). Reproductive NEUROENDOCRINOLOGY refers to the ENDOCRINE and neural processes that foster sperm and egg development and release, fertilization, PREGNANCY, PARTURITION, and LACTATION. Reproductive strategies refer to both the type of reproduction that occurs and the behaviours that make it so.

Types of reproduction differ in different species and span the genetic gamut from cloning in unisexual (parthenogenetic) species to recombination in bisexual (gonochoristic or hermaphroditic) species. Perhaps the oldest form of reproduction occurs in bacteria. Bacteria are

ASEXUAL and can CLONE themselves by simple CELL DIVISION. However, bacterial growth and survival are hastened if one bacterium can exchange genetic material with another. This occurs essentially by infection. Some bacteria are considered 'male' and contain genetic sequences in a circular chromosome that is transmitted through a long protein tube to another bacterium by means of a 'conjugation bridge' of cell membrane that connects the two. The tube pokes through the bridge into the 'female' bacterium and the chromosome is ejected, much like viral DNA is ejected into a host cell (see VIRUS). This process can be interrupted at any time, meaning that the daughter cells of the other bacterium will not necessarily be recombinations of the complete male sequence. This assures a rudimentary level of genetic diversity.

Some species, such as nematode worms or certain whiptail lizards, are unisexual 'females' who clone themselves through a process of self-fertilization. Interestingly, such self-fertilization requires 'male' copulatory stimulation from another female, which is hormonally mediated and induced by chemical or pheromonal signals (see PHEROMONES) emitted by the soon-to-be mother. Still other species, like freshwater snails and earthworms, are both hermaphroditic and bisexual, possessing the internal and external genitalia of both sexes. Although capable of self-fertilization, snails will often copulate in social circumstances. The 'male' will climb on the back of the 'female' and insert 'his' intromissive organ into 'her' vagina, after which he ejaculates. Thus, sperm from both the host and donor can compete for access to the egg. Sometimes snails mate in groups, each one behaving as both female and male at the same time. Earthworms mate in pairs and exchange both sperm and eggs through their intromissive organs. Some species of fish are hermaphroditic (for example Mediterranean serranids) and can fertilize their own eggs. Still others (labrids for instance) are functional males when young but develop functional ovaries as they mature into adulthood. These reproductive strategies challenge ideas about gender, sex role, and sex-typical sexual behaviour, or about the notion that sexual behaviour serves only reproduction.

Finally, bisexual species (in which there are 'true' males with sperm and 'true' females with eggs) can recombine their genes following internal fertilization from another individual's sperm (for example in humans and other mammals) or eggs (for example seahorses, in which males become gestational after females release eggs into the males' sperm pouches). Eggs may also be released and fertilized externally (in many species of fish for instance).

In mammals, ovulatory cycles follow three distinct patterns. In Type 1 cycles, both ovulation and PSEUDOPREGNANCY are spontaneous, with the length of the cycle being either medium (as in female great apes and humans) or long (as in canines). For these females, sexual behaviour can be either constrained to a periovulatory period (as in some rodents and guinea pigs) or not constrained (as in humans). In Type 2 cycles, ovulation occurs only following requisite copulatory stimulation (typically vaginocervical stimulation from the penis), however pseudopregnancy is spontaneous. As with Type 1 females, some cycles are of moderate duration (for example in rabbits) whereas others are of long duration (for example in ferrets). In Type 3 cycles, ovulation is spontaneous but pseudopregnancy requires prolactin release that is induced by copulatory stimulation (in rats and hamsters for instance). The process of pregnancy and subsequent parental behaviour also differs greatly in different species. Mammals maintain the fertilized egg and FOETUS within a UTERUS for the duration of pregnancy. Other species, like birds, enclose the egg within a hard shell and deposit it after copulation into a nest, where it will be incubated until the offspring hatch. Still others, like some species of fish, deposit eggs with a SEMIPERMEABLE MEMBRANE into the water or patches of mud for subsequent external fertilization.

Reproduction occurs in cycles. Some bisexual species, like rats or humans, can reproduce any time an egg is secreted, whereas for others, like dogs and some birds, ovulation and reproduction occur during breeding seasons. Still others, like prairie voles, do not ovulate until they are exposed to pheromones from male conspecifics. Different reproductive cycles, like the vast array of reproductive strategies, evolved to increase reproductive success within particular, species-specific ecological constraints.

See also: estrus; gender; menstrual cycle; sexual behaviour; sexual differentiation; sexual dimorphism

JAMES G. PFAUS

reproductive interference *see* interference

Rescorla–Wagner theory The central concept of the Rescorla–Wagner theory is that stimuli which are surprising are the subject of more intense LEARNING than those stimuli which are expected and therefore less surprising. This theory had its origins in KAMIN'S EFFECT or blocking effect but has intuitive appeal as surprising events generally signal that something important is happening and learning should occur if the organism is to better be able to cope effectively with such stimuli in the future (obviously an adaptive consideration in evolutionary thinking). In CLASSICAL CONDITIONING, the UNCONDITIONED STIMULUS (US) is a surprise when it is first presented and the occurrence of a CONDITIONED STIMULUS (CS) will help reduce future surprise if it predicts the US and if the animal learns this relationship. In this model, learning continues until the CS no longer reduces the surprise produced by the US. The Rescorla–Wagner theory is also a mathematical model that makes precise predictions.

Reference

Rescorla R.A & Wagner A.R. (1972) A theory of Pavlovian conditioning: variations in the effectiveness of reinforcement and non-reinforcement. In *Classical Conditioning: Current Research and Theory*, ed. Black A.H. & Prokasy W.F., pp.64–99, Appleton-Century-Crofts: New York.

JAMES R. STELLAR

resection (rom Latin, *resecare*: to cut off) Resection, in surgery, describes a process of cutting away; to resect is to cut away.

reserpine One of the ALKALOIDS and a potent inhibitor of CATECHOLAMINE storage within SYNAPTIC VESICLES, reserpine is derived from *Rauwolfia serpentina* (snake root). It has a hypotensive effect (it induces HYPOTENSION –

lowers blood pressure) and is a potent SEDATIVE. It binds to the VESICULAR TRANSPORTERS for DOPAMINE, NORADRENALINE and SEROTONIN, thereby blocking the accumulation of these transmitters for RELEASE. Following administration of reserpine there is an initial release of transmitter followed by profound depletion which can last for several days. It has been used to mimic, transiently, the symptoms of PARKINSON'S DISEASE in animals (since this disease involves loss of dopamine) and has been used as a pharmacological tool with which to investigate mechanisms of MONOAMINE transmitter synthesis and release.

residual symptoms *see* prodromal symptoms

resolution acuity *see* Snellen letters

respiration Respiration is used to mean two things: (i) it is used as a synonym for breathing (see BREATHING, NEURAL CONTROL OF); (ii) more fundamentally, it is an OXYGEN-dependent process in the CELL that involves three elements: GLYCOLYSIS (which takes place in CYTOSOL and produces two molecules of PYRUVATE for every one of glucose); the Krebs cycle (which takes place in MITOCHONDRIA: one molecule of pyruvate is decomposed to CARBON DIOXIDE). Each of these processes, glycolysis and the Krebs cycle, also produces ADENOSINE TRIPHOSPHATE (ATP), but most of this is produced by a third process, the ELECTRON transport chain, which takes electrons generated in glycolysis and the Krebs cycle, and uses chemical energy from this to engage in oxidative phosphorylation, which generates ATP. Cellular respiration is a phenomenally complex process.

References

Campbell N.A., Reece J.B. & Mitchell L.G. (1999) *Biology*, 5th edn, Addison-Wesley: Menlo Park CA.

respondent conditioning *see* conditioning

response The term response was once thought of as being a defined action – that is, a specific set of movements of MUSCLES. Such a strict definition is not now regarded as the most appropriate. Instead, a response is taken to be a set of actions elicited by a STIMULUS (or stimuli) which have the same effect on the effect on the internal or external environment. In a LEARNING experiment involving an OPERANT CHAMBER for example, what is important is that a lever is pressed and that this delivers a certain reinforcer. Precisely how the lever is pressed – which muscles the animal uses – though interesting, is not the main point at issue.

The term response is combined with many other terms (see for example CONDITIONED RESPONSE, DELAYED RESPONSE, STIMULUS–RESPONSE ASSOCIATION, RESPONSE GENERALIZATION, RESPONSE TOPOGRAPHY, and so on). The following terms are also encountered: *response amplitude* (or *response intensity*) is a measure of response strength (the duration of lever pressing or amount of bodily secretion for example); *response class* refers to a group of responses that all have the same effect; *response probability* refers to the likelihood of a response at a given point in a learning experiment (and is an index of response strength); *response rate* refers to the frequency with which responses are emitted; *response set* is a measure of readiness to respond to particular stimuli with particular responses (see MOTOR READINESS); *response strength* (or *response magnitude*) refers to the strength of a response, measured in some appropriate manner; and *response time* is a synonym for reaction time.

See also: emulation

response competition Response competition is a term that has been used to refer to two related processes: (i) the suppression of one action by the presence of another; (ii) the competition that occurs within the CENTRAL NERVOUS SYSTEM between different potential behavioural outputs for control of the machinery of action selection: in many instances, different responses could be selected but only one ever can be. How responses selection is achieved remains uncertain; see for example, SUPERVISORY ATTENTIONAL SYSTEM for a theoretical account of this.

See also: cognitive inhibition

response cost method A method of training in which NEGATIVE REINFORCEMENT is used: subjects lose something they value (such as a small amount of money) whenever some de-

fined, unwanted, behaviour occurs. It has been used as a method to eliminate undesirable actions in individuals with behavioural disorders.

See also: cognitive overlearning; errorless learning

Reference

Alderman N. & Ward A. (1991) Behavioural treatment of the dysexecutive syndrome: reduction of repetitive speech using response cost and cognitive overlearning. *Neuropsychological Rehabilitation* 1: 65–80.

response equivalence *see* equivalence

response generalization The ability to make different responses in order to achieve the same goal, a phenomenon most commonly seen when the original response is prevented.

See also: equivalence; stimulus generalization

response learning The learning of a specific RESPONSE to solve a problem or execute a task, as opposed to learning a more general theory and using that to guide responding in an at least potentially more flexible manner.

response topography The term response topography is typically encountered in OPERANT studies: it relates to the precise way in which a response is to be made. At one level, subjects may be required to emit different types of response; see NOSE POKE VS. LEVER PRESS for example. Alternatively, a requirement might be made for delivering the same response but in different ways: pressing a lever firmly or weakly for example.

rest–activity cycle A rhythm of alternating activity and inactivity (including SLEEP). Activity includes functions ranging from photosynthesis in plants, to nutrient intake, REPRODUCTION, and LOCOMOTION in animals. Such cycles have a 24-hour periodicity, generated by an internal BIOLOGICAL CLOCK or circadian oscillator. Because organisms are adapted to the different ecologies of day and night, such cycles ensure that ENERGY is expended at times most likely to yield benefits, while the rest phase conserves energy and restricts potentially dangerous activities. A higher-frequency basic REST–ACTIVITY CYCLE has been described in humans with a period of approximately 90 minutes, which may be continuous with the REM SLEEP – NON-REM SLEEP cycle.

BENJAMIN RUSAK

restiform body Alternative name for the INFERIOR CEREBELLAR PEDUNCLE; see CEREBELLUM – ANATOMICAL ORGANIZATION.

resting potential This is the same thing as the membrane potential; see MEMBRANE POTENTIAL.

resting tremor *see* tremor

restless leg syndrome *see* nocturnal myoclonus

restrained and unrestrained eating Terms applied to describe patterns of eating below (restrained) or at (unrestrained) a typical or desired amount. Theories of restraint arose from investigations of overeating in OBESITY. However, restrained eating occurs across weight categories and may be characterized as an eating pattern which varies between restriction and excess. The boundary model of eating regulation proposed by Peter Herman and Janet Polivy (1984) suggested that dieters (scoring high on the HERMAN & POLIVY RESTRAINT SCALE) who chronically restrict their food intake impose a cognitive limit on eating. The purpose of the diet boundary is to control eating in order to achieve weight loss or for weight loss maintenance. However, periodically this limit is crossed and the dieter may lose control and overeat. This model was forwarded to explain COUNTER-REGULATION. Thus when dieters are given a pre-load of food, they eat more than dieters given no pre-load. The pre-load serves to break the diet limit and results in overeating compared to consuming no pre-load. A series of studies has since investigated other disinhibitory factors which might result in overeating, such as consumption of ALCOHOL, imagined or believed excess calorie intake, emotional distress and social factors. Recently devised measures of restrained eating (see Gorman & Allison, 1995) isolate attempts to restrict intake from the tendency to abandon restraint, since it is proposed that some dieters fail to show counter-regulation and do not experience periods of overeating (successful dieters). A potential link between restrained eating and the development of EATING DISORDERS has been proposed using a continuity model. Dieting typically predates the onset of eating problems and could precipitate ANOREXIA or BULIMIA NERVOSA in predisposed individuals. Counterregulation has been examined as a possible template for understanding BINGE EATING in bulimia nervosa, but this proposition is controversial.

Significant differences in the eating behaviour of restrained and unrestrained eaters have been found consistently suggesting that the long-term restriction of eating below a normal or desired amount influences appetite regulation. However, it is not yet established what the psychological and physiological consequences of chronic restraint are, nor how any such effects alter eating behaviour.

See also: body weight; feeding

References

Gorman B.S. & Allison D.B. (1995) Measures of restrained eating. In *Handbook of Assessment Methods for Eating Behaviors and Weight-Related Problems*, ed. D.B. Allison, Sage: Thousand Oaks CA.

Herman C.P. & Polivy J. (1984) A boundary model for the regulation of eating. In *Eating and its Disorders*, ed. A.J. Stunkard & E. Stellar, Raven Press: New York.

MARION M. HETHERINGTON

restriction enzymes *see* DNA fingerprinting

retention (from Latin, *re*: back, *tenere*, to hold) To retain something is to hold it back. Water retention refers to the accumulation of fluid within the body. In biological psychology retention most commonly refers to the maintenance of information in MEMORY – to LEARNING and not FORGETTING.

reticular activating system *see* ascending reticular activating system

reticular formation (from Latin, *reticulum*: net) The reticular formation refers to the net-like structure in the central core of the BRAINSTEM. It is composed of nerve cell bodies lying among fascicles of myelinated nerve fibres which course longitudinally, as well as transversely, through the MEDULLA, PONS and MID-

BRAIN. The reticular neurons have long smooth dendrites (see DENDRITE) that radiate out from the cell body and through the passing fibres. They can thus receive input from multiple sources. Neurons in the lateral portion of the reticular formation are medium sized (15–25 m in diameter) and project predominantly to other brainstem sites. They are important for sensorimotor reflexes involving the cranial sensory and motor nerves. Neurons in the medial portion of the reticular formation are large (> 25 μm) or giant (> 50 μm) in size and give rise to bifurcating axons of which one major branch extends to the SPINAL CORD or to the FOREBRAIN. The large and giant reticular neurons concentrated in the caudal pons and medulla give rise to the major reticulo-spinal projections that are important in the control of POSTURE and movement (see LOCOMOTION). Medium and large reticular neurons concentrated in the ORAL PONS and midbrain give rise to the ascending projections which pass to the THALAMUS (and innervate the midline, medial and intralaminar nuclei) along a dorsal pathway, and to the HYPOTHALAMUS and BASAL FOREBRAIN, along a ventral pathway. These neurons comprise the ASCENDING RETICULAR ACTIVATING SYSTEM which via the dorsal relay to the non-specific thalamo-cortical projection system and the ventral relay to the hypothalamo- and basalo-cortical projection systems, stimulate and maintain cortical activation. Through both its descending and ascending components, the reticular formation thus plays a critical role in the generation and maintenance of behavioural and cortical responsiveness and arousal that characterize wakefulness. Particular reticular neurons are also important for the central activation that occurs during the state of REM SLEEP. Extensive lesions of the pontine and mesencephalic reticular formation in animals and humans can result in COMA, in which a loss of responsiveness and cortical activation occurs.

The reticular formation is made up of neurons containing different chemical neurotransmitters. The major population of cells contains the excitatory amino acid GLUTA-MATE. Although pharmacological studies have not yet specifically proven the importance of these glutamatergic neurons in mechanisms of activation, they must be presumed to be the most important component of the ascending reticular activating system. In addition, however, there are collections of cells containing other neurotransmitters. A large group of cells in the PONTOMESENCEPHALIC TEGMENTUM (see PEDUNCULOPONTINE TEGMENTAL NUCLEUS and LATERODORSAL TEGMENTAL NUCLEUS) contain ACETYLCHOLINE and project in parallel with other reticular neurons in this region to the thalamus and less so to the hypothalamus and basal forebrain. These cholinergic cells play an important role in mechanisms of both waking and REM sleep. Clustered in a small nucleus (LOCUS COERULEUS) dorsal to the reticular core in the pons, NORADRENERGIC neurons also serve to enhance wakefulness and cortical activation, although these cells prevent the occurrence of REM sleep. Ventral to the reticular core in the midbrain, DOPAMINERGIC cells (of the VENTRAL TEGMENTAL AREA and SUBSTANTIA NIGRA) play an important role in behavioural arousal and responsiveness of wakefulness. Finally, the inhibitory neurotransmitter GABA is contained in small (< 15 μm) to medium-sized cells that are distributed among the glutamatergic, cholinergic and catecholaminergic cells and give rise predominantly to local projections. These GABAergic neurons would have the capacity to inhibit and thus turn off the excitatory projection neurons of the reticular activating system, which maintain wakefulness. They may thus be important for the onset and maintenance of SLOW-WAVE SLEEP.

BARBARA E. JONES

reticular nucleus of the thalamus *see* thalamic reticular nucleus

reticular theory *see* neuroanatomy

reticulospinal tract A pathway from the RETICULAR FORMATION to the SPINAL CORD: see LOCOMOTION.

retina A thin layer of neural tissue lining the back of the eye. Part of the CENTRAL NERVOUS SYSTEM, it is displaced into the eye during development. The retina contains two types of photoreceptors – RODS which mediate dim light vision, and CONES which are responsible for colour vision – and four major types of neurons – HORIZONTAL, BIPOLAR, amacrine and GANGLION CELLS. One major type of GLIAL CELL (MÜLLER CELL) is present in the retina. The retinal cells are organized into three cellular (nuclear) layers separated by two synaptic (PLEXIFORM) layers. Virtually all of the retinal synapses occur within the two plexiform layers and all visual information crosses at least two synapses, one in the outer plexiform layer, the other in the inner plexiform layer before it leaves the eye via the axons of the ganglion cells. Each PHOTORECEPTOR passes on the visual signal to the second-order horizontal and bipolar cells in the outer plexiform layer, whereas the bipolar cell terminals pass on the visual signal to the third-order amacrine and ganglion cells in the inner plexiform layer.

In the outer plexiform layer, visual information is first separated into on- and off-bipolar cell channels. If on-bipolar cells are blocked pharmacologically, animals cannot see objects brighter than the background whereas they can see objects darker than the background. Furthermore, a spatial type analysis occurs in the outer plexiform layer such that both on- and off-bipolar cells demonstrate an antagonistic centre-surround RECEPTIVE FIELD organization, termed a CONTRAST-SENSITIVE RECEPTIVE FIELD. The centre response reflects direct photoreceptor–bipolar cell synaptic interactions, whereas the antagonistic surround response is mediated via the horizontal cells. Contrast-sensitive receptive fields play an important role in the detection of light-dark borders and can explain the MACH BAND PHENOMENON. In animals with good COLOUR VISION, evidence of the first stages of colour processing is observed in the receptive field properties of the bipolar cells. Centre responses of the bipolar cell receptive fields are maximally responsive to light of one wavelength whereas antagonistic surround responses are maximally responsive to another wavelength. Such a receptive field organization is termed colour opponent.

The inner plexiform layer is concerned more with the temporal aspects of the visual stimulus. Many amacrine cells respond transiently to retinal illumination and are highly responsive to moving stimuli. Many ganglion cell responses reflect primarily outer plexiform layer processing – these cells respond in a sustained fashion to appropriately positioned stimuli on the retina and show a centre-surround receptive field organization. Some of these ganglion cell receptive fields are also colour opponent. Other ganglion cells reflect inner plexiform layer processing – the cells give transient responses to static spots of light projected onto the retina but respond vigorously to moving stimuli. These cells may or may not show a centre surround receptive field organization. Furthermore, some of the movement-sensitive ganglion cells in non-primate species show directional properties. They respond vigorously to spots of light moving in one direction (preferred direction) but are inhibited by light spots moving in the other (null) direction.

Most retinas have one rod type but multiple cone types that absorb light maximally from different regions of the spectrum (for instance red, green or blue). The ability to discriminate colour relates to the light-absorbing properties of the different cone types. Within the outer segment region of the photoreceptor cells are light-sensitive molecules, the visual pigments. Red-sensitive cones contain a visual pigment that absorbs red light maximally, green cones a visual pigment that absorbs green light maximally, and so on. Loss of one or another of the cone types leads to COLOUR BLINDNESS; red blind individuals have no red-sensitive cones; green blind individuals lack green-sensitive cones, etc. Receptors, horizontal and bipolar cells respond to retinal illumination with sustained graded electrical responses – they do not generate action potentials as do amacrine and ganglion cells. These outer retinal cells also generally respond to light with hyperpolarizing (see HYPERPOLARIZATION) electrical potentials, again in contrast to amacrine and ganglion cells which generate both depolarizing (see DEPOLARIZATION) and hyperpolarizing electrical signals.

Photoreceptor and bipolar cells release L-GLUTAMATE at their synapses whereas horizontal and amacrine cells release mainly inhibitory neurotransmitters, namely GABA and GLYCINE. The retina, like other regions of the brain, contains a number of monoamines (see MONOAMINE) and NEUROPEPTIDES. These substances are found mainly in amacrine or amacrine-like cells and are thought to play a role in NEURO-MODULATION in the retina. The role of dopamine is best understood; it has been shown to modify the properties of both chemical and electrical synapses within the retina. Dopamine does this by interacting with receptors linked to the enzyme ADENYLATE CYCLASE, resulting in the synthesis of cyclic AMP. PROTEIN KINASE A (PKA) is ultimately activated and phosphorylation of MEMBRANE CHANNELS at the synapses occurs modifying their properties. This results in a modification of the retinal circuitry appropriate to the light-dark conditions.

See also: visual system

JOHN E. DOWLING

retinal cell layers The RETINA is made up five types of cells organized in five layers. Cell bodies (see CELL BODY) are found in the nuclear layers while complex synaptic interactions (see SYNAPSE) take place in the PLEXI-FORM layers. Information flow occurs between and within the layers. The cells and their layers are arranged as following:

Outer nuclear layer: contains both types of PHOTORECEPTOR (RODS and CONES).
Outer plexiform layer: contains HORIZONTAL CELLS, which spread horizontally through this layer. Horizontal cells communicate with the processes (see PROCESS) of photoreceptors and BIPOLAR CELLS, all of which penetrate this layer.
Inner nuclear layer: contains the cell bodies of bipolar cells and AMACRINE CELLS.
Inner plexiform layer: contains the processes of amacrine cells, bipolar cells and GANGLION CELLS.
Ganglion cell layer: contains ganglion cells, which give rise to the OPTIC NERVE.

See also: Muller cell

Reference

Kandel E.R., Schwartz J.H. & Jessell T.M. (1991) *Principles of Neural Science*, 3rd edn, Appleton & Lange: East Norwalk CT.

retinal disparity The difference between the position of an object as seen by the two eyes. For an object beyond the FIXATION POINT, the position seen by the left eye is further to the left (CROSSED DISPARITY); for one nearer than the fixation point, it is further to the right (UNCROSSED DISPARITY). Thus the extent and direction of the disparity is a sensitive indicator of relative distance. Neurons in VISUAL CORTEX which combine signals from the two eyes respond selectively to particular ranges of disparity and so serve as the basis of STEREO-DEPTH PERCEPTION. Disparity also serves as the control signal for changes that adjust VER-GENCE of the eyes, to enable BINOCULAR fixation on a specified object. Such changes will alter the disparity of objects in the field of view, but leave relative disparity unchanged.

See also: binocular fusion

OLIVER J. BRADDICK

retinal image see image

retinal local signs The theory of LOCAL SIGNS was first advanced in the nineteenth century. At its core is the hypothesis that the visual system preserves information about the exact place of retinal stimulation, and it is on this basis that the visual direction of objects and hence their relative position is perceived.

DAVID W. HEELEY

retinex theory The theory of the RETINEX was devised as a formal statement of the common-place observation of COLOUR CONSTANCY (Land, 1964, 1983). In general, surface colours do not change noticeably when the spectral composition of the illuminating source is altered, even though the change might be significant, such as moving from a room lit by an incandescent light bulb to full daylight. Retinex theory suggests that this constancy might be achieved by a system that compares the light reflected from the test surface in three different wavebands with the similarly band-limited average for the scene as a whole. The three coefficients derived in this way define a point in a 3-dimensional space whose location determines the perceived colour. There is some physiological evidence that neural mechanisms exist in the primate brain that function in a manner suggestive of this otherwise wholly abstract theory, and that species other than man possess forms of colour constancy. Nevertheless, colour constancy is not complete, and the range of conditions over which it might operate is not yet fully understood.

References

Land E.H. (1964) The Retinex. *American Scientist* 52: 247.

—— (1983) Recent advances in retinex theory and some implications for cortical computations – colour vision and the natural image. *Proceedings of the National Academy of Science USA* 80:5163–5169.

DAVID W. HEELEY

retinoblast A developing cell of the RETINA; see BLAST.

retinoblastoma A cell from a TUMOUR found in the RETINA.

retinohypothalamic system A subcortical VISUAL SYSTEM that carries information from the RETINA to the HYPOTHALAMUS. The LATERAL HYPOTHALAMUS receives information from this system, but of more importance is the information that travels from the retina to the SUPRACHIASMATIC NUCLEUS, which is critically involved in CIRCADIAN RHYTHM.

See also: accessory optic system

Reference

Davson H. (1990) *Physiology of the Eye*, 5th edn, Macmillan: London.

retinotectal Retinotectal describes the connections between the RETINA and the SUPERIOR COLLICULUS (which is in the TECTUM of the MIDBRAIN and is also known as the OPTIC TECTUM).

See also: visual system

retinotopic A form of receptotopic organization, in which each NEURON is organized in respect of its input from the RETINA: see LATERAL GENICULATE NUCLEUS for a description of retinotopic organization.

retrieval In biological psychology, as in computer science, retrieval refers to the recovery of information from MEMORY.

See also: on-line, off-line memory; recall; retrieval-induced forgetting

retrieval-induced forgetting Retrieval-induced forgetting refers to the phenomenon whereby information is actively inhibited during RETRIEVAL. The repeated retrieval of information from MEMORY not only facilitates the retrieval of target items but can also produce temporary FORGETTING of related items. As the retrieval CUE is often insufficiently specified, competition is set up between the target item that one wishes to retrieve and other related items of information. This competition is thought to result in the related items being inhibited, thereby making their retrieval less likely and the retrieval of target items more likely.

See also: cognitive inhibition

MALCOLM D. MacLEOD

retroactive interference *see* interference

retrograde From Latin, retro, backward and *gressus*, to go: to go back. RETROGRADE AMNESIA is a failure of memory that exists backwards in time from a defined event; a RETROGRADE TRACER is a tracing agent (see TRACT TRACING) that moves from terminal to cell body.

See also: anterograde

retrograde amnesia The loss of information acquired prior to some catastrophic event resulting in brain damage. Loss of this information is often accompanied by ANTEROGRADE AMNESIA, inability to acquire new information after a LESION. A determinant of the magnitude of retrograde amnesia is the location and size of the lesion within the brain. An interesting and important aspect of this type of MEMORY impairment is that information acquired at time points closer to the onset of AMNESIA have a greater tendency to be lost than material learned long before it, this is called temporally graded retrograde amnesia. The impairment can also be uniform across the time periods.

The observation of temporally graded impairments gave rise to the concept of CONSOLIDATION. Consolidation is a theory describing a process by which information, unstable when initially acquired and stored temporarily, is eventually encoded in a more stable permanent form. Major questions facing neuroscientists concern the processes that occur during memory ENCODING and consolidation: which neuroanatomical structures are involved, and what are the neurobiological, molecular, cellular and circuit properties of these processes? A characteristic of the extent of temporally graded retrograde amnesia is its correlation to the magnitude of the corresponding anterograde amnesia. This correlation can be explained by a description of the proposed mechanism of the consolidation process. When a structure intimately involved in the acquisition of new information is damaged, information learned just prior to the lesion, and any new material to be learned after the lesion, will be incomplete. The magnitude of this disruption will be dependent, in part, on the length of time elapsed between the time of acquisition and lesion, simply because the longer the amount of time, the more information that has been encoded into LONG-TERM MEMORY.

It has been proposed that the HIPPOCAMPAL FORMATION is intimately involved in the ACQUISITION and consolidation of information. It is this structure that interacts with various areas of the NEOCORTEX, to make more permanent newly acquired information. The nature of this interaction is still the subject of much speculation. It is proposed to involve a recurrent activation and interaction between these different regions to produce a lasting representation of the relevant information. Evidence in support of the hippocampus being a primary site of consolidation stems from the most famous patient and subject in the history of the study of learning and memory, H.M. The profound disruption to H.M.'s medial TEMPORAL LOBE and the resultant memory impairment led to intense study of the hippocampal region. H.M. was unable to remember anything within the several years leading up to his surgery. Based on this model, if the area that initially contains that material to be transferred is in some way damaged, there will be an obvious loss in the integrity of those memories. Along the same lines, if the final stage in the information transfer is disrupted, meaning a lesion of the neocortical storage sites, then the information encoded and stored at some prior time will be lost, in spite of the spared ability to acquire new information.

Since H.M., researchers have attempted to come up with animal models of retrograde amnesia based on the lesions suffered by human patients. These models, using rodents and non-human primates, are an effective method for studying the various mechanisms and neuroanatomical structures resulting in this memory impairment. It is through the use of these methods that researchers have gained the insight into brain structures such as the HIPPOCAMPUS as playing an integral role in the consolidation of newly acquired information, as well as it not being a critical long term memory storage site. Animal models allow for much more control of precisely what information is known by the animals, and therefore a more complete and accurate record of the actual information, and the time course of the LEARNING can be made. In animals highly localized lesions can be made in order that specific structures and there roles be evaluated at various time points after certain learning events. This is in contrast to the work with human amnesiac patients. It is in these cases that researchers do not have a way to control for what is learned and when. Attempts at uniformity have been made by using very public information such as television programming and highly publicized political events. This still has not allowed for researchers to account for the high individual variability in the practices of people while growing up.

HOWARD EICHENBAUM

retrograde tracers *see* tract tracers

retrograde transport Movement of a chemical from an AXON TERMINAL to CELL BODY within a NEURON; the opposite is of course ANTEROGRADE TRANSPORT.

retrosplenial The splenium is a part of the CORPUS CALLOSUM that forms a landmark in the brain: the term retrosplenial simply refers to tissue behind the splenium.

retrovirus A complex type of VIRUS that works backwards: retroviruses can make DNA from RNA (see GENE). They are used in experiments involving GENE TRANSFER IN THE CNS. The human immunodeficiency virus (HIV) responsible for acquired immunodeficiency syndrome (AIDS – see AIDS-RELATED DEMEN-TIA) is a retrovirus.

Rett syndrome (Rett's disorder) A developmental disorder affecting only females: DEVELOPMENT proceeds normally for up to 18 months, after which there follows a cascade of increasing impairments. The first to present are motor impairments, including ATAXIA and STEREOTYPY. MICROCEPHALY becomes apparent as the child grows, and MENTAL RETARDATION and DEMENTIA follow. It is a relatively rare condition affecting 1:15 000 infants. The cause is unknown.

return stroke *see* locomotion

reuptake One of the ways in which a NEURON can save energy is by re-accumulating the NEUROTRANSMITTERS (or parts of transmitters) it releases. The neurotransmitter DOPAMINE for example is recaptured whole; ACETYLCHOLINE is broken down in the SYNAPTIC CLEFT, but one of the products of this breakdown, CHOLINE, is taken back up by neuronal terminals. This process – known as REUPTAKE, or more simply as UPTAKE – requires energy and the presence of SODIUM but is nevertheless not as costly as synthesizing molecules *de novo*. There are four points of interest about reuptake processes. (1) Reuptake is often described as being HIGH or LOW AFFINITY. High affinity reuptake processes will collect molecules when they are in a relatively low concentration; low affinity uptake requires molecules to be in higher concentrations to be effective. (2) Reuptake sites can exist at many different sites on neurons, at terminals as well as on axons and at other places, and are found on GLIAL CELLS as well as on neurons. (3) Reuptake is achieved by specialized transporter mechanisms in neuronal membranes (and within neurons, specialized transporters – VESICULAR TRANSPORTERS – exist to capture molecules from the CYTOPLASM and package them into VESICLES). (4) Reuptake mechanisms have functional importance. Experimental and therapeutic drugs can act by blocking reuptake, thereby increasing the concentrations of neurotransmitter within the synaptic cleft. The neurotoxins 6-HYDROXYDOPAMINE, 5,7-DIHYDROXYTRYPTAMINE and AF-64A all act through reuptake processes, using these transport mechanisms to gain entry to specific types of neurons. Once inside a cell they produce toxic metabolites.

reverberating circuit A circuit composed of neurons (see NEURON) incorporating REENTRANT systems that enables FIRING of neurons to continue after the initial stimulus has been discontinued; see SHORT-TERM MEMORY.

reversal learning A training procedure in which, after an animal has learned a discrimination between two stimuli, one reinforced (see REINFORCEMENT) and the other not, this relationship is reversed such that the originally reinforced stimulus is now non-reinforced, and the originally non-reinforced is reinforced. The reversal task takes longer to learn than the original discrimination, as the animal has to overcome the response tendencies acquired in the first phase. However, if a series of reversals is given the animal becomes progressively better at each successive task.

See also: discrimination learning; serial reversal learning

CHARLOTTE BONARDI

reverse engineering Reverse engineering originally referred to the practice in industry of obtaining a rival's product and taking it apart to determine how it operates. It is a term now applied in many settings: any neuroscientific technique in which brains are taken apart (by a LESION for example) in order to find out how they work can be described as reverse engineering.

reverse microdialysis *In vivo* MICRODIALYSIS is typically used to take MOLECULE samples from the EXTRACELLULAR spaces of the CENTRAL NERVOUS SYSTEM. It works by perfusing a fluid through a SEMIPERMEABLE MEMBRANE implanted into brain tissue. The interface between the membrane and brain presents a CONCENTRATION GRADIENT: molecules found in a high concentration in that part of the brain will diffuse across the membrane into fluid that is being perfused through the tubing – that is, molecules will diffuse down a concentration gradient – and the fluid collected can be analysed to reveal its content. But if high concentrations of molecules are added to the perfusing fluid, they will diffuse out of the membrane, into the brain – also going down a concentration gradient. This is the process of reverse dialysis: using microdialysis to bathe an area of tissue with a drug or chemical. It has the advantage over MICROINJECTION of giving temporal control over the stimulus. Microinjected fluid will quite quickly diffuse away from the point of injection, having an effect that dissipates over time. Reverse microdialysis allows a constant level of stimulation to be maintained, or adjusted systematically.

See also: drug administration

reverse tolerance *see* sensitization (drugs)

reversible binding *see* receptor binding

reward Reward is considered by some to be a more informal version of the term REINFORCEMENT. B.F. Skinner (1904–1990) who invented the term reinforcement, cautioned against using terms which had as a connotation or part of their definition a reference to an unobservable process. EMOTION as a central hedonic state is unobservable, although informally most of us feel we can tell when someone else is happy by their facial emotions and other behaviours observed in context. Some people also felt that Skinner was opposed to psychobiological research, something that one of the editors of this Dictionary (JS) has observed by direct conversation to be untrue, at least in Skinner's later years. However, perhaps because of this perceived opposition to psychobiological research into reinforcement processes, some psychobiologists began to use the term reward to separate their interests from those researchers who were following Skinner's interests. Currently, OPERANT psychology is so well integrated into PSYCHOBIOLOGY that the perceived conflict does not exist, yet the term reward persists. If there is any current differentiation between the terms reward and reinforcement in modern usage it is the slight connotation to emotional processes in the reward term.

JAMES R. STELLAR

Rexed's laminae *see* spinal cord

Rey–Osterreith figure Also known as the Rey complex figure: developed by A. Rey & P. Osterreith in 1944, this is a complex line drawing that is shown to subjects. They are asked first to copy it and then, without warning, to reproduce it from MEMORY following its removal. It is a task that has been used to assess many cognitive functions (in for example, memory, planning and organization) types of patients, including those with SPATIAL NEGLECT, SPLIT BRAIN patients and individuals with the DYSEXECUTIVE SYNDROME. The Taylor complex figure fulfils similar functions.

See also: copying and drawing

rhinal sulcus A sulcus on the surface of the TEMPORAL LOBE; it separates the UNCUS from the remainder of the temporal lobe and is valuable in locating the ENTORHINAL CORTEX.

rhinarium An area of hairless SKIN at the tip of the nose; whether it is wet or not is one discriminating feature in the classification of PRIMATES.

rhinencephalon (from Greek, *rhinos*: nose, *enkephalon*: brain) The rhinencephalon is that part of the CENTRAL NERVOUS SYSTEM concerned with OLFACTION. It can be taken to include the OLFACTORY BULB, OLFACTORY TRACT, OLFACTORY TUBERCLE and the OLFACTORY CORTEX, most notably the PYRIFORM CORTEX. Other structures in the OLFACTORY SYSTEM can also be included.

See also: stereochemical theory of odour discrimination

rhodamine A red fluorescent dye; see FLUOROCHROME; TRACT TRACERS.

rhodopsin Rhodopsin is a VISUAL PIGMENT, the one that is contained in the RODS, the photoreceptors that subserve human vision under low light conditions.

DAVID W. HEELEY

rhombencephalon (from Greek, *rhombos*, a magic wheel [now taken to mean an equilateral parallelogram (but not a square) or an oval-shaped object], *enkephalon*: brain) The HINDBRAIN.

rhombomeres *see* neurodevelopment

rhythmic slow activity (RSA) *see* hippocampal theta

ribonucleic acid *see* RNA

ribosomal RNA (rRNA) *see* RNA

ribosomes A ribosome is a structure within a CELL: the site of synthesis of PROTEINS (and PEPTIDES), processes controlled by genes (see GENE; RNA).

Ribot's law The law of regression formulated by Theodule-Armand Ribot (1839–1916) states that new memories are lost before older memories in AMNESIA. This law came from his observations of the progression of memory loss in patients suffering from DEMENTIA. His patients first had difficulties remembering recent events, then ideas and 'intellectual acquisitions', and then began losing older memories. Later emotions could no longer be remembered, and finally automatic daily routines were forgotten.

See also: consolidation

Reference

Ribot, T. (1881) *Maladies de la Mémoire*, Baillière: Paris. (Available as: *The Diseases of Memory*, trans. J. Fitzgerald, Humboldt Library of Popular Science Literature: New York.)

HOWARD EICHENBAUM

right hemisphere Each cerebral HEMISPHERE is almost a mirror images of the other, but in the human brain there is a large degree of LATERALIZATION. The LEFT HEMISPHERE is typically specialized for speech (see SPEECH PERCEPTION; SPEECH PRODUCTION) and LANGUAGE (but despite the left usually being the dominant hemisphere for these, approximately 30% of left-handers and 4% of right-handers show right hemisphere dominance). Other functions such as READING, WRITING, calculation (see ACALCULIA; MATHEMATICS AND THE BRAIN), verbal MEMORY, generating images (see VISUAL SYSTEM), and purposeful skilled movements (see APRAXIA) are typically lateralized to the left hemisphere. Functions usually lateralized to the right hemisphere include SPATIAL COGNITION, music perception (see MUSIC AND THE BRAIN), emotional expression (see EMOTION), non-verbal memory, and FACE PERCEPTION.

right–left confusion *see* left–right confusion

righting reflex A reflex often used to determine the depth of ANAESTHESIA in rodents. Placing a rat on its back produces an immediate righting reflex. This is absent during deep anaesthesia.

rigidity (from Latin, *rigidus*: stiff) This is an everyday term that is used in various scientific contexts. For example, the BASILAR MEMBRANE is often described as being rigid, meaning that it has a certain stiffness that is important to its functions. Rigidity is a term that has been used also in PSYCHIATRY and CLINICAL PSYCHOLOGY to indicate a PERSONALITY type in which resistance to change is a principal feature. However, in biological psychology, the term rigidity encountered alone usually refers to rigidity of the MUSCLES.

Muscular rigidity appears in several forms in different conditions. These include: CATATONIC RIGIDITY: muscular rigidity present in CATATONIA (and see also SCHIZOPHRENIA); CEREBELLAR RIGIDITY: this follows damage to the VERMIS of the CEREBELLUM and is caused by increased tone in the EXTENSOR MUSCLES; CLASP KNIFE RIGIDITY: is rigidity of the extensor muscles at a joint, leading to a rigid, bent, positioning of a limb; COGWHEEL RIGIDITY: is a condition seen in PARKINSON'S DISEASE – movement of a limb has a jerkiness that appears similar to that of moving a toothed cog one space at a time; DECEREBRATE RIGIDITY: is muscular rigidity that appears following TRANSECTION through the brain at very low levels in the NEURAXIS; LEAD PIPE RIGIDITY: is a form of rigidity, sometimes seen in Parkinson's disease, in which it seems possible to gradually bend a patient's limb as if one were bending a soft lead pipe (see also WAXY FLEXIBILITY); and finally, CADAVERIC RIGIDITY – also known as *rigor mortis* – is the stiffening of the muscles that occurs after death, caused by coagulation of muscle PROTEINS.

rigor mortis *see* rigidity

risk Epidemiologists use a variety of statistics when calculating risk. These include: (1) RELATIVE RISK (the incidence of a condition in organisms exposed to particular factors, compared to the incidence in organisms not exposed to those factors); (2) ATTRIBUTABLE RISK, which is calculated as the incidence of a condition in organisms exposed to risk factors multiplied by relative risk minus one. Attributable risk is a valuable statistic for individuals to calculate since it includes information about relative risk (how likely is an organism to contract condition A?) and incidence (how common is condition A?). (3) POPULATION ATTRIBUTABLE RISK is defined as the attributable risk multiplied by the prevalence of exposure to a risk factor in the population under consideration.

Ritalin *see* methylphenidate

ritanserin An ANTAGONIST at the $5HT_{2A}$ receptor; see SEROTONIN RECEPTORS.

ritualization *see* animal communication

RNA (ribonucleic acid) A class of molecules used in translation of genetic information contained in DEOXYRIBONUCLEIC ACID (DNA) into PROTEINS. RNA differs from DNA as follows: RNA is normally single-stranded, it contains a ribose sugar backbone, and the base thymidine is substituted by uracil.

In EUKARYOTE organisms, RNA synthesis, or DNA TRANSCRIPTION, occurs in the NUCLEUS of the CELL, and is initiated by the binding of the enzyme RNA polymerase to a region of DNA called the promoter, upstream from the GENE. During transcription the DNA helix is unwound and RNA polymerase catalyses the addition of complementary ribonucleotides in a FIVE-PRIME–THREE-PRIME ($5'$–$3'$) manner. As the RNA molecule grows the DNA helix re-forms, causing release of the RNA. Several types of RNA are formed by transcription: MESSENGER RNA (mRNA), TRANSFER RNA (tRNA) and RIBOSOMAL RNA (rRNA). mRNA is a copy of a gene which will be translated into protein. Its synthesis is initiated by RNA polymerase II, which transcribes DNA to form a primary transcript of heterogeneous nuclear RNA. This molecule contains regions called EXONS (see EXON/INTRON) which code directly for AMINO ACIDS used in proteins and non-coding regions called INTRONS (see EXON/INTRON), which are removed to form mRNA. The $5'$ end of mRNA is capped with methylated guanine and a poly-adenine tail is added to the $3'$ end. These additions function to protect mRNA from breakdown and facilitate

its transport to the cytoplasm and recognition by the RIBOSOMES. The ribosome is a small structure in the cell cytoplasm which contains proteins and ribosomal RNA (rRNA). rRNA comprises two subunits, transcribed by RNA polymerase I and III. Ribosomes bind mRNA and catalyse translation of its sequence into protein. Each amino acid in a protein is encoded by a specific series of three adjacent NUCLEOTIDES, called a CODON, within mRNA. Translation of each codon into protein involves transfer RNA (tRNA), synthesized by RNA polymerase III. tRNA has a characteristic 'clover-leaf' structure, containing four loops and a stem, caused by the molecule folding and forming covalent bonds between apposing nucleotides. The $3'$ end of tRNA, located in the stem, binds a specific amino acid, while the loop opposite contains the ANTICODON, a complementary sequence to the codon for the amino acid. The anticodon of tRNA binds to the mRNA codon and the amino acid is released from tRNA and attached to a growing polypeptide chain. When a STOP CODON is reached, protein synthesis is terminated and the finished protein released.

Of these molecules, mRNA is short-lived, and its production controlled. The activity of RNA polymerase II is regulated by a large number of proteins called TRANSCRIPTION FACTORS, which recognize promoter and enhancer sites within DNA. Through these mechanisms regulation of mRNA synthesis permits control of gene expression within the cell.

FIONA M. INGLIS

RNA editing Also known as ALTERNATIVE SPLICING; see GENE.

rod monochromacy *see* colour blindness

rodent vs. primate prefrontal cortex There is no consensus regarding the HOMOLOGY between rodent and primate prefrontal cortex. Furthermore, there is considerable confusion over terminology, made more complex by the redrawing of cytoarchitectonic boundaries as chemoarchitectonic information has become available (see CYTOARCHITECTURE; CHEMOARCHITECTURE). Kreig's (1946) numbering system for rat cortex was based on BRODMANN'S AREAS, with presumed homology between rat and primate assumed from location. Zilles (1985) provided a comprehensive cytoarchitectonic mapping of rodent FRONTAL CORTEX, and this terminology was adopted in the atlas of Paxinos & Watson (1986; 2nd edn). However, recent chemoarchitectonic information has changed some of the boundaries as well as some of the labels applied to rodent frontal cortex. Using the terminology of Paxinos & Watson (1997), VENTRAL ORBITAL CORTEX (VO) corresponds to primate ORBITOFRONTAL CORTEX. The most likely homologue of primate DORSOLATERAL PREFRONTAL CORTEX is PRELIMBIC CORTEX (PrL).

Although there is no granular frontal cortex in the rodent brain (see AGRANULAR CORTEX; CORTICAL LAYERS), there are extensive projections from the DORSOMEDIAL NUCLEUS OF THE THALAMUS to rodent frontal cortex and these projections are generally assumed to define PREFRONTAL CORTEX. Nevertheless, in primate, areas other than prefrontal cortex also receive projections from dorsomedial nucleus (for example, ANTERIOR CINGULATE CORTEX). Thus, receipt of dorsomedial nucleus projections cannot be accepted as evidence that an area of rodent cortex is homologous to primate prefrontal cortex as opposed to, for example, CINGULATE CORTEX. An alternative approach to the issue is to compare the function, rather than anatomy, of frontal areas. The evolution of prefrontal cortex in the primate is, presumably, to support a degree of behavioural complexity that might not be found in the rat. However, if the rodent does demonstrate behaviour dependent on functions associated with primate prefrontal cortex, the neural substrate of such behaviour could be regarded as at least analogous, if not homologous, to primate prefrontal cortex.

Rats with a LESION of prelimbic cortex do have impaired WORKING MEMORY, although the deficits are not sufficiently severe or persistent to be considered as incontrovertible evidence that this is equivalent to a lesion of primate dorsolateral prefrontal cortex. In primates, dorsolateral prefrontal cortex has been shown to mediate shifts in attentional set (see ATTENTIONAL SET-SHIFTING). Rats with a lesion of prelimbic cortex are impaired in shifting between response rules, such as match- versus

nonmatch-to-sample, absolute place versus relative position in a maze or during FORAGING using spatial versus visual cues. They are also impaired in perceptual attentional set-shifting, and therefore there is some support for the notion of prefrontal cortex in the rat.

References

Krieg W.J.S. (1946) Connections of the cerebral cortex. I. The albino rat. A. Topography of cortical areas. *Journal of Comparative Neurology* 84: 221–275.

Preuss T.M. (1995) Do rats have prefrontal cortex? The Rose–Woolsey–Akert Program reconsidered. *Journal of Cognitive Neuroscience* 7: 1–24.

Paxinos G. & Watson C. (1986) *The Rat Brain in Stereotaxic Coordinates*, 2nd edn, Academic Press: San Diego.

——(1997) *The Rat Brain in Stereotaxic Coordinates*, compact 3rd edn, Academic Press: San Diego.

Zilles K. (1985) *The Cortex of the Rat: A Stereotaxic Atlas*, Springer-Verlag: Berlin.

VERITY J. BROWN

rodents *see* rat

rods Rod-shaped photoreceptors in the RETINA that are responsible for vision under relatively low (night-time) levels of illumination. The VISUAL PIGMENT of human rods absorbs blue-green light maximally.

See also: cones; spectral sensitivity; visual system

Rolandic fissure *see* central sulcus

rooting reflex If an object touches a human infants cheek it will make a REFLEX turn towards the stimulus. This movement is typically followed by movements preparatory to SUCKLING: the rooting reflex is one that prepares infants to feed.

rostral Forward; at the front. Rostral is contrasted to CAUDAL, at the back. The terms ANTERIOR (front) and POSTERIOR (back) are synonymous with rostral and caudal.

rostral pole *see* nucleus accumbens

rotation A behavioural response, typically in rats or mice, in which the animals turn in head to tail circles. The phenomenon is associated with imbalance in the BASAL GANGLIA, in particular following a unilateral 6-HYDROXY-DOPAMINE LESION of the NIGROSTRIATAL DO-PAMINE SYSTEM. Although suggested in earlier accounts, the phenomenon and its dependence on central dopamine systems was first clearly described in 1970 by Urban Ungerstedt.

As shown in the figure, unilateral nigrostriatal lesions produce a postural bias towards the side IPSILATERAL to the lesion. However, for rotation to become fully manifest, the animals must be activated either by STRESS, or by a pharmacological agent. AMPHETAMINE induces an increase in dopaminergic activation of the striatum on the CONTRALATERAL side, which is translated functionally into a marked ipsilateral rotation. Conversely, the dopamine receptor agonist APOMORPHINE induces rotation in the contralateral direction, even at very low doses below the threshold for behavioural activation in intact animals. In order to explain these initially unexpected results, Ungerstedt proposed that the dopamine receptors are upregulated as a compensatory response to loss

of dopamine inputs. Thus, the hypothesis of receptor SUPERSENSITIVITY was first proposed on the basis of behavioural evidence and has subsequently been confirmed in RECEPTOR BINDING studies.

Rotation is easily automated. In 1970, Ungerstedt & Arbuthnott introduced an apparatus – known as a ROTOMETER – that has been widely adopted. Animals are tested in hemispheric bowls and connected by a harness and tensile wire to a cam-and-pivot switch that transduces turning in quarter, half or full turns in clockwise and anticlockwise directions into incremental counts on an electromechanical or computerized counter. The rate of turning is found to correlate closely with the extent of dopamine loss, so that rotation provides a sensitive and non-invasive behavioural response to monitor the integrity of the underlying nigrostriatal system. As a result of its sensitivity, and the ease of objective and automated recording, rotation has been widely used to evaluate and compare the potency of

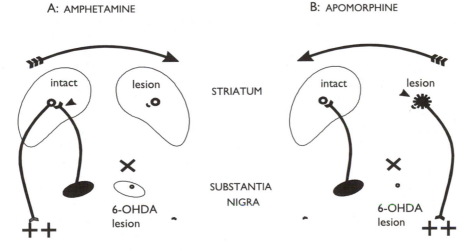

The Ungerstedt rotation model.

Notes In the illustration, the left and right NIGROSTRIATAL DOPAMINE SYSTEMS are viewed from above. A LESION (UNILATERAL) made with 6-HYDROXYDOPAMINE (6-OHDA) in the right SUBSTANTIA NIGRA removes DOPAMINE input from the ipsilateral STRIATUM.

A Spontaneous bias to the right. AMPHETAMINE induces dopamine release in the intact striatum (arrow head) and stimulates IPSILATERAL rotation.

B APOMORPHINE acts post-synaptically at RECEPTORS which have developed SUPERSENSITIVITY in the lesioned striatum (arrow head) to induce CONTRALATERAL rotation. (Based on Ungerstedt and Arbuthnott, 1970)

dopamine agonist and stimulant drugs and of novel gene transfer (see GENE TRANSFER IN THE CNS) and TRANSPLANTATION therapies. Although most research has focused on rodents, related results have also been observed in monkeys and humans. For example, patients with PARKINSON'S DISEASE (which is typically asymmetric in its early manifestation), have been fitted with electronic turning sensors, which shows that they make a predominance of turns towards the more affected side in the course of going about their daily activities.

Although the largest body of research has focused on dopaminergic systems and drugs, more modest levels of rotation can be observed following unilateral lesions and pharmacological activation in other neurotransmitter systems, including the SEROTONIN systems associated with the input from the RAPHE NUCLEI and the GLUTAMATE inputs from the CEREBRAL CORTEX to the STRIATUM, CHOLINERGIC INTERNEURONS in the striatum and output systems of the basal ganglia (see CORTICOSTRIATAL LOOPS for anatomical detail). A limited degree of rotation can also be revealed in intact animals. Although many animals are asymmetric, others show modest rates of turning in the same direction both spontaneously (when tested overnight to collect enough counts) and following injection of amphetamine. Stanley Glick has shown that these asymmetries correlate with imbalance between the two sides in striatal dopamine concentrations. Larger CONDITIONED ROTATION asymmetries can be induced in intact rats by explicit behavioural conditioning. There are also reports that patients with schizophrenia show spontaneous side biases which can be manifested as rotation.

Rotation must be distinguished from BARREL ROLLING, in which the animals make twisting rolls along a longitudinal body axis, and which is due to damage to the VESTIBULAR COMPLEX.

References

Pycock C.J. (1980) Turning behaviour in animals. *Neuroscience* 5: 461–514.

Ungerstedt U. & Arbuthnott G.W. (1970) Quantitative recording of rotational behaviour in rats after 6-hydroxydopamine lesions of the nigrostriatal dopamine system. *Brain Research* 24: 485–493.

STEPHEN B. DUNNETT

rote learning The learning of information by repeated exposure or continual REHEARSAL: rote learning implies that the meaning of what is being learnt is not important – it is the ability to remember and reproduce information that is of significance.

rotometer A device for measuring turning in animals; see ROTATION.

rough endoplasmic reticulum *see* cell

round window *see* cochlea

Roux-en-Y gastric by-pass *see* bariatric surgery

rubrospinal tract A pathway from the RED NUCLEUS to the SPINAL CORD: see LOCOMOTION.

Ruffini's endings *see* skin

rumination (from Latin, *rumen*: the gullet) Ruminants are animals that chew the cud (food brought back from the first stomach in the ruminant animals, which have more than one stomach). Rumination has two meanings: (i) the consumption of food that has been regurgitated, (as is the case, for example, with young birds); and (ii) a process in which individuals persist in contemplation of a particular thought or idea. It is a state that can become pathological and may be a feature of disorders such as DEPRESSION.

running This refers to two things: (i) it is a rapid form of LOCOMOTION in which there are specific changes in stride pattern and GAIT; (ii) in most laboratories conducting behavioural research using animals, people will talk about 'running their rats' (or whatever species they conduct experiments on): running, in colloquial lab-speak, is synonymous with testing.

running wheel A means for measuring LOCOMOTION in animals: they are wheels, typically made of wire grid or plastic (solid plastic is better for a RAT, to avoid getting its tail caught), mounted on an axle and running perpendicular to the floor (as a car wheel does). They can be enclosed, confining an animal, or open, giving access as and when the animal wishes. They have been used in the measurement of TREADMILL LOCOMOTION and in measuring activity over 24-hour cycles in CIRCADIAN RHYTHM research. In general however, spontaneous locomotion is measured in more natural environments.

runway A runway is a simple piece of apparatus: it is a straight alley with a floor and walls along which an animal can run, usually to obtain POSITIVE REINFORCEMENT. The time taken to get from one end to the other is measured and run speed taken as a measure of MOTIVATION – animals run faster, and work harder, for larger rewards.

S

saccade (saccadic) A rapid EYE MOVEMENT which serves to bring a new part of the image onto the FOVEA, and so allows any object of interest to be processed with high ACUITY. They typically occur every 250 msec – 2 sec. Neural signals from the SUPERIOR COLLICULUS, modulated by activity in cortical areas including the FRONTAL EYE FIELDS, act to initiate a saccade. Saccades are BALLISTIC responses whose duration and velocity are fixed for a given size of displacement, and are quite distinct from the smooth PURSUIT EYE MOVEMENTS used to track a moving object.

OLIVER J. BRADDICK

saccadic omission During rapid voluntary eye movements (see SACCADE) there is usually little or no impression of blurring or smearing of the retinal image. This phenomenon is referred to as SACCADIC OMISSION or SACCADIC SUPPRESSION. It has been shown experimentally to be accompanied by large increases in the detection threshold that occur in anticipation to, as well as during, the saccade indicating a central origin of the phenomenon.

DAVID W. HEELEY

saccadic suppression The reduction in visual information transmitted to the brain preceding and during a SACCADE, also known as SACCADIC OMISSION. This results from several different effects: (i) the blurring of all spatial detail by rapid image motion across the RETINA; (ii) masking of visual signals by the barrage of transient neural activity produced by this motion; (iii) a loss of sensitivity, particularly to

motion, induced in the brain by neural signals associated with the generation of a saccade. In addition, large changes in the visual scene that occur during a saccade go unnoticed if they are away from the focus of attention; this CHANGE BLINDNESS is not specific to saccades but reflects the generally short lifetime of the pre-attentive iconic store.

OLIVER J. BRADDICK

saccharin (from Greek, *sakharon*: sugar; also spelt saccharine) Saccharin is well known as an artificial sweetener. In biological psychology, saccharin is used to adulterate food and water in experiments interested in TASTE PERCEPTION (see GUSTATION) and related processes such as FINICKINESS: it has no significant nutritive content, unlike natural SUGARS, which would affect both the taste of a food or fluid and its nutritional content, a potential confound in studies of the effects of taste on intake. Saccharin is colourless and odourless, but has a characteristic sweet taste which, at appropriate concentrations (around 0.5%) causes an elevation in intake of adulterated food and water. The effects of saccharin on taste are typically contrasted with those of QUININE, which is also non-nutritive, but has a bitter taste that (in low concentrations) animals typically find unpleasant.

saccule *see* vestibular system

sacrum (from Latin, *sacrum*: holy) The bone at the base of the spinal column. It is made of five vertebral bones fused together to form one triangular element: it sits at the bottom of the spinal cord, forming a key into the pelvic girdle. Sacral describes this area; there are for example, sacral nerves (see SPINAL CORD).

sagittal section *see* planes of section

salbutamol A non-selective beta NORADRENA-LINE receptor AGONIST (also known as ALBU-TEROL); see ADRENOCEPTORS.

saline *see* isotonic saline

saliva Saliva is a clear fluid, without taste or odour, released from the salivary glands (the *parotid*, *sublingual* and *submaxillary salivary* glands – in the cheek near the ear, by the jaw and under the tongue respectively) in the MOUTH. It functions to keep the mouth moist and to lubricate food, such that it can be swallowed. It is slightly acid and contains some enzymes (such as ptyalin) to begin the process of digestion (see ENZYME; DIGESTIVE SYSTEM). Salivation is one of the CEPHALIC REFLEXES OF DIGESTION, triggered by the sensory character-istics of food. Heightened states of general AROUSAL may also be associated with altera-tions (increases or decreases) in salivation.

salt Salt can refer to a broad chemical class of substances, but is most often used to refer to the substance known as ordinary table salt: sodium chloride (NaCl). Salt has importance for biopsychology in three distinct ways: as a taste, as the target of SODIUM APPETITE, and as the source of sodium (Na^+) and chloride (Cl^-) ions that are crucial to normal physiological function.

Unlike sweet or bitter tastes, the tongue does not need specific receptor molecules in order to recognize substances that trigger the sensation of salty taste (see GUSTATION). Instead sodium salts such as sodium chloride appear able to directly activate taste cells in the tongue. In liquid solution, NaCl dissociates into separate sodium (Na^+) and chloride (Cl^-) ions (see ION). The apical membrane of taste cells contains Na^+ channels, through which Na^+ ions can enter. Na^+ ions appear directly able to trigger the sensation of salt. Evidence for this comes from the effects of a drug, AMILORIDE, which blocks Na^+ channels in cell membranes. When amiloride is applied to the surface of the tongue, it results in a temporary block of the sensation of saltiness produced by sodium

salts. This mechanism appears to be the chief way in which salty taste are recognized by the tongue, though there also appear to be second-ary mechanisms that operate in a different fashion.

The existence of a specific taste and appetite for salt (see SODIUM APPETITE) may be ex-plained by the crucial role ions play in the normal function of neurons and other cells. The generation of a neuronal RESTING POTEN-TIAL, the state in which it lies ready to process information, is maintained by active processes in the neuron that control the flow and concentration of Na^+, Cl^- and other salt ions inside the cell. The generation of an ACTION POTENTIAL, a neuronal signal and unit of information, is produced by a temporary alteration in the control of ion gates and neuron concentration. Without adequate ion supplies, neuronal function is impossible. Thus ingestion of an adequate amount of ion-con-taining salts is critical to health and function.

KENT C. BERRIDGE

salt appetite *see* sodium appetite

saltatory A type of fast electrical transmission along an AXON: see ACTION POTENTIAL.

sapid (from Latin, *sapere*: to taste) A sapid STIMULUS is one that has perceptible taste; see GUSTATION.

saporin A cytotoxic plant LECTIN. After intra-cerebral MICROINJECTION, saporin is taken up by axons and moved by RETROGRADE TRANS-PORT to the cell body, causing cell death. Saporin can CONJUGATE to antibodies that target cell surface molecules to provide a selective IMMUNOTOXIN for making a selective LESION of specific neuronal or glial popula-tions in the brain. Linked to the low-affinity p75 NERVE GROWTH FACTOR receptor or to the NORADRENERGIC enzyme DOPAMINE BETA HY-DROXYLASE it provides an effective and selec-tive toxin for CHOLINERGIC neurons in the BASAL FOREBRAIN (but not elsewhere) and noradrenaline neurons, respectively.

Reference
Wiley R.G. (1992) Neural lesioning with ribo-some-inactivating proteins: suicide transport

and immunolesioning. *Trends in Neuroscience* 15: 285–290.

STEPHEN B. DUNNETT

sarcomere *see* muscles

sarcoplasmic reticulum *see* neuromuscular junction

satiety Satiety and hunger are the opposite sides of the same coin, but satiety is not merely the absence of hunger. Satiety is itself the specific product of a cascade of active processes in the nervous system, which generate the satiety state in response to internal cues provided by food. When a meal is eaten, this cascade of satiety signals to the brain is produced by several levels of detectors that are activated in turn as food is digested. These levels are described in turn.

Stomach (gastric) level. When food enters the stomach, it stretches the walls of the stomach, activating neural receptors for mechanical stretch. These neural receptors send axons to the brain through the sensory VAGUS NERVE (one of the CRANIAL NERVES). Surgeons have attempted to harness this natural satiety cue in the operation GASTRIC STAPLING, which has been performed on some patients as a treatment for OBESITY. Gastric stapling closes off a portion of the stomach from access to food, trapping food in the remaining portion of the stomach until it can pass to the intestine. The filled portion of the stomach becomes highly stretched, since eating a normal meal becomes like trying to stuff a regular pillow into a smaller pillowcase, sending a greater satiety signal to the brain. Unfortunately, repeated overstuffing causes the walls of the stomach to physically expand, and eventually the enhanced stretch signal is lost after the operation. Food in the stomach also activates a second class of neural receptors: the CHEMO-RECEPTOR sites that detect sugars and other nutrients. These also ascend to the brain via the vagus.

Intestinal level. Gastric satiety cues by themselves are relatively weak. Food that does not reach the intestines fails to produce strong satiety even if it fills the stomach (this can be demonstrated in animals through the use of a GASTRIC FISTULA, a surgically implanted tube that allows food to escape after being processed by the stomach). The next level of satiety is stronger, and is produced by nutrient receptors in the small intestines, which receive food from the stomach. Some nutrient detectors in the intestines send their satiety signal to the brain via neural fibres in the vagus nerve, similar to gastric nutrient detectors. Other intestinal detectors use a hormonal route to send their signal to the brain, by releasing HORMONES into the bloodstream which reach the brain by circulation. The first portion of the intestine, for example, is the duodenum. The walls of the duodenum contains cells that secrete CHOLECYSTOKININ (CCK) into the blood when they are stimulated by food. CCK is a hormone that suppresses APPETITE. Injections of CCK cause animals to stop eating. Although high doses of CCK may do this partly because they cause NAUSEA and other unpleasant effects, low doses of CCK that are more similar to the levels that would be naturally secreted after a meal, appear simply to produce normal satiety.

Liver (hepatic) level. Perhaps the most important satiety cues come from the liver, an organ that produces no conscious sensation of its own, but which can markedly influence feelings of hunger and satiety. The liver normally acts as a storage site for nutrients and as a biochemical factory that can change one form of nutrient into another. Since most types of nutrients are processed by the liver, it is in an excellent position to assess the general level of nutrients available to the body. Neural detectors exist in the liver, which can monitor nutrients in the blood stream that passes from the intestines. Signals can be sent from the liver to the brain via the hepatic branch of the vagus nerve. The power of hepatic signals to influence satiety has been demonstrated by experiments in which small amounts of nutrients have been injected directly into the artery that provides blood to the liver. Although only the liver received any appreciable nutrients, the satiety signal produced was sufficient to prevent a hungry animal from eating, fooling the brain into a false state of satiety. The suppression of eating by hepatic satiety signals was eliminated if the hepatic branch of the vagus nerve had been surgically transected, which showed that the satiety signal travelled to the brain via the vagus.

Systemic long-term satiety level. BODY WEIGHT, which can be manipulated by sustained periods of dieting or overeating, can also influence feelings of satiety. Most changes in body weight are produced by reduction or growth of FAT CELLS, since fat is a chief form of long-term nutrient storage. The way by which fat stores could produce signals that would reach the brain has been difficult to understand, since there are no known neural connections to fat deposit sites and no known hormone produced by fat. However, the discovery that fat cells secrete a substance, LEPTIN, into the blood has provided the possible missing signal. Leptin can be detected by the brain, and appears to suppress eating. Higher levels of leptin are secreted when fat levels are high. Thus leptin may be a chemical signal that tells the brain about long-term nutrient storage levels, and allows body weight to contribute to the set of physiological cues that produce satiety.

See also: restrained and unrestrained eating

KENT C. BERRIDGE

saturation analysis Also known as EQUILIBRIUM ANALYSIS, this is a technique used in pharmacology to asses the degree of binding of a LIGAND to a RECEPTOR.

saxitoxin An agent that blocks activity of ion channels (see ION CHANNEL) sensitive to SODIUM (Na^+) (sodium channels) without affecting any other ion channels. Like the better-known TETRODOTOXIN it has been of great value as a neuroscientific tool, and is also a fatal paralysing agent. It is found in marine microorganisms (that accumulate to form the 'red tide', so-called because of the colouration) and can accumulate in shellfish. If not properly cooked, such contaminated shellfish can be fatal.

See also: tetraethylammonium

SB224289 An ANTAGONIST at the $5HT_{1B}$ receptors; see SEROTONIN RECEPTORS.

scala media *see* cochlea

scala tympani *see* cochlea

scala vestibuli *see* cochlea

scalp electrodes *see* electroencephalogram; electrode

Scarpa's ganglion The vestibular GANGLION; see VESTIBULAR COMPLEX; VESTIBULAR SYSTEM.

Scatchard analysis An technique used in pharmacology to assess the binding to the RECEPTOR of a DRUG that has been radiolabelled, graphically represented as a *Scatchard plot* in which the amount of bound RADIOLIGAND is plotted against bound radioligand/free radioligand). It is a method of analysis that has been replaced by more direct computer modelling procedures.

scatter hoarding The hoarding of food in widely dispersed caches.

See also: food-storing birds; hoarding behaviour

scattered light *see* straylight

Schaffer collaterals *see* hippocampus

schedule-induced polydipsia Also known as ADJUNCTIVE BEHAVIOUR (or more specifically, adjunctive drinking), this is excessive DRINKING induced by a particular SCHEDULE OF REINFORCEMENT. Hungry animals are placed in an OPERANT CHAMBER where they receive a small food pellet (typically 45 mg for a rat) on a fixed interval schedule (usually one food pellet every 60 sec). What emerges is a pattern of activity that can be divided into three phases: immediately after food presentation and consumption, *adjunctive behaviours* (such as drinking) appear, followed by what are termed *facultative behaviours* (motor activities for example – LOCOMOTION or GROOMING) and finally *terminal behaviour*, when the animals' activity is again directed toward the site at which food will be received. All of these phases are necessarily brief, but over 60 minutes, a considerable volume of fluid will be drunk – the amount should be compared to that consumed if an animal is simply presented with 60 food pellets all at once (rather than one a minute for an hour) and allowed to eat and drink as it wishes. Schedule-induced polydipsia is thought of as a laboratory analogue of DISPLACEMENT ACTIVITIES. Psychological explanations have suggested that heightened ACTIVATION might account for it: animals are motivated to eat, but the amount of food presented is insufficient at that moment to satisfy it. The thwarting of behaviour, it is argued, produces a displacement to other salient activities. The neural substrates of schedule induced polydipsia are unclear: CERE-BRAL CORTEX, STRIATUM, HIPPOCAMPUS, AMYGDALA and HYPOTHALAMUS have all been implicated – a LESION of various of these sites produce either decreases or increases in it.

See also: superstitious behaviour

schedules of reinforcement Specifications of how and when a given RESPONSE will receive REINFORCEMENT. The behaviourist B.F. Skinner (1904–1990) began formal investigations of the relationship between reinforcement sche-dule characteristics and OPERANT behaviour. Since this early work a wide variety of sche-dules have been investigated in a wide variety of subject populations. Subtle differences in reinforcement schedule requirements often pro-duce striking differences in the form of operant behaviour. Basic research on schedules of reinforcement has been applied with success in PSYCHOPHARMACOLOGY, and in clinical set-tings (see BEHAVIOUR THERAPY).

In CONTINUOUS REINFORCEMENT schedules (CRF) every response results in the delivery of reinforcement. In intermittent schedules not every response is reinforced. INTERMITTENT SCHEDULES that are based on the amount of responses produced are called RATIO SCHE-DULES. In fixed ratio schedules the number of responses necessary to produce reinforcement is constant. For example, on a fixed ratio 15 schedule (FR 15), every 15th lever press is reinforced. In VARIABLE RATIO SCHEDULES, the number of responses necessary to produce reinforcement varies over time about some specified mean number of responses. For ex-ample on a variable ratio 12 (VR 12) on average every 12 responses results in reinforcer delivery. Intermittent schedules that are based on the amount of time that has elapsed since some temporal marker (typically reinforcer delivery) are called INTERVAL SCHEDULES. In fixed interval schedules the first response pro-duced after some criterion interval of time has

elapsed produce reinforcement. For example on a fixed interval 20 (FI 20) the first response that occurs 20 seconds after the last reinforcer delivery produces reinforcement. In VARIABLE INTERVAL SCHEDULES, the criterion interval of time varies over time about some average interval. For example on a variable interval 18 (VI 18) schedule on average the first response after 18 seconds results in reinforcer delivery. Elapsed intervals and numbers of responses can be combined to create schedules of reinforce-ment in which reinforcement delivery is depen-dent on a subject responding at a criterion rate (see DIFFERENTIAL REINFORCEMENT OF LOW RATES).

Different reinforcement schedules produce markedly different patterns of responding over time. While on continuous reinforcement sche-dules subjects respond at a steady moderate rate and pauses in responding are brief and unpredictable. Well-trained subjects responding on FR schedules pause for a brief period after reinforcement delivery (the POST-REINFORCE-MENT PAUSE) and then resume responding at a high and steady rate (the RATIO RUN) until another reinforcer is obtained. This pattern of responding suggests that subjects have learned they must produce a certain amount of re-sponse to obtain each reinforcer. A similar pattern of responding is found with FI sche-dules: Immediately after reinforcement is ob-tained subjects respond at a low rate. Then as the time of reinforcer-availability approaches subjects respond at increasingly higher rates (the fixed-interval scallop). This pattern of responding suggests that well-trained subjects have learned that a set amount of time must pass before another reinforcer is available (see TIMING). On VR schedules subjects cannot predict how many responses must be produced for reinforcement. Similarly, on VI schedules subjects can not predict how much time must pass before reinforcement is available. Conse-quently, subjects respond at a roughly steady rate on VR and VI schedules. Subjects tend to respond at a higher rate on VR than VI schedules. This is true even when the timing and amount of reinforcement is the same on both schedules (see YOKED CONTROL). This likely reflects the positive feedback loop pre-sent on VR, but not VI schedules – the faster subjects respond on a VR schedule, the more reinforcers they receive which is not true of VI schedules. When an operant response no longer produces reinforcement (see EXTINCTION), a subject's response rate declines over time. However, responding may recover at the beginning of repeated extinction sessions (see SPONTANEOUS RECOVERY). Under extinction conditions, subjects who were trained on an intermittent schedule display greater persistence in responding than subjects who were trained on CRF schedule (see PARTIAL REINFORCEMENT EXTINCTION EFFECT).

Reinforcement schedules have also been used to study choice behaviour. Typically subjects are presented with two response manipulandum (typically, but not always, keys or levers – see NOSE POKE VS. LEVER PRESS) each associated with a different schedule of reinforcement. This is called a CONCURRENT SCHEDULE. Preference is measured by determining a subject's response rate on each manipulandum. A particularly striking phenomena is evident when subjects are presented with two VI schedules concurrently. In this situation a subject's response rate on each manipulandum is equal to the relative reinforcement rate for that response alternative. This is called the MATCHING LAW. Contemporary work on choice with concurrent schedules often draws on concepts in economics and OPTIMAL FORAGING THEORY. For example, animals are seen as having response budgets, experiencing energy costs, and as living in open or closed economies.

See also: appetitive conditioning; associative learning; aversive conditioning; behaviour analysis; behavioural economics; cognitive behavioural therapy; conditioned reinforcement; conditioning; contingency; cost–benefit analysis; instrumental conditioning; learning; negative reinforcement; nine-hole box; positive reinforcement; progressive ratio; shaping; Skinner box; stimulus–reinforcer association

DONALD M. WILKIE

schema (from Greek, *schema*: form; schemata is the plural although schemas is also used by those without the benefit of a classical education) A schema is a form of MENTAL SET – indeed, the term mental set is probably more frequently encountered in biological psychology than the term schema. The idea of a

schema was introduced by Frederick Bartlett (1886–1969), the first Professor of Experimental Psychology at Cambridge University. Bartlett worked on MEMORY and demonstrated how people's recollections of events were shaped by their previous experiences – that is, by the various schemata (or mental sets) they had established for dealing with information. Schema allow us to generalize our experiences: if we visit a football stadium, for example, we establish a schema that will include information on how to behave and what we are likely to experience. That schema can then be applied to later visits to other football grounds. A *high-level schema* is one that includes *low-level schemata*: a 'going to a football ground' schema for example might include lower-level ones such as 'using public transport' and 'buying a programme'. A *schema-driven error* is a misrecollection of an event in which the schema substitutes its expectations for what actually occurred. Bartlett also used the term *schema-plus-correction* for events in which the schema account for the large majority situations but not quite all. The term *schema-plus-tag* has also been used to describe similar processes, the tag serving to highlight unusual features of particular cases that do not quite match the schema.

Schild analysis A method, devised by Arunlakshana & Schild, for determining the relative potency of binding by a DRUG or chemical acting at a RECEPTOR. Data are plotted as a graph called a Schild plot; the Schild slope (that is the slope of the line plotted on the Schild plot) is of importance in determining the validity of the measures. Widely used by pharmacologists, Schild analysis is (rightly or wrongly) rarely of interest to biological psychologists.

Reference

Kenakin T.P. (1987) *Pharmacologic Analysis of Drug–Receptor Interaction*, Raven Press: New York.

Schild plot *see* Schild analysis

Schild slope *see* Schild analysis

schizoaffective disorder A disorder composed of SIGNS AND SYMPTOMS of both SCHIZOPHRENIA and MOOD DISORDER.

schizoid personality disorder *see* personality disorder

schizophrenia Common, serious psychiatric disorder, characterized by psychotic symptoms (see PSYCHOSIS), with recurrent acute episodes of illness occurring against a background of progressive, chronic disability. The aetiology of schizophrenia is at present incompletely understood: diagnosis is based on clinical examination, and rests on the recognition of clusters of SIGNS AND SYMPTOMS.

The modern concept of schizophrenia has evolved over the last century. It has its roots in the classification of mental disorders by Emil Kraepelin (1856–1926) into two broad groups based on long-term outcome. He distinguished between manic depressive insanity (see MANIC DEPRESSION), which he considered to resolve completely between episodes, and DEMENTIA PRAECOX which he believed led to either progressive impairment or only partial recovery. This latter condition is the forerunner of contemporary classifications. The term SCHIZOPHRENIA itself (it comes from Greek, *schizein*: to cleave) was coined by Paul E. Bleuler (1857–1939) who emphasized a psychological view of dementia praecox, and considered core aspects of the illness to relate to a splitting or 'loosening of associations' between such mental activities as cognition and AFFECT. (Schizophrenia does not involve a splitting of personality, but a loss of these associations.) As the concept developed, it became clear that the term schizophrenia was being used in a vague and imprecise way. Lack of agreed diagnostic criteria hampered the study of the disorder and led to wide variations in diagnostic practice. The description by Kurt Schneider (1887–1967) of proposed FIRST-RANK SYMPTOMS of schizophrenia represented a preliminary step in the development of operationalized diagnostic criteria, though Schneider himself recognized that this symptom profile was not specific to schizophrenia, and many of the symptoms occurred in other psychotic disorders.

Older classification systems used the terms HEBEPHRENIA, PARANOIA and CATATONIA to describe different types of schizophrenia. Contemporary classification systems have devel-oped from these and use a number of subtypes of schizophrenia: DSM-IV recognizes paranoid, catatonic, undifferentiated and residual types. Alternatively, the signs and symptoms were differentiated by Tim Crow into TYPE I SCHIZOPHRENIA and TYPE II SCHIZOPHRENIA. Characteristic of type I were the so-called 'positive' symptoms (signs and symptoms abnormal by their presence) including DELUSION, HALLUCINATION, disorganized speech and thinking, and disorganized or catatonic behaviour. Type II included the so-called 'negative' symptoms of schizophrenia (features abnormal by their absence) include WITHDRAWAL, APATHY, and flat or inappropriate MOOD.

Schizophrenia affects men and women equally, though men tend to have an earlier onset, with half of male sufferers being hospitalized before the age of 25. Life-time prevalence is estimated at between 1 and 1.5%. Though the aetiology of schizophrenia is poorly understood, there is little doubt that the disorder is a brain disease. Enlargement of the lateral and third ventricles (see VENTRICULAR ENLARGEMENT) with a reduction in cortical volume is a consistent finding in COMPUTERIZED AXIAL TOMOGRAPHY. FUNCTIONAL NEUROIMAGING techniques reveal reduced frontal activity (HYPOFRONTALITY), and neuropsychological investigations confirm frontal dysfunction in many cases. The ANTIPSYCHOTIC efficacy of DOPAMINE receptor blocking drugs (see DOPAMINE HYPOTHESIS OF SCHIZOPHRENIA) suggests dysfunction of dopaminergic systems. Cellular architecture abnormalities have been reported in limbic areas such as the HIPPOCAMPUS. Recent findings suggest that EXCITATORY AMINO ACID systems may be dysfunctional. Genetic factors appear to play an important role with a 10-fold increase in the prevalence of schizophrenia amongst the children of a schizophrenic parent over the general population rate. The concordance rates of MONOZYGOTIC TWINS are estimated at 47% (for DIZYGOTIC TWINS the rate is 12%). Psychosocial factors also play an important role, and families with high levels of hostility, criticism or over involvement (so-called high EXPRESSED EMOTION) may lead to high relapse rates in the condition.

The mainstay of treatment in schizophrenia is drug therapy. Traditional antipsychotics such as CHLORPROMAZINE and HALOPERIDOL have been used effectively for many years, but are increasingly being replaced by newer, so-called ATYPICAL ANTIPSYCHOTICS, which appear to have a better side effect profile, particularly with regard to EXTRAPYRAMIDAL SIDE-EFFECTS. CLOZAPINE appears to be more effective than other antipsychotics, and may have activity against negative as well as positive symptoms. This drug's propensity to cause haematological side-effects in 1–2% of patients (which may be fatal if undetected) necessitates regular blood monitoring , and restricts its use to treatment-resistant cases at present. Specific psychotherapeutic strategies (see PSYCHOTHERAPY) have met with limited success, though preliminary reports of the use of COGNITIVE THERAPY are encouraging. Novel theoretical approaches to schizophrenia based on the premise of dysfunctional METAREPRESENTATION are also generating cognitive approaches to the disorder (see Frith, 1993). Family work directed to reducing expressed emotion may reduce relapse rates. A key factor in psychosocial management is the development of a flexible therapeutic alliance with patients directed at maintaining drug COMPLIANCE and anticipating and responding to crises.

Prognosis is good for only 20–30% of sufferers – half of the patients diagnosed with schizophrenia will experience repeated relapse and hospitalization. The remaining 20–30% will experience moderate symptoms, and a significant degree of disability. It is estimated that 10–15% of patients with schizophrenia will die by SUICIDE.

References

Crow T.J. (1980) Molecular pathology of schizophrenia: more than one disease process? *British Medical Journal* 280: 66–68.
Davison G.C. & Neale J.M. (1996) *Abnormal Psychology*, 6th edn, Wiley: New York.
Frith C.D. (1993) *The Cognitive Neuropsychology of Schizophrenia*, Lawrence Erlbaum: Hove UK.

IAN C. REID

schizophreniform disorder A schizophreniform disorder can be characterized in exactly the same way as SCHIZOPHRENIA. What differentiates it from schizophrenia is its duration: a schizophreniform disorder is one that lasts only from one to six months, no longer. The term BRIEF PSYCHOTIC DISORDER is also used to describe this condition.

schizotypal personality disorder A disorder that appears to be an abbreviated form of SCHIZOPHRENIA. Individuals with schizotypal personality disorder do not show all of the features of schizophrenia and may not require hospitalization. Common SIGNS AND SYMPTOMS can include mild DELUSION, odd speech patterns, and some degree of PARANOIA. The disorder is most common amongst the children of individuals diagnosed as schizophrenic – indeed, the concept of the schizotypal personality disorder grew out of examination of the incidence of schizophrenia amongst the relatives of schizophrenics (see Kety *et al.*, 1968). Schizotypal personality disorder is thought of as being at the more extreme end of a continuum of personality disorder referred to as SCHIZOTYPY, a classification of personality in which very mild signs and symptoms of schizophrenia can be identified. In the less extreme cases schizotypy blurs into BORDERLINE PERSONALITY DISORDER, a constellation of disturbances in MOOD, self-image and interpersonal relationships. Acceptance of the concept of schizotypy, and at the most extreme, schizotypal personality disorder, indicates that many of the signs and symptoms of schizophrenia are not unique identifiers of this disease but are features present in a wider sample of the population. It is the accumulation of features in a given individual that leads to the diagnosis of schizophrenia.

Reference

Kety S.S., Rosenthal D., Wender P.H. & Schulzinger F. (1968) The types and prevalence of mental illness in the biological and adoptive families of adopted individuals who have become schizophrenic: a preliminary report based on psychiatric interviews. In *The Transmission of Schizophrenia*, ed. D. Rosenthal & S.S. Kety SS, pp. 345–362, Pergamon Press, Elmsford N.Y.

schizotypy *see* schizotypal personality disorder

Schwann cells *see* glial cells

sciatic nerve (from Latin, *sciaticus*, which is from Greek, *ischion*: hip) The sciatic nerve is major NERVE running between the hip and the foot, along the back of the thigh.

sciatica Also known as *Cotunnius' disease* or *sciatic neuralgia*: a condition involving PAIN in the back of the leg due to damage to or INFLAMMATION of the SCIATIC NERVE (though it is often used more generally to refer to any sharp stabbing pains in the legs). It is typically caused by damage to the base of the spine.

sclerosis (from Greek, *skleros*: hard) A term indicating any form of morbid hardening in body tissues. ARTERIOSCLEROSIS for example is colloquially known as hardening of the arteries. (Note though that MULTIPLE SCLEROSIS does not involve hardening of NEURONS but loss of MYELIN: it is therefore something of a misnomer.)

scopolamine A belladonna alkaloid (also known as HYOSCINE) that has action at MUSCARINIC ACETYLCHOLINE RECEPTORS. It has actions similar to those of ATROPINE: it is a CNS depressant that can produce drowsiness, EUPHORIA and AMNESIA. Medically its principal uses are as a premedication for surgical procedures (reducing mucous secretions) and as a medication to prevent MOTION SICKNESS.

scotoma (from Greek, *scotos*: dark) A scotoma is a part of the VISUAL FIELD to which the VISUAL SYSTEM is unresponsive. Everyone has a scotoma for the part of the visual field incident on the BLIND SPOT where the optic nerve exits the eye and there are no RODS or CONES. Scotomas can also be caused by a LESION in the RETINA, OPTIC NERVE, LATERAL GENICULATE NUCLEUS, or the OCCIPITAL LOBE. Although a spot of light projected from the scotoma cannot be detected, the scotoma usually does not appear as a blank spot, because the brain 'fills in' the scotoma with the surrounding visual textures.

LAWRENCE M. WARD

scotopic vs. photopic Scotopic and photopic are functional states of the RETINA. A scotopic retina is dark adapted and responsive to lower light levels. A photopic retina is light adapted and responsive to higher light levels. Exposure of a scotopic retina to a bright light results in poor vision while light adaptation occurs, while exposure of a photopic retina to dim light results in poor vision (NIGHT BLINDNESS) while dark adaptation occurs. Scotopic vision is mediated by RODS while photopic vision is mediated by CONES. Photopic vision appears as COLOUR VISION while scotopic vision appears as shades of grey.

See also: Purkinje shift

LAWRENCE M. WARD

scrapie A fatal neurodegenerative PRION DISEASE of adult sheep. Natural scrapie is associated with a GENE for the PRION PROTEIN. Scrapie appears in flocks of sheep in a pattern consistent with an autosomal RECESSIVE ALLELE inheritance but whether natural scrapie is acquired by genetically susceptible animals or is wholly genetic in origin is unresolved. Scrapie can be transmitted experimentally to sheep, goats and rodents by INTRACEREBRAL INJECTION or SUBCUTANEOUS INJECTION of the tissue from brain, or some internal organs, of affected sheep.

See also: bovine spongiform encephalopathy; Creutzfeldt–Jakob disease

Reference

Parsonson I.M. (1996) Scrapie: recent trends. *Australian Veterinary Journal* 74: 2–6.

ROSALIND RIDLEY

scratch reflex A reflex involving rhythmically repeated movements (in contrast to a STRETCH REFLEX) displayed typically by animals with fur and designed to remove an irritation. The rhythm of the movement is controlled by oscillatory activity of spinal neurons rather than by the stimulus itself.

scratchpad In everyday use, a scratchpad is a pad of paper used for scribbling notes; in computer science, it is a term used to refer to SCRATCHPAD MEMORY, a limited capacity, high-speed MEMORY used for information while being processed; in cognitive psychology, the term VISUOSPATIAL SCRATCHPAD is synonymous with VISUOSPATIAL SKETCH PAD.

SDZ 216–525 An ANTAGONIST at the $5HT_{1A}$ receptor; see SEROTONIN RECEPTORS.

season-of-birth effect A season-of-birth effect would relate to any psychological phenomenon that was known to vary dependent on season of birth. The best known is the season-of-birth effect for SCHIZOPHRENIA: individuals are most likely to be diagnosed as schizophrenic if their birth dates are in February or March and least likely if their birth dates are in August or September, though the risk associated with birth date is not high. As a predictor of schizophrenia it is rather weak: family histories and place of birth are much more strongly associated with schizophrenia than season of birth. Why there should be season of birth effects is unclear. Is it the time of birth that is important or the date of conception? It has even been argued that the effect is a statistical artefact and of not significant importance.

Reference

Mortensen P.B., Pedersen C.B., Westergaard T., Wohlfahrt J., Ewald H., Mors O., Andersen P.K. & Melbye M. (1999) Effects of family history and place and season of birth on the risk for schizophrenia. *New England Journal of Medicine* 340: 603–608.

seasonal affective disorder Possible variant of AFFECTIVE DISORDER which has controversial status. Proposed as a recurrent condition in which depression occurs during the winter months accompanied by symptoms of oversleeping, overeating and exhaustion, there is little evidence that the profile constitutes a clinical entity distinct from DEPRESSION. There is only limited support for the notion that bright LIGHT THERAPY is of specific benefit, and conventional antidepressant treatment is usually effective.

IAN C. REID

sebaceous gland *see* skin

sebum *see* skin

second messengers Molecules found within neurons that serve to propagate or distribute an incoming signal to the neuron and that mediate the biological responses of the cell. In contrast to first messengers such as NEUROTRANSMITTERS or neuroendocrine signals, which are responsible for communication *between* cells, the role of second messengers is to mediate communication *within* the cell, thus controlling the cell's physiological response to the incoming signal. The process by which an external signal is converted into an internal signal is known as SIGNAL TRANSDUCTION. There are two major second messenger systems. One employs cyclic adenosine monophosphate (CYCLIC AMP or cAMP) and the other utilizes a combination of molecules that includes CALCIUM ions (Ca^{2+}), INOSITOL triphosphate (IP_3) and DIACYLGLYCEROL (DAG). Both these pathways utilize an initial coupling mechanism requiring membrane-bound G PROTEIN, which in turn stimulates the production of second messengers. The final action of second messengers is generally to induce cellular proteins to change their structure. The most common mechanism is PROTEIN PHOSPHORYLATION; that is, second messengers activate a type of ENZYME called PROTEIN KINASE, which in turn phosphorylate (add phosphate groups) the target protein. Second messengers may also bind to proteins directly. Phosphorylation is a final common pathway of fundamental importance in regulation of neuronal activity and gene expression in the nervous system.

ANN E. KELLEY

second-order conditioning A PAVLOVIAN CONDITIONING preparation in which a CONDITIONED STIMULUS (CS) is conditioned by being paired with a previously-trained CS (that is, one capable of eliciting responding) rather than with an UNCONDITIONED STIMULUS (US). For example, rats given pairings of a light (the first-order CS) with a food US will come to show conditioned responding to that CS. In a subsequent stage of training, a tone (the second-order CS) may be paired with the light. The tone, despite never being paired directly with the US, will also come to elicit conditioned responding .

See also: higher-order conditioning

JASPER WARD-ROBINSON

secondary sensory ending *see* muscle spindle

secondary somatosensory cortex *see* primary somatosensory cortex

secretin *see* endocrine glands; hormones

section (from Latin, *secare*: to cut) The verb, to section, is the act of cutting; as a noun, a section is that which has been cut. In biological psychology the term section typically refers to a slice of tissue, only micrometres thick, that has been cut on a MICROTOME or in a CRYO-STAT, and which will be prepared for HISTOL-OGY.

See also: planes of section

sedation (from Latin, *sedare*: to still or calm) Sedate means dignified, calm, being of a slow bearing. This word existed before the SEDATIVE drugs were discovered – they take their name from this word rather than vice versa. In medical or biological terms though, SEDATION is the state induced by sedative drugs: note that it is not the same as sleep.

sedative A class of DRUG that tends to depress central nervous system function and that have a calming, sedating effect on behaviour. Seda-tives are also known as SEDATIVE-HYPNOTIC compounds, because of their ability to induce SLEEP. Sedatives comprise a variety of different drug classes, including BARBITURATES, BENZO-DIAZEPINES, ALCOHOL, and VOLATILE ANAES-THETICS. The agents from these different drug classes are remarkably varied in terms of their chemical structure and effect on brain neuro-chemistry. However, they are likely to possess at least one of three properties typical of sedative drugs: (1) ION CHANNEL disruption in the neuronal MEMBRANE such that normal electrical conduction cannot occur; (2) facilita-tion of GABA RECEPTORS such that they become more sensitive to the inhibitory effect of GABA; (3) reduction of EXCITATORY AMINO ACID neurotransmission. Most of these compounds tend to reduce ANXIETY and induce a feeling of calm and well-being in relatively low doses, whereas higher doses can promote sleep and GENERAL ANAESTHESIA. The anti-anxiety effects are thought to be due to enhancement of inhibitory transmission in brain regions med-iating EMOTION such as the LIMBIC SYSTEM; inhibition of more widespread cortical and diencephalic regions mediates the effects on sleep and CONSCIOUSNESS. Drugs in this class produce POSITIVE REINFORCEMENT and are often abused, presumably to their ability to reduce feelings of stress. COMA and death can ensue from overdose with sedatives, due to profound inhibition of BRAINSTEM respiratory and cardiovascular centres.

ANN E. KELLEY

sedative-anxiolytics *see* hypnotics

sedative-hypnotics *see* hypnotics

seizure A sudden, temporally restricted, invo-luntary change in behaviour, caused by abnor-mal electrical discharge of neurons in the central nervous system, and characterized by alterations in motor activity or CONSCIOUS-NESS. The precise symptoms depend on the location and extent of structures involved. For example, abnormal electrical activity in SEN-SORIMOTOR cortex may produce symptoms of motor dysfunction or HALLUCINATION. Seizures may be the result of diseased neurons, most commonly in EPILEPSY, but can occur as a result of acute neuronal injury. In animals, stimulating certain regions of the brain, in which GLUTAMATERGIC transmission is promi-nent, such as AMYGDALA and HIPPOCAMPUS, results in strong seizure activity. This process is called KINDLING.

See also: absence seizure; epilepsy; generalized seizure; grand mal seizure; kindling; partial seizure; petit mal seizure

FIONA M. INGLIS

selective attention The differential allocation of processing resources to a single channel of information, such as a sensory modality.

See also: attention; covert attention; dichotic listening task

VERITY J. BROWN

selective noradrenaline reuptake inhibitor A DRUG that does exactly what it says it does: it selectively inhibits the REUPTAKE of NORA-DRENALINE, (or, in American usage, NOREPI-NEPHRINE) leading to an increased concentration of noradrenaline in the EXTRA-CELLULAR spaces, outside the NEURON. Such drugs are thought to have potent ANTIDEPRES-SANT power. REBOXETINE is the best-known member of this class.

selective serotonin reuptake inhibitor A DRUG that does exactly what it says it does: it selectively inhibits the REUPTAKE of SEROTO-NIN, leading to an increased concentration of serotonin in the EXTRACELLULAR spaces, outside the NEURON. Such drugs are thought to have potent ANTIDEPRESSANT power. PROZAC is the best-known member of this class.

selegiline *see* deprenyl

self-administration Self-administration refers to the self-administration of a DRUG by an animal. Typically this is INTRAVENOUS SELF-ADMINISTRATION, though direct INTRACRANIAL SELF-ADMINISTRATION techniques are also now used. Intravenous self-administration of drug is typically achieved by implanting a permanent CATHETER into the JUGULAR VEIN. This catheter is connected by polyethylene tubing running under the skin to a pedestal either on the SKULL surface or surgically affixed to the animals back or flank. At the pedestal the polyethylene tubing connects to a metal tube to which can be attached a drug line connected to a syringe filled with whatever drug the animal is to have available. Of course, great care has to be taken of the intravenous catheter. It has to be flushed daily with heparinized saline (see HEPARIN) to keep it clean and free of blockage. Drug self-administration is achieved by mounting the drug syringe in a pump controlled by activation of a lever in an OPERANT CHAMBER. Various SCHEDULES OF REINFORCEMENT can be used for drug delivery. The simplest would be a fixed ratio in which each lever press delivered a small quantity of fluid (0.1 ml for example) containing the drug. Limits on the numbers of drug shots that an animal can take are normally set (see Caine *et al.*, 1993). A large number of studies over the last several years have examined animals' willingness to self-administer drugs, in the belief that this represents a reasonable model of drug taking by humans (see DRUG ABUSE; DRUG CRAVING; DRUG-SEEKING BEHAVIOUR). Animals are, if anything, more likely to self-administer drugs than are humans, being possessed of no moral scruples about drug abuse. Intriguingly, studies suggest that the self-administration of drugs produces different neurochemical effects to passive, involuntary delivery (see YOKED CONTROL) suggesting that having control of admin-istration produces different brain states compared to involuntary administration of the same stimulation (see DiCiano *et al.*, 1998).

Intracranial self-administration is less common than intravenous. Essentially the same sorts of procedures are used, but in this case drug is delivered directly to specific sites in brains, using a specially adapted CANNULA. This technique models less well aspects of human drug abuse, such as drug craving, but does allow one to determine which sites in brain are important for the rewarding actions of drugs in a very direct manner.

See also: intracranial self-stimulation

References

Caine S.B., Lintz R. & Koob G.F. (1993) Intravenous drug self-administration techni-ques in animals. In *Behavioural Neu-roscience: A Practical Approach*, ed. A. Sahgal, pp. 117–143, Oxford University Press: Oxford.

DiCiano P., Blaha C.D. & Phillips A.G. (1998) Conditioned changes in dopamine oxidation currents in the nucleus accumbens of rats by stimuli paired with self-administration or yoked administration of *d*-amphetamine. *European Journal of Neuroscience* 10: 1121–1127.

self concept *see* mirror test

self-stimulation Shorthand for INTRACRANIAL SELF-STIMULATION; most definitely not synon-ymous with self-abuse.

selfish gene A hypothesis developed by Ri-chard Dawkins that NATURAL SELECTION oper-ates at the level of the GENE, rather than the organism: that organisms are vehicles for the transmission of genes across generations. It is an idea that has received considerable atten-tion, much of it very positive. It has also been criticized for offering a too-simple view of the determinants of human behaviour.

Reference

Dawkins R. (1976) *The Selfish Gene*, Oxford University Press: Oxford.

selfish herd *see* sociobiology

semantic (from Greek, *semantikos*: signifi-cant) As a general term semantic relates to meaning; semantics is that branch of linguistics that deals with the meaning of words (as opposed to SYNTAX, which deals with the structure of LANGUAGE).

semantic anomia *see* anomia

semantic categorization task *see* pure alexia

semantic dementia This is a behavioural label for a neurodegenerative condition (see NEURODEGENERATION) in which the primary deficit is a deterioration of conceptual or SEMANTIC MEMORY. The most prominent early symptoms are difficulties in comprehending and producing content words (names of objects, names of people, verbs with specific meaning and so on); the disorder is not, however, restricted to the domain of words but also affects conceptual knowledge of real objects and people. Semantic dementia is distinguished from more general dementing conditions by considerable preservation of other cognitive domains, including visual-spatial processing, nonverbal problem solving and – in striking contrast to ALZHEIMER'S DEMENTIA – EPISODIC MEMORY for recent events. Age of onset is typically in the 50s or early 60s.

Semantic dementia is associated with focal atrophy of lateral and inferior areas of the TEMPORAL LOBE, usually in both hemispheres but sometimes more strikingly on the left side. Where *post-mortem* analysis has been possible, the underlying pathology is typically one of PICK'S DISEASE or non-specific spongiform encephalopathy (see PRION DISEASE). This syndrome is sometimes called PROGRESSIVE FLUENT APHASIA, because the semantic deficit yields speech that is fluent (with reasonably normal SYNTAX, PHONOLOGY and PROSODY). However, there is a marked ANOMIA in which general, high-frequency nouns like *thing* or *place* and verbs like *make* and *do* are substituted for more specific nouns and verbs. The pattern of better syntactic than lexical semantic abilities applies to speech comprehension (see SPEECH PERCEPTION) as well as production, and contrasts with the language deficit in PROGRESSIVE NON-FLUENT APHASIA, in which SPEECH PRODUCTION is characterized by phonological and syntactic errors but single-word comprehension is spared. Oral reading in semantic dementia is better preserved than

naming, although a pattern of SURFACE DYSLEXIA often emerges.

Longitudinal assessments suggest a gradual loss of specific, detailed knowledge, eroding the discrimination between semantically similar concepts. Concepts which are less generally familiar show the affects of the deficit first. In naming, a patient may progress from naming a picture of a *zebra* correctly, to naming it as a more common category coordinate like *horse*, to being able to say only that it is an *animal*. This progression is mirrored in tests of comprehension such as word–picture matching, in which correct matches give way to semantic errors and eventually to semantically unrelated choices. Tests that involve no words (such as sorting pictures of objects into conceptually related piles) also indicate an early deterioration of detailed differentiation between conceptually similar objects.

References

Patterson K.E. & Hodges J.R. (1994) Disorders of Semantic Memory. In *Handbook of Memory Disorders*, ed. A. Baddeley, D. Wilson & F. Watts, Lawrence Erlbaum: Hove UK.

Snowden J.S., Neary D. & Mann D.M.A. (1966) *Fronto-Temporal Lobar Degeneration, Fronto-Temporal Dementia, Progressive Aphasia and Semantic Dementia*, Churchill Livingstone: Edinburgh.

ELAINE FUNNELL AND KARALYN E. PATTERSON

semantic differential *see* questionnaire studies

semantic error In computer science, a semantic error is one which produces ambiguity or error in a program; see CONNECTIONIST NEUROPSYCHOLOGY for a description of semantic errors in a psychological context.

semantic memory This term was originally restricted to MEMORY for word meanings for use in LANGUAGE but is now generally extended to include conceptual knowledge about objects, places, people, facts and so forth, as well as words. Semantic memory is distinguished from the other main form of LONG-TERM MEMORY, EPISODIC MEMORY, which is the memory people have for their own personal experiences. Different people from the same culture have largely shared semantic memory (such as knowing that Paris is the capital of France, that France is famous for its wines) but clearly do not share their episodic memories for specific experiences in France. These two forms of memory are distinguished on a neuroanatomical as well as a behavioural basis. Localised damage to structures in the medial part of the TEMPORAL LOBES, especially the HIPPOCAMPAL FORMATION, disrupts the acquisition of new episodic memories but appears to leave semantic memory largely intact. By contrast, lesions to inferior and lateral areas of the temporal lobes (as in SEMANTIC DEMENTIA) disrupt semantic memory but still enable at least some degree of memory for events. However, this contrast is not a pure one, since all knowledge (semantic or episodic) must initially be acquired through episodes.

Psychological theories generally represent semantic memory as a distributed network (see DISTRIBUTED PROCESSING) of overlapping associated features. For example the concept for *bird* might be composed of a collection of features such as *has wings, beak, feathers, can fly, makes nest* together with some more specific features (such as *red breast*). Few concepts possess uniquely defining features, but instead possess a particular combination of features drawn from the pool of features shared amongst members of the category. Prototypical members of the category possess the most commonly occurring features. A conceptual hierarchy emerges from this feature network, in which the greatest overlap of attributes applies to concepts at the lowest level (for example different types of spaniel have very similar perceptual and functional features), with less overlap as one moves up the hierarchy from *spaniels > dogs > domestic animals > mammals > animals > living things*. The optimal level of distinctiveness, referred to as the basic level, occurs when there is a balance between the similarity of members within a category and the contrast with other categories. It is the level at which most object concepts are processed and named. At the top of the hierarchy, broad, superordinate categories, such as living things and man-made artefacts share, very few if any features. Likewise, words with concrete, im-

ageable referents (such as penguin, or red) share few features with the meanings of abstract words (such as *theory* or *ambiguous*). This view of the structure of semantic memory, in which categories are distinguished on the basis of overlapping featural representation, may offer a framework for explaining apparent category-specific deficits (as for example in neurological patients with impairments of comprehension for abstract relative to concrete words, or for living things relative to artefacts and so on) without postulating discretely different brain regions for each of these categories.

Reference

Saffran, E.M., and Schwartz, M.F. (1994). Of cabbages and things: Semantic memory from a neurological perspective: A tutorial review in C. Umilta and M. Moscovitch (eds.), *Attention and Performance XV*, MIT Books: Cambridge, Mass

ELAINE FUNNELL AND KARALYN E. PATTERSON

semantic paraphasia *see* anomia

semantic priming A technique for studying organization and processing within SEMANTIC MEMORY. In a typical experiment, subjects are presented with two successive stimuli, called the prime and target, respectively, and must name the target or determine that it is a word (as in the LEXICAL DECISION TASK). Usually, no response is made to the prime. Subjects' response to the target (for example, *dog*) is faster and more accurate when the target is preceded by a semantically related prime (for instance, *cat*) relative to a semantically unrelated prime (for example, *carrot*). This facilitation – the semantic priming effect – is thought to arise in part from activation spreading down associative links from the prime to semantically related items, lowering the threshold of activation necessary to activate the lexical and semantic REPRESENTATION of these related items on a subsequent trial. (see Neely, 1991 for review of the multiple processes thought to influence semantic priming).

See also: priming; semantic

Reference

Neely J.H. (1991) Semantic priming effects in visual word recognition: a selective review of current findings and theories. In *Basic Processes in Reading: Visual Word Recognition*, ed. D. Besner & G. Humphreys, pp. 264–336, Erlbaum: Hillsdale NJ.

JENNIFER A. MANGELS

semen *see* testes

semicircular canal *see* vestibular system

seminal fluid *see* testes

semiochemical (from Greek, *semeion*: sign, and chemical) A chemical that is able to transmit information, for example any of the PHEROMONES.

See also: breath; social transmission of food preferences

semipermeable membrane A membrane that is permeable to certain types of MOLECULE but not others is called semipermeable. The critical determinant of passage is the size of the molecule, indexed by MOLECULAR WEIGHT. Semipermeable membranes may be natural or artificial: the NEURON membrane is semipermeable (in ways that can be changed; see ACTION POTENTIAL). Artificial semipermeable membranes with varying degrees of permeability are used for MICRODIALYSIS.

See also: osmosis

senile dementia Any form of dementia occurring before the onset of SENILITY is described as PRESENILE DEMENTIA; forms of dementia accompanying senility are described as SENILE DEMENTIAS. The value of these terms is probably not large. ALZHEIMER'S DEMENTIA for example can occur in quite young adults (in which case it characteristically has a strong genetic component) or it can occur much later in life (when any genetic component is much less evident).

senile dementia of the Alzheimer type *see* Alzheimer's dementia

senile dementia of the Lewy body type *see* Lewy body dementia

senility The increasing proportion of incapacitated aged persons in the population has become a major social problem in several first-world countries. Diseases specific to senescence, such as ALZHEIMER'S DEMENTIA and PARKINSON'S DISEASE, may prove a lesser problem than incapacity due to simple senility. Even in the absence of specific pathology biological AGEING brings about a relentless deterioration of bone, brain and connective tissue. Cell loss in the CEREBRAL CORTEX may be surprisingly mild but there is usually a progressive shrinkage of the underlying WHITE MATTER and a loss of critical AMINERGIC and CHOLINERGIC neurons, and neurons in the HIPPOCAMPUS. The IMMUNE SYSTEM, the special senses and the endocrine system follow a similar downhill course. It is by no means obvious why mammalian somatic tissue should decay with time. Amoebae and germ line cells, for example, and some cancer cells, are immortal. Earlier explanations now seem inadequate. Cumulative damage to CHROMOSOMES during one's lifetime by background radiation, or carcinogens, or by one's own FREE RADICALS, can generally be repaired and kept in check: our DIPLOID GENOME incorporates 22 or 23 useful back-ups for the purpose; nor is there convincing support for the idea that we are born with a finite supply of some sort of metabolic potential. The true explanation seems to go deeper. There are clear evolutionary benefits – from the point of view of the GENE – to be derived from a rapid turnover of generations if subjected to continually changing selective pressures and competion for resources. Unfortunately for us this will favour the evolution of inborn genetic programmes that limit individual life spans. Hence, perhaps, Hayflick's well-known observation that cultured fibroblasts – and probably most mammalian cells – can divide a fixed number of times, and then no more. Keeping the tally of CELL DIVISION is thought to rely on TELOMERE shortening – that is, the progressive loss of NUCLEOTIDES from a fixed complement at chromosome ends, with each successive division. Another route to genetically programmed suicide (see APOPTOSIS) may be provided by the *clk-1* gene sequence identified first in *Caenorhabditis elegans* and in yeast, but conserved also in higher animals. Inactivation of this gene in *C. elegans* greatly increases lifespan. Similar interventions may well prove feasible in *Homo sapiens* but it is unclear whether the outcome would enhance the quality of later life or just prolong one's decrepitude and bankrupt the pension schemes.

Reference

Schneider E.L. & Rowe J.W. (eds.) (1996) *Handbook of the Biology of Ageing*, 4th edn, Academic Press: London.

L. JACOB HERBERG

sensation A sensation is a elementary conscious experience initiated by stimulation of sensory receptors. It also can be characterized as the simple process of detecting the presence of stimuli. It may be distinguished from perception (see SENSATION VS. PERCEPTION). For many contemporary investigators, sensations reflect: (1) the activity of receptors and the resulting activity of afferent pathways to the corresponding sensory cortical areas (in mammals – the highest point of afferent conduction in animals without significant development of cerebral cortex); and (2) (what is of most interest currently) the neural coding mechanisms underlying the analysis of sensory information and how they contribute to correspondences and discrepancies between the physical stimulus and sensations (see DOCTRINE OF SPECIFIC NERVE ENERGIES).

RICHARD C. TEES

sensation vs. perception Since Thomas Reid (1710–1796) introduced the distinction in 1785, some have advocated its use, and others have ignored it, arguing the conceptual distinction adds nothing to our understanding of either the conscious experiences initiated by stimulation of sensory receptors, or their neural substrates (see CONSCIOUSNESS). Those who do subscribe to the value of the distinction between the two argue that the study of sensation, or sensory processes, is concerned with less complex (although not less complicated) aspect of the complete experience. The study of perception or perceptual processes is seen to focus on those aspects of the experience resulting from the interpretation and elaboration of these initial sensations. In a sense, the sensory aspects are the product of the early stage, 'bottom-up' analysis of the physical stimulus (see TOP-DOWN VS. BOTTOM-UP PERCEPTUAL/NEURAL PROCESSING) – that is, the

activity of receptors and the resulting activity of afferent pathways to corresponding sensory cortical regions. Donald Hebb (1904–1985) described perception as reflecting the activity of cortical mediating processes to which sensations give rise. He argued these mediating processes involved activity of cell assemblies involving interconnected cortical neurons in and beyond primary sensory projection areas (see CELL ASSEMBLY THEORY). Thus, the perceptual aspects of our experiences (that is, which mediating processes are active when a physical object appears) depend on which processes are activated by the initial sensory analysis of what is there (that is, the physical stimulus); what sorts of mediating processes have been established as a result of previous stimulation history, and resultant PERCEPTUAL LEARNING; and which are facilitated as a result of current attentional and motivational states of a subject. Obviously these two terms reflect psychological processes and neural systems that are highly interrelated, and some of a subject's conscious stimulus-related experiences can be accounted for largely in terms of sensations or sensory processes. However, in other cases, perception or perceptual processes are clearly evident. Our conscious awareness of objects and events are convincingly an amalgam of the potentially competitive interactions between bottom-up and top-down neural processing of the sensory world by a functioning adult subject.

RICHARD C. TEES

sensitive period A biologically determined period, generally early in ONTOGENY, during which some aspect of an organism's neural and behavioural functioning is especially sensitive to a particular environmental factor. While the term CRITICAL PERIOD is often employed synonymously, a sensitive period is better characterized as an optimum period. Environmental-induced modifiability (albeit less effective) outside this 'best' time period is acknowledged as a possibility. Also possible are shifts in beginning and end of the period depending on the organism's stimulation history prior to and during the normal sensitive time period. There are usually limitations on the nature of the stimulus input that can influence the organism during the time window.

RICHARD C. TEES

sensitization (behavioural) If an animal receives a strong stimulus, it is often observed that responding to other stimuli changes. For example, presentation of an AVERSIVE STIMULUS, such as a strong shock, might enhance responding to a previously innocuous noise and might decrease the probability of appetitive responses, such as FEEDING. This quantitative change in responding to other stimuli is termed behavioural sensitization. It should be noted that the term sensitization is often used more generally to refer to any enhanced responsiveness of neurons (for example, NOCICEPTORS during nociceptive sensitization) as well as behavioural changes.

MARK A. UNGLESS

sensitization (drugs) Sensitization to the effects of drugs – also known as REVERSE TOLERANCE – is the process by which the effect of a drug increases on repeated administration. (TOLERANCE of course describes the related phenomenon in which the effect of a drug diminishes with repeated administration.) Why this process occurs is not entirely clear: behavioural, psychological and neurochemical mechanisms have been suggested.

References

Feldman R., Meyer J.S. & Quenzer L.F. (1997) *Principles of Neuropsychopharmacology*, Sinauer Associates: Sunderland MA.

sensitization (receptor) Receptor sensitization happens over a short space of time (seconds to minutes) and is produced by activation of a RECEPTOR. It is manifest as a reduction in responsivity to stimulation and is brought about by intracellular changes, principally the uncoupling of receptors from their SECOND MESSENGERS. Once stimulation has ended, a return to normal sensitivity occurs promptly.

Receptor sensitization is not to be confused with DOWN REGULATION, which occurs when receptors are exposed to stimulation over longer periods of time (hours rather than minutes). Down-regulation involves changes in

the numbers of BINDING SITES and destruction of receptor PROTEINS, over and above the changes in second messenger activation brought about by short term sensitization. UP-REGULATION can also occur. It is typically seen when a NEURON loses its normal inputs through natural or experimental degeneration. Up-regulation is typically manifest through increased numbers of receptor binding sites. The terms SUBSENSITIVITY and SUPERSENSITIVITY are also used to describe down- and up-regulation respectively. In biological psychology, the most common demonstration of supersensitivity is the behavioural response to DOPAMINE receptor stimulation in rats that bear a UNILATERAL dopamine-depleting LESION of the NIGROSTRIATAL DOPAMINE SYSTEM; see ROTATION for an explanation of this.

Changes in the sensitivity of receptors to their natural LIGAND and to DRUG action is an important consideration: long-term exposure to drugs can induce SENSITIZATION or REVERSE TOLERANCE (see SENSITIZATION [DRUGS]). Hypotheses concerning the nature of conditions such as SCHIZOPHRENIA have been built around the idea of altered receptor sensitivity.

sensorimotor Pertaining to both sensory and motor function. This term is most frequently used in psychobiology to refer to the integrative processes by which sensation comes to influence motor output. In disorders of ATTENTION, such as neglect consequent upon a LESION of right POSTERIOR PARIETAL CORTEX, primary sensory and primary motor impairments are ruled out and, therefore, the impairments are often referred to as being sensorimotor in nature. Jean Piaget (1896–1980) also used this term to refer to the first developmental period (birth to 18 months), during which a human infant is considered to have perceptual and motor skills and must acquire integrative function.

VERITY J. BROWN

sensorimotor cortex The term sensorimotor cortex is a rather vague one, used to describe large parts of the FRONTAL LOBE and PARIETAL LOBE. The parietal lobe contains SOMATOSENSORY CORTEX, and has functions that are considered more sensory than motor. The frontal lobes contain the MOTOR CORTEX (as well as systems for higher order behavioural regulation such as the PREFRONTAL CORTEX) and are thought of as rather more motor than sensory (see Kaas, 1987). However, both frontal and parietal systems have a degree of sensory and motor functions, and hence can be collectively termed sensorimotor cortex. It can be argued though that sensorimotor functions are better associated with the BASAL GANGLIA, the PUTAMEN in particular having a convergence of both sensory and motor input for the representation of sensorimotor functions.

Reference

Kaas J.H. (1987) The organization of the neocortex in mammals: implications for theories of brain function. *Annual Review of Psychology* 38: 124–151.

sensorimotor gating *see* sensory gating

sensorimotor test battery To assess sensorimotor function, ruling out primary sensory and primary motor deficits, a battery of tests is often used. An effective battery will include tests of predominantly motor skill (such as PAW PREFERENCE or foot placement), tests of predominantly sensory function (for example, a test of signal detection [see SIGNAL DETECTION THEORY] or REACTION TIME, when the reporting of signals is by a response known to be within motoric capabilities) and also tests which require integrative function (for example, making incompatible responses, such as orienting movements away from a stimulus location). The main advantage of using a multiplicity of tests is to identify a profile of preserved and impaired performance which is more informative than knowledge of performance on any individual test. Rats bearing a LESION of the NIGROSTRIATAL DOPAMINE SYSTEM made by 6-HYDROXYDOPAMINE are often tested using the sensorimotor test battery developed by John Marshall and his colleagues.

See also: behavioural checklist; Luria–Nebraska test battery

Reference

Marshall J.F. and Teitelbaum, P. (1974) Further analysis of sensory inattention following lateral hypothalmic damage in rats. *Journal of Comparative Psychological Psychology* 86: 375–395.

VERITY J. BROWN

sensory aphasia A major type of APHASIA in the classification scheme of Russian neurologist A.R. Luria (1902–1977). A form of FLUENT APHASIA associated with a LESION in the posterior first temporal gyrus (see TEMPORAL LOBE). The primary feature is a deficit of auditory comprehension secondary to a loss of the ability to discriminate the individual sounds that comprise spoken words.

See also: Wernicke's aphasia

Reference

Luria A.R. (1970) *Traumatic Aphasia*, Mouton: The Hague.

CHARLOTTE C. MITCHUM

sensory aprosodia *see* aprosodia

sensory cortex The sensory cortex consists of those parts of the CEREBRAL CORTEX that are involved in sensory function. They are located mainly in the posterior half of the cortex. The sensory regions include the SOMATOSENSORY CORTEX, VISUAL CORTEX, AUDITORY CORTEX, GUSTATORY CORTEX and OLFACTORY CORTEX. In each of these regions, the primary area directly receives sensory input from subcortical structures (usually, the THALAMUS), while the secondary and higher-order areas receive input from the primary area and other regions. The sensory cortex transforms sensory input from the periphery into meaningful patterns of perception, recognition and awareness.

KAZUE SEMBA

sensory deprivation *see* sensory enrichment vs. deafferentation/deprivation

sensory enrichment vs. deafferentation/ deprivation Deafferentation and sensory deprivation involve attempts to create laboratory circumstances in which cumulative sensory input is restricted through early development, while sensory enrichment represents an attempt to create one in which such sensory experiences are augmented, relative to that experienced by 'normally' reared animals (see ENVIRONMENTAL ENRICHMENT and ISOLATION REARING). With the publication by Donald

Hebb (1904–1985) of *The Organization of Behaviour* in 1949 not only was the significance of early postnatal (and prenatal) sensory experiences normally inevitable for all members of a species recognized as a potential antecedent of mammalian perceptual and neural development, but so was the importance of these controlled rearing techniques of deprivation, deafferentation, and enrichment in helping to provide information to assess the relative roles different kinds of experience might play in the collaboration between genetic and environmental factors (see CELL ASSEMBLY THEORY). Surgically produced deafferentation is the most radical manipulation of early sensory input and has been used to assess the impact of eliminating all early sensory input including spontaneous activity of now destroyed sensory receptors and their first order afferents on the remaining sensory neural system. The technique of early (temporary) sensory deprivation often involves a significant reduction in, rather than elimination of, stimulus input to specific receptors, but it does allow for the assessment of the effects of the early restriction on adult discriminative competencies. Although vision has been the chosen modality for almost all sensory deprivation experiments, comparable experimental designs have been used to examine the effects of auditory (for example with ear plugs, sound attenuating chambers) and tactual restrictive rearing (for example by social isolation, dewhiskering, and/or cardboard limb casts or cuffs). Deprivation of, for example, visual input by rearing from birth in total darkness allowed one to assess the visual competencies as well as the physiological and structural integrity of the visual system in an older, visually naive organism whose now mature response capabilities permit effective evaluation. The differences (or lack of differences) found in comparisons of the deprived animal with that of one raised under normal lighting conditions has been used to establish the relative contribution normally made by experiential factors in the development of specific discriminative behaviour and potentially related neural mechanisms. With respect to sensory neural mechanisms and those perceptual abilities that can be measured shortly after birth, this technique is easily adapted to help establish whether or not timing is a important feature with respect to the influence of early sensory input (see SENSITIVE PERIOD and CRITICAL PERIOD). Further, such investigations are able to specify what kind of role, if any, subsequent experience played. For example, evidence from continuous assessment throughout early ONTOGENY of, for instance, dark- and light-reared subjects can reveal whether certain aspects of the visual environment maintain (that is, sustain maturing or stable competencies) or whether they FACILITATE, sharpen, or 'fine tune' initially rudimentary perceptual ability or receptive field properties of visual neurons, or whether changes in early stimulation history induced qualitative shifts in the ontogeny of certain visual behaviours and related neural systems. Other types of restrictive and selective manipulation of early (usually visual) stimulation history have been used to test whether or not changes in perceptual functioning and/or the neural substrate can be induced in a predicted or specific way with respect to a particular controlled exposure history. For example, the effects of laboratory environments in which animals (wearing translucent contact lenses) receive diffuse, but not patterned light experience, are monocularly occluded, experience surgically induced STRABISMUS, or are exposed to selective visual input (such as vertical lines only) through goggle-masks, all have been examined. While early postnatal experience has been the focus of most of these studies, several investigators have shown the effects of manipulations of normally invariant prenatal sensory experience (for example by assessing the effects of surgically induced prenatal de-VOCALIZATION in avian foetuses on postnatal auditory competencies). Finally, a subject of some recent interest is related to the generality of the effects of unimodal manipulations of early stimulation history. In this instance, the assessment has been of the inter-modal effects of changing the early sensory input in respect to a single modality.

RICHARD C. TEES

sensory extinction *see* extinction

sensory gating A term that refers to the ability to filter (that is, to gate) sensory stimuli. The term SENSORIMOTOR GATING is often used synonymously, though it can be differentiated from the term sensory gating: whereas sensory gating just refers to the gating of sensory input, sensorimotor gating is taken to refer to the gating of sensory input as well as the suppression of inappropriate responses. Sensory (and sensorimotor) gating is thought to be measured by PREPULSE INHIBITION, and is dysfunctional in several disorders, most notably SCHIZO-PHRENIA. Schizophrenic patients, unlike control subjects, have difficulty in displaying prepulse inhibition, suggesting that they cannot effectively interrupt sensory flow.

sensory memory *see* short term memory

sensory neurons Any neuron that transmits information to the CENTRAL NERVOUS SYSTEM can be called a sensory neuron. The term is also more specifically used in direct contrast with MOTOR NEURONS. In this sense a sensory neurons is one has a CELL BODY in the GANG-LIA immediately adjacent to the SPINAL CORD. They have bifurcated AXONS, one branch contacting MUSCLES (from where they will collect information) the other entering the DORSAL HORN, sending branches in different directions. Some COLLATERALS of sensory neuron axons synapse on motor neurons in the VENTRAL HORN.

sensory preconditioning A conditioning procedure: animals are exposed to two stimuli (see STIMULUS), neither of which has any special meaning (a square and a triangle for example). No conditioning takes place at this time, but shortly afterwards, one of the stimuli is used in a conditioning procedure (for example, presentation of the triangle might be paired with food, encouraging LEARNING of a triangle–food association). In later tests, the other stimulus that was paired in the first stage (in this example the square) when now presented alone will elicit the same response as the triangle: sensory preconditioning has taken place.

See also: associative learning; countercond-itioning

sensory projection area The area of the CEREBRAL CORTEX to which specific sensory material is sent. The size of a sensory projection area reflects the degree of analytic detail required. In the human brain for example, visual areas (see VISUAL SYSTEM) are relatively large; in the RAT brain, the area representing the VIBRISSAE (the BARREL CORTEX) is relatively large.

sensory specific satiety A term used to describe the fact that an individual can be satiated and stop eating a particular food, but immediately resume if a different type of food is presented – that is, SATIETY that is sensory specific. It is of interest that there are neurons in the HYPOTHALAMUS that reflect this. Recording studies show that repeated presentation of a particular food type will be accompanied by reduced acceptance of the food as well as reduced neuron firing in the LATERAL HYPOTHALAMUS. But presentation of a novel food immediately restores both intake and neural activation.

sensory transduction The process by which a sensory stimulus is transduced into an electrical signal. Two basic sensory transduction mechanisms are known. The activation of PHOTORECEPTORS, OLFACTORY RECEPTORS and TASTE CELLS results in changes in cellular levels of SECOND MESSENGERS (such as CYCLIC GMP or CYCLIC AMP). The second-messengers gate ion channels (see ION CHANNEL) that allow ions to flow across the membrane, thereby altering membrane voltage. Auditory HAIR CELLS, TOUCH RECEPTORS and other MECHAN-ORECEPTORS possess MEMBRANE CHANNELS that are directly gated by deformation of the channels themselves or the surrounding membrane. All receptors show that property of ADAPTATION – the response declines over time to a constant stimulus.

JOHN E. DOWLING

septal nuclei A group of nuclei situated in the BASAL FOREBRAIN, comprised of medial, lateral, and triangular septal nuclei, and the septofimbrial nucleus. The medial septum forms a continuum with the vertical limb of the DIAGONAL BAND OF BROCA, located ventrally, and provides the major source of CHO-LINERGIC (Ch1 and Ch2 – see CH1–CH8) and GABAERGIC innervation to the HIPPOCAMPUS.

The lateral septum receives innervation from the hippocampus, and in turn projects to the medial septum. The loss of cholinergic neurons in the basal forebrain observed in ALZHEIMER'S DEMENTIA suggests that these neurons may be involved in LEARNING and MEMORY. However, lesions of the basal forebrain produced by NEUROTOXINS specific for cholinergic cells do not appear to disrupt learning processes in animals. The triangular septal and septofimbrial nuclei project to the medial HABENULA, which itself sends cholinergic projections to lower diencephalic structures. This pathway appears to be involved in many functions, including OSMOREGULATION, NOCICEPTION, SEXUAL BEHAVIOUR and FEEDING, and AVOIDANCE LEARNING and MAZE LEARNING.

FIONA M. INGLIS

septal rage An increased reactivity (that generally ameliorated over time) observed in animals following bilateral ELECTROLYTIC LESIONS of the SEPTAL NUCLEI. Once thought to indicate critical involvement of the septal nuclei in EMOTION, septal rage is now a forgotten phenomenon.

See also: aggression; sham rage

septohippocampal system A system of fibre connections between the septum (see SEPTAL NUCLEI) and the HIPPOCAMPUS, once the focus of much research in biological psychology. The concept of the septohippocampal system has fallen into disrepute following recognition of the more important patterns of connectivity between the hippocampus and ENTORHINAL CORTEX. However, the importance of neuromodulatory inputs to the hippocampal formation, some of which pass via the septum, are recognized as relevant to OSCILLATIONS and other aspects of information processing.

See also: Ch1–Ch8; fimbria; fornix; hippocampal theta; subiculum

RICHARD G. M. MORRIS

serial discrimination *see* discrimination

serial learning This is a form of LEARNING in which items have to be recalled in the order of presentation; it is a procedure that can be used with both humans and experimental animals.

See also: serial reversal learning

serial lesion effect A series of small lesions in a given brain area has less effect on cognitive performance and behaviour than a single large LESION; RECOVERY OF FUNCTION is more effective following several small lesions compared to a single large lesion.

serial position effect The finding that in tests of SERIAL RECALL and FREE RECALL, MEMORY performance is related to the serial position of the item in the list. Items at the beginning and end of the list are recalled better than items in the middle, resulting in a U-shaped curve when percentage of correct responses is plotted as a function of position. Higher recall performance for items at the beginning of the list is referred to as PRIMACY EFFECT. Higher recall performance for items for the end of the list is referred to as the RECENCY EFFECT. Different variables influence primacy and recency effects, indicating that they reflect the operation of different memory systems or processes.

See also: long-term memory; memory span; short-term memory

JENNIFER A. MANGELS

serial processing *see* parallel vs. serial processing

serial recall Procedure used in humans to examine the ability to RECALL from MEMORY previously encountered items in the exact order in which they were presented. It is a memory task that differs from others such as FREE RECALL and from CUED RECALL, in which RETRIEVAL cues are provided.

See also: declarative memory; episodic memory; explicit memory; recognition; serial position effect

serial reversal learning An instrumental learning paradigm in which subjects are trained on a series of two-item DISCRIMINATION problems. The pairs of cues to be discriminated remain the same, but reverse their REWARD valence from problem to problem. Depending on species and sensory modality tested, a reversal set may be formed across multiple problems such that each reversal problem comes to be solved within one trial. The adoption of a WIN–STAY, LOSE–SHIFT strategy may mediate this form of one-trial learning, as in LEARNING SET formation.

IAN C. REID

serine An amino acid with multiple biological functions; see for example INHIBITORY AMINO ACIDS.

serotonin Serotonin or 5-hydroxytryptamine is a BIOGENIC AMINE neurotransmitter (see NEUROTRANSMITTERS). Systems or cells containing serotonin are said to be SEROTONERGIC (or occasionally, serotoninergic). An INDOLEAMINE, serotonin is synthesized from TRYPTOPHAN, an essential dietary requirement. It is also present in various organ systems in the body, and released by platelets during blood clotting. Serotonin is localized in distinct cell groups in the BRAINSTEM, designated as B1–B9 (see CLASSIFICATION OF DAHLSTRÖM AND FUXE). Most of these cell groups are associated with the RAPHE NUCLEI, including the DORSAL RAPHE NUCLEUS and NUCLEUS RAPHE MAGNUS. Serotonergic neurons innervate virtually all regions of the CENTRAL NERVOUS SYSTEM, including the SPINAL CORD. Serotonin is thought to be involved in SLEEP and AROUSAL and the modulation of basic motor and sensory processes.

KAZUE SEMBA

serotonin receptors There are multiple receptor subtypes for SEROTONIN. The basic types are identified by numbers (5-HT1 to 5-HT7 – 5HT stands for 5-HYDROXYTRYPTAMINE, the chemical name for serotonin), these then being further subdivided, indicated by letters. Receptors for serotonin are found throughout the CENTRAL NERVOUS SYSTEM, as well as in the PERIPHERAL NERVOUS SYSTEM and body tissues. They are found at PRESYNAPTIC and POSTSYNAPTIC locations, and can function as AUTORECEPTORS. Many of these classes are however

The prinicpal locations of serotonin receptor subtypes

5-HT1A	HIPPOCAMPUS, SEPTAL NUCLEI, AMYGDALA, FRONTAL CORTEX, ENTORHINAL CORTEX (all postsynaptic); RAPHE NUCLEI (autoreceptors)
5-HT1B	SUBSTANTIA NIGRA, SUBICULUM, GLOBUS PALLIDUS, SUPERIOR COLLICULUS, DORSAL STRIATUM, CENTRAL GRAY
5-HT1D	low levels only in rat brain; more common in human brain where it is found in substantia nigra, globus pallidus, dorsal and VENTRAL STRIATUM
5-ht1E	the distribution of this poorly characterized receptor is unclear
5-HT1F	hippocampus, CEREBRAL CORTEX, raphe nuclei
5-HT2A 2B & 2C	CLAUSTRUM, ventral striatum, OLFACTORY TUBERCLE, PYRIFORM CORTEX, NEOCORTEX. Discrimination between 5-HT2A, 5-HT2B and 5-HT2C in the central nervous system is unclear; 5-HT2B receptors are found outside the central nervous system also (notably in the STOMACH): whether this subtype is present in brain at all is unclear.
5-HT3	AUTONOMIC NERVOUS SYSTEM; AREA POSTREMA, entorhinal cortex, amygdala, NUCLEUS OF THE SOLITARY TRACT, TRIGEMINAL NERVE nuclei
5-HT4	the distribution of this poorly characterized receptor is unclear
5-ht5A	the distribution of this poorly characterized receptor is unclear
5-ht5B	the distribution of this poorly characterized receptor is unclear
5-ht6	the distribution of this poorly characterized receptor is unclear
5-HT7	the distribution of this poorly characterized receptor is unclear

Note: when lower case is used [5ht] it indicates that although receptors have been cloned (see CLONE), expression of the receptor in whole brain has not yet been achieved.

further subdivided, as is indicated in the table below.

Serotonin receptors are typically coupled to G PROTEIN. The family of 5-HT_3 receptors however are not: activation of this receptor produces direct ION CHANNEL opening (they are LIGAND-GATED ION CHANNELS). Serotonin receptors mediate a variety of electrophysiological effects. $5HT_1$ receptors affect ADENYLATE CYCLASE activity and produce HYPERPOLARIZATION (that is, inhibition of firing). $5HT_2$ receptors affect INOSITOL systems and have depolarizing (see DEPOLARIZATION) effects (that is, they have excitatory effects). $5HT_4$ receptors affect adenylate cyclase activity also, but have depolarizing effects. Little is known for certain about the electrophysiological effects of the remaining receptor subtypes.

While it appears that individual subtypes of serotonin receptors rarely act entirely independently of each other, there are a number of drugs that show a degree of selectivity for one or other subtypes. These are catalogued in the table below. Note though that it is unusual to find a drug that has an action exclusively at one type of RECEPTOR: in most cases selectivity for a receptor subtype is relative. The agonists and antagonists listed here, unless otherwise specifically noted, show a degree of selectivity for the receptors indicated, though this selectivity may not necessarily be absolute.

Reference

Feldman R., Meyer J.S. & Quenzer L.F. (1997) *Principles of Neuropsychopharmacology*, Sinauer Associates: Sunderland MA.

Drugs acting at serotonin receptors

5-HT1A	*agonists*	8-OH-DPAT, ipsapirone
	antagonists	SDZ 216-525, WAY-100135
5-HT1B	*agonists*	CP-93,129, sumatripan
	antagonists	SB224289
5-HT1D	*agonists*	sumatripan
	antagonists	BRL15572
5-ht1E	*agonists*	BRL54443
	antagonists	*not available*
5-HT1F	*agonists*	LY334370
	antagonists	*not available*
5-HT2A	*agonists*	alpha-methyl 5-hydroxytryptamine
	antagonists	ketanserin, ritanserin
5-HT2B	*agonists*	alpha-methyl 5-hydroxytryptamine
	antagonists	LY-53857
5-HT2C	*agonists*	alpha-methyl 5-hydroxytryptamine
	antagonists	mesulergine
5-HT3	*agonists*	alpha-methyl 5-hydroxytryptamine
	antagonists	tropisetron, ondansetron, granisetron
5-HT4	*agonists*	alpha-methyl 5-hydroxytryptamine
	antagonists	GR113808

Note: Selective agonists and antagonists for the 5-ht5A, 5-ht5B, 5-ht6 and 5-HT7 receptors are not yet available. When lower case is used [5ht] it indicates that although receptors have been cloned (see clone), expression of the receptor in whole brain has not yet been achieved.

serotonin syndrome A cluster of behavioural effects induced by administration of SEROTONERGIC drugs, especially those acting at the 5-HT$_{1A}$ receptor (see SEROTONIN RECEPTORS). The effects include: TREMOR; RIGIDITY of the MUSCLES; forepaw treading; abduction of the hindlimbs (that is the hindlimbs are splayed out backwards); head movements (typically from side to side); and STRAUB TAIL. Other phenomena can occur also, including salivation, hyperactivity and a high degree of reactivity to sensory stimuli. Overdose of serotonergic drugs in humans can cause similar phenomena. While this might be an effective indicator of serotonergic activation, and while discrimination between one serotonin AGONIST and another is made possible by virtue of their ability to elicit different elements of the syndrome, the value of the syndrome in terms of understanding psychological or behavioural functions of serotonin appears limited.

Reference

Feldman R., Meyer J.S. & Quenzer L.F. (1997) *Principles of Neuropsychopharmacology*, Sinauer Associates: Sunderland MA.

serotonin–noradrenaline reuptake inhibitor The serotonin–noradrenaline reuptake inhibitors (SNRIs) are a class of DRUG that inhibit REUPTAKE of both SEROTONIN and NORADRENALINE (which is known in the United States as NOREPINEPHRINE). Their actions are often contrasted with those of the SELECTIVE SEROTONIN REUPTAKE INHIBITOR (SSRI) group of drugs (such as PROZAC). Drugs that are thought to be SNRIs include milnacipran, sibutramine and venlafaxine. These drugs are thought to have ANTIDEPRESSANT properties.

serotonergic Relating to the neurotransmitter SEROTONIN. For instance, a neuron that synthesizes and releases serotonin is said to be serotonergic.

serum (from Latin, *serum*: whey [the fluid part of milk]; plural, sera) Serum is a liquid separated from BLOOD by clotting; it is the fluid that remains after blood clotting has taken place. It is not the same as PLASMA: plasma can be considered as being the VEHICLE for blood – the fluid in which every CELL and MOLECULE normally present in blood are suspended. If taken from the body, plasma requires anticoagulants (HEPARIN or sodium citrate for example) in order to remain fluid. Without these, blood clotting occurs, producing blood clots (aggregations of cells, fibrinogen and clotting factors) and serum. Serum contains ANTIBODIES and other molecules and PROTEINS (but no clotting agents of course). Serum containing known antibodies prepared for either experimental or therapeutic use is known as ANTISERUM and is what is used to inoculate people and animals against disease (see IMMUNE SYSTEM).

servomechanism (from Latin, *servus*: a slave, and Greek, *mechane*: a mechanical device) The term servomechanism can refer to any device, biological or not, that involves a CLOSED LOOP system in which small amounts of power are used to produce larger output in a strictly proportional manner. The use of feedback is critical and as such servomechanistic processes can be contrasted with BALLISTIC and OPEN LOOP processes, where feedback is not present (see CLOSED LOOP, OPEN LOOP).

set *see* attentional set; learning set; mental set

set point In engineering, a set point is the state that a SERVOMECHANISM is intended to achieve and maintain. In biology it has featured as a mechanism for achieving HOMEOSTASIS. Set points for such things as ENERGY BALANCE and WATER BALANCE, body temperature (see THERMOREGULATION) and BODY WEIGHT have been thought to exist. However, precise set points are probably rare in nature: regulatory mechanisms are more likely to work to boundary models with upper and lower limits, but flexibility within these boundaries: see HOMEOSTASIS for further discussion of this.

set shifting *see* attentional set-shifting; extradimensional shift; intradimensional shift

sex chromosomes *see* X and Y chromosomes

sex differences Sex differences occur along several dimensions in bisexual species, from the differentiation of gonadal structure and PHENOTYPE according to gender, to patterns of hormone release, differences in brain anatomy and function, and sexually dimorphic (see SEXUAL DIMORPHISM) behaviours. Differences in phenotype, reproductive anatomy, and behaviour are probably the most obvious to detect. SEXUAL DIFFERENTIATION of the male gonadal system leads to ANDROGEN-induced organization of anatomy and physiology, ultimately generating a male external and internal form of the organism. At PUBERTY, GONADAL STEROIDS mature the phenotypic characteristics of both males and females (they produce secondary sex characteristics) and activate adult forms of sexually differentiated reproductive function and SEXUAL BEHAVIOUR.

Some non-reproductive behaviours, like the amount and type of rough-and-tumble PLAY in PRIMATES show a male bias in frequency whereas other behaviours, like the gender-specific urinary postures of domestic dogs (squatting in females, leg up in males) show a simple sex difference. As with sexual behaviours, these stereotyped, species-specific and gender-specific behaviours can be altered by perinatal androgen administration. Although there is a general male bias toward more aggressive behaviours, especially during seasonal breeding in which males defend territory and females, females are also capable of highly aggressive and violent behaviour, especially when protecting their young. Females in some species (for example, sandpipers, golden hamsters, hyenas) show far more aggression than males of the same species.

Sex differences are not pronounced in humans. Despite the fact that men have bigger brains than women (even when standardized as a ratio to body weight), reliable sex differences on standardized tests of INTELLIGENCE (for instance, IQ; see INTELLIGENCE TESTING) have never been found. However, there are a number of specific abilities in which men and women possess small relative advantages. On average, women tend to perform better than men on tests of fine motor skill, perceptual speed and accuracy, verbal ability, and SHORT-TERM MEMORY (using verbal or pictorial stimuli), whereas men tend to perform better than women on tests of quantitative ability, spatial skill, and strength. LANGUAGE abilities appear to be more lateralized to the LEFT HEMISPHERE in men than women. Sex differences in human brain structure could conceivably lead to these differences in cognitive

ability, although there is little evidence for this assumption. In males, the RIGHT HEMISPHERE tends to be larger than the left, whereas in females, differences in size and weight between the hemispheres are less marked. Although the right cortex is more developed in males, females have a larger PLANUM TEMPORALE and CUNEATE REGION of the OCCIPITAL LOBE on the right side. Several subcortical regions are larger in males than females, including the right CAUDATE NUCLEUS and nuclei of the preoptic area and anterior hypothalamus. Conversely, females appear to have larger intrahemispheric commissures among the five major INTRAHEMISPHERIC FIBRE PATHWAYS, the CORPUS CALLOSUM, ANTERIOR COMMISSURE and posterior commissure, MASSA INTERMEDIA, and HIPPOCAMPAL COMMISSURE. In fact, men with smaller intrahemispheric commissures perform better on non-verbal skills than men with smaller commissures, suggesting that brain organization during development could lead to differences in cognitive abilities in the adult.

See also: feminine; gender; organization effects of steroid hormones; sex hormones

JAMES G. PFAUS

sex drive *see* sexual behaviour

sex hormones The HORMONES that act on the HYPOTHALAMIC-PITUITARY-GONADAL AXIS (HPG), or in extra-hypothalamic sites in the brain, to potentiate sexual or reproductive functions. These include: (1) STEROID HORMONES secreted from the testes and ovaries (such as PROGESTERONE, TESTOSTERONE, and ESTROGEN); (2) certain PEPTIDES secreted from the ANTERIOR PITUITARY gland (for example FOLLICLE-STIMULATING HORMONE [FSH], LUTEINIZING HORMONE [LH], and PROLACTIN); (3) peptides secreted from the POSTERIOR PITUITARY gland (OXYTOCIN and VASOPRESSIN), and (4) NEUROPEPTIDES secreted by cells of the HYPOTHALAMUS into the pituitary blood system (such as GONADOTROPHIN RELEASING HORMONE [GnRH]). Steroid hormones secreted from the gonads into the bloodstream act on specific progestin, androgen, and estrogen receptors within cells of the hypothalamus, LIMBIC SYSTEM, and CEREBRAL CORTEX, to orchestrate a complex series of protein-synthetic events that alter the organism's AT-TENTION and behaviour toward sexual and reproductive ends. Some steroid hormones are converted to their behaviourally active meta-bolites within the brain itself. For example, circulating testosterone is converted to estra-diol within neurons of the MEDIAL PREOPTIC AREA by the hydroxylating enzyme AROMA-TASE. Estradiol then binds to estrogen receptors to activate proteins necessary for masculine sexual behaviours. In contrast, estradiol and progesterone binding in the ventromedial hy-pothalamus and medial preoptic area activates proteins necessary for feminine sexual beha-viours (for example, oxytocin receptors). Ster-oid hormones also induce growth of peripheral reproductive tissues. For example, ovarian estradiol causes the growth of the endometrial layer of the uterus, and testicular testosterone facilitates the growth and maintenance of the prostate gland. Some peptides secreted from the anterior pituitary into the bloodstream act as gonadotrophic hormones. Both FSH and LH secretion occur in response to GnRH release from cells in the preoptic area/anterior hy-pothalamus that make contact with the pitui-tary vasculature. In females, FSH acts on the ovaries to stimulate the development of the follicle, whereas in males it stimulates the development of sperm. In males, LH secretion sensitizes androgen synthesis in the testes, whereas in females it stimulates the release of the ovum. Prolactin is normally secreted in daily pulses from the anterior pituitary. How-ever, prolactin secretion increases dramatically around the time of parturition and sensitizes milk production in mammary tissues. Finally, both oxytocin and vasopressin originate in cells of the SUPRAOPTIC and PARAVENTRICULAR NU-CLEI OF THE HYPOTHALAMUS which send axons into the posterior pituitary, where they make contact with the bloodstream. These peptides play an important role in pair bond-ing, maternal bonding, and other forms of parental behaviours.

See also: estrus; hormones and cognition; maternal behaviour; organization effects of steroid hormones; pregnancy; reproduction; sex differences; sexual dimorphism

JAMES G. PFAUS

sex steroids The sex steroids are STEROID HORMONES that have an effect on sexual activity, the reproductive organs and so on. There are four major classes of steroid hor-mones: one, the CORTICOSTEROIDS, have no specific effect on sexual functions and are not classed as sex steroids. The other three are all derived from PREGNENOLONE: the PROGESTO-GENS, ANDROGENS and ESTROGENS (also spelt oestrogens). The biosynthetic pathways of these are interrelated: pregnenolone is a pre-cursor of the progestagens, the progestagens are precursors to androgens and androgens can give rise to estrogens.

See also: endocrine glands; hormones; hormones – classification; sex hormones

sexual arousal Autonomic arousal (both SYM-PATHETIC and PARASYMPATHETIC) that occurs in response to sexual stimuli. This is typically inferred from increased blood flow to the penis or vagina, and can be measured in men and women by MERCURY-IN-RUBBER STRAIN GAUGES or PLETHYSMAGRAPHS, respectively. Other erectile responses – for example, of the nipples – can also be interpreted in terms of sexual arousal, as can traditional physiological measures of increased heart rate and GALVANIC SKIN RESPONSE. Although subjective measures of sexual arousal exist, the exact definition of arousal may differ between individuals. Dis-orders of sexual arousal can occur following STRESS or DRUG ABUSE.

See also: EPOR model of sexual excitement; erection; impotence; sexual motivation

JAMES G. PFAUS

sexual behaviour Any behaviour that in-creases sexual excitement and SEXUAL AROUSAL or fulfils sexual desires. Sexual behaviour may be viewed in terms of appetitive responses that increase sexual excitement and bring animals into contact with sexually-relevant stimuli or sexually receptive partners, and consummatory responses such as masturbation or copulation, that serve to fulfil sexual desire. Although sexual behaviour plays an obvious role in REPRODUCTION, it also serves other functional endpoints, such as PLEASURE and REWARD. In fact, many 'inappropriate' appetitive and consummatory sexual responses can be conditioned by sexual reward.

For all animals, sexual behaviour occurs as a sequence or cascade of behavioural events. For copulation to occur at all, animals must be capable of responding to a variety of internal and external cues. They must be able to respond to hormonal and neurochemical changes that signal their own sexual excitement, arousal, and receptivity, to identify external stimuli that predict where potential sex partners can be found, to actively seek out or work to obtain sex partners, to distinguish pheromonal cues (see PHEROMONES) or behavioural patterns of potential sex partners from those that are not sexually receptive and to attract, solicit and pursue desired sex partners once contact has been made. Most of these appetitive responses occur before copulation is initiated and can be used to make inferences concerning such motivational variables as SEX DRIVE, LIBIDO, sexual arousal and desire, distinct from copulatory performance. An animal's ability to perform these responses requires a great deal of behavioural flexibility and the capacity to learn which stimuli or responses are the most predictable or efficacious, respectively. In fact, such learning may play an important role in the development of sexual preferences and erotic orientation.

Once contact is made, animals engage in more stereotypic, species-specific and gender-specific patterns of copulation. An exception to this is humans, in which there are no real gender-specific copulatory behaviours (except those that are culturally based). In species in which the females display ESTRUS cycles, copulation is typically under the complete control of the female. In such species, females do not show sexual receptivity until they are in behavioural estrus or HEAT, when ovarian steroids have activated the appropriate neurochemical systems and neuroanatomical pathways for FEMININE sexual behaviour (for instance in the MEDIAL PREOPTIC AREA and VENTROMEDIAL HYPOTHALAMUS). Females in estrus attract, solicit and pace the rate of sexual contact with desired males, which in turn, provides them with the requisite type of sexual stimulation (for example, vaginocervical stimulation) necessary to promote PREGNANCY

if insemination occurs. In contrast, males will pursue, mount and intromit (see INTROMISSION) one or more receptive partners in a seemingly non-discriminatory fashion until they become sexually exhausted (for example, from repeated ejaculations) or the females terminate estrus. However, males of some mammalian species (rodents for example) are capable of learning to direct their ejaculations to females that bear conditioned extroceptive cues (such as odours). For males, consummatory copulatory responses are under the control of testicular steroids which maintain the integrity of peripheral sex organs and activate the appropriate neurochemical systems and neuroanatomical pathways for MASCULINE sexual behaviour. In males of many species, the aromatization (see AROMATIC) of androgens into estrogens within certain brain regions (for instance, medial preoptic area) is crucial for copulatory responses to occur because estrogen activity in these regions promotes masculine copulatory responses. However, some male primates retain masturbation following castration long after copulatory responses have declined. Even in egg-laying species in which fertilization occurs externally, males often make contact with females (which in some cases helps to promote egg-laying) prior to ejaculation. Interestingly, in some parthenogenetic females (certain whiptail lizards for instance; see PARTHENOGENESIS) 'male' copulatory stimulation (for example mounting and clasping) by another female CONSPECIFIC is necessary to promote ovulation and self-fertilization.

Sexual reward shares many features of drug reward. Copulation activates the MESOLIMBICOCORTICAL SYSTEM in male rats in a manner similar to low, self-administered doses of AMPHETAMINE. Ejaculation in male rats also induces the release of endogenous opioids, and promotes HIPPOCAMPAL THETA rhythm, SLEEP, the modulation of PAIN, and the reduction of ANXIETY. Although intromissions alone are capable of sustaining the development and maintenance of copulatory responses in male rats, ejaculation appears necessary for the development of certain conditioned sexual responses and unconditioned parental behaviours. Until recently, there has been little evidence that females of many species find sexual behaviour rewarding. Although ovarian steroids facilitate appetitive sexual responses in females, certain types of sexual stimulation (for instance vaginocervical stimulation) lead to a faster termination of both appetitive and consummatory sexual behaviour. However, female rats show a CONDITIONED PLACE PREFERENCE for distinctive environments in which they can pace the copulatory contact, compared to other environments in which they cannot. In contrast, some female primates are capable of ORGASM and appear to derive as much pleasure and reward from it as males do.

See also: EPOR model of sexual excitement; sex differences; sex hormones; sexual motivation

JAMES G. PFAUS

sexual differentiation The biological process by which GENDER is formed. During the first trimester of prenatal development, all foetuses are sexually bipotential, having primordial GONADS and two sets of INTERNAL GENITALIA. The presence of the Y CHROMOSOME (see X AND Y CHROMOSOMES) normally differentiates a foetus into a male because it contains a GENE (*Sry*) which codes for a protein (H-Y antigen) that promotes TESTOSTERONE secretion and helps to inhibit the growth of the MÜLLERIAN INTERNAL GENITALIA (female). The result is the strengthening of the WOLFFIAN INTERNAL GENITALIA (male), and the subsequent differentiation of the gonads and other dimorphic structures (such as CENTRAL NERVOUS SYSTEM).

See also: organization effects of steroid hormones; puberty; sex differences; sexual dimorphism

JAMES G. PFAUS

sexual dimorphism Any anatomical, physiological, or behavioural difference between genders in a bisexual species. Obvious and robust gender differences exist in chromosome type (see X AND Y CHROMOSOMES), gonadal structure and function (see GONADS), BODY WEIGHT, muscle development, fat disposition, secondary sex characteristics, hormone release and action, and gender-specific behaviours (for example aggression, sexual, parental behaviours, differences in general activity, responsiveness

to certain drugs, cognitive abilities and so on). Sexual dimorphisms also exist in brain structure, for example within hormone-concentrating regions of the MEDIAL PREOPTIC AREA, BED NUCLEUS OF THE STRIA TERMINALIS, parastrial nucleus, and SPINAL CORD (spinal nucleus of the bulbocavernosus), that may underlie behavioural dimorphisms.

See also: feminine; gender; hormones and cognition; organization effects of steroid hormones; puberty; reproduction; sex differences; sex hormones; sexual behaviour; sexual differentiation

JAMES G. PFAUS

sexual motivation A concept with heuristic value that provides logical order and strength to different components of SEXUAL BEHAVIOUR, such as SEXUAL AROUSAL, INCENTIVE, DRIVE, excitement and performance. Sexual motivation reflects the theoretical sum of all internal and external processes that strengthen and weaken the likelihood of a particular sexual behaviour. For example, a male that has copulated to sexual exhaustion and ignores an incentive female is said to have less sexual motivation than a fresh male that attends to the incentive. Although by definition, all sexual behaviours are sexually motivated, an animal may possess sexual motivation without performing a sexual response.

See also: EPOR model of sexual excitement; erection; homosexual

JAMES G. PFAUS

sexual seizure *see* hypersexuality

sexually dimorphic nucleus of the preoptic area *see* preoptic area

shaking palsy An old term, not used any longer, describing PARKINSON'S DISEASE.

shallow encoding *see* levels of processing

sham feeding An experimental procedure in which animals are equipped with a CATHETER in the OESOPHAGOUS or STOMACH leading out of the body. All of the food and water that is taken into the mouth and swallowed fails to be digested. It is a technique only rarely used; it enables the contribution of oral mechanisms to the control of FEEDING to be examined.

sham lesion A control procedure: when making a chemical LESION one injects the VEHICLE only, and when making electrolytic or radio-frequency lesions one inserts the ELECTRODE but passes no current. Animals receiving sham lesions should receive all parts of the surgical procedure necessary for the production of a lesion, with the one exception being that the toxin or current itself is not delivered.

sham rage Heightened emotionality following interference with brain systems: it can be produced experimentally in animals and has been observed after brain damage in patients, where it is typically expressed as hostility. The TEMPORAL LOBE and associated LIMBIC SYSTEM structures are thought to be involved in this.

See also: aggression; septal rage

shape constancy *see* object constancy

shaping Shaping is the learning process by which animals form a new behaviour – that is, how they shape an appropriate response. There are two processes involved: first, animals can make successive approximations to the response required (or the maximally efficient response). Each improvement is positively reinforced (see POSITIVE REINFORCEMENT) thereby gradually improving the response until it reaches the required form. Second, the failure to REWARD (or provide NEGATIVE REINFORCEMENT) earlier approximations to the correct response will lead to the suppression of inappropriate forms of responding. Shaping can be used to train both OPERANT responses and UNCONDITIONED BEHAVIOUR.

See also: autoshaping; schedules of reinforcement

Reference

Domjan M. (1993) *Domjan and Burkhard's The Principles of Learning and Behavior*, revised by M. Domjan, Brooks/Cole Publishing: Pacific Grove CA.

shell (nucleus accumbens) *see* nucleus accumbens

shiverer mutant mouse *see* jimpy mutant mouse

shivering *see* thermoregulation

shivers down the spine The thrill of having shivers go up (or down) ones spine is a very common one, and is typically associated with states of high EMOTION. Both FEAR and PLEASURE are reported anecdotally to send shivers down the spine (though whether they in fact travel up or down – or both – is uncertain. Literature has it that shivers go down the spine but informal investigation suggests that many people experience them travelling upwards). Problems in controlling the initiation of these – they appear (again anecdotally) to be utterly involuntary – as well as the problem of having no means for measuring them, has meant that there is no scientific literature concerning this phenomenon. It may very well be related to PILOERECTION along the spine, a vestige of our more hairy ancestors.

short-term memory Often termed IMMEDIATE MEMORY, ICONIC MEMORY, or SENSORY MEMORY, it is essentially memory for information which has not yet left conscious processing, though some debate as to the classification of this type of memory has arisen. Short-term memory is often likened to a memory buffer, in which a very limited store of information can be held for a very brief period of time. This concept was originally proposed by William James (1842–1910) who differentiated immediate memory from a more long-lasting memory. Through further study, the definition of short-term memory became more specific and better understood on both cognitive and cellular levels. Unfortunately, the definition is not clear in all branches of psychology and neuroscience.

One widely accepted definition of short term memory comes from the neuropsychological literature (see NEUROPSYCHOLOGY). Early attempts to explain short-term memory are operational and established through the demands of tasks which tested it. This has proven an effective, in fact the most effective way to differentiate between short-term memory and other memory systems. This early definition described short-term memory as the length of time for which information could be stored without REHEARSAL. Essentially this constitutes a very brief, near AFTERIMAGE span, lasting no more than a few seconds. Since short-term memory is thought of as an active 'buffer', it is additionally limited by the capacity of the buffer. The capacity of short-term memory is seven plus or minus two chunks of information. Thus if subjects are given a DIGIT SPAN TASK in which they are asked to remember as many numbers as possible from a list of digits, they will be able to remember approximately seven digits. Short-term memory is thus limited not only by the amount of time through which a memory can be retained, but also the amount of information which can be stored. This is in contrast to LONG-TERM MEMORY which is not limited in either the length of time of retention or the amount of information which can be stored. Short-term memory is susceptible to factors in the order of presentation, the cognitive load, and the delay between presentation and test. Material which is presented first or most recently tends to be remembered better than that presented in the middle (PRIMACY and RECENCY respectively – see SERIAL POSITION EFFECT). Since subjects, by definition, are not permitted to rehearse the information in short-term memory, any substantial delay will prohibit the retention of any information. Essentially this allows for a short-lasting memory capacity for information which is not currently being processed consciously. Short-term memory is thought to be a lingering activation in specific sensory realms. If, for instance, a subject is shown a series of objects on a screen, the subject will be able to recall some of the objects for a very brief period of time after exposure, after which time memory traces will diminish. Increasing the intensity of the image causes an increased length of time through which the memory will be sustained. This is thought to be controlled by short-term changes in the sensory receptor. Another possible mechanism is the generation of a REVERBERATING CIRCUIT. In this proposal there is an excitatory input which initiates a cascade of excitatory signals within a closed neural circuit. The memory is sustained as an active interaction in the brain. Differentiated from long-term memory, short-term memory does not require new synthesis of PROTEINS, rather it depends on the modification of existing proteins.

Another memory system, WORKING MEMORY, shares similar characteristics to short-term memory. The two memory systems are distinguished through specific task requirements. Short-term memory is similar to working memory in that it involves a memory buffer which is relatively short-lasting. One major difference between the two types of memory, however, is the cognitive demands placed on the subject. Whereas in short-term memory the subjects are not permitted to rehearse the information to be retained, working memory allows a subject to use any cognitive tool available to them in order to remember the information. The investigation and differentiation of these two memory systems has been carried out through the development of several tasks. One such task is the TWO BACK TASK in which the subject is asked continuously to remember and update information in their memory buffers. Because this task places a high explicit cognitive demand on the subject, rehearsal is not possible, thus this task provides an assessment of short term rather than working memory.

Short-term memory is believed to be dependent on perceptual structures in the sensory NEOCORTEX. Thus, short-term memory is one spared domain in human AMNESIA. Human amnesia provides a dissociation between long- and short-term memory. Long-term memory is impaired in amnesia and is dependent on structures in the MEDIAL TEMPORAL LOBE and DIENCEPHALON. Short-term memory is preserved in amnesia and is presumably dependent on sensory cortical areas. Short- and long-term memory can also be differentiated through the human verbal field. PHONETIC MEMORY, or the sensory memory for sound, can be controlled short-term verbal memory. SEMANTIC MEMORY, or the memory for verbal content requires long-term memory. The sparing of short-term memory has thus become a requirement for validation of an animal model of amnesia.

Outside of the psychological literature, the definition of short-term memory is considerably more controversial. Nearly every strain of animal, and many behavioural or cellular assays depends on a different definition of short-term memory. In *Drosophila melanogaster* – the fruit fly – for instance, the characteristics of long-term memory are understood on a behavioural and cellular level. Short-term memory in these animals is often classified as anything which does not meet the requirements of long-term memory. Because long-term memory is known to depend on the creation of new proteins, and short-term mechanisms are somewhat more ambiguous, the definition of short-term memory, particularly on a cellular or molecular level, is often dependent on the absence of long-term memory. However, since protein generation required for long-term memory takes time, the span of short-term memory is considerably lengthened in these animals. Thus in some realms, short-term memory can last up to 4 hours, quite a divergence from the few seconds generously allocated in humans.

HOWARD EICHENBAUM

short-term potentiation *see* long-term potentiation

shoulder cortex An area of FRONTAL CORTEX of the RAT, located on the dorsal surface of the medial wall, medial to PRIMARY MOTOR CORTEX. Lacking granular layer 4 (see AGRANULAR CORTEX; CORTICAL LAYERS), this area is also called MEDIAL AGRANULAR CORTEX. It is designated Fr2 in the atlas of Paxinos & Watson (1986), after the nomenclature of Zilles (1985). In their more recent atlas, Paxinos & Watson (1997) designate it M2, in order to stress its homology to the secondary motor cortex and FRONTAL EYE FIELDS of PRIMATES.

References

Paxinos G. & Watson C. (1986) *The Rat Brain in Stereotaxic Coordinates*, 2nd edn, Academic Press: San Diego.
—— (1997) *The Rat Brain in Stereotaxic Coordinates*, compact 3rd edn, Academic Press: San Diego.
Zilles K. (1985) *The Cortex of the Rat: A Stereotaxic Atlas*, Springer-Verlag: Berlin.

VERITY J. BROWN

Shy–Drager syndrome Progressive failure of the AUTONOMIC NERVOUS SYSTEM. This syndrome, like OLIVOPONTOCEREBELLAR ATROPHY and PARKINSON'S DISEASE, is an instance of MULTIPLE SYSTEM ATROPHY. In this case the cells most affected are preganglionic sympathetic neurons situated in the LATERAL HORN of the SPINAL CORD, but striatonigral and olivo-

pontocerebellar cell loss is also common. The resulting autonomic impairment is marked by progressively worsening postural hypotension, urinary incontinence, impotence and loss of sweating. Onset occurs in adulthood, occasionally by inheritance as a Mendelian AUTOSOMAL DOMINANT, but its incidence is more usually sporadic. There is no effective specific treatment.

L. JACOB HERBERG

SI units Si stands for Système International (d'Unités) – the system of units used in measurement. The measures of main interest to biological psychologists are: length, measured in metres (m) and area, measured in square metres (m^2); volume, measured in litres (l); and mass (weight), measured in grams (g). The SI unit of time is the second (s) and of temperature, the kelvin (K), which has absolute zero for zero. In practice, for temperature centigrade is used (degrees C: 0 °C is the freezing point of water, 100 °C the boiling point at standard pressure). Units can all have prefixes placed in front of them to indicate multiplying factors. For example, a kilogram (kg) is 1000 g, a millilitre (ml) one thousandth of a litre. The prefixes used are as shown in the adjacent table.

These prefixes – either the full term or the abbreviation – are simply added to the unit being used, e.g. g, m, l or s. It is important to use the abbreviations in the case given here: for example, m is a milli-, a millionth; M is mega-, one million times. One would not wish to get these confused: one might, for example, order thousands times more of a chemical than one required, and have to pay for it.

Siamese twins *see* parabiosis

sibutramine *see* serotonin–noradrenaline reuptake inhibitor

side-effects *see* magic bullet

Sidman avoidance A procedure, named after its originator, which requires animals to repeat timed responses to avoid brief unsignalled FOOTSHOCK delivered at regular intervals. For example, footshock can be given every 5 seconds except if a lever press occurs. By

Orders of magnitude

Prefix	Abbreviation	Factor	Description	Number
tera	T	10^{12}	one million million times	1,000,000,000,000
giga	G	10^{9}	one thousand million times	1,000,000,000
mega	M	10^{6}	one million times	1,000,000
kilo	k	10^{3}	one thousand times	1000
deci	d	10^{-1}	one tenth	0.1
centi	c	10^{-2}	one hundredth	0.01
milli	m	10^{-3}	one thousandth	0.001
micro	μ	10^{-6}	one millionth	0.000001
nano	n	10^{-9}	one thousand millionth	0.000000001
pico	p	10^{-12}	one million millionth	0.000000000001
femto	f	10^{-15}	one thousand million millionth	0.000000000000001
ato	a	10^{-18}	one million million millionth	0.000000000000000001

making regularly spaced lever presses the animal avoids the shock.

See also: animal models of anxiety

Reference

Sidman M. (1953) Avoidance conditioning with brief shock and no exteroceptive warning stimulus. *Science* 118: 157–158.

sign language A gestural LANGUAGE used by the deaf and hearing-impaired. Many sign languages exist, having developed separately from spontaneous gestural systems of deaf people in different lands, and sign languages are, unless related, not mutually intelligible. The GRAMMAR of sign language is as abstract and complex as that of spoken language; its realization in space exhibits structure analogous to the PHONOLOGY of spoken language; and sign languages possess universal characteristics found in all natural languages. Early exposure to sign language exploits the deaf child's language-learning abilities and can avoid cognitive development being slowed by the unavailability of auditory language input.

See also: auditory perception; deafness

ANNE CUTLER

sign tracking Synonym for AUTOSHAPING.

signal detection theory Signal detection theory proposes that sensory thresholds estimated experimentally do not simply depend on the strength of the stimulus, but also on the criterion (the willingness to state 'yes, a signal has occurred') that the observer may adopt. This criterion in turn is influenced by the payoff for a correct detection and the penalty for a false positive.

DAVID W. HEELEY

signal-to-noise ratio The relative strengths of the signal and the sum of the extraneous factors which may be caused by random events that are uncorrelated with the presentation of the signal, collectively referred to as NOISE.

DAVID W. HEELEY

signal transduction *see* transduction

signs and symptoms Disorders can have signs and symptoms: signs are overt observable behaviours; symptoms are reported experiences.

silent synapse A SYNAPSE which is present but not participating in signaling. If LONG-TERM POTENTIATION (LTP) is induced, any RECEPTOR which was inactive can be activated. This is thought to involve the recruitment of previously silent synapses.

simple reaction time *see* reaction time

simple, complex and hypercomplex cells
Neurons of the PRIMARY VISUAL CORTEX are exquisitely sensitive to the orientation of a stimulus. Only bars within 15 to 30° of the optimal orientation for a given neuron are capable of eliciting a response, while different neurons respond best to different orientations. These orientation selective cells can be divided into three different classes on the basis of their spatial structure. Simple cells are defined by the presence in their receptive fields of two or more adjacent ON or OFF sub-regions. Each sub-region is elongated parallel to the cell's preferred orientation, and adjacent sub-regions are displaced from one another in the direction perpendicular to the orientation axis. Properly oriented bright bars flashed in an ON region excite the cell, and dark bars inhibit it. Dark bars flashed in an OFF region excite the cell, and bright bars inhibit it. Simple cell responses to moving stimuli are related to the sub-field structure: a moving bright bar will evoke a response as it moves out of an OFF region or into an ON region. The RECEPTIVE FIELD of complex cells cannot be subdivided in the way that simple receptive fields can. If a flashing bright bar excites the cell in one part of its receptive field, then it will do so throughout. Thus the entire receptive field will be ON, OFF or ON/OFF in character. Unlike simple cells, complex cells' responses to moving bars cannot be predicted from the receptive field structure: ACTION POTENTIAL activity is evoked during the entire traverse of the receptive field by the stimulus. Both simple and complex cells can be sensitive to the direction of motion of a stimulus (see DIRECTION SELECTIVITY), to BINOCULAR DISPARITY, and to stimulus length. In length sensitive, or end-inhibited cells, the response increases with stimulus length up to a point. But once the stimulus length exceeds the optimal, the response will fall. Complex cells that exhibited length selectivity were once called hypercomplex cells, but since length selective simple cells were found this term has gradually fallen into disuse. In the cat, simple cells receive strong input from neurons of the LATERAL GENICULATE NUCLEUS. The elongated ON and OFF sub-regions are created by excitatory input from groups of relay cells whose receptive fields are arranged in rows, rows of ON-centre cells giving rise to ON sub-regions, and OFF-centre cells to OFF regions. Some complex cells, in turn receive excitatory input from other simple cells of the same preferred orientation, but of slightly offset positions.

See also: motion perception object recognition; retina

DAVID L. FERSTER

simultagnosia An inability to perceive more than one object at a time. For example, if two objects were shown to a patient with simultagnosia they would only be able to recognize one of them at a time. Either could be recognized independently. The existence of such a phenomenon implies that different objects are processed independently in the brain and that it is possible to restrict the numbers of simultaneously recognized objects.

See also: ataxia; Balint's syndrome; object agnosia; object recognition

simultaneous extinction Used interchangeably with EXTINCTION to refer to a deficit of visual, auditory or tactile perception due to lateralized brain damage. The term simultaneous links the symptom with the standard assessment method of presenting simultaneous stimulation bilaterally to left and right ears, body parts, or each VISUAL FIELD. Extinction can be evoked across modalities (for example, left hand, right hemifield) and it can occur between stimuli presented to the same side of the body: Left extinction can manifest when a right visual field stimulus is extinguished by another stimulus presented further to the right in that same hemifield.

See also: contralateral neglect

PATRICIA A. REUTER-LORENZ

sine wave gratings A visual stimulus comprising a series of alternating light and dark 'fuzzy' bars. The luminance profile is a sinusoid. Stimuli of these type have been used extensively in the development of the theory of SPATIAL FREQUENCY CHANNELS, and in physiological investigations of NEURON properties in the vertebrate VISUAL SYSTEM.

DAVID W. HEELEY

single blind study *see* double blind study

single photon emission tomography *see* SPECT

single spiking A state in which a NEURON produces an individual ACTION POTENTIAL, in contrast to BURST FIRING.

single unit A single NEURON; see SINGLE-UNIT ELECTROPHYSIOLOGICAL RECORDING

single unit electrophysiological recording (or more simply, single unit recording) A technique used to examine the ACTION POTENTIAL activity of a single NEURON (or SINGLE UNIT). The purpose is to characterize the conditions responsible for producing action potentials in that neuron. For example in a sensory system the stimulus can be altered to produce an increase or a decrease in firing. These changes in firing rate can be analysed to determine the neuron's RECEPTIVE FIELD and the relationship between stimulus intensity and neuronal response, as in the classic experiments of Vernon Mountcastle in the SOMATO-SENSORY system and of David Hubel and Torsten Wiesel in the VISUAL SYSTEM (for which they received the Nobel Prize for Medicine in 1981). Comparison of receptive fields with other nearby neurons can be used to determine the organization of a particular brain region (see MAPS). Comparison of response properties within one region can be compared with those of its inputs to determine how that region processes or transforms information. The use of single-unit recordings in the motor regions of awake animals was introduced by Edward Evarts. Correlation of cell firing with the contraction of various muscles or with movement in space can be used to determine how different brain regions contribute to the production of movement

The technique consists of inserting a high impedance MICROELECTRODE (see ELECTRODE) into the CNS: electrodes can be repeatedly inserted through surgically implanted guide tubes or more permanently implanted (see STEREOTAXIC SURGERY). If conscious, behaving animals are used, permanent implantation is not recommended. The high impedance ensures that the action potentials of only one or a few neurons that are close to the microelec-

trode tip will be recorded. The electrical potential recorded at the microelectrode tip must be amplified several thousand times and filtered. This signal can then be monitored visually on an oscilloscope or made audible via a stereo speaker. This signal can be stored on various analogue tape recorders or on computer for later analysis. The size and shape of the action potential from a given neuron depend on several factors, the most important of which are the size of the neuron and the distance between the microelectrode tip and the neuron. It is often possible, therefore, to record from several neurons at once (MULTI-UNIT RECORDING) and separate the action potentials from different neurons either at the time of recording (on-line analysis) or after the experiment (off-line analysis).

The recording of neurons from human patients before or during brain surgery is often carried out. Indeed, because different neurons in the brain have characteristic firing patterns it is possible to record these as an electrode travels slowly down through brain. By listening for these neuronal signatures, neurosurgeons can identify very accurately where the electrode is in the brain. This can help them target exactly the tissue they might wish to excise from brain (by making an ELECTROLYTIC LESION using the electrode they have been recording with – see PALLIDOTOMY for example).

DOUGLAS D. RASMUSSON

sinistral (from Latin, *sinister*: left) Left-handed (see HANDEDNESS).

See also: dextral

sinus A sinus is either a cavity in bone or a blood vessel; see BLOOD.

sissy boy syndrome *see* gender identity disorder of childhood

size constancy *see* object constancy

skeletal muscle *see* muscles

skeleton The system of bones or other hard tissue that provides a framework for an organism; an animal may have an *endoskeleton* (inside the body; as humans and all vertebrates) or an *exoskeleton* (outer casings covering the body tissues; as beetles, etc.). The

CYTOSKELETON is an internal frame supporting individual cells.

See also: skull

skill learning The acquisition of coordinated perceptual–motor mechanisms dedicated to accomplishing a specific task. Skills research in psychology, MOTOR CONTROL and ergonomics have investigated tasks ranging from relatively simple routines such as opening a can or tracking a visual target with a hand-held stylus, to the more complex SENSORIMOTOR activities required in high-level sports. Central research questions in skill learning include the degree to which sensorimotor routines require CLOSED LOOP or OPEN LOOP movements (that is, how sensory feedback about movements are used to control task performance; see CLOSED LOOP, OPEN LOOP); the degree of automaticity of a an acquired skill; and attentional/cognitive factors in acquisition and successful task performance.

DAVID P. CAREY

skin (from Old Norse, *skinn*) Skin is the outer covering of an animal (though of course the term is also used to describe a variety of other coverings). It is a body's first line of defence against infection (see IMMUNE SYSTEM); important in RESPIRATION and THERMOREGULATION; involved in the excretion of fluids and salts; important in the formation of certain VITAMINS (skin is the main source of vitamin D, which requires PHOTIC energy for its formation); skin pigmentation helps protect against the damaging effects of ultraviolet light; and is the largest sensory organ – 3 to 6 square metres for a human – primarily through its processing of HAPTIC information (relating to TOUCH) and PAIN processing.

Skin is made of three layers, each composed of various types of CELL. The outer layer is the EPIDERMIS. This is relatively thin compared to the other layers, though its exact texture depends on location: the palms of the hands or soles of the feet have a relatively thick epidermis compared to more delicate structures. Despite being thin in comparison with other skin cell layers, the epidermis is still complex. It has distinct layers of cells, some further divided: the horny layer (divided into

stratum corneum and *stratum lucidum*), granular layer (or *stratum granulosum*), squamous cell layer (or *stratum spinosum*) and basal layer (or *stratum basale*). (These layers together are known as SQUAMOUS EPITHELIUM.) Cells of the epidermis are constantly shed, new cells replacing sloughed off dead ones. (It is a rather queasy fact that most household dust is in fact dead skin cells which forms the food for house dust mites.) A line of cells – the EPIDERMAL BORDER or DERMAL-EPIDERMAL JUNCTION – separates the epidermis from the DERMIS, a broader layer of tissue which divides into the papillary dermis and reticular dermis. It contains NERVE fibres, CONNECTIVE TISSUE (it is especially rich in COLLAGEN), BLOOD vessels, SWEAT GLANDS (which connect, via ducts through the epidermis, to sweat pores on the skin surface) and SEBACEOUS GLANDS (which secret sebum, a fatty, lubricating, substance: it is this that produces 'greasiness' in skin and hair). The specialized growths of skin – hair, feathers, claws and so on – originate in the dermis. Below the dermis is a third layer, SUBCUTANEOUS TISSUE, mainly containing FAT CELLS. (Note that the term subcutaneous indicates tissue below the cutis, this being more or less synonymous with dermis. The cutis is contrasted with the *cuticle*, or outermost layer of dead skin in MAMMALS or the hard shell that covers many INVERTEBRATES. *Cutaneous* is an adjective relating to skin: CUTANEOUS SENSATION is sensation arising from the skin.)

Hair originates in the skin, and most skin can be characterized as hairy skin. GLABROUS SKIN is the term given to those parts of the skin that have no hairs – the palms of the hands and soles of the feet. Hairs originate in HAIR FOLLICLES, found deep in the dermis near the subcutaneous layer. In the human, there are thought to be about 5 million of these. They are complex structures that give rise to cells that become coated in keratin (they are *keratinized*): it is the keratinized portion that protrudes out of the skin. The principal function of hair is to protect against loss of heat, which it does by trapping air, though specialized hairs (such as the hairs in the nose) may have other protective functions, and the VIBRISSAE of rodents have specialized sensory functions. Hair follicles have a neural input (and there are HAIR FOLLICLE RECEPTORS, divisible into *hair-guard*, *hair-tylotrich* and *hair-down* sub-types) that allow motor control of the hairs (important in thermoregulation) and transmit sensory information, working in much the same way as HAIR CELLS in other sensory systems: it is the degree of bending of the hair that can generate an ACTION POTENTIAL.

Within skin are various types of sensory RECEPTOR. In the epidermis this is the FREE NERVE ENDING, important in transmitting information relating to pain. Within the dermis are five types of receptor: MEISSNER'S CORPUSCLES and MERKEL'S DISKS (just below the epidermal border); PACINIAN CORPUSCLES, RUFFINI'S ENDINGS and KRAUSE'S END BULBS (deeper in the dermis). These are discriminated by location, function, the relative sizes of their RECEPTIVE FIELD and by the type of neural activation they produce (see table).

Information from these receptors is transmitted to the CENTRAL NERVOUS SYSTEM via SOMATOSENSORY PATHWAYS. The qualities of skin sensation that can be discriminated by humans are very varied, ranging from simple pressure, through tickle to pain. Qualities such as 'smooth' and 'wet' can also be discriminated. The relationships between our psychological experiences of skin sensation and the activation of particular receptor types is not a straightforward one in which activation of one type of receptor produces one pure form of sensation. Skin sensation is much more a product of higher-order integration and interoperation.

Theories concerned with information from the skin have been described as either SPECIFICITY THEORIES or PATTERN THEORIES. Specifity theorists have argued that separate qualities of skin sensation (touch, temperature and pain for example) are mediated by different types of

Sensory receptors of the skin

Receptor	Function	Location	Receptive field	Activation pattern	Fibre type
Meissner's corpuscle	Spatial discrimination; flutter	Epidermal border	Small, with clear edges	Fast adapting	A fibres (beta)
Merkel's disc	Touch - steady pressure	Epidermal border	Small, with clear edges	Slow adapting	A fibres (beta)
Pacinian corpuscle	Vibration	Dermis	Large, with indistinct edges	Fast adapting	A fibres (beta)
Ruffini's ending	Temperature Touch - steady pressure	Dermis	Large, with indistinct edges	Slow adapting	A fibres (beta)
Krause's end bulb	Temperature	Dermis			
Free nerve endings	Pain	Epidermis			A fibres C fibres
Hair follicle receptors	Touch Temparature	Dermis (hair follicles)			A fibres (beta) A fibres (delta)

Notes: Fast adapting responses: action potentials at the onset and offset of stimulation, but not necessarily in between. *Slow adapting responses:* action potentials present throughout stimulation.

receptor. Pattern theorists have argued that the type of receptor is less important and that the pattern of activation is what gives rise to discriminably different sensations. Both receptor type and activation pattern are probably of importance.

See also: dermatome; homunculus; mechanoreceptors; muscles; piloerection; skin conductance; somatosensory cortex

skin conductance Skin resistance refers to the electrical resistance of SKIN to electric current; SKIN CONDUCTANCE is the reverse of this, being a measure of electrical transmission across the skin. The term GALVANIC SKIN RESPONSE (after Luigi Galvani [1737–1798]) is synonymous with skin conductance. Skin conductance is typically measured on the palms of the hand (*palmar conductance*) but can also be measured on the forehead or elsewhere. It varies throughout the day, but increases when individuals are perspiring. It is taken to reflect activity in the SYMPATHETIC NERVOUS SYSTEM and is thought of as part of the FIGHT-OR-FLIGHT response. Psychologists have in the past used skin conductance as a measure of emotional AROUSAL (see also EMOTION), but considerable caution has to be exercised in doing this. Skin conductance is a crude measure, responsive to changes in a wide variety of psychological states and as such a poor measure with which to understand emotional states. See Grossman (1967) for discussion of the history of skin conductance.

See also: lie detection; polygraph

Reference

Grossman S.P. (1967) *Physiological Psychology*, Wiley: New York.

Skinner box Experimental chamber designed by B.F. Skinner (1904–1990) to study instrumental behaviour (see INSTRUMENTAL CONDITIONING) in animals. The chamber typically has two operandi (which may be retractable or fixed levers for a rat or lighted keys for a pigeon). There may be lights in the chamber which can be used, for example, as a DISCRIMINATIVE STIMULUS or a CONDITIONAL STIMULUS. There will also be a method for delivering REINFORCEMENT. This might be in the form of a food or liquid dispenser, or PUNISHMENT, such as a current generator to deliver FOOTSHOCK. The chambers are controlled and the responses are recorded automatically, usually by computer.

See also: learning; nine-hole box; nose poke vs. lever press; operant chamber

VERITY J. BROWN

skull (from Middle English, *scolle*) The term skull is in fact a rather colloquial term for what is more strictly called the CRANIUM (from Greek, *kranion*). The cranium is that part of the SKELETON associated with the head, face and lower jaw (the mandible). It forms part of the axial skeleton, which includes the cranium, vertebral column (the spinal column), ribs and sternum (breastbone), this being in contrast to the appendicular skeleton, which includes those parts associated with the arms and legs.

The cranium is not a solid box but an integrated selection of individual bones (see the adjacent table, 'The bones of the human skull'). The CRANIAL BONES are those that enclose the brain (forming the CRANIAL CAVITY, where the brain resides), while the FACIAL BONES are those that underlie the face and do not form part of the braincase (that is, the part of the cranium enclosing the brain: it is also known as the NEUROCRANIUM). The term CALVARIA is also used to describe the cranium without the facial bones (and the term CALOTTE refers to the calvaria without its base) and the term SPLANCHNOCRANIUM refers to the facial bones alone. The various bones of the cranium may be paired or unpaired: paired bones are obviously found on either side of the head, while the unpaired bones cross the MIDLINE. The lines where bones meet are plainly visible; they are known as SUTURES. The table lists the principle bones of the skull, indicating their approximate position.

The cranium is obviously intended to protect the brain, which is suspended within the MENINGES inside the cranial cavity. As such it is rarely of particular interest to biological psychologists. However, note that during STEREOTAXIC SURGERY, skull landmarks – BREGMA and LAMBDA – are used in order to locate positions in the underlying brain tissue. Any STEREOTAXIC ATLAS will also use these

The bones of the skull

Paired cranial bones

PARIETAL BONES | top of the cranium, paired right and left, covering approximately the area of the PARIETAL LOBE

TEMPORAL BONES | to the sides, paired left and right, covering approximately the area of the TEMPORAL LOBE: the AUDITORY MEATUS is present

Unpaired cranial bones

FRONTAL BONE | covering the FRONTAL LOBES from the parietal bones behind to the tops of the ORBITS OF THE EYE (the eye sockets)

OCCIPITAL BONE | covering the OCCIPITAL LOBES at the back of the head; contains the FORAMEN MAGNUM, through which the spinal cord joins the brain

SPHENOID BONE | at the base of the brain; connects facial and cranial bones

ETHMOID BONE | at the base of the brain; forms the CRIBRIFORM PLATE

Paired facial bones

LACHRYMAL BONES | (also spelt *lacrimal bones*); form the medial part of the orbits of the eye, by the tear ducts

NASAL BONES | form the bridge of the nose

ZYGOMATIC BONES | form part of the cheek, connecting frontal and temporal bones

MAXILLAE | form the upper jaw and teeth and the area immediately above, below the nose

PALATINE BONES | form part of the palate and nose

INFERIOR NASAL CONCHAE | form the lateral part of the nose

Unpaired facial bones

VOMER BONE | forms the nasal septum; see VOMERONASAL ORGAN

MANDIBLE | the lower jaw and teeth

HYOID BONE | found at the front of the throat above the LARYNX; does not connect to any of the other bones of the cranium

---

landmarks in presenting the anatomy of the brain section by section.

Reference

Technology and Learning Program of the California State University at Chico: see the website at http://www.csuchico.edu/anth/Module/skull.html

skull screws Small precision screws used to anchor a HEADCAP created from DENTAL ACRYLIC to the SKULL surface. Skull screws sit in bone and do not penetrate to the tissue below.

sleep Sleep is a BEHAVIOURAL STATE in mammals that is defined by recumbent postures, elevated sensory threshold and distinct polygraphic (see POLYGRAPH) signs. During sleep, there is little motor activity, the eyes are usually closed, and responses to external stimuli are greatly diminished compared to during wakefulness. There is also a loss of CONSCIOUSNESS and occasional DREAMING in humans. Unlike COMA, however, these conditions are reversible, and sleeping individuals or animals can be awakened by sufficiently strong stimuli. Sleep is not a homogeneous state but consists of two basic states: non-rapid eye movement sleep (NON-REM SLEEP, or SLOW-WAVE SLEEP) and REM SLEEP (rapid eye movement sleep). Non-REM sleep is classified further into four stages. These states and stages are best characterized by polygraphic recordings including the ELECTROENCEPHALOGRAM (EEG), ELECTROMYOGRAM (EMG) and ELECTRO-OCULOGRAM (EOG). Nocturnal sleep is organized in cycles, with a period of about 90 minutes in humans. Each cycle starts with wakefulness, which can be very brief or absent between cycles, and evolves through the stages of non-REM sleep and then REM sleep. REM sleep occurs only directly after stage 4 of non-REM sleep, and it will not occur if awakening follows non-REM sleep. Otherwise, reverse transitions between adjacent stages are not uncommon. In humans, the proportion of REM sleep in each cycle increases towards dawn. Dreaming occurs mostly during REM sleep, but some occurs during non-REM sleep.

Sleep is regulated by neuronal mechanisms located in both the BRAINSTEM and FOREBRAIN. REM sleep is thought to be induced by the activation of CHOLINERGIC neurons in the MESOPONTINE TEGMENTUM and ACETYLCHOLINE release in the PONTINE RETICULAR FORMATION, which in turn triggers ATONIA and the phasic components of REM sleep. MONOAMINERGIC neurons in the LOCUS COERULEUS and DORSAL RAPHE NUCLEUS are thought to have a permissive role in REM sleep induction, by disinhibiting the cholinergic neurons. At the same time, ascending pathways from the reticular formation activate the THALAMUS and forebrain structures to induce AROUSAL of the CEREBRAL CORTEX. The mechanisms for non-REM sleep are less well understood than for REM sleep. However, the PREOPTIC AREA in the HYPOTHALAMUS and the dorsal reticular formation of the MEDULLA including the NUCLEUS OF THE SOLITARY TRACT are thought to have a role in non-REM sleep. Humoural factors such as HORMONES, CYTOKINES and ADENOSINE have also been implicated in promotion of sleep. Sleep and wakefulness also show daily rhythms, and are controlled by the circadian clock (see BIOLOGICAL CLOCK; CIRCADIAN RHYTHM) located in the SUPRACHIASMATIC NUCLEUS of the hypothalamus. The

circadian pacemaker does not appear to affect sleep and arousal equally, but rather, promotes and maintains wakefulness at particular times in the circadian cycle.

The function of sleep remains speculative. The function of non-REM sleep is thought to be the restoration of bodily functions. In support of this notion, non-REM sleep represents the largest portion of sleep time, and is associated with decreases in autonomic functioning such as heart rate, blood pressure and rate of respiration, as well as increased release of GROWTH HORMONE, PROLACTIN and other hormones. In contrast, much less is known about the function of REM sleep. Unlike non-REM sleep, REM sleep is associated with elevated AUTONOMIC activity, although temperature regulation is lost. Penile erection occurs in males. Subjects awakened during REM sleep often report dreaming. These observations suggest that the brain is active during REM sleep. One hypothesis is that REM sleep helps to maintain the excitability of the cerebral cortex. This might have a role in the CONSOLIDATION of MEMORY in adults, and in stimulating the developing brain, as new-born babies sleep about 16 hours a day about half of which is spent in REM sleep. This cortical HOMEOSTASIS hypothesis is consistent with the view that REM sleep represents evolutionarily a more recent phenomenon than non-REM sleep because it is seen only in mammalian species.

KAZUE SEMBA

sleep apnoea Sleep apnoea is a form of APNOEA (American: apnea) that occurs during SLEEP. Individuals lose control of their breathing (see BREATHING, NEURAL CONTROL OF) due to abnormal accumulation of CARBON DIOXIDE in the BLOOD. This accumulation is registered by sensory mechanism in brain, triggering rapid waking.

See also: narcolepsy; sleep disorders

sleep attack A cardinal symptom of NARCOLEPSY, a sleep attack is an unpredictable bout of SLEEP during the daytime. Typically brief (less than 5 minutes), it involves what is apparently normal sleep that is not unpleasant. Sleep attacks are made dangerous if accompanied by CATAPLEXY – an involuntary loss of muscle power.

sleep disorders Sleep remains a somewhat mysterious phenomenon. Its importance is undoubted. During the course of EVOLUTION some animals have lost or substantially downgraded one or other of their special senses: bats and naked mole rats have lost vision for example, adapting to life at night or life underground. Sleep on the other hand is never lost. Indeed, animals will develop special means for retaining the ability to sleep. Dolphins and porpoises are known, for example, to be able to sleep with one HEMISPHERE of their brain at a time. The Indus dolphin, which lives in and around the estuary of the river Indus (which has muddy waters and much dangerous debris), sleeps in very brief bursts each lasting not much more than a minute, but cumulating to about 7 hours per day. That special mechanisms have evolved to accommodate sleep indicates its importance. However, despite this, the amount of sleep individuals require varies enormously: some humans must have a minimum of 8 hours per night to function effectively, others manage with much less. Similarly, sleep disorders can have exceptionally debilitating effects on an individuals cognitive and behavioural performance. Sleep disorders can be divided into three general categories. (1) There are two main disorders of REM SLEEP (rapid eye movement sleep): first, the inappropriate induction of bursts of sleep – NARCOLEPSY (which includes SLEEP ATTACK, CATAPLEXY, HYPNAGOGIC HALLUCINATION and HYPNOPOMPIC HALLUCINATION, and SLEEP PARALYSIS). Second, REM SLEEP BEHAVIOUR DISORDER (also known as REM WITHOUT ATONIA) in which the normal muscular inactivation (atonia) associated with REM sleep is absent, leading to often quite complex and significant movements. (2) Disorders of SLOW-WAVE SLEEP include BEDWETTING (NOCTURNAL ENURESIS), NIGHT TERRORS (*pavor nocturnis*) and SOMNAMBULISM (SLEEP-WALKING). These disorders are associated with the later stages of slow-wave sleep and are much more marked in children rather than in adults; they can in some instances though persist into adulthood. (3) INSOMNIA is a problem associated with the proper induction or maintenance of sleep and has several forms (DRUG DEPENDENCY INSOMNIA; MAINTENANCE INSOMNIA; ONSET INSOMNIA; TERMINATION INSOMNIA). SLEEP APNOEA is a form of insomnia in which individuals have difficulty breathing, causing them to wake up.

sleep paralysis One of the symptoms of NARCOLEPSY; sleep paralysis is an inability to move as SLEEP is either beginning or ending. When accompanied by HYPNAGOGIC HALLUCINATION or HYPNOPOMPIC HALLUCINATION it is rather frightening. Sleep paralysis is not the same as CATAPLEXY.

sleep spindles *see* electroencephalogram; K complex; sleep; slow-wave sleep

sleep–wake cycle This term refers to the alternation between SLEEP and wake states. In mammals, there are two distinct sleep states, SLOW-WAVE SLEEP and REM SLEEP (RAPID EYE MOVEMENT SLEEP, also called PARADOXICAL SLEEP) in addition to the wake state. One complete cycle passes through these three states, beginning for example in wake, passing through slow-wave sleep and ending with REM sleep, which always follows a period of slow-wave sleep. The length of this cycle differs across species and is correlated with both weight and metabolic rate, being short in mice (~10 minutes), intermediate in cats (~30 minutes), long in humans (~90 minutes) and the longest in elephants (~120 minutes). The cycle has an ULTRADIAN RHYTHM (occurring more than once per day). Young mammals sleep the majority of time with brief awakenings in each cycle. With maturity, sleep decreases, and sleep and waking become organized as a CIRCADIAN RHYTHM, with waking being concentrated in the night in nocturnal animals, like rodents and cats, or in the day in diurnal animals, like humans and elephants. In adult humans, approximately 5–6 cycles of sleep with brief AROUSAL or lightening in each cycle are completed in the night. Within each 90-minute cycle, a long period of slow-wave sleep precedes a shorter period of REM sleep. The length of REM sleep episodes increases during the night into early morning, attaining lengths of up to 45 minutes. Although adults (of Northern cultures) do not usually sleep during the day, they manifest changes in vigilance over a ~90-minute cycle, which is thus considered to represent a basal rest–activity cycle upon which the sleep–wake cycle rides.

Although much is understood concerning the organization and mechanisms of circadian rhythms, little is understood concerning ultradian rhythms such as the sleep–wake cycle. Circadian rhythms are entrained through the eye by light in mammals, however they depend upon AUTOCHTHONOUS rhythmic activity within the SUPRACHIASMATIC NUCLEUS that cycles in absence of light entrainment with a period of approximately one day. In recent years, genes (see GENE) have been isolated which may determine this ENDOGENOUS circadian activity. Given the strong correlation of metabolic rate and length of the sleep–wake cycle across species, it would appear that this ultradian rhythm must also be controlled by a cycle of gene expression determined by metabolic needs and establishing a basal rest–activity cycle of the brain and organism.

BARBARA E. JONES

sleep walking *see* somnambulism

slice In neuroscience the term slice refers to a section of fresh tissue (typically BRAIN) that has been cut on a VIBRATOME for use in *in vitro* experiments that will allow analysis of dynamic functions. Much electrophysiological work (see ELECTROPHYSIOLOGY; NEUROPHYSIOLOGY) is carried out in slice preparations: they allow experimenters considerable degrees of control over brain tissue.

slips of the tongue Speech errors, involving mis-selection, misordering or misformation of parts of an intended utterance. Slips of the tongue are not intentional (as puns or word play), nor do they result from deficits in articulatory (as a lisp) or linguistic competence (as misuse of a word); they arise through temporary malfunction of the normal processes of SPEECH PRODUCTION. They can involve linguistic units at any level – sound, MORPHEME, word, SYNTAX, meaning. Slips of the tongue do not necessarily provide evidence of underlying states of mind, although intense

EMOTION, fatigue and drunkenness may render malfunction in speech production more likely.

ANNE CUTLER

slow muscle fibres *see* muscles

slow neurotransmission Slow neurotransmission is a contrast to FAST NEUROTRANSMISSION. It takes place over seconds or even minutes rather than milliseconds. Various classes of NEUROTRANSMITTERS and neuromodulators (see NEUROMODULATION) can be considered as slow neurotransmitters, although NEUROPEPTIDES and the MONOAMINE group are thought to be the most common. Slow neurotransmission may operate through normal SYNAPTIC TRANSMISSION, or may involve VOLUME TRANSMISSION.

slow potential sweep voltammetry *see* voltammetry

slow release One often wishes to have a DRUG released into the BLOOD slowly. For example, one might wish to have a small amount of drug present over an extended period for therapeutic purposes (as is the case with a NICOTINE patch designed to eliminate the craving to smoke TOBACCO – see TRANSDERMAL DRUG DELIVERY) or one might wish simply to examine the effects of a drug in an experimental animal present over a long period of time. Slow release can be achieved using a device (see OSMOTIC MINIPUMP) or by coating a drug in a substance that will dissolve very slowly in the body, limiting drug diffusion (as is the case with a DEPOT INJECTION – see DRUG ADMINISTRATION). Different methods of drug delivery also change the speed at which drugs will diffuse into the bloodstream. For example, an INTRAPERITONEAL INJECTION produces much faster uptake of drug than a SUBCUTANEOUS INJECTION.

See also: drug administration

slow scan voltammetry *see* voltammetry

slow-wave sleep Slow-wave sleep refers to quiet sleep in the mammal during which slow waves are recorded from the ELECTROENCEPHALOGRAM (EEG). These slow waves range in frequency from 0.1 to 4 Hz. The waves from 1 to 4 Hz are termed DELTA WAVES, whereas more recently the waves below 1 Hz have been termed the slow oscillation. In fact, the delta waves ride on top of the slow oscillation. Slow waves increase in incidence and amplitude in a progression from sleep onset to the full development of slow wave sleep and thus in what has been divided into four stages in humans. In addition, another activity which occurs at a higher frequency (12–14 Hz) and with increasing then decreasing amplitude to form a spindle-like shape evoking the name SLEEP SPINDLE, occurs in the early stages of sleep. Thus in humans, a loss of alpha activity (marking relaxed wakefulness) occurs in stage 1, spindles riding on slower waves in stage 2 and a progressive increase in delta riding on slower waves in stages 3 and 4. Slow-wave sleep is referred to as QUIET SLEEP because there are few movements in deep slow-wave sleep, in contrast to REM SLEEP, when the eyes move and the extremities twitch or move. In addition, it was originally believed that no mental activity occurred during slow-wave sleep, in contrast to REM sleep, when DREAMING was shown to occur. However subsequent studies found that mental activity does occur in slow-wave sleep. This sleep mentation is reported as dream-like but described as less vivid and bizarre than the dreams of REM sleep.

The slow-wave activity that occurs during slow-wave sleep corresponds to a different mode of neuronal discharge than that during wakefulness by neurons in the THALAMUS and CEREBRAL CORTEX. Whereas thalamo-cortical neurons fire in a TONIC, repetitive mode during waking, they fire in a PHASIC, bursting mode (see TONIC–PHASIC) during slow-wave sleep. The frequency of this bursting varies with spindles, delta and the slow oscillation. The rhythm of the bursting is determined in part by intrinsic properties of the individual neurons and also by properties of the thalamo-cortical-thalamic network (see THALAMUS). Thus certain cells in the circuit drive certain frequencies of the NETWORK OSCILLATION. The thalamo-cortical relay neurons and cortico-thalamic feedback neurons contain the excitatory neurotransmitter, GLUTAMATE. GABAERGIC neurons are inserted between the cortico-thalamic and thalamo-cortical neurons in a shell-like nucleus surrounding the thalamus and termed the THALAMIC RETICULAR NUCLEUS (due to its net-like appearance similar to, but not to be confused with, the RETICULAR FORMATION of the BRAINSTEM). The GABAergic thalamic reticular neurons discharge in bursts in association with spindles in the early stages of slow wave sleep and accordingly both inhibit and entrain the thalamo-cortical neurons onto which they project into first a spindle then a delta rhythm riding on the slow oscillation. Though entrained (see ENTRAINMENT) in the rhythmic discharge, the thalamo-cortical neurons become progressively hyperpolarized and inhibited, giving rise to fewer and fewer spikes per burst with the progression into slow wave sleep. Transmission through the thalamus, which occurs with high fidelity during waking, is accordingly progressively decreased during slow-wave sleep. The afferent gateway to the cerebral cortex thus progressively closes during this state. In addition, the non-specific thalamo-cortical projection system is also being inhibited, blocking the widespread cortical activation produced by this system during wakefulness. This thalamic inhibition may thus underlie the decrease in sensory awareness and loss of CONSCIOUSNESS that occur during slow-wave sleep.

The changes that occur in thalamo-cortical activity and transmission are in part the result of a decrease in the activating influence arising from the brainstem ASCENDING RETICULAR ACTIVATING SYSTEM. Indeed neurons in the reticular formation decrease their rate of discharge prior to the onset of slow wave sleep, resulting in a decrease in the facilitatory influence on (or a disfacilitation of) the thalamic neurons. The PROJECTION NEURONS of the reticular formation contain glutamate or ACETYLCHOLINE (or possibly glutamate and acetylcholine), both of which normally excite thalamic neurons. In addition, NORADRENERGIC neurons also excite (and depolarize; see DEPOLARIZATION) the thalamic cells. These depolarizing influences maintain a tonic discharge of the thalamic cells during waking, and their withdrawal results in a slight HYPERPOLARIZATION and subsequent burst discharge of the thalamic cells during slow wave sleep. The initial cause of the decrease in firing by the brainstem neurons has not been identified. It is likely that it could be produced by active inhibition by GABAergic neurons, which are co-distributed with the other projection neurons in the brainstem reticular formation. No specific chemical substances have been discovered which can produce natural sleep. Substances, which are used to facilitate the onset of sleep and also to produce ANAESTHESIA, are drugs that act to enhance the activity of GABA at its receptors. These drugs also tend to produce slow wave and/or spindle wave activity on the EEG probably by damping neuronal discharge in the reticular formation and enhancing inhibition in the thalamus.

BARBARA E. JONES

small intestine *see* digestive system

smart drug More correctly known as a NOOTROPIC drug.

See also: cognitive enhancers

smell The sense of smell (properly called OLFACTION) is one of the primary senses, critical for awareness of olfactory stimuli and taste.

See also: gustation; social odours; social transmission of food preferences; stereochemical theory of odour discrimination

smell prism *see* olfactory prism

smooth endoplasmic reticulum *see* cell

smooth eye movement A movement of the EYE which, unlike a SACCADE, is smooth and controlled by feedback processes. There are three basic types of smooth eye movement: COMPENSATORY EYE MOVEMENTS, SMOOTH FOLLOWING MOVEMENTS and VERGENCE.

smooth following movement A movement of the EYE: following FIXATION on a moving object, they eyes move smoothly, maintaining fixation on that object. Smooth following movements are not made across a stationary scene: they are only used for tracking moving objects.

smooth muscle *see* muscles

snapshot memory Snapshot memory has been proposed as a special form of SPATIAL MEMORY: it is understood as a form of panoramic view identifying spatial relations between salient landmarks. It is suggested that current position can be compared to the snapshot memory, allowing targets to be located. However, as with FLASHBULB MEMORY, whether a special mechanism of 'snapshot memory' is required, or whether other forms of MEMORY can satisfactorily account for NAVIGATION remains unclear.

See also: cognitive map; dead reckoning

snare proteins *see* mobilization

Snellen acuity *see* 6/6 notation; grating acuity; Snellen letters

Snellen letters A form of test chart used in the assessment of eyesight (see 6/6 NOTATION). The underlying assumption is that a normal individual with optically corrected vision is just able to read letters that subtend 5 minutes of arc (5/60th of a degree) at the eye. The letters on the chart are drawn with stokes of constant width and therefore for a letter E 5 minutes of arc high, the horizontal strokes would each subtend 1 minute of arc separated from each other by 1 minute of arc. The chart contains rows of letters of different sizes. The observer views that chart from a standardized distance (for example 6 metres) and the smallest letters that can be read reliably is determined. RESOLUTION ACUITY is the ratio of the distance of the observer from the chart to the distance that the observer would have to stand in order for the minimally resolvable letters to subtend 5 arc minutes. For example, the observer might have poor ACUITY and be able to read only some of the largest letters. In this case they might subtend 5 minutes of arc at 12 metres. The SNELLEN ACUITY would then be expressed as 6/12. Conversely, an observer with better-than-normal resolving power might have an acuity of 6/4.

DAVID W. HEELEY

Snellen test *see* Snellen letters

SNRI An abbreviation used to indicate (confusingly) either SEROTONIN–NORADRENALINE REUPTAKE INHIBITOR or SELECTIVE NORADRENALINE REUPTAKE INHIBITOR.

social behaviour A term to describe those behaviours which mediate specific functions relating to the establishment and maintenance of relationships, usually with others of the same species. Social behaviours generally refer to those concerned with communication (see VOCALIZATION) and frequently are elicited by stimuli produced by others of the same species. Specific social behaviours include courtship behaviours, parental behaviours, those which maintain position within hierarchical social structures (see ALPHA MALE; DOMINANCE) and those which demonstrate co-operation between individuals for a shared goal. The degree to which animals exhibit social behaviours varies widely from species to species. For some, existence is solitary, with social contact (see SOCIAL ISOLATION) only at times of territorial dispute (see TERRITORIAL BEHAVIOUR), courtship, COPULATION and during the provision of parental care (see MATERNAL BEHAVIOUR). For others, highly complex social relationships maintain coordinated social structures with shared responsibilities for crucial survival tasks such as food gathering, the care of offspring and the deterrence of predators. As a general rule, the most complex social behaviours are found in species with the most complex social structures. Although these species are often those with evidence of the greatest development of the NEOCORTEX and cognition, there are exceptions – the social insects for example.

Ethologists (see ETHOLOGY) have defined a number of so-called social behaviour systems. These include FEAR and ESCAPE systems (see FIGHT-OR-FLIGHT), AGGRESSION systems, sexual systems (see SEXUAL BEHAVIOUR), parental and filial systems and maternal systems (see MATERNAL BEHAVIOUR). These putative systems are operationally defined, restricted patterns of behaviour which are elicited by specific stimuli generated by others of the same species, often within a specific environmental context. The presence of specific perceptual capabilities to recognize the appropriate stimuli is inferred, as is that of a neural circuitry to process and execute the necessary actions. One of the most studied social behaviour systems is that which underlies the maternal care of offspring. Depending on the species studied, maternal behaviours that are entirely unique to the period following birth can be elicited by highly specific stimuli. These may either be related to the process of birth itself (and often hormonal in nature) or may be provided by the offspring by, for example, visual, auditory or olfactory cues. Such processes are probably influential in the subsequent development of so-called ATTACHMENT behaviours. Attachment is also considered to exist between some animals outwith the parent–offspring relationship and responses to social separation (see SOCIAL ISOLATION and MATERNAL SEPARATION/DEPRIVATION), or the disruption of inferred attachment bonds, can be demonstrated in a variety of mammalian and bird species. The disruption of such affectional bonds in primates and laboratory rodents have been explored as potential ANIMAL MODELS for human DEPRESSION.

One specific category of social behaviour which seems to be almost unique to those species with highly developed cognitive processes is that of PLAY. Although difficult to define, play consists of apparently purposeless activity, with no immediate goal of obvious adaptive significance, involving the execution of species-specific motor programmes. Although solitary play is observed, it is most often a social activity seen in immature members of a species. There are at least three major benefits to be obtained from play. In addition to the obvious role in the development of cognitive and motor skills, play also facilitates the development of a wider range of behavioural capabilities which are responsive to the environment. Furthermore, it promotes LEARNING about social interactions. Play permits the development and refinement of such capabilities in a safe environment, usually whilst still vulnerable and dependent upon adults of the species.

Observation and manipulation of social behaviour has proven particularly valuable in the fields of PSYCHOPHARMACOLOGY and in the development of animal models of PSYCHOPATHOLOGY. The social interaction test of ANXIETY exploits the reliable generation of a fearful emotional state (see CONDITIONED FEAR) by placing a male rat in an unfamiliar or brightly lit environment and recording the amount of time spent in active social contact with another, unfamiliar, male rat. Duration of social interaction is inversely related to the familiarity with the arena and to the intensity of lighting. The administration of drugs which have a marked anti-anxiety effect (ANXIOLYTIC drugs) leads to a greater time spent in contact with the other rat. This procedure has proven valuable as a behavioural assay for screening drugs for anxiolytic activity. The procedure is much less reliable if female rats or mice are used. Similarly, the provision of ideal circumstances in which to observe the reliable induction of aggression in rats or mice has proven valuable as a behavioural assay for the testing of drugs for anti-aggression properties. Observation of the behavioural, physiological and neurochemical consequences of social defeat in laboratory rodents has provided information on subsequent biological adaptations such as STRESS-induced ANALGESIA and ANHEDONIA.

See also: birdsong; comparative psychology

KEITH MATTHEWS

social cognition Social cognition is the term used to describe a general theoretical and methodological approach to the study of social behaviour. It is not simply, however, the wholesale importation of methods and principles from COGNITIVE PSYCHOLOGY as social psychological research has always retained an interest in cognition, even at times when the remainder of the discipline was dominated by BEHAVIOURISM. The identifying feature of social cognition is the importance it attaches to MENTALISM and psychological processes either from the point of view of how mental events affect social behaviour or how social behaviour affects mental events. Basically stated, social cognition is concerned with how people perceive, remember and interpret information about themselves and others. This general approach has given rise to a number of influential metatheories, the most dominant of which remains the cognitive miser model. This model embodies the idea that people are capacity-limited information processors and, as such, adopt strategies to simplify complex tasks or take cognitive short-cuts wherever possible. Thus, any errors or biases that occur are considered to be inherent features of our information-processing systems and that the underlying goal of such systems is to provide rapid solutions that are adequate for the task in hand but not necessarily accurate.

MALCOLM D. MacLEOD

social isolation A term to describe the state engendered by placing a social animal in a situation where it is denied interaction with others of the same species. The state in which an animal is denied: (1) the opportunity to DISPLAY the full repertoire of behaviours that are required for communication (see ANIMAL COMMUNICATION) and interaction with others of the same species; (2) the opportunity to EXPERIENCE the full repertoire of behaviours that are required for communication and interaction from others of the same species. The term is used to describe a variety of experimental manipulations of the environment (see ENVIRONMENTAL ENRICHMENT) of social laboratory animals (see SOCIAL BEHAVIOUR) in addition to its colloquial use to describe the degree to which an individual human has contact with other humans. An isolation experience can have widely differing behavioural and neurochemical consequences, critically dependent upon the species studied, the developmental stage and upon the detail of the isolation procedure. Social isolation manipulations during the early neonatal period are often referred to as MATERNAL SEPARATION/DEPRIVATION experiences, where it is assumed that the critical component of the procedure is that of the absence of availability of the mother. The effect of isolation at later stages of development is believed to be due to the absence of the capacity to interact with other, non-parent animals. Absence of the opportunity to make tactile contact with others appears to be a particularly influential component of the experience. Social isolation has been studied in some detail in both laboratory rodents and in non-human PRIMATES and there is substantial commonality in the behavioural consequences. Such ISOLATION REARING of young animals leads to an enhancement of central DOPAMINE activity with exaggeration of the response to PSYCHOMOTOR STIMULANTS such as AMPHETAMINE. The neurochemical changes are not confined to dopamine systems however, and there are widespread effects across multiple transmitter systems in many areas. The effects of social isolation seem less potent with increasing age, probably reflecting resultant changes in brain PLASTICITY. Isolation experiences at different developmental stages in the rat have generated considerable interest as potential models for human PSYCHOPATHOLOGY, reflecting an increasing clinical focus on the interactions between the genes (see GENE) and early environment in disease processes.

See also: sensory enrichment vs. deafferentation/deprivation

KEITH MATTHEWS

social odours Animals emit odours which other animals, usually CONSPECIFIC but occasionally members of other species, can recognize. In VERTEBRATES, PHEROMONES (chemical messengers secreted to the outside environment) have been suggested to serve in SEXUAL BEHAVIOUR, MATERNAL BEHAVIOUR and in other ways. However, the concept of pheromonal action has been criticized by some, and SOCIAL ODOURS has been mooted as a replacement term.

social transmission of food preferences The principal component of rats' breath is CARBON DIOXIDE, as is the case with all MAMMALS. However rats' breath – which comes exclusively from their noises: rats do not breathe through their mouths – contains a variety of other chemicals, including CARBON DISULPHIDE (CS2) and CARBONYL SULPHIDE (COS). These are all forms of SEMIOCHEMICAL – chemicals that can transmit information to other animals. It has been shown that rats can learn from CONSPECIFIC contacts. This can be shown as follows: one rat (the demonstrator) is allowed to eat a novel, flavoured, nutritious food. This rat is then housed for a period with another rat (the observer) with whom it will interact socially. The observer can then be isolated and offered a range of flavoured, novel, foods, one of which is that same as that eaten by the demonstrator, which is the one that is most usually chosen: information about diet choice has been communicated by associating particular foods with the presence of carbon disulphide. Such social transmission of food choice is very valuable, allowing rats effectively to communicate the information

that particular foodstuffs are safe to eat. This appears to be a valid basic effect, but further complexities involving the use of interactions between an observer and two demonstrators, and the use of 'trustworthy' and 'untrustworthy' demonstrators, has revealed that there are, for rats at least, limitations on the amount and nature of the information that can be transferred.

See also: observation learning; olfaction; social behaviour; social odours

References

Galef B.G., Mason J.R., Preti G. & Bean N.J. (1988) Carbon disulfide: a semiochemical mediating socially-induced diet choice in rats. *Physiology and Behavior* 42: 119–124.

Galef B.G., Whiskin E.E. & Horn C.S. (1999) What observer rats don't learn about foods from demonstrator rats. *Animal Learning and Behaviour* 27: 316–322.

sociobiology Many behavioural traits are influenced by inheritance and are appropriately viewed as adaptations (see NATURAL SELECTION). Indeed, in some species, almost every aspect of behaviour is under rather tight genetic control. Behavioural adaptations must have conferred fitness benefits on individuals possessing them, or they could not have been selected, yet some traits of social species seem at first sight to benefit other individuals – as well as, or instead of, the one with the trait (see ALTRUISM). The development of a proper understanding of how natural selection applies to SOCIAL BEHAVIOUR has largely resolved these puzzles, immensely increasing the power of evolutionary theory to account for social tendencies and social structures. In the process, a new discipline – sociobiology – has been created, concerning the adaptive value and evolution of all aspects of social behaviour, with implications for the origin of animal (and human) societies. Inevitably, this has trespassed on other subject areas (such as social psychology, sociology, social anthropology) some of which have long held that biology has no relevance to their subject-matter. Sociobiology has thus been subject to controversy.

Social grouping may confer direct individual benefit without any interaction among group members. W.D. Hamilton showed that under many circumstances, joining other potential victims is an appropriate strategy when threatened by a predation risk (Hamilton, 1971): the probability of the particular individual becoming victim is thereby decreased. Previous accounts, claiming that such behaviour evolved 'for the good of the species' are flawed and unnecessary. Hamilton's SELFISH HERD principle remains valid even if the probability of some individual falling victim is increased. For instance, the response of a fish school to dolphin predation is to associate closer and closer, which clearly makes the dolphin's life simpler. Some animal groupings are evidently based on affiliative interactions and even helpful behaviour among group members (see ALTRUISM). However, in most cases, the members are not unrelated. Hamilton showed that apparently altruistic traits could become established genetically, if their net beneficial effect on kin – which share genetic material, and thus a probability of possessing any given gene – outweighs their direct cost (Hamilton, 1964). Here, costs and benefits are in the currency of fitness (see NATURAL SELECTION). The crucial variable for calculating a trait's adaptive effect is its INCLUSIVE FITNESS rather than its INDIVIDUAL FITNESS: this measure adds in components from relatives, each weighted by a coefficient expressing the closeness of the relationship, in cases where kin are affected by the trait. The approach is often called KIN SELECTION, but it is a consequence of, not an alternative to, natural selection. The great majority of long-term social groupings among animals have since proved to be kin-based, showing the power of kin selection to explain the origin of societies. Since biological kinship ('blood') is important also to humans, and humans traditionally live in groupings partly composed of relatives, the relevance of kin selection to human society is clear.

An additional way by which traits, which do not advantage their possessor, can nevertheless evolve is where the help is later reciprocated by the individual helped. Provided a group is long-lasting, individuals can recognize each other and remember past interactions – and thus discriminate against cheats – RECIPROCAL ALTRUISM can spread genetically (Trivers, 1971). One way of looking at this is as a form of SYMBIOSIS, with a time-delay before the mutual benefit arrives. Relatively few cases of reciprocal altruism have been verified in non-humans (blood-donation in vampire bats is a notable example); most often, kinship or immediate benefit prove also to be involved. However, this may simply reflect the greater ease of establishing reciprocation among relatives, where genetical costs of altruism are lower, rather than the irrelevance of the concept. In humans, complex forms of reciprocation are found, but here genetically-based reciprocation is augmented by the power of LANGUAGE to enable arrangements to be agreed and remembered; the relative contributions are hard to disentangle.

References

Hamilton W.D. (1964) The genetical theory of social behaviour. I & II. *Journal of Theoretical Biology* 7: 1–52.
—— (1971) Geometry for the selfish herd. *Journal of Theoretical Biology* 31: 295–311.
Trivers R.L. (1971) The evolution of reciprocal altruism. *Quarterly Review of Biology* 46: 35–57.

RICHARD W. BYRNE

sodium (Na^+) Sodium is an ALKALI metal; sodium ions (Na^+) (see ION) are critical for the proper functioning of brain tissue (see for example ACTION POTENTIAL) and there are specific mechanisms in brain to detect sodium and stimulate intake in the face of depletion (see SODIUM APPETITE). The principal salt of sodium is sodium chloride (NaCl) which is of course table salt.

See also: periodic table of the elements

sodium amobarbital Short-acting drug, one of the BARBITURATES; similar to PENTOBARBITAL in structure and pharmacotherapeutic use as a hypnotic agent in humans and general ANAESTHETIC in animals.

See also: phenobarbital; thiopental

CHARLES D. BLAHA

sodium amytal This is the same as SODIUM AMOBARBITAL.

See also: Wada test

sodium appetite A SPECIFIC HUNGER for SALT that is triggered by an insufficiency of sodium chloride in the body. Sodium chloride is ordinary table salt, and its component ions (see ION) are essential for neurons and other cells to function. Although in Western society, there is more than enough sodium chloride available in foods, this may not be true in other societies, and salt was often lacking in our evolutionary history. Hence a special appetite has evolved for obtaining it as a specific nutrient. In states of insufficiency, the kidney secretes ALDOSTERONE. This hormone, together with other causes, makes the brain instigate a psychological craving for salt. In this state, even the taste of seawater (approximately 3% sodium chloride), which is normally perceived as distasteful, may instead be perceived as pleasant. Salt at any concentration is sought out for consumption during salt appetite.

See also: gustation

KENT C. BERRIDGE

sodium channel *see* ion channel

sodium nitroprusside One of a group of compounds known as NITRIC OXIDE (NO) donors: nitric oxide can be synthesized by a process involving enzymatic reactions (in which NITRIC OXIDE SYNTHASE [NOS] converts L-ARGININE to L-CITRULLINE) or by a chemical process involving the NO donors. In high concentrations sodium nitroprusside is a neurotoxin (see NEUROTOXINS), lending support to the hypothesis that dysfunctional NO activity could be involved in conditions in which there is neuronal cell death.

sodium pentobarbitone *see* pentobarbital; pentobarbitone

sodium–potassium ATPase *see* sodium–potassium pump

sodium–potassium pump One of several membrane pumps – consisting of a specialized MOLECULE embedded in a MEMBRANE – that actively pumps ions across membranes against the CONCENTRATION GRADIENT. An ION can exist in different concentrations on either side of neuronal membranes, and even when neurons are at rest (see MEMBRANE POTENTIAL) there is a flow of these ions across membranes. However, ACTION POTENTIAL generation causes very significant changes in the concentrations of ions on either side of neuronal membranes: principally, sodium ions flow in and potassium ions out. In order to restore the appropriate balance and prevent accumulation of sodium ions within neurons, the sodium–potassium pump is activated. The relative concentrations of sodium (Na^+) and potassium I (K^+) ions activates SODIUM–POTASSIUM ATPASE, an ENZYME that degrades ADENOSINE TRIPHOSPHATE (ATP) which in turn leads to the production of energy to fuel the pump. The sodium–potassium pump does not simply exchange the one ion for the other: approximately three sodium ions are pumped out of the neuron for every potassium ion that is pumped in. Since the action potential sweeps along an axonal membrane, sodium–potassium pumps exist in considerable density: approximately 750 sites per square micrometer.

See also: ouabain

sodium pump *see* sodium–potassium pump

sodium valproate One of the most commonly used ANTICONVULSANT drugs, commercially available as Depakene. It is thought to act by inhibition of VOLTAGE-SENSITIVE ION CHANNELS for sodium (Na^+) and possibly calcium (Ca^{2+}) in neuronal membranes.

soft neurological sign A soft neurological sign (see SIGNS AND SYMPTOMS) is one that is not in itself diagnostic of a particular condition but is suggestive. These are perhaps best considered in the following way. (1) In order to diagnose a condition it is typically the case that one must see a certain number of defined signs or symptoms – not necessarily all of the possible signs and symptoms, but at least a given proportion of them. (2) Around this core can be a cluster of soft signs (and symptoms) that are indicative of a condition but not necessary or specific for diagnosis. Soft neurological signs both suggest options to consider in diagnosis and help confirm diagnosis. Such things as disordered GAIT, BALANCE or coordination (see MOTOR CONTROL; MOVEMENT DEFICITS; TREMOR), as well as conditions such as GRAPHESTHESIA and STEREOGNOSIS are typically encountered soft neurological signs. These signs are usually associated with neurological conditions but are observed also in psychiatric disorders such as SCHIZOPHRENIA.

solution A solution is composed of a solute dissolved in a solvent. For instance one might make a salt solution by dissolving sodium chloride (NaCl) (the solute) in water (the solvent).

soma (plural: somata) Soma is an alternative term for a CELL BODY; see NEURON.

somaesthesia *see* somatosensory

somata *see* soma

somatic Relating to the body: in cellular terms, referring to a CELL BODY (the SOMA). One speaks of the somatic portion of a NEURON, meaning its cell body. In gross anatomical terms, somatic refers to the whole body of an animal. For example, somatic sensations are those sensations arising from the body.

See also: somatosensory

somatic cell *see* cell division

somatic marker hypothesis The somatic marker hypothesis is a framework to explain the enigmatic changes in social conduct, planning, and DECISION-MAKING which typify neurological patients who suffer damage to the lower front portion of the brain (ventromedial PREFRONTAL CORTEX). Such patients, whose personalities were normal prior to the brain damage, pursue courses of behaviour that repeatedly lead to adverse outcomes, including loss of occupational, interpersonal and social status. What makes this behaviour especially puzzling is the fact that the patients have normal intellectual function, MEMORY, speech (see SPEECH PERCEPTION; SPEECH PRODUCTION) and LANGUAGE and perception (see SENSATION VS. PERCEPTION) and ATTENTION. What they have lost, and what causes problems with planning and decision-making, is the capacity to use emotions and feelings (somatic states) to help guide behaviour. The somatic marker hypothesis provides a neurobiological explanation for this phenomenon, proposing that the patients do not have access to somatic guideposts that normally mark various behavioural alternatives as positive or negative, and thereby facilitate advantageous decision-making. The basic idea of the hypothesis is that when we are confronted with a complex decision, especially in a social situation, we activate somatic states that mark various response options as good or bad for us. Some options are associated with positive somatic states, while others are associated with negative somatic states. Using this information (either consciously or non-consciously), we make a decision and choose a course of behaviour that is in our overall best interest. The ventromedial prefrontal cortex provides a key link between brain regions involved in emotions and feelings, brain regions that process sensory information, and body control mechanisms in lower parts of the central nervous system. When the ventromedial prefrontal region is damaged, this link cannot operate, and body states cannot be used to help guide decision-making. The somatic marker hypothesis goes against popular and scientific lore that reasoning and decision-making are optimal when a person is cool, calm, and calculated – in short, un-emotional. The hypothesis is supported by studies of patients with ventromedial prefrontal damage, which have shown that absence of emotion is just as bad for decision-making as too much emotion. In fact, based on psychophysiological measurements, research has shown that people develop somatic markers that help guide behaviour even before they have conscious knowledge about which choices might be good and which might be bad. To make good decisions, we need our emotions and feelings, the somatic markers that help us navigate the course that is in our best long-term interests.

See also: frontal lobe; frontal cortex; Phineas Gage; social behaviour

Reference

Damasio A.R. (1994) *Descartes' Error: Emotion, Reason and the Human Brain*, Putnam: New York.

DANIEL TRANEL

somatic nervous system A division of the PERIPHERAL NERVOUS SYSTEM: in contrast to the AUTONOMIC NERVOUS SYSTEM, which principally targets the internal the body, the somatic nervous system is mainly concerned with initiating movement in and receiving information from the SKIN, MUSCLES and joints of the body. The sensory neurons are in the DORSAL ROOT and dorsal ganglia that innervate skin, muscle and joints: although the cell bodies may be in the CENTRAL NERVOUS SYSTEM, they are classified as part of the peripheral nervous system by virtue of their function

somatization disorders Apparent physical disorders for which medical help is sought but for which no organic cause can be found. Such disorders are often associated with ANXIETY and DEPRESSION; they form a part of what once was known as NEUROSIS.

somatocrinin *see* growth hormone releasing hormone

somatoform disorders Somatoform disorders are psychological disorders with physical symptoms but no physical cause. BODY DYSMORPHIC DISORDER is an example.

Reference
Davison G.C. & Neale J.M. (1996) *Abnormal Psychology*, Wiley: New York.

somatofugal SOMATOFUGAL is movement away from a body: either from the whole body – that is from the body tissues towards the CENTRAL NERVOUS SYSTEM; or away from a neuronal CELL BODY towards AXON TERMINALS. SOMATOPETAL is movement in the reverse direction: away from a body; see FUGAL; PETAL.

somatomedin *see* growth factors

somatoparaphrenia A condition in which patients refuse to acknowledge that a particular body part – a limb for example – belongs to them, even to the extent of claiming that it belongs to someone else.

See also: anosagnosia

somatopetal *see* somatofugal

somatosensory (from Greek, *soma*: body, and sensory) Sensations arising from the body. Somatosensory information includes such things therefore as the external senses of TOUCH, PAIN and TEMPERATURE as well as internal sensations from the VISCERA and KINAESTHESIA. In general, when people talk of somatosensation, they are generally referring to sensations of touch arising from the SKIN. An older term encompassing all of these sensations, external and internal, is SOMAESTHESIA (or somaesthesis).

somatosensory cortex The somatosensory cortex is located posterior to the CENTRAL SULCUS of the CEREBRAL CORTEX, and includes the primary (BRODMANN'S AREAS 1, 2 and 3) and secondary areas. It receives information regarding touch, PROPRIOCEPTION, PAIN and temperature (see THERMOREGULATION). The somatosensory cortex on one side receives input largely from the opposite side of the body. Each point on the body maps to a specific location in each somatosensory area, and body parts requiring high sensitivity and fine discrimination have larger representations, as for the lips and fingertips in humans, VIBRISSAE in rodents, and digits in racoons.

See also: homunculus; topography

KAZUE SEMBA

somatosensory homunculus *see* homunculus

somatosensory pathways Somatosensory information is relayed from the various types of RECEPTOR in the SKIN to the SPINAL CORD. Information ascends via two pathways: the DORSAL COLUMN – MEDIAL LEMNISCAL SYSTEM and the ANTEROLATERAL SYSTEM (which is alternatively known as the SPINOTHALAMIC TRACT). The dorsal column–medial lemniscal system carries HAPTIC and PROPRIOCEPTION information (about TOUCH and activity in the MUSCLES) while the anterolateral system carries information about PAIN and TEMPERATURE.

In both cases information enters the spinal cord via the DORSAL HORN from CUTANEOUS NERVES (which receive information directly from receptors in the SKIN). Cutaneous nerves synapse on neurons of the dorsal column. Information ascending in the dorsal column does not cross the midline at this level, but ascends ipsilaterally to make synaptic connection in the brain at the GRACILE NUCLEUS and CUNEATE NUCLEUS. From here FIBRES ascend via the medial lemniscus, having crossed the MIDLINE, travelling to the THALAMUS (to the ventral posterior lateral nucleus and posterior nuclei of the thalamus). From the ventral posterior lateral nucleus of the thalamus, information is relayed (via the INTERNAL CAPSULE) to the PRIMARY SOMATOSENSORY CORTEXand POSTERIOR PARIETAL CORTEX. The anterolateral system involves DECUSSATION in the spinal cord: the cutaneous nerves, having entered via the dorsal horns, synapse on neurons which cross and ascend on the CONTRALATERAL side of the spinal cord. The anterolateral system provides input to the RETICULAR FORMATION, PONS and MEDULLA, MIDBRAIN and directly to the thalamus. The same pattern of thalamic input and cortical connection is seen as with the dorsal column-medial lemniscal system, though in addition there is input to intralaminar thalamic nuclei which projects to various areas of ASSOCIATION CORTEX.

See also: dermatome; homunculus

Reference

Kandel E.R., Schwartz J.H. & Jessell T.M. (2000) *Principles of Neural Science*, 4th edn, McGraw-Hill, New York.

somatostatin Somatostatin is one of the NEUROPEPTIDES, with multiple RECEPTOR subtypes (classified as sst1 – sst5) all G PROTEIN coupled. It was first found in the HYPOTHALAMUS where it is able to inhibit the release of GROWTH HORMONE (and was initially called GROWTH HORMONE RELEASE INHIBITING HORMONE). Subsequent research identified somatostatin in many parts of the body, including the PANCREAS and GASTROINTESTINAL TRACT. It is also found widely distributed in CENTRAL NERVOUS SYSTEM, most notably within the CEREBRAL CORTEX where it is found within INTERNEURONS. Somatostatin has attracted interest because it is markedly diminished in the brains of patients with PARKINSON'S DISEASE. There is an apparent association between the extent to which somatostatin is lost in these patients and the incidence of DEMENTIA – the greater the loss, the greater the degree of dementia.

somatotopic A form of RECEPTOTOPIC REPRESENTATION: in which each NEURON is placed in respect of the input from the body surface.

See also: homunculus; somatosensory pathways; touch

somnambulism Somnambulism is sleep walking. It is one of several motor behaviours that interrupt the sleep of about 15% of adolescents. The episodes arise from the deep stage 4 NON-REM SLEEP periods that occur early in the night. Sleep laboratory studies reveal that high-voltage slow ELECTROENCEPHALOGRAM (EEG) waves may persist through the sleep-walking bouts indicating a dissociation between upper and lower brain–body arousal systems and explaining why the subjects may engage in complex automatic motor behaviours but are verbally unresponsive to the communications of roommates and parents. Somnambulism is usually harmless and subjects can be guided safely back to bed but common-sense safeguards against physical harm like window locks and stairway gates may sometimes need to be instituted. Because stage 4 sleep declines after age 30 and disappears by age 40, somnambulism is also self-limited. In extreme cases the BENZODIAZEPINE sedative, CLONAZEPAM may be helpful, probably because it both suppresses stage 4 and induces muscle relaxation.

J. ALLAN HOBSON

somnolence Sleepiness is the normal subjective experience of SLEEP-ready or sleep-deprived subjects. It is characterized by a lack of physical energy, an inability to maintain attention to external events and difficulty maintaining internal mental processes. Even before the eyes close and muscle tone declines precipitately, somnolent individuals may experience lapses of CONSCIOUSNESS lasting from seconds or even minutes especially if they are engaged in semi-automatic behaviours like walking or driving. Somnolence is thus not only subjectively unpleasant and socially undesirable but may also be fatally dangerous. Fortunately it is readily reversible if subjects are capable of normal sleep and allow themselves to get it. When somnolence persists or is disabling, it is called excessive daytime sleepiness and should be evaluated by a sleep disorders specialist to rule out NARCOLEPSY, SLEEP APNOEA, and NOCTURNAL MYOCLONUS.

See also: arousal

J. ALLAN HOBSON

sonic hedgehog Sonic hedgehog is a PROTEIN critical in DEVELOPMENT, including that of the CENTRAL NERVOUS SYSTEM; *see* NEURODEVELOPMENT

sound localization Sound localization is the perceptual ability to locate an acoustic event in space, using only auditory information. For normal listeners, sound localization is a BINAURAL task. This is because the sounds arriving at the two ears do so at different times and with different spectra, depending on the eccentricity of the sound source with respect to the head's midline plane; it is the neural computation of these disparities in the timing and spectra of the signals at the two ears that results in the spatial percept. Interaural disparities in the timing of sounds arise because of differences in the path length to the two ears from the sound source. Interaural disparities in the spectra of the sound arise from the shadowing effect of the head (and PINNAE) for sound frequencies with wavelengths shorter than the head diameter (or pinna height). The absolute magnitude of interaural disparities depends on both the eccentricity of the source, and the frequency of the sound. Disparity magnitudes are close to zero for sources near the midline, increase with increasing source eccentricity, and plateau in the lateral hemifields.

The neural coding of interaural disparities is done on a frequency-specific basis. Neurons of the MEDIAL SUPERIOR OLIVE receive phase-locked inputs from each ear (see HEARING THEORIES) and execute a coincidence detection on them for the analysis of interaural phase differences of low frequency components. Neurons of the LATERAL SUPERIOR OLIVE receive an intensity dependent excitatory signal from one ear and an inhibitory one from the other; the neurons execute a summation of these to encode the relative amplitudes of the sounds at the two ears. The neural coding is most unambiguous for relatively small disparities, and it is relatively small disparities which themselves most unambiguously specify sound source eccentricity. It is probably for this reason that behavioral localization ACUITY is greatest for sound sources near the midline. Noisy sounds are more accurately localized than pure tones. This is because each frequency in the noisy sound generates its own interaural disparities; these are encoded independently in the nervous system, with the consequence that more information is available for the localization judgement. Monaural listeners are able to learn to localize sounds with some accuracy using spectral cues from the head and pinna on the intact side.

Reference

Phillips D.P. & Brugge J.F. (1985) Progress in neurophysiology of sound localization. *Annual Review of Psychology* 36: 245–274.

DENNIS P. PHILLIPS

source amnesia Source amnesia refers to AMNESIA for where and when particular information was acquired. For example, one may remember that Sally went on vacation last week, but not remember who it was that furnished this information. Source memory abilities depend importantly on FRONTAL LOBE integrity. Source memory errors are especially common in young children and in AGEING, and are thought to be an important cause of errors and distortions in MEMORY. If the source of a FACT MEMORY is lost or confused, then it becomes more difficult to know whether the memory refers to an AUTOBIOGRAPHICAL MEMORY or to an image, a fantasy, or a story told by another.

LARRY R. SQUIRE

source memory *see* source amnesia

Southern blotting *see* blotting

space Space is an abstraction, a physical characterization of a system of location of n objects in x dimensions. Euclidean space or 'real' space is the actual arrangement involving a finite number of objects in three dimensions and cognitive space, an internal representation of this space in the nervous system. Some theories of spatial behaviour find it useful to divide this conceptual space into focal space (the part of space we are looking directly at) and global space (the space that lies outside this focused region). Global space includes our own body and appears to provide a framework in which we monitor our own movements and that of other objects (see ALLOCENTRIC SPACE; EGOCENTRIC SPACE). In focal space the details, the identities of objects (their colours and shapes for example) rather than their movement and location are primary concern as far as analysis is concerned. Mishkin and his co-workers have proposed that there are at least two neural systems that process information about objects in visual space (see GENICULOSTRIATE AND TECTOPULVINAR VISUAL PATHWAYS) and a number of theories associate global and focal vision with these two neural systems. It is thought that the MAGNOCELLULAR cells in the VISUAL SYSTEM which project to visual areas V5 to 7a of the PARIETAL CORTEX and then to DORSOLATERAL PREFRONTAL CORTEX are responsible for processing movement and location information and executing actions (such as orienting responses) within global space. The PARVOCELLULAR system which projects to visual areas V3 and V4 (see AREAS VI–V5) then to INFERIOR TEMPORAL CORTEX, and from there to midlateral FRONTAL CORTEX, is thought to be responsible for processing information about the identity (pattern and colour for instance) of the objects and executing actions in focal space.

Reference

Mishkin, M., Ungerleider, L.G. and Macko, K.A. (1983) Object vision and spatial vision: two cortical pathways. *Trends in Neuroscience* 6: 414–417.

RICHARD C. TEES

spaced trial *see* trial

span tasks Tasks that require animals to hold information in memory; the experimenter makes an attempt to determine how much information (that is, the span of memory) can be held.

Reference

Dudchenko P.A., Wood E.R. & Eichenbaum H. (2000) Neurotoxic hippocampal lesions have no effect on odor span and little effect on odor recognition memory but produce significant impairments on spatial span, recognition, and alternation. *Journal of Neuroscience* 20: 2964–2977.

sparse coding *see* neural coding

spasm (from Greek, *spaein*: to draw or convulse) The term spasm is derived from the same Greek root as the term SPASTICITY. A spasm is an abnormal contraction of MUSCLES, that can be relatively brief or sustained over a period of time. There are various causes for spasm, including damage to the nervous system and local muscle effects.

spasticity (from Greek, *spaein*: to draw or convulse) The term spasticity is derived from the same Greek root as the term SPASM. Spasticity is a term used in clinical practice to indicate a dysfunction of the MUSCLES produced by damage to the CENTRAL NERVOUS SYSTEM. Spasticity in patients is distinct from other muscle disorders, such as DYSTONIA or RIGIDITY, by virtue of the velocity-dependent increase in stretch resistance of a muscle: essentially it involves exaggeration of the STRETCH REFLEX, causing abnormal muscle contractions. Damage, induced by various means including STROKE and CEREBRAL PALSY, to any part of the MOTOR SYSTEM, from the MOTOR CORTEX downwards, can cause spasticity.

spatial attention The allocation of ATTENTION to a region of space to enhance processing of information at the attended location.

See also: covert attention; covert orienting

VERITY J. BROWN

spatial behaviour Spatial behaviours are those where an animals' actions are guided primarily by EGOCENTRIC or ALLOCENTRIC spatial cues in the environment. For example, FORAGING on a spatially-cued RADIAL ARM MAZE requires the animal to keep track in MEMORY of which spatial locations on the maze the animal has visited, and use allocentric spatial cues in the environment to guide the animal towards the arms that it had not yet entered during the trial. Behaviours which are considered spatial include EXPLORATION, foraging, hoarding and DEAD RECKONING (see MAPS; NAVIGATION).

Spatial behaviours can be classified in terms of the sensory-motor response that an organism engages in (see Kolb & Wishaw, 1996). Position responses are movements made with the body as a reference point, where no external cue is required. These responses are referred to as egocentric. Left–right discriminations are an example of position responses. CUE responses are referred to as allocentric; these are movements guided by an external cue. Landmark navigation is an example of a cue response. Place responses are those which can guide an organism to a particular place or object, even if the target is out of the organisms' immediate perception. The relational properties of the surrounding cues guide the behaviour. Place responses are thought to require the consultation of a COGNITIVE MAP of the animals environment. Locating the hidden platform in a WATER MAZE is an example of a place response. There is ample evidence that the HIPPOCAMPUS is important for spatial behaviours, particularly place responses. Lesions to the hippocampus proper or associated cortical structures impair spatial behaviours. Lesions to the HIPPOCAMPAL FORMATION decrease accuracy on a radial arm maze task and increase ESCAPE latencies on a water maze task. Electrophysiological recordings in freely moving animals further support the notion of hippocampal involvement in spatial behaviours. One subset of hippocampal neurons which have been labelled PLACE CELLS increase their activity when an animal is oriented to a particular region in SPACE. Another subset of hippocampal neurons, termed THETA CELLS exhibits rhythmic activity when an animal is engaged in exploratory locomotion through a spatially cued environment. It is believed that the hippocampus integrates visuo-spatial and movement related information of an organisms' surroundings to form a cognitive map which is used to guide an animals' behaviour when it must use spatial cues to navigate through its environment.

References

Kolb B. & Wishaw I.Q. (eds.) (1996) *Fundamentals of Human Neuropsychology*, 4th edn, W.H. Freeman: New York.

STANLEY B. FLORESCO

spatial cognition Cognition can be viewed as the use of a neural representation, or 'mental record' of some past experience as a basis for action (Domjan, 1998). SPATIAL COGNITION refers to the broad subset of cognitive functions that deals with the storage, manipulation and processing of information pertaining to the characteristics of SPACE in an organism's environment, resulting in GOAL-DIRECTED BEHAVIOUR. Different types of spatial cognition can be differentiated either by the type of spatial information that is being processed, or the way in which the spatial information is manipulated and used for the purpose of goal-directed behaviours. The processing of EGOCENTRIC or ALLOCENTRIC spatial information (see EGOCENTRIC SPACE; ALLOCENTRIC SPACE) or the consultation of a spatial map (see SPATIAL MAPPING) are some examples of different forms of spatial cognition characterized by the type of spatial information used. Likewise, different ways that spatial information can be used include SPATIAL MEMORY, NAVIGATION, EXPLORATION and HOARDING BEHAVIOUR. Spatial memory may be the most frequently discussed form of spatial cognition because other types of spatial functions are though to work in concert with this type of MEMORY. An example is exploration. An organism acquires spatial memory of predictable stimulus events within its environment. When the organism encounters a novel environment, current environmental stimuli are compared to the existing representation stored in spatial memory. When a discrepancy exists between the immediately perceptible environment and the one stored in memory, the organism becomes activated to either approach or withdraw, in order to eliminate the discrepancy. During the course of ongoing behaviour, different spatial cognitive functions may interact dynamically. When searching for one's car in a parking lot, one may initially consult a cognitive map of the environment in order to plan the shortest route to a landmark that is not visible initially. Upon arriving at this landmark, one may then use a simpler allocentric strategy, and go immediately left of the landmark towards the goal. Once the goal has been located and approached, egocentric spatial localization can be used to find one's car keys in one's pocket.

See also: hippocampus

Reference

Domjan M. (1998) *The principles of Learning*

and Behavior, 4th edn, Brooks Cole: Pacific Grove CA.

STANLEY B. FLORESCO

spatial frequency channels Hypothetical neural circuits selectively responsive to variations of light intensity on the RETINA. There is much evidence that the VISUAL SYSTEM analyses the distribution of light intensity on the retina into parts, and then, after further processing of the parts, recombines them into the seen percept, which is a representation of the distal stimulus. In one theory, the functionally relevant parts of visual stimuli are the SINE WAVE GRATINGS, the elementary components produced by a spatial FOURIER ANALYSIS of the retinal image of the stimulus. Spatial Fourier analysis is mathematically related to temporal Fourier analysis with which complex sound stimuli are described in AUDITION. In temporal Fourier analysis, complex waves varying in time are analysed into a sum of several simple sine (and cosine) waves of appropriate frequencies and amplitudes. The AUDITORY SYSTEM analyses complex sounds in a similar way and seems to respond to the sine wave components rather than to any other features of the complex sounds. In spatial Fourier analysis, the role of time is taken by 2-dimensional space, and the resulting components are sine wave gratings. Any visual scene, and the retinal image it produces, can be analysed into a series of sine wave gratings oriented at various angles to the vertical and with different spatial frequencies and amplitudes. The visual system has been shown to be differentially sensitive to sine wave gratings of various spatial frequencies. The spatial modulation transfer function (a plot of the inverse of threshold contrast ratio, the ratio of most to least intense light level in the bars of a grating, versus spatial frequency) that describes the functioning of the visual system looks like an upside-down letter V, with a peak at around 6 cycles per degree (a cycle of a sine wave goes smoothly from 0 to a maximum, back past 0 to a minimum, and then to 0 again), indicating that the visual system is most sensitive to that spatial frequency. The modulation transfer function changes with age, with the peak sensitivity decreasing to about 1 cycle per degree by age 80. The spatial modulation transfer function and its changes with experimental conditions, age, and other factors, can be explained by assuming that the visual system is organized into a set of spatial frequency channels that act like filters, with each channel 'tuned' to a specific spatial frequency, and variations in sensitivity of the various channels explaining variations in the amount of contrast between light and dark regions of the visual stimulus required for above threshold responding. One striking result is the decrease of sensitivity of a particular channel with prolonged exposure to its preferred spatial frequency grating. Such selective ADAPTATION can change the apparent contrast of other gratings and also change their apparent spatial frequency, since many channels, with different preferred frequencies, typically respond to any visual stimulus. Adaptation to a sine wave grating can alter visual response to non-grating stimuli, implying that the processing of all visual stimuli can be viewed in spatial frequency terms.

Known properties of neurons in the visual system are sufficient to explain how such a spatial frequency analysis could be accomplished by the visual system. Retinal GANGLION CELLS and LATERAL GENICULATE NUCLEUS neurons have a centre-surround RECEPTIVE FIELD on the retina, with central regions to which the neuron responds in one way (excited either by onsets or by offsets of light stimuli) and concentric surrounding regions to which the neuron responds in the opposite way. These receptive fields vary in size, with those of neurons in the central retina smaller than those of neurons in the periphery, and those of neurons in the retina smaller than those of neurons in the lateral geniculate nucleus. Such neurons respond best to a grating when a light or dark bar completely fills the central region of the receptive field. Thus, neurons with larger receptive fields, and thus larger central regions, are tuned to lower spatial frequencies, while neurons with smaller receptive fields are tuned to higher spatial frequencies. Presumably, groups of such neurons combine to create spatial frequency channels and other kinds of visual system filters, for example those specialized to detect edges and lines.

More generally, spatial frequency channels are one among several sets of analysers, including also those for orientation, direction of motion, spatial position, extent, and phase, and temporal frequency, position, extent and phase, that break down the retinal image of a visual stimulus into parts. These analysers are thought to be located in areas V1 and V2 (see AREAS V1–V5). Several of these dimensions, including spatial frequency, are served by multiple analysers that inhibit one another, act as independent detectors, and produce labelled output (see LABELLED LINE THEORY). The outputs of these analysers both inform responses to visual stimuli and, when combined appropriately, form the visual percept.

See also: motion perception; object recognition

Reference

Graham N. (1989) *Visual Pattern Analyzers*, Oxford University Press: New York.

LAWRENCE M. WARD

spatial frequency vs. feature theory The two most prominent theories that attempt to explain how visual perceptual objects are formed and identified from the fragmented visual information detected by the RETINA. It is generally agreed that the VISUAL SYSTEM first breaks the retinal image into parts, processes these parts, and then reassembles the parts into the visual percept, which is a representation of an object in the world. Further analysis of the visual percept may also take place in order to inform a response to the object represented, or such responses may be based on processing of the not-yet-resynthesized parts. The remaining deep question concerns the nature of the functionally relevant parts of the visual stimulus: are they spatial frequency components, *ad hoc* features, or some other type of part, such as GEONS (see below).

One useful way to see this problem is in the context of visual OBJECT RECOGNITION. A generic theory would include the following stages of information processing: (1) from the input retinal image the visual system generates a set of parts; (2) this 'input part set' is compared (correlated) with various remembered sets of parts that characterize previously encountered objects; (3) the label associated with the remembered object whose set of parts is the most similar to the input part set is selected as the identity of the object that generated the input retinal image. The problem is: exactly what are the parts in the input and remembered part sets? There is empirical evidence and argument for both of the two major contenders: spatial frequency components (SINE WAVE GRATINGS generated by SPATIAL FREQUENCY CHANNELS) and features detected by each FEATURE DETECTOR. Both types of parts are consistent with the physiology of the visual system. Neurons in the VISUAL CORTEX are selectively responsive ('tuned') both to the spatial frequency of gratings and to various types of *ad hoc* features, such as bars, angles, edges, curves, line length, width and orientation, and relative retinal position. Both types of parts can be used to account for variations in performance in tasks involving visual objects. For example, confusions between briefly exposed alphabetic characters can be accounted for either in terms of the similarities of the letters' spatial frequency components (including local phase) or the similarities of the letters' features, such as line orientation, curvature, closure, and relative location of the lines.

Interestingly, the two approaches have reciprocal benefits and drawbacks. Spatial frequency components are universal (every visual pattern can be analysed into a subset of the same superset of sine wave gratings) and thus not *ad hoc*, but they are not available to our conscious perception (we don't see the sine wave gratings when we look at a scene – we see the scene). In contrast, the most popular and useful feature sets are *ad hoc* (they cannot be derived from universal principles but must be created anew for each new set of stimulus objects) but they are available to conscious perception – we can easily see the lines, angles, curves, etc. The two points of view seem to be roughly equivalent in both consistency with known facts and explanatory power.

A possible resolution to the impasse would involve finding a set of parts that is both universal and available to CONSCIOUSNESS, as well as being consistent with visual physiology and experimental data. One possibility is geons. The set of geons is the set of variants of generalized cylinders constrained by the properties of visual geometry that remain relatively constant under various transformations (such as motion and angle of view). This is a universal set, and it is easy to see the geons that make up 3-dimensional objects (for example, drawing of the human body is taught by pointing out that the body is roughly composed of 'cucumbers, sausages, and melons'). When the parts of the visual image that specify the geons of 3-dimensional objects are hidden, the objects become difficult to identify, while when an equal number of parts that are not involved in specifying geons are hidden, identification performance is unimpaired. However, physiologists have not yet found 'geon detectors' in the visual system, so the case for geons is not complete.

Finally, it should be pointed out that parts like geons, or lines and angles, or spatial frequency components, comprise only one of several aspects of visual objects that are analysed by the visual system. Colour, motion, position, texture and temporal properties, even association with sounds or tactile stimuli, for example, all contribute to the identification of real world objects. Analysers for these dimensions are always involved in both generating the percept and in identifying the object it represents. Moreover, top-down effects, such as those of ATTENTION and expectancy, generally interact with these bottom-up effects on object identification, especially under degraded conditions (see TOP-DOWN VS. BOTTOM-UP PERCEPTUAL/NEURAL PROCESSING).

LAWRENCE M. WARD

spatial mapping The process of acquiring spatial information about an organisms' environment, storing that information, and using that MEMORY to form a COGNITIVE MAP of the spatial cues of that environment. The acquisition of a REPRESENTATION usually requires an animal to move through an environment and engage in exploratory behaviors see EXPLORATION to acquire enough information about the spatial arrangements in the area. One advantage of acquiring a spatial map is that it enables the animal to be aware of properties of the environment that are beyond its field of perception, thereby allowing for more flexible

and efficient interactions with an animals surroundings.

See also: hippocampus; spatial memory; spatial cognition

STANLEY B. FLORESCO

spatial memory Spatial memory refers to the ENCODING, storage and retrieval of information regarding the characteristics of SPACE in an organism's environment. Spatial memory is crucial for a number of adaptive behaviours, such as FORAGING, ESCAPE and EXPLORATION. There are different memory systems that process different types of spatial relationships among environmental stimuli. For example, egocentric spatial memory (see EGOCENTRIC SPACE) refers to information about spatial relationships relative to ones body. Remembering whether a goal is situated to the left or right of ones current position is an example of egocentric spatial memory. In contrast, allocentric spatial memory (see ALLOCENTRIC SPACE; EGOCENTRIC SPACE) refers to information about the significance of specific external stimuli that are available in an environment. Using a landmark to navigate towards a goal, or beacon homing, is an example of allocentric spatial memory. Another form of spatial memory requires the consultation of a COGNITIVE MAP: an organism using a cognitive map is able to navigate towards a goal even when the goal is not directly perceptible to the animal, or take novel routes to reach the goal. Locating a hidden platform in the WATER MAZE requires the use of a cognitive map to reach a goal that is not directly visible.

It has been posited that different memory systems, including spatial memory, emerged as adaptive specialization (see ADAPTATION) to deal with specific problems animals were required to solve in order to survive. An adaptive specialization of a memory system is characterized by rules of operation that makes it especially suitable for a solution of a particular environmental problem, while poorly suited for the solving of other problems (see Sherry & Schacter, 1987). Thus, it is possible that different forms of spatial memory emerged in response to different problems of NAVIGATION, each of which required a specialized memory subsystem to solve the particular type of problem. There is evidence to suggest that different forms of spatial memory are subserved by distinct and largely independent neural systems. For example, the HIPPOCAMPUS appears to be involved in cognitive-map-based spatial memory, but not in egocentric or allocentric spatial memory. Likewise, the CAUDATE NUCLEUS may be more involved in egocentric and simple allocentric spatial memory, but not in the use of a cognitive map. Moreover, it appears that these different memory systems can learn to solve a spatial memory task simultaneously and independently of each other. In one study (Packard & McGaugh, 1996), rats were trained on a task that could be solved using either an allocentric spatial strategy or an egocentric strategy. On a probe day, rats were given reversible LIDOCAINE-induced inactivation (see TRANSIENT LESIONS) of either the hippocampus or the caudate nucleus. Inactivation of the hippocampus biased rats to use an egocentric strategy, while similar inactivation of the caudate nucleus biased rats to use an allocentric spatial strategy. These data suggested that separate spatial memory systems that govern egocentric and cognitive map-based spatial learning are able to solve spatial problems independently, and in parallel to each other.

See also: spatial behaviour

References

Sherry D.F. & Schacter D.L. (1987) The evolution of multiple memory systems. *Psychological Review* 94: 439–454.

Packard M.G. & McGaugh J.L. (1996) Inactivation of hippocampus or caudate nucleus with lidocaine differentially affects expression of place and response learning. *Neurobiology of Learning and Memory* 65: 65–72.

STANLEY B. FLORESCO

spatial neglect The neurological syndrome of spatial neglect consists of a group of symptoms which are partially dissociable from each other, and which occur most frequently following a STROKE or other form of brain disease that affects the region surrounding the junction between OCCIPITAL LOBE, TEMPORAL LOBE and PARIETAL LOBE of the RIGHT HEMISPHERE. In most cases, these symptoms recover with days or weeks, but in some cases they persist for long periods. The most striking constituent of the syndrome is often known as HEMISPATIAL NEGLECT, though the terminology is inconsistent. Here the patient will ignore items in the left side of SPACE (whether explored visually or through TOUCH). This failure is not due to BLINDNESS in the left half of the VISUAL FIELD, since that is not always present, and in any case many patients who do have such blindness do not show neglect. The classic demonstrations of Bisiach and his colleagues provide graphic evidence that hemispatial neglect is a rather high-level disorder. For example, an abstract shape passing behind a vertical slit is perceived as a whole by normal observers; and hemispatial neglect patients make errors in recognizing the leftward parts of such shapes. Thus part of a shape can be neglected *despite never having appeared as an image on the retina*. A more famous example is given by the efforts of hemispatial neglect patients to describe from memory the buildings around the famous Cathedral Square in Milan, from each of two opposite perspectives. They only named buildings on the right side of their imaginary view, even when their viewpoint was reversed by the examiner. It is difficult to understand these high-level neglect phenomena other than as a distortion of, or other form of interference with, representational processes in the brain.

More recent work has shown that information on the left side of a display, and which is therefore not reported, described or acknowledged by a patient, may nevertheless influence the person's behaviour. For example, a patient may see no difference between two pictures of a house which are identical apart from the presence of flames coming out of the left side of one of them. Yet if asked which she would prefer to live in, the patient will have a strong preference. In other studies, neglect patients have been shown to process the meaning of information presented on the neglected side in that their reaction times to categorize drawings on the 'good' side were affected by unacknowledged semantically related drawings on the neglected side. These observations show that rather deep visual information processing can occur without awareness in hemispatial neglect. Hemispatial neglect can sometimes be more pronounced within objects than within the person's visual space as a whole. For example, in copying a scene with trees, houses and people in it, a patient may draw all of the items, but in each case omit those parts lying to the left, such as the branches on the left side of each tree. Other patients will show the opposite tendency, neglecting the items on the left side of the picture altogether. These observations show that neglect does not affect only a single kind of mental representation. Indeed cases have been described whose neglect selectively affects particular categories of visual patterns, such as faces. In the light of all this, it is not surprising that it has proved difficult to demonstrate hemispatial neglect in an animal model. It may be that the substrates that are damaged are scarcely present in non-human animals, perhaps even in our relatives among the PRIMATES. Another reason is that animal brains are approximately symmetrical (see ASYMMETRY), at least in relation to perceptual processing: it may be that this protects them from suffering hemispatial neglect.

The other well-known symptom that is frequently associated with hemispatial neglect is EXTINCTION. This refers to a failure to detect one of two stimuli (lights, touches to the skin, or sounds) when both are presented simultaneously (see SIMULTANEOUS EXTINCTION). The stimulus that goes undetected is the one on the side opposite to the brain LESION – that is, the one on the left in a typical neglect patient. Since by definition a single stimulus on either side *can* be detected, this again cannot be explained as a simple sensory failure. Yet extinction can occur without hemispatial neglect, and vice versa. It is also relatively common after LEFT HEMISPHERE lesions, indeed after a wide range of lesions in the brain, unlike hemispatial neglect. Extinction can be readily studied in animals, and has been frequently reported following unilateral experimental lesions. Visual and tactile extinction occurs, for example, after damage to the SUPERIOR COLLICULUS, and after damage to the POSTERIOR PARIETAL CORTEX. Such observations suggest that extinction in both animals and man may be the result of a shift in the balance between sensorimotor orienting mechanisms on the two sides of the brain which

normally maintain equilibrium through mutual inhibition.

Reference

Bisiach E. & Vallar G. (1988) Hemineglect in humans. In *Handbook of Neuropsychology*, vol. 1, ed. F. Boller & J. Grafman, pp. 195–222, Elsevier: Amsterdam.

DAVID MILNER

spatial primitives A key concept in the computational approach to understanding biological visual systems (see COMPUTATIONAL VISION) is the notion of a spatial primitive. A spatial primitive is a localized feature in the image that will generally correspond to a single discrete spatial event in the scene (such as a small piece of an edge). The feature is primitive, in the sense that it is to be regarded as indivisible for further processes. Thus once, a number of points on an edge or a patch of texture have been identified as belonging together, they can be compiled into a spatial primitive and will not thereafter be processed separately.

See also: feature detector; spatial frequency vs. feature theory

ROGER J. WATT

spatial scale Spatial scale is an important concept in the computational approach to understanding biological visual systems (see COMPUTATIONAL VISION). Images have different structures at different spatial scales. For example, a tree has one sort of structure at a coarse spatial scale (the overall shape of the tree) and another structure at a fine spatial scale (the shape of the individual leaves). Different spatial scales are generally appropriate for different visual tasks, so that avoiding the tree as an obstacle requires coarse scale information, but picking the apples, requires much finer scale information. It is thought that vision proceeds by analysing coarse spatial scales before fine.

ROGER J. WATT

spatial summation *see* summation

species In biology, a species is a group of individuals – animals or plants – with, for example, common anatomical and morphological features, and an ability to interbreed. The term species is however also used more generally to indicate any group showing similarities. For example, one speaks of molecular species to indicate groups of molecules (see MOLECULE) with common characteristics.

See also: hominid; taxonomy

specific anosmia Insensitivity to a specific ODORANT: around 90 kinds of ANOSMIA specific to individual odorants have been described. It is frequently tested using STEROID HORMONES found in human body odour (such as androstenone). There are suggestions that (1) specific anosmia is more common in women than in men; and (2) that repeated exposure to odorants might be able to induce olfactory detection – the stability of the phenomenon has been questioned.

See also: olfaction; stereochemical theory of odour discrimination

specific appetites *see* malnutrition; sodium appetite

specific hungers *see* malnutrition; sodium appetite

specific language impairment *see* language

specificity theories As relating to SOMATOSENSORY experience, see SKIN.

SPECT (single photon emission tomography) A FUNCTIONAL NEUROIMAGING method with relatively low resolution compared to other techniques. It is widely used to measure cerebral BLOOD flow, offering a relatively inexpensive and straightforward means for making a 'first pass' assessment of brain state. It predates techniques such as positron emission tomography (PET), which was developed to improve image resolution.

spectral sensitivity The spectral sensitivity of a PHOTORECEPTOR results from the presence of light-sensitive molecules, termed VISUAL PIGMENT, contained within the cells' outer segments. Visual pigments consist of a light-absorbing CHROMOPHORE bound to a protein (termed OPSIN). The chromophore is always 11-cis retinal (11-cis vitamin A aldehyde) whereas the protein varies somewhat, resulting in visual pigments that absorb light maximally

from different regions of the spectrum. The visual pigment of human RODS absorbs blue-green light maximally (~500 nm), whereas the pigment in human CONES absorbs maximally in the blue (~420 nm), green (~530 nm) or red-yellow (~560 nm) regions of the spectrum.

See also: retina

JOHN E. DOWLING

spectral sensitivity curves Functions describing the relative response to different wavelengths of light. They may be used to characterize the responses of light sensitive neurons in the VISUAL SYSTEM, or the ability of an animal or human subject to detect lights from different regions of the visible spectrum. The measurements of spectral sensitivity functions in human and non-human primates have been used to reveal the three different types of cones in the retina and to reveal the presence of missing or anomalous cone types, as in the inherited colour vision deficiencies (see DICHROMATIC COLOUR BLINDNESS). Spectral sensitivity measurements also reveal the presence of cone opponent processing in colour vision.

See also: opponent process theory of colour vision; Purkinje shift; trichromatic theory of colour vision

KATHY T. MULLEN

speech deficits SPEECH DEFICITS can be used as a very general term to indicate a variety of conditions in which SPEECH PRODUCTION is impaired, either through disturbance of the musculature and the machinery of speech production (in structures such as the LARYNX) or through dysfunction in the CENTRAL NERVOUS SYSTEM. Speech deficits include, for example, STUTTERING, STAMMERING, DYSARTHRIA and MUTISM.

speech perception This term refers to the process which transforms the auditory representation derived by peripheral AUDITORY PERCEPTION into a representation which can be used to access the LEXICON. The acoustic signal corresponding to a particular lexical representation is highly variable: the length and shape of vocal tracts differ as a function of age, sex and body size; speakers can be nearer or further away, tired or excited or angry, speaking slowly or rapidly; they can have a cold in the nose or a mouthful of food; there may be barriers intervening between speaker and hearer, or background noise. This extreme variability motivates the assumption that speech perception converts the acoustic input into a relatively abstract (or normalized) form to use for lexical access. Since the lexicon is very large, it is also attractive to propose that this conversion process makes use of a small set of sub-lexical units. Candidate sub-lexical units have been the units of analysis used by linguistics, with the PHONEME the most popular choice because (by definition) it is the smallest unit into which speech can be sequentially decomposed. However phonemes do not possess constant, invariant properties. They are variable due to the factors described above; and they are subject to co-articulation – that is, the acoustic form of phonemes conveys information not only about the phonemes' own identity but also about the nature of their phonetic context. Other candidate units include (below the phonemic level) featural representations or spectral templates, and (above it) SYLLABLES, DEMI-SYLLABLES AND DIPHONES (the syllable 'keep', phonetically [kip], consists of two demi-syllables: [ki], [ip], and four diphones: when 'keep' is uttered in isolation these are silence-to-[k], [k]-to-[i], [i]-to-[p], [p]-to-silence). Research in speech perception has chiefly addressed the factors determining listeners' identification of phonemes. Phoneme identification tends to be categorical; this can be shown with a continuum of sounds progressing in equal steps from a clear realization of one phoneme to a clear realization of another. (For example, a continuum from [pi] to [bi] formed by shortening the voice onset time – time between release of the lip closure and beginning of the vowel.) Listeners will identify the sounds as belonging to one category or the other, not as between the categories. Phoneme perception also involves sensitivity to the contextual variability of phonemes, in that listeners adjust their expectations of different cues for a phoneme according to the context in which it occurs. For example, voice onset time can be evaluated in relation to the duration of adjacent vowels.

See also: motor theory of speech perception;

phonology; speech production; word recognition

Reference

Nygaard L.C. & Pisoni D.B. (1995) Speech perception: new directions in research and theory. In *Handbook of Perception and Cognition*, ed. E.C. Carterette & M.P. Friedman, vol. 11, *Speech, Language and Communication*, ed. J.L. Miller & P.D. Eimas, pp. 63–96, Academic Press: New York.

ANNE CUTLER

speech production To produce speech, the speaker expels air from the lungs through the vocal tract, and modulates the airflow by changing the vocal tract's shape and moving the tongue against the lips, teeth, alveolar ridge (behind the upper teeth) and palate, thus creating speech sounds. Voiced sounds (vowels, many consonants – for example [d], [l], [m] and [v]) involve audible vibration produced by the vocal folds in the LARYNX; unvoiced sounds (other consonants – for example [t] and [f]) are produced without such vibration. The speech sounds are produced in a smooth continuous manner which has the effect that the articulation of a sound overlaps with the articulation of adjacent sounds (known as co-articulation). One result of this is that the same PHONEME can be produced differently in different phonetic contexts (compare the [k] in 'key' and 'caw'). The production of sounds is the final stage of a process that begins with the planning of a message to be spoken, and continues via the selection of words and syntactic structure to convey this message, the determination of the appropriate phonological structure (including prosodic form) of the chosen sequence of words, and the specification of the precise phonetic form to be articulated. The selection of words from the mental LEXICON in speech production proceeds in two stages: first conceptual representations are mapped onto the meaning representation of words, then the phonological forms linked with these meaning representations are activated. The construction of syntactic form is in part dependent on the precise words chosen and in part on the conceptual content of the message. Speech production sometimes goes wrong, and such SLIPS OF THE TONGUE can occur at any level of production: choosing the concept ('Pass the dog' instead of 'pass the salt' when the speaker is looking at the dog), selecting the words (instead of 'Sunday' the semantically related 'Monday' or the phonologically related 'summer'), constructing the syntax ('the boys who I saw the boys'), determining the phonological form ('Lunday sunch' for 'Sunday lunch'); and many more. Slips can thus provide evidence about the processes and stages involved in speaking. During speech production speakers monitor their output and may repair infelicitous or faulty utterances; this monitoring can also apply to any aspect of the output – style, content, words, syntactic form, pronunciation. What aspects of the output are monitored depends however on where the speaker's attention is directed (a non-native speaker may concentrate on careful monitoring of pronunciation, a witness in court may concentrate on correct choice of formal style, etc.)

See also: grammar;　phonology;　prosody; speech perception

References

Fowler C.A. (1995) Speech production. In *Handbook of Perception and Cognition*, ed. E.C. Carterette & M.P. Friedman, vol. 11, *Speech, Language and Communication*, ed. J. L. Miller and P.D. Eimas, pp. 29–61. Academic Press: New York.

Levelt W.J.M. (1989) *Speaking: From Conception to Articulation*, MIT Press: Cambridge MA.

ANNE CUTLER

speed Street name for AMPHETAMINE.

spelling Spelling is, in a curious sense, a relatively recent phenomenon. Before the publication of Dr Samuel Johnson's magisterial *Dictionary of the English Language* in 1755 there was no accepted and standardized way of spelling words, nor common agreement on the meaning of many words. Johnson's Dictionary was incomplete but prepared the ground for later works, culminating in the authoritative *Oxford English Dictionary* (see Winchester, 1999). There are various disorders of spelling: see AGRAPHIA for discussion of these.

See also: reading; speech production; writing

Reference

Winchester S. (1999) *The Surgeon of Crowthorne*, Penguin Books, London.

spermatozoa *see* testes

sphenoid bone *see* skull

sphingolipid *see* lipids

spike; spiking A spike is a common term for a single ACTION POTENTIAL; spiking is the term given to the generation of action potentials. FIRING is a term synonymous with spiking.

See also: burst firing; single spiking

spike frequency adaptation A process of modification of an ACTION POTENTIAL. It can be produced by a slow afterhyperpolarization CURRENT (that is an ION flow that occurs after HYPERPOLARIZATION has been initiated), an effect that involves a calcium (Ca^{2+}) activated potassium (K^+) current into the NEURON. The net effect of the afterhyperpolarization current is to reduce the generation of action potentials when neurons are in a state of constant depolarization: in crude terms it is a braking mechanism. It is a process that has been associated with beta ADRENOCEPTORS, which can increase firing in neurons that are already excited.

Reference

Feldman R., Meyer J.S. & Quenzer L.F. (1997) *Principles of Neuropsychopharmacology*, Sinauer Associates: Sunderland MA.

spinal cord The spinal cord is that part of the CENTRAL NERVOUS SYSTEM encased in the vertebral column – the spine or backbone. It is continuous with the MEDULLA OBLONGATA rostrally. The gross anatomical and internal microscopic features of the spinal cord vary over its length as a consequence of differences in the degree of innervation of the limbs and viscera. The spinal cord is divided into segments grouped according to the relationships of the SPINAL NERVES to the vertebrae. In humans, there are 31 segments divided among 8 cervical, 12 thoracic, 5 lumbar, 5 sacral and 1 coccygeal spinal nerves. Because of the differential growth of the vertebral column and the spinal cord, the DORSAL and VENTRAL ROOTS of the lower spinal cord are elongated in the vertebral canal forming the CAUDA EQUINA (Latin, horse's tail). Two spinal cord enlargements are related to innervation of the limbs. The cervical enlargement (C4–T1) innervates the arms (the corresponding spinal nerves form the brachial PLEXUS) and the lumbosacral enlargement (L2–S4) innervates the legs and PERINEUM (the corresponding spinal nerves form the lumbar and sacral plexuses). The thoracic spinal cord has a smaller cross-section because it innervates the skin and muscles of the thorax and back, and the internal organs, which are less densely innervated than the limbs. In cross-section, the spinal cord consists of WHITE MATTER surrounding grey matter resembling the shape of a butterfly, a shape that varies at different segmental levels. The white matter is divided into dorsal, dorsolateral, lateral and ventromedial funiculi or columns consisting of myelinated and unmyelinated (see MYELIN) ascending and descending axons that connect the spinal cord with higher levels of the NEURAXIS.

The different functional pathways in the white matter cannot be distinguished microscopically but they are segregated within specific areas. The DORSAL FUNICULUS contains ascending sensory axons that originate in the periphery and synapse in the DORSAL COLUMN NUCLEI OF THE MEDULLA OBLONGATA (the GRACILE NUCLEUS and the CUNEATE NUCLEUS). These axons carry sensations of fine, discriminative TOUCH and vibration. The DORSOLATERAL FUNICULUS contains afferent sensory fibres mediating PAIN and temperature sensations and descending axons from the BRAINSTEM. The periphery of the lateral funiculus contains axons ascending to higher levels of the neuraxis including the brainstem (spinoreticular pathways), CEREBELLUM (spinocerebellar pathways) and THALAMUS (spinothalamic pathways). The inner parts of the lateral funiculus contain axons descending from the CEREBRAL CORTEX (the lateral corticospinal tract) and RED NUCLEUS of the MESENCEPHALON (rubrospinal tract) that modulate spinal cord activity, especially movements of the DISTAL limb musculature. The ventral funiculus contains axons descending from several structures, including the cerebral cortex, the

RETICULAR FORMATION, VESTIBULAR COMPLEX and TECTUM. These latter pathways are important in regulating basic movements and posture. PROPRIOSPINAL pathways that interconnect different levels of the spinal cord, especially between the cervical and lumbar enlargements, are located around the borders of the GREY MATTER. In the region of the CENTRAL CANAL, the remnant of the spinal ventricular system (see VENTRICLES), the anterior white commissure is formed by crossing axons of the spinothalamic tract.

The grey matter of the spinal cord is divided into dorsal and ventral horns with an intermediate zone in between and, at thoracic levels, a lateral horn containing sympathetic preganglionic neurons. Two main schemes are regularly used to describe the organization of the grey matter. In the classical neuroanatomical approach, differences in their CYTOARCHITECTURE are used to define nuclei. In a second approach, the grey matter is divided into 10 layers (REXED'S LAMINAE). This system is popular because of the ease with which it can be correlated with physiological and functional differences within the spinal cord and because it is applicable across species. The 10 laminae and the equivalent spinal nuclei are from dorsal to ventral: I – posteromarginal nucleus, II – substantia gelatinosa, III and IV – nucleus proprius, V and VI – deeper layers of the dorsal horn, VII – intermediate zone, VIII – non-motoneuronal areas of the ventral horn, IX – motor neurons and X – grey matter surrounding the central canal of the spinal cord. Two groups of neurons are present only at thoracic levels of the cord: the sympathetic preganglionic neurons of the intermediolateral and intermediomedial nuclei in lamina VII and the nucleus dorsalis of Clarke which projects to the cerebellum. Sacral parasympathetic preganglionic neurons are found in lamina VII of the sacral cord.

The functions of the many descending and PROPRIOBULBAR pathways of the spinal cord are best understood by considering how they terminate in relationship to SENSORY NEURONS, INTERNEURONS and MOTOR NEURONS. Thus, axons terminating in the dorsal horn modulate sensory processing. Axons terminating in the ventromedial grey matter regulate posture and gross locomotion, those in the ventrolateral grey matter of the ventral horn regulate proximal movements of the limbs, and those in dorsolateral regions of the ventral horn regulate distal movements, according to the somatotopical organization of motor neurons.

DAVID A. HOPKINS

spinal lemniscus (from Greek, *lemniskos*: a ribbon or bandage) A pathway of FIBRES made up of ascending axons (see AXON) coming from the spinal cord travelling into the central nervous system.

See also: dorsal column – medial lemniscal system; hindbrain; lateral lemniscus

spinal nerves Spinal nerves are formed by the axons of dorsal (posterior) and ventral (anterior) roots that arise throughout the length of the spinal cord. DORSAL ROOTS contain sensory axons and aggregations of cell bodies (DORSAL ROOT GANGLIA) of sensory neurons. Ventral roots contain axons of somatomotor neurons and, at thoracic and sacral levels, they also contain autonomic preganglionic axons. The roots unite to form segmentally arranged, mixed spinal nerves. In humans, there are 31 pairs grouped and numbered according to the corresponding vertebrae, thus forming 8 cervical, 12 thoracic, 5 lumbar, 5 sacral pairs and 1 coccygeal pair of spinal nerves.

See also: cranial nerves; peripheral nervous system; spinal cord

DAVID A. HOPKINS

spinal reflex A reflex contained entirely in the SPINAL CORD.

See also: reflex arc

spinal tap Synonymous with LUMBAR PUNCTURE.

spinalization Transection of the SPINAL CORD. It is an operation rarely performed, but used in certain circumstances to examine neural processing in the spinal cord (and associated SPINAL NERVES). Spinalization is achieved under general ANAESTHESIA: the dura (see MENINGES) around the spinal cord is exposed, LOCAL ANAESTHETIC applied, BLOOD vessels cauterized and the cord then cut using surgical scissors. Spinalized rats that have had transec-

tions at relatively low levels (the lower THORACIC SPINAL CORD for example) will maintain themselves well, eating and drinking normally, though bladder activity is poor and rats will have to have their bladders emptied twice daily by the application of manual pressure. However, with operations such as this, a very careful consideration of the likely costs (to the rat) and benefits (in terms of knowledge gained for medical and veterinary practice) has to be made.

See also: locomotion

spinocerebellum *see* cerebellum – anatomical organization

spinothalamic tract *see* anterolateral system

spiral ganglion *see* auditory pathways

spiroperidol *see* antipsychotic

splanchnic nerve (from Greek, *splanchna*: entrails) In general the term splanchnic refers to the VISCERA and anything pertaining to them (though the Latin term *viscera* is far more commonly used). The splanchnic nerve is one of the SPINAL NERVES, originating in thoracic and LUMBAR SPINAL CORD and connecting to internal organs. It has been suggested that it carries information about the state of the stomach (see DIGESTIVE SYSTEM).

splanchnocranium *see* skull

splenium *see* corpus callosum

splice variants *see* gene

split brain The term split brain refers to a neurological condition when the main COMMISSURES connecting the two CEREBRAL HEMISPHERES have been surgically disconnected (see COMMISSURE; HEMISPHERE). The term initially described an animal preparation used in the classic work of Ronald Myers and Roger Sperry. It was subsequently applied to a small group of patients – split-brain patients – in whom, as a last resort, the CORPUS CALLOSUM (and in some cases also the ANTERIOR COMMISSURE) was sectioned in order to reduce the spread of EPILEPSY from one cerebral hemisphere into the other. Myers' studies on cats and monkeys were important because they established new and hitherto unexploited methods. There had been previous attempts to cut these main pathways between the two cerebral hemispheres but the outcome, whether in humans or animals, had seemed to be trivial with seemingly few consequences from such a major change in brain structure. With carefully controlled studies, maintaining orienting and preventing information exchange between the hemispheres through transactions with the external world, Myers & Sperry found that the split-brain animals appeared to have totally divided perception and learning. At the same time, their movements and alertness when moving about freely and their general motivation seemed to be unchanged.

The split-brain patients showed profound changes in some of their mental activities. Direct awareness was no longer whole. An object placed in the left hand out of sight could not be matched to the same object felt separately and unseen in the right hand. As long as the eyes remained stationary, something seen just to the left of the fixation point could not be accurately compared to something seen on the right side. Similar divisions in olfactory and auditory awareness were also demonstrated. By far the most dramatic finding of the early tests was the total failure of the RIGHT HEMISPHERE on its own to express itself in speech. It was unable to produce words to explain that of which it was aware or which it thought it knew. By contrast, when stimuli were given to the LEFT HEMISPHERE, the subject could say perfectly well what the experience had been like. Subsequent, more detailed testing has shown that some transfer of information is possible through subcortical pathways but the basic dramatic findings of the surgical split-brain remain well established. In the case of human commissurotomy patients, Sperry argued that there were 'two minds in one brain'.

See also: callosal agnesis; consciousness; spatial neglect

References

Myers R.E. & Sperry R.W. (1958) Interhemispheric communication through the corpus callosum. *Archives of Neurology and Psychology* 80: 298–303.
Sperry R.W. (1982) Some effects of disconnect-

ing the cerebral hemispheres. *Science* 217: 1223–1226.

MALCOLM A. JEEVES

spongiform encephalopathy *see* bovine spongiform encephalopathy; Creutzfeldt–Jakob disease; prion disease

spontaneous alternation A test used to examine EXPLORATION and WORKING MEMORY without use of REWARD. It relies on the fact that rodents and other animals will spontaneously alternate their choices of locations to visit if allowed to do so – an effective form of FORAGING. Spontaneous alternation can be examined in a T MAZE, PLUS MAZE, Y MAZE or RADIAL ARM MAZE, each one offering an umber of different locations to visit following introduction to the maze either in a start arm (as one would do with the T maze) or at a central location (as one would do with the other mazes). Spontaneous alternation is scored simply by counting the arms visited and computing the number of different arms visited out of the total number entered.

spontaneous recovery Responding can be diminished or lost completely following, for example, HABITUATION or EXTINCTION: SPONTANEOUS RECOVERY describes the resumption of responding after a period of habituation or extinction.

See also: schedules of reinforcement

Sprague-Dawley rats *see* rat

spreading depression A transient inactivation of responsiveness in the CEREBRAL CORTEX that appears as a series of waves of silence on the ELECTROENCEPHALOGRAM that spread slowly (3–6 mm/sec) from a site of local stimulation or injury. The underlying disturbance, investigated especially by A.A.P. Leão, probably involves extrusion of potassium ions (K^+) from hyperactive cortical neurons, serving to pass on a chain of DEPOLARIZATION BLOCKADE to adjacent cortical cells. The phenomenon has been exploited especially by I. Steele Russell as a means of producing reversible HEMIDECORTICATION in rats, and a similar process has been implicated, controversially, in the prodromal aura of MIGRAINE in man.

L. JACOB HERBERG

spritzing A technique, relatively rarely used, for making lesions of the outermost tissues by dusting the surface of the brain with a neurotoxin; see LESION.

sprouting The re-development of axons (see AXON) following non-fatal damage induced by any means to a NEURON; see, for example, NERVE CRUSH.

squamous epithelium *see* skin

SQUID magnetometry SQUID (an acronym for superconducting quantum interference device) magnetometry is a specialized form of MAGNETOENCEPHALOGRAPHY – the measurement of weak magnetic fields in brain tissue. The best-known example is MAGNETIC RESONANCE IMAGING (MRI). FUNCTIONAL NEUROIMAGING, achieved most commonly by FUNCTIONAL MRI and by POSITRON EMISSION TOMOGRAPHY (PET), has produced significant advances in understanding the actions of living brain tissue. Both of these techniques are able to resolve images of the brain to within millimetre accuracy, but both suffer from the same significant drawbacks: the temporal resolution is very poor (requiring considerable periods of time for a subject within the measuring equipment) and neither is a direct measure of neuronal activity. Both measure BLOOD flow, a metabolic index of neural activity, but necessarily one step removed from the neural activity itself. Measures of electrical activity that give excellent temporal resolution – EVENT-RELATED POTENTIALS – can be combined with functional MRI to give an overall impression of both the location and timing of events in the brain, but SQUID magnetometry offers the hope of being able to make direct measurements of neuronal activity in real time with a spatial resolution of millimetres (though at present this is restricted to only the outer tissues of the brain, to a depth of no more than 3 cm, meaning that subcortical structures cannot be investigated).

SQUID magnetometry is used to overcome the general problems of magnetoencephalography, which are the weakness of the magnetic fields generated by biological tissue (more so in brain tissue than in other tissues of interest, such as the heart) and the strength of the magnetic sources in the environment. SQUID

magnetometry addresses these problems by allowing for the accurate detection of very low magnetic field strengths. It measures the quantum mechanical tunnelling current that passes through a link in a superconducting loop, this current being dependent on the magnetic flux through the loop. An individual SQUID magnetometer can be used to detect localized magnetic fields. An array of SQUIDs allows one to build a tomographic image of brain tissue in exactly the same way as other functional neuroimaging techniques do.

Reference

Singh K.D. (1995) Functional imaging of the brain using superconducting magnetometry. *Endeavour* 19: 39–44. (This paper is also available on a website: http://psyserver.pc.rhbnc.ac.uk/vision/MAGRESpaper/final4web.html)

squint *see* strabismus

stains When tissue is processed by HISTOLOGY, sections are stained in any of several ways in order to colour structures or chemical such that they can be seen and discriminated using MICROSCOPY. Common forms of staining include CRESYL VIOLET (to stain NISSL BODIES, allowing visualization of a NEURON and of GLIAL CELLS – THIONIN and TOLUIDINE BLUE also do this), LUXOL FAST BLUE (which stains MYELIN) and ALIZARIN RED (which stains CALCIUM). Stains are in fact types of DYE that literally stain certain types of tissue or chemical. The use of stains is to be discriminated from HISTOCHEMISTRY which involves chemical reactions with coloured end products. The range of staining procedures available is in fact quite enormous.

Reference

Bancroft J.D. & Stevens A. (1982) *Theory and Practice of Histological Techniques*, Churchill Livingstone: Edinburgh.

staircase test A simple but effective test developed by Steven Dunnett and his colleagues to examine the ability of a RAT to reach (see REACHING) for and to GRASP food pellets. Rats are placed in a box on a raised plinth: the box does not constrict them but they cannot turn round on the plinth or jump down. On either side of the plinth a series of steps – the staircase – descends. All the rat has to do is to reach down and grasp the pellets: the number of steps cleared of pellets gives an index of the rat's reaching abilities; the number of pellets that disappear (that is, are eaten) gives an index of the rat's skill in grasping. Pellets that are grasped properly are eaten, but those that are not properly grasped fall to the bottom of the staircase, out of reach.

Reference

Montoya C.P., Campbell-Hope L.J., Pemberton K.D. & Dunnett S.B. (1991) The staircase test: a measure of independent forelimb reaching and grasping abilities in rats. *Journal of Neuroscience Methods* 36: 219–228.

stammering *see* stuttering

stance phase *see* locomotion

standard metabolic rate *see* metabolic rate

Stanford–Binet scale *see* intelligence testing

stapes ossicles

startle reflex A reflex 'jump' in response to sudden stimulation. HABITUATION normally occurs to startling stimuli over time and warning signals can be used to minimize the startle response – PREPULSE INHIBITION. Prepulse inhibition of the startle reflex has been used to investigate SENSORY GATING mechanisms in experimental animals, normal human subjects and in patients with SCHIZOPHRENIA.

state dependency A phenomenon that describes the dependence of a behavioural or cognitive effect (usually MEMORY or LEARNING) on a particular stimulus setting. The most well-known example of state dependency is STATE-DEPENDENT LEARNING, in relation to a state produced by a PSYCHOACTIVE drug. In this situation, information that is acquired under the influence of a drug is not transferred to the non-drug state, and vice versa. For example, if a rat learns to run a MAZE under the influence of the drug, it may perform substantially worse when tested in the non-drug state, even though the drug may actually impair performance in a naive animal. It is theorized that in cases like this, the drug becomes part of the environment 'set' – that is, it is a critical and salient stimulus cue, much as familiar spatial cues would serve

to guide performance. It is important to be aware of state-dependent effects and their influence on drug-related behaviour in many behavioural testing paradigms. An example of how state dependence can influence interpretation of a behavioural effect is illustrated by the PLACE CONDITIONING paradigm. In this task, a drug is given on multiple occasions paired with one environment and on other occasions, no drug is paired with another environment. On the test day, the animal's 'preference' for each environment is recorded, and it is assumed that the drug treatment was rewarding if the animal spends more time in the drug-paired environment. This could be the case, but it could also be due to state dependence. In this interpretation, the animal prefers the drug-paired environment because it appears novel, due to the fact that it is experiencing a stimulus situation quite different from that perceived during drug treatment. Factors like these must be accounted for when evaluating the effects of psychoactive drugs on behaviour.

ANN E. KELLEY

state-dependent learning *see* state dependency

status epilepticus *see* epilepsy

steady state The term steady state can be applied in very many different contexts. In biological psychology there are two common usages: (i) pharmacological: the *steady state plasma level* of a DRUG is the concentration achieved between the phase of absorption and distribution around the body, and the phase of metabolism and excretion. Typically, therapeutic drugs are taken at intervals and so the concentration in PLASMA fluctuates over time: the achievement of a steady state is desirable but difficult. Longer-term forms of administration are valuable in helping achieve this; see for example TRANSDERMAL DRUG DELIVERY. (ii) In OPERANT psychology, *steady state responding* refers to a constant level of performance maintained by a definable set of conditions which provide just enough REINFORCEMENT to maintain responding. Typically, small fixed ratio SCHEDULES OF REINFORCEMENT are used to achieve this. There is minimal session-to-session variability and sessions can be extended without change for hundreds of hours. A *steady state baseline* of responding represents a valuable BASELINE for comparing the effects of further experimental manipulations.

stearic acid (stearate) White fatty acids (see FATTY ACIDS) found in animal fats and many vegetable oils. Also used to modify the recording surface of a CARBON PASTE ELECTRODE used in VOLTAMMETRY.

See also: drug ionization

CHARLES D. BLAHA

Steele–Richardson–Olzewski disease *see* progressive supranuclear palsy

stellate cells (stellate NEURON) These are NON-PYRAMIDAL NEURONS, found in the CEREBRAL CORTEX and cerebellum (see CEREBELLUM – ANATOMICAL ORGANIZATION) which function as INTERNEURONS. They are called star cells because their dendritic organization gives the impression of the cells being star-shaped.

See also: basket cells

stem cells Embryonic stem cells are able to give rise to all types of cells in the body: they are the precursors of all cells. In the adult body there are various types of stem cells – intestinal stem cells, skin stem cells and neural stem cells – that are involved in the regeneration and repair of tissues (though note that different tissues contain different amounts of stem cells: the heart for example has relatively few, the intestine a relatively large number). When stem cells divide, some of the progeny differentiate into specialized cells, others remain as stem cells. The discovery of stem cells – a recent event – has opened the possibility that neurodegenerative diseases such as PARKINSON'S DISEASE could be treated by administration of stem cells to replace those that had been lost, though of course, whatever process was causing NEURON destruction in the first place would need to be understood and controlled to prevent the possibility of replacement cells being destroyed as the originals had been.

See also: transplantation

Reference

Pedersen R.A. (1999) Embryonic stem cells for medicine. *Scientific American* 280: 44–49.

stem completion A technique used in cognitive psychology experiments, in which subjects are given part of a word and are required to complete it; see, for an example, ERRORLESS LEARNING.

stenin *see* neurin

Stent–Singer rule *see* Hebbian synapse

stereochemical theory of odour discrimination Odour detection depends exclusively on the interaction of chemical cues with the olfactory receptor neurons and is signalled when an odorant molecule is bound to a RECEPTOR on the cilium (see CILIA). Over the years, mechanisms for odour discrimination have been formulated from electrophysiological recordings of individual olfactory receptor cells, and more recently from the molecular genetics of olfactory receptor coding. A mechanism hypothesized to be fundamental to olfactory discrimination has been the selective sensitivity of individual receptor cells to different odorants. However, electrophysiological recordings from individual receptor units have failed to show specificity to single odorants. A given unit is responsive to a large number of different odorants, but they are usually of the same chemical grouping. Nevertheless, the grouping of specificities is not consistent from one receptor cell to another; very few receptor cells respond to exactly the same set of chemicals. How then are particular odours identified by the OLFACTORY SYSTEM?

A molecular basis for odour discrimination has been provided by the sequencing and cloning of a large family of genes, approximately 1000 in rats, that encode for odorant receptor proteins which belong to the seven-transmembrane-domain family of receptors coupled to G PROTEIN. Olfactory neurons expressing a given receptor are located in one of four broad parallel zones, each occupying 25% of the mucosal surface area. However, within a given zone there appears to be no further patterning of neurons expressing a given receptor. The current opinion is that only one of the 1000 receptor genes is expressed in a single olfactory neuron, and the axons from each of these widely dispersed neurons converge into a single GLOMERULUS in the OLFACTORY BULB, thereby achieving a spatial organization at the first synaptic relay. But if a given olfactory neuron only expresses one receptor type, why do electrophysiological recordings fail to show specificities? Clearly, the receptor protein has the capacity to bind more than one type of chemical LIGAND. Whether or not these different ligands have structural features in common is a distinct possibility. By monitoring the response specificity of a single mitral cell (see MITRAL CELL) whose apical dendrites (see APICAL DENDRITE) project to a single glomerulus, information can be obtained on those receptor neurons that converge into this glomerulus. It would appear that an individual mitral cell is activated by a range of odour molecules with a similar stereochemical structure (see STEREOCHEMISTRY). When stimulated with a range of ALIPHATIC ALDEHYDES, individual mitral cells are selectively responsive to odorants with similar hydrocarbon chain lengths and similar functional groups, especially if these occupy a similar molecular position. Increasing or shortening the hydrocarbon chain length may produce an inhibitory response.

Assuming that a single odour molecule has several molecular conformations and can activate several different receptor types, the question arises as to whether the neurons for these different receptor types are divergently spaced in the bulb or cluster in selected regions. Mapping of odour-evoked responses in the olfactory bulb using C-FOS expression, VOLTAGE-SENSITIVE DYE RECORDING, and 2-deoxyglucose uptake (see METABOLIC MAPPING) shows that single odour molecules activate more than one glomerulus, but the spatial patterns of glomerular activation are regionalized. Electrophysiological recordings confirm that odour receptors that map to neighbouring glomeruli may have a similar structure in their receptive sites since they respond to similar classes of odour molecules. It is possible that the large seven-transmembrane olfactory receptor possesses more than one binding site. The olfactory mucosa contains diverse, functionally distinct odorant-binding proteins which recognize and bind separate classes of odorants. These odorant-binding proteins probably act as transporter molecules for hydrophobic odorants, and may themselves interact with the receptor for ligand presentation. In addition to this complication, recent advances in our understanding of olfactory transduction suggest that the capacity to integrate chemical signals may occur in the olfactory receptor neuron. Two systems of SECOND MESSENGERS, INOSITOL phosphate (Ins P3) and CYCLIC NUCLEOTIDE (cyclic AMP) signalling pathways mediate olfactory transduction. Both pathways can target multiple ION CHANNEL effectors and can localize to the same receptor neuron, mediating opposing conductances. This allows the olfactory neuron to encode bipolar information and presents possibilities for integration of odour cues.

Whatever the mechanism might be at the molecular level, a pattern of multiple receptor firing must provide the code for odour discrimination. This would account for cross-adaptation, the alteration in the perceived discrimination of one odour according to the identity of a preceding odour. When more than one odour is presented simultaneously, we are often unable to identify the components of the mixture. Again the pattern of receptor neuron activation generated by each individual odour is lost in the total pattern produced by the odour complex. It is well known that skilled perfumers are able to analyse odour complexes, but it is likely that they have learnt through experience to recognize the sensations that given odours produce when mixed.

See also: across-fibre pattern theory; gustation; olfaction

BARRY KEVERNE

stereochemistry (from Greek, *stereos*: solid, *chemeia*: the Egyptian art, i.e., chemistry) Stereochemistry is that branch of chemical analysis concerned with the organization of atoms in a MOLECULE – the organization that gives a molecule its 3-dimensional shape; stereochemical is an adjectival form of this. The stereochemical structure of a molecule is an important consideration in determining its ability to show BINDING to a specific RECEPTOR.

See also: stereochemical theory of odour discrimination

stereodepth perception see depth perception; stereopsis

stereognosis Stereognosis is knowledge of an object – particularly OBJECT RECOGNITION – that has been obtained by TOUCH.

stereoisomer *see* isomer

stereology A procedure for estimating parameters of CENTRAL NERVOUS SYSTEM cells or nuclei. Introduced in the early 1990s, stereology provides efficient algorithms for counting cells in defined areas of the brain (such as discrete nuclei), measuring the volumes of those nuclei, or the diameter, area or volume of neuronal or glial cells themselves. Stereology is based on rigorous statistical principles for unbiased sampling. It allows automation of the microscopic sampling procedures, and the algorithms are both more accurate and much more efficient than conventional procedures based on ABERCROMBIE CORRECTION of total or randomly sampled cell counts in serial sections.

See also: cavalieri principle; disector stereology; image analysis; optical fractionater

Reference

Gundersen H.J.G., Bendtsen T.F., Korbo L., Marcussen N., Møller A., Nielsen K., Nyengaard J.R., Pakkenberg B., Sørensen F.B., Vesterby A. & West M.J. (1988) Some new, simple and efficient stereological methods and their use in pathological research and diagnosis. *Acta Pathologica, Microbiologica et Immunologica Scandinavica* 96: 379–394.

STEPHEN B. DUNNETT

stereopsis Stereopsis is, literally, 'solid sight' and is the impression of depth derived from the combination by the brain of the two different views of the visual world enjoyed by the two eyes. Because the two eyes are horizontally displaced, one from another, the retinal images differ and are said to be DISPARATE. One of the most remarkable feats of the VISUAL SYSTEM is to combine these two images to deliver a unitary impression of the visual world, interpreting the disparity as depth. It has been shown that disparity on its own is a sufficient cue to depth. This phenomenon was exploited commercially in the Victorian era with the production of stereoscopic photographs, and there has been a recent resurgence of interest in depth-from-disparity with the common avail-

ability of virtual-reality headsets, 3-dimensional movie films and the so-called 'Magic Eye' pictures. A similar impression of solidity and depth results from MONOCULAR PARALLAX.

DAVID W. HEELEY

stereoscopic depth *see* depth perception; stereopsis

stereoscopic perception For us to interact efficiently with the world of objects, the brain needs to transform a 2-dimensional visual array on the retina into a 3-dimensional representation. This feat is known as DEPTH PERCEPTION. The single most powerful depth cue lies in the differences between the two views received through BINOCULAR vision. These are encoded by neurons in the VISUAL CORTEX responsive to similar visual elements but located in slightly disparate locations within each eye's field of view. Depending on each neuron's favourite disparity, it will respond to objects at different distances in front of or behind the current FIXATION POINT.

A. DAVID MILNER

stereoscopic vision *see* depth perception; stereopsis

stereotaxic atlas An atlas of the BRAIN, or parts of the brain, mapped out in serial sections and typically providing both pictures of brain tissue and schematic representations of it. The brain tissue may have been processed by specific histological techniques (see HISTOLOGY) to illustrate features (fibres and cell bodies for example) or to show particular cells identified by their NEUROCHEMISTRY. Adult or developing brains can be mapped. The brain is mapped out into coordinate systems (see COORDINATE SYSTEMS, STEREOTAXIC) by atlases and are invaluable when conducting STEREOTAXIC SURGERY. Atlases are available for many different species, including most of the typical species of experimental animal and humans.

References

Paxinos G. & Watson C. (1997) *The Rat Brain in Stereotaxic Coordinates*, compact 3rd edn, Academic Press: San Diego.
Paxinos G. & Huang X.-F. (1995) *Atlas of the Human Brainstem*, Academic Press: San Diego.

Paxinos G., Ashwell K.W.S. & Tork I. (1999) *Atlas of the Developing Rat Nervous System*, Academic Press: San Diego.

Paxinos G., Kus L., Ashwell K.W.S. & Watson C. (1999) *Chemoarchitectonic Atlas of the Rat Forebrain*, Academic Press: San Diego.

Swanson L.W. (1992) *Brain Maps: Structure of the Rat Brain*, Elsevier: Amsterdam.

stereotaxic coordinates *see* coordinate systems, stereotaxic; stereotaxic atlas; stereotaxic surgery

stereotaxic frame *see* stereotaxic surgery

stereotaxic surgery (from Greek, *stereos*: solid, *tassein*: to arrange) The term *stereotaxic* (also spelt *stereotactic*) refers to the location of an object within a 3-dimensional space. In the neurosciences, stereotaxic surgery involves the placement within the brain of devices of various sorts, with 0.01 mm precision in each dimension. It is not species-specific: stereotaxic surgery can be performed experimentally on animals or therapeutically on humans. In the following text, a standard stereotaxic surgical operation on an experimental animal is described, this serving to illustrate the basic principles involved. The operation involves several stages.

All experimental stereotaxic surgery is carried out on anaesthetized animals. (1) The first step in the operation therefore is the induction of general ANAESTHESIA, using an anaesthetic agent (usually combined with an analgesic; see ANALGESIA) that will maintain anaesthesia throughout the surgical procedure. Once this has been achieved the animal's head is shaved on the top surface, where a scalp incision will be made. As with human surgery, hair is cleared away from the site of the operation to maintain cleanliness. Prior to making an incision in the scalp it will be swabbed with an appropriate cleansing agent. (2) The animal is placed in a STEREOTAXIC FRAME. This is a device that has two functions: it holds the subject's head in a fixed position, and it permits manipulation of one or more arms (also called [micro-]manipulators or [micro-] positioners) in three dimensions: ANTERIOR–POSTERIOR, MEDIAL–LATERAL and DORSAL–VENTRAL. Normally any arm is at right angles to the stereotaxic frame in each dimension. An animals undergoing stereotaxic surgery has its head held by two devices: EAR BARS and INCISOR BARS. The ear bars should always be appropriate for the species being used, and be ATRAUMATIC: that is, they should penetrate the AUDITORY CANAL only to the degree necessary for supporting the animal's head. No damage to the auditory apparatus should be produced. The incisor bar (or TOOTH BAR) is a bar over which the front teeth are placed. These two devices do not produce any TRAUMA, but do hold the animal's head in a fixed position. For human stereotaxic surgery, ear and incisor bars are not appropriate. Nevertheless, the same principles operate: the head is held in a fixed position using clamps. While on the stereotaxic frame, animals body temperature can be maintained, if necessary, using a HOMEOTHERMIC BLANKET. (3) Once the animal has been fitted in the stereotaxic frame, and its scalp cleaned, an incision along the midline is made; the scalp is reflected (folded back) and the membranes (the fascia) between the scalp and skull exposed. Cutting directly through these invariably produces bone bleeding, which is not helpful, but blunt dissection (literally, scraping the fascia away) avoids bone bleeding and has the benefit of producing a 'raggy wound': these heal more quickly than clean cuts. Once the incision is made and the fascia removed, the surface of the SKULL is exposed and cleaned. If bone bleeding is produced, it can be controlled using BONE WAX (a rather old-fashioned approach), cauterization (a rather dramatic approach) or, for preference, by the application of a surgical gelatin sponge which absorbs blood and provides a gelatin-based matrix to facilitate blood clotting. (4) The manipulators on the stereotaxic frame can be moved to an appropriate position in 3-dimensional space within the animal's brain: a STEREOTAXIC ATLAS provides coordinates for brain structures. These coordinates are expressed in terms of distance in three dimensions from a zero reference point. Typically these reference points are: (a) anterior–posterior: either BREGMA (a skull landmark) which is best suited for structures relatively anterior in the brain; or EAR BAR ZERO, more properly referred to as the INTERAURAL LINE (a hypothetical line that runs, literally right between the ears: it is measured from the position of the ear bars before the animal is placed in the frame). This is best suited for locating structures relatively anterior in the brain. (b) Medial–lateral: the midline SUTURE along the skull is typically used. (c) Dorsal–ventral: either skull surface or the surface on the midline at the anterior–posterior level at which surgery will be conducted; or the DURA MATER (see MENINGES)(a reading of the depth of this can be taken once the appropriate portion of skull has been removed). (Note: when rats or other small animals are being operated on their heads are typically held at one of two orientations: LEVEL SKULL, which is as it says (and is determined by ensuring that the dorsal–ventral measurement at two skull landmarks, bregma and LAMBDA, are identical: typically the incisor bar will be ~3.3 mm below the interaural line); or the DE GROOT ORIENTATION, in which the incisor bar is set 5 mm above the interaural line. Typically, level skull is chosen, being a more direct route to any given structure.) The manipulator will be carrying a device: an ELECTRODE for recording, a CANNULA for making infusions, a GUIDE CANNULA carrier for implanting cannulae or whatever. This device can be used to locate the chosen zero reference points – for example, bregma, the midline suture and skull surface. For each of these three points, a numerical value can be taken from vernier scales on the manipulators. These three numbers – one for each direction – represent the zero reference point. A stereotaxic atlas will provide coordinates for each structure. These can be added to or subtracted from the zero reference point coordinates. Moving the manipulator in the anterior–posterior and medial–lateral planes to these new coordinates will position the manipulator above the skull at an appropriate point for the structure of interest. (5) Having determined the point on the skull surface that lies directly above the structure of interest, a small hole is drilled, usually using a dental drill. Once this has been done, and any necessary coordinate taken from the surface of the dura mater, the dura can be cut (to permit smooth access of whatever is to be inserted in brain). The instrument attached to the manipulator – electrode, cannula or whatever – can be lowered slowly and carefully into position and the

appropriate operation performed: passage of fluid for example (see MICROINJECTION), or electrical recording (see SINGLE-UNIT ELECTRO-PHYSIOLOGICAL RECORDING), MICRODIALYSIS, or the induction of a LESION. (6) Once this is done, the device is retracted and the wound cleaned and sealed. The hole made by the dental drill can be packed with sterile gelatin foam, or left clean for tissue to grow in and fill, and the scalp wound sealed, either with suture silk (stitches) or with specialized wound clips (Michel clips). The animal is then removed from the frame, incisor bar before ear bars to prevent accidental damage to the teeth, and allowed to recovered from the general anaesthetic (while of course being carefully monitored).

This has described in general terms, the typical approach to experimental stereotaxic surgery using animals. Clearly, specific operations might need to adapt this. For example, operations that run close to the cerebral VENTRICLES or aqueducts might require a cannula or electrode to approach the brain not at 90° but at a more acute angle, in order to avoid penetrating the ventricle. However, the basic principles remain the same in the vast majority of cases.

See also: aseptic technique

stereotrode *see* electrode

stereotyped In biological psychology, the adjective stereotyped is descriptive of an activity that is produced invariantly and repetitiously. It might relate to the rather pathological process of STEREOTYPY or it might simply describe a response that is relatively invariant – the patterns of SEXUAL BEHAVIOUR in many SPECIES follow a fixed pattern that can be called stereotyped, though this does not have the overtones of PERSEVERATION that use of the term stereotypy implies.

stereotypy Stereotypy describes behaviour which is both repetitive and excessive and with no obvious function. It differs from PERSE-VERATION in being excessive in quantity as well as restricted in repertoire. The term is usually used to describe repetitive motor acts such as hand-flapping, head-banging, and pacing up and down, but it can also refer to excessive and repetitive thoughts known as RUMINA-TIONS. Stereotypy can be induced in healthy people by physical confinement under conditions of high AROUSAL, for example, by imprisonment especially in conjunction with solitary confinement and SENSORY DEPRIVATION. Such stereotypy typically involves LOCOMOTION and disappears when the constraint is removed. Clinically, stereotyped behaviour is seen in people who have received limited sensory input in childhood because of sensory disability (for example BLINDNESS, or DEAFNESS), limited meaningful sensory input in childhood because of MENTAL HANDICAP or AUTISM or, rarely, severe SOCIAL ISOLATION. This type of stereotypy does not involve locomotion but does involve repetitive movements such as rocking, jumping up and down, head-banging, hair-pulling and hand-flapping. Such behaviour can be self-injurious. Prolonged efforts at rehabilitation may be required to 'unlearn' these behaviours, suggesting that they develop because of a failure to integrate motor output with sensory input through interaction with the environment during a SENSITIVE PERIOD of childhood. In captive mammals (especially large cats and bears), confinement in small cages induces locomotor, CAGE STEREOTYPIES. Higher mammals (especially monkeys and apes) reared in social and sensory isolation exhibit non-locomotor, DEPRIVATION stereotypies which may be self-injurious and incurable (Berkson, 1967). OBSESSIVE COMPULSIVE DISORDER is characterized by stereotyped behaviours and thoughts. Motor stereotypy, in the form of mannerisms and rituals, and stereotypy of thought, in the form of lack of variability in language production and content, is seen in SCHIZOPHRENIA.

Chronic ingestion of large amounts of AMPHETAMINE in humans produces a psychotic, schizophreniform reaction which includes stereotyped behaviour known as PUNDING. Such behaviour may involve dismantling and reassembling bits of machinery or sorting and rearranging collections of small items. Large, chronic doses of amphetamine given to monkeys produces stereotyped behaviour which evolves from complex sequences, such as grooming routines, into more restrictive fragments of behaviour, such as poking the skin on one part of the body. Rodents treated with large doses of amphetamine exhibit stereotyped head movements, sniffing, and rearing (standing up on the back legs) at low doses and licking, gnawing and grooming behaviours at higher doses. As the acute dose of amphetamine in rodents is increased 'the repetition rate of all motor activities will increase with the result that the organism will tend to exhibit increasing response rates within a decreasing number of response categories'. This description is known as the LYON–ROBBINS HYPOTHESIS. Amphetamine increases DOPAMINE release in the brain. It is supposed that increasing levels of dopamine in the brain, increase the probability of the production of possible motor routines, which compete with each other for behavioural expression. As the dose of amphetamine is increased, the 'stronger' (more probable) responses become ever more dominant over 'weaker' (less probable) responses so that the number of different motor routines becomes progressively more restricted to only the very strongest responses. Animals reared in conditions of social isolation, or subjected to acute stress immediately prior to drug treatment, show exaggerated behavioural sensitivity to amphetamine, suggesting an influence of environmental conditions on dopamine receptor sensitivity or dopamine release in the brain. Experimental lesion studies in rats indicate that the production of restricted, stereotyped behaviours may be dependent on levels of dopamine activity in the STRIATUM, whereas production of stereotyped locomotor activity may be dependent on levels of dopamine release in the MESOLIMBIC DOPAMINE SYSTEM (which projects to wider parts of the rat forebrain) (see Kelly et al., 1975) .

Reference

Berkson G. (1967) Abnormal stereotyped motor acts. In *Comparative Psychopathology*, ed. J. Zublin & H.F. Hunt, Grune & Stratton: New York.

Kelly P.H., Seviour P.W. & Iversen S.D. (1975) Amphetamine and apomorphine responses in the rat following 6-OHDA lesions of the nucleus accumbens septi and corpus striatum. *Brain Research* 94: 507–522.

ROSALIND RIDLEY AND CHRISTOPHER FRITH

steroid hormones A class of HORMONES: steroids are synthesized from CHOLESTEROL in the GONADS and the ADRENAL GLAND. (The term steroid is derived from sterol – itself derived from Greek, *stereos*: solid – this being a solid form of ALCOHOL). Receptors for steroids are found in several brain areas, including the HYPOTHALAMUS, PREOPTIC AREA and HIPPOCAMPUS (see ADRENAL GLAND for discussion of the effects of GLUCOCORTICOIDS on the hippocampus).

See also: activational effects of steroid hormones; endocrine glands; hormones; hormones – classification; organizational effects of steroid hormones; pregnancy; sex hormones

sticky labels test A test of motor ability used in rodents: a small sticky label is attached to one forepaw and the task the animal has is simply to remove it: the time taken to do this is measured. The sticky labels test often forms part of a SENSORIMOTOR TEST BATTERY. Rats bearing a unilateral LESION of the NIGROSTRIATAL DOPAMINE SYSTEM made by 6-HYDROXY-DOPMAINE are often assessed with this task and show marked lateralized deficits, having difficulty using the paw CONTRALATERAL to the lesion.

stimulants Drugs that stimulate the central nervous system and generally produce activating effects on MOOD and behaviour. Every day, millions of people use stimulating drugs. Although COCAINE and AMPHETAMINE are considered the prototypical illicit stimulants, stimulating drugs are found in TEA AND COFFEE, soft drinks, cigarettes (see TOBACCO), chocolate and in many non-prescription medicines. If one includes all these sources, stimulants are by far the most commonly used psychoactive substances in the world. A common property of stimulant drugs is that they stimulate the brain and produce activation of behaviour, thought and mood. Although stimulant drugs are classified in this way, the diverse substances which belong to this class may differ markedly in their chemical structure, pharmacological action, and behavioural effects. Strictly speaking, this class is divided into (1) PSYCHOMOTOR STIMULANTS (for example, amphetamine, cocaine, METHYLPHENIDATE); (2) the METHYL-

XANTHINE group (compounds found in coffee and tea, such as CAFFEINE): (3) the CONVULSANT group (strychnine, picrotoxin); (4) the clinical ANTIDEPRESSANT group; and (5) NICOTINE. The most typical stimulants are the psychomotor stimulants, caffeine, and nicotine. Convulsants block inhibitory synapses in the brain and induce excitation at every level of the nervous system; however they are generally not self-administered or abused. Antidepressants have complex pharmacological effects and seem to have a potent elevating effect on mood, without the motor component of the psychomotor stimulants or the attentional effects of caffeine or nicotine. Psychomotor stimulants, nicotine and methylxanthines, all of which are commonly used (and abused) drugs share a number of behavioural and pharmacological properties. These drugs all produce a feeling of well-being and generally enhanced AROUSAL and they can act as SYMPATHOMIMETICS (drugs that activate the SYMPATHETIC NERVOUS SYSTEM). Amphetamine and cocaine are potent activators of central DOPAMINE, and it thought that this property underlies that main euphoriant or rewarding effects that these compounds produce. Amphetamine also stimulates central NORADRENALINE, and this may mediate the ATTENTION-enhancing effects of certain stimulants. Caffeine and nicotine also stimulate central dopamine pathways, but additionally have other complex effects on the brain. All of these compounds, which are self-administered in animal tests, have high ABUSE POTENTIAL and can be addictive, although in the case of caffeine it is unlikely to be deleterious to health.

See also: addiction

ANN E. KELLEY

stimulating electrode *see* electrode

stimulus (from Latin, *stimulus*: a goad) The term STIMULUS appears barely to need definition: a stimulus is something – an object, action, sound or whatever – that produces a response. In a broad sense this is clearly correct. However, for scientists interested in analysing behaviour in terms of relationships between stimuli and responses (see for example

CONDITIONING), a critical task is to define the EFFECTIVE STIMULUS. Stimuli are very rarely pure: they are composites of many features – texture, size, orientation, movement, colour, sound and so on. Which element is important in establishing an association between a stimulus and a response or REINFORCEMENT? That is, what is the effective stimulus? For example, during the breeding season, male sticklebacks will defend their territory against other breeding males. Breeding male sticklebacks have red bellies. The defending male will attack any more or less fish-shaped object that has a red underbelly, but will leave a non-breeding male (lacking the red coloration) alone. The effective stimulus to TERRITORIAL BEHAVIOUR is clearly very specific. It is also worth noting that stimulus properties may appear to be different under different circumstances, though in fact the stimulus never changes. Hall cites the example of moon rock, which appears to be very dark, almost as black as coal, even under bright illumination. The brightness of the moon seen in the sky (as opposed to a piece of it in a lab) is due to its illumination by the sun, but the extraordinary degree of brightness it seems to possess is a product of the contrast between it and the blackness of the night sky surrounding it.

Evidently, a stimulus is something that produces a response: but the effective component of a stimulus must be properly clarified, and one must be aware that stimulus properties may not be constant across all conditions.

See also: stimulus generalization

Reference

Hall G. (1983) *Behaviour*, Academic Press: London.

stimulus-bound behaviour In biological psychology, a stimulus-bound behaviour is one that is tied temporally to a STIMULUS: as long as a stimulus is present, a behaviour will occur, but as soon as the stimulus is absent, the behaviour will cease. (Note that stimulus-bound has other meanings in other contexts: in personality theory it refers to someone who is inflexible in their behaviour; and in psychophysics, stimulus-bound relates to perceptions that are determined entirely by stimulus characteristics with little or no interpretation re-

quired.) Two classic examples in the physiological psychology literature are: (1) ELECTRICAL BRAIN STIMULATION directed at the LATERAL HYPOTHALAMUS will elicit a specific behaviour: FEEDING, DRINKING or GROOMING for example. These activities will persist for as long as the electrical stimulation is maintained. When it ceases, so will the activity: the behaviour is bound by the stimulus. (2) TAIL-PINCH of a rat can induce a similar range of behaviours: while the pinch is on, behaviour is elicited; when the stimulation is off, the activity stops. However, stimulus-bound behaviour need not involve such obvious experimental stimulation. Any stimulus that has the power to 'bind' behaviour can be considered as generating stimulus bound behaviour.

See also: perseveration

Reference

Valenstein E.S., Cox V.C. & Kakolewski J.W. (1970) Re-examination of the role of the hypothalamus in motivation. *Psychological Review* 77:16–23.

stimulus dimension The class of features, attributes or properties by which stimuli may be classified and discriminated is called a STIMULUS DIMENSION. A dimension might be a physical attribute of a stimulus, such as the colour of a visual object, or a semantic attribute, such as words and non-words. Variations within a stimulus dimension are called exemplars. Thus, yellow is an exemplar of the dimension colour.

See also: attentional set-shifting; extradimensional shift; intradimensional shift

VERITY J. BROWN

stimulus enhancement The enhancement of a STIMULUS by having ATTENTION drawn to it; LOCAL ENHANCEMENT is a similar phenomenon in which attention is drawn to a particular place or location, rather than to a specific stimulus. These are thought to be important features of OBSERVATION LEARNING and examples can be found in a variety of natural settings and among a very wide variety of species. Note that PLACE CONDITIONING (in which an animal learns that a particular place is associated with a REINFORCER) is not the same as local enhancement, which involves having attention drawn to a location rather than just associating a location with REINFORCEMENT.

stimulus equivalence *see* equivalence

stimulus generalization The ability to respond in a similar manner to stimuli that are generally similar. Stimuli are generally very complex (see STIMULUS) and it is clearly important to be able to generalize a response to all members of some relevant class. Experiments using colour as a stimulus for example have shown that animals trained to respond in a particular way to presentation of a coloured stimulus will show the same response to closely matching colours. As the stimulus colour becomes increasingly distant from the original however, it loses its power to control behaviour. Such functions are called STIMULUS GENERALIZATION gradients.

Reference

Domjan M. (1993) *Domjan & Burkhard's The Principles of Learning and Behaviour*, 3rd edn, Brooks Cole: Pacific Grove CA.

stimulus–reinforcer association. An association between the mental representation of a STIMULUS and that of a REINFORCER. Its existence allows subsequent presentation of the stimulus to activate the representation of the reinforcer, and thus elicit any responses normally elicited by that reinforcer; this is known as a CONDITIONED RESPONSE. Formation of such an association results from training procedures in which presentation of the stimulus accompanies or precedes presentation of the reinforcer (provided that reinforcer is not concurrently predicted by any other event). CLASSICAL CONDITIONING is one such training procedure, and classically conditioned responses are typically thought to be the product of the formation of stimulus-reinforcer associations. This contrasts with the now-outdated view that classical conditioning is the product of a STIMULUS–RESPONSE ASSOCIATION. Stimulus–response associations might also form during pairings of a stimulus and a reinforcer, as the animal would experience the stimulus in conjunction with the response elicited by the reinforcer. Subsequent presentations of the

stimulus would then elicit the response directly, rather than via activation of the reinforcer representation. Evidence that this account is incorrect comes from experiments in which the reinforcer representation is changed in value. If the reinforcer representation were not involved in performance of the conditioned response, as the stimulus–response association interpretation predicts, then a change in its value should have no effect on conditioned responding. Typically, however, manipulations of reinforcer value do affect conditioned responding, suggesting that the stimulus-response interpretation is incorrect.

See also: associative learning; learning; stimulus–stimulus association

CHARLOTTE BONARDI

stimulus–response association *see* instrumental conditioning; stimulus–reinforcer association; stimulus–stimulus association

stimulus–stimulus association In a standard PAVLOVIAN CONDITIONING experiment, the subject is presented with a neutral CONDITIONED STIMULUS (CS) paired with some motivationally significant UNCONDITIONED STIMULUS (US). During training the CS comes to elicit the conditioned response, usually that originally produced only by the US. Two possible associative accounts of this are available: (1) The subject may form an association between central representations of the CS and the US (a STIMULUS–STIMULUS ASSOCIATION); the presentation of the CS will then generate sufficient activity in the representation of the US to elicit conditioned responding. (2) The alternative is that the CS becomes associated with the response representation (the US representation is then unimportant in generating the conditioned response; STIMULUS–RESPONSE ASSOCIATION). Both analyses have their advantages. The stimulus–response analysis is certainly parsimonious: learning involves the minimum required account for learning, the CS and the conditioned response. However, it seems doubtful that an organism whose learning was restricted to stimulus–response associations would be very well adapted to its environment. Fortunately, this speculation is unnecessary: experimental evidence is available which allows discrimination between the two accounts of Pavlovian conditioning. Most experimenters who have investigated this question have exploited the fact that the two accounts emphasize different roles of the US representation. For example, rats trained with a tone CS and a food US will come to show responding (for instance, an increase in general activity) during the tone. If the value of the food is modified (such as by allowing the rat to satiate itself with the food, or by pairing it with poison), the activity responding to the tone is reduced. Apparently, and contrary to the stimulus–response analysis, the representation of the food US is important in the control of conditioned responding – precisely what would be anticipated by the stimulus–stimulus analysis.

It should be noted, however, that while much evidence, like that described above, supports the stimulus–stimulus analysis, under certain circumstances (such as in some SECOND-ORDER CONDITIONING preparations) post-conditioning modifications of the US leave responding unaffected. It seem, then, that under some conditions stimulus–response associations play a crucial role in Pavlovian conditioning.

See also: associative learning; learning; stimulus-reinforcer association

JASPER WARD-ROBINSON

stimulus substitution hypothesis *see* Pavlovian conditioning

stockings of Cambridge *see* tower of Hanoi

stoichiometry (from Greek, *stoicheion*: an element) A branch of chemistry of interest to pharmacologists, including those interested in NEUROPHARMACOLOGY: stochiometry is concerned with determining the quantities of chemicals that react together: how much of this needs to be added to that to produce the other?

stomach *see* digestive system

stop codon *see* codon

strabismus An incorrect alignment of the eyes, better known as cross-eyes or SQUINT. Strabismus typically occurs in childhood and is caused by weakness of the MUSCLES of the eye. BINOCULAR FUSION will fail to develop and, unless treated (which it can be) AMBLYOPIA will result.

Straub tail An effect seen in rodents, induced typically by a DRUG (see for example SEROTONIN SYNDROME). It involves the tail being held rigidly and in an arched position. Although drugs can induce this effect (and as such its appearance can help discriminate between the effects of different drugs) its psychological or behavioural function is, at best, obscure.

straylight Light that is scattered across the RETINA beyond the imaging area. Such light may be important in the detection of visual events by cortically blind patients; see BLINDSIGHT.

stress A state of threatened HOMEOSTASIS brought on by repeated exposure to an AVERSIVE STIMULUS or other threat. Stress-inducing stimuli are commonly referred to as STRESSORS and include physical (for example, extreme cold or heat) and psychological threat (for example, dismay at the loss of one's job). Walter Cannon (1871–1945) introduced the term stress response in the early 1900s to refer to an animal's response to stressors. Animals, including humans, react to stressors by activating a complex array of responses in the body which include a combination of cognitive (negative emotions), physiological, endocrine, and immunological responses (McEwen & Sapolsky, 1995). Alterations in the ability of the organism to respond to stressors, with the responses being either excessive or inadequate in magnitude and duration, may lead eventually to a myriad of different disease states including psychiatric risk (for instance acute onset SCHIZOPHRENIA), cardiovascular disorders, GASTRIC ulcers, and reduced resistance to infections (for instance autoimmunity diseases). The magnitude of stress responses are determined by a multiplicity of factors, including the type of stressor and length of exposure, the individual's developmental history and genetic makeup, and strategies that the individual adopts to cope with the stress.

Threatening stressful situations generally evoke vigorous activity and activate various

AUTONOMIC and ENDOCRINE responses that assist to mobilize the body's ENERGY resources. Under these conditions, activation of the autonomic SYMPATHETIC NERVOUS SYSTEM results in the secretion of the HORMONES, ADRENALINE (epinephrine) and (norepinephrine) from the medulla (core) of the ADRENAL GLAND. Adrenaline affects GLUCOSE metabolism, causing nutrients stored in muscles to become available as an energy source for strenuous exercise. Adrenaline, together with noradrenaline, also increases blood pressure and blood flow to muscles. Over the long term, stress-related elevations in circulating blood concentrations of these hormones may contribute to cardiovascular disease. Stressors can also activate neurons in the central nucleus of the AMYGDALA, a component of the LIMBIC SYSTEM known to play a role in EMOTION. The central nucleus of the amygdala sends a projection to the PARAVENTRICULAR NUCLEUS OF THE HYPOTHALAMUS to signal the secretion of the peptide neurohormone CORTICOTROPIN RELEASING FACTOR (CRF). CRF may act as a neuromodulator/neurotransmitter (see NEUROMODULATION/NEUROTRANSMITTERS) at sites in the brain involved in emotional responses, such as the PERIAQUEDUCTAL GREY and the LOCUS COERULEUS, including the central nucleus of the amygdala. Secretion of CRF from the paraventricular nucleus of the hypothalamus stimulates the anterior PITUITARY GLAND to secrete ADRENOCORTICOTROPIC HORMONE (ACTH). In turn, ACTH enters the circulatory system to activate the release of steroid stress hormones called GLUCOCORTICOIDS (such as CORTISOL) from the cortex (shell) of the adrenal gland. Glucocorticoids assist in the catabolism of PROTEINS and conversion to glucose, help in utilization of FAT as an energy source in the body, increase blood flow, and stimulate behavioural responses. The increased fuel supply to cells enables them to sustain a high level of activity in the face of stress. They also decrease the sensitivity of the GONADS to LUTEINIZING HORMONE which, in turn, suppresses the secretion of steroid SEX HORMONES.

Experimental evidence suggests that prolonged secretion of glucocorticoids represents the most harmful effects of stress. Long-term effects of glucocorticoids on the body include increased blood pressure, damage to muscle tissue, steroid DIABETES, infertility, acceleration of the AGEING process, inhibition of developmental growth, inhibition of the inflammatory responses, and the suppression of the IMMUNE SYSTEM. Stress-induced elevations in brain levels of glucocorticoids has also been linked to damage to brain regions involved in LEARNING and MEMORY (cells in the CA1 field of the HIPPOCAMPUS for example). These cells appear highly susceptible to changes in energy metabolism. Cortisol treatments effectively decrease the ability of these neurons to utilize glucose, such that when blood flow decreases to a critical level these cells die. Animal investigations of stress have also implicated central DOPAMINE systems in the neurochemistry of the stress response. Stress-inducing procedures used in the rodent model include IMMOBILIZATION, TAIL-PINCH, and inescapable electric FOOTSHOCK. These procedures have been paired with previously neutral stimuli (a tone for example) which after several pairings can elicit a stress response on its own – this is fear conditioning. These procedures have proven useful for studying neurochemical correlates of stress apart from physical PAIN and have been shown to decrease activity of TUBEROHYPOPHYSEAL DOPAMINE SYSTEM and the TUBEROINFUNDIBULAR DOPAMINE SYSTEM. In contrast, midbrain dopamine neurons projecting to the OLFACTORY TUBERCLE, amygdala, NUCLEUS ACCUMBENS, STRIATUM and PREFRONTAL CORTEX are activated by mild stressors. The selective response of MESOLIMBICOCORTICAL SYSTEM to mild stressors may be 'associated with either an emotional state of anxiety or a coping response in reaction to that emotional state' (Horger & Roth, 1996).

See also: fight-or-flight; learned helplessness; post-traumatic stress disorder; stress cascade

References

Horger B.A. & Roth R.H. (1996) The role of mesoprefrontal dopamine neurons in stress. *Critical Reviews in Neurobiology* 10: 395–419.

McEwen B.S. & Sapolsky R.M. (1995) Stress and cognitive function. *Current Opinion in Neurobiology* 5: 205–216.

CHARLES D. BLAHA

stress (linguistic) Accentuation of syllables within words, or words within sentences.

ANNE CUTLER

stress cascade A term that describes the varied changes in NEUROCHEMISTRY and activation of HORMONES that occur in response to STRESS.

stress hormones HORMONES involved in the behavioural and physiological responses to STRESS; see ENDOCRINE GLANDS; FIGHT-OR-FLIGHT; HORMONES – CLASSIFICATION; PREGNANCY.

stressor Something – an event, object or state for example – that produces STRESS is a stressor.

stretch receptors Proprioceptors (see PROPRIOCEPTION) that respond to stretching of MUSCLES.

stretch reflex A muscular contraction in response to muscle stretching. An example is the ever-popular 'tap on the knee' REFLEX. Tapping below the kneecap (on the patellar tendon) causes the quadriceps muscle (on the top of the thigh) to contract, causing a forward kick. These are spinal reflexes: the speed of action makes brain system involvement impossible.

See also: reflex arc

stretching–yawning syndrome A modestly titled syndrome involving stretching of the body and yawning as well as penile erection and excessive GROOMING of the body (including the penis); see YAWNING.

stria medullaris (stria medullaris of the fourth ventricle; stria medullaris of the thalamus; nucleus of the stria medullaris) An older literature (see Grossman, 1967; Pellegrino *et al.*, 1979) describes this as a bundle of FIBRES running across the brain, marking the division between the PONS and MEDULLA OBLONGATA. These fibres lie below the FOURTH VENTRICLE and COCHLEAR NUCLEUS, but above the INFERIOR CEREBELLAR PEDUNCLE. This pathway is best identified as the *stria medullaris of the fourth ventricle* because later authors (see Risold & Swanson, 1995; Swanson, 1992) use the term stria medullaris to identify the *stria*

medullaris of the thalamus, a FOREBRAIN pathway. It is worth noting the etymology of this term: *stria* is Latin for a narrow strip (a furrow, or the fluting on a stone column) and *medulla* means marrow or core. Thus stria medullaris does not have to refer to tissue belonging to the medulla oblongata: in this context it means a fine strip in the core of the brain. While this describes the position and appearance of the stria medullaris of the thalamus very well, it is rather confusing, for one expects medulla, in the context of brain, to relate to the medulla oblongata. Clearly the qualifiers are useful: stria medullaris of the fourth ventricle and stria medullaris of the thalamus identify the structures of interest.

The *nucleus of the stria medullaris* (also known as Cajal's nucleus of the stria medullaris), which has been described as a BED NUCLEUS for the stria medullaris of the thalamus, contains densely packed small neurons containing high levels of ENKEPHALIN (which discriminates them from surrounding neurons). It is thought that these receive input from the FORNIX and the fibres they gives rise to – the stria medullaris of the thalamus – carry input around the anterior pole of the THALAMUS from the SEPTAL NUCLEI, PREOPTIC AREA, anterior thalamic nuclei, and GLOBUS PALLIDUS to the HABENULA. Psychologically, the stria medullaris has been associated with REWARD, though its functions have been little investigated.

References

Blander A. & Wise R.A. (1989) Anatomical mapping of brain stimulation reward sites in the anterior hypothalamic area – special attention to the stria medullaris. *Brain Research* 483: 12–16.

Grossman S.P. (1967) *A Textbook of Physiological Psychology*, 1st corrected printing, Wiley: New York.

Pellegrino L.J., Pellegrino A.S. & Cushman A.J. (1979) *A Stereotaxic Atlas of the Rat Brain*, 2nd edn, Plenum Press: New York.

Risold P.Y. & Swanson L.W. (1995) Cajal's nucleus of the stria medullaris: characterization by in situ hybridization immunohistochemistry for enkephalin. *Journal of Chemical Neuroanatomy* 9: 235–240.

Swanson L.W. (1992) *Brain Maps: Structure of the Rat Brain*, Elsevier: Amsterdam.

stria terminalis A major projection connecting the AMYGDALA with, among other places, the PREOPTIC AREA and anterior parts of the HYPOTHALAMUS. As with most other projection systems of the hypothalamus, information flow is in both directions.

See also: bed nucleus of the stria terminalis; extended amygdala

striate cortex The area of the visual cortex (see VISUAL CORTEX) that contains the primary visual area. The striate cortex corresponds to BRODMANN'S AREA 17. The name derives from the fact that this part of the cerebral cortex has a conspicuous white line, known as the BAND OF GENNARI, which is visible to the naked eye in fresh sections of the human cortex. The line is due to dense fibres in the middle sub-layer of the unusually thick cortical layer 4. This band is not present in the higher-order visual areas in the extrastriate regions of the cortex.

KAZUE SEMBA

striate muscle *see* muscles

striatonigral degeneration A form of MULTIPLE SYSTEM ATROPHY involving loss of tissue in the STRIATUM and related structures (see BASAL GANGLIA). It shares some of the features of PARKINSON'S DISEASE.

striatonigral pathway The striatonigral pathway is a complement to the NIGROSTRIATAL DOPAMINE SYSTEM. It is composed of neurons (see NEURON) each with the CELL BODY in the CAUDATE–PUTAMEN and with AXON projections to the SUBSTANTIA NIGRA (principally the pars reticulata, though there is some contact with the dopamine containing neurons of the pars compacta also). Chief of the NEUROTRANSMITTERS of this pathway is GABA. Loss of these neurons is seen in BASAL GANGLIA disorders such as SHY–DRAGER SYNDROME and HUNTINGTON'S CHOREA.

See also: direct and indirect striatal output pathways

Reference

Smith A.D. & Bolam J.P. (1990) The neural network of the basal ganglia as revealed by the study of synaptic connections of identified neurons. *Trends in Neurosciences* 13: 259–265.

striatum The striatum is comprised of the CAUDATE NUCLEUS, PUTAMEN, NUCLEUS ACCUMBENS and OLFACTORY TUBERCLE. The caudate and putamen are anatomically and functionally closely related and are grouped as the DORSAL STRIATUM. The nucleus accumbens, olfactory tubercle and the most ventral parts of the caudate and putamen are grouped as the VENTRAL STRIATUM. The dorsal striatum is characterized by receiving cortical afferents arising from the NEOCORTEX and DOPAMINERGIC afferents arising in the SUBSTANTIA NIGRA pars compacta. Dorsal striatal neurons project to the internal and external segments of the dorsal GLOBUS PALLIDUS. The ventral striatum is characterized by receiving allocortical (see ALLOCORTEX) afferents arising from the basolateral AMYGDALA, HIPPOCAMPAL FORMATION and prelimbic parts of the PREFRONTAL CORTEX and dopaminergic afferents arising from the medial VENTRAL TEGMENTAL AREA. Ventral striatal neurons project to the VENTRAL PALLIDUM and also to the LATERAL HYPOTHALAMUS (the latter arising especially from neurons in the nucleus accumbens shell).

See also: corticostriatal loops; patch and matrix organization of the striatum

BARRY J. EVERITT

striosomes *see* patch and matrix organization of the striatum

stroke The clinical syndrome of abrupt onset of temporary or permanent loss of focal nervous system function due to blood vessel disease. Focal malfunction results from the inadequate delivery of nutrients necessary for electrical and biochemical operations of neurons and glial cells. Any region of nervous system tissue can be affected including the CEREBRAL HEMISPHERES, BRAINSTEM, CEREBELLUM, SPINAL CORD or PERIPHERAL NERVOUS SYSTEM. Arterial blood vessel disease occurs most commonly, but disease of veins can also lead to strokes.

The characteristic clinical feature that alerts one to the vascular aetiology of stroke is the sudden onset of focal loss of neurologic function. The severity of the deficit can vary from barely noticeable to life-threatening. The deficit may be maximal at onset or may progress over a period of minutes to hours. The clinical presentation depends on the vascular territory of the diseased blood vessel. Patients may come to medical attention complaining of weakness of one side of the body (HEMIPLEGIA), sensory loss on one side of the body (HEMIANAESTHE-SIA), visual loss (MONOCULAR or HEMIVISUAL FIELD), APHASIA, dizziness, double vision (DI-PLOPIA), slurred speech (DYSARTHRIA), confusion, agitation and other more subtle focal deficits. In some patients the deficit lasts only a few minutes and the event is termed a TRANSIENT ISCHAEMIC ATTACK (TIA). By definition TIAs resolve within 24 hours of onset although typically they last less than 30 minutes. TIAs may be isolated events or recur (sometimes hundreds of times) over weeks to months. Focal neurologic events that persist for more than 24 hours are termed STROKES. In many individuals TIAs are an indicator of cerebrovascular disease and are a harbinger of stroke.

The narrowing or occlusion of diseased arteries leads to an inadequate delivery of OXYGEN and GLUCOSE to neurons and glial cells necessary for their normal function. Lack of blood flow leading to tissue insult is termed ISCHAEMIA. If the ischaemic insult is not severe, permanent tissue injury may be avoided and presents clinically as a TIA. Complete absence of blood flow for 4 to 5 minutes causes irreversible injury referred to as infarction (see INFARCT). Infarction of neuronal tissue typically causes a clinically detectable and permanent focal neurologic deficit. The nature of the blood vessel disease is diverse and may or may not involve intrinsic blood vessel pathology. Common intrinsic blood vessel diseases include ATHEROSCLEROSIS, ARTERITIS, DISSECTING ANEURYSM, and inherited, developmental or IDIOPATHIC disease of the vessel wall. Whether or not tissue ischaemia occurs depends on the rapidity of progressive lumenal narrowing and the extent of collateral circulation. Vessel narrowing may be accompanied by the formation of a THROMBUS and this combination typically causes tissue insult because of the relatively quick change in haemodynamics. Thrombi are composed of hematologic elements such as red blood cells, platelets and fibrin. Arterial thrombosis leading to stroke

may also occur in the absence of obvious blood-vessel disease. In hypercoaguable states such as polycythaemia or advanced malignancy, the development of arterial thrombosis may cause stroke. In the absence of intrinsic blood-vessel disease, a primary pathologic process occurring elsewhere in the body may cause stroke. A stroke may occur when a thrombus floating in the arterial circulation lodges in a blood vessel feeding nervous system tissue. The obstructing material is the EMBOLUS and the tissue infarction that results is referred to as an EMBOLIC STROKE. Emboli frequently originate from thrombi that have formed in the heart or the aortic arch. The clinical presentation of an embolic stroke can mimic precisely a stroke that results from intrinsic blood vessel disease.

Pathologically, strokes can be pale (or bland) or contain a HAEMORRHAGE. In a bland infarction the lack of tissue perfusion leads to a whitish appearance on gross inspection. During the evolution of some strokes, blood vessel damage within the vascular territory of the infarct leads to EXTRAVASATION of blood. The degree of haemorrhagic transformation of the infarction can vary from microscopic to massive. In general, the greater the haemorrhage the worse the clinical outcome. With the routine application of clinical imaging technologies, some degree of haemorrhagic transformation of a stroke is not uncommon, although bland infarctions are still the most common. Brain haemorrhages can also result from either rupture of a small deep blood vessel damaged by long-standing hypertension or rupture of an intracranial aneurysm or arterio-venous malformation.

Until the 1990s, there was no treatment for acute stroke. Breaking up an intra-arterial clot (thrombolysis) is now a treatment option. If thrombolytic agents are administered early to select patients, the size of the infarcted tissue is reduced with a concomitant beneficial clinical effect. For prevention of stroke in high-risk individuals, anti-platelet agents such as aspirin or anticoagulation with warfarin are useful. Under certain circumstances, surgical removal an atherosclerotic plaque in the extracranial carotid artery (endarterectomy) is beneficial in preventing recurrent stroke. In general, both the treatment of acute stroke and the prevention of future strokes must be individually tailored to the underlying pathophysiologic process.

See also: aneurysm; hypertension

ROBERT G. KALB

Stroop effect In the classic form of the Stroop effect, colour names are written in coloured ink. The subject's task is to name the colour of the ink. Subjects are slower to name the ink colour if it conflicts with the colour name. That is, if the ink colour is RED, it takes longer to say 'red' if the word is GREEN than if the word is RED. Effects of this sort are of interest because they indicate that some processes (here READING) are sufficiently automatic that they cannot be stopped even when stopping them would be beneficial.

Reference

Stroop J.R. (1935) Studies of interference in serial verbal reactions. *Journal of Experimental Psychology* 12: 242–248. (Reprinted in *Journal of Experimental Psychology: General* (1992), 121: 15–23.)

JEREMY M. WOLFE

strychnine Strychnine is an ANTAGONIST at the GLYCINE receptor. One of the ALKALOIDS, it is found naturally in the seeds of an Indian plant, *Strychnos nux vomica*. It was known in Europe in medieval times and was used as a rat poison but it is known also to kill humans. It can act at a variety of sites in the SPINAL CORD, MEDULLA, PONS, MIDBRAIN and in the RETINA. It produces CONVULSIONS that are exacerbated by sensory stimulation.

See also: psychomotor stimulants

Reference

Feldman R., Meyer J.S. & Quenzer L.F. (1997) *Principles of Neuropsychopharmacology*, Sinauer Associates: Sunderland MA.

stupor (from Latin, *stupere*: to be amazed) A state not of unconsciousness or SLEEP, but extreme lethargy and drowsiness; typically associated with the use of a DRUG such as ALCOHOL or NARCOTICS.

See also: addiction

stuttering A defect of SPEECH PRODUCTION in which there is repetition of parts of a word (typically the initial portion). STAMMERING is a related disorder in which there are repetitions of or hesitations within the production of individual words. The terms TONIC and CLONIC are applied to both conditions: the pauses are said to be tonic while the repetitions themselves are clonic. Both stuttering and stammering often occur during DEVELOPMENT; and both are more common (by four times) in males than in females. The precise causes of these conditions are not clear. Some evidence for the involvement of disordered brain LATERALIZATION exists but there is no clear and unambiguous evidence in favour of this. There is a body of opinion that suggests stuttering to be the product of dysfunctional control of the vocal cords, which might be the product of any one of several processes, all of which could affect vocal cord tension. In addition there is a suggestion that stuttering might be a product of psychological forces (STRESS) and from FATIGUE or illness. Treatment tends to focus on behavioural and psychological processes.

stylet *see* microinjection

subarachnoid space *see* meninges

subcallosal gyrus A gyrus identified as part of the limbic system; it is in effect an extension of the CINGULATE GYRUS, the subcallosal gyrus being anterior and inferior to the cingulate gyrus.

subcellular fractionation A technique for examining the composition of cells. Tissue is homogenized (ground up) and suspended in a fluid. This fluid is then centrifuged (spun): at relatively low speeds the heaviest cellular components fall to the bottom of the tube forming what is known as a PELLET. The liquid above the pellet is the SUPERNATANT. This supernatant can be drawn off and spun again, repeatedly. Each pellet extracted will contain different cellular elements: SYNAPTOSOMES, MITOCHONDRIA and other SUBCELLULAR ORGANS. Eventually CYTOSOL is all that remains: this contains only small molecules and PROTEINS from the tissue, all the identifiable components having been extracted in the various pellets.

subcellular organs Within cells are various structures suspended in the CYTOSOL: some examples are ROUGH ENDOPLASMIC RETICULUM, MITOCHONDRIA, VESICLES. These are literally subcellular organs, or ORGANELLES. Just as a human body contains identifiable parts – organs like the heart, brain and liver – so individual cells also contain subcellular organs with specific functions; see CELL.

subcommissural ventral pallidum That part of the VENTRAL PALLIDUM that lies ventral to the DECUSSATION of the ANTERIOR COMMISSURE. Its afferents arise in the NUCLEUS ACCUMBENS and ventral pallidal neurons project variously to the DORSOMEDIAL NUCLEUS OF THE THALAMUS, SUBTHALAMIC NUCLEUS and PEDUNCULOPONTINE TEGMENTAL NUCLEUS.

See also: basal ganglia; corticostriatal loops

BARRY J. EVERITT

subcortical A rather imprecise and general word used in describing a variety of things, it refers simply to tissue in the CENTRAL NERVOUS SYSTEM below the CEREBRAL CORTEX, most particularly the NEOCORTEX. Properly, 'subcortical' should refer to all tissue in the central nervous system other than that of the neocortex, ALLOCORTEX and JUXTALLOCORTEX. In practice, allocortical structures such as the AMYGDALA and HIPPOCAMPUS are often referred to as subcortical.

subcortical dementia A general term used to describe DEMENTIA that is associated with SUBCORTICAL damage rather than damage to the CEREBRAL CORTEX. Such conditions as KORSAKOFF'S SYNDROME, PARKINSON'S DISEASE and HUNTINGTON'S CHOREA can be considered under this heading, since all involve subcortical PATHOLOGY and can all show (amongst many other things) dementia to at least some degree. However, it is unclear how useful a term this really is. The best-known form of dementia, ALZHEIMER'S DEMENTIA, clearly involves damage in both cortical and subcortical tissue. Moreover, even disorders such as Parkinson's disease that have clear subcortical pathology have a profound impact on cortical functioning. The notion that cortical and subcortical functions can be neatly separated is false and

terms such as subcortical dementia are probably best avoided.

subcortical plate A layer of cells in the developing CEREBRAL CORTEX of mammals. Also known as the SUBPLATE, its neurons (see NEURON) are among the first to be generated during cortical development, and they extend axons to the THALAMUS and MIDBRAIN well before the appearance of the main PROJECTION NEURONS of the cerebral cortex in the overlying layers. Subplate axons appear to provide a scaffold for the guidance of these later-projecting axons, when the distances from the cerebral cortex to other brain regions are relatively large. Remarkably, the subplate is almost entirely removed by APOPTOSIS in early postnatal life.

See also: neurodevelopment

ROGER J. KEYNES

subcutaneous injection *see* drug administration

subcutaneous tissue *see* skin

subdiaphramatic vagotomy A surgical operation performed to isolate the lower branches of the VAGUS NERVE (the tenth cranial nerve; see CRANIAL NERVES) from the brain (a vagotomy being a transection of the vagus). This prevents sensory signals from the stomach, liver, kidneys and other visceral organs from reaching the brain. It also prevents AUTONOMIC commands to these organs from the brain, releasing them from neural control and leaving them autonomous. The operation has been performed in biopsychology experiments typically to examine the role of neural communication between brain and visceral organs in motivations such as HUNGER and THIRST. The vagus nerve is cut in this procedure immediately below the diaphragm, at the top of the abdominal cavity. This isolates the lower viscera while preserving the neural control of breathing and heartbeat performed by upper branches of the vagus.

KENT BERRIDGE

subdural space *see* meninges

subfornical organ A small structure in the centre of the brain, which hangs below the FORNIX into the third ventricle (see VENTRI-

CLES). The subfornical organ plays a special role in the control of THIRST. Angiotensin II (see ANGIOTENSIN) is a hormone created when the body is in a state of HYPOVOLAEMIA: depleted of water, blood pressure drops, and this hormone results. The presence of angiotensin II in the blood is sensed by receptors in the subfornical organ. The subfornical organ is especially able to sense this hormone because, as one of the CIRCUMVENTRICULAR ORGANS, it is one of the few parts of the brain to lack a BLOOD–BRAIN BARRIER. Activation of the subfornical organ by angiotensin II appears to be a crucial step in the elicitation by hypovolaemia of thirst and DRINKING behaviour.

KENT BERRIDGE

subiculum A component structure of the hippocampal formation (see HIPPOCAMPUS) which receives a major and topographical input from area CA1, but is also reciprocally connected to the ENTORHINAL CORTEX. There are also major output projections to the MAMMILLARY BODIES of the diencephalon via the post-commissural FORNIX and to other regions (AMYGDALA, midline thalamic nuclei [see THALAMUS] and NEOCORTEX). Its PYRAMIDAL NEURONS have a columnar organization. The function is unknown, but single-cell recordings from the adjacent pre-subiculum in rats suggest the subicular complex may be part of a brain system monitoring an animal's head-direction (see HEAD DIRECTION CELLS).

RICHARD G. M. MORRIS

subjective contour see contour perception; pattern completion

subpeduncular tegmental nucleus see caudal cholinergic column

subplate see subcortical plate

subsensitivity see sensitization (receptor)

substance abuse see abuse potential; addiction

substance dependence disorder see addiction

substance P One of the NEUROPEPTIDES and one of the transmitters most widely distributed in the CENTRAL NERVOUS SYSTEM and the PERIPHERAL NERVOUS SYSTEM. It was discovered in 1931 by Von Euler (who was co-winner of the Nobel Prize for Physiology or Medicine in 1970). It is unclear why it is called substance P: the apocryphal story is that it was first synthesized in (P for) powder form. There are three RECEPTOR types, NK1, NK2 and NK3, all G PROTEIN coupled, that bind substance P and NEUROKININ A and NEUROKININ B. (The NK1 receptor is most strongly activated by substance P; NK2 is better activated by the neurokinins, and NK3 is best activated by neurokinin B.) Substance P is co-localized with other neurotransmitters (for example, with ACETYLCHOLINE in some neurons of the PEDUNCULOPONTINE TEGMENTAL NUCLEUS) and has been associated with many different functions, depending on the anatomical localization. It is found in many sites, including the STRIATUM, FRONTAL CORTEX, HYPOTHALAMUS, MIDBRAIN and in many nuclei in the brainstem. It is perhaps best known for its actions in the SPINAL CORD, where it is closely involved in the processing of PAIN. Blockade of substance P action on the C FIBRES of the spinal cord blocks pain perception; GENE KNOCKOUT mice lacking the NK1 receptor in the spinal cord similarly have reduced sensations of pain.

substantia gelatinosa (from Latin, *substantia*: substance, and Italian, *gelatina*: jelly, derived from Latin, *gelare*: to freeze or solidify) The substantia gelatinosa – literally gelatinous substance – is an alternative name for layer II in Rexed's classification (REXED'S LAMINAE) of the SPINAL CORD. It is one of the layers with integrative (rather than purely sensory or motor) functions.

See also: gate control theory of pain

substantia nigra The substantia nigra lies above the CEREBRAL PEDUNCLES in the MIDBRAIN ventro-lateral tegmentum, extending from the rostral border of the PONS into the SUBTHALAMIC AREA. The neurons in the cell-rich part are called collectively the *pars compacta*, and contain the black pigment NEUROMELANIN that is visible to the naked eye in the sectioned fresh human brain. These neurons synthesize and use DOPAMINE as their neurotransmitter and project heavily onto the dorsal striatum (see NIGROSTRIATAL DOPAMINE SYS-

TEM; STRIATUM). Dopaminergic neurons lying more medially (that is, between each substantia nigra) are referred to as the VENTRAL TEGMENTAL AREA dopamine neurons, but are continuous with the neurons of the substantia nigra pars compacta; they project to the ventral striatum (see MESOLIMBIC DOPAMINE SYSTEM), AMYGDALA and PREFRONTAL CORTEX. The dopaminergic neurons of the substantia nigra are among the first to degenerate in PARKINSON'S DISEASE and the resultant dopaminergic denervation of the striatum is associated with AKINESIA and a variety of cognitive deficits. The cell-sparse part of the substantia nigra is called the *pars reticulata* and is found ventral and adjacent to the cell groups of the pars compacta. This region of the substantia nigra shares many, but not all, cytoarchitectonic (see CYTOARCHITECTURE) and connectional characteristics with the internal segment of the GLOBUS PALLIDUS. Both structures together represent the major output nuclei of the dorsal striatopallidal system. Pars reticulata neurons invariably contain the neurotransmitter GABA and project to the THALAMUS, SUPERIOR COLLICULUS, PEDUNCULOPONTINE TEGMENTAL NUCLEUS and the PONTINE RETICULAR FORMATION. (Note: the terms pars compacta and pars reticulata are synonymous with zona compacta and zona reticulata. Most authors use pars, but many use zona; some mix the two and refer to pars compacta and zona reticulata.)

See also: corticostriatal loops

BARRY J. EVERITT

subthalamic nucleus This lens-shaped nucleus is located medial to the INTERNAL CAPSULE at the border between the MIDBRAIN and DIENCEPHALON, where it overlies rostral parts of the SUBSTANTIA NIGRA. This nucleus is a key structure within BASAL GANGLIA circuitry. Its primary afferents arise from the external segment of the GLOBUS PALLIDUS and also direct afferents from motor areas of the NEOCORTEX. Its GLUTAMATERGIC outputs are directed to the internal pallidal segment and substantia nigra pars reticulata. Together this striatal-external pallidal segment-internal pallidal segment/substantia nigra pars reticulata circuitry has become known as the *indirect path*, to

distinguish it from the *direct path* – the GABAERGIC projections from the dorsal striatum to the internal pallidal segment/substantia nigra pars reticulata (see DIRECT AND INDIRECT STRIATAL OUTPUT PATHWAYS). Lesions of the subthalamic nucleus, usually caused by a STROKE, result in the motor disorder HEMIBALLISMUS, characterized by involuntary wild flailing movements of the contralateral limbs.

See also: corticostriatal loops

BARRY J. EVERITT

subtraction methodology Subtraction methodology refers to an experimental technique for isolating specific sensory and cognitive process which is widely employed in FUNCTIONAL NEUROIMAGING studies of brain function.

MICHAEL D. RUGG

subtractive logic F.C. Donders applied a subtractive logic to the study of mental operations. He reasoned that by comparing the REACTION TIME in tasks which differed in their composition by exclusion of one or more processing stages, one could infer the timing of those processing stages. This is a procedure that has been quite widely use in psychology. More recently a similar SUBTRACTION METHODOLOGY has been applied in FUNCTIONAL NEUROIMAGING studies. Essentially this involves scanning two sets of brains, either the brain of an individual in both control and test conditions (during quiet rest and the performance of a psychological task for example) or the brains of subjects from control and experimental subjects (often involving comparison of patients suffering from a disease or BRAIN INJURY with matched control subjects). The principle applied is the same in both cases: subtract the control activation from the experimental activation in order to determine what the difference is. While this has considerable appeal, it can be a dangerous procedure. It rests on the assumption that specific psychological functions are localizable in brain and that any system activated by both the control and experimental procedure is not selectively involved in the process of interest. It may be the case that a structure is not *selectively* involved in a process, but it may be *necessarily* involved: it might be critical to activate a particular area of the brain in all sorts of different processes. By extension, it is clear from studies using ELECTROPHYSIOLOGY that neurons in some parts of the brain can respond to various inputs: a subtractive approach would likely remove them from every computational analysis made.

subventricular zone *see* cortical development

succinate *see* GABA

suckling Suckling refers to the act of sucking milk from a breast or any other appropriate thing; an animal that is known as a suckling is one that has not been weaned (see WEANING) from its mother's milk. Suckling appears to be an innate action (see ROOTING REFLEX) and has considerable power to stimulate the production of HORMONES in the mother. Hormonal activity during PREGNANCY stimulates milk production (LACTATION) in mothers. When suckling occurs, mechanical stimulation of the of the nipple or teat produces a neural signal to the HYPOTHALAMUS that triggers release of OXYTOCIN, which in turn will trigger release of milk. This process is very rapid, the entire sequence being completed within 40 seconds.

sucrose (from French, *sucre*: sugar) One of the DISACCHARIDE SUGARS. Sucrose is table (or cane) sugar, a mix of one MOLECULE of GLUCOSE and one of FRUCTOSE. Sucrose solutions or sucrose pellets are often used in experiments in which one wishes to motivate the performance of animals.

sudden infant death syndrome Also known as COT DEATH or CRIB DEATH: the unpredicted death of an infant during SLEEP which remains unexplained after (i) an AUTOPSY (which will differentiate SIDS from what has become known as *shaken baby syndrome*, a condition associated with a pattern of pathology never seen in SIDS); (ii) examination of the location and circumstances of the infants death (which will eliminate, for example, bed-sharing as a cause of death); and (iii) examination of infants' medical history (and that of the family). Infants are at risk between the ages of one month and a year, with two to four months being the high point of risk (accounting for over 50% of cases in the United States of America). It is more common in males than females and there is a tendency for it to be associated with low birth weight. The children of mothers under 20 years old are at greater risk, and parental use of drugs (notably TOBACCO) has been linked in a proportion of cases (see DRUG EFFECTS *IN UTERO*). Many medical organizations have suggested that infants should sleep on their backs (the '*back to sleep*' regime) rather than face down, and the adoption of this practice has had considerable benefit. However, although there is a belief that it might be associated with failure of the neural control of BREATHING or of THERMOREGULATION, no cause has been identified.

sugars A class of simple CARBOHYDRATES. The simplest are MONOSACCHARIDES, such as GLUCOSE or FRUCTOSE. Glucose is the chief fuel used by the brain, and can be created out of other carbohydrates. Fructose is a natural component of fruits. Slightly more complex are DISACCHARIDES. For example, sucrose, or common table sugar, is a disaccharide formed of one molecule of glucose and one molecule of fructose. Sugars share in common their sweet taste, which they produce by activating metabolic processes within taste receptor cells on the tongue.

See also: energy

KENT C. BERRIDGE

suicide The deliberate taking of one's own life. Suicide is a significant public-health problem, and while there are geographic and cultural variations in rates, suicide represents one of the top 10 causes of death in all age groups in most countries. Amongst young adults, suicide represents the second or third most common cause of death. Suicide rates are difficult to estimate accurately because ascertainment is not always straightforward, and the grounds for classification of death as suicide vary even within the component nations of the UK. For this reason, suicide rates tend to be underestimated, and a significant proportion of undetermined deaths will, in fact, have been suicides. Not all suicides occur amongst the psychiatrically ill, and cultural, social and other demographic factors are important. Suicide is more common in males, rates increase with age, and suicide occurs more often amongst the single, separated, divorced or widowed. Social isolation and unemployment appear to be important background determinants. At time of writing, rates have been increasing, particularly among younger males, while there is no evidence of a corresponding increase in psychiatric disorder in this group. None the less, there are significant associations between suicide and psychiatric disorder. AFFECTIVE DISORDER is implicated in particular, with perhaps 15% of sufferers of major depressive disorder dying ultimately by their own hand. SCHIZOPHRENIA is also associated with significant mortality by suicide, with estimates ranging between 10% and 15%. ALCOHOLISM and DRUG ABUSE are commonly found amongst those who subsequently commit suicide. Suicide is notoriously difficult to predict and therefore to prevent. Availability of method is, perhaps counterintuitively, an important consideration. For example, the detoxification of the domestic gas supply in Britain in the 1960s reduced suicide rates by about one-third – there was no compensatory increase in the use of other methods at the time. Suicide prevention strategies therefore need to consider methods available (such as the ease with which paracetamol can be obtained and used in overdose) as well as the identification and effective treatment of psychiatric disorder. Completed suicide must be distinguished from deliberate self-harm or attempted suicide. The latter is much more common, and has different characteristics. While the suicide rate amongst those harming themselves is considerably greater than that found amongst the population overall, only a proportion of those harming themselves will go on to die by suicide (estimates range between 1% and 12%).

IAN C. REID

suicide transporters Suicide transporters are agents that can be taken up by a NEURON, which then transports them internally: they are lethal: for an example, see SAPORIN.

sulcus *see* gyri and sulci

sulfonterol An beta-2 noradrenaline receptor AGONIST; see ADRENOCEPTORS.

sulpiride An atypical antipsychotic with potent DOPAMINE receptor binding properties. It is an ANTAGONIST at dopamine receptors: binding is greater to D1 rather than D2 dopamine receptors; see ANTIPSYCHOTIC.

sumatripan An AGONIST at the $5HT_{1B}$ and $5HT_{1D}$ receptors; see SEROTONIN RECEPTORS.

summation An increase in neuronal ACTIVATION achieved by adding together of a number of postsynaptic potentials (SPATIAL SUMMATION), or by increasing the frequency of individual SYNAPSE discharge (TEMPORAL SUMMATION).

See also: EPSP/IPSP; excitatory postsynaptic potential; inhibitory postsynaptic potential

superior *see* inferior

superior cerebellar peduncle A large fibre tract carrying information between the CEREBELLUM, RED NUCLEUS and THALAMUS; see HINDBRAIN.

superior colliculus Also referred to as the OPTIC TECTUM, the superior colliculus is part of the VISUAL SYSTEM. It is composed of distinct layers of neurons and fibres: (from dorsal to ventral) *zonal, superficial grey, optic, intermediate grey, intermediate white, deep grey, deep white*. RETINOTOPIC visual input comes from the RETINA: slow-conducting fibres terminate in the upper part of the superficial grey layer while faster-conducting fibres terminate in the lower parts of this layer, and in the optic layer. Inputs also arrive from the THALAMUS and ZONA INCERTA, cholinergic neurons in the PEDUNCULOPONTINE TEGMENTAL NUCLEUS and PARABIGEMINAL NUCLEUS, and there is a substantial input from the SUBSTANTIA NIGRA pars compacta (the NIGROTECTAL PATHWAY) that uses GABA and tonically inhibits the superior colliculus. Outputs of the colliculus are directed to a variety of motor sites in the BRAINSTEM and to the thalamus (see GENICULOSTRIATE AND TECTOPULVINAR VISUAL PATHWAYS).

The superior colliculus is evolutionarily old. It has important functions for amphibia: the frog superior colliculus operates as a BUG DETECTOR, the sight of an insect moving across the visual field triggering a reflexive tongue extension for prey capture. In more advanced VERTEBRATES, the superior colliculus retains an important aspect of this process: it has direct visual input and direct output to motor systems, enabling it to activate behaviour very rapidly in response to stimulation. Indeed, in the mammalian superior colliculus, while there are no bug detectors, there are neurons whose firing is graded according to the salience of the visual stimuli being processed. It has been argued that what the superior colliculus does is provide a first-pass analysis of visual input and activate orienting movements, approach or avoidance behaviour as required, and there is evidence to suggest that these processes are served by distinct anatomical systems (see Redgrave *et al.*, 1993). There is also evidence that the superior colliculus is involved in NOCICEPTION, serving a similar function of altering behaviour promptly in response to stimulation that requires immediate attention.

See also: blindsight

Reference

Redgrave P., Westby G.W.M. & Dean P. (1993) Functional architecture of rodent superior colliculus – relevance of multiple output channels. *Progress in Brain Research* 95: 69–77.

superior olivary complex The superior olivary complex is a group of auditory relay nuclei located in the ventral part of the caudal PONTINE TEGMENTUM. The TRAPEZOID BODY, a conspicuous bundle of horizontal fibres, is part of this complex. The superior olivary complex receives second-order axons convergently from the two sides of the COCHLEAR NUCLEI. This binaural input provides cues for sound localization. The superior olivary complex then projects to the inferior colliculi (see INFERIOR COLLICULUS) via the LATERAL LEMNISCUS. TONOTOPIC REPRESENTATIONS are preserved at each level of the central AUDITORY PATHWAYS.

KAZUE SEMBA

superior parietal lobule *see* inferior parietal lobule

superior temporal gyrus The TEMPORAL LOBE has three principal gyri (see GYRI AND SULCI) clearly visible on its outer surface: the inferior, middle and superior temporal gyri (the inferior being most ventral, the superior most dorsal); see MUSIC AND THE BRAIN.

superior temporal sulcus A major sulcus (see GYRI AND SULCI) of the TEMPORAL LOBE; neurons in this area are important components of the VISUAL SYSTEM; see FACE PERCEPTION; PATTERN PERCEPTION.

supermarket diet Also known as CAFETERIA DIET, this is a means for inducing BODY WEIGHT gain in laboratory animals. It involves the provision of a palatable and varied (in taste, texture and composition) diet from which animals can select items to eat. Females gain more weight than males during exposure to the diet, but also shed weight more readily when diets return to normal. Duration of exposure to the diet appears to be a major factor in determining the degree of persistence of the weight gain. Supermarket diet is important for two reasons: first, it demonstrates that, given the opportunity, animals will overeat and put on weight, contrary to the idea that there is a predetermined SET POINT for body weight that must be adhered to. Second, the amount of excess energy consumed does not match the amount of energy stored. Much of the energy taken on board is burned as heat by BROWN ADIPOSE TISSUE.

supernatant *see* subcellular fractionation

superoxide A superoxide anion is an oxygen free radical (see FREE RADICALS) that can damage neurons by mutating their DNA and initiating a catastrophic series of reactions leading to breakdown of LIPIDS. These anions are produced naturally in the CENTRAL NERVOUS SYSTEM (though not equally across all structures within it) but various enzymes can transform them, rendering them harmless. SUPEROXIDE DISMUTASE is such an enzyme, existing in at least two forms: a copper- and zinc-dependent form, found in CYTOPLASM, and a manganese-dependent form found in MITOCHONDRIA. Overproduction, or failure properly to control, superoxides have been associated with neurodegenerative disorders such as PARKINSON'S DISEASE.

References

Zhang P., Anglade P., Hirsch E.C., Javoy-Agid F. & Agid Y. (1994) Distribution of manganese-dependent superoxide dismutase in the human brain. *Neuroscience* 61: 317–330.

superoxide dismutase *see* superoxide

superposition Superposition (also known as INTERPOSITION) describes the condition in which an object is placed between an observer and a target object; the object in the super-position partially conceals the target. This gives a cue in DEPTH PERCEPTION, though superposition gives no information about depth *per se*, except that one can be clear that one object is behind another and therefore further away.

supersensitivity *see* sensitization (receptor)

superstitious behaviour A term used to de-scribe the inadvertent acquisition of a re-sponse, such as lever pressing, that is not productive or meaningful. Animals trained on random SCHEDULES OF REINFORCEMENT will often show superstitious behaviours, and cer-tain brain lesions can produce superstitious effects.

See also: schedule-induced polydipsia

Reference

Devenport L.D. (1979) Superstitious bar press-ing in hippocampal and septal rats. *Science* 205: 721–723.

supervised learning *see* backpropagation; neural networks

supervisory attentional system The central component of a mechanism described by Shal-lice to account for the selection of any one action from a range of possible actions (an action being identified as a goal-directed re-sponse). In this model, sensory information flows into the CENTRAL NERVOUS SYSTEM and undergoes CONTENTION SCHEDULING. This de-scribes a process in which, through mutual inhibition, one RESPONSE is selected and all other responses are suppressed. This is a mechanism that allows for simple STIMULUS–response processing: all stimuli are assessed and the most potent and appropriate response selected. Contention scheduling mechanisms then activate effector mechanisms which gen-erate appropriate behaviour. The process of contention scheduling has three possible out-comes: in the presence of stimulation from the environment (both the external environment [the world] and the internal environment [the body]) an appropriate response will be selected and inappropriate responses inhibited. In the absence of stimulation from the environment the system will do one of two things: it will persist with the last selected response (that is, show PERSEVERATION), or it will cease activity , producing no output. The supervisory atten-tional system is a mechanism that is proposed to intervene on the processes of contention scheduling, biasing it in particular directions. It may be, for example, that the response most likely to be activated by environmental stimuli is, for some superordinate reason, not desired and should, at that time, be suppressed. The suppression of food intake by an individual on a diet is an example of this: environmental stimuli (both internal and external) can make eating the most highly selected response by a contention scheduling process, but the super-visory attentional system can suppress or divert this. As well as biasing contention scheduling, the supervisory attentional system has another important function: it can generate responses when none is being selected by environmental stimuli, thus avoiding the problems of perse-veration or inactivation. This model of action selection has been influential in apparently diverse areas, including explanation of the effects on behaviour of AMPHETAMINE (see Robbins, 1982) and in explaining some of the behavioural difficulties expressed by patients with SCHIZOPHRENIA or FRONTAL LOBE da-mage (see Frith, 1992). Note also that the actions of the supervisory attentional system have an intimate relationship with the CENTRAL EXECUTIVE described by Alan Baddeley and his colleagues. (Indeed, Baddeley has made it explicit that the supervisory attentional system was a model for the central executive and has described how the functions of these equate). The actions of the supervisory attentional system are also clearly bound with the concept of EXECUTIVE FUNCTIONS and, as with execu-tive functions, there is debate about the rela-tionship between the functions of the supervisory attentional system and CONSCIOUS-NESS. Some authors believe that the super-visory attentional system requires in some way conscious processing, while others argue that it does not. This is a particularly interesting point when considering whether animals other than humans operate a supervisory attentional system.

References

Frith C.D. (1992) *The Cognitive Neuropsychology of Schizophrenia*, Lawrence Erlbaum: Hove UK.

Robbins T.W. (1982) Stereotypies: addictions or fragmented actions? *Bulletin of the British Psychological Society* 35: 297–300.

Shallice T. (1988) *From Neuropsychology to Mental Structure*, Cambridge University Press: Cambridge.

supplementary motor area Synonymous with SUPPLEMENTARY MOTOR CORTEX; see MOTOR CORTEX.

supplementary motor cortex Synonymous with SUPPLEMENTARY MOTOR AREA; see MOTOR CORTEX.

suprachiasmatic nucleus A nucleus in the HYPOTHALAMUS functioning as the primary circadian clock in mammals, and probably other vertebrates (see BIOLOGICAL CLOCK; CIRCADIAN RHYTHM). The suprachiasmatic nuclei (SCN) comprise unusually small, densely packed neurons and glial cells that lie immediately dorsal to the OPTIC CHIASM, in the midline near the base of the THIRD VENTRICLE. The SCN are innervated by retinal ganglion cells that convey light information and are responsible for ENTRAINMENT to day–night cycles. They also receive prominent projections from the INTERGENICULATE LEAFLET of the THALAMUS, containing NEUROPEPTIDE Y, and from the RAPHE NUCLEI, containing SEROTONIN. SCN cells are remarkable for the variety of neurochemicals they contain. Most or all SCN cells contain GABA, while ventral cells also contain VASOACTIVE INTESTINAL POLYPEPTIDE (VIP), and dorsal cells contain VASOPRESSIN. SCN neurons also have, for example, SOMATOSTATIN, GASTRIN RELEASING PEPTIDE, MELATONIN receptors, CALBINDIN, NERVE GROWTH FACTOR receptors, and SUBSTANCE P. SCN cells respond to photic input (that is, light) by changes in firing rates and by rapid increases in the expression of several IMMEDIATE EARLY GENES, including C-FOS, which may be important in mediating light effects on rhythms (see ENTRAINMENT). The evidence that the SCN are a major circadian clock or pacemaker in mammals is overwhelming. Destruction of the SCN results in severe disruption or loss of most physiological and behavioural circadian rhythms (see BIOLOGICAL CLOCK). Activation of the SCN by electrical or chemical stimulation can shift circadian rhythms in ways that mimic the effects of light. SCN cells show circadian oscillations of electrical activity and neurochemical release *in vivo*, and these rhythms are remarkably preserved in slice preparations or cell culture. These rhythms persist for several cycles *in vitro* and can be phase-shifted by neurochemical manipulations. Even single, isolated SCN neurons show circadian firing-rate rhythms. Transplantation of a foetal SCN into the hypothalamus of an SCN-lesioned, arrhythmic rodent can restore circadian activity rhythms, with characteristics typical of the SCN donor GENOTYPE. Some circadian mechanisms exist outside the SCN, but their locations are unknown. Circadian anticipation of restricted daily FEEDING cycles survives SCN ablation, as does a rhythm in photic sensitivity (possibly retinal). The efferent mechanisms by which the SCN control rhythms involve neural pathways that regulate neuroendocrine rhythms, including the prominent rhythm of melatonin secretion from the PINEAL GLAND, and a humoural agent that may mediate control of some behavioural rhythms. The evidence in other vertebrates is less complete, but indicates that the SCN, the eyes and the pineal gland are phylogenetically ancient components of the vertebrate circadian system.

BENJAMIN RUSAK

supraoptic nucleus of the hypothalamus A nucleus in the HYPOTHALAMUS containing MAGNOCELLULAR neurons that synthesize OXYTOCIN (important in the regulation of LACTATION and other aspects of SEXUAL BEHAVIOUR) and VASOPRESSIN (important in OSMOREGULATION and the initiation of DRINKING). It sends projections to the PITUITARY GLAND, where it releases both of these HORMONES. It receives a strong innervation from the VENTRAL NORADRENERGIC BUNDLE, PREOPTIC AREA, SUBFORNICAL ORGAN and several hypothalamic nuclei.

See also: paraventricular nucleus of the hypothalamus

surface dysgraphia *see* agraphia

surface dyslexia An ACQUIRED READING DIS-ORDER particularly affecting the oral reading and comprehension of previously familiar written words. The ability to read aloud novel written material (such as written nonsense words) is relatively well preserved. Words with irregular spelling-to-sound correspondences (for example, *pint*, *yacht*) are often mispronounced using more regular correspondences (for example *pint* to rhyme with *mint*; *yacht* to rhyme with *hatched*). Words with regular spelling-to-sound correspondences (for example *mint*, *throng*) are usually read correctly. Written words that are mispronounced are not usually read correctly. Written words that are mispronounced are not usually understood and the meanings of written HOMOPHONES (for example *pear*, *pair*, *pare*) – with pronunciations that sound identical – are often confused.

Surface dyslexia occurs with a variety of LESION sites but in most cases TEMPORAL LOBE structures of the dominant HEMISPHERE are affected. Theoretical models of normal reading can account for surface dyslexia as an impairment to the lexical processes involved in reading previously familiar words. A variety of lexical impairments can give rise to surface dyslexia. Successful therapies for surface dyslexia using VISUAL IMAGERY and PHONEMIC CUEING strategies have been reported.

See also: central dyslexia; deep dyslexia; developmental dyslexia; phonological dyslexia

Reference

Patterson E., Marshall J.C. & Coltheart, M. (ed.) (1985) *Surface Dyslexia*, Lawrence Erlbaum: Hove UK.

ELAINE FUNNELL

surmountable/unsurmountable antagonists *see* antagonist

suspensory ligaments Ligaments connecting the CILIARY MUSCLE and LENS of the EYE: extension or contraction cause the lens to change shape.

sustained attention A state of alert readiness which is maintained, particularly during the performance of tasks not under automatic control. In the laboratory, continuous perfor-mance tasks (usually the monitoring of a continuous stream of input for target signals) are used to measure sustained attention.

See also: attention; vigilance

VERITY J. BROWN

suture (from Latin, *sutura*: seam) There are two meanings for the term suture: (i) the verb 'to suture' means to stitch a wound (either with suture silk or specialized wound clips); and as a noun, SUTURE can refer to the stitches themselves; and one can speak of a wound having been sutured (that is, closed with sutures); see STEREOTAXIC SURGERY. (ii) As a noun, suture can also refer to the points where bones meet. For example, the various bones of the SKULL meet at sutures and the skull landmarks BREGMA and LAMBDA represent points where sutures intersect.

sweat gland *see* skin; thermoregulation

sweetness The sensation of sweetness, once thought to arise primarily only from the tip of the tongue, is now recognized to be generated by receptors distributed equally over the tongue. Unlike certain other taste qualities, such as sour or salt, which can activate neural fibres in the tongue directly, sweet tastes need an intermediary receptor. Specialized molecules in the surface membrane of taste cells function as sweet receptors. Activation of these receptors produces metabolic changes within the nucleus of the taste cell, which stimulate ADENYLATE CYCLASE. This in turn causes ION CHANNEL closure in the cell MEMBRANE, trapping the positively charged potassium (K+) ions within the cell, and producing DEPOLARIZATION that can lead to a neuronal ACTION POTENTIAL signal. For some taste cells, a second sweetness receptor mechanism has been implicated, which operates by sodium (Na+) rather than by K+ channels. In this case, since positively-charged sodium is primarily outside of cells, the mechanism may work by opening Na+ channels, allowing the positive ions to enter and depolarize the cell. This has been called the amiloride-sensitive sweetness channel, because it can be blocked by application of the chemical, amiloride, to the tongue. If that is done, the intensity of sweetness perception diminishes. Regardless of receptor mechanism, the sensation of sweet, like other taste qualities, is finally conveyed to the brain primarily by sensory fibres of the FACIAL NERVE (the seventh cranial nerve; see CRANIAL NERVES) AND GLOSSOPHARYNGEAL NERVE (THE NINTH CRANIAL NERVE). THERE IT ACTIVATES NEURONS FIRST IN THE NUCLEUS OF THE SOLITARY TRACT, WHICH IN TURN ACTIVATE HIGHER NEURONS IN FOREBRAIN STRUCTURES SUCH AS THE THALAMUS, THE HYPOTHALAMUS, AND THE GUSTATORY CORTEX AT THE BOTTOM OF THE POSTERIOR EDGE OF THE FRONTAL LOBE.

See also: gustation

KENT C. BERRIDGE

swim bladder *see* vestibular system

swimming *see* locomotion; water maze

swing phase *see* locomotion

switching In the context of biological psychology, the term switching (or sometimes more fully, *behavioural switching* or *response switching*) is the description given to the change an animal makes from one activity to another. How this is achieved remains a matter of debate. Various models have been proposed to account for the organization of response choice (the most widely cited being Shallice's SUPERVISORY ATTENTIONAL SYSTEM) and various systems of NEUROTRANSMITTERS and brain structures suggested to be involved in switching. Emphasis has been given to the role of SEROTONIN systems (see for example Al Ruwaitea et al., 1997) and to DOPAMINE systems, particularly with regard to the operation of the BASAL GANGLIA (see Redgrave *et al.*, 1999).

References

Al Ruwaitea A.S.A., Al Zahrani S.S.A., Ho M.Y., Bradshaw C.M. & Szabadi E. (1997) Effects of central 5-hydroxytryptamine depletion on performance in the 'time left' procedure: further evidence for a role of the 5-hydroxytryptaminergic pathways in behavioural 'switching'. *Psychopharmacology* 134: 179–186.
Redgrave P., Prescott T.J. & Gurney K. (1999) The basal ganglia: A vertebrate solution to the selection problem? *Neuroscience* 89: 1009–1023.

syllable A word or part of a word, further divisible into the elements DEMI-SYLLABLE and DIPHONE, suitable for linguistic analysis; see SPEECH PERCEPTION.

Sylvian fissure *see* lateral fissure

Sylvian sulcus *see* lateral sulcus

symbiosis (from Greek, *syn*: together, *bios*: livelihood) A mutually beneficial relationship in which members of different SPECIES live together at the same time. (Were it not at the same time the relationship would be better described as RECIPROCAL ALTRUISM.) The benefiting partners could live directly one on another (*ectoparasitism*); or one species could live within the other (*endoparasitism*). It is contrasted with the life of a PARASITE: parasitism involves one species living off another, to its own exclusive benefit, though without necessarily (in the short term at least) being detrimental to the host. (A better contrast for symbiosis might be the more specific form, MUTUAL PARASITISM, in which two species live off each other to the long-term detriment of both.) A related term is COMMENSAL (from Latin, *con*: together, *mensa*: table – commensal literally means sharing a table). Commensalism is where two species share an environment, but without necessarily bringing either harm or benefit to each other: foxes and badgers are often commensal.

While symbiosis, as a biological construct, was originally concerned with the cooperation of two species, it as come to be used more liberally in everyday talk to describe mutually beneficial associations between CONSPECIFIC animals; it should not be so improperly used.

See also: sociobiology

Reference

Campbell N.A., Reece J.B. & Mitchell L.G. (1999) *Biology*, 5th edn, Addison-Wesley: Menlo Park CA.

symmetric synapses *see* synapse

symmetry perception Perception of VISUAL SYMMETRY in patterns is an interesting example of direct pattern matching within the visual field without requiring access to MEMORY for pattern recognition (see PATTERN PERCEPTION). Both humans and other species have been shown to be sensitive to bilateral and other types of symmetry of the visual scene. Humans are able to detect symmetry within presentations of less that 100 msec in otherwise random patterns, even when the symmetric regions are widely separated across the visual field. A preference for the vertical axis of bilateral symmetry is often found, but this preference can be eliminated or even reversed when knowledge of axis position is controlled.

Reference

Tyler C.W. (ed.) (1996) *Human Symmetry Perception and its Computational Analysis*, VSP Press: Utrecht.

CHRISTOPHER TYLER

sympathectomy Destruction of the SYMPA-THETIC NERVOUS SYSTEM. It is a procedure that does not involve destruction of the entire sympathetic nervous system, but selected portions of it, achieved either by surgical removal of particular ganglia or by administration of chemical NEUROTOXINS that will destroy particular neurons.

sympathetic In biological psychology, use of this term generally indicates not a sharing of EMOTION but activity or involvement of the SYMPATHETIC NERVOUS SYSTEM in an effect or process.

sympathetic arousal A term indicating a state of AROUSAL activated by the SYMPATHETIC NERVOUS SYSTEM; see, for example, ORGASM.

sympathetic ganglia *see* parasympathetic ganglia

sympathetic nervous system One of the major divisions of the autonomic nervous system, the others being the PARASYMPATHETIC NERVOUS SYSTEM and the ENTERIC NERVOUS SYSTEM; see AUTONOMIC NERVOUS SYSTEM for a comprehensive description.

sympathomimetic Sympathomimetic drugs are those that stimulate the SYMPATHETIC NERVOUS SYSTEM. The sympathetic nervous system (a division of the AUTONOMIC NERVOUS SYSTEM) uses NORADRENALINE (NOREPINEPHRINE) as its neurotransmitter: drugs that mimic the actions of noradrenaline in the sympathetic nervous system can therefore be called sym-

pathomimetic. The term is often used in rather more expanded form to include related drugs – those that stimulate DOPAMINE activity for example.

See also: psychomotor stimulants; stimulants

symptoms *see* signs and symptoms

synaesthesia (American spelling: synesthesia) (from Greek, *syn*: together, *aisthesis*: sensation) Perceiving in one sensory modality a stimulus presented in another sensory modality: hearing music in terms of colour for example. It is a phenomenon associated with the use of a DRUG, most notably PSYCHEDELIC DRUGS; see LSD.

synapse The synapse is the site for interneuronal signalling in the nervous system. The adjectival form of synapse is synaptic. Synapses are either chemical or electrical. The CHEMICAL SYNAPSE consists of the PRESYNAPTIC TERMINAL, SYNAPTIC CLEFT and POSTSYNAPTIC neuron. The presynaptic terminal contains SYNAPTIC VESICLES with NEUROTRANSMITTERS. Upon the arrival of action potentials and the opening of CALCIUM (Ca^{2+}) ion channels (see ACTION POTENTIAL; ION CHANNEL), these vesicles fuse with the cell membrane, and the transmitters are released into the synaptic cleft, which is about 10 nm in width. The released transmitters diffuse in the synaptic cleft and then bind to postsynaptic as well as presynaptic receptors (see RECEPTOR). In the postsynaptic membrane, binding of transmitters to IONOTROPIC receptors immediately opens ion channels, inducing a current flow and causing excitation or inhibition of the cell. In contrast, their binding to METABOTROPIC receptors is followed by a cascade of events leading to activation of SECOND MESSENGERS. This may or may not lead to induction of current flow, but could result in long-term changes in cellular functions. Morphologically, chemical synapses are defined by three criteria: (1) synaptic vesicles in the presynaptic profile; (2) pre- and postsynaptic densities; and (3) widening of the cell membranes to form the synaptic cleft. Depending on the relative thickness of pre- and postsynaptic densities, synapses are either asymmetric or symmetric. Synapses can also be classified according to the pre- and postsynaptic components. AXODENDRITIC and AXOSOMATIC synapses are the most common. AXOAXONIC synapses are present in certain regions of the nervous system, and are thought to the anatomical substrate of presynaptic inhibition. Dendrites (see DENDRITE) may contain neurotransmitters and form DENDRODENDRITIC synapses, as in the OLFACTORY BULB and RETINA. TYPE I and TYPE II SYNAPSES have been identified by E.G. Grey. Type I synapses have round, clear synaptic vesicles and asymmetric densities, whereas type II synapses are associated with flattened vesicles with symmetric densities. It is often thought that type I synapses are excitatory whereas type II are inhibitory. In addition to chemical synapses, ELECTRICAL SYNAPSES are present in various regions of the nervous system. At electrical synapses, a current flows directly from one neuron to another in either bi- or unidirectional manner. The anatomical basis for electrical synapses is thought to be GAP JUNCTION channels, which are known to pass ions and other small molecules. Electrically coupled neurons can fire in synchrony, and such coupling is thought to play a role in stereotypic, all-or-none type behaviour in invertebrates, as well as brain maturation during development.

KAZUE SEMBA

synaptic cleft The gap between the PRESYNAPTIC TERMINAL and the POSTSYNAPTIC membrane. The gap varies dependent upon the location of the SYNAPSE, but in the CNS is generally between 10 and 50 nm. The synaptic cleft appears to contain substances more dense than the surrounding extracellular fluids – the so-called SYNAPTIC GAP SUBSTANCE composed of complex PROTEINS and SUGARS. The function of this is probably twofold: to impair the movement of transmitters away from the synapse (and inhibit entry of transmitters from outside the synapse; see VOLUME TRANSMISSION) and to help the presynaptic terminal bind to the postsynaptic membrane. Some of the contents of the synaptic cleft may serve as recognition markers during SYNAPTOGENESIS.

See also: neurotransmission

synaptic gap substance *see* synaptic cleft

synaptic pruning Stage of development of the nervous system in VERTEBRATES after synapse formation (SYNAPTOGENESIS), typically during the postnatal period, when neurons retract some of their SYNAPTIC TERMINALS but preserve others. First described in synapses at the NEUROMUSCULAR JUNCTION, it has been detected widely throughout the developing CNS, and is thought to ensure quantitative matching of synaptic connections between PRESYNAPTIC and POSTSYNAPTIC cell populations, and to remove errors of axon targeting. It may also be important in determining a CRITICAL PERIOD of development of the CEREBRAL CORTEX, when synaptic patterning is influenced by electrical activity. The mechanism is unclear; presynaptic nerve endings may compete for TROPHIC MOLECULES derived from the postsynaptic cell.

See also: Hebbian synapse; neurodevelopment

ROGER J. KEYNES

synaptic terminals The presynaptic portion of a SYNAPSE, typically an AXON TERMINAL.

synaptic transmission Neurotransmission that occurs at a morphologically identified SYNAPSE, involving the release of chemical NEUROTRANSMITTERS or neuromodulators (see NEUROMODULATION). It is contrasted with VOLUME TRANSMISSION, which involves the release of chemicals diffusely into the EXTRACELLULAR spaces, without specialized synaptic connections being present; and with EPHAPTIC TRANSMISSION, which involves the passage of electrical current between neurons.

See also: fast neurotransmission; slow neurotransmission

synaptic vesicles Packages of neurotransmitter within SYNAPTIC TERMINALS. Synaptic vesicles are formed either in the PERIKARYON (from where they are transported to synaptic terminals) or by PINOCYTOSIS in the terminals themselves. The MEMBRANE from which they are constructed is thin (< 8 nm thick) and does not have the same composition as the neuronal membrane. Various types of vesicle have been described: (1) small clear (agranular) vesicles (40–60 nm diameter), often containing ACETYLCHOLINE or AMINO ACID NEUROTRANS-

MITTERS; (2) medium granular vesicles (80–100 nm), usually containing MONOAMINE neurotransmitters. Their granular appearance comes from a dense material at the core. (3) Larger granular vesicles (100–160 nm) most commonly associated with NEUROPEPTIDES. The same terminal may contain more than one type of vesicle.

See also: mobilization; synapse

synaptogenesis The process of SYNAPSE formation between the presumptive PRESYNAPTIC and POSTSYNAPTIC cell MEMBRANE, best understood at the neuromuscular synapse. Here, the first step is the rapid migration within the muscle membrane of pre-existing ACETYLCHOLINE receptors, which accumulate at the nerve ending under the influence of molecular complexes formed by nerve-muscle interaction. The muscle membrane simultaneously becomes refractory to further innervation at adjacent sites, while the motor axon stops growing and differentiates into a mature nerve terminal under the control of molecules in the synaptic BASAL LAMINA. Less is known about synaptogenesis in the CENTRAL NERVOUS SYSTEM, but the main principles are likely to be similar. Many individual synaptic sites are initially multiply innervated by presynaptic terminals, and undergo subsequent SYNAPTIC PRUNING.

See also: neurodevelopment

ROGER J. KEYNES

synaptophysin *see* mobilization

synaptosomes SUBCELLULAR FRACTIONATION is a preparation used in biochemistry: neural tissue is ground and suspended in fluid. Centrifuging this separates out the cellular contents, heavier elements falling to the bottom. Repeated spinning and drawing off yields identifiable fractions of cells, one of which contains most of the synaptic material (see SYNAPSE): synaptosomes.

synaptotagmin *see* mobilization

synchrony/desynchrony A description of the activity in the ELECTROENCEPHALOGRAM (EEG). The defining feature of synchrony is the relatively large AMPLITUDE waves in the EEG, whereas desynchrony is marked by low-amplitude activity. Modulation of cortical EEG in different BEHAVIOURAL STATES is due to the underlying influence of SUBCORTICAL structures, particularly in the RETICULAR FORMATION. Since EEG activity mainly results from extracellular current flow associated with summated EXCITATORY POSTSYNAPTIC POTENTIAL and INHIBITORY POSTSYNAPTIC POTENTIAL, synchronized activity occurs through massive summation of synaptic events or intrinsic currents from large ensembles of neurons. Synchrony is commonly considered to be the hallmark of SLOW-WAVE SLEEP (or NON-REM SLEEP), when 'slow' high-amplitude DELTA WAVES (1–4 Hz) and bursts of spindle activity are recorded across the entire CORTEX. Such synchronized activity across the entire cortex manifests itself gradually as an animal moves from wakefulness to slow wave sleep. During relaxation and drowsiness (stage 1), the eyes close and the EEG shows a moderately slow, synchronous activity of 8–14 Hz (ALPHA WAVES). At this stage, synchrony is not generally recorded over the entire cortex, but specifically on the back of the head over the occipital lobes (see OCCIPITAL LOBE). As sleep becomes progressively deeper during stages 2 and 3, the EEG waves become slower and larger, occasionally interrupted by bursts of fast spindle-like activity, and can be recorded over wide regions of the cortex. The delta frequency is characteristic as sleep deepens further to stage 4, with very large and slow EEG waves. When subjects open their eyes or when a light is flashed over the closed eyelids, slow synchronous activity is replaced by a faster, desynchronous wave pattern of > 14 Hz (beta waves). Beta waves are often present in frontal areas of the brain, and are associated with AROUSAL, alertness, and mental activity. EEG desynchrony – low amplitude 'fast' activity – is typical of wakefulness, as well as REM SLEEP. The conventional distinction between synchrony (slow-wave sleep) and desynchrony (waking or paradoxical sleep) is however an oversimplification, since high-amplitude synchronized rhythms can be observed during both wakefulness and REM sleep. The unique feature of synchrony in slow-wave sleep is that it is found across the entire cortex, rather than in distinct cortical foci. For example, in wakefulness, high-amplitude synchronized rhythms have been recorded during states of HYPERVI-GILANCE, such as experimental hunting conditions: a rhythm of 14 Hz has been localized over the anterior limb zone of the primary SOMATOSENSORY CORTEX when a cat is waiting for an unseen mouse to reappear from a hole. A fast but synchronized rhythm of 35–45 Hz can be recorded over motor and parietal cortices when a cat is watching a visible, but out of reach, mouse. Similarly, synchronized 40Hz oscillations have been recorded over the primary VISUAL CORTEX of a cat in response to moving light bars. Finally, synchronized THETA WAVES (4–10 Hz), consisting of high-amplitude activity in the SEPTOHIPPOCAMPAL SYSTEM, can be recorded in sub-primate mammals during exploratory activity, as well as during REM sleep.

See also: burst firing

WENDY L. INGLIS

syncope *see* fainting; synergistic muscles

synergistic muscles *see* muscles

syntax (i) Grammar, or the structure of permissible sentences in a language; (ii) a branch of linguistic science: the study of [i].

ANNE CUTLER

syntaxin *see* mobilization

synuclein This is a protein (see PROTEINS) found in the PRESYNAPTIC TERMINAL. It is also found accumulated in LEWY BODIES and in PLAQUES both of which are markers for neuro-degenerative conditions. PARKINSON'S DISEASE, ALZHEIMER'S DEMENTIA, LEWY BODY DEMEN-TIA, MULTIPLE SYSTEM ATROPHY and AMYO-TROPHIC LATERAL SCLEROSIS all show accumulation of alpha synuclein. It also is found in certain BRAIN TUMOURS. Alpha synuclein is clearly associated with these conditions: other

variants (beta synuclein and gamma synuclein) have been less investigated, but evidence is accumulating suggesting that these may be associated with neuronal degeneration also.

syphilis Infection by the spirochaete *Treponema pallidum*, resulting in a characteristic painless swelling (primary chancre) at the site of entry, followed by widespread secondary lesions of skin and lymph nodes. Degenerative changes affecting especially the larger blood vessels or brain VASCULATURE (tertiary syphilis) follow some years later. Stage 4 (neuro)syphilis, now rare, affects the CNS either as *tabes dorsalis* (wasting of spinal sensory tracts), characterized by a splayed stamping gait, or as GENERAL PARESIS OF THE INSANE (GPI), an ORGANIC PSYCHOSIS with DEMENTIA and DELUSION. Syphilis is diagnosed serologically by a positive Wasserman reaction, and early stages respond well to penicillin.

L. JACOB HERBERG

systemic A term typically encountered with reference to DRUG ADMINISTRATION: systemic injections (that is, injections being made systemically) are injections into any body system other than the brain. Injections made into the brain are referred to as INTRACEREBRAL INJECTIONS.

systemic circuit *see* blood

systemic injection Injection of a DRUG or chemical into any body system other than the CENTRAL NERVOUS SYSTEM, for which the term INTRACEREBRAL INJECTION (or, more loosely, INTRACRANIAL INJECTION) is used: systemic and intracerebral injections are typically regarded by biological psychologists as contrasting routes of administration.

See also: drug administration

systole *see* blood

T

T cell *see* immune system

T maze Literally, a maze shaped like a capital letter T: animals are typically placed at the base of the column of the T (the start arm) and allowed to make either a left or a right choice of arms to enter at the junction of the column and cross part of the T. T mazes have been used in a wide variety of experiments looking at LEARNING and MEMORY and many other processes. Salamone and his colleagues for example, trained rats to go to one arm of a T maze for a high-density REWARD, the other arm having a low density of reward. Once this routine was established, barriers were placed in the way of the high-density reward to test rats' willingness to expend effort in order to obtain the high-density reward. Using this technique it was possible to measure COST–BENEFIT ANALYSIS in rats.

See also: plus maze; radial arm maze; spontaneous alternation; water maze; Y maze

Reference

Cousins M.S., Atherton A., Turner L. & Salamone J.D. (1996) Nucleus accumbens dopamine depletions alter relative response allocation in a T-maze cost–benefit task. *Behavioural Brain Research* 74: 189–197.

tachycardia (from Greek, *tachos*: speed, *kardia*: heart) Literally, an abnormally high heart rate.

tachykinin The tachykinins are a family of peptides that includes SUBSTANCE P, NEUROKININ A and NEUROKININ B; NEUROPEPTIDE K and NEUROPEPTIDE GAMMA. All of these except neurokinin B are derived from PREPROTACHYKININ, coded by a single GENE. By far the most closely investigated is substance P.

tachyphylaxis Tachphylaxis is the term given to a decrease in the effect a DRUG has even though it is present continuously. It is in effect a form of TOLERANCE. For example, the response to a drug might depend upon that drug binding to a RECEPTOR, with that binding then triggering a second chemical process in order to produce the required response. If that second process was exhausted for some reason (by running down a cellular store for example) then even though the drug was still present in maximal concentration and receptors fully occupied, the response would not be present: the response would decline despite the drug being present. Tachyphylaxis is a form of tolerance that is often associated with a sudden very large demand on a system, rather than repeated small demands.

Reference

Feldman R., Meyer J.S. & Quenzer L.F. (1997) *Principles of Neuropsychopharmacology*, Sinauer Associates: Sunderland MA.

tacrine (tetrahydroaminoacridine) An ACETYLCHOLINESTERASE inhibitor (or ANTICHOLINESTERASE), administration of which will work to enhance the actions of ACETYLCHOLINE by preventing its enzymatic destruction. It has been used in the treatment of ALZHEIMER'S DEMENTIA, where it is thought possibly to have NOOTROPIC actions.

See also: cognitive enhancers

tact *see* tacting

tactile (from Latin, *tactilis*: touch) Tactile is an adjective relating to the sense of TOUCH. The term HAPTIC has the same meaning.

tactile agnosia Tactile agnosia is a modality-specific disorder characterized by an impaired ability to recognize objects tactually in the absence of basic somaesthetic insensitivity. It is distinguished from tactile object recognition deficits produced by ANOMIA, APHASIA, APRAXIA, HEMIPARESIS, DEMENTIA, neglect, or reduced levels of alertness. Tactile agnosia is indicated by asymmetric tactile object recognition performance between the hands. Patients with tactile agnosia have intact visual and auditory OBJECT RECOGNITION.

Tactile agnosia results from a unilateral LESION affecting the contralesional hand. Although reported cases are rare, several brain regions have been implicated in tactile agnosia: the left INFERIOR PARIETAL LOBULE including BRODMANN'S AREAS 40 and perhaps 39 as well as secondary somatosensory contex (S-II). Primate studies suggest that the posterior insula is important for tactile learning and object recognition in which it serves to connect S-II to MESIAL temporal limbic structures. Tactile agnosia may be distinguished from basic sensory impairment through extensive somatosensory testing. Tactile agnosics can draw objects they are feeling, and often recognize the drawn object, thereby indicating adequate sensory input. In addition, tactile agnosics display normal ability to move their hands and explore objects. People without brain damage use stereotypical forms of exploration to identify objects by TOUCH. Tactile agnosics often use the same forms of exploration without success. None the less, exploration is not critical for basic object recognition. Hemiparetic patients, without damage to primary somatosensory cortical areas, have normal tactile object recognition despite non-existent exploration. Although parts of the body other than the hands can be used to recognize objects, tactile agnosia appears to affect the hands only. No evidence for asymmetric object recognition performance was found when using the feet to feel objects or for GRAPHESTHESIA on the forearms and cheeks. When asked to recognize objects with their 'agnosic' hand, tactile agnosics are typically 50–80% accurate. Because their sensory input is unaffected, they can combine the raw sensory input with their knowledge about objects to reason about the object's identity. Errors in recognition often share structural similarity with the to-be-identified object (for example, mistaking a safety pin for a paper clip). They may also get the supraordinate category correct but misjudge the specific subordinate category (for example, identify small, wiry pin-like items for a paper clip) or identify an object generically (identifying a wrench as a tool for example). Cases of tactile agnosia point to a deficit in tactile shape processing. The severity of the deficit depends upon the demands of the task. Recognition of familiar objects and simple shapes is less impaired than unfamiliar objects and complex shapes. In contrast, a similar visual deficit in shape processing produces severe VISUAL AGNOSIA. This difference may indicate that the tactile system relies on properties (such as texture and hardness) other than shape to identify objects, but the visual system relies primarily on shape. Tactile agnosia appears to occur at a higher-level processing stage where perceptual information is integrated. Tactile agnosics can demonstrate intact memory for tactile properties of objects through intact HAPTIC IMAGERY (for example, asking 'Which is smoother, a teaspoon or a marble?'). Unlike patients with PROSOPAGNOSIA, they can associate tactually defined objects and their parts with EPISODIC MEMORY. (So for instance, personal items such as the patient's wallet can be recognized with greater success than other non-personal items.)

Tactile agnosia can also be dissociated from a more general problem of supramodal spatial processing. In one case study, a patient who was impaired on tactile object recognition displayed normal performance on tactile spatial tasks, visual spatial tasks, visual integration tasks and environmental navigation tasks. These findings suggest that there may be an analogous object and spatial pathways in somatosensory cortex as in visual cortex. Although tactile object recognition cannot rival visual object recognition in its speed or accuracy, normal humans are nevertheless able to recognize most common objects after a few PALPATIONS in under 2 seconds. Furthermore, tactile object recognition plays a regular, if not highly frequent role in everyday life. Whenever we retrieve keys from our pocket or awake at night to answer a phone, we must identify by touch the desired objects as distinct from other objects on which our hands might alight. Despite our proficiency at tactile object recognition and our reliance on it in daily activities, tactile agnosia does not produce a great disability. Since tactile agnosia is a modality-specific disorder, visual and auditory systems can be recruited to help identify an unknown felt object. Thus, although tactile agnosia is probably as common as visual agnosia and AUDITORY AGNOSIA, the reported frequency of occurrence is low because patients do not often report problems and neurologists do not often investigate tactile agnosia in favour of more debilitating problems. Nonetheless, tactile agnosia has important implications for understanding the functional organization of cortical processes. It suggests that there are modality-specific tactile object recognition processes that are not shared by vision.

See also: astereoagnosia; object regognition; object agnosia; parietal cortex

CATHERINE REED

tacting A TACT is a verbal response which is controlled by a non-verbal antecedent or discriminative stimulus (see DISCRIMINATIVE CUE). For example a child sees a four-legged animal and points to it, uttering the word 'dog'. According to the theory of B.F. Skinner (1904–1990) (see BEHAVIOUR ANALYSIS) the child learns to tact in this way – that is, to say the word 'dog' in the presence of dogs, because of a history of generalized REINFORCEMENT. In the past the child has received praise and acknowledgement for saying 'dog' under such circumstances. A tact is a typical example of a discriminated OPERANT, and childrens' behaviour is shaped (see SHAPING) by their verbal community so that increasingly finer discriminations can be made. Having correctly labelled a four-legged creature as a dog, children may then label other four-legged creatures as a dog. They will be corrected, and will then learn to discriminate between dogs and cats. This

process is one of the essential elements of behaviour analysis.

Skinner first described tacts as functional units in his 1957 book *Verbal Behavior*. Another functional unit is the MAND, which is a verbal operant in which the response is reinforced by a characteristic consequence and which is therefore under the control of relevant conditions of deprivation or aversive stimulation. Examples are the utterance 'milk' when the child wants a drink of milk. Clinical behaviour analysts have utilized mands and tacts to teach people with severe MENTAL RETARDATION to communicate. First they have been taught to tact food and beverage items and the utensils required to access these items by pointing to line drawings, and then by utilizing specific stimulus control (see STIMULUS GENERALIZATION) procedures they are taught to mand (that is, ask for) those food and beverage items at a later time. Tacting plays an important role in Skinner's theory of how people come to be able to describe their private events, their feelings, emotions, thoughts and so on. According to Skinner when we talk about our inner states we are tacting conditions of our body, no more and no less. The reason we are often poor at describing private events is because the verbal community which would usually provide reinforcement for correct tacting does not itself have access to the events or states being tacted. Put simply the verbal community does not have direct access to our thoughts, feeling and other bodily states to know whether or not we are describing them accurately.

CHRIS CULLEN

tail-flick test *see* analgesia

tail-pinch Mild sustained pinching of a rats' tail will reliably elicit organized behaviour. The pinch must not be painful, since this, not unreasonably, encourages 'pinch-directed behaviour'. It should be constantly applied, about an inch from the tip of the tail. A specialized clamp, accurately regulated by compressed air, can be used for absolute scientific precision or, more economically, a paper clip can serve adequately. The behaviour most commonly elicited is eating, though other forms of activity can also be produced. Tail-pinch-induced eating is of interest because it demonstrates that something other than food palatability or an internal deprivation state can elicit food consumption. The mechanism involved was initially thought to be the generation of a STRESS or ANXIETY-like state, the consumption of food serving to reduce the stress or anxiety. These stress–anxiety reduction hypotheses appear implausible for two reasons. First, as Robbins & Fray argued, if the effect of eating was to reduce the stress–anxiety, then eating should decline as the state was ameliorated. However, eating does not decline, but persists in a stimulus-bound manner (see STIMULUS-BOUND BEHAVIOUR). Second, an ANXIOLYTIC does not *reduce* tail-pinch-induced eating but *increase* it. This does indeed suggest that tail-pinch has an aversive component, but removal of this by drug treatment gives full rein to an appetitive component of the stimulation. It is important to note also that the response to tail-pinch appears to be learnt. The first time rats are exposed to tail-pinch they typically do not engage in any form of behaviour, merely appearing generally activated. On subsequent tests however, rats begin to organize their behaviour, reacting to relevant features of the environment.

For a brief period in the late 1970s and early 1980s, tail-pinch-induced behaviour was intensively studied. Almost no work on it is now conducted, though the body of extant literature does serve to illustrate neatly the clear fact that eating can be elicited by factors other than those one would expect – food palatability and food deprivation.

References

Robbins T.W. & Fray P.J. (1980) Stress-induced eating: fact, fiction or misunderstanding? *Appetite* 1: 103–133.
Robbins T.W., Phillips A.G. & Sahakian B.J. (1977) Effects of chlordiazepoxide on tail pinch induced eating in rats. *Pharmacology, Biochemistry and Behaviour* 6: 297–302.

tangles *see* neurofibrillary tangles

tanycyte *see* blood–brain barrier

tapetum (from Greek, *tapetos*: carpet) A layer of pigmented cells on the RETINA that reflect light, possession of which is thought to indicate nocturnal adaptation in PRIMATES.

tardive dyskinesia A motor side effect of the prolonged administration of any ANTIPSYCHOTIC (that is, DOPAMINE ANTAGONIST) drug. The dyskinetic movements (see DYSKINESIA) often involve the orofacial region, although other body areas can be involved. By definition, tardive dyskinesia occurs with a late onset – tardive means delayed – typically, after years of administration. In most patients the condition worsens upon drug withdrawal, and in many patients the condition is permanent.

JOHN D. SALAMONE

taste aversion learning *see* food aversion learning

taste buds The taste buds are clusters of 50–150 individual cells which are able to bind substances and generate taste sensations; these clusters are located on PAPILLAE (from Latin, *papula*: pimple) The TASTE CELLS are replaced at a more or less constant rate: most will be replaced every 10–14 days. There are three different types of papillae, discriminated by form and location. FUNGIFORM PAPILLAE (from Latin *fungus*: mushroom – these papillae have a mushroom shape) are found mainly at the front of the tongue. They are numerous and each posses only one taste bud. CIRCUMVALLATE PAPILLAE are less numerous but each has multiple taste buds; they are found at the back of the tongue. FOLIATE PAPILLAE are located at the side of the tongue at the rear; they also contain multiple taste buds. There is a degree of coding on the tongue: at the front, sweet is better detected than the other tastes, while at the back bitter is the most strongly detected. But this separation is only relative: taste buds on all parts of the tongue can detect all of the PRIMARY TASTES. Most of the receptors in taste buds signal taste (that is sweet, sour, salt or bitter – see GUSTATION for a description of the processing involved in taste) but information relating to heat (both physical heat and the 'hotness' of spices such as chilli pepper) and PAIN is detected on the taste buds.

taste cells *see* sensory transduction; taste buds

taste perception *see* gustation

taurine Taurine is found in the CENTRAL NERVOUS SYSTEM and might be an inhibitory amino acid neurotransmitter (see INHIBITORY AMINO ACIDS).

taxis (Not the plural of 'taxi', a vehicle for hire; this one is pronounced *tax-is*: tax as in tax, with the '-is' sounded as the '-is' in 'kiss'.) In biology, taxis refers to the movement of an organism following presentation of a STIMULUS.

taxon (from Greek, *tassein*: to arrange) A taxon (plural: taxa) is a biological group or category, for example a family or SPECIES.

See also: evolution; taxonomy

taxon learning *see* dispositional memory

taxon memory *see* memory

taxonomy Taxonomy is a system for organizing biological categories or taxa (singular, TAXON). The method used to name and classify living organisms was provided by Carolus Linnaeus (1707–1778), a Swedish naturalist, in his book *Systema Naturae* (1735). His system – the Linnaean system – is a binomial classification (each species has two names, which are in Latin) though this is arrived at through a hierarchical sequence involving the following (with the classification for human beings given):

> Kingdom *Animalia*
> Phylum (phyla) *Chordata*
> Class *Mammalia*
> Order *Primates*
> Family *Hominidae*
> Genus (plural: genera) *Homo*
> Species *sapiens*

Further subdivision using the terms sub-, super- and infra- may also be used to further group or divide levels within this classification. Groups of animals are defined by traits and important characteristics that are shared by all members of the group but not by others. A common evolutionary lineage should also be present and, increasingly, biochemical and genetic markers are used to identify members of particular species. It is important to note that this classification is an abstraction: it does not occur naturally and was developed in order to allow classification and delineation of species

to take place. The only level of the classification that can be thought to have 'natural' meaning is the binomial species name, which identifies an individual species, discriminating it from all others.

See also: evolution; clade; rat

TD50 The toxic dose, 50%; that is, the dose of a DRUG that produces a toxic response on 50% of the occasions on which it is administered. Such statistics help one decide what drug dose to use in experiments.

See also: EC50; IC50; LD50; therapeutic index

tea and coffee Tea and coffee are both consumed in very large quantities world-wide, though the proportion of each consumed varies from place to place. Coffee contains CAFFEINE, one of the PSYCHOMOTOR STIMULANTS, while tea contains caffeine (only about one-third as much as coffee) and THEOPHYLLINE, another of the XANTHINES, which is also a psychomotor stimulant. Tea and coffee are not the only source of these drugs: cola drinks typically contain caffeine, as do chocolate and, perhaps more surprisingly, several analgesic (see ANALGESIA) drugs. Taking a cup to contain 5 fluid ounces (150 ml), one cup of fully brewed coffee contains about 85 mg caffeine while a cup of tea contains a little under 30 mg, the same as a cup of hot chocolate. Regular cola drinks contain, depending on brand, around this much also. An ounce (28.3 g) of milk chocolate contains about 6 mg caffeine while plain chocolate (baking chocolate) not surprisingly, given its darker nature and more bitter taste, can contain as much as 35 mg per ounce (28.3 g). The caffeine intake of an American adult is estimated at 400 mg caffeine per day: the amount children consume in chocolate and cola may be larger than this. Tea and coffee both have psychological properties. Improved REACTION TIME, ATTENTION, MEMORY and other cognitive tasks. Caffeine has ABUSE POTENTIAL and some individuals may develop a pattern of tea and coffee use that could be described as DRUG ABUSE, developing DEPENDENCE. WITHDRAWAL symptoms are experienced by regular users denied access to tea and coffee. Altered blood pressure may lead those with very high tea and coffee intake to be at risk for heart disease, and heavy use is not recommended for pregnant women.

Reference

Feldman R.S., Meyer J.S. & Quenzer L.F. (1997) *Principles of Neuropsychopharmacology*, Sinauer Associates: Sunderland MA.

tectorial membrane *see* organ of Corti

tectospinal tract *see* motor system

tectum (rom Latin, *tectum*: roof) The upper part of the MIDBRAIN is known as the tectum: it includes the SUPERIOR COLLICULUS and INFERIOR COLLICULUS. The term OPTIC TECTUM is synonymous with the superior colliculus.

tegmentum (from Latin, *tegumentum*: a cover) Like the TECTUM, the tegmentum is regarded as part of the MIDBRAIN. The midbrain tegmentum lies immediately above the CEREBRAL PEDUNCLES (with the tectum, the other division of the midbrain) and contains the VENTRAL TEGMENTAL AREA and the SUBSTANTIA NIGRA. The term tegmentum however also covers an area of the PONS, containing a variety of fibre pathways and nuclei such as the PEDUNCULOPONTINE TEGMENTAL NUCLEUS.

telemetry (from Greek, *tele*: far, *metron*: measure) Telemetry is measurement made at a distance, typically involving a signalling device that transmits electrical signals to a remote recording device. While not particularly common in the laboratory, telemetry has many uses in field studies (see ETHOLOGY) where tracking animals over distances in their natural habitat is of importance. This relies on the placement on an animal of a transmitter which one hopes will not interfere with its normal behaviour.

telencephalon The telencephalon is the most rostral structures of the CENTRAL NERVOUS SYSTEM, and is represented by the CEREBRAL HEMISPHERES (see HEMISPHERE). The term CEREBRUM is usually used synonymously with the cerebral hemispheres. The two sides of the cerebral hemispheres are interconnected via the CORPUS CALLOSUM. The superficial part of the cerebral hemispheres is the CEREBRAL CORTEX, thought to be the most important site of cognitive and other higher functions. Deep in

the cerebral hemispheres are the BASAL GANGLIA, which are involved in motor co-ordination (and other processes to do with behavioural control). The structures that line the inner border of the cerebral hemispheres comprise the LIMBIC SYSTEM, which is important in emotional behaviours.

KAZUE SEMBA

telergones *see* pheromones

telodendria A rarely used term: the telodendria are the small branches that occur at the end of an AXON as it ramifies, each AXON TERMINAL making synaptic contacts (see SYNAPSE) with other neurons.

telomere A protective structure at the ends of CHROMOSOMES; see SENILITY.

temperature *see* thermoregulation

temperature regulation *see* thermoregulation

temporal bone *see* skull

temporal contiguity A term that indicates the closeness (CONTIGUITY) in time ('temporal' is derived from Latin, *tempus*: time) of two or more events. The temporal contiguity of events is important in LEARNING; see CLASSICAL CONDITIONING.

temporal lobe One of the four principal lobes of the mammalian BRAIN, located on the lateral aspect. They are apparently named TEMPORAL (from Latin, *tempus*: time) because this is the part of the head – the temples – on which the passage of time is indicated: one's hair turns grey here first. It has complex functions including, in humans, SPEECH PRODUCTION and SPEECH PERCEPTION, the understanding of LANGUAGE and MEMORY (see TEMPORAL LOBE AMNESIA for example) have all been associated with the temporal lobe. Sensory functions are also present: the AUDITORY CORTEX is in the upper part of the temporal lobe and olfactory functions are represented in the MEDIAL TEMPORAL LOBE (see OLFACTORY SYSTEM); visual functions are present also (see for example ACHROMATOPSIA). Higher-order associative sensory functions (see for example FACE PERCEPTION) are also represented in the temporal lobe. In humans, its functions show a strong degree of LATERALIZATION. Clinically, the temporal lobe has been associated with AGNOSIA (see also PROSOPAGNOSIA), AMNESIA and with the production of EPILEPSY (TEMPORAL LOBE EPILEPSY), two conditions unfortunately united in patient H.M. who had bilateral LOBECTOMY of the temporal lobes in order to control epilepsy – the operation was successful in controlling the seizures but left H.M. with a permanent amnesic condition.

The anatomy of the temporal lobe is complex, with boundaries between component parts often being indistinct and controversial. At the posterior edge the temporal lobe is bordered by the OCCIPITAL LOBE (more particularly, number 19 of BRODMANN'S AREAS). At the dorsal edge the SYLVIAN FISSURE marks a clear border, though at the point where this ends, the transition from temporal to PARIETAL LOBE is indistinct and defined better by connectivity (principally to the THALAMUS) rather than by gross surface features. The temporal lobe is marked by banks of tissue, with sulci running parallel to the Sylvian fissure. The three main sulci are the superior (at the top) middle and inferior temporal gyri (INFERIOR TEMPORAL GYRUS, MIDDLE TEMPORAL GYRUS and SUPERIOR TEMPORAL GYRUS), with the SUPERIOR TEMPORAL SULCUS and middle temporal sulcus and INFERIOR TEMPORAL CORTEX separated by them. The HIPPOCAMPUS, AMYGDALA and RHINAL SULCUS are embedded in the MEDIAL TEMPORAL LOBE.

See also: entorhinal cortex; Heschl's gyrus; inferotemporal cortex; planum temporale; uncus; Wernicke's area

temporal lobe amnesia When bilateral injury or disease occurs to the medial aspect of the TEMPORAL LOBE of the brain, an AMNESIC SYNDROME results. The syndrome includes the loss of FACT MEMORY and EVENT MEMORY from the period prior to the onset of amnesia, usually in a temporally graded fashion, such that recently acquired information is more affected than remote information (see ANTEROGRADE AMNESIA and RETROGRADE AMNESIA). In addition, amnesia involves a loss of new learning ability for both facts and events. The amnesia affects DECLARATIVE MEMORY but leaves intact the capacity for a variety of non-declarative, implicit forms of memory. The critical structures include the HIPPOCAMPAL FORMATION, including the entorhinal cortex, and the adjacent, anatomically related PERIRHINAL CORTEX and PARAHIPPOCAMPAL CORTEX, which are part of the PARAHIPPOCAMPAL GYRUS.

LARRY R. SQUIRE

temporal lobe epilepsy Epilepsy with a focus in a TEMPORAL LOBE; see EPILEPSY.

temporal summation *see* summation

temporal visual hemifield *see* hemifield

temporary lesions *see* transient lesions

tension headache *see* headache

tension tremor *see* tremor

tensor network theory A mathematical process that allows vectors of one coordinate system to be integrated with those of another. (Vectors are defined in mathematics as a quantity having direction and magnitude; in computing, vectors involve a one-dimensional sequence of elements in a matrix, with a single identifying code.) It neuroscience, theorists have argued that the BRAIN operates using tensor analysis: it is suggested that the activities of a NEURON can be expressed in terms of vectors and that NEURAL NETWORKS transform inputs in a tensor-like manner.

Reference

Pellionisz A. & Llinas R. (1982) Space–time representation in the brain: the cerebellum as a predictive space–time metric tensor. *Neuroscience* 7: 2949–2970.

tentorium A brain landmark close by the CEREBELLUM: it is an extension of the DURA MATER (see MENINGES) stretched between the cerebellum and the OCCIPITAL LOBE; see COMA.

TEO A commonly used abbreviation for the temporal occipital area: a subdivision of the INFERIOR TEMPORAL CORTEX proximal to area V4 (see AREAS V1–V5). It has been associated with the processing of COLOUR VISION.

tera Prefix indicating a factor of 10^{12}, or one million million times; see SI UNITS.

teratology (from Greek, *teratos*: monster) The prefix terato- indicates, literally, the formation of monsters, but in modern practice the term monsters is substituted by abnormal growths or malformations (a TUMOUR or cancer, for example). So TERATOLOGY is the study of such growths; a *teratogen* is an agent promoting such malformation; *teratogenesis* is the act of creating such malformations.

terminal A word that has many meanings and uses, from railways to electrical circuitry: in neuroscience, TERMINAL typically refers to the ending of an AXON – that is, where the axons of one NEURON make synaptic contact (see SYNAPSE) with another; see SYNAPTIC TERMINALS; AXON TERMINAL.

termination insomnia The state of INSOMNIA in which, having fallen asleep, an individual wakes early and is unable to resume sleeping.

See also: maintenance insomnia; onset insomnia; sleep; sleep disorders

territorial behaviour Territorial behaviour, or *territoriality*, involves the recruitment and defence of an area of space (land, water or air) by individuals, typically defending it against any CONSPECIFIC attempting to gain access to and exploit the resources of the territory. Some animals maintain a specific territory throughout their lives, while others will change and adapt as time goes by. Factors that influence territorial behaviour and the size of territories are the quality of available resources, their distribution across space and their distribution across time (reflected typically is seasonal availability of food). Territories are often marked out, by the deposition of urine or faeces which contain distinctive odours (see PHEROMONES) that serve to warn intruders of the presence of occupied territory. It is thought that AGGRESSION can be produced by overcrowding as an 'over-expression' of territorial behaviour. While overcrowding does produce aggression in rodents and other species, the relationship is much less clear in humans and primates.

See also: animal communication; social behaviour

tertiary cortex A term given to the area where the association cortices (see ASSOCIATION CORTEX) of the PARIETAL LOBE, TEMPORAL LOBE and OCCIPITAL LOBE meet.

See also: left hemisphere

testes The testes are the male gonads. They produce (in the Leydig cells) TESTOSTERONE (a process controlled by LUTEINIZING HORMONE secreted from the ADENOHYPOPHYSIS; the secretion of this is controlled by GONADOTROPHIN RELEASING HORMONE) and (in the Sertoli cells) SPERMATOZOA (male sex cells which, in MAMMALS, will combine with egg cells in the OVARIES to initiate the development of offspring). These are transported to the VAS DEFERENS where they are stored. (Male reproductive capacity can be halted by closing off the vas deferens – this is what a vasectomy does.) For EJACULATION from the PENIS into the female VAGINA during COPULATION, spermatozoa are suspended in SEMINAL FLUID; the term SEMEN is given to the combination of spermatozoa and seminal fluid.

See also: androgens; reproduction; sex hormones

Reference

Johnson M. & Everitt B.J. (1980) *Essential Reproduction*, Blackwell Scientific Publications: Oxford.

testosterone *see* androgens

tetanus Tetanus is a disease, the major feature of which is TONIC spasms of MUSCLES. However, in neuroscience, tetanus also refers to a sustained ACTION POTENTIAL burst, which can either occur spontaneously of be induced by stimulation.

See also: long-term depression; long-term potentiation; post-tetanic potentiation

tetraethylammonium (TEA) An agent that blocks activity of ION CHANNELS sensitive to POTASSIUM (K^+) (potassium channels; see ION CHANNEL). It was once thought to have particular effects on the AUTONOMIC NERVOUS SYSTEM, but it transpires that this is so only because the autonomic nervous system is very sensitive to potassium channel disruption: TEA can in fact work anywhere in the nervous system. It would be a grave error to confuse TEA with tea.

See also: tetrodotoxin; saxitoxin

tetrahydroaminoacridine *see* tacrine

tetrahydrocannabinol Δ9-tetrahydrocannabinol (THC) is the principal active ingredient of CANNABIS. It binds to specific THC receptors in brain, for which ANANDAMIDE is the natural LIGAND.

See also: marijuana

tetrodotoxin An agent that blocks activity of ION CHANNELS sensitive to SODIUM (Na$^+$) (sodium channels; see ION CHANNEL) without affecting any other ion channels. It has been of great value as a neuroscientific tool. It is also known as a fatal paralysing agent. It is found in the ovaries and liver of Japanese puffer fish. Such fish are considered a delicacy but if not properly prepared can, since they contain tetrodotoxin, cause fatal poisoning.

See also: saxitoxin; tetraethylammonium

Texas red *see* tract tracers

textons Textons are local pattern elements suggested to be the basic units from which the perception of texture is assembled; see TEXTURE PERCEPTION.

texture perception Most natural and artificial surfaces are covered with regular or irregular repetitive elements that form a texture. The ability to register visually the shape and distribution of these texture elements serves several important perceptual functions. (1) The nature of the surface (for example wood or gravel, smooth or rough) can be recognized. (2) Boundaries between differently textured surfaces can be located, yielding a SUBJECTIVE CONTOUR and aiding the segmentation of the field of view into distinct objects. (3) Perspective projection produces a gradient of texture density and element size across the retinal image of a surface; this gradient carries information about the angle of the surface to the line of sight and hence the relative distance of surface points from the observer (see DEPTH PERCEPTION). For all these reasons, there need to be patterns of neural activity in the VISUAL SYSTEM that represent texture properties explicitly. Experimental studies of texture perception have mostly concentrated on the second of these processes, texture segmentation. If a pair of textures can readily be segmented, this provides evidence that they have distinct neural representations.

One way in which textures may have distinct neural representations is if they activate different SPATIAL FREQUENCY CHANNELS; texture is a natural area for this approach because it is a property of an extended region which, unlike a single location, can be analysed in spatial frequency terms. Indeed, spatial frequency differences can lead to highly distinctive textures. However, Julesz and co-workers (see Julesz, 1981) devised pairs of textures that, despite identical spatial frequency content, could be immediately segregated in perception. They used this strategy in experiments to identify candidate TEXTONS – types of local pattern element hypothesized to be the primitives out of which visual representations of texture are constructed. Two textures could be segmented if they differed in the density of one or more texton types. (This theory implies that spatial frequency content provides a second basis for texture representation which does not depend on discrete textons.) However, if texton densities were equal, their detailed distribution (for instance, pairings of two textons close together) did not provide a basis for texture discrimination. Texture perception does not require the exact location of each texture element to be registered or retained in processing. Thus in PERIPHERAL VISION, or PRE-ATTENTIVE VISION, texture properties may be represented without the detailed geometrical relationships that define a complex shape and which require focal ATTENTION for processing. Controversies on the set of textons or texture primitives used in the human visual system have not yet been fully resolved. However, two kinds of texture primitive have been widely accepted: oriented line and edge segments, and the endings or 'terminators' of such segments. Both these are signalled by the activity of specific classes of cells in early areas of VISUAL CORTEX, V1 and V2 (see AREAS V1–V5): simple and complex cells (see SIMPLE, COMPLEX AND HYPERCOMPLEX CELLS) respond to oriented lines or edges, and end-stopped cells are activated by such segments with terminators. Furthermore, edge segments and terminators (or corners) are taken as low-level primitives by most theories of shape perception. Thus it appears that both texture and shape perception depend on a common set of primitive elements, represented in the activity of neurons at the level of V1. On this view, shape and texture processing diverge in that they depend on different grouping processes: the representation of shape depends on continuous outline contours which result from grouping together aligned edge segments, while a texture is defined when similar primitives are grouped together over a 2-dimensional region rather than along a contour. Both kinds of grouping require information to be combined from neurons with similar types of RECEPTIVE FIELD in different locations, a function which may be served by long-range horizontal connections that have been identified in visual cortex. Such connections are presumably also necessary for the spatial comparison that identifies the places where textures differ, enabling texture segmentation, and the immediate detection of a discrepant element from a uniformly textured background. However, no distinct neural bases has yet been identified for the different kinds of processing involved in shape and texture.

See also: contour perception; pattern perception

Reference

Julesz B. (1981) Figure and ground perception in briefly presented isodipole textures. In *Perceptual Organization*, ed. M. Kubovy & Pomerantz J. R., Erlbaum: Hillsdale NJ.

OLIVER J. BRADDICK

texture primitives *see* texture perception

thalamic reticular nucleus The reticular nucleus of the thalamus (TRn) presents as a band of tissue at the outermost edge of the THALAMUS. In the rodent brain it sites on the inner surface of the INTERNAL CAPSULE at the lateral aspect of the thalamus. It is more or less continuous with the ZONA INCERTA, which travels from the end of the reticular nucleus towards the MIDLINE, immediately above the HYPOTHALAMUS. The thalamic reticular nucleus is divisible into functionally distinct

territories (visual, auditory and somatosensory for example). It is intimately connected to other thalamic nuclei, to the CEREBRAL CORTEX and has input from neurons in the ASCENDING RETICULAR ACTIVATING SYSTEM, these various inputs and outputs existing in a highly structured, complex interaction (see Guillery *et al.*, 1998). Functionally, the thalamic reticular nucleus is thought to be critically involved in ATTENTION, and in the modulation of SLOW-WAVE SLEEP.

Reference

Guillery R.W., Feig S.L. & Lozsádi D.A. (1998) Paying attention to the thalamic reticular nucleus. *Trends in Neurosciences* 21: 28–32.

thalamic stimulation *see* deep brain stimulation

thalamotomy Surgical removal of the THALAMUS, or part of it. Specific nuclei may be surgically lesioned to provide relief from intractable PARKINSON'S DISEASE.

See also: pallidotomy; psychosurgery

thalamus A complex nucleus in the DIENCEPHALON, comprising a number of different cell groups. It is subdivided into three component parts – the dorsal thalamus, ventral thalamus and epithalamus – on the basis of differences in connectivity and development. A major function of the thalamus is the relay of incoming information from major sensory, motor or limbic nuclei to specific regions within the CEREBRAL CORTEX; this is carried out by the principal neurons of the dorsal thalamus. The thalamus is also intimately involved in the control of BEHAVIOURAL STATE, as a result of its major input from the CHOLINERGIC, NORADRENERGIC and SEROTONERGIC cell groups in the BRAINSTEM RETICULAR FORMATION.

The dorsal thalamus comprises principal (or relay) nuclei and INTRALAMINAR NUCLEI. The classical organization of principal thalamic nuclei is that they receive a well-defined subcortical input, relay these signals to the middle layers of a restricted cortical region, and receive a reciprocal corticothalamic projection from the same region of cortex. Each principal thalamic nucleus also receives an input from a restricted area of the THALAMIC RETICULAR NUCLEUS, from a specific region of the pallidum as part of the systems of CORTICOSTRIATAL LOOPS, and from the reticular formation. The intralaminar nuclei, found within the fibre LAMINAE of the dorsal thalamus, form an integral system of their own, but also have an organization which implies separable sensory, motor and limbic functions. The ventral thalamus includes the reticular nucleus of the thalamus, a thin sheet of neurons surrounding the lateral and rostral aspects of the dorsal thalamus. It is a 'non-specific' thalamic nucleus, which does not project to the cortex, but receives COLLATERALS of the cortical projections to dorsal thalamic nuclei. It also has reciprocal interactions with all nuclei in the dorsal thalamus and receives efferents from the brainstem reticular formation. The EPITHALAMUS contains the medial and lateral HABENULA, and is unique in relation to other thalamic systems because it has strong functional links with the BASAL GANGLIA, ventral STRIATUM and brainstem rather than with the cortex.

Within the dorsal thalamus, the principal sensory nuclei are the LATERAL GENICULATE NUCLEUS (vision), MEDIAL GENICULATE NUCLEUS (hearing) and ventroposterior (somatic sensation), relaying information to the primary visual, auditory and somatosensory cortices respectively. The ventrolateral nucleus is a comparable motor nucleus relaying activity from the CEREBELLUM to the MOTOR CORTEX. The anterior nuclei and DORSOMEDIAL NUCLEUS OF THE THALAMUS are the principal limbic nuclei (see LIMBIC SYSTEM) and have a particular relationship with the PREFRONTAL CORTEX and CINGULATE CORTEX. Of this diverse group of nuclei, only the dorsolateral geniculate shows a 'classical' relationship with the cortex, as described above: it receives a well-defined input from the RETINA and has organised reciprocal connections with the middle layers of the primary VISUAL CORTEX. Other principal nuclei may receive a less clearly defined input pattern, or interact with a number of related cortical areas.

The AFFERENT connections from the reticular nucleus are inhibitory – the only inhibitory outputs from any thalamic nucleus. The nucleus is so-called as a result of its long and relatively non-divergent output neurons, which are similar to those arising from the brainstem reticular formation. In the thalamic reticular nucleus, the profuse GABAERGIC collaterals form a mesh around passing fibres, and together with electrophysiological evidence suggest a role in gating the activity of thalamocortical relay neurons, in a similar manner to the PURKINJE CELLS in the cerebellum. The interplay between the brainstem reticular formation, thalamus and cortex, has been implicated in the regulation of levels of ATTENTION, VIGILANCE and MOTIVATION during waking, as well as the control of SLOW-WAVE SLEEP and rapid eye movement sleep (REM SLEEP). Efferents to the principal and reticular thalamic neurons from the reticular formation have STATE-DEPENDENT firing patterns (see STATE DEPENDENCY): they operate in distinct modes, which depend on the state of arousal. Their thalamic targets also show differences in activity which are dependent on behavioural state. During alert wakefulness, principal and reticular neurons have similar firing patterns, characterized by spontaneous single-spike tonic discharges which are thought to promote the transfer of information to the cortex. As vigilance moves towards drowsiness, reticular neurons become exceptionally active, firing exceedingly long spike barrages which phasically hyperpolarize (see HYPERPOLARIZATION) principal thalamic neurons; during this stage, principal neurons are characterized by spontaneous oscillations in a 7–14 Hz 'spindle' rhythm. Spindle waves in the dorsal thalamus herald the appearance of slow-waves in the cortical ELECTROENCEPHALOGRAM (EEG) during sleep. Although the interactions between thalamic reticular and principal neurons in different states are now relatively well understood in electrophysiological terms, the precise role of other structures such as the brainstem reticular formation – or indeed forebrain structures such as the HYPOTHALAMUS or cholinergic BASAL FOREBRAIN – in modifying thalamic activity, is still not clearly understood.

WENDY L. INGLIS

thebaine *see* opium

theme analysis A procedure developed by Magnusson to perform a structural analysis of real time behaviour. It was intended for use with humans (and has been used in clinical settings; see Lyon *et al.*, 1994) but in fact is well suited to analysis of animal behaviour also. There are many techniques for the analysis of spontaneous behaviour, but most classify either acts (see BEHAVIOURAL CHECKLIST) or notate the actual structure of movement (see ESHKOL–WACHMAN NOTATION). Theme analysis differs from other methods by looking for patterns in activity over time, rather than simply categorizing behaviour.

References

Lyon M., Lyon N. & Magnusson M.S. (1994) The importance of temporal structure in analysing schizophrenic behavior: some theoretical and diagnostic implications. *Schizophrenia Research* 13: 45–56.

Magnusson M.S. (1999) Discovering hidden time patterns in behavior: T-patterns and their detection. *Behavior Research Methods: Instruments and Computers* 32: 93–110.

theobromine *see* xanthines

theophylline Theophylline is one of the XANTHINES: it is one of the PSYCHOMOTOR STIMULANTS found in tea (see TEA AND COFFEE). It has a variety of mild psychological properties similar to CAFFEINE. The name theophylline derives from Greek, *thea*: goddess, *phyllon*: leaf; the accepted translation is 'divine leaf'. Thea is also the name given to the genus of tea plants.

theory of mind This refers to the ability to attribute mental states to self and others in order to predict and explain behaviour. Predicting behaviour based on a false belief has been seen as a key test, where own belief and true state of affairs will not suffice to predict action. For example, a child is asked to predict where a character who has not seen her ball moved, will look for the ball – the correct answer being the original, now empty, location. Most children pass standard false-belief tests between 3 and 4 years old, and this seems to be broadly true in different cultures. There is considerable debate concerning the theory-of-mind abilities of children under 3 years (there are, for instance, naturalistic examples of deception, teasing). Young children's failure on false-belief tests has been attributed variously to problems in understanding the representational nature of beliefs, to pragmatic elements of the task, or to difficulties inhibiting a response towards the real location of the object. The 18-month-old's ability to understand and engage in pretend play has been linked by some authors to theory of mind, with the suggestion that both require METAREPRESENTATION – thoughts about thoughts. Along with JOINT ATTENTION (such as pointing and showing) pretend play may be among the first signs of sensitivity to other people's independent mental states. The evolutionary value of theory of mind has been discussed, both for competition (so-called MACHIAVELLIAN INTELLIGENCE) and cooperation and pedagogy. Despite considerable research, there is as yet no compelling evidence that non-human PRIMATES attribute mental states to others. A possible modular basis has been proposed for theory of mind (see MODULES AND MODULAR ORGANIZATION), although environmental factors such as mental state talk in the family may be crucial, and certainly play a part in individual differences in age of passing theory of mind tests. There is current interest in theory of mind in the deaf and in the blind, as researchers postulate necessary social experiences such as gaze monitoring, embedded grammatical forms, or conversations about internal states. Recent FUNCTIONAL NEUROIMAGING studies of theory of mind ability in adults have implicated different candidate regions in the FRONTAL LOBE, including left medial frontal gyrus and right orbitofrontal regions. The notion that theory of mind has a dedicated brain basis has found support from the existence of AUTISM, a developmental disorder characterized by failure to represent mental states in experimental tasks and everyday life, despite sometimes good general INTELLIGENCE.

See also: consciousness

Reference

Carruthers P. & Smith P.K. (eds.) (1996) *Theories of Theories of Mind*, Cambridge University Press: Cambridge.

FRANCESCA G. HAPPÉ

therapeutic index The therapeutic index (TI) of a DRUG is the TD50 divided by the ED50: that is, the toxic dose 50 divided by the effective dose 50. If the TD50 and the ED50 are the same dose one would have a TI of 1, which would not be good. If the TD50 was very high (that is, toxic effects required administration of massive doses) while the ED50 was very low (that is, tiny amounts of drug were very effective in producing a desired effect) then the TI would be very much greater than 1, which would be good.

thermogenesis The production of heat: see THERMOREGULATION.

thermoneutrality The environmental temperature at which an organism need not adjust their body temperature – that is, the temperature of the environment is the same as the organism's internal milieu; see THERMOREGULATION.

thermoregulation Animals need to maintain body temperature to prevent CELL damage caused by overheating or freezing: heat changes the structure of PROTEINS and kills neurons – even the high temperatures (HYPERPYREXIA) associated with FEVER can sometimes do this, while cold leads to ice formation in LIPID BILAYER MEMBRANE sites. Some species that live in extremely cold conditions have developed intracellular chemical processes (effectively the production of antifreeze molecules) to avoid this. Certain species in HIBERNATION can also withstand body temperatures below freezing, though how they do is not clear. To maintain body temperature, animals either recruit heat from the environment (they are known as poikilothermic or ectothermic – 'cold-blooded' animals) or they generate heat (THERMOGENESIS) internally (they are endothermic or HOMOIOTHERMIC – 'warm-blooded' animals). METABOLIC RATE and body size are important determinants of thermoregulation: small animals tend to have higher metabolic rates and to maintain higher body temperatures than larger animals, while low surface-to-volume ratio makes for more efficient thermoregulation.

Both endotherms and ectotherms use a variety of mechanisms to affect body temperature. (1) Altered heat exchange with the environment: increasing BLOOD flow (VASODILATION) of vessels near the body surface (in the SKIN) produces heat loss; VASOCONSTRICTION helps retain heat. A mechanism known as counter-current heat exchange is used by many endotherms – warmer blood in arteries travelling from the body core heats cooler blood in veins returning. In addition many animals have fur or feathers which insulate them: PILOERECTION (adjustment of the position of individual hairs) aids heat loss. (2) Evaporation: water is lost during BREATHING (either normal breathing or panting; dogs for example lose heat in this way) and by perspiration – SWEAT GLANDS in the skin allow evaporation of water which produces heat loss. (3) Behavioural responses: moving to warmer or cooler environments helps regulate temperature. SOCIAL BEHAVIOUR (for example huddling together to share and conserve heat) is also important. The construction of clothing or specialized dwellings (burrows, nests and so on) is also a behavioural adaptation to aid thermoregulation. MIGRATION, HIBERNATION and AESTIVATION are all behavioural adaptations to enable animals to deal with changed environmental temperatures. All of these processes can be used by endotherms and ectotherms. (4) In addition, endotherms have another mechanism: endogenous heat production. Muscle activity is important in this, as is SHIVERING (which is caused by neural impulses causing muscles to contract desynchronously) a response triggered by the brain's detection of lowered body temperature. NON-SHIVERING THERMOGENESIS is the production of heat by other endogenous means, principally through the action of BROWN ADIPOSE TISSUE (popularly known as BROWN FAT) and in the LIVER – some 20% of the body's heat is generated here.

The neural mechanisms involved in thermoregulation appears to depend on monitoring of blood temperature and skin. Thermoregulatory systems appear to be distributed across a large part of the CENTRAL NERVOUS SYSTEM and to be organized hierarchically: there appear to be mechanisms in the SPINAL CORD, BRAINSTEM and the HYPOTHALAMUS and PREOPTIC AREA, with increasing refinement as one moves higher up the system. As with other sensory systems, the higher level processes are more finely tuned, triggering physiological and behavioural changes in response to a narrower range of changes in temperature. It was once thought that body temperature was maintained to a strict SET POINT and a rather rigid homeostatic manner (see HOMEOSTASIS) but this does not appear to be quite the case: there is more flexibility in temperature regulation than had been supposed: a BOUNDARY MODEL probably provides a better account; see Satinoff (1983) for further discussion of this.

See also: goosebumps; REM sleep; thermo-neutrality

Reference

Satinoff E. (1983) A re-evaluation of the concept of homeostatic organization of temperature regulation. In: *Handbook of Behavioral Neurobiology*, vol. 6, *Motivation*, ed. E. Satinoff & P. Teitelbaum, pp. 443–472, Plenum Press: New York.

theta cell Theta cells are cells in the medial septum (see SEPTAL NUCLEI) responsible for the maintenance of THETA WAVES (see ELECTROEN-CEPHALOGRAM) in the HIPPOCAMPUS. The term theta cell has also been applied (rarely) to a type of GANGLION CELL the RETINA. This is a more unusual use of the term: where there is no clear context, it should be assumed that theta cell refers to a cell type in the hippocampus.

theta waves *see* electroencephalogram

thiamine Thiamine (vitamin B1) is one of the essential VITAMINS.

See also: Korsakoff's syndrome; malnutrition

thick filaments *see* muscles

thigmotaxis (from Greek, *thigma*: touch, *taxis*: arrangement) Movement by an organism in response to SOMATOSENSORY experience – that is, TOUCH (see also HAPTIC). An animal is said to be thigmotaxic if it maintains contact with an object. For example, rats in a WATER MAZE, before they have learned what is required of them, will often swim around the perimeter of the pool, keeping contact with the wall: such rats can be said to be swimming in a thigmotaxic manner.

thin filaments *see* muscles

thionin *see* stains

thiopental (Pentothal) Ultrashort-acting barbiturate and most widely used intravenous pre-anaesthetic (see ANAESTHETICS) for inducing a hypnotic state in humans and experimental animals.

See also: pentobarbital; phenobarbital; sodium amobarbital

CHARLES D. BLAHA

thioxanthines *see* antipsychotic

third ventricle *see* ventricles

thirst Thirst, like hunger, is a subjective EMOTION: it is an attributional label (see ATTRIBUTION) that humans apply to states they experience. As an expression made by humans 'thirst' has value as a predictor of behaviour, but does not necessarily reveal what physiological state a person is in; see DRINKING; OSMOREGULATION.

thoracic spinal cord *see* spinal cord

thought disorder A feature of SCHIZOPHRENIA and, to a lesser extent, of DEMENTIA. Schizophrenia was characterized by Bleuler as a loosening of associations, a process made manifest as thought disorder and DELUSION. Features of thought disorder can be categorized as follows.

Disorganized speech
Deviance in thought as it is produced
   incoherence – literally, incoherent speech
   loose associations – the association of unrelated ideas
   derailment – losing the track of a thought; veering from one thought to another

Delusions
Delusions to do with the content of thought
   thought insertion – having thoughts placed by an external agent
   thought broadcast – the belief that others are privy to one's thoughts
   thought withdrawal – the belief that one's thoughts are being stolen

Delusions to do with feelings and actions
   somatic passivity – being an unwilling host

to bodily feelings imposed by an external agency

made feelings – feelings are projected into one from outside

made volitional acts – others are controlling one's actions

made impulses – impulses to act caused by others

threshold The THRESHOLD or LIMEN is the minimum stimulus magnitude that can just be detected. This is not a single, fixed value but varies over time and therefore is usually defined statistically (for example, the value that can be detected with a probability of 0.75).

DAVID W. HEELEY

thrombus (from Greek, *thrombos*: a clot) Literally, a THROMBUS is a blood clot. 'Thrombosis' refers to the formation of blood clots, 'thrombolysis' refers to the ability to dissolve blood clots.

thymidine One of the nucleotides; see DNA and RNA.

thymidine tracing Thymidine is a NUCLEO-SIDE of thymine, one of the bases of DNA. It can be taken up into a NEURON as it is developing but not into a post-mitotic (see CELL DIVISION) CELL of any kind. As such, if thymidine with a RADIOLABEL (usually tritiated thymidine – [3H]thymidine) is given to pregnant animals, it will be taken up by all of the developing neurons of every FOETUS being carried. Sacrifice of the foetuses at specific times following injection of [3H] thymidine will allow one to track the progress of developing neurons by examining AUTORADIOGRAMS of brain sections. This technique has been used successfully to study the development of brain structures (see Altman & Bayer, 1986). In adult rats the technique is not normally used, neurons being post-mitotic. However, if a VIRUS has been introduced (as a TRANSNEUR-ONAL TRACER using, for example, ALPHA HERPES VIRUS) DNA replication will have occurred and the progress of the virus can be monitored using [3H]thymidine.

References

Altman J. & Bayer S.A. (1986) *The Develop-ment of the Rat Hypothalamus* (Advances in Embryology and Cell Biology, vol. 100), Springer-Verlag: Berlin.
Bolam J.P. (1992) *Experimental Neuro-anatomy: A Practical Approach*, IRL Press at Oxford University Press: Oxford.

thymosin One of the HORMONES released by the THYMUS GLAND.

See also: endocrine glands; hormones – classification

thymostatin One of the HORMONES released by the THYMUS GLAND.

See also: endocrine glands; hormones – classification

thymoxin One of the HORMONES released by the THYMUS GLAND.

See also: endocrine glands; hormones – classification

thymus gland *see* endocrine glands; immune system; lymphatic system

thyroid gland *see* endocrine glands

thyroid stimulating hormone (also known as THYROTROPIN) One of the HORMONES released by the ADENOHYPOPHYSIS.

See also: endocrine glands; hormones – classification

thyroid stimulating hormone releasing hormone *see* thyrotropin releasing hormone

thyrotropin *see* thyroid stimulating hormone

thyrotropin releasing hormone A hormone involved in the control of the release of other HORMONES from the PITUITARY GLAND.

See also: adenohypophysis; endocrine glands; hormones – classification

thyroxine (T4) One of the HORMONES released by the THYROID GLAND.

See also: endocrine glands; hormones – classification

tic douloureux Also known as trigeminal neuralgia; see NEURALGIA.

tickle Tickling is a phenomenon most commonly associated with PLAY in its various forms. It is of interest to biological psycholo-gists not so much because of its social functions, but because of the observation that it is virtually impossible to tickle oneself: tickle relies on being touched by an external stimulus of some sort. The implication of this is that the (predictable and known) act of self-tickling produces a cancelling signal that eliminates the sensation of tickling. This phenomenon has been recently investigated using controlled procedures that allow the same type and intensity of stimulus to be used in producing self-tickle and externally generated tickle (Blakemore *et al.*, 1998). The SOMATOSENSORY CORTEX was shown to be activated by externally generated tickle but not self-tickle. The activity of the CEREBELLUM indicated that it was implicated in predicting the consequences of self-initiated movements, and could therefore be involved in the process of cancelling signals that otherwise would signal tickle.

See also: laughter

Reference

Blakemore S.T., Wolpert D.M. & Frith C.D. (1998) Central cancellation of self-produced tickle sensation. *Nature Neuroscience* 1: 635–640.

tics Brief, repetitive, purposeless, involuntary movements, usually involving the head and neck. Tics usually take the form of blinking, grimacing, or making brief sounds. Most tics are transient and of no pathological significance. They are particularly common in preadolescent boys. Rarely, tics may be severe and disabling, extending to trunk and limbs and associated with complex vocal abnormalities (for example COPROLALIA) as in TOURETTE'S SYNDROME.

See also: perseveration; stereotypy

IAN C. REID

timbre (from Latin, *tympanum*: a drum) Timbre is the perceived quality of the sound, as opposed to its PITCH and its LOUDNESS. Two sounds with the same pitch and loudness could still sound different to an individual – timbre depends upon the ACOUSTIC SPECTRUM and temporal characteristics and distribution of the harmonic frequencies. Timbre is a term most often applied to music and speech rather than to other everyday sounds.

timing Many organisms possess a BIOLOGICAL CLOCK that enables them to anticipate temporally graded biologically important events. There are two main types of timing. PHASE TIMING provides organisms with information about their current position in an oscillatory process (see OSCILLATION). INTERVAL TIMING enables organisms to measure the amount of time that has elapsed since a temporal marker. Most organisms experience periodic environmental changes including the daily light–dark cycle, tides and seasons. Phase timing allows animals to track these rhythms. Most animals display a CIRCADIAN RHYTHM in their SLEEP–WAKE CYCLE. Additionally, many animals display an increase in LOCOMOTION and DRINKING before a regular daily feeding. These rhythms may allow animals to concentrate their activities during the portion of the day when they are most efficient (as a result of sensory specialization or increased prey availability) and/or restrict their activity to the period of the day when they face a reduced probability of predation. A variety of animals can learn to obtain food at different places at different times of day. Many insects and birds use the sun as a compass, a process that involves the use of circadian phase information to compensate for the movement of the sun throughout the day. Some crabs and birds use circalunar phase information to track the tidal cycle, and the restlessness displayed by migratory birds is controlled by a circannual rhythm (see MIGRATION). Phase timers are synchronized by periodic cues called ZEITGEBERS (see ENTRAINMENT; ZEITGEBER). The light–dark cycle and daily periods of food availability are major circadian zeitgebers. When a zeitgeber is removed circadian rhythms persist but often attain a periodicity slightly different from 24 hours (see FREE RUNNING RHYTHMS). This self-sustaining rhythmicity reflects the periodicity of the circadian pacemaker.

Interval timing allows animals to anticipate events that occur a fixed amount of time after some temporal marker. Interval timers operate like stopwatches as significant external cues stop, reset, and restart timing. This type of temporal discrimination is evident in the behaviour of animals on fixed interval SCHEDULES OF REINFORCEMENT and in the behaviour of hummingbirds that time their flower revisits to match the timing of nectar replenishment. Interval timing also underlies the anticipatory aspect of the CONDITIONED RESPONSE that is evident in many demonstrations of CLASSICAL CONDITIONING. Interval timing obeys WEBER'S LAW as the error in interval timing is a fixed proportion of the length of the interval timed.

See also: diurnal; endogenous rhythm; infradian rhythm; jet lag; melatonin; nocturnal; pineal gland; ultradian rhythm

DONALD M. WILKIE

Timm's stain *see* zinc

tingling A prickling sensation caused by any of various events: cold and nerve excitation (either due to some pathological process or to mechanical stimulation) are the most common causes. Perhaps the most common occurrence is when one strikes one's elbow (the 'funny bone'), thereby mechanically stimulating the ULNAR NERVE and inducing a tingling sensation. The presence of tingling can indicate the presence of certain medical conditions; see for example RAYNAUD'S SYNDROME.

See also: skin; shivers down the spine; tickle

tinnitus A constant ringing or buzzing sound in the ears, without any external sound source causing it. Various forms are known to exist: tinnitus aurium is a ringing sound in both ears associated with the AUDITORY SYSTEM *per se*. It may be caused by disturbance at any level of the auditory system, though its exact cause is unclear. OTOACOUSTIC EMISSIONS may have a causal role; irritation of the AUDITORY NERVE may also play a part. Tinnitus cerebri is a ringing noise in the head rather than the ears; clicking TINNITUS is a noise that is produced by the opening and closing of the EUSTACHIAN TUBE, and which may be audible to others in addition to the patient; and Leudet's tinnitus is a spasmodic click present sometimes during INFLAMMATION of the Eustachian tube, and which also is externally audible.

tip links The cilia present on HAIR CELLS have tip links: that is, the tip of one hair cell is linked by a rather elastic filament to the cilia on either side of it. The point of contact is known as an INSERTIONAL PLAQUE, and it is

from here that activation is generated. Tip links are important in regulating ion channel opening in the hair cells.

See also: cochlea

tissue culture Tissue culture involves growing cells (see CELL) taken from multicellular animals (rather than just cultivating single-celled animals) *in vitro* in the laboratory. While there is little to be gained from such studies of a psychological or behavioural nature, tissue culture is important for NEUROSCIENCE. Questions about the regulation of cell growth, DEVELOPMENT and interactions can be answered using culture methods, and tissue can be grown for use in TRANSPLANTATION studies. Tissue culture also reduces the need for so many animals to be used in research: one animal can provide a stock of tissues that can then be maintained in culture; see ANIMAL WELFARE.

tissue fixation *see* fixation

tissue tortuosity Tortuosity is a term that refers not to torture (though derived from the same Latin root, *tortuosus*: twisted) but to the twisting or winding nature of something. Tissue tortuosity refers therefore to organization of a piece of tissue and is an important consideration when injecting fluid into the brain. Some tissue is very densely packed with cells, other tissue is relatively cell-poor (see CELL). Some tissue has FIBRES running through, that will offer a line of least resistance to fluids, other tissue has fibres running above or over, which will serve to contain and direct fluid flow. Tissue tortuosity is a factor that needs to be borne in mind when infusing substances in to brain because it will directly affect spread of fluid. Adjusting the volume of injection is a straightforward means of correcting for tissue tortuosity, though if a very large type of MOLECULE is being injected, volume may be less important in determining spread.

See also: drug administration; microdialysis; microinjection

titration In chemistry, the addition of small amounts of one substance to another in incremental steps until a reaction occurs. In general, titration refers to the gradual, progressive, measurement or determination of a volume or quantity of any sort; see TITRATION SCHEDULE.

titration schedule A SCHEDULE OF REINFORCEMENT similar to a PROGRESSIVE RATIO schedule. With a progressive ratio schedule, subjects have to make a progressively greater RESPONSE, in incremental steps, until BREAKING POINT is reached; this being in effect the point at which the individual refuses to pay the cost of obtaining REINFORCEMENT (see SCHEDULES OF REINFORCEMENT). A similar procedure is adopted with a titration schedule, with the difference that once responding has stopped, the schedule is reset to a point significantly below breaking point, allowing the subject to resume responding. This procedure is repeated, gradually titrating responding until one finds the maximal level at which responding will be steadily maintained. It is therefore a means of defining the maximal schedule at which responding will be maintained, rather than the point at which it stops.

tobacco Dried leaves of the plant *Nicotiana tabacum*. Tobacco is smoked in cigarettes or cigars, chewed, or taken intranasally as snuff. The active ingredient in tobacco is NICOTINE, a mild stimulant (see STIMULANTS) that is responsible for tobacco's addictive properties. Tobacco has been used by humans for several thousand years. Indigenous peoples in North and South America were the first to grow the tobacco plant and smoked its leaves for its PSYCHOACTIVE effects. New World explorers first observed tobacco smoking in the time of Christopher Columbus, and it was introduced into Western cultures and other parts of the world in the sixteenth century. In our present society, smoking tobacco is a common and legal form of psychoactive drug consumption. Aggressive anti-smoking campaigns have reduced the levels of smoking, but smoking tobacco continues to be a major health risk and a significant factor in causing death and disease.

ANN E. KELLEY

token economy A form of BEHAVIOUR THERAPY involving OPERANT principles. Hospitalized patients with behavioural disturbances can have appropriate and desired actions (both self-directed actions such as feeding and dressing, as well as social interactions) rewarded with tokens that have an assigned value – they can be exchanged for goods, services or privileges. To work successfully token economies have to be systematic and require clear rules describing the relationships between behaviour and REWARD. Such procedures have been quite extensively used, though perhaps not as often as might be expected, and have even been found to have benefit when applied to patients with severe SCHIZOPHRENIA.

Reference

Davison G.C. & Neale J.M. (1996) *Abnormal Psychology*, 6th edn, Wiley: New York.

token test Used to examine patients with APHASIA: subjects are required to use tokens representing elements of LANGUAGE in order to discriminate patients who have no comprehension of language from those who have only a motor impairment in the production of language (see SPEECH PRODUCTION).

tolerance The central feature of tolerance, in the context of biological psychology, is the reduced reaction a DRUG produces following its repeated administration. Tolerance can be seen to have developed when the original effect of the drug can only be achieved using larger (and progressively larger) doses. With ABSTINENCE though, tolerance will decline. A single drug may have more than one psychological or behavioural effect: tolerance may develop to one of these but not the other. The BENZODIAZEPINE drug, CHLORDIAZEPOXIDE, is both a SEDATIVE and ANXIOLYTIC. The sedative effect shows tolerance, while the anxiolytic effect does not, a property of considerable therapeutic value. The opposite of tolerance is SENSITIZATION (or REVERSE TOLERANCE). There are many different types of tolerance (see BEHAVIOURAL TOLERANCE; CELLULAR TOLERANCE; CONTINGENT TOLERANCE; DRUG DISPOSITION TOLERANCE; METABOLIC TOLERANCE; PHARMACODYNAMIC TOLERANCE) and different types of drugs can show different types of tolerance. MORPHINE for example shows both cellular and drug-disposition tolerance, while AMPHETAMINE shows cellular but not drug disposition tolerance.

See also: overdose

Reference

Feldman R., Meyer J.S. & Quenzer L.F. (1997) *Principles of Neuropsychopharmacology*, Sinauer Associates: Sunderland MA.

toluidine blue *see* stains

tomboy syndrome *see* gender identity disorder of childhood

tone In acoustics, the term tone is used to describe a musical sound of a particular PITCH: the contrast to a tone is often thought of as NOISE. The term tone is also used to describe the firmness or elasticity of body tissues, most obviously of course, MUSCLES.

tongue *see* gustation

tonic The term tonic is used in various ways: it is an adjective describing acoustic TONE; it describes a healthy drink; and it is used in other specific ways: see TONIC–CLONIC and TONIC–PHASIC.

tonic–clonic (from Greek, *tonos*: pitch or tension, *klonos*: tumult) These adjectives are often descriptive of CONVULSIONS (*clonic–tonic convulsions*) but in fact refer to muscle spasms. Tonic spasms of the musculature are those that are long-lasting and more or less invariant in intensity. Clonic spasms involve rapid and repeated muscular contractions and relaxations, giving an on–off flicker effect.

See also: epilepsy; generalized seizures; kindling; stuttering

tonic–phasic (from Greek, *tonos*: pitch or tension, *phaein*: to shine). These adjectives are used in a variety of contexts: *tonic* is an adjective used to describe something that has a tone (that is, occurs continuously); *phasic* describes something that occurs in phases or bursts (that is, occurs discontinuously).

tonotopic representation Tonotopic representation is the expression of RECEPTOTOPIC REPRESENTATION in the auditory system. It refers to the spatial arrangement of neurons within a nucleus (or cortical field) according to the tone frequency (or COCHLEAR place) which provides the most sensitive excitatory input. This results in the generation of neural MAPS of preferred tone frequency. It is the central neural expression of the peripheral PLACE CODE for stimulus frequency. Tonotopic representations form the structural framework within which other stimulus dimensions (such as sound location, amplitude, bandwidth) are processed.

DENNIS P. PHILLIPS

tool use This is of interest in biological psychology for two reasons: the initiation of tool use marks an important point in the EVOLUTION of *Homo sapiens* (see HOMINID); and tool use by non-human animals is thought to reflect a degree of INTELLIGENCE. Tool use does not include behaviours shown by many animals in which specialized body adaptations are used in a quasi-tool like manner – many birds for example have beaks designed to achieve specific goals. Instead, tool use requires the operation of an object as an extension of one's body in pursuit of a particular and immediate end. Various PRIMATES have been observed to use tools in the laboratory (Wolfgang Köhler [1887–1967] observed laboratory chimpanzees using sticks to obtain otherwise unreachable food rewards) and in the wild. Chimpanzees use sticks and leaves in gathering food and, famously, macaques on Koshima island washed sand from sweet potatoes before eating them. The many examples of primate tool use have generated further appreciation of their intelligence, but it is clear that other animals can also use tools. For example, birds with their wings clipped have been shown to be able to move wooden blocks to use as steps in order to obtain food placed at an otherwise unreachable height.

See also: emulation; observation learn-ing

tooth bar *see* stereotaxic surgery

top-down vs. bottom-up perceptual/neural processing In any hierarchical information processing (see INFORMATION THEORY) system, processing of input information by fixed analysers that take as their input the output of the next lower level and give output to the next higher level is called bottom-up processing, while any influence of higher levels on the processing carried out by the lower levels is called TOP-DOWN PROCESSING. In perception, the registration of elementary features of stimulus input, such as colour, shape, or motion of visual stimuli, is considered to be mostly bottom-up, or data-driven, while the effects of such things as ATTENTION, expectancy, MEMORY, context and goals on perception are considered to be top-down, or conceptually driven. In neural processing, responses of neurons to inputs from more peripheral neurons (see PERIPHERAL NERVOUS SYSTEM) that are unaffected by inputs from more central neurons (see CENTRAL NERVOUS SYSTEM) would be considered to be bottom-up neural processing, while input from more central neurons that modulates the responses of more peripheral neurons to other inputs would be considered to be top-down neural processing.

In addition to top-down and bottom-up influences on the activity of processing units at a given level of a hierarchy, there can also be lateral interactions (MIDDLE-IN/OUT PROCESSING) among the units that can profoundly influence their responses to inputs from both lower and higher levels. All such interactions depend on the connections between processing units. Bottom-up connections will be from lower to higher level units, top-down connections will be from higher to lower level units, and middle-in/out connections will be among units at the same level. The activity of each unit in such a hierarchy depends on the confluence of inputs to that unit. Top-down, bottom-up and middle-in/out processing refer to occasions when a particular set of connections is under consideration. If certain connections do not exist for some units, that type of processing does not occur for those units – that is, if top-down and middle-in/out connections do not exist for a set of units, they are capable of only bottom-up processing (see NEURAL NETWORKS). It is doubtful if any neural or perceptual processing is purely top-down, middle-in/out, or bottom-up in humans or other animals. Most processing is a blend of all three types. Even the appearance of elementary properties of objects can be influenced by 'psychological' factors such as attention, expectancy and context. For example, the length of the line enclosed by the arrowheads in the display < —————————— > can be influenced by whether one attends to the arrow-

heads or to the line; it appears to be shorter if one attends to the arrowheads. On the other hand, the perception of the existence of the arrowheads and the line cannot usually be affected by such factors that aspect results from bottom-up processing of the retinal image by the VISUAL SYSTEM. In neural processing, there seem to be ascending (peripheral to central) and descending (central to peripheral) connections between every pair of brain areas that communicate, as well as ubiquitous lateral connections (see LATERAL INHIBITION) within each functional and structural area. The activity of each neuron seems to be influenced by that of other neurons at all levels of the neural hierarchy, and in many cases the arrangement of neurons is heterarchical rather than hierarchical (especially within brain areas). However, on various occasions and for particular neurons the influence might be strongest from a particular direction. In these cases, it is both justified, and useful, to talk of top-down, bottom-up, or middle-in/out processing.

There do seem to be many perceptual analysers that operate predominantly in a bottom-up way, especially under optimal conditions. The lines, edges, textures and colours of typical visual scenes seem to be detected in the same, data driven way by the visual system regardless of such things as peoples' previous experiences and goals. For example, regardless of the variations in the words available for naming colours (hues), people of all languages and cultures group hues into four basic categories: red, yellow, green and blue. However, people vary widely in their preferences for hues and hue combinations and their affective reaction to a given visual scene will depend strongly on such top-down (conceptual) influences. Similarly, in neural processing, many peripheral neurons seem to operate in a largely bottom-up way, detecting energy fluctuations or the presence of particular molecules regardless of neural activity in more central regions. However, there are many examples of more central neural circuits that modulate the activity of more peripheral neurons, such as the connection from the OLIVOCOCHLEAR BUNDLE to outer HAIR CELLS that affects the response of the inner hair cells to incoming sounds, possibly by adjusting the tension of the BASI-

LAR MEMBRANE whose motions stimulate those cells.

See also: artificial intelligence; binding problem; neural coding

LAWRENCE M. WARD

topical In biological sciences, this refers to a method of DRUG ADMINISTRATION or some other form of treatment: topical application is the application of something to only one part of the outer surface of the body. It is typically used in relation to the administration of an agent to a limited area of the SKIN, though other surfaces can present themselves for topical application – the surface of the SKULL for example, during STEREOTAXIC SURGERY.

topographical memory This can be treated as synonymous with SPATIAL MEMORY.

See also: prosopagnosia

topography (from Greek, *topos*: a place, *graphein*: to describe) Topography is the study of the features of a place or object. In biological psychology, the term topography has particular uses: topography can for example relate to RESPONSE TOPOGRAPHY or to TOPOGRAPHICAL MEMORY. Note though that the term topographically organized is occasionally used in a synonymous manner.

topology (from Greek, *topos*, a place, and *logos*, discourse) Topology is the study of the relationships between places. (More specifically, in mathematics, topology is the systematic study of connected or adjacent points of a plane or space which remain present regardless of separating: this is most easily grasped by thinking of the study of stretching or knotting objects, rather than cutting them.) In biological psychology, the term TOPOLOGY is used more in an anatomical sense, indicating that two or more structures connect in precise topological ways: that is, neurons at points A and B in one structure project their axons to equivalent points A′ and B′ in another structure. In complex systems, the neurons at A′ and B′ may further project to equivalent points A″ and B″ in a third structure: such a system would be said to be topologically organized. Topology is also used, in abbreviated form, in terms such as RETINOTOPIC, RECEPTOTOPIC REPRESENTATION, TONOTOPIC REPRESENTATION and SOMATOTOPIC.

torsion *see* eye position

torticollis (from Latin, *tortus*: twist, *collum*: neck) An abnormal position of the head, with the neck twisted to one side; it is caused by contraction (or spasm) of the MUSCLES in the neck on one side of the body and not the other. It is colloquially known as 'wryneck'.

See also: convulsions; tonic–clonic

touch Touch is the class of sensations produced by mechanical disturbances of the skin from physical contact or thermal stimulation. Vibration, PAIN, pressure, and TEMPERATURE are encoded via fine nerve endings and the MECHANORECEPTOR system. The most sensitive body regions (tongue, lips, fingers) have the greatest density of mechanoreceptors and the largest cortical representation. Impulses travel along sensory nerve fibres to SOMATOSENSORY PATHWAYS, the THALAMUS, and SOMATOSENSORY CORTEX (Kaas, 1988). Somatosensory cortex maintains somatotopic organization. Primary somatosensory cortex (S-I) processes primary sensations; damage to S-I produces numbness. Secondary somatosensory cortex (S-II) processes complex tactile information; damage to S-II or higher-level association areas may produce TACTILE AGNOSIA.

See also: haptic; homunculus; sensory transduction;

Reference

Iwamura Y. (1998) Hierarchical somatosensory processing. *Current Opinion in Neurobiology* 8: 522-528.

CATHERINE L. REED

touch receptors These are mechanoreceptors present in the skin that respond to such things as pressure and vibration (that is, all forms of TOUCH); see SKIN for a description of the various types of touch receptor.

Tourette's syndrome Relatively rare movement disorder characterized by multiple TICS and associated with involuntary vocalization, first described by Georges Gilles de la Tourette (1857–1904). The condition is more commonly seen in males, and onset is rare after the age of

11. Once believed to be very rare, the incidence is now thought to be 1 in 2000. There may be a familial component to the illness, though no clear genetic association has been demonstrated. Initial manifestations of the disorder usually comprise isolated tics, affecting the head and neck. They take the form of rapid, purposeless, stereotyped movements (see STEREOTYPY). The movements can be withheld for short periods, though sufferers usually become increasingly tense while doing so. Later movements can spread throughout the body, and in severe cases may take the form of complex, multiple tics which can be very disabling. Involuntary vocalization and related phenomena may take the form of grunting, sniffing and spitting. Full vocalization is often obscene in nature (COPROLALIA), with either aggressive or sexual content. Both movements and vocalizations may mimic the movement or speech of others (ECHOPRAXIA or ECHOLALIA respectively). The syndrome is often severely disabling socially, resulting in considerable embarrassment and ANXIETY, though many cases are very mild. Though the syndrome may be associated with other disorders, often DEPRESSION and may be related to OBSESSIVE COMPULSIVE DISORDER, sufferers are not in any sense 'out of touch with reality' and remain cognitively intact. Without treatment, Tourette's syndrome persists throughout life, though the intensity of the symptoms may wax and wane, or one constellation of tics may replace another. Psychosocial and pharmacological interventions form the mainstay of treatment. HALOPERIDOL and other DOPAMINE-blocking drugs are often very effective in attenuating symptoms. Other drug treatments which have been explored with rather more limited success include ANTIDEPRESSANT drugs, CLONIDINE and NICOTINE. The aetiology of Tourette's syndrome remains unknown: contemporary investigation centres on genetic and FUNCTIONAL NEUROIMAGING studies. The response of the condition to dopamine-blocking agents has led to speculation that dopaminergic systems are abnormal in the disorder, but no conclusive evidence has yet emerged.

IAN C. REID

tower of Hanoi A computational puzzle devised by Édouard Lucas (1842–1891), a French mathematician. It is familiar to two disparate groups of scientists: mathematicians and computer scientists, who use it to investigate mathematical questions; and to neuroscientists and psychologists, who use the tower of Hanoi (and tasks derived from it) to probe DECISION-MAKING strategies and problem solving in both normal and brain damaged individuals. The tower of Hanoi is composed of three upright poles parallel to each other (*source* at one end, *auxiliary* in the centre and *destination* at the other end). On the source pole are placed four rings: a large one at the bottom, followed by the other three in descending order of diameter. The task a subject has is simple: to move all of the rings from the source pole to the destination pole, using the auxiliary pole as an intermediate. However, a larger ring can never be placed on a smaller ring. Some psychologists have argued that while the tower of Hanoi is a well-defined computational problem that has value in assessing abstract problem-solving, it has much less value in assessing 'real-life' problem-solving, which necessarily involves more uncertainty and less clear computations. Moreover, it involves a degree of TRIAL-AND-ERROR LEARNING and it has been suggested that the need constantly to inhibit responses (see INHIBITION) makes it a difficult instrument with which to assess PLANNING. The tower of London task is a related task, widely used in NEUROPSYCHOLOGY research, which is thought to overcome some of the problems of the tower of Hanoi by reducing the number of rings from four to only three: normal subjects learn this task quickly while patients with various forms of neural injury or functional impairment do not. The STOCKINGS OF CAMBRIDGE is a task that forms part of the CANTAB battery and is analogous to the tower of London task. It is a computerized task which involves moving balls from one stocking to another (the stockings being hung in a 'Christmas stocking' manner). The essential planning component of tasks such as the tower of London or the stockings of Cambridge can be made even more clear by having subjects look at two different arrays and report the number of moves it would take to transform one into the other. The Tower of Toronto is a further variant, having three pegs and, like the tower of Hanoi, four rings. In this case though the rings are coloured and there is an additional rule: one cannot move a darker disc onto a lighter one. Having the extra rule makes the task much harder to acquire (involving considerable trial and error learning) but giving the experimenter more material with which to assess the subjects' acquisition of a formula for solving the task; a period of stable performance; and the subjects move toward making the solution an AUTOMATIC ACTION.

All of these tasks – towers of London and Toronto, stockings of Cambridge – are used to examine EXECUTIVE FUNCTIONS and spatial abilities (see SPATIAL BEHAVIOUR; SPATIAL COGNITION; SPATIAL MEMORY). Patients with functional disorders (such as SCHIZOPHRENIA) and with various forms of brain damage, including degenerative disorders such as Parkinson's disease, and damage to the FRONTAL CORTEX (see FRONTAL SYNDROME) all find these tasks difficult. Patients with DYSEXECUTIVE SYNDROME are often assessed with these tasks.

See also: attentional set-shifting; Wisconsin card-sort task

tower of London *see* tower of Hanoi

tower of Toronto *see* tower of Hanoi

toxic; toxicity; toxin From Greek, *toxon*, a bow; *toxikon*, arrow poison: toxic is synonymous with poison, toxicity with poisonous and toxin with a poison. There are very many different types of toxin used either accidentally or deliberately (and either naturally or experimentally) against the nervous system; *see* NEUROTOXIN.

trace conditioning A PAVLOVIAN CONDITIONING preparation in which a gap occurs between conditioned stimulus (CS) termination and unconditioned stimulus (US) onset: the trace of the CS (rather than the CS itself) is paired with the US. It typically produces weaker conditioned responding than delay conditioning; and sufficiently long trace intervals produce no conditioning at all.

See also: backward conditioning; delay conditioning

JASPER WARD-ROBINSON

tracers *see* tract tracers

trachea *see* mouth

tracheotomy An incision into the windpipe (the trachea); used to enable INTRATRACHEAL INJECTIONS; see DRUG ADMINISTRATION.

tract tracers Tract tracers are used to map neuronal pathways within the nervous system. Four main categories of tracing agent can be identified: FLUORESCENT TRACERS, ANTEROGRADE TRACERS, RETROGRADE TRACERS and TRANSNEURONAL TRACERS. A fifth – RADIOACTIVE TRACER – is described here though it is rarely used now. Such techniques have been very powerful in describing connections within the nervous system.

Fluorescent tracers. Tracing using fluorescent material (that is by using a FLUOROCHROME – a chemical that emits light [fluoresces] when light of a specific wavelength is shone on to it) can be done in several ways. Fluorescent agents such as TEXAS RED, TRUE BLUE or DIAMIDINO YELLOW can be delivered by MICROINJECTION or MICROIONTOPHORESIS into specific brain areas, where they will be taken up by neurons and spread throughout those neurons. Fluorochromes can also be combined with immunohistochemical procedures (IMMUNOFLUORESCENCE – see IMMUNOHISTOCHEMISTRY), though this is a relatively rare procedure. Another use of fluorescent agents is in intracellular injection (a procedure referred to as NEURONAL FILLING). With this, agents such as LUCIFER YELLOW are injected directly into neurons (on tissue sections rather than in whole brain) in which they spread out colouring the entire cell and giving a vivid picture of its complete MORPHOLOGY.

Anterograde tracers. An anterograde tracer is one which is transported anterogradely along a neuron: that is from CELL BODY to AXON TERMINAL. The most commonly used is *PHASEOLUS VULGARIS*-LEUCOAGGLUTININ (PHA-L – a LECTIN derived from the red kidney bean; other plant lectins have also been used), which is usually delivered by microiontophoresis into brain tissue. Cell bodies and dendrites take it up and transport it along axons to terminals, a procedure that takes 7–12 days typically. An alternative anterograde tracing agent is BIOCYTIN (biotinyl-lysine), which is also taken up by cell bodies but transports in 24–48 hours. There are a number of advantages and disadvantages to weigh up when deciding whether to use PHA-L or biocytin; these are discussed in Bolam (1992).

Retrograde tracers. A retrograde tracer is one which is transported retrogradely along a neuron: that is from AXON TERMINAL TO CELL BODY. The first to be widely used was HORSERADISH PEROXIDASE (HRP), though this is in fact taken up by axon terminals as well as by cell bodies and dendrites. Making a conjugate of HRP and wheatgerm agglutinin (WGA – a plant lectin) to produce WGA-HRP, or producing a conjugate of CHOLERA TOXIN SUBUNIT B (CTB) and HRP to produce CTB-HRP improves the selectivity of retrograde transport. Both WGA and CTB can also be used independently of HRP. COLLOIDAL GOLD can also be used in conjunction with these (WGA-HRP-gold or CTB-HRP-gold). The significant advantage of this is that colloidal gold preparations are taken up by intact neurons but not by the cut ends of damaged fibres, which of course yields a better representation of tracing from the neurons in the injected regions. This is a general problem when using tracing agents, and anything that can help obviate it is of value.

Transneuronal tracers. These are agents that can cross a SYNAPSE, making it possible to deliver them to one part of the brain and then determine what the trans-synaptic connections of that area are. WGA-HRP is in fact to a very limited degree a transneuronal tracer (it does not present a significant problem of interpretation), but the most commonly used agents are ALPHA HERPES VIRUSES. The presence of these in tissue can be detected using immunohistochemistry, antibodies for herpes viruses being commercially available.

Radioactive tracers. These are tracing agents – typically one of the AMINO ACIDS such as LEUCINE – that have been tagged with a RADIOLABEL. Amino acids injected into brain are taken up by cells and used in the formation of PROTEINS at various points within them.

Since they are radiolabelled they can be detected using AUTORADIOGRAPHY. Such techniques were valuable, but because it lacks the anatomical or functional specificity of other techniques it is now rarely used.

These techniques are widely used in NEUROANATOMY. They do not have to be used singly: DOUBLE or even TRIPLE LABELLING allows one to combine different procedures. For example, one could combine the use of tract tracers with immunohistochemistry to examine the relationships between specifically identified neurons in one structure (using immunohistochemistry) and projections from another structures (using an anterograde tracer). Alternatively, one could use two different fluorescent tracers, each injected into different structures, and attempt to detect neurons in a third structure that show either single or double labelling. Some care has to be exercised when attempting double or triple labelling, to make sure that the different labels can be effectively processed (they may for example require different forms of tissue fixation) and effectively visualized, showing clear differentiation between each type of label.

See also: chemical neuroanatomy; fluorogold; histochemistry; *in situ* hybridization; metabolic mapping; thymidine tracing

Reference

Bolam J.P. (1992) *Experimental Neuroanatomy: A Practical Approach*, IRL Press at Oxford University Press: Oxford.

trade-off function A general principle that indicates the extent to which the maximum efficiency with which one function is performed (or occurs) must be reduced in order that a second function can be performed (or occur). It is a function that operates at both physiological and behavioural levels.

trail-making test Also known as the REITAN TRAIL-MAKING TEST; see HALSTEAD–REITAN NEUROPSYCHOLOGICAL BATTERY.

training Animals undertaking psychological or behavioural tests will often need to be trained to perform a task: to work in an OPERANT CHAMBER or to run MAZES for example. Other tests require no training but just examine spontaneous behaviour of one sort or another measurement of LOCOMOTION or OPEN FIELD behaviour for example. In LESION or DRUG studies, training can be given *before* some brain manipulation or *after*. In the former case one therefore examines the effects of brain manipulation on ACQUISITION of a learnt task while in the latter one examines how a treatment affects RETENTION of a task.

See also: entrainment; reacquisition

tranquillizer Any DRUG that has a SEDATIVE effect on the nervous system. The term does not denote a specific drug class, but rather applies to a range of drugs that have the ability to depress activity in the nervous system or to calm behaviour. Older usage of this term included the terms MINOR TRANQUILLIZER and MAJOR TRANQUILLIZER. Minor tranquilizers referred to drugs such as BARBITURATES and the BENZODIAZEPINE group, which have a relaxing, calming effect and in higher doses cause SLEEP. Major tranquilizers were the ANTIPSYCHOTIC drugs such as CHLORPROMAZINE, RESERPINE, and HALOPERIDOL. These drugs have the ability to reduce PSYCHOSIS and severe ANXIETY, without strong sedative effects. The terms are used less in more recent terms; minor tranquilizer has been replaced by the terms SEDATIVE-HYPNOTIC and ANXIOLYTIC, and major tranquilizer by the term NEUROLEPTIC.

ANN E. KELLEY

transcardial perfusion A technique used to aid extraction of the BRAIN and SPINAL CORD from a dead animal prior to histological analysis. The standard procedure is to inject the animal with a lethal dose of BARBITURATE (what is colloquially known as 'putting to sleep'). Immediately after death, the HEART is exposed and a CANNULA inserted into the left ventricle; the right auricle is cut. Fluid passed through the cannula will circulate around the body, exiting via the open right auricle. A neutral fluid is initially perfused: phosphate buffered saline (see PHOSPHATE BUFFER), or PHYSIOLOGICAL SALINE, or some other appropriate fluid. This removes the BLOOD from the body (HEPARIN can be added to prevent clotting). After this, a fixative (see FIXATION) appropriate to the histological procedures (routine HISTOLOGY or IMMUNOHISTOCHEMISTRY for example) to be a employed is perfused. This has the effect of fixing the brain in place: it can then easily be removed from the SKULL.

transcortical motor aphasia A clinical syndrome of APHASIA. The essential feature of this syndrome is a striking disparity between spontaneous speech and repetition. Spontaneous speech is undermined by a pathological disinclination to initiate. When produced, speech is well-articulated and fluent, but limited to short phrases of two or three words; sentences are incomplete. In striking contrast, repetition may be flawless for long and complicated sentences. This syndrome is associated with the occurrence of a LESION in the area just anterior or superior to BROCA'S AREA along with SUBCORTICAL sites. It is hypothesized that lesions in the SUPPLEMENTARY MOTOR CORTEX, or along its path may prevent the LIMBIC SYSTEM from communicating with the cortical speech areas.

Reference

Goodglass H. & Kaplan E. (1983) *The Assessment of Aphasia and Related Disorders*, 2nd edn, Lea & Febiger: Philadelphia.

CHARLOTTE C. MITCHUM

transcortical sensory aphasia A clinical syndrome of APHASIA. The essential feature of this syndrome is fluent, but meaningless speech like that observed in WERNICKE'S APHASIA. Preserved ability to repeat sentences distinguishes this aphasia syndrome from Wernicke's aphasia. Repetition may be sensitive to errors of GRAMMAR produced in the model whereas SEMANTIC distortion of sentences may go undetected. The LESION associated with this syndrome is found in the cortical areas posterior to the ROLANDIC FISSURE around WERNICKE'S AREA. BROCA'S AREA and the ARCUATE FASCICULUS are spared.

Reference

Goodglass H. & Kaplan E. (1983) *The Assessment of Aphasia and Related Disorders*, 2nd edn, Lea & Febiger: Philadelphia.

CHARLOTTE C. MITCHUM

transcranial magnetic stimulation A technique for inducing electical activation within the CEREBRAL CORTEX: a pulse of electricity is delivered to a coil placed over a subjects head. This has the effect of inducing a magnetic field of some strength in the tissues immediate beneath the coil (that is, the cerebral cortex) which has a stimulating effect. Structures beneath the cortex are not directly activated, though of course activation of the cortex will have consequential effects on SUBCORTICAL tissue. It has, like ELECTROCONVULSIVE THERAPY (ECT), been used in the treatment of DEPRESSION. Attempts to use it in the alleviation of the SIGNS AND SYMPTOMS of other disorders have also been made.

See also: SQUID magnetometry

transcription The process by which a genetic sequence contained in DNA is used as a template to produce a strand of mRNA (messenger RNA) which will be used subsequently to form a PROTEIN; not to be confused with TRANSLATION.

FIONA M. INGLIS

transcription factor A protein which enters the NUCLEUS of a CELL and binds to a region of DNA, initiating or regulating the TRANSCRIPTION of a GENE into MRNA (messenger RNA).

FIONA M. INGLIS

transcutaneous Across the skin: for example, transcutaneous electrical nerve stimulation is a treatment for several chronic pain states (see GATE CONTROL THEORY OF PAIN) that involves electrical stimulation of nerve endings across the skin.

transcutaneous electrical nerve stimulation *see* gate control theory of pain

transdermal drug delivery Transdermal drug delivery involves, as the name implies, delivery of a DRUG across the skin and from there into the bloodstream. Some drugs will do this on contact, and often this presents a hazard. Many insecticides can be delivered in this way and great care must therefore be taken when using them. Better known is the deliberate use of this technique to administer drugs therapeutically. This involves the application of a patch (a DRUG PATCH, with an appearance much like a conventional Band-Aid) which will deliver a drug transdermally. Drug delivery is slow,

occurring at a known rate. Patches are constructed of a drug reservoir separated from the skin by a microporous membrane (these being covered by the adhesive patch); or they are made of a polymer based matrix in which the drug has been saturated (this again being held by the adhesive patch). This means of drug delivery is useful when administering agents that are absorbed through the skin, which of course, many drugs are not. The use of NICOTINE PATCHES to control WITHDRAWAL from ADDICTION to NICOTINE is well known.

See also: drug administration

transdermal patch *see* transdermal drug delivery

transduction Transduction is synonymous with transfer: it is a term commonly encountered in biological psychology and refers to the conversion of a signal in one form into another – the conversion of sound or light into neural activity for example. SECOND MESSENGERS engage in SIGNAL TRANSDUCTION, in which extracellular signals are converted to intracellular signals. Transduction can also refer to the transmission of genetic material between bacteria.

See also: sensory transduction

transection A cut through; KNIFE CUT LESIONS work by making transections, which can be small and discrete – cutting through a particular pathway in brain for example – or they can be large and gross, cutting through the brain at a particular level; see PRECOLLICULAR–POSTMAMMILLARY TRANSECTION; *CERVEAU ISOLÉ.*

transfer appropriate processing A view of MEMORY processing which states that the greater the similarity between mental operations conducted at ENCODING and RETRIEVAL, the more likely information will be successfully 'transferred' from study to test. For example, a rhyming (non-semantic) orienting task at encoding produces better RETENTION on a test for rhymes of the studied words than does a semantic orienting task. A semantic orienting task, however, produces superior performance, relative to a rhyming orienting task, on a tests that emphasize semantic processing (such as CUED RECALL or FREE RECALL). Transfer appropriate processing is one of a class of memory principles stressing the importance of the relationship between study and test situations.

See also: context-dependent learning; state-dependent learning

JENNIFER A. MANGELS

transfer of training *see* transfer test

transfer RNA *see* RNA

transfer test A transfer test is an evaluation of whether or not the experience of LEARNING one version of a task, or of learning to discriminate one specific object from another, has an effect (either positive or negative) on subsequent performance with different versions of the task or different objects (see DISCRIMINATION LEARNING). The term is general and often qualifiers are used to denote specific types of transfer under consideration (for example, cross-modal transfer). The term TRANSFER OF TRAINING is best reserved when transfer of learned motor skills from one situation to another is at issue. TRANSFER TEST represents a much broader category which encompasses follow-up assessment of an original test.

RICHARD C. TEES

transferrin (also known as siderophilin) One of the PROTEINS present in PLASMA; it can transport IRON in BLOOD.

transgenic Term for an organism containing a foreign GENE, or transgene, inserted into the chromosomal DNA, which will code for a protein novel to that organism. In animals, a fertilized egg cell will contain a male and a female pronucleus, which fuses to form the NUCLEUS. In the mouse, a transgene injected into the larger male pronucleus will sometimes be incorporated into the genome, and can be detected in a DNA sample from the fully-developed mouse. These founder mice contain a single copy of the gene. Mice in which copies of the gene are found in both chromosomes are created by interbreeding founder mice and should express the gene product, or protein, encoded by the transgene. Transgenic techniques permit functional analysis of abnormal genes linked to disease processes, such as HUNTINGTON'S CHOREA. Transgenic technology may also allow animals to be used in large

scale production of human factors such as INSULIN, needed to treat disease.

See also: gene knockout; gene transfer in the CNS

FIONA M. INGLIS

transient global amnesia A form of AMNESIC SYNDROME with complete but temporary loss of memory (featuring both ANTEROGRADE AMNESIA and RETROGRADE AMNESIA). The exact cause of this is not known: it occurs more often in older people and in MIGRAINE sufferers; and it is thought possibly to involve ISCHAEMIA.

transient ischaemic attack *see* stroke

transient lesions (Also known as TEMPORARY LESIONS) Most experimental brain lesions (see LESION) are permanent, induced by passage of current at an ELECTRODE tip or by induction of NEUROTOXINS into discrete brain regions. Lesions may be made before or after training on some task, to determine what the effects are on the acquisition or retention of a task. An alternative strategy is to make transient lesions – temporary lesions – that allow one to gauge the performance of an individual animal before the lesion is made, while it is present, and after it has gone. Two techniques have been used to induce transient lesions. One is by cooling a part of the brain to a point at which neural activity ceases. BRAIN COOLING – a CRYO-LESION – is achieved using a CRYODE, a loop that can be inserted in brain and cool liquid passed through. The more common method though is by microinjection of LOCAL ANAES-THETIC (such as LIDOCAINE) into a brain region, to inactivate it. The advantage of these techniques over permanent lesions is the flexibility they introduce into experimental designs: being able to test an individual animal before, during and after a lesion is of considerable benefit. The disadvantage is in the lack of specificity. Brain cooling or local anaesthetics stop neurons, glial cells and fibres of passage through an area of tissue working: they are effectively transient ELECTROLYTIC LESIONS. However, neuroscientists making permanent lesions have been assiduously trying to produce more and more selective lesions, destroying whenever possible only specific, neurochemically identified groups of neurons within a given brain area.

transitive inference Test of reasoning in which an inferential judgment is made about items that are only indirectly related based on overlaps between other known relations. For example, when paired, stimulus A bears a specific relation to B; stimulus B, when paired with stimulus C, bears the same relation. A and C have never been paired, and therefore their relationship has not been explicitly taught. Upon subsequent pairing of stimulus A and stimulus C, one would have to rely on previous experience and the ability to make transitive judgements to know about their relationship. The ability to make a transitive inference exists in rodents, pigeons and primates.

HOWARD EICHENBAUM

translation The process by which the CODON sequence within a molecule of MRNA (messenger RNA) is used as a template in the production of a protein (see PROTEINS) from individual AMINO ACIDS; not to be confused with TRANSCRIPTION.

FIONA M. INGLIS

transmission In biological psychology transmission typically refers to communication between neurons, but it is also used to indicate transmission of material or information between animals: see CABLE TRANSMISSION; CHEMICAL TRANSMISSION; COTRANSMISSION; ELECTRICAL TRANSMISSION; EPHAPTIC TRANSMISSION; FAST NEUROTRANSMISSION; NEUROTRANSMISSION; NON-SYNAPTIC TRANSMISSION; PARASYNAPTIC TRANSMISSION; SLOW NEUROTRANSMISSION; SOCIAL TRANSMISSION OF FOOD PREFERENCES; SYNAPTIC TRANSMISSION; WIRING TRANSMISSION.

transmittance *see* reflectance

transneuronal tracers *see* tract tracers

transplantation Neuronal tissues can survive transplantation into the brain, and the brain is in certain respects particularly suitable as a target organ for transplantation. For transplantation of CENTRAL NERVOUS SYSTEM (CNS) neurons, it is necessary to use embryonic or (at the latest) neonatal donor tissues. In particular, neurons only survive transplantation at the stage in their DEVELOPMENT when they are undergoing final cell division and are just beginning active and directed NEURITE outgrowth. There is a brief developmental time window for each neuronal population that needs to be determined empirically. By contrast GLIAL CELLS and PERIPHERAL NERVOUS SYSTEM (PNS) tissues (such as ADRENAL GLAND or other endocrine ganglia) can survive transplantation even in adulthood, which is believed to be related to the fact that these cell populations can also undergo cell division throughout life. The brain is an efficient transplantation target, provided the graft is placed in a position that will permit rapid and efficient vascularization and incorporation into the host blood and CEREBROSPINAL FLUID circulation. IMMUNOLOGY factors are less important than for organ transplants since the brain is an immunologically privileged site, at least relatively. Embryonic neural ALLOGRAFTS (that is, grafts within the same species) survive well when grafted in the brain, whereas skin or organ transplantation across the same barriers results in rapid rejection. Although XENOGRAFTS (that is, grafts between different species) are generally rejected, they can be effectively maintained with standard IMMUNOSUPPRESSION. Grafts of embryonic neuronal tissues not only survive, but have been shown to grow, and establish reciprocal connections in a number of different model systems in the brain. They can also provide functional restoration of damage in the CNS by a number of distinct mechanisms (each of which have been demonstrated to apply in different model systems). These mechanisms include: (1) non-specific aspects of surgery; (2) TROPHIC stimulation of restorative processes in the host brain; (3) provision of bridges or growth substrates for regeneration of host axons; (4) diffuse release of specific NEUROTRANSMITTERS or neuromodulators (or NEUROHORMONES); (5) glial replacement for reconstruction of brain environment, including remyelination (see MYELIN) and restoration of conductance of axons; (6) REINNERVATION and reactivation of denervated targets; (7) reciprocal connections and repair of damaged circuits.

Clinical applications of neural transplantation are under active development for a variety of neurological and neurodegenerative disorders. Transplantation of embryonic DOPAMINE cells is now demonstrated to be effective in PARKINSON'S DISEASE. The grafts can alleviate both akinetic and rigid symptoms (see AKINESIA and RIGIDITY), reduce the required levels of L-DOPA medication and abolish many of the most troubling dyskinetic (see DYSKINESIA) side-effects. The grafts are typically less effective on TREMOR and AXIAL symptoms. Active trials are in development for several other diseases: embryonic cells from the STRIATUM in HUNTINGTON'S CHOREA, PRECURSOR CELLS of oligodendrocytes for MULTIPLE SCLEROSIS, and encapsulated cells engineered to secrete CILIARY NEUROTROPHIC FACTOR (CNF) in AMYOTROPHIC LATERAL SCLEROSIS (ALS). Each of these diseases involves a circumscribed degeneration of identified populations of cells. Present transplantation techniques hold less prospect of finding clinical application in diseases that involve more widespread damage of multiple cell types, such as in ALZHEIMER'S DEMENTIA or MULTI-INFARCT DEMENTIA, STROKE or TRAUMA.

Whereas embryonic neurons have proved effective for functional transplantation in experimental animals, and initial clinical trials are promising, widespread clinical application is likely always to be limited by both ethical and practical constraints on the availability of human foetal cells. There is therefore active investigation of alternative sources of suitable tissues for clinical transplantation. These include: (1) improvements in the methods of cell preparation, HIBERNATION, CRYOPRESERVATION and implantation that allow better survival and more efficient use of available embryonic tissues. (2) Expansion of STEM CELLS and precursor cells *in vitro*, so that limited supplies of embryonic tissue can generate large quantities of cells that can be banked for use as and when required rather than just as and when available. (3) GENETIC ENGINEERING of ethically neutral cells, in particular allografts for *ex vivo* gene transfer. This has so far proceeded to the first clinical trials in ALS of spinal implantation of encapsulated baby hamster kidney cells engineered to secrete CNTF. The critical problems still to be resolved for both *in vivo* or *ex vivo* gene transfer relate to safety issues and the stability of long-term expression of the gene inserts. Moreover, this strategy is only likely to prove effective (at least in the foreseeable future) for delivery of diffusible neurotransmitters (see VOLUME TRANSMISSION), HORMONES or TROPHIC FACTORS, and not for neuronal reconstruction. (4) XENOGRAFTS of (for example, porcine) foetal cells. Although this provides the best long-term prospect for easily available neuronal tissues, problems related to long-term immunosuppression and the safety factors related to risks of cross-species transfer of new viruses are yet to be fully resolved.

Reference

Dunnett S.B. & Björklund A. (eds.) (1994) *Functional Neural Transplantation*, Plenum Press: New York.

STEPHEN B. DUNNETT

transport The term transport in biological psychology refers to the movement of molecules. For example, there are active transport mechanisms that move molecules across a MEMBRANE (see for instance BLOOD–BRAIN BARRIER and REUPTAKE); and there are transport mechanisms within the CELL (see AXOPLASM) that can be exploited using anterograde or retrograde TRACT TRACERS.

transsexualism Better described as GENDER IDENTITY DISORDER, transsexualism is the belief an individual has that they are not of the GENDER that their bodies express. It is a condition that causes intense distress. It is resolved in many cases by hormonal treatment and reconstructive genital surgery, to effect a sex change (better described as sex reassignment surgery). The biological causes of the condition are not known (and indeed may not exist: a search for psychological causes may be more appropriate than biological). However, two points are worth making: first, the disorder often has a history reaching back into childhood, transsexuals reporting that their belief in gender misassignment had a very early onset. Second, the seriousness of the condition is underlined by the fact that, whatever else an individual may feel about themselves, belief in their identity as a man or woman is typically unshakeable. It is unusual, even in the most severe cases of mental disturbance (such as SCHIZOPHRENIA) when psychological processes are profoundly affected, for gender identity to be questioned. Finally, transsexualism is not to be confused with *transvestism*, in which sexual pleasure is derived from wearing the clothes of the opposite sex.

See also: bed nucleus of the stria terminalis

Reference
Davison G.C. & Neale J.M. (1996) *Abnormal Psychology*, 6th edn, Wiley: New York.

transverse patterning A task used to challenge CONFIGURAL LEARNING: subjects have to solve three concurrent discriminations: A+ vs. B; B+ vs. C and C+ vs. A (in which + represents the correct discrimination). Each stimulus, A, B and C is presented as both the correct and incorrect stimulus to choose – none is a unique predictor of the correct solution – establishing a demand for configural representations of the stimuli.

transverse section *see* planes of section

transvestism *see* transsexualism

tranylcypromine A monoamine oxidase inhibitor; it is rarely used because, unlike other monoamine oxidase inhibitors such as PARGYLINE, it is a *suicide substrate* – that is, it binds irreversibly to MONOAMINE OXIDASE, rendering it permanently inactive. Such binding is rarely of value and usually unhelpful to an experiment or therapeutic regime.

trapezoid body *see* superior olivary complex

trauma (from Greek, *trauma*: a wound) Trauma refers to a wound or an injury. It can refer both to physical and psychological injuries, though in everyday talk it is more likely now to be associated with psychological shocks, events or states rather than physical ones.

travelling wave Auditory stimulation produces a travelling wave along the BASILAR MEMBRANE (from the OVAL WINDOW to the apex – that part of the COCHLEA that is at greatest distance from the oval window). With high frequency sound, the amplitude of the travel-ling wave is greatest at its point of origin nearest the STAPES; with low frequency, amplitude is greatest at the apex.

See also: auditory system

treadmill locomotion Literally locomotion on a treadmill, either a circular treadmill or on a device similar to a conveyor belt. Treadmill locomotion has been used by neuroscientists interested in the control of locomotion, since it allows recordings to be made from the BRAIN, SPINAL CORD and MUSCLES of animals actually engaged in locomotion at a constant rate. While it has undoubted value for such studies, one needs to be careful in assessing psychological states using this: forced (as opposed to voluntary) locomotion on a treadmill is likely to be affected by NEGATIVE REINFORCEMENT.

trefine *see* trepanning

tremor (from Latin, *tremor*: tremor) This involves the involuntary, rhythmic movements of a single muscle or groups of MUSCLES. They are more severe and longer-lasting than TICS and are commonly associated with damage to parts of the MOTOR SYSTEM, the exact form and nature of the tremor depending on the precise location of damage within the brain. There are however also forms of tremor that do not involve brain damage at all. The following types of tremor can be identified: a RESTING TREMOR is a cardinal symptom of PARKINSON'S DISEASE, which is the commonest cause of pathological tremor. As its name implies, resting tremor is present when patients are at rest, and it often takes the form of a PILL ROLLING nature, involving rhythmic movements of the fingers and hands. Tremor in the muscles of the head and neck is also very common in Parkinson's disease. Such small tremors – seen as an inability to keep the head absolutely still – are often seen in the elderly, including many who are not formally diagnosed as Parkinsonian. However, such cases are often indicative of a developing Parkinsonian pathology. Damage to the DENTATE NUCLEUS of the CEREBELLUM is associated not with a resting tremor but with INTENTION TREMOR. Patients with damage here appear normal when at rest but display increasing degrees of tremor in the hands as they reach for objects – that is, the tremor depends on patients attempting an action. This is also known as ACTION TREMOR or KINETIC TREMOR. In WILSON'S DISEASE, a rather bizarre type of BATSWING TREMOR is seen: it is a form of tremor in which wing-beating movements of the arms are present (and is also called WING-BEAT TREMOR). Wilson's disease involves liver damage and, rather curiously, other forms of advanced liver damage are also associated with tremors, often involving movements of the wrist. All of these forms of tremor, discriminated by their form, nature and intensity, are the product of damage to the brain. ESSENTIAL TREMOR, PHYSIOLOGICAL TREMOR and TENSION TREMOR are not associated with brain damage or dysfunction, but are the product of excessive muscle activation – lifting heavy objects for long periods can, when the action is terminated, be followed by a brief tremor. FAMILIAL TREMOR is similarly a muscle condition that is present within families.

Tremor can be induced experimentally in animals, though with difficulty. Attempts to mimic Parkinsonian conditions in rats using the neurotoxin 6-HYDROXYDOPAMINE, while producing degrees of DOPAMINE depletion similar to Parkinsonism, do not produce tremor. Similarly, use of the neurotoxin MPTP in primates does not reliably elicit tremor. In both cases, many other features of Parkinson's disease are reproduced in the ANIMAL MODELS, but not tremor. It is not clear why this should be, though it may indicate that Parkinsonian tremor is the product of more than just loss of dopamine. Certain drugs, most notably CHOLINERGIC stimulants, can induce tremor: OXOTREMORINE is particularly effective in doing this. Tremor in rodents, induced by oxotremorine, can be measured on a JIGGLE PLATE.

tremor control therapy *see* deep brain stimulation

tremorogenic Having the ability to induce TREMOR.

trepanning (from Greek, *trypanon*: an auger) A trepan is a circular saw or drill bit that will cut a round hole. Such a device can be used to produce a hole in the SKULL – the act of trepanning – giving access to the brain. A TREPHINE (or TREFINE) is a smaller version of

a trepan: a fine, hollow, drill bit that will cut a circular hole in the skull. In ancient times, trepanning was used to liberate demons from the heads of individuals presumably suffering from some disorder. Skulls from, for example, Inca peoples in South America have been found showing evidence of trepanning.

trephine *see* trepanning

trial (from Anglo-French, *trier*: to try) In biological psychology the term trial is used to refer to a single attempt by a subject (animal or human) at a particular task. Trials may occur singly or in multiples; and they may be in the form of MASSED TRIALS (where a subject repeatedly attempts the task) or SPACED TRIALS (in which there is a greater temporal delay: a subject may have one trial per day for example, or may be one of a group of subjects who all take turns at a task).

trial-and-error learning Trial-and-error learning is as it says: a task is approached and a RESPONSE made at a venture. If on a particular trial the outcome is not correct – an error – that response is not repeated, leading to elimination of incorrect responses. Initially behaviourists (see BEHAVIOURISM) thought that all LEARNING began as trial-and-error learning, but this is not thought now to be the case. Previous experience can be brought to bear on a novel task that allows an individual to eliminate certain responses before starting the task.

triangular septal nucleus *see* septal nuclei

trichromatic theory of colour vision (also called the YOUNG–HELMHOLTZ THEORY OF COLOUR VISION) Proposed by Thomas Young in the early nineteenth century and subsequently championed by Hermann von Helmholtz. The theory states that human COLOUR VISION depends on three receptoral mechanisms each with a different SPECTRAL SENSITIVITY. The theory was proposed on the basis of colour-mixing experiments in which an observer is asked to match the colour of one light by mixing together three others. (For example, red, green and blue lights when added together in equal proportions match a white light.) These experiments demonstrate that the mixture of three suitably chosen lights (or *pri-*

maries) in the appropriate proportions can generate the appearance of any colour. The choice of possible primary lights is very wide, but because three are always required human colour vision is called trichromatic. Colour mixing may also be done using pigments or paints and is referred to as a *subtractive colour mixing* as opposed to the *additive* mixing of lights.

The principle of trichromacy is exploited in colour technology because it allows any colour to be specified in terms of the proportions of three primary lights required to match it, providing a convenient means of quantifying a colour and allowing its exact replication. Furthermore, the manufacture of colour television also relies on this property of human vision since only three light emitting phosphors (red, green and blue) are required to generate to the satisfaction of the normal human visual system a full range of naturally occurring colours. It is important to note that the mixture of three primaries is not physically identical to the light being matched, since the two matching test fields have different spectral power functions. Rather, the identity between the two is a perceptual one, arising because they set up an equivalence in the visual system of the observer. Such an identity is called a METAMERIC MATCH. The colour-mixing experiments are governed by the rules of linear algebra (GRASSMANN'S LAWS), and because of this they imply the presence of three underlying receptoral mechanisms in human vision. Subsequent physiological and behavioural experiments have identified these as the three types of light-absorbing CONES of the human retina. Each cone type has a different spectral sensitivity, absorbing light from a slightly different but overlapping regions of the VISIBLE SPECTRUM. They are termed the short wavelength (S), medium wavelength (M) and long wavelength (L) absorbing cones. Coloured surfaces or lights usually stimulate all three cone types, but to different relative degrees. Thus each colour is coded uniquely in the nervous system by its own special ratio of activity in the L, M and S cone mechanisms.

See also: colour blindness; colour constancy; dichromatic colour blindness; opponent process theory of colour vision

KATHY T. MULLEN

tricyclic antidepressants *see* antidepressant; monoamine hypothesis of depression

trifluoperazine One of the PIPERAZINE drugs with ANTIPSYCHOTIC activity.

trigeminal nerve The fifth cranial nerve (see CRANIAL NERVES), having three major branches – ophthalmic, maxillary and mandibular – receiving sensory information from, and directing muscular activity of, the musculature of the face and head; involved in mastication.

trigeminal nucleus The trigeminal nucleus is in the PONS, below the fourth ventricle (see VENTRICULAR SYSTEM). It has input from the a variety of motor systems and gives rise to the motor fibres of the TRIGEMINAL NERVE (see CRANIAL NERVES). Sensory information flows through the TRIGEMINAL GANGLION (also known as the semilunar or Gasserian ganglion) and is associated with nuclei in the pons. The trigeminal nucleus, with input from all of the areas of the head and face associated with the trigeminal nerve, has a SOMATOTOPIC organization. This is reflected in the presence of several subnuclei within the trigeminal system: the mesencephalic trigeminal nucleus (abbreviated Me5), the principal sensory nucleus (Pr5), the oral subnucleus (also referred to as the ORAL PONS), interpolar subnucleus and caudal subnucleus.

See also: hindbrain

triglycerides The complex molecules contained within FAT CELLS (see ADIPOSE TISSUE). A triglyceride molecule itself contains two types of component. One is GLYCEROL, a CARBOHYDRATE molecule that can be converted into GLUCOSE by the LIVER. The other component is one of the FATTY ACIDS, of which there are three types (STEARIC ACID, oleic acid and PALMITIC ACID). Triglycerides may be broken down into their components and released by fat cells, especially when the hormone GLUCAGON has been released into the blood by the PANCREAS. Fatty acids can be used as fuel by most body cells but typically not by brain neurons.

KENT C. BERRIDGE

triiodothyronine (T3) One of the HORMONES released by the THYROID GLAND.

See also: endocrine glands; hormones – classification

trimester *see* pregnancy

triple dissociation As DOUBLE DISSOCIATION, but with three factors, not two.

triple labelling *see* tract tracers

triple X syndrome (Also written as XXX SYNDROME) A very rare chromosome abnormality in which a female has three X CHROMOSOMES rather than two. It is associated with a degree of MENTAL RETARDATION.

See also: chromosome abnormalities; X and Y chromosomes

trisomy 21 Trisomy 21 refers to the acquisition of an extra copy (there are three not two – hence trisomy) of chromosome 21 at MEIOSIS (see CELL DIVISION;). The most common condition this leads to is DOWN SYNDROME, though there is also evidence for trisomy 21 occurring in ALZHEIMER'S DEMENTIA; see DOWN SYNDROME for more detail.

tritanomaly *see* colour blindness

tritanopia *see* dichromatic colour blindness

triune brain A concept devised by the noted anatomist Paul MacLean (who was influential in defining the LIMBIC SYSTEM), the triune brain was a hypothesis concerning the organization and EVOLUTION of the BRAIN in VERTEBRATES. He characterized three stages in brain evolution: reptilian, palaeomammalian and neomammalian ('old mammal' and 'new mammal'). Each type of brain was thought of as having its own distinct type of properties: the reptilian brain had 'lowest common denominator' properties and could organize effectively such things as basic processes of MOTIVATION and AGGRESSION; the palaeomammalian brain added emotion to this (MacLean equated the palaeomammalian brain with the limbic system) while the neomammalian brain (represented by the neocortex) pursued intellectual

functions. Obviously, reptiles only have the reptilian brain, but primitive mammals were suggested to have the reptilian brain and the palaeomammalian brain, and more recent mammals – PRIMATES – have all three types. The idea of the triune brain generated considerable debate – and has survived in the popular concept of humans having a deep reptilian brain – but more recent anatomical studies have not always supported the idea. For example, greater HOMOLOGY between the various areas of cortex present in reptiles and mammals has discouraged the idea of clear separation between evolutionary levels present in the triune hypothesis.

trochlear nerve The fourth cranial nerve (see CRANIAL NERVES); it controls activity of the musculature of the eyes .

troncoencephalon (from Spanish, *troncoencefálico*, from *tronco*: trunk, *encéfalo*: brain) An alternative term for BRAINSTEM.

trophic Trophic is derived from Greek, *trophe*: food; it is used biologically to indicate growth – see for example TROPHIC FACTORS. TROPIC is often taken to mean the same, but it does not: though it occurs, the term 'tropic factors' should not be substituted for 'trophic factors'. Tropic is derived from Greek *tropos*: a turning, and has the same root as the geographical terms tropic and tropical; *tropism* also has the same root and means a tendency to turn towards a stimulus – plants that turn towards the sun are *heliotropic*.

trophic factors Trophic factors are chemicals essential for CELL survival. Strictly, they are contrasted with GROWTH FACTORS which are essential for cell division and growth but have no role in survival. However, the first discovered trophic factor is known as NERVE GROWTH FACTOR. More recently discovered trophic factors are BRAIN-DERIVED NEUROTROPHIC FACTOR and *ciliary neurotrophic factor*.

See also: apoptosis; neurodevelopment; synaptic pruning

trophic molecules Synonymous with TROPHIC FACTORS.

tropic *see* trophic

tropisetron An ANTAGONIST at the 5HT₃ receptor; see SEROTONIN RECEPTORS.

tropomyosin *see* neuromuscular junction

troponin complex *see* neuromuscular junction

true blue *see* tract tracers

truth drug A term used to describe a pharmacological agent that purportedly increases the willingness of a person to tell the truth (also called TRUTH SERUM). It has its origins in the early part of the twentieth century, when it was believed that administering a SEDATIVE during PSYCHOTHERAPY would relax a person and induce more talking. Drugs used for this included the BARBITURATES (for example SODIUM PENTOTHAL and amobarbital) and SCOPOLAMINE, an ANTICHOLINERGIC. It was believed that by reducing inhibitions, repressed thoughts would be brought out. These drugs (as well as BENZODIAZEPINES and ALCOHOL) certainly have the ability to cause disinhibitions of EMOTION or thoughts; whether they induce telling of the truth is open to conjecture.

ANN E. KELLEY

truth serum *see* truth drug

tryptophan An amino acid and precursor of the neurotransmitter SEROTONIN. A series of studies have examined the relationships between the tryptophan content of the diet and concentrations of serotonin in brain. Meal composition does appear able to influence brain neurochemistry, but the relationships and transport systems involved are complex.

Reference

Feldman R.S., Meyer J.S. & Quenzer L.F. (1997) *Principles of Neuropsychopharmacology*, Sinauer Associates: Sunderland MA.

tuberohypophyseal dopamine system *see* classification of Dahlström and Fuxe; dopamine

tuberoinfundibular dopamine system A system of short-axoned DOPAMINE neurons found in the region of the HYPOTHALAMUS. The cell bodies of this system originate in the ARCUATE NUCLEUS and PERIVENTRICULAR NUCLEUS of the HYPOTHALAMUS and project to the MEDIAN EMINENCE and PITUITARY GLAND (intermediate and posterior lobes). The dopaminergic terminals regulate the secretion of the lactating hormone PROLACTIN, exerting an inhibitory effect upon secretion.

ANN E. KELLEY

tuberomammillary nucleus A small nucleus that lies at the posterior pole of the LATERAL HYPOTHALAMUS, adjacent to the MAMMILLARY BODIES. It contains HISTAMINERGIC neurons which project extensively to the CEREBRAL CORTEX, OLFACTORY TRACT, AMYGDALA, SEPTAL NUCLEI, THALAMUS and wide areas of the BRAINSTEM and SPINAL CORD.

See also: ascending reticular activating system

tubulin *see* cytoskeleton

tumescence *see* erection

tumour (from Latin *tumere*: to swell) tumours are inappropriate growths of cells. (The term NEOPLASM is used to describe the formation of new morbid tissue.) Intracranial tumour is the term given to such growths within the nervous system; BRAIN TUMOUR is the more colloquial term. Tumours may grow at very different rates, faster growth being associated with more debilitating consequences. The damage they produce tends to be localized – the LESION is FOCAL – unlike the damage that is produced by neurodegenerative diseases such as PARKINSON'S DISEASE or ALZHEIMER'S DEMENTIA.

Tumours can be generated from and in a variety of tissues within the CENTRAL NERVOUS SYSTEM: the most common are ASTROCYTOMAS (formed from ASTROCYTES); GLIOMAS can originate in any type of the GLIAL CELLS; MENINGIOMAS are associated with the MENINGES; HAEMATOMAS are formed from a composite of BLOOD and CONNECTIVE TISSUE. ANGIOMAS and HEMANGIOBLASTOMAS are tumours of the vascular system (see BLOOD) – these terms can be qualified using the term cerebral (cerebral angioma) to indicate that they are in brain rather than other tissues. ADENOMAS from in glands: those that form in the PITUITARY GLAND are closest to the central nervous system. METASTASES are secondary tumours (formed by displaced cells moving away from primary tumours); metastatic tumours with their origins in the breast, testicles or other sites can be found in brain. Tumours may be described as benign or malignant: benign tumours are those that do not produce especially harmful effects; malignant tumours are those which by their growth or by their ability to metastasize can have damaging, or even fatal, effects.

Tumours are treated by a combination of surgery and radiation treatment (to kill cells that survive surgery). Clearly, the nearer the surface of the brain a tumour is the better the likelihood of being able to remove it successfully without causing structural damage to unaffected parts of the brain.

See also: closed head injury; headache; neurinoma

tumour necrosis factor One of many types of CYTOKINE; see IMMUNE SYSTEM.

TUNEL method The TUNEL method involves histochemical (see HISTOCHEMISTRY) detection of terminal deoxynucleotidyl transferase-mediated dUTP biotin nick-end labelling. It is a technique used to detect neurons undergoing APOPTOSIS.

tuning Tuning is a term derived from music, in which the verb *to tune* refers to an accurate adjustment of PITCH. It is used more generally in all of the sensory systems to describe the degree to which a NEURON responds to a particular stimulus. In the gustatory system for example (see GUSTATION), neurons in the BRAINSTEM are responsive to any taste stimulus applied to the tongue. At cortical levels neurons are present that respond maximally to particular stimuli (one of the PRIMARY TASTES): these neurons can be said to be highly and selectively tuned.

tunnel vision A condition in which PERIPHERAL VISION is restricted (or non-existent) leading to dependence on information projected onto central regions of the RETINA, which naturally produces a narrowing of the VISUAL FIELD. The term tunnel vision has also been used metaphorically to refer to narrow mindedness or to a fixation of ATTENTION on a specific object; such metaphorical use is not particularly helpful.

turbinate bones Delicate bones in the nasal cavity that guide the flow of air through the nasal passages; the bones are given individual numbers (in Roman numerals) to distinguish them; see OLFACTION.

Turner's syndrome A chromosome abnormality in women produced by loss of an X CHROMOSOME (characterized as XO therefore rather than XX). AMENORRHOEA is a major feature, as is short stature and defects in the CARDIOVASCULAR SYSTEM; also known as gonadal dysgenesis (see GONADS; DYSGENESIS).

See also: chromosome abnormalities; X and Y chromosomes

turning behaviour *see* rotation

turnover In pharmacology, turnover refers to the use of NEUROTRANSMITTERS (or some other chemical). Various measures of turnover can be adopted: the rate of synthesis (see METABOLISM), RELEASE or CATABOLISM are all used.

twin studies Twin studies have been used to estimate the degree with which certain traits and conditions are genetically transmitted (that is, their HERITABILITY). Two different procedures have been used: comparison of MONOZYGOTIC TWINS with DIZYGOTIC TWINS; and the comparison of twins separated in early life and raised apart. Monozygotic twins are IDENTICAL TWINS who share a common GENOME: they are the product of a single ZYGOTE (a fertilized egg) that, for reasons that are not entirely clear, divides to produce two developing individuals. Dizygotic twins are FRATERNAL TWINS: they are the product of two eggs being fertilized separately and this always involves development in separate chorions. The degree of generic relatedness of fraternal twins is the same as for normal siblings (that is, 50%) though of course they do share a common INTRAUTERINE environment and more closely share developmental experiences. Comparison of monozygotic and dizygotic twins can reveal information about the degree to which traits are heritable: the difference in relatedness between twins indicates the degree to which a trait under study is heritable. Similarly, the differences on a particular trait or characteristic shown by twins (especially monozygotic twins) raised apart can reveal the extent to which the environment influences the development of particular traits. Twin studies have been used extensively in studies of the heritability of INTELLIGENCE, and in assessment of the heritability of conditions such as SCHIZOPHRENIA. Controversy stills surrounds both of these topics (see Eysenck & Kamin, 1981 for a typical debate about these).

References

Eysenck H.J. & Kamin L. (1981) *Intelligence: The Battle for the Mind*, Pan Books: London.

Plomin R., DeFries J.C., McClearn G.E. & Rutter M. (1997) *Behavioral Genetics*, 3rd edn, W.H. Freeman: New York.

two-back task *see* short-term memory

two cortical visual streams The primate CEREBRAL CORTEX contains very many visual areas each doing slightly different jobs. Their interconnections form them into two quasi-separate 'streams', each emanating from PRIMARY VISUAL CORTEX – one terminating in POSTERIOR PARIETAL CORTEX, the other in INFERIOR TEMPORAL CORTEX. Ungerleider & Mishkin (1982) hypothesized that the function of the occipito-parietal stream was for spatial vision (*where*) and the occipito-temporal for object vision (*what*). The currently favoured view (Milner & Goodale, 1995), based on more recent evidence from physiology and from neuropsychology, is that the occipito-parietal stream processes vision for guiding action (*how*) and the occipito-temporal for perception (*what*).

See also: object recognition; visual system; visuomotor control

References

Milner A.D. & Goodale M.A. (1995) *The Visual Brain in Action*, Oxford University Press: Oxford.

Mishkin M., Ungerleider L.G. and Macko K.A. (1983) Objective Vision and Spatial Vision: two cortical pathways. *Trends in Neurosciences*, 6: 414–417.

Ungerleider L.G. & Mishkin M. (1982) Two cortical visual systems. In *Analysis of Behavior*, ed. Ingle D.J., Goodale M.A. & Mansfield R.J.W., pp. 549–586, MIT Press: Cambridge MA.

A. DAVID MILNER

two-factor learning theory An account of AVOIDANCE LEARNING: first, CLASSICAL CONDITIONING mechanisms are proposed to account for the association of a FEAR with a particular STIMULUS; second, INSTRUMENTAL CONDITIONING processes are used to account for the avoidance response, reduction of fear being the REINFORCER. Although this is the origin of two-factor learning theory, the term has been used in other situations where classical and instrumental conditioning operate.

two-point threshold A technique for examining SOMATOSENSORY coding on the SKIN: two points – pins or just the tips of pencils – are placed on the skin at separate points: they are brought closer together until such time as the individual being investigated cannot discriminate between them, believing them now to be only point. The two-point threshold gives an indication of spatial sensitivity. On sensitive skin, such as the tips of fingers or lips, two points can be discriminated even when quite close. On less sensitive areas of the body, the threshold is much greater.

See also: dermatome; receptive field

two-process theory *see* two-factor learning theory

two visual streams The two visual streams are the dorsal stream and the ventral stream: the dorsal stream manipulates visual information that is used to guide actions on-line. The ventral stream manipulates visual information that is to be stored in, and recalled from, MEMORY (see DORSAL STREAM and VENTRAL STREAM for further details).

two-and-a-half-D sketch (2.5 D sketch) *see* Marr's computational theory of vision

tympanic membrane The eardrum: see COCHLEA; OSSICLES

type A and type B behaviour These types of behaviour are symptomatic of certain personality traits. Type A behaviour is characterized by the following traits and terms: competitive, driven, urgent, aggressive, hostile, impatient, eager for material and quantifiable success. It has been suggested that such traits are the product of insecurity and low self-esteem. Type B behaviour either does not feature such traits, or features the opposite traits. Type A behaviour is of concern because it is associated with a variety of PSYCHOPHYSIOLOGICAL DISORDERS, most notably heart disease (see CARDIOVASCULAR PSYCHOPHYSIOLOGY). PSYCHOTHERAPY of some form is usually indicated for individuals displaying type A behaviour patterns. The essentials of type A behaviour were described in the early years of the twentieth century, but the use of this construct came into vogue in the 1970s and 1980s. Concern has been expressed about its validity and usefulness, but while some degree of diagnostic clarification and refinement might be of value, some elements of the category being rather vague, it remains the case that we can all identify colleagues who can be classified in this way. As these individuals are at very much greater risk for certain types of (often fatal) illness, it seems necessary to persist with the central conception of these traits.

Reference

Davison G.C. & Neale J.M. (1996) *Abnormal Psychology*, 6th edn, Wiley: New York.

type I schizophrenia A form of SCHIZOPHRENIA defined by T.J. Crow and typified by the so-called positive symptoms.

type I synapse; type II synapse *see* synapse

type II schizophrenia A form of SCHIZOPHRENIA defined by T.J. Crow and typified by the so-called negative symptoms.

tyramine The action of aromatic acid decarboxylase on TYROSINE produces tyramine. CA-TECHOLAMINE neurons can take this up and release it as a false neurotransmitter.

tyrosine One of the AMINO ACIDS, it is a precursor of the CATECHOLAMINE neurotransmitters DOPAMINE and NORADRENALINE. It is supplied by the diet and can in addition be synthesized in the liver. The enzyme TYROSINE HYDROXYLASE catalyses the conversion of tyrosine to DOPA.

tyrosine hydroxylase An ENZYME, tyrosine hydroxylase catalyses the conversion of TYROSINE to DOPA (see L-DOPA) which is converted to DOPAMINE by amino acid decarboxylases. Dopamine can be further converted to NORADRENALINE and ADRENALINE. It is the RATE-LIMITING STEP in the synthesis of catecholamines.

tyrosine kinase A protein KINASE; one of the SECOND MESSENGERS.

tyrosine kinase receptors (trk) These are subunits of the RECEPTOR for TROPHIC FACTORS. The NERVE GROWTH FACTOR receptor was identified as having two subunits: the p75 subunit (with low affinity for nerve growth factor) and a larger subunit, first identified as the *trk* ONCOGENE, which can bind nerve growth factor on its own or in combination with the p75 subunit. The PROTEINS coded for by *trk*, TrkB and TrkC are though to be receptors for BRAIN-DERIVED NEUROTROPHIC FACTOR and NEUROTROPHIN-3.

U

UK14,304 An alpha-2 noradrenaline receptor AGONIST; see ADRENOCEPTORS.

ulnar nerve *see* tingling

ultradian rhythm A biological rhythm with a period less than 24 hours (the prefix ultra- indicating a high frequency).

See also: biological clock; overt rhythm

ultrastructure (from Latin, *ultra*: beyond) Ultra- is a prefix that indicates that something is at an extreme. Ultrastructure indicates the most microscopic level of structure that can be analysed. It is a term used when describing, for example, the detailed organization of SUBCELLULAR ORGANS, and is typically assessed using ELECTRON MICROSCOPY.

umami *see* primary tastes

unconditioned behaviour This is a term applied to the natural and spontaneous behaviour of an animal: it indicates a response that has not been the subject of a CONDITIONING procedure or learnt in a specific situation (see LEARNING). Of course one might argue that all behaviour is learned in one way or another, and so the possibility of there being an unconditioned behaviour is, at best, limited. However, in a laboratory setting, one can differentiate between those behavioural acts that have been specifically conditioned (such as pressing a lever in an OPERANT CHAMBER) and those behavioural acts that are spontaneously emitted by an animal (a rat DRINKING water in its home cage for example).

unconditioned reinforcer *see* reinforcer

unconditioned response This is a term applied to an animal's natural and spontaneous responses to a STIMULUS, as opposed to responses that are produced following a CONDITIONING procedure or that have been learnt in a specific situation (see LEARNING). For example, in a laboratory setting, one can differentiate between responses that have not been learned – a STARTLE REFLEX for instance – and those responses that have been trained, such as pressing a lever in an OPERANT CHAMBER in response to the presentation of a light.

unconditioned stimulus *see* classical conditioning

uncrossed disparity *see* retinal disparity

uncus (from Latin, *uncus*: a hook) The uncus is the name given to the anterior portion of the *hippocampal gyrus*, one of the gyri of the TEMPORAL LOBE.

See also: H.M.

unfeeling touch A somatosensory equivalent to the phenomenon of BLINDSIGHT; see CONSCIOUSNESS.

unilateral Affecting or present on one side only: the BRAIN has two hemispheres (see HEMISPHERE) so, for example, a unilateral LESION of a particular structure would be one that was present in that structure in one hemisphere only. A BILATERAL lesion would be present in that structure in both hemispheres.

unilateral neglect A term used to describe NEGLECT SYNDROME. It is a somewhat pointless term (though nevertheless used) since its opposite, bilateral neglect, would involve failures to detect or respond to stimuli bilaterally. Such conditions exist but go under other names: BLINDNESS for example.

unipolar *see* bipolar

unipolar depression Recurrent episodes of clinical DEPRESSION, without intervening episodes of MANIA – as distinct from BIPOLAR DISORDER. Unipolar depression is much more common than bipolar disorder, and most clinical depressive disorders will take this form. A proportion of patients who appear to have a unipolar disorder will, of course, eventually have a manic episode, thus reclassifying their illness as bipolar.

IAN C. REID

unipolar neuron *see* bipolar, multipolar and unipolar neurons

unique hues Red, green, blue and yellow cannot be described in terms of any other colour: they are therefore called UNIQUE HUES; see OPPONENT PROCESS THEORY OF COLOUR VISION.

unmyelinated *see* myelin

unsupervised learning *see* backpropagation; neural networks

upregulation *see* sensitization (receptor)

uptake *see* reuptake

uracil One of the NUCLEOTIDES; see RNA.

Urbach–Wiethe disease A very rare disease (also know as *lipid proteinosis*) which involves CALCIFICATION (accumulation of calcium deposits) in a variety of tissues, including within the brain. The TEMPORAL LOBE, HIPPOCAMPUS and AMYGDALA have all been known to be damaged bilaterally. AMNESIA has been reported, as have difficulties in the perception of specific EMOTIONS, especially FEAR.

ureter *see* osmoregulation

uterus The Latin term for the womb, in which a foetus will develop (see DEVELOPMENT). Uterine describes the property of belonging to the uterus. Clearly, what happens to a foetus within the uterus will have a profound effect on physical development. The extent to which intra-uterine events determine psychological states in childhood and later life is uncertain. Postnatal effects are of more consequence for these.

See also: drug effects in utero; pregnancy

utility A concept taken from economics forming part of what is known as BEHAVIOURAL ECONOMICS. Utility describes the assumption that animals will prefer states or conditions that are associated with *more* of a desired goal object to states or conditions that provide *less*. It describes the estimate an animal makes about the value a given goal object – an assessment of value in terms of usefulness. It is assumed that animals must have a mechanism that allows them to assess the utility of disparate goal objects, but how the computation is made is the subject of debate.

Reference

Shizgal P. & Conover K. (1996) On the neural computation of utility. *Current Direction in Psychological Science* 5: 1–7.

utricle *see* vestibular system

V

vacuole (from French, *vacuole*: a little vacuum) A vacuole is a small sac or cavity within a CELL. In plants vacuoles are subcellular elements containing a variety of chemicals with important functions relating to growth, development and reproduction. But if one describes vacuoles in animal tissues one will not be describing the same thing as plant vacuoles. Instead, the formation of vacuoles – fluid-filled inclusions – in brains may be evidence of a disease process at work. *Vacuolization* describes the formation of vacuoles.

vacuous chewing *see* jaw movements

vacuous jaw movements *see* jaw movements

vagina Female genitalia – a passage joining the VULVA (the opening of the vagina – the female external genitalia) and the UTERUS.

See also: copulation; penis

vagus nerve (from Latin, *vagus*: wandering) The vagus nerve, the tenth cranial nerve (see CRANIAL NERVES), is named for its extensive distribution and many sensory and motor branches in the neck, thorax and abdomen. It is the primary brainstem nerve controlling the upper gastrointestinal tract, respiratory system and the heart. As well, the vagus nerve innervates the pancreas, liver and gall bladder. Functionally, it is involved in the coordination of swallowing, respiration, cardioinhibition, and secretomotor function of the DIGESTIVE SYSTEM. The vagus nerve has two sensory ganglia, containing PSEUDOUNIPOLAR NEURONS, located immediately external to jugular foramen via which the nerve reaches the

periphery. The superior JUGULAR GANGLION contains general somatic afferent neurons that innervate the DURA MATER (see MENINGES) and skin of the ear and external acoustic meatus. Neurons of the inferior NODOSE GANGLION provide general visceral afferent input from the upper alimentary tract (oesophagus, stomach, small intestine), respiratory system (larynx, trachea, lungs) and heart. Vagal sensory information from CHEMORECEPTOR, BARORECEPTOR and MECHANORECEPTOR systems is relayed primarily to the nucleus of the solitary tract and area postrema in the BRAINSTEM. A few special visceral afferent neurons relay taste information from the epiglottis. General visceral efferent (PARASYMPATHETIC) axons originate mainly in the dorsal motor nucleus of the vagus nerve which has a longitudinal columnar viscerotopic organization. The parasympathetic preganglionic neurons project to parasympathetic ganglia in most of the viscera that have vagal sensory innervation. Preganglionic neurons in the dorsal motor nucleus of the vagus also project to interlobular ganglia of the pancreas to regulate insulin secretion. Special visceral efferent (branchiomotor) neurons originate in the NUCLEUS AMBIGUUS and project to the striated muscles of the pharynx, larynx and esophagus. The nucleus ambiguus also contains preganglionic cardioinhibitory neurons that course in cardiopulmonary nerves to intrinsic cardiac ganglia on the heart. Their function is to reduce heart rate and force of contraction of the myocardium. The exact location of cardiac preganglionic neurons remains somewhat controversial but the preponderance of evidence indicates that they originate primarily in the external formation of the nucleus ambiguus and, possibly, to a lesser extent, in the dorsal motor nucleus of the vagus nerve. Vagal motor neurons serve as a final common pathway for autonomic regulation, especially subserving visceral responses to EMOTION and PAIN. The vagus nerve also mediates satiety signals and sensations of gastric pain. Fever and sickness behaviour induced by activation of the IMMUNE SYSTEM by proinflammatory cytokines are mediated by vagal afferents associated with intra-abdominal vagal paraganglia.

DAVID A. HOPKINS

valid cue *see* Posner effect

validity effect *see* Posner effect

Valium The brand name of DIAZEPAM, a DRUG in the BENZODIAZEPINE class. Valium was developed at the drug company Hoffman-LaRoche, and was first synthesized and introduced in the early 1960s. During that time there was considerable research aimed at developing safer alternatives to the BARBITURATES, which were used as sedatives and relief of anxiety. Librium was developed first, followed soon after by Valium. Prescriptions for Valium were extremely popular in the 1970s, when it was the most prescribed drug worldwide. The rate of use has decreased since then, as it gradually became apparent the benzodiazepines had fairly high ABUSE POTENTIAL, and could be associated with a WITHDRAWAL syndrome with chronic use. Nevertheless, Valium is still a very useful therapeutic treatment of anxiety, seizures, sleep disorders, muscle spasms, and as an adjunct treatment in certain surgical procedures. Like other benzodiazepines, Valium works by enhancing the action of the inhibitory neurotransmitter GABA. Lower doses of the drug relieve anxiety and induce a sense of well-being; higher doses cause sedation.

ANN E. KELLEY

Vandenbergh effect The Vandenbergh effect describes the accelerated onset of puberty in female rodents following exposure to adult male pheromones.

See also: Bruce effect; Lee–Boot effect; Whitten effect

vanillymandelic acid *see* noradrenaline

variable interval schedule *see* schedules of reinforcement

variable ratio schedule *see* schedules of reinforcement

vas deferens *see* testes

vascular cuffing This is a term that has been used in two different ways: (i) to describe an accumulation of cells around a BLOOD vessel. This has been observed in the CENTRAL NERVOUS SYSTEM following breakdown of the BLOOD–BRAIN BARRIER (induced by EXCITOTOXIC LESION) and after transplantation of tissue into the adult central nervous system. (ii) It has been used in studies of tumour formation to describe a process in which small blood vessels surround (cuff) tumour cells.

vascular dementia DEMENTIA caused by loss of BLOOD flow to the brain. In older medical literature it is referred to as MULTI-INFARCT DEMENTIA, which describes a form of vascular dementia in which there are multiple infarcts in the brain, the total loss of tissue being great enough to produce serious psychological dysfunction – dementia. The more general term VASCULAR DEMENTIA reflects a growing awareness that a variety of assaults upon the blood flow to the brain can cause profound impairment.

vasculature (from Latin, *vas*: a vessel) The VASCULATURE is the system of blood vessels in a body. 'Vascular' is the adjective describing the body's blood vessels; see BLOOD.

vasectomy *see* testes

vasoactive (from Latin *vas*: a vessel) The prefix vas- always indicates the vascular system – the system of veins, arteries and capillaries in the body (see BLOOD). A VASOACTIVE substance is one that causes contraction or dilation of blood vessels.

vasoactive intestinal polypeptide One of the NEUROPEPTIDES; it is a GUT–BRAIN PEPTIDE, often associated with CHOLINERGIC neurons in the PERIPHERAL NERVOUS SYSTEM. There are two RECEPTOR subtypes (VPAC1 and VPAC2), both G PROTEIN coupled. Its functions in the CENTRAL NERVOUS SYSTEM are not especially well characterized.

See also: hormones

vasoconstriction Vasoconstriction is constriction of blood vessels; VASODILATION is the reverse; see BLOOD.

vasodilation *see* vasoconstriction

vasopressin Also known as ANTIDIURETIC HORMONE, vasopressin is one of the NEURO-PEPTIDES transmitter and a hormone with potent actions concerned with OSMOREGULA-TION. There are two forms: VASOPRESSIN and ARGININE vasopressin. Arginine vasopressin (AVP) has an arginine residue and is the form found in most MAMMALS. Vasopressin has a lysine residue and is found in pigs and hippopotami. It is closely related to OXYTOCIN and formed from pre-propressophysin. Both arginine vasopressin and oxytocin act at the same RECEPTOR group, classified as V_{1A}, V_{1B}, V_2 and OT: vasopressin is more active at the first three, oxytocin at the last, though all act at each one. All these receptors are G PROTEIN coupled.

In the CENTRAL NERVOUS SYSTEM, vasopressin is synthesized by the MAGNOCELLULAR and PARVOCELLULAR neurons of the PARAVENTRICU-LAR NUCLEUS OF THE HYPOTHALAMUS and the supraoptic nucleus of the hypothalamus. The magnocellular neurons project to the PITUI-TARY GLAND, where AVP is released into the BLOOD stream. The parvocellular neurons use AVP as a neurotransmitter with projections to a variety of sites, including other nuclei in the HYPOTHALAMUS, the SEPTAL NUCLEI, AMYG-DALA, HIPPOCAMPUS and several sites in the BRAINSTEM. Dehydration is the most effective stimulant to pituitary release of vasopressin: it stimulates the retention of water by the kidney and, in through its actions in brain, is involved in the initiation of DRINKING. It thus helps preserve existing water in the body and triggers behaviour appropriate to recruitment of more water. It has also been suggested to have a role in LEARNING and MEMORY, though the evidence for this is a little controversial. Some authors have suggested that vasopressin injections can prolong EXTINCTION of learning. BRATTLEBORO RATS, genetically MUTANT animals that are vasopressin deficient, have some learning and memory deficits. However, other authors have suggested that the effects of AVP on learning and memory are secondary effects of osmoregulatory disturbance.

See also: neurophysin

vasopressor *see* pressor

vection Vection is the illusion of self-motion opposite in direction to motion of visual surroundings as experienced, for example, in the widescreen cinema. Motion of the more distant scene induces vection, as when one observes a moving train from a stationary train. Foreground movement does not induce vection when the background is stationary. When we rotate or translate at constant velocity, the vestibular organs stop responding; only the relative motion of the visual scene indicates that we are moving. When we see the background move we believe it is due to self motion, since the background is normally stationary.

See also: motion perception

IAN P. HOWARD

vehicle The SOLUTION in which a DRUG is dissolved, usually used as the treatment given to a control group in an experiment. The choice of vehicle solution will depend on the route of injection and the solubility of the drug to be dissolved. Artificial CEREBROSPINAL FLUID, ISOTONIC SALINE or PHOSPHATE BUFFER are most commonly used. A term often used in PSYCHOPHARMACOLOGY research, the vehicle can be a number of different types of solutions. In EXPERIMENTAL DESIGN, it is important to have a vehicle control group, in order to eliminate non-specific factors, not related to the drug itself, that might contribute to an observed effect. For example, one might be interested in testing the behavioural effects of a drug that only dissolves in a solution that is slightly acidic. Suppose that the treatment, which is given subcutaneously, appears to lower motor activity. This may be the effect of the drug, or it could be due to an adverse effect of the acidic solution under the skin (or perhaps, simply to the stress of the injection itself). The only way to dissociate these effects to include a vehicle control group.

ANN E. KELLEY

vein *see* blood

Veith–Muller circle *see* horopter

venlafaxine *see* serotonin–noradrenaline reuptake inhibitor

ventral *see* dorsal

ventral bundle *see* dorsal noradrenergic bundle; ventral noradrenergic bundle

ventral horn A part of the SPINAL CORD: this has a VENTRAL and a DORSAL HORN and, at thoracic levels, a LATERAL HORN also.

See also: ventral root

ventral noradrenergic bundle *see* dorsal noradrenergic bundle; ventral noradrenergic bundle

ventral orbital cortex Following the terminology of Paxinos & Watson (1997), ventral orbital cortex (VO) corresponds to primate ORBITOFRONTAL CORTEX.

See also: rodent vs. primate prefrontal cortex

Reference

Paxinos G. & Watson C. (1997) *The Rat Brain in Stereotaxic Coordinates*, compact 3rd edn, Academic Press: San Diego.

ventral pallidum The ventral pallidum is the major target for the efferent projections from the ventral STRIATUM, especially the NUCLEUS ACCUMBENS. It lies in the BASAL FOREBRAIN, ventral and posterior to the nucleus accumbens as well as ventral to the dorsal striatum and dorsal pallidum. Much of the ventral pallidum lies underneath lateral parts of the decussation of the ANTERIOR COMMISSURE and is therefore called the SUBCOMMISSURAL VENTRAL PALLIDUM. The ventral pallidum, together with the MAGNOCELLULAR neurons of the nucleus basalis of Meynert and the cell columns of the extended AMYGDALA comprise the substantia innominata region of the basal forebrain. The ventral pallidum is a direct continuation of the dorsal part of the pallidal complex and appears to be a mix of both internal and external

pallidal segments, receiving both a SUBSTANCE-P positive and ENKEPHALIN-positive innervation from the ventral striatum (these inputs arrive separately from the dorsal striatum to reach the internal and external segments of the globus pallidus, respectively). FIBRES from the core of the nucleus accumbens mainly terminate in the dorsolateral ventral pallidum, whereas fibres from the shell of the nucleus accumbens mainly terminate in the ventromedial parts of the ventral pallidum. The EFFERENT projections of the ventral pallidum are rather limited in their distribution. Those from the dorsolateral part project to the SUBTHALAMIC NUCLEUS and SUBSTANTIA NIGRA, whereas those from the ventromedial part project mainly to the mediodorsal nucleus of the THALAMUS, and also to the internal segment of the GLOBUS PALLIDUS (entopeduncular nucleus in the rat), LATERAL HYPOTHALAMUS and VENTRAL TEGMENTAL AREA.

See also: corticostriatal loops

BARRY J. EVERITT

ventral root A body of nerves extending from the ventral portion of the SPINAL CORD. These roots arise bilaterally, at each segment of the spinal cord, from the ventrolateral surface of the cord. They are composed of the axons of MOTOR NEURONS whose cell bodies form nuclei within the ventral horns of the spinal cord. These motor neurons innervate skeletal musculature. In the thoracic and upper lumbar region of the spinal cord, ventral roots also contain processes from sympathetic preganglionic neurons. These synapse within ganglia of the SYMPATHETIC NERVOUS SYSTEM. In the sacral region, ventral roots carry fibres of PARASYMPATHETIC NERVOUS SYSTEM neurons which innervate the bladder, parts of the colon and rectum, and the sexual organs.

See also: dorsal root

FIONA M. INGLIS

ventral stream The primary visual cortex (area V1; see AREAS V1–V5) receives fragmented information about the optic array, and distributes this selectively to other cortical areas. These include visual areas V2 and V3, which themselves pass information via areas

V4 and V4A to TEO and area TE in the INFERIOR TEMPORAL CORTEX TEO and area TE. This occipito-temporal pathway – the VENTRAL STREAM – is anatomically distinct from the other main visual pathway, the DORSAL STREAM. The ventral stream passes high-resolution visual information for the inferior temporal cortex to categorize useful objects and places for storage in memory, and to gain access to these memories at a later time.

See also: two cortical visual streams; visuo-motor control

A. DAVID MILNER

ventral striatopallidal system The ventral striatopallidal system parallels the DORSAL STRIATOPALLIDAL SYSTEM (see CORTICOSTRIA-TAL LOOPS) and is represented by the circuitry that originates in limbic cortical structures (HIPPOCAMPAL FORMATION, basolateral AMYG-DALA, PRELIMBIC CORTEX), projects to the ventral STRIATUM and thence to the VENTRAL PALLIDUM, mediodorsal nucleus of the THALA-MUS and back, as re-entrant circuitry, to the PREFRONTAL CORTEX.

BARRY J. EVERITT

ventral striatum *see* striatum

ventral tegmental area The ventral tegmental area (VTA) is literally the floor of the MID-BRAIN and contains such structures as the INTERPEDUNCULAR NUCLEUS, the ventral tegmental area of Tsai both of which are in the medial VTA, and the SUBSTANTIA NIGRA, which lies ventrolaterally. Common usage associates the VTA rather specifically with the group of DOPAMINE neurons lying between the two substantiae nigrae which give origin to the MESOLIMBIC DOPAMINE SYSTEM and MESOLIM-BICOCORTICAL SYSTEM that innervate the NU-CLEUS ACCUMBENS, AMYGDALA and cortical areas, especially the PREFRONTAL CORTEX. These DOPAMINERGIC projections distinguish them from the nigrostriatal dopamine pathway that arises in the more lateral substantia nigra pars compacta. The VTA dopaminergic cell group is often called the A10 cell group (see CLASSIFICATION OF DAHLSTRÖM AND FUXE).

BARRY J. EVERITT

ventral tegmental area of Tsai *see* ventral tegmental area

ventricles (i) *Cardiovascular system*: chambers of the heart; see BLOOD.

(ii) *Brain*: The ventricles of the brain are cavities inside the brain that are filled with the CEREBROSPINAL FLUID (CSF). They are lined with the ependyma consisting of a single layer of EPENDYMAL CELLS. The ventricular system is comprised of a pair of the lateral ventricles located in the CEREBRAL HEMISPHERES, the third ventricle located at the midline in the DIENCEPHALON, and the fourth ventricle located between the lower BRAINSTEM and CERE-BELLUM. The lateral ventricle is the largest and is composed of the anterior horn, the body, the inferior horn and the posterior horn. The lateral ventricles communicate with the third ventricle through narrow passages called the interventricular FORAMINA OF MONRO. These foramina are used as reference points in radiographic studies. The slit-like third ventricle narrows into the CEREBRAL AQUEDUCT (AQUE-DUCT OF SYLVIUS) in the MIDBRAIN, and then opens up as the fourth ventricle, a flat and diamond-shaped ventricle between the lower brainstem and cerebellum. At its widest part, a lateral recess communicates with the CISTERNA MAGNA or CEREBELLOMEDULLARY CISTERN, a large SUBARACHNOID SPACE (space between the ARACHNOID MEMBRANE and PIA MATER [see MENINGES]) posterior to the cerebellum. There is also a small median opening called the FORAMEN OF MAGENDIE. Caudally, the fourth ventricle is continuous with the CENTRAL CA-NAL of the SPINAL CORD. The CIRCUMVENTRI-CULAR ORGANS are present in the third and fourth ventricles. They usually lack the BLOOD–BRAIN BARRIER and have a role in mediating direct actions of blood-borne substances on neurons.

The CSF protects the brain from mechanical shocks, and provides an optimal chemical environment for neuronal signalling. It also has a role in circulating HORMONES and NEUROTRANSMITTERS (see VOLUME TRANSMIS-SION) and removing waste products and drugs. CSF is formed in the CHOROID PLEXUS on ventricular walls via chemical filtering of the blood across the blood–cerebrospinal fluid barrier. The CSF passes through the ventricles, central canal of the spinal cord, and the surface of the brain and spinal cord and is then absorbed back into the blood through the arachnoid villi located in the superior sagittal sinus, a large superficial vein. Normally, the rate of formation matches the rate of reabsorption of CSF. However, an obstruction of the normal drainage, excess formation of CSF, or any space-occupying conditions such as a TUMOUR or haematoma could result in an abnormal increase in the CSF pressure, causing damage to brain tissues and nerves. This condition is called HYDROCEPHALUS. CSF can be sampled in patients by LUMBAR PUNCTURE – insertion of a needle into the central canal of the spinal cord and drawing off of fluid. Chemical analysis of CSF can provide important clues to dysfunction in the state of the brain.

KAZUE SEMBA

ventricular enlargement As it says, this term indicates that the cerebral VENTRICLES are enlarged. This is a condition that is associated with HYDROCEPHALUS and MACROCEPHALY but it is a phenomenon that has received more attention in recent years by virtue of an association with SCHIZOPHRENIA. The introduction of modern neuroimaging methods such as COMPUTERIZED AXIAL TOMOGRAPHY (CAT scanning – see also FUNCTIONAL NEUROIMAGING) led to the discovery that in schizophrenia there appeared to be enlargement of the lateral ventricles. This was associated principally with negative symptoms (TYPE II SCHIZOPHRENIA) and with a resistance to standard ANTIPSYCHOTIC drug medication. It appeared to suggest that the two types of schizophrenia identified by T.J. Crow – type I and type II – were different in their basic pathology. However a number of problems have become apparent with this hypothesis: (1) ventricular enlargement commonly occurs in disorders in which there is loss of brain tissue – the ventricles simply expand to fill the space available. However, the evidence for brain pathology in schizophrenia is at best inconclusive. There is no evidence of massive NEURODEGENERATION (as there is in ALZHEIMER'S DEMENTIA for example) and REACTIVE GLIOSIS is not prominent. (2) The cerebral ventricles do

not become progressively larger over time in schizophrenic patients as they do in other neurodegenerative disorders. (3) Ventricular size is known to be increased before symptoms are present in schizophrenia. (4) It seems possible that the variability in ventricular size within the normal population is greater than that between schizophrenic patients and the normal population.

ventricular system The various ventricles and connecting aqueducts are sometimes referred to as the ventricular system; see VENTRICLES.

ventricular zone *see* cortical development

ventromedial hypothalamic syndrome (VMH syndrome) Bilateral electrolytic lesions (see LESION) of the ventromedial area of the HYPOTHALAMUS produce a characteristic syndrome, first described in 1942 by Hetherington & Ranson, featuring behavioural and metabolic disturbances. Metabolic dysfunction include HYPERINSULINAEMIA (the first feature to develop, and the degree of which predicts the severity of the syndrome *en masse*), increased GASTRIC ACID section, increased FAT deposition, decreased OXYGEN consumption and decreased utilization of AMINO ACIDS. Behavioural problems include elevated BODY WEIGHT (in an initial *dynamic phase* of rapid gain and a *static phase* in which a stable, elevated, weight is maintained), HYPERPHAGIA (which is dissociated from the weight gain: animals gain weight even if fed the same amount as controls), FINICKINESS, heightened reactivity to stimuli and a reluctance to work for food on high SCHEDULES OF REINFORCEMENT. The VMH syndrome was an integral part of Stellar's DUAL CENTRES HYPOTHESIS: it appeared to provide evidence of a brain centre that normally inhibited feeding (that is, controlled SATIETY). Later theories emphasized the regulation of body weight or metabolic dysfunctions rather than the control of feeding itself, but no account satisfactorily explained all the signs until Powley developed a hypothesis around the CEPHALIC REFLEXES OF DIGESTION. However, even this all-embracing theory was ultimately undermined. For example, it was suggested that the VMH syndrome produced hyperinsulinaemia that was not responsive to cephalic phase modulation. More importantly it became clear that the VMH syndrome was dissociable. For example, Gold demonstrated that discrete lesions of the VEN-TROMEDIAL NUCLEUS OF THE HYPOTHALAMUS (as distinct from the larger ventromedial *area* of the hypothalamus) did not produce the syndrome while various authors showed that elements of the syndrome were accounted for by damage to the VENTRAL NORADRENERGIC BUNDLE or the PARAVENTRICULAR NUCLEUS OF THE HYPOTHALAMUS. That the VMH syndrome should lack anatomical distinctiveness is perhaps not surprising. Research on the syndrome was triggered by clinical observations in the late nineteenth and early twentieth century by neurologists such as Babinski and Frohlich that patients with damage – typically TUMOURS – in the ventromedial area of the hypothalamus presented with a complex syndrome involving changes in metabolism and behaviour. But the damage produced by hypothalamic tumours very rarely localizes to particular nuclei, and the damage produced by electrolytic lesions is never specific, destroying both the neurons in a given area and FIBRES OF PASSAGE. The syndrome is now of scant academic interest but persists in the continuing popular, but erroneous, belief that feeding and drinking are controlled by 'brain centres'.

See also: lateral hypothalamic syndrome

References

Gold R.M. (1973) Hypothalamic obesity: the myth of the ventromedial nucleus. *Science* 182: 488–490.
Hetherington A.W. & Ranson S.W. (1942) The spontaneous activity and food intake of rats with hypothalamic lesions. *American Journal of Physiology* 136: 609–617.
Powley T.L. (1977) The ventromedial hypothalamic syndrome, satiety and a cephalic phase hypothesis. *Psychological Review* 84: 89–126.

ventromedial nucleus of the hypothalamus
A nucleus in the core of the HYPOTHALAMUS. It has AFFERENT and EFFERENT connections with a variety of sites in the brain: other nuclei of the hypothalamus, GLOBUS PALLIDUS, HIPPO-CAMPUS, AMYGDALA, PREOPTIC AREA, PERIA-QUEDUCTAL GREY, VENTRAL NORADRENERGIC BUNDLE all send inputs, while outputs travel

to the SEPTAL NUCLEI, other hypothalamic sites, MAMMILLARY BODIES, DORSOMEDIAL NU-CLEUS OF THE THALAMUS (and other sites in the THALAMUS), periaqueductal grey, RAPHE NUCLEI and VENTRAL TEGMENTAL AREA. It has been implicated in the control of SEXUAL BEHAVIOUR and FEEDING. Note however that its involvement with the VENTROMEDIAL HY-POTHALAMIC SYNDROME is not as clear as originally thought. Gold showed that discrete lesions confined to only the ventromedial nucleus of the hypothalamus, not expanding into the more general ventromedial area of the hypothalamus, did not produce the syndrome. Several various authors showed that elements of the syndrome were accounted for by damage to the ventral noradrenergic bundle or the PARAVENTRICULAR NUCLEUS OF THE HY-POTHALAMUS.

Reference

Gold R.M. (1973) Hypothalamic obesity: the myth of the ventromedial nucleus. *Science* 182: 488–490.

venule *see* blood

verbal paraphasia *see* anomia

vergence An EYE MOVEMENT which alters the angle between the lines of sight of the two eyes, as opposed to a conjugate movement in which the eyes move together. The eyes may either converge so that both fixate on a near object, or diverge to fixate at a greater distance. Vergence movements occur in response to RETINAL DISPARITY and/or in conjunction with changes in accommodation.

See also: stereodepth perception; strabismus

OLIVER J. BRADDICK

vermis Short for CEREBELLAR VERMIS; see CEREBELLUM – ANATOMICAL ORGANIZATION

vernier acuity *see* visual acuity

vertebral artery blood

vertebrates A term that covers all the members of the subphylum *Vertebrata*: an animal with a vertebral column – a backbone composed of individual vertebrae – including fish, amphibia, reptiles, birds, mammals.

See also: taxonomy

vertex The vertex is effectively the crown of the SKULL – the high point as one moves along the MIDLINE. It is important in research using SCALP ELECTRODES (for example, when making ELECTROENCEPHALOGRAM recordings). Because the vertex lies on the midline it is electrically neutral with respect to each HEMISPHERE and the scalp electrode at the vertex can be used as a REFERENCE ELECTRODE.

vertical limb of the diagonal band of Broca *see* diagonal band of Broca

vertigo (from Latin, *vertere*: to turn) A sensation of dizziness or giddiness caused by disturbance to the mechanisms of BALANCE.

See also: oscillopsia; vestibular system

vesicle (from Latin, *vesica*: a bladder) A vesicle describes any bodily or cellular component that is bag-like. In general when the term is used by neuroscientists it refers to SYNAPTIC VESICLES.

vesicular transporters SYNAPTIC VESICLES are packaged with neurotransmitter molecules that are synthesized within neurons. The passage of NEUROTRANSMITTERS from the CYTOPLASM into vesicles is achieved using vesicular transporters, GLYCOPROTEIN molecules embedded in the vesicle membranes. ANTIBODIES to a number of these – the vesicular ACETYLCHOLINE transporter for example – now exist, enabling immunohistochemical localization studies (see IMMUNOHISTOCHEMISTRY) to plot the locations of terminals containing specific vesicular transporters (that is, terminals capable of releasing particular neurotransmitters).

vessels This term will usually refer to BLOOD vessels (or, less commonly, to vessels in the lymphatic system). It will often be accompanied by other terms (such as cerebral vessels, microvessels and so on).

vestibular complex The vestibular complex is a term used to describe the vestibular nucleus in the MEDULLA OBLONGATA, and its connections. Sensory information for the vestibular complex is collected from HAIR CELLS in the vestibular labyrinth by neurons in the VESTIBULAR GANGLION (also known as SCARPA'S GANGLION). There are approximately 20 000 bipolar neurons per ganglion: they connect to hair cells (recruiting information) and to nuclei in the BRAINSTEM (sending information centrally). The vestibular ganglion is divided into two portions: the superior division (connected to the UTRICLE) and the inferior division (connected to the SACCULE and AMPULLA). Axons from the ganglion join the VESTIBULAR NERVE, a branch of the VESTIBULOCOCHLEAR NERVE (the eighth cranial nerve) to innervate the VESTIBULAR NUCLEUS.

See also: vestibular system

Reference

Kandel E.R., Schwartz J.H. & Jessell T.M. (2000) *Principles of Neural Science*, 3rd edn, McGraw-Hill: New York.

vestibular ganglion *see* vestibular system

vestibular labyrinth *see* vestibular system

vestibular nerve With the COCHLEAR NERVE (or AUDITORY NERVE) one of the principal branches of the vestibulocochlear nerve (the eighth cranial nerve); see VESTIBULAR SYSTEM.

vestibular nucleus The vestibular nucleus is divided into four: (1) the lateral vestibular nucleus (also known as DEITER'S NUCLEUS), important for the control of posture; it has inputs from CEREBELLUM (the VERMIS), SPINAL CORD and VESTIBULAR LABYRINTH; and has output (via lateral vestibulospinal tract) to the VENTRAL HORN. (2 and 3) The medial vestibular nucleus and the superior vestibular nucleus, both important for vestibulo-ocular interactions; there is input from the AMPULLAE of the SEMICIRCULAR CANALS; and output via the medial vestibulospinal tract (to the cervical spinal cord) from where control of the neck muscles can be established. There is also output via the MEDIAL LONGITUDINAL FASCICULUS to sites of control of EYE MOVEMENTS (including the cranial nerve nuclei involved in controlling the musculature of the eye (the third [OCULOMOTOR NERVE], fourth [TROCHLEAR NERVE] and sixth [ABDUCENS NERVE] CRANIAL NERVES). (4) The inferior vestibular nucleus, important for integration of information from the VESTIBULAR SYSTEM and the cerebellum. It has inputs from the semicircular canals, UTRICLE and SACCULE, and from the cerebellum (the vermis); and it has outputs that travels via the

VESTIBULOSPINAL and VESTIBULORETICULAR PATHWAYS to influence other sites in the BRAIN-STEM and in the THALAMUS.

vestibular sac *see* vestibular system

vestibular system The vestibular system monitors gravity and acceleration of the body through space, and maintains balance. The sensory mechanisms of the vestibular system are found in the EAR, by the COCHLEA. The principal organs of the vestibular system are the series of fine bone tubes known as the SEMICIRCULAR CANALS and the VESTIBULAR SAC, containing the UTRICLE (from Latin, *utriculus*, diminutive of *uterus*: a small womb) and the SACCULE (from Latin, *sacculus*, diminutive of *saccus*: a small sack). These are collectively known as the VESTIBULAR LABYRINTH. The semicircular canals detect acceleration in any direction while the vestibular sac organs monitor the static position of the head.

The receptor mechanisms of the semicircular canal and vestibular sac are organized as follows. Within the semicircular canal there are three tubes, each one oriented in a principal plane, and filled with fluid (known as ENDOLYMPH). The three tubes are joined at their ends to the utricle and below this, to the saccule. The receptors within these organs operate as do those of the auditory system. Within the semicircular canals, an area known as the AMPULLA (from Latin, *amphora*: a flask) contains the cilia of HAIR CELLS, whose cell bodies are found in the adjacent CUPOLA (from Latin, *cupula*, diminutive of *cupa*: a cask). The hair cells are arranged in order of their length and take up precise positions, much as the hair cells of the BASILAR MEMBRANE do – and of course, the hair cells are connected to nerve fibres which will aggregate to form the VESTIBULAR NERVE. Movement of the fluid within the semicircular canals reflects acceleration through space in any direction: because the three canals are organized in each of the three principal planes of orientation, the degree of movement, integrated across all three canals, gives an accurate index of acceleration and direction. Fluid movement in the semicircular canals changes the activity of the hair cells, which transduce mechanical energy into neural activity. The receptor mechanisms of the ves-

tibular sac – the utricle and saccule – are not the same as those of the semicircular canal. Both utricle and saccule contain hair cells bedded into a gelatinous mass. The cilia of the hair cells extend out of this mass, above which is the otolithic membrane, with OTOLITHS (or OTOCONIA) on top. Head movement causes small changes in the distribution of the otoliths: the shifting of the weight of these produces movement in the underlying hair cell cilia, movement that is transduced into neural impulses by the hair cells.

The neurons of the semicircular canals and vestibular sac project to the VESTIBULAR GANGLION (also known as SCARPA'S GANGLION), which contains the bipolar neurons that give rise to the vestibular nerve (which, with the COCHLEAR NERVE [or AUDITORY NERVE], forms the VESTIBULOCOCHLEAR NERVE, the eighth cranial nerve; see CRANIAL NERVES). The vestibular branch of the vestibulocochlear nerves terminate in two places: most arrive at the vestibular nuclei in the MEDULLA OBLONGATA, but a proportion terminate in the CEREBELLUM, where they provide important sensory information related to the control of movement. The vestibular nuclei have complex projections to many places, including the THALAMUS and CEREBRAL CORTEX, as well as to the cranial nerve nuclei involved in controlling the musculature of the eye (the third [OCULOMOTOR NERVE], fourth [TROCHLEAR NERVE] and sixth [ABDUCENS NERVE] CRANIAL NERVES). These connections with the muscles of the eye are important for what are known as VESTIBULO-OCULAR INTERACTIONS. As the head moves it is of obvious importance to maintain stability of the eye, so that the information transmitted from the retina is not disrupted unnecessarily. Linkage of information about head movement with mechanisms of ocular motor control allow for rapid and precise adjustments, ensuring that the retinal image remains stable. Damage to this machinery leaves patients able to form stable visual images only when their heads are not moving.

A final curiosity to note is that the EVOLUTION of the auditory and vestibular systems has been easier to track than that of other sensory systems because the receptors are encased in, and made of, bone, which fossilizes, unlike soft tissue (in the eye for example). The vestibular and auditory systems appear to have evolved from the lateral line system of fish and amphibia (a mechanism for detecting movement of water) and from the swim bladder (a mechanism that fish have to aid balance); see Rosenzweig *et al.*, 1996 for a discussion of this point.

See also: macula; motion sickness; vection; vestibular complex

References

Carlson N.R. (1998) *Physiology of Behavior*, 6th edn, Allyn & Bacon: Boston.

Kandel E.R., Schwartz J.H. & Jessell T.M. (2000) *Principles of Neural Science*, 4th edn, McGraw Hill: New York. (This book contains an extensive and advanced discussion of the vestibular system.)

Rosenzweig M.R., Leiman A.L. & Breedlove S.M. (1996) *Biological Psychology*, Sinauer Associates: Sunderland MA.

vestibular-ocular interactions When a person rotates in the dark, the eyes move in the opposite direction at about the same velocity, with periodic quick returns. This vestibular-ocular response is evoked by signals from the semicircular canals, vestibular organs – sensitive to head rotation. The response is horizontal, vertical or around the visual axis, depending on which canals are in the plane of body rotation. The vestibular-ocular response is also evoked by vestibular organs sensitive to linear body motion. With eyes open, the vestibular-ocular response is supplemented by visually evoked optokinetic nystagmus and stabilizes the retinal image of stationary surroundings as the head rotates or translates.

IAN P. HOWARD

vestibulocerebellum *see* cerebellum – anatomical organization

vestibulocochlear nerve The eighth cranial nerve (see CRANIAL NERVES); involved in auditory processing and balance.

vestibuloreticular pathway *see* vestibular complex

vestibulospinal tract *see* vestibular complex

Viagra Viagra is the trade name of sildenafil citrate, an agent that stimulates CYCLIC GMP formation and enables ERECTION of the PENIS.

It has been used in the treatment of male IMPOTENCE, though it does have other effects: it has an action in the RETINA (creating in some users increased light sensitivity) and is mildly hypotensive (see HYPOTENSION). Already in the clinical literature are reports of deaths following use of Viagra, caused by cardiovascular problems, and there have been reports of cardiovascular accidents in the eye. As yet the risk in taking Viagra appears to be quite low.

vibratome In older literature this was known as a vibrating knife MICROTOME. The advantage of having a vibrating knife in the microtome is that it can cut sections of tissue that has not been fixed (see FIXATION) or processed in any other way. It is important therefore for use in experiments where slices of fresh tissue are taken for *in vitro* electrophysiological examination.

vibrissae (from Latin, *vibrissa*: nostril hair) A term that is applied to several types of stiff bristly hair, and to certain types of feather. Most commonly it is used to refer to the long whiskers that many animals (cats and rats for example) have on their snouts. For rodents, the vibrissae are important sources of sensory information; see BARREL CORTEX.

vibrotactile stimulus A vibrating pad that can be touched; a vibrotactile STIMULUS involves a subject (human) touching with a finger a small pad which can be made to vibrate. Initially the pad is at rest, vibration being initiated remotely by an experimenter. The subject's task is to remove their finger as quickly as possible. Vibrotactile stimuli elicit faster reaction times than other forms.

vigilance A state of attentive preparedness for the detection of anticipated but unpredictable events. Vigilance is required for any detection task, but there are greater vigilance demands when signals are rare, difficult to detect or occur unpredictably.

See also: attention; sustained attention

VERITY J. BROWN

viral encephalitis An infection of the BRAIN brought about by a VIRUS; see ENCEPHALITIS LETHARGICA; HERPES ENCEPHALITIS.

viral vector A modified VIRUS used to introduce genes into cells or tissues. Viral vectors are usually altered so that they are defective in their capacity to replicate, while still able to infect cells and induce the CELL to manufacture PROTEINS encoded by the viral genes (see GENE). Novel genes, inserted into the viral GENOME, are also expressed. Some viral vectors are constructed in viruses which do not need CELL DIVISION in order for their genetic material to be incorporated into the cell genome, such as adenovirus, or herpes simplex virus. Others require cell division in order to be expressed. Viral vectors are useful because a gene which is normally absent may be expressed in a localized manner, and the functional consequences of expression of the protein product, for example a RECEPTOR or a GROWTH FACTOR, may be observed. Viral vectors may prove useful in treating diseases, in a method called GENE THERAPY. For example, viral vectors may provide genes in disorders characterized by lack of a functional gene, such as cystic fibrosis. Such a virus would be required to be non-toxic to the target cell. Viral vectors may also be useful in treating some tumours (see TUMOUR), in which cells are rapidly and abnormally dividing to produce new tissue. In this case, viruses which require cell division to replicate may be useful, and may be targeted against the tumour, inferring toxicity only against those cells which are actively dividing.

See also: gene transfer in the CNS; transgenic

FIONA M. INGLIS

virtual reality A 'catch-all' term for computer-generated simulated environments with which subjects may interact via sensory and motor interfaces. At present these include head-mounted display systems that can generate illusion of 3-dimensional stereoscopic images and sensor gloves which permit the apparent manipulation of the artificial environment. It is likely that such interface systems will become increasingly sophisticated, enhancing the degree to which subjects can become immersed in the virtual world. There are many potential applications, ranging from the study of perceptual psychology to, with the use of robots, the virtual exploration of dangerous environments

and the practice of surgery 'at a distance'. Some commentators have raised ethical questions about the use of virtual environments and the disabled.

IAN C. REID

virus (plural: viruses) A virus is a curious thing: it is a particle, very much smaller than a normal animal CELL or even bacteria, constructed from a protein coating (called a CAPSID) inside which is nucleic acid. Sometimes the protein coat is covered in a membrane, sometimes not. Viruses lack the structure of cells (they are in fact the size of SUBCELLULAR ORGANS such as RIBOSOMES) and are capable of aggregating into crystals, which no animal cells can do. The nucleic acid they contain is a GENOME: it may be a double or single strand of DNA or RNA – viruses with RNA are called *RNA viruses*, those with DNA, *DNA viruses*. The number of genes they have can vary from only four to hundreds. Viruses cannot reproduce on their own: they must infect a host cell to do so. For some, the host is very specific – particular cell types in particular species – but for other viruses, a variety of cells from a variety of species are satisfactory hosts. What a virus does is always the same though: they infect cells, placing their own DNA or RNA into the host, using the cellular machinery to reproduce their DNA or RNA, before assembling new capsids which form new viruses that exit the cell. This process is likely to destroy the host cell.

Viruses are of interest to neuroscience in respect of three things: first, there are NEUROTROPIC viruses that infect the CENTRAL NERVOUS SYSTEM. Rabies virus is an example of this. Second, modern molecular biology has provided tools with which to control viral expression. A VIRAL VECTOR is a powerful tool with which to manipulate gene expression experimentally in cells (see GENE TRANSFER IN THE CNS). Third, viri are used as TRACT TRACERS.

See also: encephalitis; prion disease

Reference
Campbell N.A., Reece J.B. & Mitchell L.G. (1999) *Biology*, 5th edn, Addison-Wesley: Menlo Park CA.

viscera (The term VISCERA is plural; the singular is *viscus*, directly from Latin) The viscera are the internal organs contained within the chest and the abdomen: heart, lungs, liver, stomach, kidneys and so on; *visceral* is the adjectival form, and is often used not just to describe body organs but in the sense of being opposite to cerebral or rational. A *visceral reaction* would be one that was spontaneous and immediate, not thought about at all.

viscerotopic The VAGUS NERVE has a viscerotopic organization, meaning that the various VISCERA controlled by the vagus have systematically organized connections through the vagus nerve: there is a segregated portion that relates to each organ, rather than the connections being mixed.

visible spectrum The range of electromagnetic energy that can be perceived by the VISUAL SYSTEM. In humans this covers light of wavelengths from 400 to 700 nm (violet to red). Other species are able to detect different ranges.

DAVID W. HEELEY

20/20 vision *see* 6/6 notation

visual acuity Visual acuity is the fundamental measure of the ability of the VISUAL SYSTEM to partition space and as such represents the basic yardstick by which form vision is assessed. The key concepts that have driven quantification of this ability were derived initially from measurements of resolving power – that is, the ability of the visual system to resolve two closely spaced small stimuli such that they are seen as separated rather than as a single object. When the two stimuli are small points of light or thin lines, this measure is referred to as the minimum separable and is usually expressed in terms of the minimum angular subtense of the two stimuli at the nodal point of the eye that permits them to be seen as separate. As a sensitivity measure, VISUAL ACUITY is defined as the reciprocal of the minimum resolvable angle.

In general, three factors are considered to dictate the resolving power of the eye at a given retinal eccentricity. (1) Even for point-like stimuli and optimum-sized pupils, the retinal image of two closely spaced stimuli is not the same as the stimuli themselves (that is, point-like) but instead the light distribution on the RETINA is spread over a finite distance and appears as two peaks separated by a trough. (2) Appreciation of the separateness of the two stimuli requires that the retinal illuminance difference between the peaks and troughs of the light distribution on the retina exceeds the threshold for detection of small intensity differences at the prevailing state of adaptation. (3) The sampling grain of the retina must be such that separate sampling elements are stimulated by the peaks and troughs of the light distribution on the retina. Under optimum testing conditions the minimum separable is about 30–35 seconds of arc for stimuli imaged in the centre of the human FOVEA, a value that fits closely with predictions based on the sampling density of foveal CONES. On the other hand, in the peripheral retina, the resolving power is considerably poorer than that predicted on the basis of the density of cone photoreceptors, but instead fits closer to predictions based on the receptive field dimensions of specific classes of retinal ganglion cells.

Contemporary testing of visual acuity in laboratory settings typically employs grating patterns or grating patches in which the edges of the grating are smoothed according to a Gaussian or related function. Such stimuli also permit measurement of the minimum contrast required to detect gratings of any size (spatial frequency) in order to generate contrast sensitivity functions. The visual acuity for gratings, equivalent to the finest grating of maximum contrast that can be resolved, represents an extreme point on this function. In clinical settings the most common targets are the familiar SNELLEN LETTERS that are typically presented in rows with letters in each row having the same size but graded in size between rows. The dimensions of the letters are constructed on the assumption that the average minimum resolution angle amongst the population at large is 1 min (as opposed to half that value in young adults in laboratory settings). A letter that can just be resolved by a normal subject so defined has limbs and spaces between limbs that subtend a visual angle of 1 min and has an overall angular subtense of 5 min. By convention, testing is conducted at either 6 m or 20 feet and so the letter size that is just resolvable by a normal subject would have linear dimensions such that its angular subtense is 5 min when viewed from 6 m. Subjects with reduced vision will recognize only letters having larger dimensions. The acuity is defined as a fraction in which the numerator is the testing distance (usually 6 m) and the denominator is the distance at which the letter read by the subject would subtend 5 min (or its limbs 1 min). A person with normal vision will have a Snellen acuity of 6/6 or better, while a person who reads only the top letter on a conventional eye chart will have an acuity score of 6/60 (see 6/6 NOTATION).

The ability to partition space may also be assessed by measures of the smallest discriminable difference in the position of stimuli. The prime exemplar of this is VERNIER ACUITY that measures the minimum displacement that permits perception of misalignment. This amazing ability (5 sec of arc or better) is exploited practically in vernier scales or in slide-rules. Other measures that probe the ability to assign location include the ability to perceive differences in width, length or orientation of two stimuli. In principle, the location of a stimulus requires only the detection of the centroid of the distribution of the RETINAL IMAGE of that feature, a task that can be achieved with arbitrary precision provided that sufficient quanta are available. As such, location acuities (collectively referred to as HYPERACUITIES) are not limited by the sampling densities of receptors as is the case for resolution acuity.

DONALD E. MITCHELL

visual agnosia *see* agnosia; apperceptive agnosia; associative agnosia; integrative agnosia; prosopagnosia

visual cortex The visual cortex is located in the occipital lobes (see OCCIPITAL LOBE). Because the visual pathway is partially crossed, the left visual cortex receives from the left side of each retina and represents the right visual field. The term visual cortex refers strictly to area V1 (see AREAS VI–V5) in PRIMATES. Also known as PRIMARY VISUAL CORTEX, or STRIATE CORTEX or area 17 (see BRODMANN'S AREAS), it contains a complete map of its half of the

visual field. The higher-order visual areas are located in areas 18 and 19 and other regions. The term VISUAL CORTEX is often used to refer to the collection of areas including both the striate cortex and the EXTRASTRIATE CORTEX which have been heavily implicated in the processing of visual information (such as and are concerned with motion, depth, colour and orientation of edges). There are at least 25 such areas expanding over all four lobes of the CEREBRAL CORTEX, with several hundred connections between them and may account for over 50% of the primate cortical area.

KAZUE SEMBA AND ROBERT J. SNOWDEN

visual defect A visual defect refers to subnormal vision that cannot be attributed to an abnormality of either the optics of the EYE or the oculomotor system. More specifically, the condition is defined by reduced performance on detection or discrimination tasks that probe the efficacy of processing of one or more of the major visual stimulus attributes of brightness, motion (see MOTION PERCEPTION), colour (see COLOUR VISION), stereodepth (see DEPTH PERCEPTION), or form (see PATTERN PERCEPTION). The magnitude of the defect is usually indexed by the extent of elevation of either or both an absolute or differential threshold. Since thresholds and sensitivity are reciprocally related, visual defects can also be quantified in terms of the loss of sensitivity. Visual defects can be either general, affecting all stimulus attributes, or specific, when the defect is confined to a single attribute as occurs with the common inherited forms of defective colour vision. Here, the visual defect is restricted to colour and is manifested by elevation of the absolute thresholds for certain wavelengths of light and by even larger increases in differential thresholds that measure the smallest change in wavelength that produces a perceptible alteration of hue (colour). Visual defects should be distinguished from visual agnosias (see AGNOSIA) which are characterized by an inability to identify or name particular classes of objects. Agnosias are not usually accompanied by changes in visual thresholds and for this reason are thought to result from defects of higher levels of processing than the impairments of (low-level) processing that result in visual deficits. Visual deficits can result from a variety of causes such as from disease, damage due to mechanical or circulatory injury, or from abnormalities of neural development. Defects may be evident in the vision of only one eye or in parts of the visual field of both eyes. Indeed, the localization of the visual deficit in the visual field can provide diagnostic clues to the level in the visual pathway that may be affected. Unless quite circumscribed in extent, visual deficits that result from a LESION or disease are profound and affect the processing of all stimulus attributes. However, circumscribed lesions to certain brain regions may produce specific defects. A case in point is provided by subject X, who has acquired a visual deficit specific to the perception of motion. Visual deficits that can be linked to abnormalities of neural development can also be specific. For example, the visual defects associated with the common developmental disorder, amblyopia, are most evident in tests of form vision.

See also: achromatopsia; blindsight; quadrantanopsia; scotoma

visual development Studies of human infants show that the newborn, starting with very limited visual behaviour, develops over the first months of life many of the complex visual processes of pattern perception and depth perception. Neurophysiological and anatomical evidence, and clinical observations, show that this is achieved by a programmed sequence of maturation interacting closely with activation by the environment.

At birth, the infant can orient with saccadic (see SACCADE) eye movements towards high contrast targets, a function probably mediated by the SUPERIOR COLLICULUS, but function of the VISUAL CORTEX is at the best rudimentary. Behavioural and evoked potential measurements show the onset after birth of cortical visual processes: orientation selectivity around 3–6 weeks of age; directional motion selectivity (see MOTION PERCEPTION) around 7–8 weeks; and binocular interaction yielding stereodepth perception (see DEPTH PERCEPTION) around 10–15 weeks. The infant can use perspective information for depth perception by about 6 months. Alongside the qualitative emergence of

these functions, there are steady quantitative improvements in vision. The VISUAL ACUITY of the newborn is 2–4% of the adult's, improves rapidly in the early months, but approaches adult levels asymptotically only after 2–3 years. The range of velocity for motion perception, and the range of RETINAL DISPARITY for stereo vision, also expand quantitatively after the initial onset of these processes. Control of EYE MOVEMENTS improves over the first few months. Infants become able to shift their fixation point by voluntary saccades, rather than the reflex capture of gaze by conspicuous targets. Smooth pursuit of moving targets is seen from about 2 months. This control is believed to reflect increasingly effective modulation, by the cortex, of the subcortical systems that direct eye movements.

Even the immature visual processes of the young infant can be effectively exploited for specific perceptual needs. Specific responses to face-like patterns, and discrimination between faces (see FACE PERCEPTION) have been demonstrated in the first week of life. Infants can use directional motion information to group and segment visual objects, to recognize 3-dimensional structure, and to distinguish characteristically human action patterns, within 1–2 months of the first demonstrated directional discriminations. Maturation of the RETINA is one factor limiting infants' visual function. At birth, the cone photoreceptors (see CONES) of the fovea centralis are small and sparsely spaced. Although this imposes a serious limit on acuity and contrast sensitivity, overall visual development probably depends more critically on neural changes, especially in the cortex. Well before birth, all cortical neurons have been formed and migrated to their final positions, and fibres from the LATERAL GENICULATE NUCLEUS have entered the cortex. However, the number of synapses in visual cortex greatly increases during the first six postnatal months, presumably establishing the organization of cortical receptive fields required for orientation- and direction-selectivity, binocular interaction, and high acuity. A significant decline in the number of synapses after 6–9 months implies that the initially established neural connections are selectively pruned to refine this organization (see SYNAPTIC PRUNING).

The establishment and selection of connections in the visual system is determined by the pattern of neural activity. Even before birth (and thus before any true visual experience), blocking activity in the optic nerve disrupts the organization of the lateral geniculate nucleus: synchronous action potentials arising from orderly waves of spontaneous activity in the foetal retina appear to play a part in determining the pattern of inputs to lateral geniculate nucleus cells. Activity-dependent modifications of connections, in lateral geniculate nucleus and in visual cortex, are believed to depend on the HEBBIAN SYNAPSE which becomes stronger when presynaptic and postsynaptic activity coincide. Activity-dependent plasticity in connections has been most fully explored in the development of binocular interaction. If a kitten or young monkey is deprived of vision through one eye, there is a shrinkage of the ocular dominance columns in area V1 (see AREAS V1–V5) which receive input from that eye. Cortical cells become exclusively connected to the other eye, reflecting a competition between inputs in which the more active eye wins. If the two eyes receive uncoordinated input (for example, because they are looking in different directions in STRABISMUS), then each eye retains connections to a group of cortical cells, but no single cell becomes connected to both eyes. This is consistent with Hebbian theory (see HEBB'S POSTULATE), which predicts that binocular connections to a cell will only survive if input activity from the two eyes coincides. These synaptic changes can only be produced during a critical period in early life, after which cortical connections become relatively fixed. The experimental effects in animals are a model for the AMBLYOPIA and loss of stereoscopic vision which occur in humans with early strabismus or deprivation of pattern vision in one eye. Experiments in which kittens are deprived of visual exposure to certain contour orientations, or to smooth image motion, have shown that orientation- and direction-selectivity of cortical cells, like binocular interaction, depend on an appropriate pattern of input activity. As yet, little is known about the development of the more complex patterns of connectivity which determine the properties of cells in EXTRASTRIATE CORTEX. However, it seems certain that these properties also must become established by activity-dependent selection among the synapses which are made potentially available in the genetic programme for cortical development. In this way, the visual system becomes sensitive to the specific types of stimulus encountered in the environment in which it develops.

Reference

Daw N.W. (1995) *Visual Development*, Plenum Press: New York.

OLIVER J. BRADDICK

visual direction The visual direction of one object relative to another is coded by the positions of their RETINAL IMAGE – their retinal local signs. The smallest detectable difference in direction is VISUAL ACUITY. At the FOVEA, acuity is about 2 seconds of arc, considerably less than receptor spacing. In judging directions relative to the head we take eye position into account and for directions relative to the body we take head position into account. We judge the position of an isolated point of light relative to the head with a precision of about 1°. A small light in dark surroundings appears to wander about at random – the AUTOKINETIC EFFECT. Muscular factors can be demonstrated by straining eyes or head to the left for a minute, returning to the straight ahead position and noting that a point of light straight ahead appears displaced to the right. After an eye movement it takes about 0.1 second to recompute perceived directions. When the eyes are moved rapidly to and fro, perception fails to keep up and the world appears unstable – we experience OSCILLOPSIA. People with unstable gaze experience oscillopsia constantly. Also, the world appears unstable when we push an eye with a finger or when we visually pursue a moving finger. We achieve visual stability in the rest intervals between eye movements. We allow for the eyes being in different positions by judging visual directions as if from a cyclopean eye midway between the eyes. This can be demonstrated by holding a horizontal card to the eyes with a line extending from the centre of each pupil to an apex on the opposite side of the card. When the eyes converge on the apex the two lines appear as one line pointing towards the cyclopean eye. A single line directed to the bridge of the nose appears as two lines intersecting where the eyes converge. The line appears single and in its correct direction relative to the cyclopean eye only at the point of image intersection. This is because the images of this point fall on corresponding retinal points in the two eyes. At all other points the line appears double and subject to errors of reaching because the images fall on non-corresponding points.

References

Howard I.P. (1982) *Human Visual Orientation*, Wiley: Chichester.

Howard I.P. & Rogers B.J. (1995) *Binocular Vision and Stereopsis*, Oxford University Press: New York.

IAN P. HOWARD

visual efficiency An experimental technique, often based on SIGNAL DETECTION THEORY, that compares the sensory performance of an observer with that of a so-called 'ideal observer' whose theoretical performance is limited solely by the signal-to-noise ratio inherent in the stimulus. Ideal observers are assumed to use all of the information in the stimulus that is available to them. Visual efficiencies that have been measured vary widely and depend critically on the nature of the task. Cases of nearly 100% efficiency have been reported, whereas other processes such as stereoscopic vision have been shown to have efficiencies that are below 10%.

DAVID W. HEELEY

visual field The field of view is described as the envelope of positions in space that denote the maximum distance that an object can be displaced in any direction from the FIXATION point and still be reported as visible. In the horizontal meridian the boundary of the field of view of each eye on its own is limited in one direction (the nasal side) by the nose to approximately 45° from the fixation point. However, on the other (temporal) side, the boundary extends more that 90° from the fixation point, to about 95°. When both eyes are open the nose no longer provides a barrier, since objects blocked from view of one eye by the nose can still be seen by the other eye. As a consequence, when both eyes are open the full field of view in the horizontal meridian is about 190° as compared to about 140° for each eye on its own. With binocular viewing the field of view can be divided into three parts, a central region referred to as the BINOCULAR field of view in which objects are visible simultaneously to both eyes, flanked on either side by two monocular segments within which objects are visible exclusively to the ipsilateral eye. Certain species of animals, such as horses, with eyes positioned laterally in the head, possess small binocular but large monocular fields so that the total field of view can exceed 300°. Damage at any level of the visual system can result in visual field defects representing regions of the visual field where objects cannot be seen. Such a region, a SCOTOMA, can be either absolute, in which case objects of any intensity are not visible, or relative, where only dim stimuli are invisible, Even normal subjects possess a small absolute scotoma in the visual field of each eye (the blind spot) representing the projection into space of the optic nerve head. Because the limits of the visual field are determined in response to conscious reports by the subject, they are thought to probe the efficacy of the geniculostriate pathway (see GENICULOSTRIATE AND TECTOPULVINAR VISUAL PATHWAYS), a conclusion supported by the condition referred to as BLINDSIGHT. Certain rare subjects with extensive lesions of the striate cortex and profound absolute scotomata, nevertheless can make saccadic eye movements (see SACCADE) in the direction of objects presented in the scotoma as well as make forced choice judgements as to their colour, orientation and position in the absence of conscious awareness of the stimuli.

DONALD E. MITCHELL

visual form agnosia An inability to recognize objects with preserved ability to use those same objects.

See also: agnosia

visual imagery Visual imagery refers to the phenomenal experience that goes along with visual perception. When we look at something, there are two logically distinct types of mental event that happen. First, readinesses to act are set up: if one sees a glass of water then a series of visual measurements are made that can provide the information that would be required to allow one to pick the glass up. In this sense, one has a readiness in response to the glass. Second, one has a phenomenal experience of the glass. This phenomenal experience is rather like a picture, in that the spatial layouts of different things seem directly analogous to their actual layout in the scene. In this way, vision can appear to place us in a mental analogue of the scene. A simple case to illustrate this point is found with the sensations of colour. Imagine that another person exists, for whom the experience of two colours, red and green, is reversed compared with you. This person will still call grass green and roses red, because that is how they will have learned the meanings of the colour words. This person will still understand red as the complementary colour to green. In short to any third party there will seem to be no difference between you and the other person in all respects of behaviour. The readiness for behaviour in the two people is identical and it would be impossible to establish whether there was any difference in their experience because that experience can only be expressed through readiness to act. As will be appreciated from this, experimental study of visual imagery has proven very difficult. An important line of approach has been concerned with situations where the analogue nature of visual imagery has been exploited. If subjects are shown two patterns, one being a spatial rotation of the other and asked to verify their similarity, then the amount of time that their response takes depends on the size of the angle of rotation. The implication of this result is that subjects are rotating one of the two inside their head, just as an analogy of real rotation, until the two match. The larger the rotation, the longer it takes to accomplish the process. As well as being involved, somehow, in perception, visual imagery is also involved in processes that require spatial memory or can benefit from the application of spatial memory. Thus, when asked to report how many windows their home has, most if not all subjects will generate a memory visual image of their home and then proceed to inspect this image to count the windows.

See also: illusions

ROGER J. WATT

visual pigment The visual pigments are contained within the outer segments of the photoreceptors in the RETINA. They comprise a large opsin molecule which links through the membranes of the discs of the outer segment, and attached to which is a much smaller, light-sensitive retinal molecule (or CHROMOPHORE), an ALDEHYDE of vitamin A (see VITAMINS). Absorption of a photon of light induces a change in the shape of the chromophore which is followed by a cascade of chemical reactions that are the initial phases of the visual process. Differences in the exact molecular structure of the opsin lead to differences in the wavelength of light that is absorbed most strongly. The combination of different chromophores and opsins is therefore the basis of the family of differing photopigments.

See also: spectral sensitivity curves

DAVID W. HEELEY

visual search In visual search tasks, subjects look for a target item among a variable number of distractor items. For example, subjects might be asked to look for the letter 'F' in a display filled with other letters. There are several visual search literatures using the basic method for different, if related purposes. Three of these are: (1) an applied literature, concerned with search strategies in specific, real-world tasks (such as driving, interpretation of photo-reconnaissance or radiologic images); (2) studies of control of EYE MOVEMENTS (for example in reading). Most real-world search tasks involve eye movements because, even if the target is present in the visual field, limitations on visual processing in peripheral parts of the field require that items be fixated before they can be identified. (3) Studies of basic processes in visual perception. In the perception studies, an effort is made to distinguish between visual properties that can be identified without search and those properties requiring search. In a standard experiment, the number of items in a display (set size) is varied from trial to trial and the time to respond 'yes' or 'no' to the presence of the target is recorded (see REACTION TIME). For some tasks, reaction time does not increase with set size (for example, finding a red item among green items). This suggests parallel processing (see PARALLEL VS. SERIAL PROCESSING) of all items. This is possible for targets defined by a set of perhaps a dozen pre-attentive features (colour, orientation, size, various depth cues and so on). These features are similar to those that produce effortless segmentation of different regions in texture perception. In other cases, reaction time increases as a linear function of set size (for example, finding a T among Ls of various orientations). In these cases, the slope of the reaction time by set size function is roughly twice as great for trials with the target absent as for trials where the target is present. This pattern of results suggests serial, item-by-item search that terminates when the item is found. Alternatively, items may be processed in parallel but with a limited processing capacity so that the amount of processing per item declines as the number of items increases. Most real-world searches are hybrids in which some pre-attentive feature information can be used to aid search even if the target is not defined by a unique feature.

See also: attention; Stroop effect

Reference

Wolfe J.M. (1997) Visual search. In *Attention*, ed. H. Pashler, pp. 13–73, University College London Press: London.

                                                    JEREMY M. WOLFE

visual senescence The decline in visual performance that accompanies AGEING. Senescent changes range from a loss of the elasticity of the capsule of the eye lens, to more subtle decrements in acuity, losses of contrast sensitivity and alterations of colour perception.

                                                    DAVID W. HEELEY

visual suppression *see* saccadic omission

visual symmetry Symmetry is a mathematical concept concerning the presence of two or more copies of the same feature in an image, distinguished by some transformation. In its most restricted sense, symmetry refers to the bilateral symmetry derived from mirror reflection of features about a linear axis (such as the frontal view of a human face). More generally, symmetry refers to multiple copies of features after any spatial transformation, such as lateral translation, rotation, expansion, contraction or shear (in addition to reflection), or any combination of such transformations. In concert with these spatial transformations, visual symmetry encompasses transformations of local qualities such as contrast reversal and shifts of luminance and colour.

Reference

Washburn D.K. & Crowe D.S. (1988) *Symmetries of Culture*, University of Washington Press: Seattle.

                                                    CHRISTOPHER TYLER

visual system The visual system is the part of the BRAIN that receives information from the eyes and processes that information to facilitate actions and decisions. The information received and processed can be used to control directly undertaken actions, such as walking or grasping an object, but can also be used to facilitate the planning of future actions. The first stage of the visual system is to be found in the EYE itself. An image of the scene is focused by the lens of the eye on to the RETINA, the layer of photosensitive cells or receptors which lines the back of the eye. The light causes a pattern of electrical activity in the receptor cells. This pattern is converted into a pattern of neuronal impulses at the stage of the retinal ganglion cells. These cells send axons up the OPTIC NERVE and into the brain proper. The information first gets processed at the LATERAL GENICULATE NUCLEUS (LGN) and is then passed on to the VISUAL CORTEX. These early stages of the visual system are generally concerned with ensuring that the best quality of information is recovered from the image as possible. For example, the range of luminances in a scene can be extremely high – much beyond the capacity of the bandwidth of the visual system. Some parts of the image are very dim and the luminance differences are very small, but at the same time, other parts of the image can be very bright and have relatively large luminance differences. The early stages of the visual system are concerned with making sure that, whatever the local image luminance is, the important contrast information is received at the visual cortex, where the bulk of the visual processing occurs.

After the lateral geniculate nucleus, some of the visual information is passed on to the SUPERIOR COLLICULUS, where it is responsible for controlling eye movements. The majority of the information however, gets passed up into the visual cortex. In the visual cortex, the information from the retinal image is analysed in a variety of different ways to extract information about spatial luminance pattern (mainly edges and texture), motion, depth and colour. The visual cortex is split up into a number of different visual areas, each with its own retinotopic mapping of the visual field (see AREAS V1–V5). Within each visual area, there is a considerable degree of specialization of function. A major feature of most visual areas is that the cells in these areas tend to have receptive fields that are considerably smaller than the whole visual field. This means that each cell is processing information from a small part of space. The whole visual field is covered by arranging for a large number of cells to process the information at each stage, each covering a slightly different part of the visual field. In the first visual area, V1, cells have receptive fields that indicate that they are each individually sensitive to a bar or edge of a particular size and orientation light and moving in a particular direction. These cells are organized into a column of cells, within which all orientations and spatial scales from the one retinal region are processed. The output of these cells in V1 can be thought of as comprising a register of the local structures within the image. There are various classes of cells, differing in the extent to which the pattern they are optimally sensitive to is contrast specific (so-called simple cells, are tuned to an edge or bar of a particular contrast direction, whereas so-called complex cells are tuned to an edge or bar of any contrast direction – see SIMPLE, COMPLEX AND HYPERCOMPLEX CELLS).

Later stages of processing in the visual pathway are involved in processing higher level aspects of the visual stimulus. One of these, the sensation of colour, has been studied to some considerable extent (see COLOUR VISION). The colour of a surface is a property of that surface that does not vary significantly with changes in how the surface is illuminated, even though the intensity of the light at different wavelengths will change. Thus a red surface looks red whether it is illuminated with light that has a reddish or a bluish tinge to it. This phenomenon is referred to as COLOUR CONSTANCY. Cells in V1 are typically sensitive to the wavelength of the light that they receive and are thus not colour constant, whereas cells at a later stage of processing in V4 tend to show responses that are related to the colour of the surface that falls within their receptive field, irrespective of the wavelength composition of the light involved. Other visual areas at this stage of processing are involved in similar complex computations, such as the MIDDLE TEMPORAL REGION (area MT), which is concerned with spatial aspects of motion processing and spatial form.

The visual system projects information, after processing to this level, onwards in at least two different directions (see TWO CORTICAL VISUAL STREAMS). One projection is up through the TEMPORAL LOBE towards sites in the brain where memory information of various types is held. This projection is thought to be much involved in object recognition. Another projection is forwards in the brain towards the MOTOR CORTEX areas, where the information from vision is used to control actions, such as LOCOMOTION.

ROGER J. WATT

visuomotor control When you carry out an action under visual guidance, whether it be an eye movement towards a sudden light or an arm movement to pick up a cup or catch a ball, the visual information you use may not necessarily correspond with the visual percept you have of the stimulus. There are many examples of dissociations, usually brought about by the use of visual illusions. A light flash may appear in a place shifted from its real location, due to the displacement of a surrounding frame; but one's eye movement or arm reach is generally carried out correctly to the true location. In recent experiments, geometric ILLUSIONS have been used that cause the size of one object to appear different from that of another, identical, object. Yet despite the perceptual system being deceived, the visuomotor system was not; the hand grip opened correctly in anticipation of grasping the object, irrespective of the illusion. It is now realized that visual processing is not done by a single monolithic system in the brain. Indeed a lesion to the posterior part of the PARIETAL LOBE in humans and monkeys will cause impairments in the visual control of action (REACHING, EYE MOVEMENTS, GRASP and so on) while frequently not affecting the ability to perceive or discriminate the very visual cues that cannot guide action. Conversely, bilateral damage that affects the inferior OCCIPITAL LOBE and TEMPORAL LOBE may cause profound difficulties in the perception and discrimination of shape and form, while leaving intact the control of actions with respect to those same visual properties.

These behavioural findings are supported by electrophysiological recordings from single neurons in the visual areas of the brain (see SINGLE-UNIT ELECTROPHYSIOLOGICAL RECORDING). In the occipitotemporal system (the VENTRAL STREAM) neurons are selectively responsive to a range of object properties, such as their colour, size, orientation, shape, and texture. Some cells in the temporal lobe can even learn about different patterns. But none respond differentially according to the current behaviour of the animal. In contrast, many neurons in the occipitoparietal system (the DORSAL STREAM) are selectively activated by a visual stimulus not so much by what it looks like, but instead according to the action that the animal makes with respect to the stimulus. Visuomotor control is not achieved purely by cortical systems. These have evolved to sharpen and modulate specialized visuomotor systems located throughout the NEURAXIS from the PONS and CEREBELLUM, through the MIDBRAIN (the SUPERIOR COLLICULUS for example) and THALAMUS, up to the BASAL GANGLIA.

A. DAVID MILNER

visuospatial scratch pad *see* visuospatial sketch pad

visuospatial sketch pad (Also known under an older name, VISUOSPATIAL SCRATCH PAD) The visuospatial sketch pad is a component of WORKING MEMORY, as detailed by Alan Baddeley and his colleagues. It is involved in processing the MEMORY for recently seen information – that is, what things look like and where they are in space relative to each other, and to the viewer. Its operations are supervised by the CENTRAL EXECUTIVE, to which it is a slave system, operating in parallel with the ARTICULATORY LOOP (which is also known as the PHONOLOGICAL LOOP).

References

Baddeley A.D. & Hitch G. (1974) Working memory. In *The Psychology of Learning and Motivation*, ed. G.A. Bower, pp. 47–90, Academic Press: New York.

vitamins A neologism from Latin, *vita*: life and amine (which is not correct: vitamins are organic molecules but not amines). Small quantities of specific vitamins are essential for proper body functioning – vitamin deficiencies are associated with a wide variety of specific disorders (see MALNUTRITION). Vitamins A, D, E and K are fat-soluble; those of the vitamin B complex (there are many subtypes of vitamin B) and vitamin C are water-soluble. The vitamins essential for humans are: B1 (thiamine), B2 riboflavin, B6 (pyroxidone), B12, vitamin C (ascorbic acid), niacin, pantothenic acid, folic acid and biotin (these are all water-soluble); and A (retinol), D, E (tocopherol) and K (phylloquinone). Of special interest to biological psychologists are vitamin B1 (thiamine), which is associated with KORSAKOFF'S SYNDROME, and vitamin A (retinol) which is associated with the VISUAL SYSTEM. Ascorbic acid (ascorbate) is used as an anti-oxidant (see OXIDATION) in drug solution preparation and folic acid has been reported possibly to act as an excitotoxin (but only in exceptionally large doses) (see EXCITOTOXINS).

Reference

Campbell N.A., Reece J.B. & Mitchell L.G. (1999) *Biology*, 5th edn, Addison-Wesley: Menlo Park CA.

vitreous humour The substance lying between the LENS and RETINA in the EYE.

vocalization *see* alarm call; animal communication; birdsong; distress call; laughter; social behaviour

Vogel conflict A CONFLICT TEST in which an appetitive UNCONDITIONED BEHAVIOUR such as licking for water is simultaneously punished by an unconditioned aversive event such as FOOT-SHOCK.

See also: animal models of anxiety; aversive conditioning; Geller–Seifter conflict

A. SIMON KILLCROSS

volatile anaesthetics Volatile organic liquids composed typically of halogenated hydrocarbons and applied as inhalational general anaesthetic agents – for example halothane, enflurane, methoxyflurane, and isoflurane.

See also: anaesthesia

CHARLES D. BLAHA

volition (from late Latin, *volitio*: an act of will) Volition is the act of willing. A difference is drawn between willed actions – volition acts – and those that are automatic or reflex.

See also: voluntary

voltage *see* voltage clamp

voltage clamp A voltage clamp is a technique used in NEUROPHYSIOLOGY for studying ION CHANNEL activity in membranes. One records the voltage required to prevent the MEMBRANE POTENTIAL from changing to obtain a measure of current across the membrane. The technique was used in the 1950s by Alan Hodgkin and Andrew Huxley in their classic experiments on the squid giant axon which established much of what is now known about neuronal membrane activity. The work of Hodgkin and Huxley was rewarded by the Nobel Prize for Physiology or Medicine in 1963.

What a neurophysiologist can do with a voltage clamp is hold the voltage of a membrane constant and measure the current; with a current clamp, it is possible to do the reverse – to hold the current constant and measure the voltage across the membrane. Current (the SI unit of current is the amp, symbol A) is a flow of electricity; voltage (the SI unit of voltage is the VOLT, symbol V) is a measure of potential difference – that is the difference in electrical potential between two points. In neurophysiological terms, measures of CURRENT represent the movement of ions across a membrane (in

effect, the degree of ion channel opening) while measures of VOLTAGE represent the difference in electrical potential (that is, how positively charged one side of a membrane is with respect to the other side). Action potentials are expressed as voltage; single unit electrophysiological recording is in effect a current clamp.

See also: extracellular recording; intracellular recording

voltage-dependent ion channels *see* voltage-sensitive ion channels

voltage-gated ion channels *see* voltage-sensitive ion channels

voltage-sensitive dye recording These are dyes (see STAINS) that show fluorescence. Changes in MEMBRANE POTENTIAL affect the fluorescence (that is, the degree of fluorescence is voltage sensitive) which can be visualized, allowing one to track neuronal activity in a dynamic manner. Questions about which neurons respond to activation can be examined using this anatomical technique

voltage-sensitive ion channels The permeability of axon membranes to SODIUM (Na^+) and POTASSIUM (K^+) ions is dependent on the voltage across the membrane. That is, the opening of these ion channels is *voltage sensitive* (or *voltage dependent*, or *voltage gated*: all of these terms are more or less synonymous). Voltage-sensitive channel activity is critical in ACTION POTENTIAL conduction. This is in contrast to ion channels on cell bodies and dendrites which are generally ligand-gated – that is, the opening and closing of ion channels is dependent on the biding of a LIGAND (normally a neurotransmitter) to a receptor molecule (see IONOTROPIC and METABOTROPIC). Ligand-gated ion channel opening is critical in the generation of EXCITATORY POSTSYNAPTIC POTENTIAL and INHIBITORY POSTSYNAPTIC POTENTIAL (EPSP/IPSP) activity. Voltage-sensitive and ligand-gated ion channels are independent, in the sense that they are clearly discriminable processes, but interdependent in that the generation of action potentials, mediated by the actions of neurotransmitters at ligand-gated receptors, triggers the axon DEPOLARIZATION upon which voltage-sensitive ion channels depend.

The mechanisms through which voltage-sensitive ion channels work are complicated. Sodium channels are normally kept closed by a voltage-sensitive gating process, but when the membrane is depolarized they open. However, if this is all there was, then sodium would continuously flow inwards – some other mechanism must act to close the channel. There are two mechanisms for this: first, each sodium channel itself appears to self-regulate; and second the opening of other channels has an effect on the membrane also. The self-regulation appears to come about by each sodium channel behaving as if it had two gates: an *activation gate* and *inactivation gate*. At the resting potential neither gate is operational. When the membrane is depolarized the activation gate opens and the inactivation gate slowly closes. The channel remains open until closed by a combination of inactivation channel operation and by potassium channel opening, which causes a reduction in membrane potential.

The operations of voltage-sensitive channel opening and closing are much more complex than can be described here; see Kandel *et al.* (1991) for an introduction to this topic.

See also: neurophysiology; patchclamp; voltage clamp

Reference

Kandel E.R., Schwartz J.H. & Jessell T.M. (2000) *Principles of Neural Science*, 4th edn, McGraw-Hill: New York.

voltammetry Several related electrochemistry techniques used to measure the concentration in animals – either anaesthetized or awake and behaving – of electroactive compounds, such as MONOAMINE NEUROTRANSMITTERS (for example DOPAMINE, NORADRENALINE and SEROTONIN) or their metabolites (see METABOLISM), that overflow into extracellular space during release from neurons. Commonly referred to as IN VIVO VOLTAMMETRY, these recording techniques include potential scanning (for example DIFFERENTIAL PULSE, SLOW POTENTIAL SWEEP, and RAPID SCAN VOLTAMMETRY) and potential pulse procedures (for example CHRONOAMPEROMETRY and CHRONOCOULOMETRY). Voltammetry provides the means to measure both slow and rapid changes in neurotransmitter

EFFLUX, such as those following drug administration or behavioural stimulation (Blaha & Phillips, 1996) and those occurring as a result of brief electrical stimulation of neuronal fibres or local application of potassium ions (K^+) (Kawogoe *et al.*, 1993). Most voltammetric procedures employ one of several types of carbon-based electrochemical recording microelectrodes (such as CARBON PASTE ELECTRODES and microcarbon fibres), in combination with an auxiliary and reference electrode. These microelectrodes are relatively small (10–200 m diameters) permitting measurements within very small brain areas. A potentiostat circuit is utilized to control and apply the various voltage waveforms across the auxiliary-microelectrode pair to induce the oxidation or reduction of a compound at the microelectrode surface. In the case of anodic potential scanning procedures, a ramped positive-going voltage is applied to the microelectrode resulting in a flow of oxidation current that is measured and plotted with respect to the applied voltage resulting in a peak-shaped wave, a VOLTAMMOGRAM. Reversal of the waveform in the negative-going cathodic direction may result in the re-REDUCTION of the species at the microelectrode surface. In the case of anodic potential pulse procedures, a positive-going voltage pulse (0.1–1 sec duration) is applied at relatively brief intervals (0.1–60 sec). OXIDATION current is integrated over a significant duration of the applied pulse (chronocoulometry) or at the end of the pulse (chronoamperometry) with the resulting current displayed as a function of time. Thus, as an applied potential is varied, an electroactive species such as dopamine oxidizes near the microelectrode surface and loses electrons to the microelectrode. The resulting current flow thereby serves as a direct quantitative measure of the concentration of the electroactive species in solution.

See also: dialysis

References

Blaha C.D. & Phillips A.G. (1996) A critical assessment of electrochemical procedures applied to the measurement of dopamine and its metabolites during drug-induced and species-typical behaviours. *Behavioural Pharmacology* 7 : 675–708.

Kawagoe K.T., Zimmerman J.B. & Wightman

R.M. (1993) Principles of voltammetry and microelectrode surface states. *Journal of Neuroscience Methods* 48: 225–240.

CHARLES D. BLAHA

voltammogram Oxidation/reduction current profiles of electroactive substances recorded with respect to applied voltages at an electrode surface using, for instance, RAPID SCAN VOLTAMMETRY.

See also: voltammetry

CHARLES D. BLAHA

volume conduction Volume conduction is the flow of ionic (see ION) currents or the propagation of electric potentials through the extracellular space. Its properties are determined by the electrical characteristics of the source and the extracellular space. Volume conduction is the basis of the ELECTROENCEPHALOGRAM (EEG), which is recorded by relatively large electrodes (see ELECTRODE) and reflects the activity of neurons at a distance. The human EEG recorded on the scalp is based on volume conduction through both the brain tissue and the skin. The HIPPOCAMPAL THETA activity can be recorded via volume conduction from the CEREBRAL CORTEX overlying the HIPPOCAMPUS due to its unusually large amplitude in animals.

KAZUE SEMBA

volume transmission A means of long-distance communication between neurons. Following synaptic or somatic release (the signal source), neuroactive substances may diffuse through extracellular space several millimetres away from their site of origin to interact with receptors (see RECEPTOR), the signal targets. Volume transmission differs from classical neurochemical communication confined within nerve terminal synapses (WIRING TRANSMISSION). Separate forms of volume transmission are: (1) *private-coded signals*, exemplified by neurotransmitters released by nerve cells and recognized by specific receptors and activating SECOND MESSENGERS or cytosolic enzymes. These are neurotransmitters that may be released from sites on a neuron that are not opposite specialized postsynaptic membranes (that is, non-synaptic or PARASYNAPTIC TRANSMISSION) or may be 'overflow' from specia-

lized synapses. However, given the presence of degradative enzymes and specialized reuptake processes at synapses the amount of neurotransmitter that can escape from within a synaptic cleft is probably very limited. Non-synaptic transmitter release works in essentially the same way as hormones do: they are released from a specific site but are able to diffuse to any other site, however distant, that has appropriate receptors present. (2) *Accessible-coded signals*, such as electrical signals conveyed by all neuronal cells and recognized by almost every cell type in the central nervous system (see VOLUME CONDUCTION).

Reference

Fuxe K. & Agnati L.F. (1991) *Volume Transmission in the Brain*, Raven Press: New York.

CHARLES D. BLAHA

volumetric thirst *see* osmoregulation

voluntary (from Latin, *voluntarius*: willing, derived from *volontas*: choice, in turn derived from *velle*: to will) In biological psychology, the terms voluntary and INVOLUNTARY are applied to actions or processes that are either free and spontaneous (voluntary) or automatic and reflexive (involuntary). The voluntary MUSCLES are those striate muscles that can be controlled by an independent act of will or choice; the VOLUNTARY NERVOUS SYSTEM is an alternative term for the SOMATIC NERVOUS SYSTEM (which controls the striate muscles); and the INVOLUNTARY NERVOUS SYSTEM is an alternative term for the AUTONOMIC NERVOUS SYSTEM (which controls the internal organs in a manner that is thought to be largely automatic and without independent control).

However, use of these terms continues to generate debate. There are several broad questions that can be identified. (1) To what degree are actions dichotomized into voluntary and involuntary? The earliest theorists assumed that there was clear separation, but it is now thought that this is much less likely to be the case. For example, studies using BIOFEEDBACK have shown that it is possible to obtain a degree of voluntary control over such apparently involuntary processes as heart rate. (2) Are all voluntary actions genuinely 'voluntary'? It is not the case that all movement of the striate musculature involves voluntary control – many reflexes for example are not under voluntary control. Indeed, some authors have argued that all actions are composed of complex chains of innate reflexes and learnt actions (see for example MOTOR PROGRAMMING) that have become in a sense reflexive. As such, the very idea of a voluntary movement comes into doubt: if all movements have antecedent causes and can be decomposed into constituent parts, no account of independent volition ('free will') is required (see Prochazka et al., 2000) Such accounts are however, limited in their capacity to explain such things as the synthesis of new motor programmes in the face of novel tasks and environments, or the active suppression of behaviour which should be automatically selected. (3) Is there a distinction between voluntary and willed actions? The distinction between willed actions (actions being 'purposeful, goal-directed behaviours, usually involving movement' – see Jahanshahi & Frith, 1998) and automatic actions was drawn by William James (1842–1910). James distinguished willed acts, requiring conscious control, from what he called IDEOMOTOR ACTIONS, which were automatic actions. Jahanshahi & Frith identify willed actions in three ways: by the involvement of attention and conscious awareness (see CONSCIOUSNESS); by choice and control; and by intentionality (see INTENTION). This is a much more interesting approach to the notion of 'voluntary actions', leading to consideration of a hierarchy of types of actions. At the highest levels are willed actions that require attention in order to be properly devised and executed. But willed actions can become automatic actions – that is, they can become learnt motor programmes. Handwriting is initially effortful and requires attention, but becomes automatic; driving a motor car similarly begins as a frightening and complex process needing one's full attention, but in the course of time, this too can become automatic. Below these are actions that are more or less reflexive: catching sight in peripheral vision of an approaching object will lead to an avoidance movement – ducking for example – that is automatic, not conscious. Such actions probably depend upon

a degree of learning but are nevertheless classifiable as reflexes because of the simplicity of the neural connections between sensory input and motor output. Very basic reflexes – such as the monosynaptic STRETCH REFLEX – are the simplest form of these. Clearly, willed actions and automatic actions can be seen as forming part of a continuum from, at the one end, actions requiring a high degree of control by various psychological processes, though to actions that are automatic and require little or no cognitive processing.

The psychological processes involved in controlling willed actions are complex: Shallice's SUPERVISORY ATTENTIONAL SYSTEM is such a mechanism. Others have used the term EXECUTIVE FUNCTIONS to describe these processes. With regard to both of these processes, and now in respect of willed actions, there is some debate about the involvement of consciousness. The definition of willed action as involving attention, choice, control and intention could apply as well to a rodent as to a human. The involvement of consciousness however clouds this, since there is debate over the nature of consciousness in animals other than humans. While they are evidently conscious (they are awake and alert) are they necessarily self-aware in the same way as humans?

Clearly the terms voluntary and involuntary are the tips of conceptual icebergs. The term FOLK PSYCHOLOGY refers to those terms used in everyday language that describe our psychological states as we experience them (as opposed to the scientific terms with which we hope to dissect the machinery of our psychological states). Perhaps the best way to consider the terms voluntary and involuntary is to think of them as a type of 'folk science' term: terms without precise meaning but conveying broad ideas.

References

Jahanshahi M. & Frith C.D. (1998) Willed action and its impairments. *Cognitive Neuropsychology* 15: 483–533.
Prochazka A., Clarac F., Loeb G.E., Rothwell J.C. & Wolpaw J.R. (2000) What do reflex and voluntary mean? Modern views on an ancient debate. *Experimental Brain Research* 130: 417–432.

voluntary nervous system An alternative name for the SOMATIC NERVOUS SYSTEM.

vomer bone *see* skull

vomeronasal nerve This connects the VOMERONASAL ORGAN to the ACCESSORY OLFACTORY BULB; see OLFACTION.

vomeronasal organ The vomer (from Latin, *vomer*: a plough) is a thin bone that runs along the middle of the nasal cavity, or nose; hence vomeronasal is the term that describes this region) The vomeronasal organ is a second source of olfactory input (see OLFACTION) in addition to the OLFACTORY EPITHELIUM and is present in all mammals (except the marine mammals). Situated in the nasal passageway, it has sensory receptors which transmit to the ACCESSORY OLFACTORY BULB. It is notably important in the detection of PHEROMONES, amongst other things.

vomiting (from Latin, *vomere*: to vomit) The Greek root is *emeein*, from which the term EMESIS (a synonym for vomiting) derives. The term emesis gives rise to emetic, an agent that produces vomiting, and ANTIEMETIC, the general term given to a DRUG or other agent that suppresses the urge to vomit. NAUSEA (from Greek, *nausia*: seasickness, derived from *naus*: a ship) is a feeling of sickness leading to the likely occurrence of vomiting.

The ability to vomit food out of the GASTROINTESTINAL SYSTEM is advantageous for an organism, in that it enables it to remove poisons inadvertently eaten. FOOD-AVERSION LEARNING then helps avoid the poisoned food being eaten again. (Food-aversion learning is the only defence that animals which cannot vomit – such as rats – have against poisoning.) Stimulation of the AREA POSTREMA can trigger ejection reflexes, and it been argued that this structure functions as a vomiting centre. However, the idea that there is a unique vomiting centre reflects rather dated thinking about the control of FEEDING and DRINKING which used to be thought of in terms of specific brain centres (see DUAL CENTRES HYPOTHESIS). A single operational centre for vomiting is unlikely because of the wide variety of sensory stimuli and a complex effector mechanisms involved. Nigel Lawes (1988) suggested instead that control of the internal environment might depend on a complex system of tissue, the PARAVENTRICULAR SYSTEM, which recruits information widely and is capable of effecting various changes to body state. Simulation or lesion of various parts of this system, from the area postrema to the AMYGDALA, can trigger vomiting.

Reference

Lawes I.N.C. (1988) The central connections of area postrema define the paraventricular system involved in antinoxious behaviors. In *Nausea and Vomiting: Recent Research and Clinical Advances*, ed. J. Kucharczyk, D.J. Stewart & A.D. Miller, pp. 77–101, CRC Press: Boca Raton FL.

von Restorff effect In LEARNING, when one particular STIMULUS among a set of stimuli is distinct from all the others, information about that stimulus will be learned more quickly and retained better.

vulva *see* vagina

W

Wada test This is a test, named after its developer, that allows one to anaesthetize one cerebral HEMISPHERE. Anaesthetic – SODIUM AMYTAL has typically been used – is injected into the branch of the carotid artery, left or right, that serves one or the other hemisphere. This effectively inactivates that hemisphere temporarily, allowing psychological tests to be used to assess the functions of the non-anaesthetized hemisphere. The test was originally developed as an aid to neurosurgery: if a patient was to receive a UNILATERAL LESION of a structure (destruction of one TEMPORAL LOBE for the relief of EPILEPSY, for example) it would be important to know that the same structure on the CONTRALATERAL side could function normally.

See also: H.M.; lateralization

Reference

Wada J. & Rasmussen T. (1960) Intracarotid injection of sodium amytal for lateralization of cerebral speech dominance. *Journal of Neurosurgery* 17: 266–282.

walking *see* locomotion

Wallerian degeneration A process of neuronal degeneration described in the nineteenth century by Augustus Waller (1856–1922). When an AXON is damaged, several degenerative changes occur. The precise nature of these changes of course depends on exactly where along its length the axon is cut. Almost immediately, the ability to conduct an ACTION POTENTIAL and to engage in synaptic transmission (see SYNAPSE; NEUROTRANSMISSION) is

lost, as synthesis of PROTEINS synthesis and AXONAL TRANSPORT fail. The NEURON may however survive. For example, if the neuron has extensively collateralized axons (see COLLATERALS) with many branches, and only one branch is cut, then that branch will no longer work but the others may remain viable. The cut segment of axon – the DISTAL axon segment – degenerates slowly after the injury, and it is the degeneration of this that is known as Wallerian degeneration. About a week following the injury, gross morphological changes are apparent in the damaged axon segment: the MYELIN sheath (if present) will break down and NEUROFILAMENTS and MICROTUBULES will occupy an increasing amount of space within the axon which will begin to break up into segments. The debris created by this degeneration will gradually be cleared away by phagocytosis, a process that takes a few days in the PERIPHERAL NERVOUS SYSTEM but rather longer in the CENTRAL NERVOUS SYSTEM.

See also: lesion; nerve crush; transplantation

Reference

Kandel E.R., Schwartz J.H. & Jessell T.M. (2000) *Principles of Neural Science*, 4th edn, McGraw-Hill: New York.

water balance *see* osmoregulation

water maze A widely used apparatus for studying spatial and other types of LEARNING in rodents. Introduced by Morris (1981), it consists of a large circular pool of opaque water in which animals swim to find a hidden escape platform located at one place underneath the water surface. The platform itself offers no local cues to guide NAVIGATION but, once found, the rat or mouse can stand on it to learn its relation to extra-maze cues. The animals rapidly learn to take relatively direct escape paths and, if the platform is removed, search persistently in its former location. Modifications of this training have been introduced to study spatial event MEMORY. The task is sensitive to disruption by a variety of drugs and lesions, notably lesions of the HIPPOCAMPUS, and is now used as a screening task for learning in studies of TRANSGENIC animals.

Reference
Morris, R.G.M. (1981) Place navigation does not require the presence of local cues. *Learning and Motivation* 12: 239–260.

RICHARD G. M. MORRIS

water of crystallization The water trapped in crystals when a solution crystallizes. This is included in the MOLECULAR WEIGHT, but not the FORMULA WEIGHT. A large volume of water of crystallization will change the molecular weight significantly. When making molar solutions (see MOLARITY) it is appropriate always to use the molecular weight.

waterfall illusion *see* opponent processes

watershed areas of cortex An area of the CEREBRAL CORTEX at the junction of the middle, anterior and posterior cerebral arteries that include parts of the occipital, parietal and temporal cortices.

See also: anoxia

waxy flexibility An unusual condition described in CATATONIA, in which it is possible to place an individual's limbs in positions that will then be held; it is synonymous with LEAD PIPE RIGIDITY; see RIGIDITY.

WAY-100135 An ANTAGONIST at the $5HT_{1A}$ receptor; see SEROTONIN RECEPTORS.

WB4101 An alpha-1 noradrenaline receptor ANTAGONIST; see ADRENOCEPTORS.

weaning The verb to wean means to accustom an organism to a novel event: it typically refers to the change an animal makes in infancy from dependence on mother's milk to independent eating, although it does have more general use. (Addicts are described as being weaned off drugs, for example.) An animal described as a weanling or weaner is one that is undergoing weaning. In Scotland, *wean* is the term used to describe a child – it is derived from Scots, *wee ane*: small one.

See also: lactation; suckling

Weber's law A fundamental principle in PSYCHOPHYSICS formulated in 1834 by Ernst Weber (1795–1878): the just noticeable difference (between two categorically similar stimuli) is proportional to the magnitude of the difference. Formulaically it is expressed as:

$$\Delta I = kI \, (or \, alternatively, \, \Delta I/I = k)$$

where ΔI is the just noticeable difference; k is the relative change (substituting $100 \, k$ gives the percentage change); and I is the intensity of the standard stimulus. Weber's law generally holds good, though it breaks down when extreme values are involved.

See also: Fechner's law

Wechsler Adult Intelligence Scale *see* intelligence testing

Wernicke–Geschwind theory Neurologist Norman Geschwind revived the classical typology of APHASIA described a century earlier by Carl Wernicke (1848–1904). These classic works are the foundation of clinico-anatomic explanations of the major syndromes of aphasia.

See also: Wernicke's aphasia

Reference
Geschwind N. (1965) Disconnection syndromes in animals and man, I and II. *Brain*: 88, 237–294, 585–644.

CHARLOTTE C. MITCHUM

Wernicke–Korsakoff syndrome The commonest cause of MEMORY loss, characterized by ANTEROGRADE AMNESIA and variable RETROGRADE AMNESIA. The condition results from MALNUTRITION leading to THIAMINE deficiency. This is often a concomitant of severe ALCO-

HOLISM, but may follow any disorder resulting in impaired nutritional status. The illness starts with WERNICKE'S ENCEPHALOPATHY, an acute organic state with clouding of CONSCIOUSNESS and focal neurological signs. If this is untreated (by the administration of thiamine), the KORSAKOFF'S SYNDROME supervenes, and patients are left with persistent, largely irreversible, neurological damage. Pathologically, lesions are found in the DORSOMEDIAL NUCLEUS OF THE THALAMUS and the MAMMILLARY BODIES.

IAN C. REID

Wernicke's aphasia A major clinical syndrome of APHASIA (see Goodglass & Kaplan, 1983). Named for the nineteenth-century neurologist Carl Wernicke (1848–1904), who first described the classical syndrome, it is a common form of FLUENT APHASIA with impaired auditory comprehension. Speech is usually marked by frequent PARAPHASIAS. Sentences are poorly formed syntactically with a relative lack of substantive words. ANOMIA is often severe in relation to the flow of fluent speech and thus the use of grammatical words may be disproportional to the production of meaningful content words. Hence, the speech of these patients is often described as 'empty'. Nevertheless, the relative preservation of intonation, often with accompanying gesture and facial expression are deceptive to the naive listener. Some degree of accurate auditory comprehension is present. Patients with relatively mild comprehension impairments can be quite masterful in conveying a false appearance of understanding what is said to them, particularly in casual conversation. Wernicke's aphasia is distinguished from ANOMIC APHASIA by the presence of impaired auditory comprehension. The strikingly intact ability to repeat differentiates TRANSCORTICAL SENSORY APHASIA from Wernicke's aphasia, in which repetition ability is poor.

See also: sensory aphasia

Reference

Goodglass, H. & Kaplan, E. (1983) *The Assessment of Aphasia and Related Disorders*, 2nd edn, Lea & Febiger: Philadelphia.

CHARLOTTE C. MITCHUM

Wernicke's area An area of the posterior TEMPORAL LOBE named after Carl Wernicke who, in 1876 at the age of only 26, described a patient who had a LESION in this area: the patient was able to speak properly but had difficulty comprehending language; see WERNICKE'S APHASIA.

See also: aphasia; arcuate fasciculus; Broca's area

Wernicke's encephalopathy *see* Wernicke–Korsakoff syndrome

Wernicke's syndrome *see* Korsakoff's syndrome; Wernicke–Korsakoff syndrome

Western blotting *see* blotting

white matter *see* grey matter and white matter

white noise *see* noise

Whitten effect In groups of females exposed to male PHEROMONES or odours, the synchronization of the MENSTRUAL CYCLE.

See also: Bruce effect; Lee–Boot effect; Vandenbergh effect

willed action *see* voluntary

Williams syndrome *see* mental retardation

Wilson's disease Rare genetic disorder of copper metabolism affecting liver and central nervous system. Abnormal copper accumulation in tissues leads to cell damage and appears to be associated with defective caeruloplasmin expression in sufferers. Caeruloplasmin is a copper binding and transporting protein. The BASAL GANGLIA are particularly affected, and motor symptoms, such as TREMOR (which often appears as BATSWING TREMOR), RIGIDITY and writhing movements may be presenting features. Alternatively, signs of liver disease, or psychiatric disturbance may be the first features of the illness to become apparent. Age of onset is usually in childhood or adolescence, but may be delayed to middle age. Treatment centres on the use of chelating agents (such as penicillamine) to remove copper.

IAN C. REID

win–shift *see* win–stay, lose–shift

win–stay, lose–shift This term describes a common strategy adopted by organisms to repeat a RESPONSE that receives POSITIVE REINFORCEMENT and to change response in the absence of REINFORCEMENT (or the presence of NEGATIVE REINFORCEMENT). The reverse strategy is WIN–SHIFT. The principle of win–stay, lose–shift is entirely compatible with Thorndike's LAW OF EFFECT, which indicates that animals will repeat responses that are associated with what were then called satisfiers, but which are known now as POSITIVE REINFORCERS. However, SCHEDULES OF REINFORCEMENT can be used that challenge this. A schedule can be arranged with two levers in an OPERANT CHAMBER, only one of which delivers reinforcement (a food pellet for example) at any one time. Once a REINFORCER has been delivered, a random selection is made to determine which lever will deliver the next reinforcer. It is impossible to predict which lever will deliver reinforcement, although it is clear that over time each can be expected to deliver reinforcement on half of all trials. Under these circumstances rats show a marked win–stay, lose–shift strategy despite the fact that it confers no advantage. In contrast, in other tests, rats have been shown to display marked win–shift tendencies. Evidently, the nature of the reinforcers on offer and the specific conditions under which tests are conducted influence the degree to which either win–stay or win–shift will be seen. Win–stay and win–shift procedures have been frequently used in biological psychological research. They are of particular interest in the study of how animals choose responses, and have been used in research concerned with PERSEVERATION.

See also: radial maze; supervisory attentional system

Reference

Evenden J.L. & Robbins T.W. (1984) Win stay behaviour in the rat. *Quarterly Journal of Experimental Psychology (B)* 36: 1–26.

Wing's triad A cluster of deficits that occur together in AUTISM and ASPERGER'S SYNDROME: they include socialization difficulties, communication problems and impairments of imagination.

Reference

Wing L. & Gould J. (1979) Severe impairments of social interaction and associated abnormalities in children: epidemiology and classification. *Journal of Autism and Developmental Disorders* 9: 11–30.

wingbeat tremor *see* tremor

wiring transmission An alternative (and not widely used) term for classical NEUROTRANSMISSION, achieved by the liberation of neurochemicals at specific SYNAPSES (see NEUROCHEMISTRY; SYNAPSE). It stands in contrast to VOLUME TRANSMISSION, which involves the liberation of NEUROTRANSMITTERS diffusely into the EXTRACELLULAR spaces.

Wisconsin card-sort task The Wisconsin card-sort task involves the presentation to subjects of cards that require sorting into a particular category: cards are discriminated by form (that is, they may have shapes on them – circles, squares or triangles for example), colour (the shapes may be yellow, green or red for instance) or number (there may be one, two or three exemplars of each shape on the card). Subjects have to sort the cards into sets (for example, 'all the cards with triangles', 'all the yellow cards' or 'all the cards with three shapes on') discovering the rule that governs sorting from the feedback that the examiner gives. In this form, this is a test of concept formation. However, it can also be used as an ATTENTIONAL SET-SHIFTING task. It has been widely used in NEUROPSYCHOLOGY, particularly to assess the abilities of patients with FRONTAL LOBE damage or DYSEXECUTIVE SYNDROME.

See also: executive functions; extradimensional shift; intradimensional shift

Wistar rats *see* rat

withdrawal In literal terms withdrawal means removing or taking back. There are at least three ways in which the term is used in biological psychology. (i) One uses the term *withdrawal* to indicate the removal of a hypodermic syringe from a subject once the injection has taken place; or one uses it in respect of the removal of fluids from a body. (ii) It is often used as shorthand for the term WITHDRAWAL SYNDROME. (iii) It is used in a clinical context to indicate a loss of social contact and a state of apathy (see for example, SCHIZO-PHRENIA).

withdrawal reflex *see* pedal reflex

withdrawal syndrome (abstinence syndrome) A complex state, involving both physical and psychological features, that appears when individuals who show DEPENDENCE on a DRUG have their drug supply terminated. The effects of withdrawal vary with the types of drug that has been abused. Sweating, diarrhoea, tremors, temperature changes and weight loss are relatively common features of withdrawal. DRUG CRAVING is often present also. The symptoms of withdrawal may be so bad that the avoidance of them becomes a motivating factor in drug use.

See also: addiction

Reference

Feldman R., Meyer J.S. & Quenzer L.F. (1997) *Principles of Neuropsychopharmacology*, Sinauer Associates: Sunderland MA.

Wolffian internal genitalia *see* Müllerian internal genitalia

womb *see* uterus

word deafness *see* auditory aphasia

word recognition Perceiving language is a RECOGNITION process: perceivers cannot know in advance what an incoming message will be, but must understand it via recognition of the parts of which it is made up – the WORDS which they already know and have stored in their mental LEXICON. Any language user knows tens of thousands of different words; but these are constructed of only a handful (on average, 30 to 40) different sounds in the PHONETIC repertoire of the language (and represented in written form by only a handful of elements, for example, the 26 letters in the alphabet used for English). The consequence of this is that words inevitably resemble other words, and may have other words embedded within them (thus 'great' sounds like 'grape' and 'crate', and contains 'grey' and 'rate' and 'eight'; its written form looks like 'greet', and contains 'eat'). Word recognition therefore involves identifying the correct form among a large number of competing forms. The recog-

nition of spoken words takes place in time – words are not heard all at once, but from beginning to end. Further, words usually occur in longer utterances of continuous speech, in which there are no reliable cues to where one word ends and the next begins. Thus listeners must segment utterances into the portions which correspond to individual words. Research on spoken-word recognition has addressed the temporal course of the activation of lexical representations, competition between similar and overlapping words, and the effects of unclear or distorted speech sounds. The recognition of written words is, in most orthographies, facilitated by explicit coding of the boundaries between lexical units – for example the spaces between words in written English, or the separation of characters in written Chinese. Research on written-word recognition has addressed the question of whether a written form is recognized directly or activates the phonological (see PHONOLOGY) form of the word, and on the way in which different orthographies are read. Finally, the form of words varies widely across languages; some languages (such as Turkish) construct words from stems with very many morphological affixes, while other languages (such as Chinese) use virtually no affixes but allow many cases of a single form encoding multiple meanings; some languages distinguish between closely related words, such as different forms of a verb, by means of affixes (English for example), while others vary the sounds within the word (Hebrew for example); and there are many other types of variation, so that word recognition necessarily involves some language-specific aspects.

References

Cutler A. (1995) Spoken word recognition and production. In *Handbook of Perception and Cognition*, ed. E.C. Carterette & M.P. Friedman, vol. 11, *Speech, Language and Communication*, ed. J.L. Miller & P.D. Eimas, pp. 97–136, Academic Press: New York.

Seidenberg M.S. (1995) Visual word recognition: an overview. In *Handbook of Perception and Cognition*, ed. E.C. Carterette & M.P. Friedman, vol. 11, *Speech, Language and Communication*, ed. J.L. Miller & P.D.

Eimas, pp.138–179, Academic Press: New York.

ANNE CUTLER

words Independently combinable units contributing meaning and/or function to a sentence.

See also: lexicon; grammar; phoneme

ANNE CUTLER

working memory A MEMORY system which allows for the maintenance of incoming information in a readily accessible memory store that can be easily manipulated. This allows for the active manipulation and expansion of information necessary for performance of cognitive tasks. Essentially working memory is composed of several memory stores which are individually responsible for the maintenance of a specific subset of information (visuospatial, phonological, organizational for example). Incoming information can be integrated from separate pathways, and associations about novel and previously stored information can be made. In this way, working memory allows for the simultaneous representation of several modalities of information. Further, working memory allows for enriched perception because it permits the integration of diverse information. Working memory was differentiated from SHORT-TERM MEMORY as a result of short-comings of the initial short-term memory model. Short-term memory was originally considered to be a unitary memory system. However, when subjects were asked to perform multiple short-term memory tasks simultaneously, such as performing a DIGIT SPAN TASK while retaining visual images, they were not as impaired as would have been predicted from a unitary system. This ability to perform multiple tasks at once suggested that short-term memory is composed of many working memory components. Thus working memory explains the ability to maintain accessibility to many distinct types of information at a given time. This information can span modalities, including perceptual outputs, motor plans, retrieval of preexisting knowledge and management of processing (organization or bookkeeping). The term working memory, then, is the overarching heading under which these more distinct categories of working memory fall.

Though there is some controversy about the definition of working memory, one widely accepted definition was developed by Alan Baddeley. In this definition, working memory is broken down into three basic subcategories, VISUOSPATIAL SKETCHPAD, PHONOLOGICAL LOOP and executive. Visuospatial working memory deals with the memory for recently-seen information and information about objects. Phonological memory temporarily encodes information about words and recently heard information. The executive allows for the maintenance of the incoming information, the building of the associations and the bookkeeping functions which enrich the associations and cause the formation of longer lasting memories.

A more functionally oriented working memory definition was proposed by David Olton (1943–1994). This type of working memory (also termed EPISODIC MEMORY) described the memory for what the subject is working with in a given situation. Because many pieces of information are repeated across situations (digits, letters, words and so on), the inability to differentiate any specific episode of use from any other would be devastating. Thus working memory allows for the memory of what happens in a given situation. Olton distinguished this from REFERENCE MEMORY, which is the knowledge about the information being used in working memory (for instance what a '4' is, what 'dog' means and so on).

Working memory and short-term memory can be differentiated functionally and through task specificity. One major difference between the two types of memory is the cognitive demands placed on the subject. Whereas in short-term memory the subject is not permitted to rehearse the information to be retained, in working memory the subject is permitted to use any cognitive tool available to them in order to remember the information. Thus tasks that are typically used to assess working memory include digit span task, word recall task, and paired associate task. These tasks are influenced by cognitive load, delay and other cognitive demands. Working memory allows for the coherence of conversation, the maintenance of information 'in mind' for use in a given situation. In order to maintain this information however, an organism must initially perceive the information. In addition to relying on perception, however, working memory can also bolster the perceived stimulus. For instance, the ability to maintain information about an object in the temporary store can allow for the enrichment of the perception through association with other previously stored information, or through the simultaneous association with other incoming information. The perception of a stimulus can then be maintained in working memory long enough for an association to be formed (for example in aversion training tone-shock pairing; see ASSOCIATIVE LEARNING).

See also: central executive; phonological store

References

Baddeley A.D. (1994) Working memory. In *Memory Systems*, ed. D. Schacter & E. Tulving, MIT Press: Cambridge MA.
Olton D.S., Becker J.T. & Handlemann G.E. (1979) Hippocampus, space, memory. *Brain and Behavioral Sciences* 2: 313–365.

HOWARD EICHENBAUM

writing The formation of characters (letters of the alphabet, numerals, symbols) on a surface or using an implement or machine; writing is of major importance in human development because it permits a significantly deeper transmission of cultural information than an oral mechanism alone. Writing provides a good example of MOTOR PROGRAMMING: initially effortful, requiring conscious ATTENTION, the production of writing rapidly becomes automatic. What appears to be registered in the programme is the concept of writing rather than a definitive mechanism of production. Appropriate written output can be produced holding a pen in different ways – normally, at arms length, with the non-dominant hand – or even moving paper across a stationary pen. Such phenomena indicate that the motor programme for writing does not have embedded specific patterns of muscular activation: different MUSCLES can be activated in order to produce appropriate writing.

See also: agraphia; grapheme; micrographia; reading; spelling

X

X and Y chromosomes Non-autosomal CHROMOSOMES (see AUTOSOMAL CHROMOSOME) in the CELL nucleus of sexually reproducing organisms, which determine the sex of the organism (hence they are also known as SEX CHROMOSOMES). Females have two X chromosomes, whereas males have one X and one Y chromosome. Since each organism receives one sex chromosome from each parent, it will receive an X chromosome from the mother, and either an X or Y chromosome from the father. Thus the type of sex chromosome present in the gamete from the father (see GAMETES) will determine the sex of the offspring.

FIONA M. INGLIS

X cells An older term for the small GANGLION CELLS now recognized as the P (or P-beta) ganglion cells; see LATERAL GENICULATE NUCLEUS; RETINA; RETINAL CELL LAYERS.

X-ray X-rays are used in medicine and science diagnostically in the production of the familiar 2-dimensional images and the more complex images generated by COMPUTERIZED AXIAL TOMOGRAPHY. In very large doses (measured in rads) irradiation with X-rays destroys cells, especially haematopoietic and LYMPHATIC SYSTEM cells involved in IMMUNE SYSTEM functions. For an example of this use, see Coffey *et al.* (1990).

Reference
Coffey P.J., Perry V.H. & Rawlins J.N.P. (1990) An investigation into the early stages of the inflammatory response following ibo-

tenic acid-induced neuronal degeneration. *Neuroscience* 35: 121–132.

xamoterol A beta-1 noradrenaline receptor AGONIST; see ADRENOCEPTORS.

xanthines Name of a class of DRUG including CAFFEINE, THEOPHYLLINE and THEOBROMINE, though these are in fact methyl derivatives of a specific drug, xanthine. All are PSYCHOMOTOR STIMULANTS: caffeine and theophylline and are found in TEA AND COFFEE.

xenografts Grafts between different species; see TRANSPLANTATION. These are contrasted with ALLOGRAFTS, grafts of tissue within the same species (rat to rat, human to human and so on).

XXX syndrome *see* triple X syndrome

XXY syndrome *see* Klinefelter's syndrome

xylazine A potent SEDATIVE with analgesic (see ANALGESIA) properties. ANAESTHESIA for rats can be produced by administration of a combination of xylazine and KETAMINE.

Reference
Flecknell P.A. (1987) *Laboratory Animal Anaesthesia*, Academic Press: London.

XYY syndrome A very rare chromosome abnormality (see CHROMOSOME ABNORMALITIES) in which a male has an extra Y chromosome. It has been rather sensationally associated with criminality, but there is now considerable doubt as to the validity of this controversial association.

See also: X and Y chromosomes

Y

Y cells An older term for the large GANGLION CELLS now recognized as the M (or P-alpha) ganglion cells; see LATERAL GENICULATE NUCLEUS; RETINA; RETINAL CELL LAYERS.

Y maze Literally, a maze shaped like a capital letter Y. To start, animals can either be placed at the centre (giving them a choice of three arms to enter) or at the end of one of the arms, allowing them to proceed to the centre of the maze, at which point they will have a choice of the remaining two arms to enter. Y mazes have been used in a wide variety of experiments looking at LEARNING and MEMORY and many other processes. Reid & Morris used a Y maze in an olfactory discrimination task. Rats were placed in one arm and approached the centre: here they were able to detect a smell in one of the remaining arms and a different smell in the other. One of the odours would be paired with REWARD, presenting the rats with a discrimination task.

See also: mazes; plus maze; radial arm maze; spontaneous alternation; T maze; water maze

Reference

Reid I.C. & Morris R.G.M. (1992) Smells are no surer – rapid improvement in olfactory discrimination is not due to the acquisition of a learning set. *Proceedings of the Royal Society of London series B – Biological Sciences* 247: 137–143.

yawning Yawning is a ubiquitous behaviour, typically associated with drowsiness or with boredom. It has been suggested that yawning, like other simple activities such as swallowing or coughing, is a FIXED ACTION PATTERN. Its function, however, unlike coughing or swallowing, remains obscure, though it is often assumed that yawning has something to do with RESPIRATION and BREATHING. A STRETCHING–YAWNING SYNDROME in rats has been described.

Yerkes–Dodson law R.M. Yerkes and J.D. Dodson formulated what became their law in 1908: it provided the first major attempt to provide an account of the effects of AROUSAL on performance. It has two basic principles: (1) that the relationship between arousal and performance on a task describes an inverted U-shaped function, with tasks being performed optimally at a moderate level of arousal – not enough arousal and task efficiency is low, too much and task performance falls away; and (2) that the optimal level of arousal is inversely related to the difficulty of the task being performed – lower levels of arousal are optimal for more difficult tasks. The Yerkes–Dodson law has maintained interest across the century and is still favourably regarded, though there are some well-known problems associated with it. For example, when arousal is produced by using an AVERSIVE STIMULUS the law appears to hold good, but when arousal is increased using POSITIVE REINFORCEMENT, the relationships between arousal and performance are less convincing. A second problem concerns the assessment of task difficulty: the law rather assumes that this can be measured in a single dimension, but in fact most tasks are complex and not well suited to such simple analysis.

See also: Lyon–Robbins hypothesis

References

Eysenck M.W. (1982) *Attention and Arousal*, Springer-Verlag: Berlin.

Yerkes R.M. & Dodson J.D. (1908) The relation of strength of stimulus to rapidity of habit formation. *Journal of Comparative Neurology and Psychology* 18: 459–482.

yohimbine A commonly used DRUG, an ANTAGONIST at alpha-2 noradrenaline receptors (see ADRENOCEPTORS).

yoked control A yoked control is one slaved to exactly the same conditions as a subject receiving a particular treatment or working under particular conditions. Subjects are matched as closely as possible in all relevant dimensions. In rats, these would include sex, age, training experience and BODY WEIGHT (a crude indicator of general physiological state). Yoking could then occur in a number of different ways. For example, two rats could be placed in their own OPERANT CHAMBER, similarly fitted with levers, but only for one rat would the levers deliver POSITIVE REINFORCEMENT. However, whatever (and whenever) the rat in control got, so would the yoked control. The reinforcement could be food or water, or a DRUG delivered by SELF-ADMINISTRATION. This would allow the effects of precisely the same drug, given at precisely the same time, to be examined in rats *voluntarily delivering* them or *involuntarily receiving* them. Alternatively, NEGATIVE REINFORCEMENT could be delivered: one rat of the pair would be able to operate a lever to turn off FOOTSHOCK, while the yoked control would be unable to regulate the duration of negative reinforcement. This procedure has shown dramatic effects – see LEARNED HELPLESSNESS. Operant techniques need not be used. For example, one might wish to compare the effects of food intake on body weight gain in two groups of rats, one group bearing a LESION, the other not. In this case, the amount of food consumed by one group would determine the amount of food given to the other.

See also: instrumental conditioning; schedules of reinforcement

Young–Helmholtz theory of colour vision
see trichromatic theory of colour vision

Z

zeitgeber (from German, *Zeitgeber*: time-giver or time-cue) This term describes an external cycle which entrains (see ENTRAINMENT) an endogenously rhythmic BIOLOGICAL CLOCK and thus any OVERT RHYTHM it controls. The most often studied and most important zeitgeber for CIRCADIAN RHYTHMS is the day–night cycle. Another potent zeitgeber for POIKILO-THERMS (see THERMOREGULATION) is an oscillation in temperature. Other effective non-photic zeitgebers for some daily rhythms in mammals include temporal restriction of food availability and a variety of social (perhaps pheromonal; see PHEROMONES) cues. MELATO-NIN has been suggested to serve as an internal zeitgeber for circadian systems, and other HORMONES may have limited, internal entraining effects.

BENJAMIN RUSAK

zinc The metal ION zinc (Zn) is found free in many SYNAPTIC VESICLES. It has been associated with synaptic functions in many parts of the brain, including the CEREBRAL CORTEX, HIPPOCAMPUS, RETINA and HYPOTHALAMUS. It is very possibly involved throughout the BRAIN and SPINAL CORD. It is thought to act as a neuromodulator (see NEUROMODULATION), and has been reported to affect NEUROTRANS-MISSION at synapses using GLYCINE and GABA. It has also been associated with a particular family of genes, the metallothionein family (see GENE). TIMM'S STAIN (see HISTOLOGY; STAINS) is known to show the presence of zinc in neural tissues and, more recently, zinc has been imaged successfully in live brain slices. Clearly it is present and active in the mammalian brain, but exactly what it is doing there is not known. Zinc is also involved in the regulation of DNA: zinc ions form a critical part of the so-called ZINC FINGER, involved in TRANSCRIP-TION.

Reference

Budde T., Minta A., White J.A. & Kay A.R. (1997) Imaging free zinc in synaptic terminals in live hippocampal slices. *Neuroscience* 79: 347–358.

zinc finger *see* zinc

zona incerta A narrow structure situated between the THALAMUS and the HYPOTHALA-MUS that contains scattered neurons and intermixed fibres. The anterior part of zona incerta is continuous with the RETICULAR NUCLEUS OF THE THALAMUS. The zona incerta receives a projection from the MOTOR CORTEX, and projects to the RED NUCLEUS, SUPERIOR COLLICU-LUS and the pretectal (see PRETECTUM) area, suggesting its role in visuomotor coordination. The zona incerta also appears to be involved in limbic (see LIMBIC SYSTEM) and AUTONOMIC functions, as some of its neurons project to the MIDBRAIN PERIAQUEDUCTAL GREY and the PARABRACHIAL NUCLEI in the PONS.

KAZUE SEMBA

Zucker rats A strain of genetically obese RAT, carrying the recessive allele *fa* in the homozygous condition (*FA/FA*). Rats carrying the dominant allele (*Fa*), either heterozygous (*Fa/fa*) or homozygous (*Fa/Fa*) will be lean, not obese. Zucker rats have massively enlarged fat depots, with more and larger adipocytes (see ADIPOSE TISSUE). They eat about one-third as much again as their lean littermates and deposit a greater proportion of their ENERGY intake as FAT. Obese Zucker rats also tend, surprisingly, to have a shorter NASAL–ANAL LENGTH than normal and have a variety of smaller problems, such as a greasy fur and skin.

See also: leptin; obesity; *ob/ob* mouse

zugunruhe A period of restlessness prior to MIGRATION.

zygomatic bone *see* skull

zygote A fertilized egg. In species that engage in sexual REPRODUCTION, the zygote is the DIPLOID outcome of the fusion of GAMETES that are HAPLOID.